* New exam!

March 11 Tuesday for Bact T

Two hour exam.

All

All

A lot of 7

Some 9

Some 13

The illustration on the facing page is an adaptation of a figure that appears in Chapter 9, "Cell-mediated Reactions." The intent is to indicate the complexity of the immune response and the interrelationships and interdependencies of various cellular and humoral components of the immunoregulatory network. It also illustrates the pivotal role of the T-lymphocyte in this immunoregulatory network and in the various expressions of cell-mediated and humoral immune responses.

"Rebuck-skin window"

The illustration on the cover is an adaptation of a figure that appears in Chapter 5, "Antibody and Immunoglobulins: Structure and Function." The figure illustrates schematically one of the most exciting recent developments in immunology, hybridoma technology, and the production of monoclonal antibodies, which are finding diagnostic and therapeutic applications in medicine today.

W.B. Saunders Company
Philadelphia London Toronto Mexico City Rio de Janeiro Sydney Tokyo

IMMUNOLOGY III

Joseph A. Bellanti, M.D.

Professor of Pediatrics and Microbiology
Director, International Center for
Interdisciplinary Studies of Immunology
Georgetown University School of Medicine
Washington, D.C.

W. B. Saunders Company: West Washington Square
Philadelphia, PA 19105

1 St. Anne's Road
Eastbourne, East Sussex BN21 3UN, England

1 Goldthorne Avenue
Toronto, Ontario M8Z 5T9, Canada

Apartado 26370—Cedro 512
Mexico 4, D.F., Mexico

Rua Coronel Cabrita, 8
Sao Cristovao Caixa Postal 21176
Rio de Janeiro, Brazil

9 Waltham Street
Artarmon, N.S.W. 2064, Australia

Ichibancho, Central Bldg., 22-1 Ichibancho
Chiyoda-Ku, Tokyo 102, Japan

Library of Congress Cataloging in Publication Data

Bellanti, Joseph A., 1934–

Immunology III

Rev. ed. of: Basic immunology. 2nd ed. c1984. Includes index.

1. Immunologic diseases. 2. Immunology. I. Title.
[DNLM: 1. Immunity. QW 504 I33]

RC582.B45 1985 616.07′9 84–1253

ISBN 0–7216–1668–2

Listed here is the latest translated edition of this book together with the language of the translation and the publisher.

Italian (*1st Edition*)—Piccin Editore, Padova, Italy

Portuguese (*2nd Edition*)—Editora Interamericana Ltda., Rio de Janeiro, Brazil

Spanish (*1st Edition*)—Nueva Editorial Interamericana S.A. de C.V., Mexico 4 D.F., Mexico

Spanish (*2nd Edition*)—Nueva Editorial Interamericana S.A. de C.V., Mexico 4 D.F., Mexico

Cover illustration by Margaret Siner and Jane Hurd

Immunology III ISBN 0-7216-1668-2

Last digit is the print number: 9 8 7 6 5 4 3 2

This edition is dedicated with affection to my parents, my wife Jacqueline, and my children Dawn, Lisa, Jeannine, Loretta, Maria, Joseph (who was born during the First Edition), and little Tony (who was born during the Second Edition) and to my grandchildren Jeannine, Shannan, Mark, and Kristen (who were born during the preparation of the Third Edition).

A set of 35 mm. teaching slides of drawings and photographs from this book is available through the publisher.

Contributors

Joseph A. Bellanti, M.D.
Professor of Pediatrics and Microbiology, and Director, International Center for Interdisciplinary Studies of Immunology, Georgetown University School of Medicine, Washington, D.C.
Introduction to Immunology; General Immunobiology; Immunogenetics; Antigen-Antibody Interactions; Cell-Mediated Immune Reactions; A Unifying Model for Immunologic Processes; Host-Parasite Relationships; Mechanisms of Immunity to Bacterial Diseases; Mechanisms of Immunity to Viral Diseases; Mechanisms of Immunity to Fungal Diseases; Immune Defense Mechanisms in Tumor Immunity; Immunologically Mediated Diseases; Immunoprophylaxis: The Use of Vaccines; Immunotherapy: The Use of Passive Immunization; Diagnostic Application of Immunology

George M. Bernier, M.D.
Joseph M. Huber Professor and Chairman of Medicine, Dartmouth Medical School; Chairman of Medicine, Dartmouth-Hitchcock Medical Center, Hanover, New Hampshire.
Antibody and Immunoglobulins: Structure and Function; Monoclonal Gammopathies

John J. Calabro, M.D.
Professor of Medicine and Pediatrics, University of Massachusetts Medical School; Director, Division of Rheumatology, Saint Vincent Hospital, Worcester, Massachusetts.
Immunologically Mediated Disease Involving Autologous Antigens

Lynn H. Caporale, Ph.D.
Assistant Professor of Biochemistry, Georgetown University Medical Center, Washington, D.C.
The Complement System

Joseph A. Church, M.D.
Associate Professor of Clinical Pediatrics, University of Southern California School of Medicine; Associate Attending Physician, Division of Allergy–Clinical Immunology; Consultant, Department of Laboratories, Children's Hospital, Los Angeles, California.
Immune Deficiency Disorders

Jeffrey Cossman, M.D.
Senior Investigator, National Cancer Institute, National Institutes of Health, Bethesda, Maryland.
Lymphomas and Leukemias

Raymond H. Cypess, D.V.M., Ph.D.
Professor of Parasitology and Epidemiology, Cornell University, Ithaca; Adjunct Professor of Parasitology, School of Public Health, University of Pittsburgh; Adjunct Professor of Preventive Medicine, Upstate Medical School, Syracuse, New York.
Mechanisms of Immunity to Parasitic Diseases

Anthony S. Fauci, M.D.
Chief, Laboratory of Immunoregulation, National Institute of Allergy and Infectious Diseases, National Institutes of Health, Bethesda, Maryland.
Clinical Aspects of Immunosuppression: Use of Cytotoxic Agents and Corticosteroids

Michael C. Gelfand, M.D.
Associate Professor of Clinical Medicine, Georgetown University School of Medicine, and Co-Director, Hemodialysis, Transplantation, Hemoperfusion, and Plasmapheresis Unit, Georgetown University Hospital, Washington, D.C.
Organ Transplantation; Immunologically Mediated Disease Involving Autologous Antigens

Peter M. Henson, Ph.D., B.V.M.&S., M.R.C.V.S.
Professor of Pathology and Medicine, University of Colorado School of Medicine; Office of Biomedical Affairs, National Jewish Hospital and Research Center, Denver, Colorado.
Mechanisms of Tissue Injury Produced by Immunologic Reactions

Ronald B. Herberman, M.D.
Acting Associate Director, Biological Response Modifiers Program, National Cancer Institute, Frederick, Maryland.
Immune Defense Mechanisms in Tumor Immunity

Herbert B. Herscowitz, Ph.D.
Professor of Microbiology, Georgetown University Schools of Medicine and Dentistry, Washington, D.C.
Immunophysiology: Cell Function and Cellular Interactions in Antibody Formation

Anne L. Jackson, Ph.D.
Becton-Dickinson Monoclonal Center, Mountain View, California.
Antigens and Immunogenicity

Josef V. Kadlec, S.J., M.D.
Assistant Professor of Pediatrics and Microbiology, Georgetown University Medical School; Member, International Center for Interdisciplinary Studies of Immunology, Georgetown University Hospital, Washington, D.C.
Introduction to Immunology; General Immunobiology

Paul Katz, M.D.
Associate Professor of Medicine, and Director, Division of Rheumatology, Immunology, and Allergy, Georgetown University School of Medicine; Attending Physician, Georgetown University Hospital, Washington, D.C.
Immunomodulation: Immunopotentiation, Tolerance, and Immunosuppression

Steven L. Kunkel, Ph.D.
Assistant Professor, Department of Pathology, University of Michigan Medical School, Ann Arbor, Michigan.
The Complement System

Stephen M. Peters, Ph.D.
Assistant Professor of Pediatrics, Georgetown University School of Medicine; Associate Director, Division of Immunology and Virology, Department of Clinical Laboratories, Georgetown University Hospital, Washington, D.C.
Diagnostic Applications of Immunology

John B. Robbins, M.D.
Chief, Laboratory of Developmental and Molecular Immunity, National Institute of Child Health and Human Development, National Institutes of Health, Bethesda, Maryland.
Immunoprophylaxis: The Use of Vaccines; Immunotherapy: The Use of Passive Immunization

Ross E. Rocklin, M.D.
Professor of Medicine, Tufts University School of Medicine; Chief, Allergy Division, New England Medical Center, Boston, Massachusetts.
Cell-Mediated Immune Reactions

Robert T. Scanlon, M.D.
Clinical Professor of Pediatrics, Georgetown University School of Medicine, Co-Director, Allergy Training Programs, Georgetown University Hospital, Washington, D.C.
Immunologically Mediated Disease Involving Allogeneic Antigens

Robert J. Schlegel, M.D.
Professor and Chairman, Department of Pediatrics, Martin Luther King, Jr./Charles R. Drew Medical Center (UCLA); Physician-in-Chief, Department of Pediatrics, Martin Luther King, Jr. General Hospital, Los Angeles, California.
Immune Deficiency Disorders

Kenneth W. Sell, M.D., Ph.D.
Clinical Professor of Pediatrics, Georgetown University School of Medicine, Washington, D.C.; Scientific Director, National Institute of Allergy and Infectious Diseases, National Institutes of Health, Bethesda, Maryland.
Immunogenetics

John P. Utz, M.D.
Professor of Medicine, Georgetown University School of Medicine, Washington, D.C.
Mechanisms of Immunity to Fungal Diseases

Carl-Wilhelm Vogel, M.D.
Assistant Professor of Biochemistry and Medicine; Member, International Center for Interdisciplinary Studies of Immunology, and Vincent T. Lombardi Cancer Center, Georgetown University Schools of Medicine and Dentistry, Washington, D.C.
The Complement System

Peter A. Ward, M.D.

Professor and Chairman, Department of Pathology, University of Michigan Medical School, Ann Arbor, Michigan.

The Complement System; Inflammation

James N. Woody, Capt., MC., U.S.N., M.D., Ph.D.

Professor of Pediatrics and Microbiology, Georgetown University School of Medicine, Washington, D.C.; Director, Transplantation Research Program Center, Naval Medical Research Institute, Bethesda, Maryland.

Immunogenetics

Chester M. Zmijewski, Ph.D.

Associate Professor, Department of Pathology and Laboratory Medicine; Associate Director, Department of Pathology and Laboratory Medicine; Director, Immunology, University of Pennsylvania, Philadelphia, Pennsylvania.

Antigen-Antibody Interactions

Preface

Immunology is the study of those processes used by the host to maintain constancy in his internal environment when confronted with foreign substances. Implicit in this definition is the fact that immunology embraces and discusses contributions made by both basic and clinical research observations. Thus, in the current text, contributions have come from collaborators in both the basic and the clinical sciences. *Immunology III* continues to emanate from an interdisciplinary center whose mission of research, education, and patient care is based upon the symbiotic relationship among individuals engaged in a multitude of scholarly disciplines. Moreover, since the source of the book is an international center, there is also the influence of the perspectives of the large number of visiting scientists, physicians, and students from various parts of the globe, who have greatly added to the scope and depth of the knowledge therein.

The book is directed to students at many levels: the undergraduate, the graduate, and the postgraduate. The first and second editions have been useful not only for teachers of a variety of subspecialty areas of medicine, including allergy, immunology, rheumatology, nephrology, infectious diseases, hematology-oncology, otolaryngology, and dermatology, but also for practicing physicians in need of a current overview of the state of the art in immunology to assist in the clinical management of patients. The text has also been applied to the teaching of dentistry, nursing, medical technology, and undergraduate biology. Certainly, it has been the intent of the author and his collaborators in all three editions to provide a comprehensive introductory text in immunology while maintaining a fidelity to a clinical theme.

Immunology III is organized like the previous editions—Principles, Mechanisms, and Clinical Applications. However, all chapters have been completely updated and revised to incorporate the most current information. In addition, several chapters have been expanded and new sections have been added in some, including Chapters 3 (Immunogenetics), 6 (The Complement System), 7 (Immunophysiology: Cell Function and Cellular Interactions in Antibody Formation), 10 (Immunomodulation: Immunopotentiation, Tolerance and Immunosuppression), 19 (Immune Defense Mechanisms in Tumor Immunity), and 21 (Neoplasms of the Immune System: Monoclonal Gammopathies and Lymphomas and Leukemias). Considerable basic knowledge has been stressed throughout the text, including the genetic diversity of antibody and immunoglobulins as well as the exciting applications of hybridoma technology. Also included in the present text is the most current knowledge of cells and subsets of cells based upon identification through monoclonal antibodies that identify new antigenic and cell surface receptors.

Many persons have contributed to the preparation of the third edition, and I wish to express my indebtedness to them. First, I would like to thank Dr. Philip L. Calcagno, who has been most generous and gracious in his support and encouragement of this endeavor. I would like to express my sincere appreciation to Miss Jane Hurd and Miss Margaret Siner for the continued development of the imaginative figures that illustrate the concepts of the chapters of this book so vividly. Others who have read sections of the manuscript or who have made helpful suggestions include the following: Mrs. Barbara Zeligs, Dr. Lata Nerurkar, Dr. Anne Morris Hooke, Dr. Daniel Sordelli, Dr. Cristina Cerquetti, Dr. Robert M. Chanock, Dr. Robert H. Purcell, Dr. John Gerin, Dr. Anthony Fauci, Dr. Lawrence D. Frenkel, Dr. John Dwyer, and Dr. David M. Asher.

Particular appreciation is owed to a special friend who stayed at my side throughout the revision of *Immunology III* and who made this oftentimes tedious task a joy with his uplifting spirit and steadfast and gentle determination as the book progressed through its many drafts, illustrations, and galley and page proofs. Father Josef Kadlec, priest, physician, ethicist, microbiologist, immunologist, and friend: Thank you for persevering with me in this endeavor.

My appreciation is also extended to other colleagues at Georgetown and to my clinical and research fellows and house staff who have contributed to my intellectual life and to the life of the Immunology Center. I owe a special debt of gratitude to students of all ages for whom the book is written. Learning represents a joy of discovery shared between the student and the teacher, and it is in this spirit that *Immunology III* was written. The book is a product of conversations that I have had with every student I have met. It is the questions they ask in the lecture hall, the laboratory, and the clinic and at the bedside that have provided me with the incentive to write. Although many individuals have contributed information to this text, I alone assume responsibility for any errors found within these pages.

I wish also to thank Diane Hargrave Goldstein for her diligent typing of the entire manuscript.

Finally, I wish to express my thanks and appreciation to Mr. Albert Meier, to Ms. Constance Burton, and to Mr. Frank Polizzano and other colleagues at W. B. Saunders Company for their patience, support, suggestions, and inspiration during the lengthy preparation of this third revision.

JOSEPH A. BELLANTI

Contents

Section One

THE PRINCIPLES OF IMMUNOLOGY

Chapter 1

Introduction to Immunology

Joseph A. Bellanti, M.D., and Josef V. Kadlec, S.J., M.D.

HISTORICAL BACKGROUND

The concepts of immunology are ancient and pragmatic and are derived primarily from the study of resistance to infection. It was known for centuries before the discovery of the germ theory of infectious disease that recovery from illness was accompanied by the ability to resist reinfection. Thus, the elements of classical immunology preceded bacteriology and contributed to it. In more recent years, contributions to immunology have come from both the basic sciences, e.g., biochemistry, anatomy, developmental biology, genetics, pharmacology, and pathology, as well as from the study of clinical entities, e.g., allergy, infectious diseases, organ transplantation, rheumatology, immune deficiency diseases, and oncology. These fields, in turn, have been enhanced by the application of immunologic principles. Shown in Figure 1–1 is a schematic representation of some major milestones important in the development of immunology.

Preceding modern medicine, Chinese physicians in the eleventh century observed that the inhalation of smallpox crusts prevented the subsequent occurrence of the disease. Later, the technique of variolation, the intradermal application of powdered scabs, was used in the Middle East, where its primary intent was esthetic—"preserving the beauty of their daughters." This primitive immunization reached England in the eighteenth century through Pylarini and Timoni and was later popularized by Lady Mary Wortley Montagu (Fig. 1–2). Wide variations in vaccination procedures, however, occasionally led to death, which prevented the full acceptance of this form of therapy.

The future of modern immunobiology was assured when Edward Jenner (Fig. 1–3), as a medical student, made the surprisingly sophisticated discovery that inoculation with cowpox crusts protected humans from smallpox. This important finding resulted from Jenner's observation that milkmaids who had contracted cowpox were resistant to infection with smallpox.

The enhancement and further development of preventive immunization were made possible by Louis Pasteur (Fig. 1–4), who coined the term "vaccine" (from *vacca*: L., cow) in honor of Jenner's contribution. Pasteur's researches led to the development of the germ theory of disease, from which he developed techniques for the *in vitro* cultivation of microorganisms. This work produced material that could now be used for vaccines: living, heat-killed, and attenuated (living but with reduced virulence). During these investigations, Pasteur observed that old cultures (attenuated) of fowl cholera organisms when inoculated into fowl produced no disease. Surprisingly, these fowl were resistant to subsequent infection with the organism and were

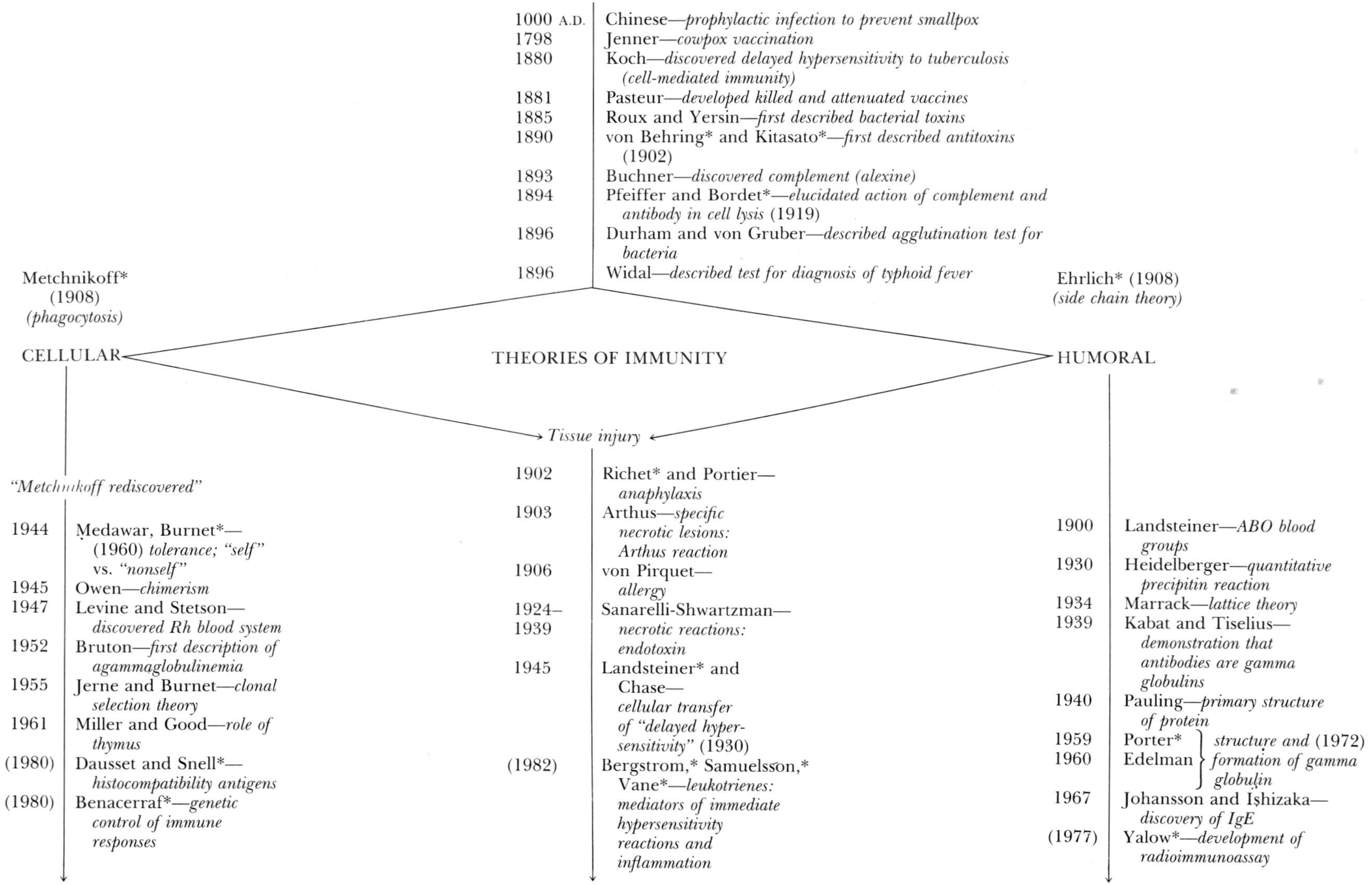
1000 A.D. Chinese—*prophylactic infection to prevent smallpox*
1798 Jenner—*cowpox vaccination*
1880 Koch—*discovered delayed hypersensitivity to tuberculosis (cell-mediated immunity)*
1881 Pasteur—*developed killed and attenuated vaccines*
1885 Roux and Yersin—*first described bacterial toxins*
1890 von Behring* and Kitasato*—*first described antitoxins* (1902)
1893 Buchner—*discovered complement (alexine)*
1894 Pfeiffer and Bordet*—*elucidated action of complement and antibody in cell lysis* (1919)
1896 Durham and von Gruber—*described agglutination test for bacteria*
1896 Widal—*described test for diagnosis of typhoid fever*
Metchnikoff* (1908) (*phagocytosis*)
Ehrlich* (1908) (*side chain theory*)
CELLULAR
THEORIES OF IMMUNITY
HUMORAL
Tissue injury
"*Metchnikoff rediscovered*"
1944 Medawar, Burnet*—(1960) *tolerance; "self" vs. "nonself"*
1945 Owen—*chimerism*
1947 Levine and Stetson—*discovered Rh blood system*
1952 Bruton—*first description of agammaglobulinemia*
1955 Jerne and Burnet—*clonal selection theory*
1961 Miller and Good—*role of thymus*
(1980) Dausset and Snell*—*histocompatibility antigens*
(1980) Benacerraf*—*genetic control of immune responses*
1902 Richet* and Portier—*anaphylaxis*
1903 Arthus—*specific necrotic lesions: Arthus reaction*
1906 von Pirquet—*allergy*
1924–1939 Sanarelli-Shwartzman—*necrotic reactions: endotoxin*
1945 Landsteiner* and Chase—*cellular transfer of "delayed hypersensitivity"* (1930)
(1982) Bergstrom,* Samuelsson,* Vane*—*leukotrienes: mediators of immediate hypersensitivity reactions and inflammation*
1900 Landsteiner—*ABO blood groups*
1930 Heidelberger—*quantitative precipitin reaction*
1934 Marrack—*lattice theory*
1939 Kabat and Tiselius—*demonstration that antibodies are gamma globulins*
1940 Pauling—*primary structure of protein*
1959 Porter*
1960 Edelman
structure and (1972) *formation of gamma globulin*
1967 Johansson and Ishizaka—*discovery of IgE*
(1977) Yalow*—*development of radioimmunoassay*

Nobel Prize winners in immunology are indicated by an asterisk,* and the date of award is shown in parentheses.

Figure 1–1. Major milestones in immunology.

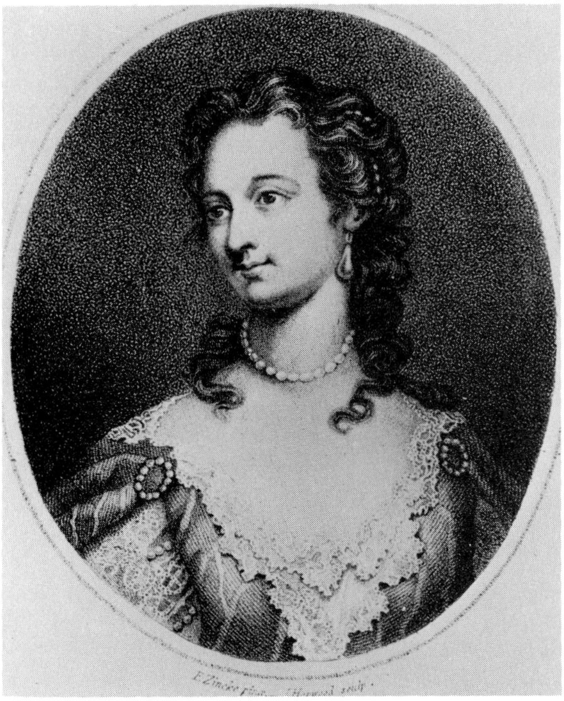

Figure 1–2. Lady Mary Wortley Montagu. (Courtesy of National Library of Medicine.)

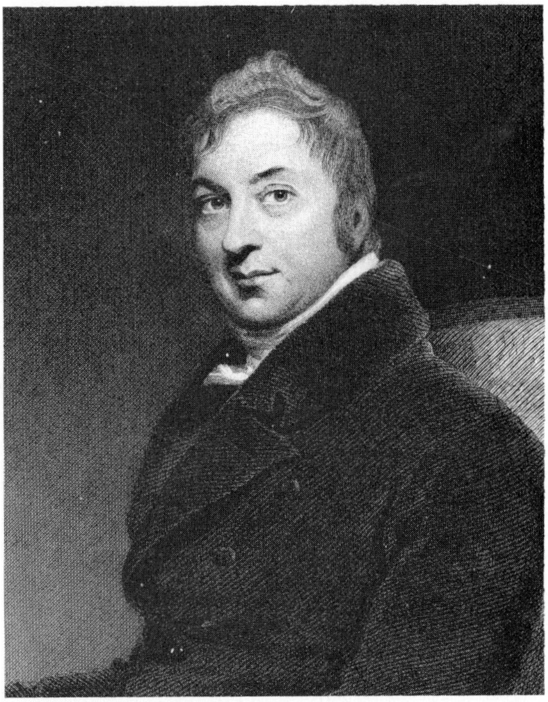

Figure 1–3. Edward Jenner (1749–1823). (Courtesy of National Library of Medicine.)

solidly immune. This use of living, attenuated, or heat-killed cultures is still our therapy of choice in the prophylaxis of many infectious diseases (Fig. 1–5), a process referred to as *active immunization* (Chapter 23).

Later, Robert Koch (Fig. 1–6) discovered the tubercle bacillus during his studies of the bacterial etiology of infectious diseases. While attempting to develop a vaccine for tuberculosis, he observed the phenomenon known today as delayed hypersensitivity or cell-mediated immunity (Chapter 9).

Following the isolation of the diphtheria bacillus, Roux and Yersin demonstrated the existence of a potent soluble exotoxin elaborated by this organism (Fig. 1–7). This toxin was used by von Behring (Fig. 1–8) and Kitasato to inoculate animals that produced in their serum a toxin-neutralizing substance called *antitoxin.* This neutralizing capability

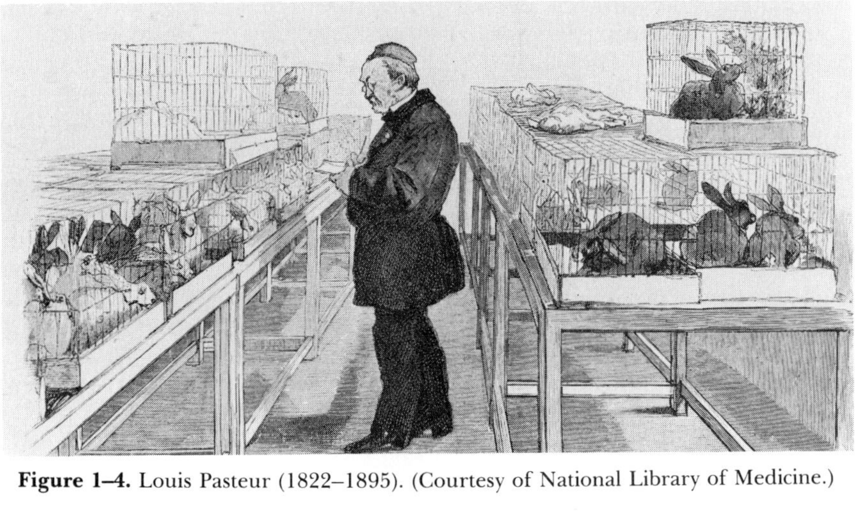

Figure 1–4. Louis Pasteur (1822–1895). (Courtesy of National Library of Medicine.)

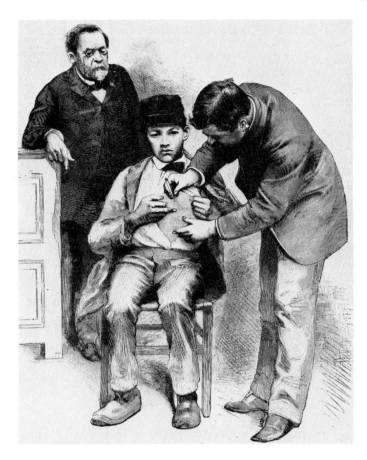

Figure 1–5. Louis Pasteur, to left, watches as an assistant inoculates a boy for "hydrophobia" (rabies). (Wood engraving in "L'Illustration" from Harper's Weekly *29*:836, 1885; courtesy of National Library of Medicine.)

could be transferred by the serum to uninoculated animals, a process called *passive immunization.* Their work formed a model for the modern techniques of preventing disease through passive immunization (immunotherapy). Pfeiffer and Bordet's work differentiated a substance in serum, distinct from antibody, called *complement* that also participates in the destruction of bacteria. The observations of Durham and von Gruber that serum could clump or agglutinate bacteria formed the basis for tests for the diagnosis of infectious specific agglutination reactions, such as the test described by Widal for the diagnosis of typhoid fever (Widal test).

Up to the turn of the century, the French and German schools dominated these areas of immunologic research. At that time there emerged two divergent vantage points from which immunology was observed and later developed: (1) the *humoral,* whose emphasis was the study of chemical products (i.e., antibodies) elaborated by cells, and (2) the *cellular,* whose emphasis was the biologic effects of intact cells involved in the host's response to foreignness (see Fig. 1–1). Paul Ehrlich (Fig. 1–9) proposed the humoral theory of antibody formation, and Elie Metchnikoff (Fig. 1–10) almost simultaneously developed the cellular theory of immunity. Both were correct, since in the individual both cellular and humoral factors are intimately interwoven and interdependent.

Ehrlich's side-chain theory proposed the pre-existence of receptors on the living cell surface that reacted with toxins; the excess receptors eventually could be released into the circulation as antibody (Fig. 1–11). It is ironic that one of the major areas of immunologic research today is the study of receptors on immunocompetent cells (Chapter 7). Subsequently, the major emphasis in immunology was directed at the identification, characterization, and biologic function of humoral factors (see Fig. 1–1).

Metchnikoff's theories of cellular immunity held that the body's scavenger cells, the phagocytes, were the prime detectors of foreign material as well as its primary defense system. His concepts went unrecognized for several decades but today represent an area of intensive immunologic research. Both cel-

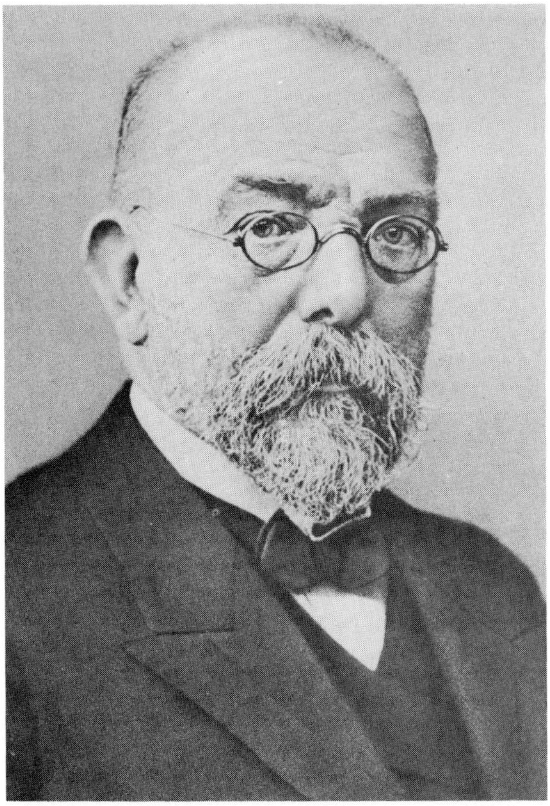

Figure 1–6. Robert Koch (1843–1910). (Courtesy of National Library of Medicine.)

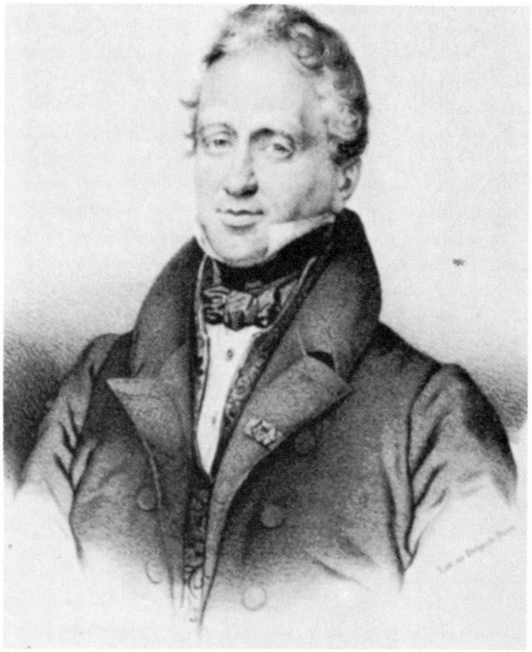

Figure 1–7. Pierre Paul Emile Roux (1853–1933). (Courtesy of National Library of Medicine.)

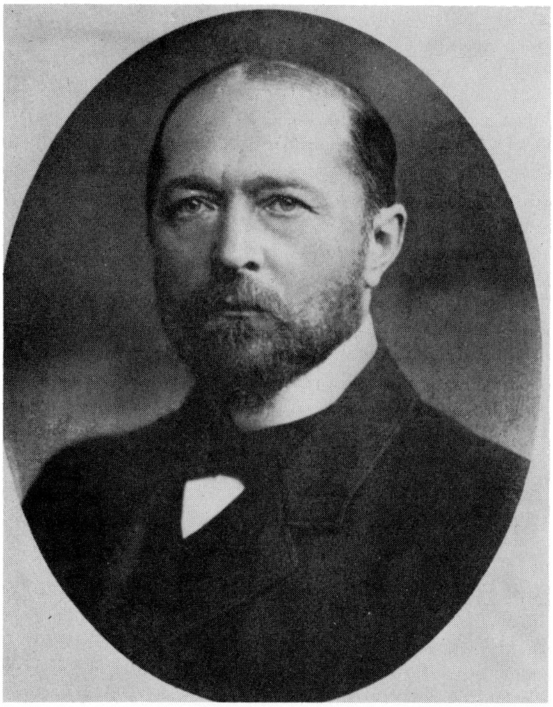

Figure 1–8. Emil Adolf von Behring (1854–1917). (Courtesy of National Library of Medicine.)

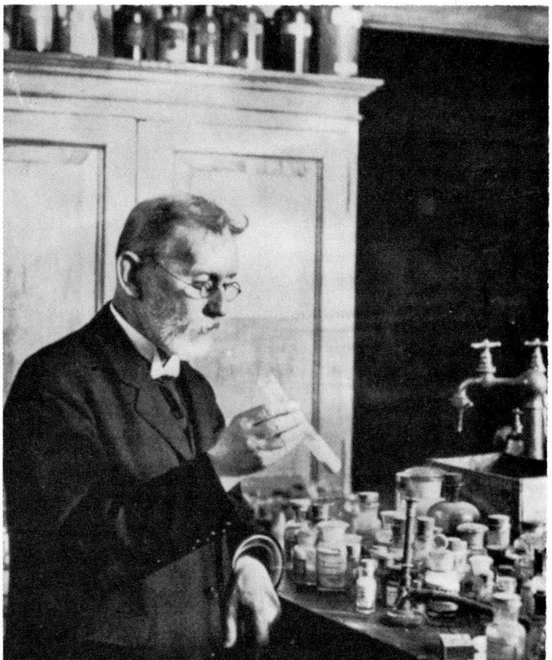

Figure 1–9. Paul Ehrlich (1854–1915). (Courtesy of National Library of Medicine.)

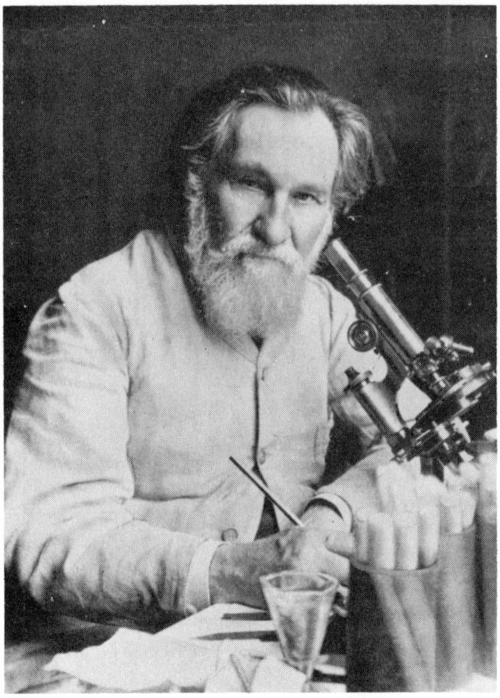

Figure 1–10. Elie Metchnikoff (1845–1916). (Courtesy of National Library of Medicine.)

lular and humoral factors are involved in understanding the principles underlying the immunologic processes that result in protection or tissue injury.

Today, there still remain two schools of immunologic investigation. The humoral school reached its peak with the discovery and characterization of the protein molecules that contain antibody activity, the *immunoglobulins* (Chapter 5). This work has culminated in the elucidation of the total amino acid sequence of almost all antibody molecules. At the same time, the cellular area is now being actively investigated from the standpoint of protection against infectious agents and graft rejection as well as immunity to tumors in man. The cellular-humoral dichotomy is also illustrated by the clinical observations of increased susceptibility to infection seen in individuals with congenital defects of the immunologic system (Chapter 22). Some lack the humoral protective function but retain the cellular; others are deficient in cellular but have normal humoral activity; still others are defective in both humoral and cellular functions. Clearly, both

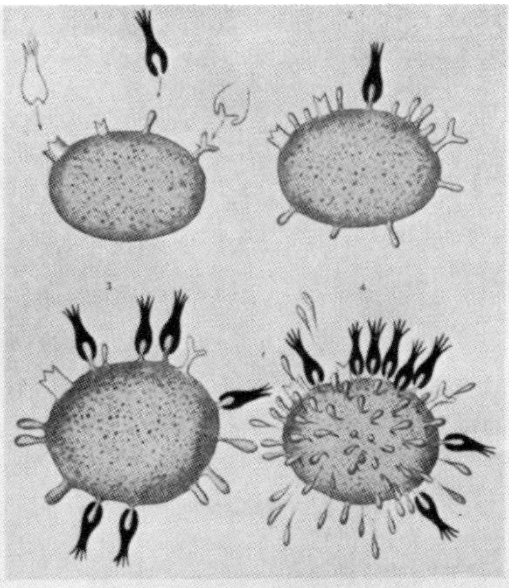

DIAGRAMMATIC REPRESENTATION OF THE SIDE-CHAIN THEORY
(PLATES I AND II)

Fig. 1 "The groups [the haptophore group of the side-chain of the cell and that of the food-stuff or the toxin] must be adapted to one another, *e.g.*, as male and female screw (PASTEUR), or as lock and key (E. FISCHER)."

Fig. 2 ". . . the first stage in the toxic action must be regarded as being the union of the toxin by means of its haptophore group to a special side-chain of the cell protoplasm."

Fig. 3 "The side-chain involved, so long as the union lasts, cannot exercise its normal, physiological, nutritive function . . ."

Fig. 4 "We are therefore now concerned with a defect which, according to the principles so ably worked out by . . . Weigert, is . . . [overcorrected] by regeneration."

Figure 1–11. Diagrammatic representation of the side-chain theory, showing the presence of pre-existing receptors on the cell surface *(A)*, which when produced in excess *(B)* could be released as antibody. (From Croonian Lecture, "On Immunity with Special Reference to Cell Life," Proc. R. Soc. Lond. (Biol.), *66*:424, 1906; courtesy of National Library of Medicine.)

Illustration continues on opposite page

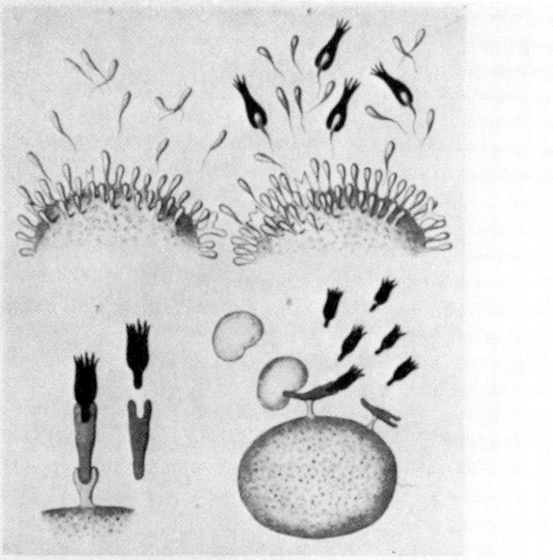

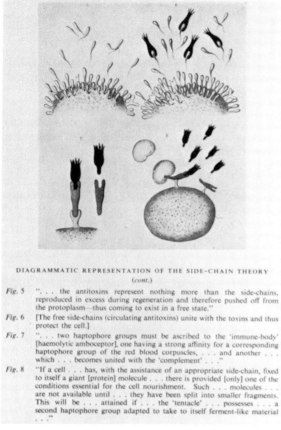

DIAGRAMMATIC REPRESENTATION OF THE SIDE-CHAIN THEORY
(*cont.*)

Fig. 5 ". . . the antitoxins represent nothing more than the side-chains, reproduced in excess during regeneration and therefore pushed off from the protoplasm—thus coming to exist in a free state."

Fig. 6 [The free side-chains (circulating antitoxins) unite with the toxins and thus protect the cell.]

Fig. 7 ". . . two haptophore groups must be ascribed to the 'immune-body' [haemolytic amboceptor], one having a strong affinity for a corresponding haptophore group of the red blood corpuscles, . . . and another . . . which . . . becomes united with the 'complement' . . ."

Fig. 8 "If a cell . . . has, with the assistance of an appropriate side-chain, fixed to itself a giant [protein] molecule . . . there is provided [only] one of the conditions essential for the cell nourishment. Such . . . molecules . . . are not available until . . . they have been split into smaller fragments. This will be . . . attained if . . . the 'tentacle' . . . possesses . . . a second haptophore group adapted to take to itself ferment-like material . . ."

Figure 1–11. *Continued.*

areas are of profound importance to man. Although one or the other aspect will be stressed at times throughout this book, cellular and humoral factors of immunity are interrelated and interdependent.

Immunity and Hypersensitivity

The term *immune* is derived from the Latin *immunis* (free from taxes or free from burden). In classical usage, immunity referred to the relative resistance of the host to reinfection by a given microbe. It is now evident that immune responses are not always beneficial, nor are they associated solely with resistance to infection. On the contrary, they can even confer unpleasant and harmful effects on the host. The noxious effect has been called *hypersensitivity* or *allergy*. Listed in Figure 1–1 are some of the pioneers who contributed to this field of tissue injury. The immunologic system is equipped not only to perform a *defense* function against infectious agents but also to concern itself with the more diverse biologic functions of *homeostasis* and *surveillance* (Table 1–1).

At the turn of the century, von Pirquet put forward a hypothesis to explain the multifaceted aspects of the immune response. He coined the term "allergy" to mean "altered reactivity" of the host; one change was recognized as immunity, and the other as hypersensitivity (Chapter 20A). Von Pirquet made no distinction between beneficial and harmful responses and suggested that they were all manifestations of a common biologic process of sensitization, which he encompassed by the term "allergy". He restricted the use of the term "immunity" to mean protection from infectious agents and the term "allergy" for a more generalized reactivity of the host to foreign substances. Over the years, allergy and immunity have become reversed in their meanings; immunity has come to mean that which von Pirquet defined originally as allergy, and allergy has come to mean hypersensitivity. Nevertheless, von Pirquet's concepts of the broad scope of the immune response are now accepted in immunology.

IMMUNOLOGY IN THE MODERN SENSE

A contemporary definition of immunity would include "all those physiologic mecha-

Table 1–1. Functions of the Immune System

Function	Nature of Immunologic Stimulus	Example	Aberrations	
			Hyper-	Hypo-
Defense	Exogenous	Microorganisms	Allergy	Immunologic deficiency disorders
Homeostasis	Endogenous or exogenous	Removal of effete and damaged cells	Autoimmune disease	—
Surveillance	Endogenous or exogenous	Removal of cell mutants	—	Malignant disease

nisms that endow the animal with the capacity to recognize materials as foreign to itself and to neutralize, eliminate, or metabolize them with or without injury to its own tissues." The responses of immunity may be classified into two categories: (1) *nonspecific* immunologic responses and (2) *specific* immunologic responses. Specific immune responses depend upon exposure to a foreign configuration and the subsequent recognition of and reaction to it. Nonspecific responses, on the other hand, occur following initial and subsequent exposure to a foreign configuration, and while selective in differentiating "self" from "nonself," they are not dependent upon specific recognition.

In the modern view, immunologic responses serve three functions—defense, homeostasis, and surveillance (see Table 1–1). The first is involved in resistance to infection by microorganisms, the second in removal of worn-out (effete) "self" components, and the third in perception and destruction of mutant cells.

The first function, defense against invasion by microorganisms, has occupied the thinking of immunologists for more than 100 years. If the cellular elements of defense are deployed successfully, the host will emerge victorious in the struggle with microorganisms. However, when these elements are *hyperactive,* certain undesirable features, such as allergy or hypersensitivity, may be seen (Chapter 20). Conversely, when these elements are *hypoactive,* there may be an increased susceptibility to repeated infections, as seen in the immunologic deficiency disorders (Chapter 22).

The second function, homeostasis, fulfills the universal requirement of all multicellular organisms to preserve uniformity of a given cell type. It concerns itself with normal degradative or catabolic functions of the body charged with the removal of damaged cellular elements, such as circulating erythrocytes or leukocytes. These may be damaged during the course of a normal life span or may arise as a consequence of injury. Aberrations of homeostasis are exemplified by the autoimmune diseases, in which these mechanisms are unduly enhanced (Chapter 20C).

The third function of the immune system is the most recently recognized and concerns itself with surveillance. This function monitors the recognition of abnormal cell types, which constantly arise within the body. These mutants may occur spontaneously or may be induced by certain viruses and chemicals (Chapter 19). The immune system is charged with the recognition and disposal of newly acquired configurations, most of which occur on cell surfaces. Failure of this mechanism has recently been assigned a causal role in the development of malignant disease (Chapter 19). Since it is becoming increasingly apparent that all three functions are under genetic control (Chapter 3), an understanding of the pathogenesis of many immunologically mediated diseases (Chapter 20) must take into account these genetic principles.

Modifying Factors

There are a number of factors that modify immune mechanisms: genetic, age, metabolic, environmental, anatomic, physiologic, and microbial (Table 1–2). The host immune mechanisms may be viewed *in toto* as a composite protective umbrella consisting of various components that shield the host from the injurious effects of noxious environmental agents (Fig. 1–12). Defects may be seen in any one facet, e.g., phagocyte dysfunction, or in all facets, e.g., malnutrition (Chapter 22).

Genetic Factors. The whole of the immune response is under genetic control (Chapter

Table 1–2. Elements Involved in Immunologic Processes

Modifying Factors	Type of Response	Type of Encounter	Examples
Genetic Age Metabolic Environmental and nutritional Anatomic Physiologic Microbial	Nonspecific immunity	All	Phagocytosis, inflammatory response, cellular immunity, fever, acute phase phenomena (CRP, sedimentation rate)
	Specific immunity	Initial and subsequent	Humoral, cell-mediated immunity (delayed hypersensitivity)

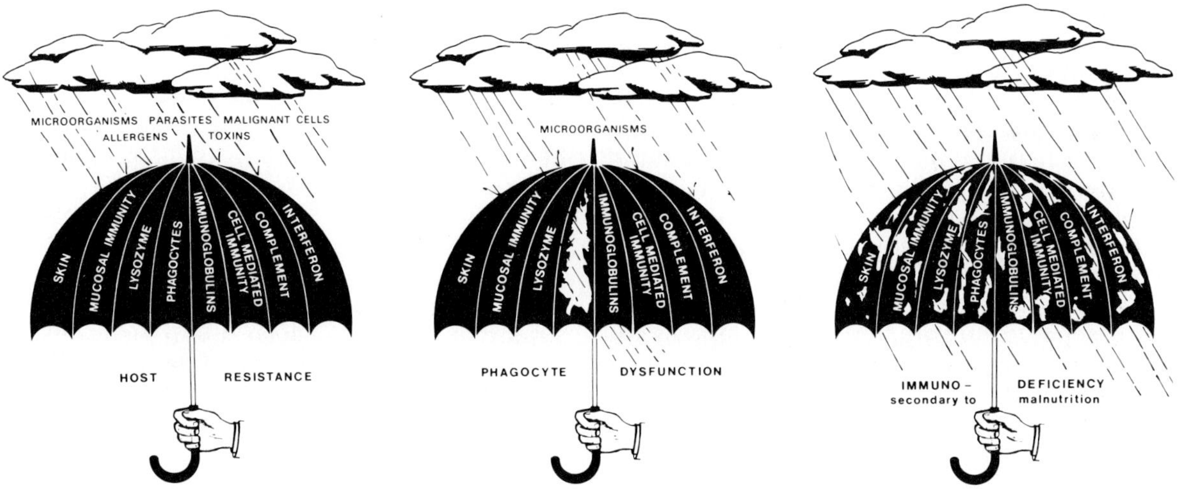

Figure 1–12. Host protective factors and examples of primary and secondary immunodeficiency. A concert of nonspecific barriers and antigen-specific immune responses protect man from extraneous and internal injurious agents *(left panel).* Primary, often inherited, deficit of a protective mechanism, for example, phagocyte defect, results in repeated infections *(center panel).* Malnutrition robs the host of many host defenses *(right panel).* Some bulwarks of immunity are impaired more often and to a greater extent than others. (From Chandra, R. K.: Malnutrition and immunocompetence: An overview. *In* Bellanti, J. A. (ed.): Acute Diarrhea: Its Nutritional Consequences in Children. New York, Raven Press, 1983. Reproduced with permission of the publisher.)

3). For example, certain strains of guinea pigs are capable of responding to a given antigen (responders), whereas others are not (nonresponders). In addition, there are genetic differences in susceptibility to infection that may have similar bases. Strains of rabbits have been bred, one susceptible, the other resistant, to infection with *Mycobacterium tuberculosis.* In man, moreover, there are racial differences in susceptibility to tuberculosis. One of the exciting recent developments in immunology has been the identification of a genetic complex (i.e., the major histocompatibility complex [MHC]) that controls both immune responsiveness and the expression of histocompatibility antigens on cells (Chapter 3). The identification of these genetic markers is finding clinical application in the diagnosis and treatment of many diseases whose pathogenesis has been unclear in the past, e.g., ankylosing spondylitis (Chapter 20C) and lymphomas (Chapter 19).

Age Factors. Chronologic age influences immunity, and direct evidence is accumulating that a hypofunctional state of the immune system occurs in the very young and the very old. For example, these two age groups are uniquely susceptible to the ravages of infection. Generalized sepsis due to *Escherichia coli* is not an uncommon event in the newborn period. Presumably, this is the result of a number of factors, including an incompletely developed specific immune system and deficiencies of nonspecific immunity, such as a thin integument and a poor inflammatory response. Similarly, fatal pneumonia due to *Streptococcus (Diplococcus) pneumoniae* and influenza is a common event during old age. Underlying cardiac, pulmonary, and metabolic derangements (e.g., diabetes mellitus) as well as a primary hypofunction of the immune system predispose this group to infection with these pathogens. This provides the rationale for immunization of this group with pneumococcal and influenza vaccines (Chapter 23). Also, the decrease in many of the immunologic functions, such as immunoglobulin concentrations and cell-mediated immunity, in the elderly may be associated with the known higher incidence of autoimmune phenomena and malignancy in this age group.

Metabolic Factors. In addition to the well-recognized susceptibility of the patient with uncompensated diabetes mellitus to bacterial infection, certain hormones have been shown to affect the host immune response. In both hypoadrenal and hypothyroid states there is an increased susceptibility to infection. Moreover, patients treated with steroids are unduly susceptible to bacterial diseases (e.g., staphylococcal infection) as well as to certain viral diseases (e.g., varicella). Steroids appear to affect many modalities of the immune response, having an inhibitory effect on phagocytosis and inflammation as well as on humoral and cellular immunity (Chapters 10 and 25).

Environmental and Nutritional Factors. The increased rate of infectious diseases due to poor living conditions is well known. An increased rate of infection may be related to a greater exposure to pathogens as well as to diminished resistance caused by malnutrition. In studies conducted in children in the developing countries, nutritional deprivation at an early age has been shown to be associated with developmental failure of the immune response, predominantly the cell-mediated immune response which presents as recurrent infections, particularly respiratory and gastrointestinal. Recently, a new acquired immune deficiency syndrome (AIDS) has been described in homosexual males and other groups, which has been associated with recurrent opportunistic infections and malignancy (Chapters 14 and 22). Although at present the precise cause of the syndrome as well as its therapy is unknown, the most plausible etiology is a transmissible agent (e.g., a variant of human T-cell leukemia virus family, HTLV-III) that may be destroying the immune system, particularly its cell-mediated component. The occurrence of the syndrome also points to the contribution of other factors, e.g., lifestyle, environment, intravenous drug use, and transfusions. The solution of these complex problems will require the broader consideration of many factors, e.g., social, economic, and political as well as medical.

Anatomic Factors. The first line of defense against invasion by microbes is usually provided by the *skin* and the *mucous membranes*. These tissues act in nonspecific immunity by providing a physical barrier to invasion. The intact skin appears to be a more effective barrier than the mucous membranes. The increased susceptibility to infections following burns or secondary to eczema is a well-known clinical finding. The skin and the mucous membranes may allow penetration by certain pathogens, e.g., the tubercle bacillus, which can pass across the intact gastrointestinal mucosa after ingestion, leading to local infection and regional lymph node enlargement.

Microbial Factors. Following colonization of the body surfaces, both internal and external, a "normal" flora develops. Not only is this flora essential for the production of metabolites, e.g., vitamin K, but it also contributes to the production of "natural" antibodies to these organisms. The flora also acts to suppress the overgrowth and the subsequent infection by pathogenic and possibly virulent organisms. The well-recognized overgrowth of virulent staphylococci in patients treated with so-called broad-spectrum antibiotics illustrates the effect of a disturbed ecologic microbial balance in man.

Physiologic Factors. The gastric juice is an unfavorable milieu for many pathogenic strains of bacteria, which are destroyed in the stomach following ingestion. Some bacteria, such as the typhoid bacilli, are not affected, survive digestion, and produce disease. Ciliary action in the respiratory tract is another important physiologic mechanism of resistance. Normal urine flow clears bacteria from the urinary tract, preventing infection. It is well known that the obstructed urinary tract or respiratory tract (e.g., cystic fibrosis) is more susceptible to infection, probably owing to the absence of this clearing action.

Certain skin secretions of normal individuals have been shown to be bactericidal. This is believed to be due in part to the acidity of the skin produced by *lactic acid.* After puberty the skin appears more resistant to infection with certain fungi (dermatophytes). This may result from an increase in saturated fatty acids in the skin. In postpubertal skin, there are also increased amounts of unsaturated fatty acids known to be bactericidal.

Lysozyme is an enzyme that has been shown to have bactericidal activity. The enzyme is found in many types of cells and body fluids and functions by virtue of mucolytic properties that cleave acetylamino-sugars, the backbone of both gram-positive and gram-negative bacteria. Certain basic polypeptides (with large amounts of lysine) have been shown to kill anthrax. There are other chemical substances in the body that kill, injure, or inhibit bacteria and viruses.

The blood contains a number of protective substances that act in a nonspecific manner. Bactericidal substances in blood have been demonstrated that do not appear to be specific antibody, since they are present without prior exposure to a foreign configuration. These have been called *natural antibodies.* Their precise origin is not known, and, indeed, the concept of preformed antibodies has been a subject of controversy. One explanation is that these antibodies are stimulated following exposure to closely related materials. It is known, for example, that isohemagglutinins—the antibody to blood groups—

(Chapter 3) may develop as a result of exposure to enteric bacilli containing blood group—like substances in their structure.

Another set of protective functions are derived from the complement system, a cascading group of serum proteins with biologic functions (Chapter 6). Deficiency of a number of the complement components may be associated with a variety of clinical disorders, including recurrent infection, edema, or autoimmune diseases (Chapters 20A, 20C, and 22).

Still another set of protective functions are provided by tissue mucoproteins with viricidal activity, which prevent attachment of certain viruses to host cells. A family of proteins, the *interferons,* originally thought to inhibit viral replication by protection of host cells (Chapter 16), are now known to have much broader cellular effects and are receiving increasing attention in the autoimmune diseases (Chapter 20C) and malignancy (Chapter 19).

Nonspecific Immune Responses: Inflammation and Phagocytosis

The first encounter of the host with a foreign configuration leads to a stereotyped response that consists of mobilization of phagocytic elements into areas where the foreign configuration has been introduced (Table 1–2). This may occur as an isolated event or as part of the inflammatory response.

Inflammation. Following any one of a variety of tissue injuries, a spectrum of cellular and systemic events occur in which the host attempts to restore and maintain homeostasis under the adverse environmental influences. This reaction is referred to as inflammation and is described in greater detail in Chapter 12. Accompanying the inflammatory response are a number of systemic events that involve fever as well as a series of hematologic phenomena. The febrile response is believed to reflect enhanced metabolic activity following injury. One mechanism is believed to be the release of endogenous pyrogen from host leukocytes. An increased leukocyte count occurs during bacterial infections or tissue injury. Tissue necrosis, for example, with myocardial infarction, is associated with a "left shift," i.e., a predominance of polymorphonuclear leukocytes with many young forms, e.g., bands. In general, bacterial products cause more tissue injury than do viruses and induce the greatest febrile response.

Increased blood fibrinogen, activation of the Hageman factor, and increased fibrinolytic activity and erythrocyte rouleaux formation are each associated with one of the most useful indices of the acute-phase response—the erythrocyte sedimentation rate (ESR). This parameter is affected by any factor causing erythrocyte rouleaux formation, such as increased gamma globulin, e.g., multiple myeloma (Chapter 21). A rapid sedimentation rate is most commonly associated, however, with a raised fibrinogen level.

Other changes in serum globulins occur during illness, such as an increase in the alpha and beta globulins. One of these, the C-reactive protein (CRP), is elevated in the early phases of many illnesses. It was originally discovered by virtue of its interaction with the C, or carbohydrate, substance of *Streptococcus (Diplococcus) pneumoniae,* but it is now recognized that CRP is released from many types of tissues following injury.

Phagocytosis. Once mobilized, the phagocytic cells mount an attack on their target by a process called phagocytosis (cell-eating), a multiphasic act requiring the following steps: recognition of the material to be ingested, movement toward the object (chemotaxis), attachment, ingestion, and subsequent intracellular digestion by a number of antimicrobial mechanisms (Chapter 2). A series of complex biochemical reactions occur involving utilization of certain humoral factors (e.g., opsonins) as well as complement, a maze of interacting serum proteins which, when triggered, lead to the generation of a number of products active in each of these functions (Chapter 6). Knowledge of these steps has assumed great clinical importance with the recent discovery that there occur in the human inborn errors of leukocyte function. This family of neutrophil dysfunction syndromes may involve deficiencies in complement, antibody, or intracellular enzymes concerned with antimicrobial activity (Chapter 22).

Specific Immune Responses

Definitions. The specific immune responses are concerned with the recognition and ultimate disposal of foreignness in a highly discriminatory fashion. The final outcome of the encounter between host and a foreign configuration is dependent upon the properties of the substance (size, structure, chemical nature, amount) and also upon properties of the host (age, genetic constitution) (Fig. 1–13). The foreign material may interact with the host in a number of ways. It may become localized or completely removed nonspecifically by phagocytes, e.g., inert carbon particles, without any further response. It may also lead to a specific immune response in which the material is referred to as an *immunogen* or *antigen* (Chapter 4). On the other hand, after interaction with the host the material may induce a state of unresponsiveness, in which case it is referred to as a *tolerogen.* The resulting condition, *immunologic tolerance,* will be considered in Chapter 10.

General Characteristics of the Specific Immune Response. The *specific immune response* is the reaction of the host to a foreign substance and encompasses a series of cellular interactions expressed by the elaboration of specific cell products. There are three general characteristics of the specific immune response that distinguish it from the nonspecific responses: (1) *specificity,* (2) *heterogeneity,* and (3) *memory.*

Specificity is the highly discriminatory selectivity by which the products of the immune response will react solely with the configuration identical or similar to that which initiated the response. Landsteiner first demonstrated specificity and showed that antibody could distinguish closely related substances; it is this property of the specific immune response that distinguishes one antigen from another. Operationally, the immune response can distinguish and differentiate antigens originating from different species *(species specificity),* from different individuals *(individual specificity),* or from different organs *(organ specificity).*

The second characteristic of the specific immune response is heterogeneity, in which a vast array of cell types and cell products are induced to interact with a diversity of response commensurate with the variety of cell types. The heterogeneity of cell types gives rise to the elaboration of an equally heterogeneous population of cell products, e.g., antibody. This heterogeneity of antibody contributes a fine degree of homeostatic control with which the host can respond in a highly variable and specific manner to foreign structures.

The third hallmark of the specific immune response is memory. Memory is the property that results in an accelerated and augmented specific response through proliferation and differentiation of sensitized cells upon subsequent exposure to an immunogen. This leads to an enhanced elaboration of cell products.

Nonspecific responses, on the other hand, represent the initial encounter with foreignness, and upon subsequent encounter merely repeat the same general response to the substance. Unlike the specific responses, the nonspecific responses include a limited number of pre-existent cell types. The specific responses are characterized by the induction and interaction of a variety of new cell types specific for the inducing antigen. The nonspecific immune responses do not include the property of memory.

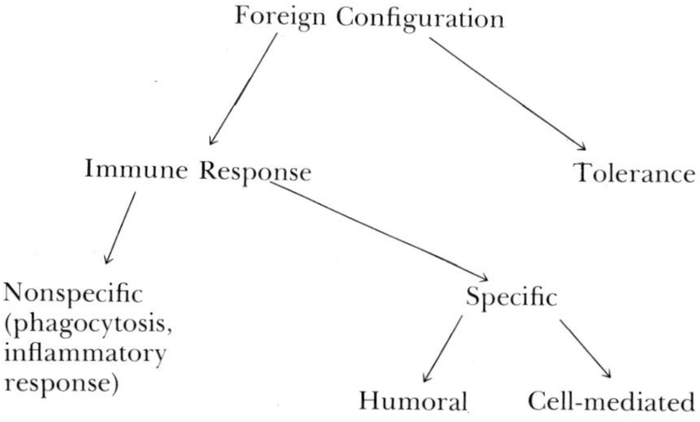

Figure 1–13. Possible outcome of an encounter of the host with a foreign configuration.

Specific Immune Responses: Humoral and Cell-Mediated

There are two types of effector mechanisms that mediate specific immune responses (Fig. 1–14): (1) those mediated by a cell product of the lymphoid tissues referred to as antibody *(humoral immunity)* and (2) those mediated by specifically sensitized lymphocytes themselves *(cell-mediated immunity).*

Following an immunogenic stimulus a series of cellular events occur prior to the expression of the *specific immune response.* For ease of discussion, we may divide these events into two general areas: (1) the *afferent limb,* in which there takes place the processing of the immunogen by macrophages and cellular interactions between lymphocytes and macrophages culminating in the activation of lymphocytes, and (2) the *efferent limb,* in which the specifically activated lymphocytes proliferate and differentiate in the expression of specific humoral and cell-mediated immunity. These events are described in detail in Chapter 7.

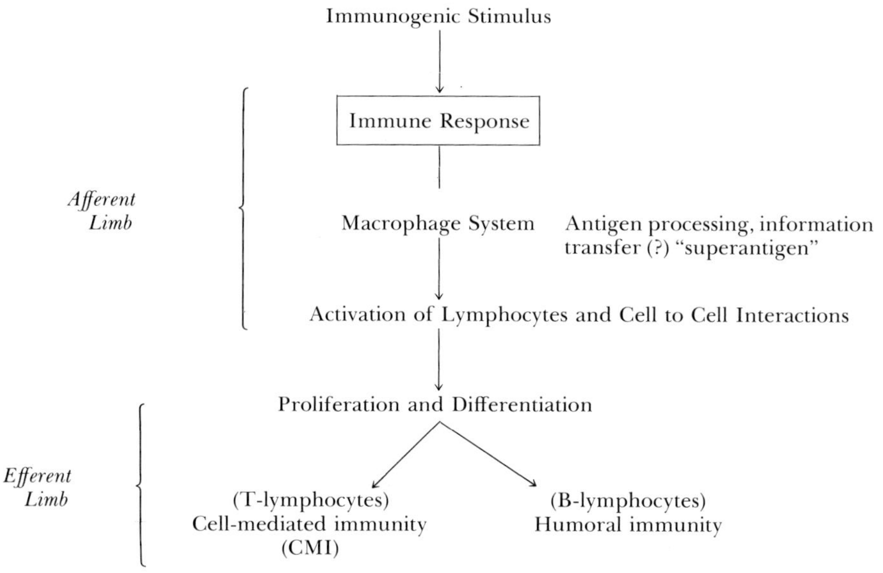

Figure 1–14. Effector mechanisms that mediate specific immunologic responses.

Humoral Immunity. Humoral immunity is mediated by a group of lymphocytes that differentiate in bone marrow and are referred to as bone marrow–derived or B-lymphocytes. Antibody is a product of B-cell elements (B-lymphocytes and plasma cells) and is either cell-bound or secreted as an extracellular product. It has the capability of reacting with the configuration responsible for its production (immunogen or antigen) (Chapter 4). In the human, antibody is associated with five major classes of proteins (immunoglobulins) that can be differentiated from one another on the basis of size, biologic function, or biochemical properties (Chapter 5). The presence of antibody is determined by measuring some functional parameter of the interaction between antigen and antibody (Chapter 8). For example, some antibodies can neutralize the effect of a toxin (antitoxin), others can punch holes in cell membranes (cytolytic antibodies), and still others are measured *in vivo* by eliciting a hypersensitive reaction (anaphylactic antibody) such as the IgE. It is believed that the humoral effector mechanism is derived embryologically in the chicken from the bursa of Fabricius. In the human, the location of this tissue is not known with certainty, but it is nevertheless referred to on occasion as the gut-associated lymphoid tissue (GALT).

Other Humoral Factors: Biologic Amplification Systems. Immunologic reactions may also involve other humoral factors that can augment or amplify the response without the direct participation of cells. The best known example is the complement system, in which a variety of factors, both cell-bound and soluble, come into play and set the stage for protective mechanisms and, in some cases, detrimental events. Most complement factors act by triggering the inflammatory response. Under certain conditions this leads to the removal of infective agents; however, under other conditions the result is tissue damage. The complement system will be described in detail in a later section (Chapter 6).

The kallikrein system is yet another component of the amplification system and represents a well-defined system of proteins in plasma, activated by a reaction of antigen with antibody. Presumably through the activation of the Hageman factor and the permeability factor of Miles, the enzyme kallikrein interacts with its substrate, an alpha-2-macroglobulin, to produce different vasoactive peptides, e.g., the bradykinins. Another humoral factor, slow-reacting substance (SRS-A), is a humoral factor liberated by the interaction of antigen with sensitized cells and has recently been identified as one of the arachidonic acid metabolites, i.e., leukotriene (Chapters 13 and 20A). All these agents increase capillary permeability.

Certain proteins of the coagulation sequence also may act to amplify the immune response during the interaction of antigen with antibody. Increase in the rapidity of clotting in plasma following such interaction has been attributed to activation of the Hageman factor, although an earlier step in the coagulation sequence may be directly activated by an antigen-antibody complex. Finally, there is some evidence that the fibrinolytic system may be activated in plasma by the antigen-antibody interaction, but the precise mechanism for the conversion of plasminogen to plasmin is unknown.

Cell-Mediated Immunity. Cell-mediated immunity is the second major type of effector mechanism underlying specific immune responses (see Fig. 1–13). This is mediated by a group of lymphocytes that differentiate under the influence of the thymus and are therefore referred to as T-lymphocytes. This effector arm of specific immunity is carried out directly by specifically sensitized lymphocytes or by specific cell products that are formed upon interaction of immunogen with specifically sensitized lymphocytes. These specific cell products, the lymphokines, include migration inhibitory factor (MIF), cytotoxin, interferon, and several others and are believed to be the effector molecules of cellular immunity (Chapter 9).

CONCEPT OF IMMUNOLOGIC BALANCE

In order to understand immunologically mediated disease, the immunologic system may be viewed as a dynamic multicompartmental network of elements with ever-changing morphologic components and functions (Chapter 11). It should be kept in mind that much of the work in experimental immunology has been performed with nonreplicating antigens. Normally, many immunologic stimuli are self-replicating, such as bacteria, viruses, and organ transplants. Thus, data obtained in the laboratory may not be directly applicable to natural phenomena occurring in humans. A second point is that not all configurations confronting the host are immunogenic, i.e., lead to a specific immune response. Some substances are taken up by phagocytic cells and may be completely degraded before they can lead to a specific immune response (Chapter 20A).

As with all physiologic mechanisms, the immunologic response may be viewed as an adaptive system in which the body attempts to maintain homeostasis between the internal body environment and the external environment.

Following confrontation of the host with a foreign configuration (stimulus) there is a period of disequilibrium. Immunologic balance is restored by the appropriate immunologic response. A pertubation occurs if the stimulus and the response are inappropriate for each other. Any derangement in homeostasis results in the production of undesirable sequelae referred to as immunologic imbalance. The clinical appearance of immunologic imbalance is manifested as immunologically mediated disease (Chapter 20).

Overwhelming sepsis is an example of a situation in which the amount of replicating antigen exceeds the capacity of lymphoreticular tissue response. Immunologic unresponsiveness or paralysis may also occur when the host is confronted with antigen in a form not easily catabolized, e.g., the pneumococcal polysaccharide. The net result is referred to as high-zone paralysis (Chapter 10). This may be the mechanism by which the host maintains nonreactivity to its own bodily constituents, i.e., "self-tolerance."

The converse is also seen and occurs when too little antigen leads to an immunologic imbalance. This is known as low-dose tolerance. The clinical counterpart of low-dose interaction is perhaps best exemplified by the interaction of certain microorganisms with the host. Certain fungi, e.g., dermatophytes, can establish a type of infection in which insufficient replication occurs to stimulate the immunologic apparatus. Consequently, these organisms live in peaceful coexistence with the host, usually at body surfaces, and persist in this relationship for many years. Disordered homeostasis due to the magnitude or type of antigen is at present a subject of intense interest in relation to organ transplantation and maternal-fetal interactions.

The second major cause of immunologic imbalance is related to aberrancy of cells of the immunologic system, e.g., immune deficiency disorders (Chapter 22) or products of the immune response. There may be a failure to produce sufficient numbers of effector cells or cell products, or they may be functionally defective in type. Failure may be genetic (e.g., congenital agammaglobulinemia) and may be controlled by certain loci in the major histocompatibility complex (MHC), e.g., immune response (Ir) locus, which specifies the synthesis of certain cell surface antigens that control cellular interactions. Failure also may be acquired, e.g., acquired immune deficiency syndrome (AIDS). The recent discovery of subpopulations of T-cells that regulate the immune response, e.g., T-helper and T-suppressor cells, and imbalance in ratios in certain disease states further exemplify the importance of an understanding of the host's immunologic system in balance. The net result is immunologic imbalance, recurrent infections, and a predisposition to malignant tumors and autoimmune disease. These aberrations also occur as a consequence of acquired cases of immunosuppression, e.g., chemical immunosuppressive agents.

Aberrations may involve the production of cell products. There may be overproduction of a product normally present in trace amounts. An example of this is the allergic individual who produces too much IgE immunoglobulin and manifests immediate-type hypersensitivity. Qualitative aberrations may also occur with natural infection; for example, following streptococcal tonsillitis, antigen-antibody complexes may be produced that damage the kidney (acute glomerulonephritis). Lastly, these aberrations may be produced iatrogenically as a complication of vaccines. Certain vaccines may produce hypersensitivity rather than protective immunity.

Suggestions for Further Reading

History of Immunology

Bulloch, W.: The History of Bacteriology. London, Oxford University Press, 1938.

Burnet, F. M.: Cellular Immunology. Cambridge, Melbourne University Press, 1969.

Edsall, G.: What is immunology? J. Immunol., *67*:167, 1951.

Ehrlich, P.: On immunity with special reference to cell life. Proc. Soc. Lond. (Biol). *66*:424, 1906.

Grabar, P.: The historical background of immunology. *In* Stites, D. P., Stobo, J. D., Fudenberg, H. H., et al. (eds.): Basic and Clinical Immunology. 4th ed. Los Altos, Lange Medical Publications, 1982.

Marx, J. L.: Strong new candidate for AIDS agent. Science *224*:475, 1984.

Metchnikoff, E.: Immunity in Infective Diseases. London, Cambridge University Press, 1905.

Immunology in the Modern Sense

Bellanti, J. A., and Dayton, D. H.: The Phagocytic Cell in Host Resistance. New York, Raven Press, 1975.

Chandra, R. K.: Malnutrition and immunocompetence: An overview. *In* Bellanti, J. A. (ed.): Acute Diarrhea: Its Nutritional Consequences in Children. New York, Raven Press, 1983.

Davis, B. D., Dulbecco, R., Eisen, H. N., et al.: Immunology. *In* Davis, B. D., et al. (eds.): Microbiology. New York, Harper & Row, 1973.

Gell, P. G. H., Coombs, R. R. A., and Lachman, P. T.: Clinical Aspects of Immunology. Oxford, Blackwell Scientific Publications, 1975.

Humphrey, J. H., and White, R. G.: Immunology for Students of Medicine. Philadelphia, F. A. Davis, 1970.

Kabat, E. A.: Structural Concepts in Immunology and Immunochemistry. New York, Holt, Rinehart and Winston, 1975.

Roitt, I. M.: Essential Immunology. Oxford, Blackwell Scientific Publications, 1974.

Rose, N. R., Milgrom, F., and van Oss, C. J.: Fundamentals of Immunology. New York, Macmillan Publishing Company, 1973.

Sell, S.: Immunology, Immunopathology and Immunity. Hagerstown, Md., Harper & Row, 1975.

Samuelsson, B.: Leukotrienes: Mediators of immediate hypersensitivity reactions and inflammation. Science, *220*:568, 1983.

Stites, D. P., Stobo, J. D., Fudenberg, H. H., et al. (eds.): Basic and Clinical Immunology. 4th ed. Los Altos, Lange Medical Publications, 1982.

Chapter 2

General Immunobiology

Joseph A. Bellanti, M.D., and Josef V. Kadlec, S.J., M.D.

ANATOMIC ORGANIZATION OF THE IMMUNE SYSTEM

Cell Types and Effector Mechanisms Involved in Nonspecific Immune Mechanisms

In order to carry out the functions of immunity, a ubiquitous immunologic cell system has appeared within the vertebrates: the *lymphoreticular system.* This collection of cellular elements is distributed strategically throughout the tissues as well as lining lymphatic and vascular channels. Its cells are housed within the *blood, tissues, thymus, lymph nodes,* and *spleen* (internal secretory system), and in those body tracts exposed to the external environment—the *respiratory, gastrointestinal,* and *genitourinary* systems (external secretory system) (Fig. 2–1).

The tissues contain a variety of cell types, each performing a separate function either directly or through the elaboration of a cell product(s). The system may be activated by a variety of stimuli that have the common characteristic of being recognized as foreign by the host. The stimuli may be presented to the host either exogenously (e.g., microorganisms) or endogenously (e.g., effete cells or transformed neoplastic cells).

Following activation, a spectrum of cellular and humoral events occurs that constitutes the nonspecific and specific immune responses (Chapter 1). The nonspecific immune responses consist of phagocytosis and the inflammatory response; if the stimulus leads to the production of specific cell products (e.g., antibody, lymphokines) by specialized groups of lymphocytes, the foreign configurations are referred to as immunogens or antigens (Chapter 4). A number of effector mechanisms involving several cell types, cell products, and soluble serum factors may be called into play by the host following the encounter and recognition of a foreign configuration (Table 2–1). The cellular constituents include *mononuclear phagocytes, granulocytes, platelets,* and *lymphocytes.* The origins of these cells are pluripotential hematopoietic stem cells located within the bone marrow, fetal liver, and yolk sac of the fetus. The cell types, differentiation, and tissue localization of these cells are shown in Table 2–2. For ease of discussion, these cells will be grouped into a functional classification according to the following categories: *phagocytic cells, mediator cells,* and *lymphocytes.*

PHAGOCYTIC CELLS

The process of phagocytosis is part of the nonspecific immune response (Chapter 1) and represents the host's initial encounter with foreignness. Endocytosis is a more general term and includes both *phagocytosis* (ingestion of particles) and *pinocytosis* (uptake of nonparticulates, e.g., fluid droplets). Both represent the process of engulfment and uptake of particles or fluid from the environment, and those groups of specialized cells that carry out these functions are commonly referred to as phagocytic cells. In some cases, subsequent digestion of these materials into smaller fragments facilitates their elimination (Fig. 2–2). In the human, phagocytosis is carried out primarily by *mononuclear phagocytes, neutrophils,* and, to a lesser extent, *eosinophils.*

Mononuclear Phagocytes. The mononuclear phagocyte system (MPS) consists of a generalized group of cells that are widely distributed throughout the body where they can effectively eliminate foreign materials and debris from the blood, lymph, and tis-

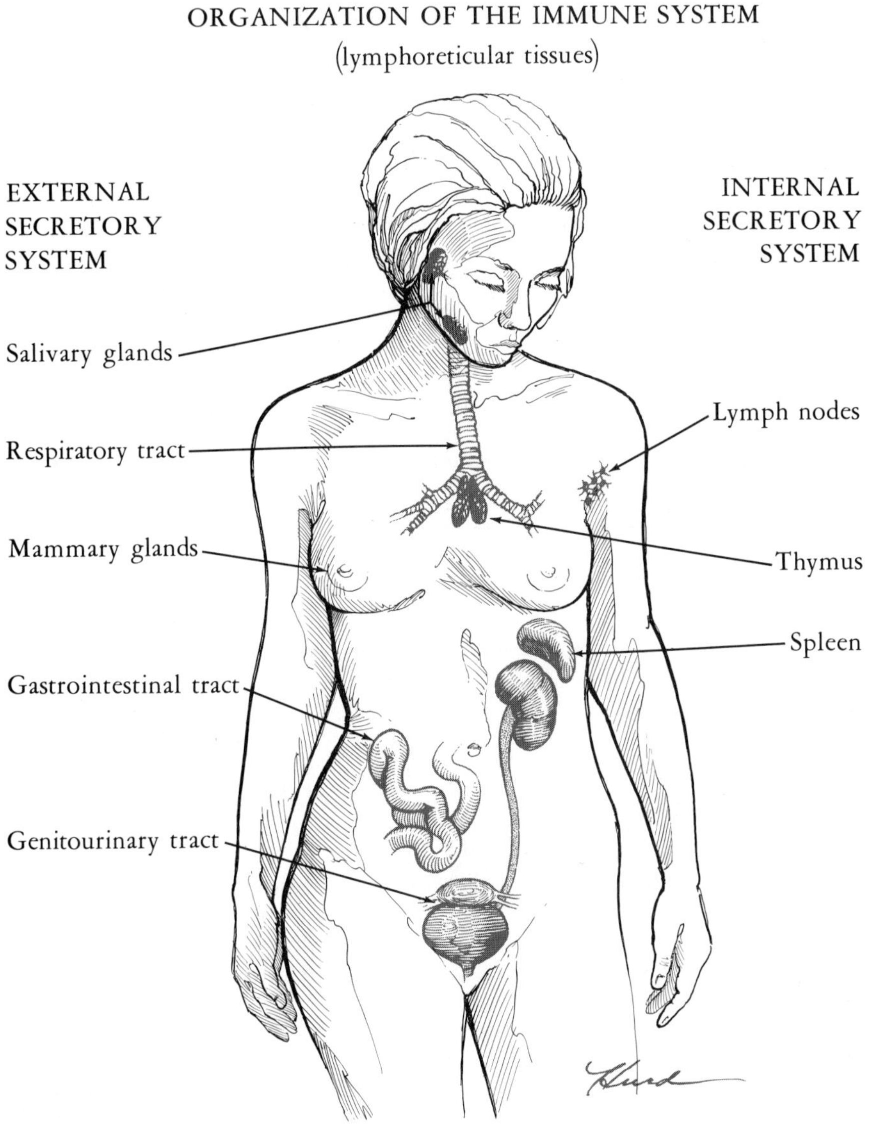

Figure 2–1. Schematic representation of the lymphoreticular tissues.

Table 2–1. Cell Types and Effector Mechanisms Triggered by or Involved in Immune Reactions

Cell Type	Humoral Factors: Agents Responsible for Mobilization of Cells	Humoral Factors: Cell Product
Nonspecific	monocytes – circulating blood macrophages – tissues	
Mononuclear phagocytes	Chemotactic factors, macrophage activating factor (MAF)	Processed immunogen
Granulocytes		
Neutrophils	Chemotactic factors (complement-associated and bacterial factors) lymphocyte-derived	Kallikreins (producing kinins). SRS-A, basic peptides
Eosinophils	Specific chemotactic factors (e.g., ECF-A), and other chemotactic factors as for neutrophils	Histaminase, aryl sulfatase, phospholipase D, eosinophil-derived inhibitor (EDI)
Basophils	?	Vasoactive amines
Platelets	Factors producing platelet aggregates (thrombin, collagen)	Vasoactive amines
Specific		
B-lymphocytes	Antigen	Antibody
T-lymphocytes	Antigen	Lymphokines, e.g., MIF, interferon, cytotoxin, "transfer factor," and others

Table 2–2. Differentiation and Localization of Cells Involved in Immune Processes*

	Bone marrow, liver, yolk sac	→ Blood	→ Lymphoid organs and connective tissue
Hematopoietic stem cell	B-cell precursor	→ B-lymphocyte	→ B-lymphocyte or → Plasma cell
	T-cell precursor	→ T-lymphocyte	→ T-lymphocyte
	T-cell precursor; Monocyte (?)	→ NK cell	→ NK cell
	Monoblast ↓ Promonocyte ↓ Monocyte	→ Monocyte	→ Free macrophage; → Fixed macrophage
	Granulocyte series	→ Neutrophils	→ Tissue neutrophils
		→ Eosinophils	→ Tissue neosinophils
		→ Basophils	
	Megakaryocyte series	→ Platelets	

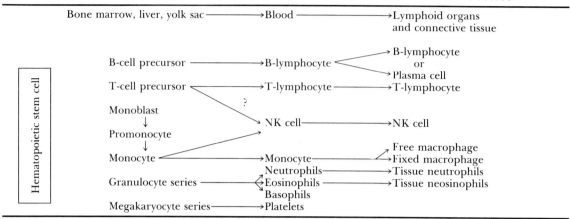

*(Adapted from van Furth, R.: Mononuclear Phagocytes in Immunity, Infection and Pathology. Oxford, Blackwell Scientific Publications, 1975.)

sues. The term MPS has been suggested to replace the less precise term reticuloendothelial system (RES), which was coined by Aschoff to define those morphologic elements of the immune system that are phagocytic as determined by clearance of particles (Fig. 2–3). The mononuclear phagocytes include both monocytes of the circulating blood (Fig. 2–4) and macrophages found in various tissues of the body.

The mononuclear phagocytes are produced from a stem cell in the bone marrow. Here they undergo proliferation and are delivered to the blood after a period of maturation through a *monoblast → promonocyte → monocyte* phase. Following a brief time in the blood (approximately one to two days), the monocytes migrate to the main site of their action in the tissues where they differentiate further into macrophages. Here they can divide, thus differing from granulocytes. The blood monocyte serves as an intermediate cell in the monocyte-macrophage transition.

The transition of monocyte to macrophage is also accompanied by morphologic, biochemical, and functional changes. During

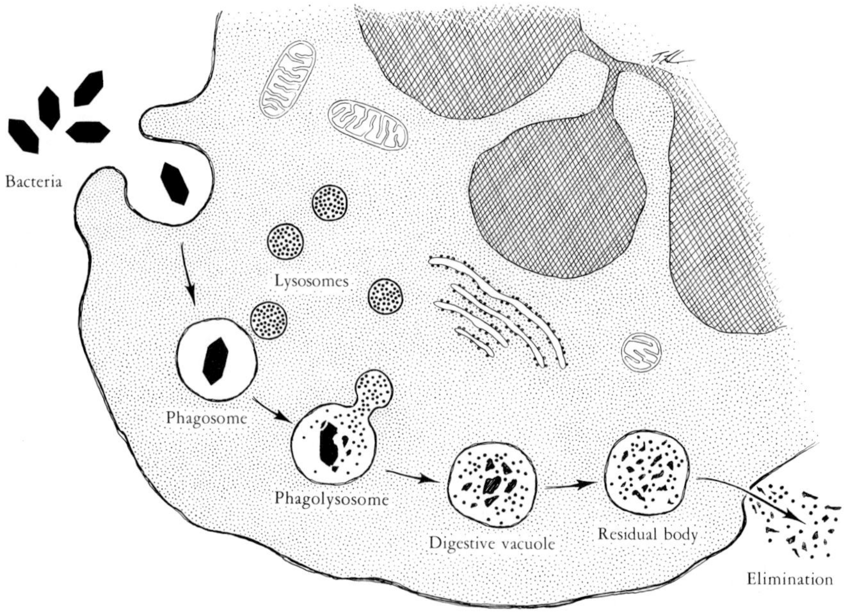

Figure 2–2. Schematic representation of phagocytosis showing ingestion process and intracellular digestion.

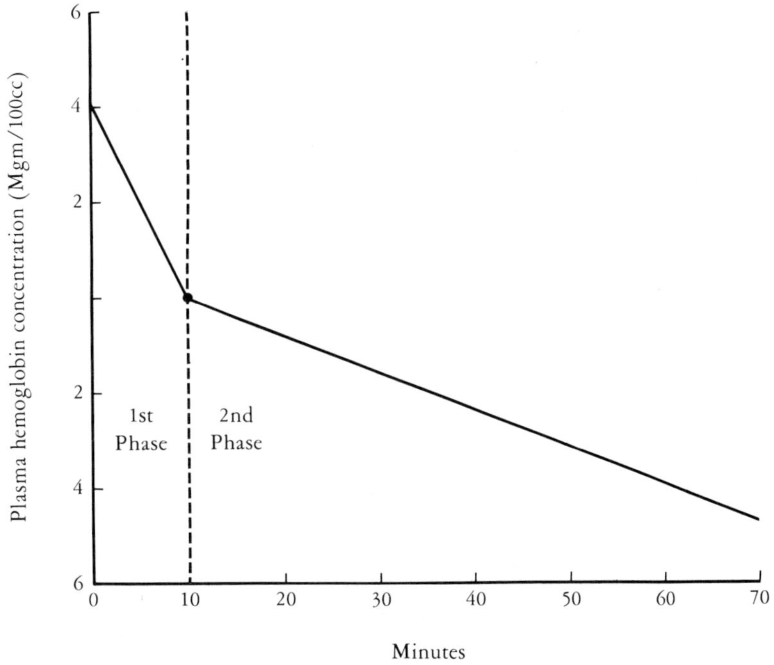

Figure 2–3. Plasma hemoglobin clearance in a group of 40 apparently healthy human subjects. (After Gabrieli, E. R., and Snell, F. M.: Reflection of reticuloendothelial function in studies of blood clearance kinetics. J. Reticuloendothel. Soc., *2*:141, 1965.)

differentiation, the cell enlarges in size and in the number and complexity of intracellular organelles (e.g., Golgi apparatus, mitochondria, lysosomes, and lipid droplets). In addition, during maturation, the cell increases in the content of lysosomal enzymes, such as acid phosphatase, beta-glucuronidase, cathepsin, lysozyme, and aryl sulfatase, as well as related mitochondrial enzymes, e.g., cytochrome oxidase. The energy sources for the cells of the MPS are dependent upon the degree of cellular maturity, the level of endocytic activity, and the environment. With the notable exception of the alveolar macrophage, which derives its energy primarily from aerobic metabolism, all other cells of the MPS derive their energy for particle uptake through the glycolytic pathway.

The macrophages are highly specialized to carry out their function in the ingestion and destruction of all particulate matter by the process of endocytosis. These cells remove and destroy certain bacteria, damaged or effete cells, neoplastic cells, colloidal materials, and macromolecules. The phagocytic process is sometimes facilitated by antibody, since particles coated with antibody are ingested more efficiently; complement, a series of sequentially reacting serum proteins, may also be involved as an amplifier of phagocytosis (Chapters 5 and 6). The term *opsonin* is used to describe this phagocytic-enhancing principle of both antibody and complement. The circulating monocytes are attracted to an area of injury (chemotaxis) by a number of factors, some of which are derived from the complement system or secreted by the T-lymphocytes (Table 2–1). Here they may further differentiate into macrophages and may be activated in a variety of ways—either following endocytosis or through humoral substances, including antibody, complement, or products of lymphocytes (lymphokines) (Chapter 9). Once activated, the cells assume heightened metabolic activity (activated macrophages) and display enhancement of function, e.g., microbicidal activity. Some workers believe that, in addition to a role in defense and surveillance, the macrophage system is important in the initial recognition and processing of antigen, steps that may be necessary for the induction of specific immunologic responses (Chapter 7).

Neutrophils or Polymorphonuclear Leukocytes. In the human the circulating granulocytes comprise three varieties of morphologically identifiable cells that are involved in a number of immunologic reactions in tissue; these include the neutrophil, the eosinophil, and the basophil (Table 2–1). Of these three, only the neutrophil and, to a lesser extent, the eosinophil are primarily phagocytic.

Neutrophils or polymorphonuclear (PMN) leukocytes (Fig. 2–5) normally account for 60 to 70 per cent of the total leukocyte count in

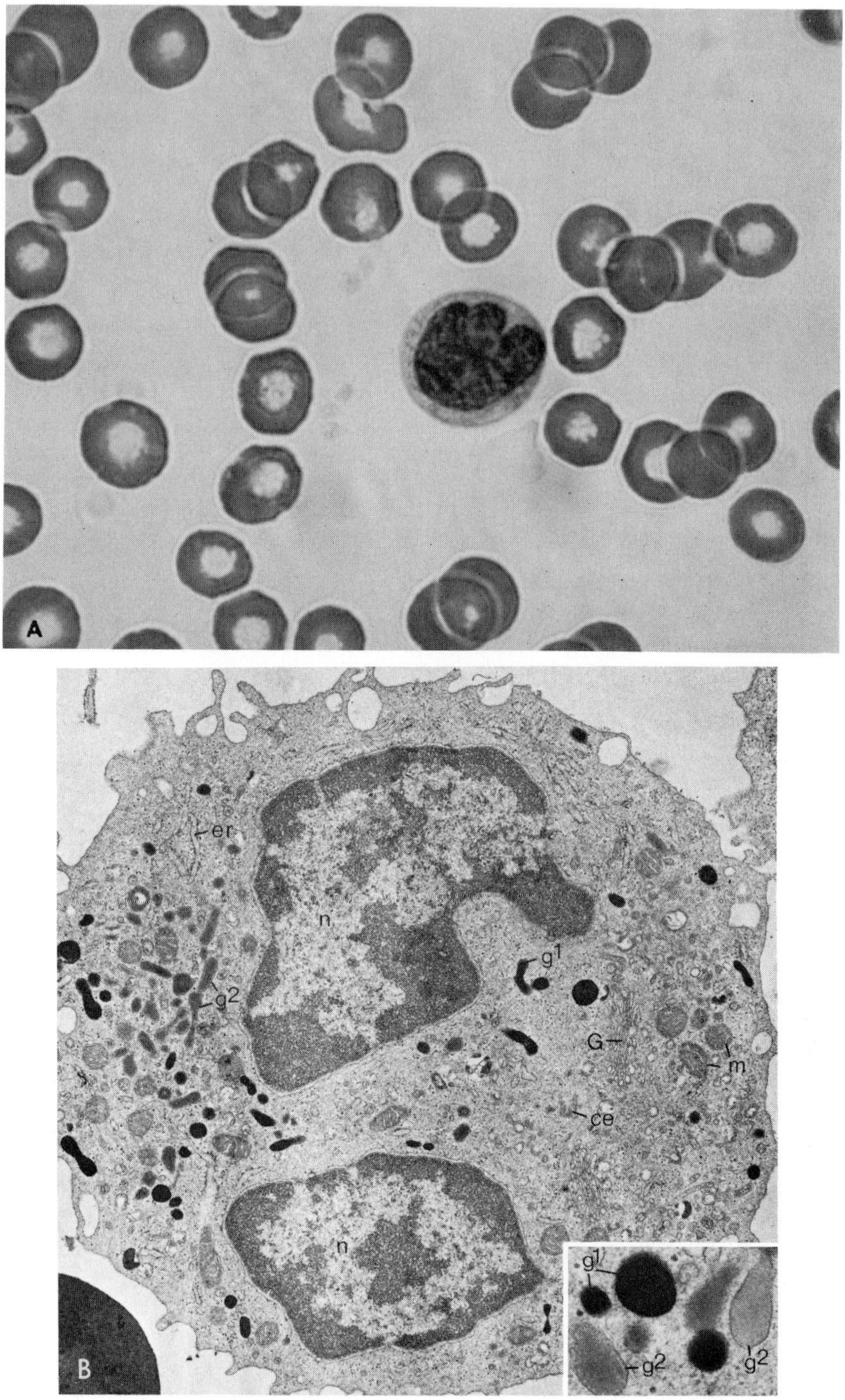

Figure 2–4. Monocyte from peripheral blood. *A,* Light micrograph, Wright-Giemsa stain, × 1400. Note the lobulated nucleus. (Courtesy of Dr. Theodore I. Malinin.) *B,* Electron micrograph, × 16,200 examined for peroxidase. Note the presence of two types of granules (g^1), peroxidase-positive and (g^2) peroxidase-negative; the endoplasmic reticulum (er); Golgi complex (G); the mitochondria (m); the centriole (ce); and the nucleus (n). (From Bainton, D. F.: *In* Dingle, J. T. (ed.): Lysosomes in Biology and Pathology. Vol. 5. New York, North-Holland, 1976.)

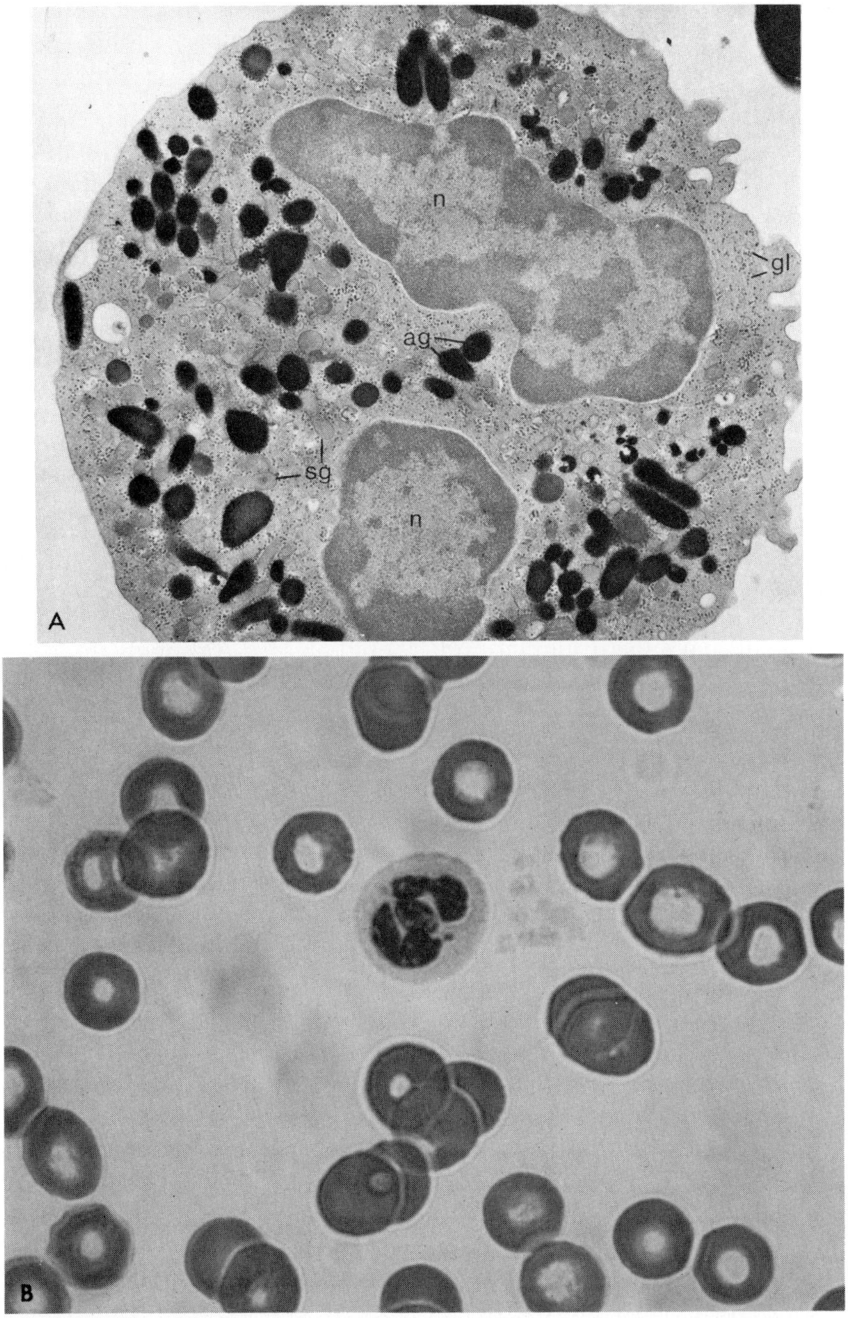

Figure 2–5. Polymorphonuclear leukocyte from peripheral blood. *A,* Electron micrograph, × 13,500, showing a lobulated nucleus (n) and cytoplasmic granules reacted for peroxidase. Note the presence of two types of granules: the peroxidase-positive azurophilic (ag) and the peroxidase-negative specific granules (sg); and the glycogen particles (gl) that are dispersed throughout the cytoplasm. (From Bainton, D. F.: *In* Dingle, J. T. (ed.): Lysosomes in Biology and Pathology. Vol. 5. New York, North-Holland, 1976.) *B,* Light micrograph, Wright-Giemsa stain, × 1400, showing fully segmented nucleus. (Courtesy of Dr. Theodore I. Malinin.)

the peripheral blood of the adult human. Unlike the macrophage, the neutrophil is an end cell of myeloid differentiation and does not divide. The neutrophils arise in the bone marrow from a common ancestral stem cell and, after a series of divisions, undergo a maturation through various stages—myeloblast → promyelocyte → metamyelocyte → band cell → mature PMN. Unlike the situation with the monocyte-macrophage series, however, there appears to be a large storage compartment in the bone marrow that can be called upon as needed to replenish cells in the circulation. After a short period in the blood (about 12 hours), the PMN's enter the tissues, where they complete their life span of a few days. Normally, there is no return of these cells from the tissues back to the blood. Some of the cells in the vascular pool do not circulate freely, presumably because they are temporarily sequestered in small blood vessels or adhere to the walls of larger vessels (marginal pool).

With maturation of the cells, there is a sequential appearance of two distinct classes of granules: the primary (azurophilic) and the secondary or specific granules (Fig. 2–5). The primary granules are electron-dense structures approximately 0.4 micron (μ) in diameter that appear early in maturation and have many features in common with lysosomes of other tissues. They contain myeloperoxidase, arginine-rich basic (cationic) proteins, sulfated mucopolysaccharides, acid phosphatase, and several other acid hydrolases. The secondary or specific granules are not truly lysosomes; they are smaller (about 0.3 μ in diameter) and are less dense than the primary granules. They are rich in alkaline phosphatase, lysozyme, and aminopeptidase. In the intermediate stage of neutrophil maturation, both populations of granules are seen. As maturation proceeds, however, the secondary granules increase in number and appear to predominate. Both types of granules are important in the breakdown of ingested material and in the killing of microorganisms. Granulocyte production and release appear to be under the control of cellular and humoral factors.

The Eosinophils. The eosinophilic granulocytes make up 1 to 3 per cent of the circulating blood leukocytes and are distinguished by large cytoplasmic granules that stain intensely red with eosin (Fig. 2–6). They share many features with the neutrophil, arise from a common progenitor cell, and display a similar morphogenesis. In contrast to the neutrophil, however, the eosinophils mature in the bone marrow in three to six days before release into the circulation, following which they circulate with a half-life of approximately 30 minutes. The eosinophils have a half-life of 12 days in tissues, where they fulfill their major function. Like the neutrophil, the eosinophils do not return from tissues to the circulation but are eliminated through the mucosal surfaces of the respiratory and gastrointestinal tracts. With maturation of these cells, there occurs a transition from primary (azurophilic) granules to large cytoplasmic granules, which have a crystalloid substructure (Fig. 2–6). The granules of the eosinophil do not contain lysozyme and phagocytin as found in PMN's. They are rich in acid phosphatase and peroxidase activity. In addition, the eosinophil granule contains in its crystalline core a unique protein, the eosinophilic basic protein (EBP), of approximately 11,000 daltons, found to be toxic to certain parasites (e.g., *Schistosoma*), as well as to normal host cells (e.g., tracheal epithelium). Although the cells have the capacity to phagocytose a variety of particles, including microorganisms and soluble antigen-antibody complexes, the process appears to be less efficient than with neutrophils. In spite of its well-known association with allergic and parasitic diseases, the specific role of the eosinophil is not known with certainty. Major roles postulated include the ingestion of immune complexes and their involvement in limiting inflammatory reactions, presumably by antagonizing the effects of certain mediators. For example, aryl sulfatase B from eosinophils has been shown to inactivate SRS-A released by mediator cells (Chapter 13). Furthermore, the eosinophil has been implicated directly as a putative cell of tissue injury, possibly through the release of its toxic components, e.g., EBP. The eosinophils have been found to participate in antibody-mediated cytotoxicity reactions of importance in the clearance of certain parasitic organisms, e.g., *Schistosoma*. The regulation of eosinophils involves a complex set of mechanisms, including products of T-lymphocytes, complement components, mast cell products (e.g., ECF-A) as well as a variety of arachidonic acid metabolites (e.g., HETE's). As a general rule, eosinophilia is more common in atopic diseases in which increased levels of IgE are found than in other immunologically mediated disorders (Chapter 20A).

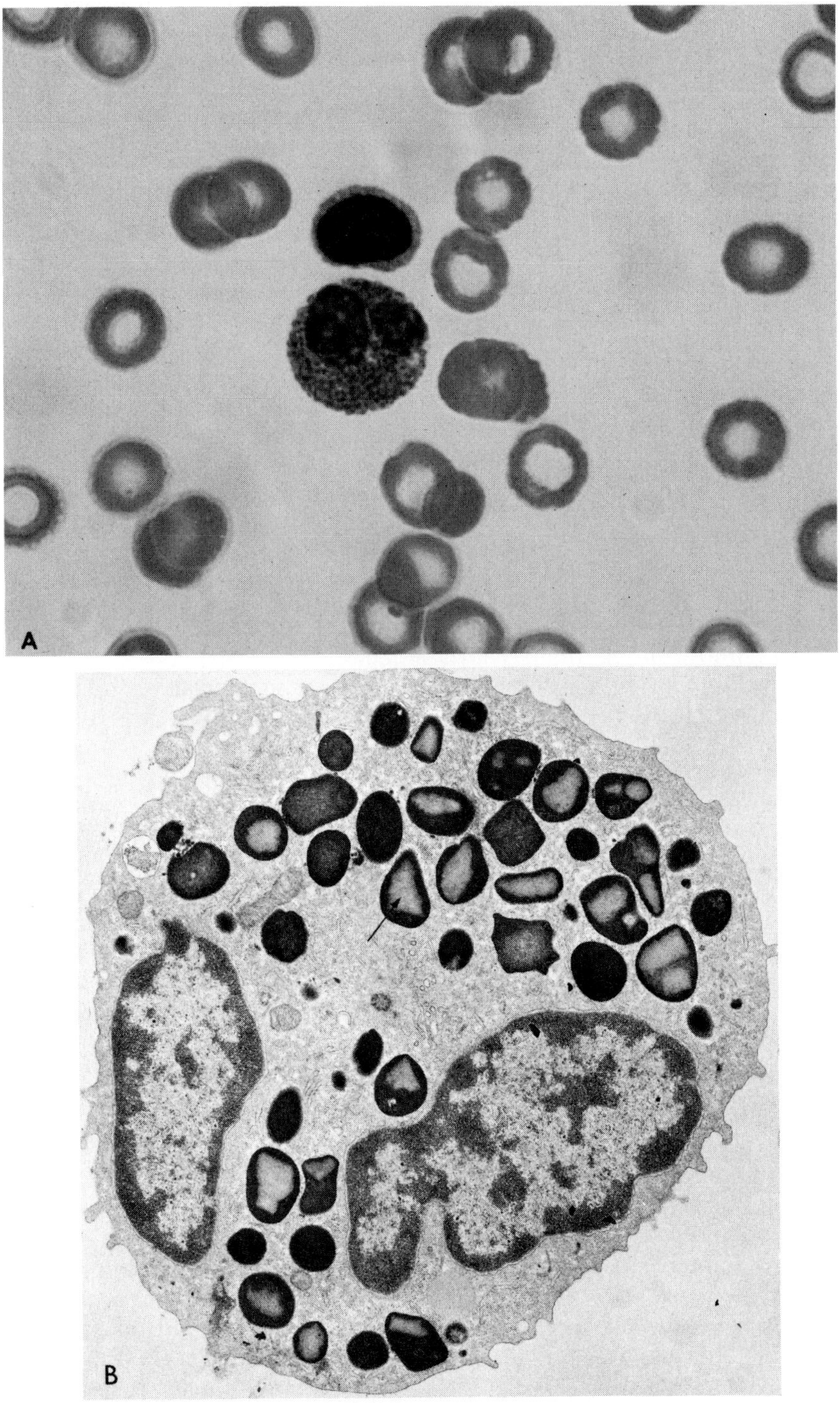

Figure 2–6. *A,* Eosinophilic leukocyte and a small lymphocyte from peripheral blood. Light micrograph, Wright-Giemsa stain, × 1400. (Courtesy of Dr. Theodore I. Malinin.) Note the bilobed nucleus and the prominent granules of the eosinophil. *B,* Electron micrograph of a human eosinophil from normal bone marrow, × 33,000, reacted for peroxidase. Note the presence of large granules that have a predominance of peroxidase staining filling the granule contents except for the area occupied by the crystalline core (*arrow*). (From Bainton, D. F.: *In* Dingle, J. T. (ed.): Lysosomes in Biology and Pathology. Vol. 5. New York, North-Holland, 1976.)

MEDIATOR CELLS

Certain cells of the body also participate in immunologic reactions through the release of chemical substances (mediators) that have a variety of biologic activities, including increased vascular permeability, contraction of smooth muscle, and enhancement of the inflammatory response. These cells are referred to as mediator cells and constitute a heterogeneous collection of morphologic types, including *mast cells, basophils, platelets, enterochromaffin* cells, and certain of the phagocytic cells, e.g., neutrophils.

Basophilic granulocytes (Fig. 2–7), which make up only 0.5 per cent of the blood leukocytes, and the platelets, the non-nucleated hemostatic elements of the blood, are the two major mediator cells in the circulation. They have been shown to contain a variety of vasoactive amines, such as histamine and serotonin (Chapter 13). The basophils are distinguished by their large purple or blue-black granules that ultrastructurally are electron-dense and homogeneous and that, when mature, show a characteristic banded pattern. These granules contain acid mucopolysaccharides (e.g., heparin), which are responsible for the tinctorial phenomenon of metachromasia. Little is known of their production, distribution, or life span. Although they resemble the mast cells morphologically, they differ in several respects.

The basophil and mast cell are important sources of mediators, e.g., histamine, which are involved in immediate hypersensitivity (Chapters 13 and 20A). The elaboration of these agents is thought to be triggered by contact of these cells with antigen-antibody complexes through complement-dependent or complement-independent mechanisms (Chapter 13). The release of these mediators can occur by direct impact of an environmental agent (e.g., compound 48/80) or indirectly through the interaction of antigen with membrane-bound IgE (Chapter 13). The release appears to be mediated by cyclic 3′,5′-adenosine monophosphate (cyclic AMP) (Chapters 7 and 20A). Substances that increase cyclic AMP lead to a decrease in the release of mediators; substances that decrease intracellular levels of cyclic AMP lead to an increased release. These vasoactive amines appear to be involved in tissue injury. Following interaction of antigen with antibody in tissues such as the renal glomerulus, for example, there is a release of these substances that results in permeability changes that lead to accelerated deposition of circulating soluble antigen-antibody complexes. The release of histamine and serotonin therefore appears to be involved in an immunologic cascade, in which there may be amplification of injury mediated by antigen-antibody complexes. The mechanism by which the accumulation of these complexes leads to tissue injury is described in greater detail in Chapter 13. Findings of this nature may have important clinical implications. In animals undergoing experimental forms of immunologic injury (serum sickness), treatment with antihistamines or serotonin antagonists leads to a protection of the animals from immune complex-induced type nephritis (Chapter 13).

Chemotaxis, Phagocytosis, and Metabolic Changes and Antimicrobial Systems of Phagocytic Cells

The primary role of the phagocytic cells in the body economy is the localization and removal of foreign substances, such as microorganisms. Several integrated functions may be required to achieve these goals. First, the cells must reach the site of the foreign configuration (chemotaxis). They must then ingest the foreign substance (phagocytosis). Finally, after a series of metabolic steps, they must destroy the foreign substance or inhibit the replication of the microorganism (microbial killing).

- epinephrine, cortisone ↑ PMN count. mobility.

CHEMOTAXIS

There are three phenomena involved in cell movements: *motility, locomotion,* and *chemotaxis.* Motility refers to a cell that moves; locomotion refers to movement from one place to another; and chemotaxis refers to unidirectional locomotion toward an increasing gradient of attractant (chemoattractant). A phagocytic cell adherent to glass, for example, can be a highly motile cell but may not be exhibiting locomotion or chemotaxis. A cell that is undergoing random locomotion may not be exhibiting chemotaxis. There are a variety of *in vivo* and *in vitro* techniques for measurement of locomotion and chemotaxis (Chapter 26).

The polymorphonuclear leukocyte responds to at least three different chemotactic

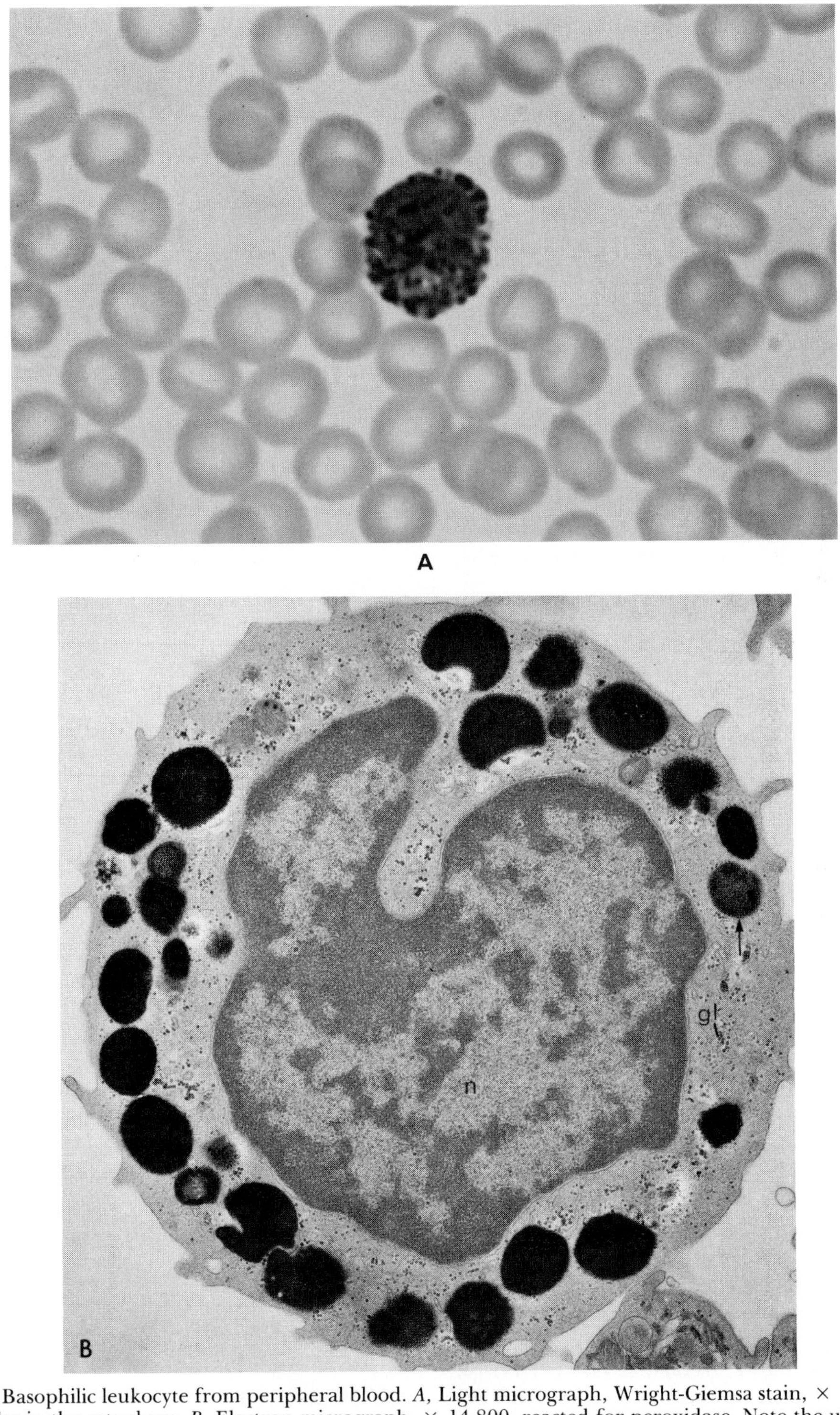

Figure 2–7. Basophilic leukocyte from peripheral blood. *A,* Light micrograph, Wright-Giemsa stain, × 1400, showing large granules in the cytoplasm. *B,* Electron micrograph, × 14,800, reacted for peroxidase. Note the unusually large nucleus (n), scattered glycogen particles (gl), and peroxidase-positive granules, some of which may appear speckled (*arrow*). (From Bainton, D. F.: *In* Dingle, J. T. (ed.): Lysosomes in Biology and Pathology. Vol. 5. New York, North-Holland, 1976.)

stimuli derived from the complement system, as well as bacterial and lymphocyte-derived factors (Table 2–1). The neutrophils also are directly or indirectly involved in the production of a substance known as slow-reactive substance (SRS-A), now identified as leukotrienes C_4, D_4, and E_4, humoral factors capable of causing the contraction of smooth muscle (Chapter 13). Other factors produced by the granulocyte include the kinins, small polypeptides that are vasoactive. These substances are important pharmacologic mediators of immediate hypersensitivity reactions (Chapters 13 and 20A).

A number of substances chemotactic for monocytes and macrophages have also been described (Table 2–1). These include products of the complement system as well as of the lymphocyte series, e.g., macrophage-activating factor (MAF). Moreover, a substance that is inhibitory for chemotaxis of monocytes has been described in extracts of tumor tissues.

There are a number of substances that are chemotactic for eosinophils that are similar to those for neutrophils. These include antigen-antibody complexes; complement-derived chemotactic factors; products of the lymphocyte series, e.g., lymphokines; and an eosinophilic chemotactic factor of anaphylaxis (ECF-A), a substance released from tissue mast cells and peripheral basophils that may be very important in the pathogenesis of immediate-type hypersensitivity reactions (Chapters 13 and 20A). ECF-A has also been shown to be released from PMN leukocytes.

PHAGOCYTOSIS

The next step in the sequence is phagocytosis, the process by which a particle is ingested by a cell. This process can be divided into two steps: the *attachment phase* and the *ingestion phase*.

During the attachment phase, firm contact is established with the particle. This can occur between the particle and phagocyte directly through unenhanced processes, in which case it is largely dependent upon surface properties of the particle to be phagocytosed, e.g., hydrophobicity and surface tension. In other cases, attachment involves the participation of two types of receptors on the plasma membrane of the phagocyte: (1) a receptor for the Fc fragment of an immunoglobulin molecule; and (2) a receptor for the C3b, a

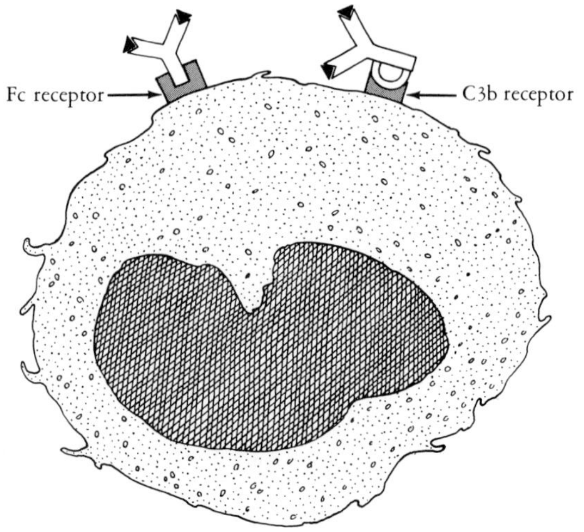

Figure 2–8. Schematic representation of the Fc and C3b receptors.

component of complement. These are shown schematically in Figure 2–8.

Many bacteria that are unencapsulated are rapidly taken up by phagocytes and destroyed. Encapsulated strains such as the pneumococcus, however, are taken up poorly and hence not destroyed. This resistance to engulfment is related to the protective capsule of the bacterium and ensures its survival within the host. When certain serum proteins, e.g., complement or antibodies (opsonins), are present, the attachment of the coated bacterium is facilitated by the surface receptors and the phagocytic uptake is enhanced (Chapter 15).

The ingestion process is the next step of phagocytosis and represents the engulfment of the particle. The phagocyte invaginates its plasma membrane and the particle is then taken up into the cytoplasm and enclosed within a vacuole (phagosome), the wall of which is made up of inverted plasma membrane (see Fig. 2–2). In addition, actin- and myosin-like proteins that appear to participate in the ingestion process through the formation of microfilaments have been isolated.

MORPHOLOGIC EVENTS ASSOCIATED WITH PHAGOCYTOSIS

Following the formation of the phagosome, the membrane enclosing the particle gradually pinches off from the surface membrane and is internalized within the cell, forming the phagocytic vacuole (see Fig. 2–2). The

Table 2–3. Enzymes and Other Substances Found Within Neutrophils*

Acid phosphatase	Hyaluronidase
Acid ribonuclease	Lysozyme
Acid deoxyribonuclease	Collagenase
Cathepsins B, C, D, E	Aryl sulfatases A and B
Phosphoprotein phosphatase	Phospholipases
Organophosphate-resistant esterase	Acid lipase
β-Glucuronidase	Lactoferrin
β-Galactosidase	Phagocytin and other related bactericidal proteins
β-N-acetylglucosaminase	Endogenous pyrogen
α-L-fucosidase	Plasminogen activator (?urokinase)
α-1,4-glucosidase	Hemolysin(s)
α-mannosidase	Mucopolysaccharides and glycoproteins
α-N-acetylglucosamidase	Basic proteins: (a) Mast cell-active (b) Permeability-inducing independent mast cells
α-N-acetylgalactosaminidase	
Myeloperoxidase	

*(Adapted from Cochrane, C. G.: Immunologic tissue injury mediated by neutrophilic leukocytes. Adv. Immunol., *9*:97, 1968.)

lysosomal granules within the leukocytes come into apposition with this phagosome, and the membranes of the two structures fuse into a phagolysosome. The granules rupture, discharging their enzymatic contents into the vacuole, and come into contact with the ingested particle. This process has been termed degranulation and represents the morphologic counterpart of the transfer of enzymes from the lysosomal granule to the phagosome. The leukocyte granules (primary) are analogous to the lysosomes of other cells and contain several hydrolytic enzymes and other bactericidal substances (Table 2–3). First, these ranges of acidity are achieved by the cell during the "respiratory burst" associated with phagocytosis as described below. Second, most of the enzymes found within the primary granules have pH optimum within this acid range. These facts suggest that the fall in pH during phagocytosis might trigger the digestive process by liberating hydrolytic enzymes that function best at a low pH.

METABOLIC EVENTS ASSOCIATED WITH PHAGOCYTOSIS

Following the formation of the phagocytic vacuole, a series of biochemical reactions is initiated in phagocytic cells. The metabolic pathways that are primarily involved include the glycolytic pathway and the hexose monophosphate (HMP) shunt (Fig. 2–9). In addition, alveolar macrophages utilize the tricarboxylic acid pathway, which provides

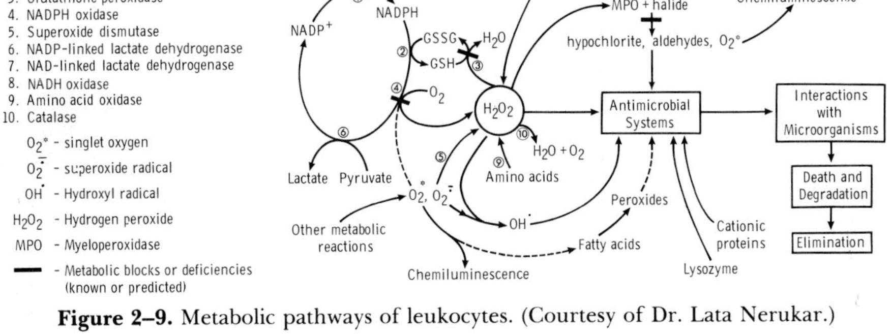

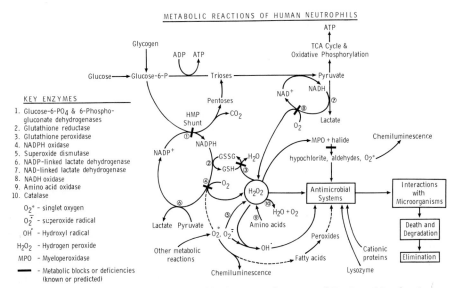

Figure 2–9. Metabolic pathways of leukocytes. (Courtesy of Dr. Lata Nerukar.)

their main energy source. Collectively, the stimulation of these pathways is termed the respiratory burst and consists of the following: (1) an increase in glycolysis; (2) a marked increase in HMP shunt activity; and (3) an elevation in oxygen consumption and H_2O_2 and lactic acid production. The increase in lactic acid production is in part responsible for the fall in pH within the phagosome, as previously described. Accompanying the respiratory burst is an enhanced RNA and phospholipid turnover, events important in protein synthesis and membrane formation. These changes are most prominent in neutrophils but also are seen to a lesser extent in the mononuclear phagocytes.

The biologic significance of the preferential utilization of these pathways by certain phagocytic cells, e.g., PMN's, may be to facilitate their function in tissues in which oxygen may be limited. In contrast, the utilization of the TCA cycle by other phagocytic cells, e.g., alveolar macrophages, may be an adaptation to their aerobic environment.

The precise initiating events that result in the metabolic changes following particle uptake are not known, but appear to involve perturbations of the plasma membrane. Several surface-active agents such as deoxycholate, digitonin, and concanavalin-A can also induce a respiratory burst similar to that seen following particle uptake. The extraordinary feature of this phenomenon is that the initiation of the respiratory burst is detectable within seconds after particle uptake and actually precedes the morphologic events, suggesting that the biochemical changes may be required for subsequent events to occur. In addition, the activation of the macrophages can be produced by several other agents, e.g., adjuvants, microorganisms, lymphokines, and bacterial products (Chapter 14). The features of the enhanced metabolism of this "activated macrophage" are the same as those described with particle uptake.

One of the proposed key enzymes involved in the metabolism of phagocytic cells is NADPH oxidase (Fig. 2–9). This enzyme may serve a twofold function: (1) It provides a source of NADP, which may be the limiting factor regulating HMP shunt activity; or (2) it may be involved in the formation of H_2O_2, which is an essential component in the microbicidal reactions. In addition, NADP also participates in many other metabolic functions, such as glutathione production, RNA and lipid metabolism, and membrane formation, events essential for phagocytic cell function. Other enzyme systems are involved in the conversion of NADPH to NADP, including glutathione peroxidase, which oxidizes reduced glutathione (GSH) to its oxidized form (GSSG) in the presence of H_2O_2. The GSSG is further reduced to GSH and in turn converts NADPH to NADP (Fig. 2–9).

With the respiratory burst there occurs an enhanced production of H_2O_2 or superoxide anion ($O_2^{\overline{\cdot}}$). The superoxide anion undergoes dismutation in the presence of an enzyme, superoxide dismutase, with further production of H_2O_2 (Fig. 2–9). The production of H_2O_2 is more prominent in PMN's than in tissue or alveolar macrophages and appears to be extremely important in microbicidal function of PMN's. Defects in H_2O_2 production associated with failure in the induction of the respiratory burst have been observed in the leukocytes of children with a variety of neutrophil dysfunction disorders, e.g., chronic granulomatous disease (CGD) (Chapter 22). A useful diagnostic test of phagocytic function has been developed based upon these biochemical considerations. The reduction of nitroblue tetrazolium (NBT) to a blue formazan derivative provides a useful functional test of leukocyte HMP activity and is abnormally low in CGD.

ANTIMICROBIAL MECHANISMS OF PHAGOCYTIC CELLS

In order to successfully destroy and eliminate microorganisms, e.g., bacteria, following their ingestion, the next step in the process is the killing and destruction of the microorganism by the phagocytic cell. The observation that anaerobic conditions only partially impair bactericidal activity led to the discovery that both oxygen-dependent and oxygen-independent antimicrobial mechanisms exist within phagocytic cells. Klebanoff has proposed a classification of these antimicrobial systems on the basis of their oxygen requirements. The oxygen-dependent mechanisms can be further subdivided on the basis of their utilization of myeloperoxidase. This classification of antimicrobial systems of phagocytic cells is shown in Table 2–4.

A system consisting of H_2O_2, halide, and MPO has been shown to have powerful microbicidal activity contributing to the microbicidal action of phagocytic cells, primarily the PMN's (Fig. 2–9). The role of this system in mononuclear phagocytes is less clear. The

Table 2–4. Antimicrobial Systems of Phagocytic Cells*

I. *O_2-dependent*	II. *O_2-independent*
a. Myeloperoxidase (MPO)-mediated	a. acid
b. MPO-independent	b. lysozyme
1. H_2O_2	c. lactoferrin
2. superoxide anion ($O_2^{\bar{\cdot}}$)	d. granular cationic proteins
3. hydroxyl radical ($OH^{\cdot}$)	
4. singlet oxygen (O_2*)	
5. ascorbate-peroxide-metal ion	
6. amino acid oxidation	

*(After Klebanoff, S. J.: *In* Bellanti, J. A., and Dayton, D. H. (eds.): The Phagocytic Cell in Host Resistance. New York, Raven Press, 1975.)

proposed mechanism of action of the MPO-H_2O_2-halide complex is thought to involve the formation of aldehydes and hypochlorite or halogenation of bacterial proteins, the net effect of which leads to the death of the microorganism. The significance of this reaction is apparent in several clinical disorders of neutrophil function in which a failure of production of H_2O_2 leads to defective bacterial killing and the clinical spectrum of recurrent infection, e.g., CGD, which suggests that there are mechanisms other than the MPO-H_2O_2-halide system operative in antimicrobial activity. These other systems have been referred to as back-up systems. In the case of low concentrations of H_2O_2, the action of MPO can be replaced by catalase. Such alternate pathways may be important in macrophages, in which the role of MPO is less clear. It is of interest that in children with CGD the characteristic spectrum of bacteria causing infection includes those that are catalase-positive and peroxide-negative, e.g., *Staphylococcus aureus.* In contrast, organisms that are catalase-negative and peroxide-positive, e.g., *Haemophilus influenzae,* do not cause serious infection in these children. It has been postulated that these latter organisms can provide an alternative source of H_2O_2, which in effect can partially correct the cellular defects (Chapter 22).

Among the MPO-independent systems, H_2O_2 itself exhibits antimicrobial activity, and since it is produced during the phagocytic event it may in part contribute to the overall killing capacity of the phagocytic cell (Table 2–4). The superoxide radical ($O_2^{\bar{\cdot}}$) that is generated during phagocytosis is formed by the univalent reduction of molecular oxygen and is an extremely toxic and reactive moiety important in bactericidal activity. Subsequent dismutation of $O_2^{\bar{\cdot}}$ by superoxide dismutase (SOD) leads to the formation of H_2O_2.

$$O_2 \xrightarrow{e} O_2^{\bar{\cdot}}$$

$$O_2^{\bar{\cdot}} + O_2^{\bar{\cdot}} + 2H^+ \xrightarrow{SOD} O_2 + H_2O_2$$

The superoxide radical, in addition to its own bactericidal activity, may through dismutation produce H_2O_2, which is microbicidal. This indicates that $O_2^{\bar{\cdot}}$ acts as an intermediate to H_2O_2 production and indirectly contributes to the MPO-mediated system. Singlet oxygen (O_2*) is an electronically excited state of molecular oxygen that emits light (chemiluminescence) when it reverts to the triplet ground state (O_2). This biochemical finding has also been used in the functional assessment of phagocytic cells. The source of this singlet oxygen (O_2*) may be an MPO-mediated reaction involving the formation of hypochlorite. Singlet oxygen might also react with certain unsaturated chemical groups, e.g., ethylene groups, forming dioxytanes across double bonds that are unstable, and may be toxic to microorganisms

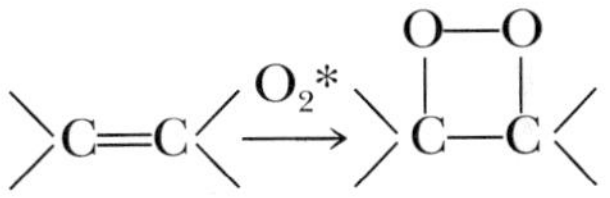

and thus responsible for the killing by MPO-mediated systems. Other proposed antimicrobial mechanisms include an ascorbate-peroxide system, which may function in synergism with lysozyme and may even be more potent in the presence of metallic ions such as cobalt and copper. The oxidation of amino acids may also add to the generation of H_2O_2.

The mononuclear phagocytes lack significant myeloperoxidase activity and must therefore resort to other microbicidal mechanisms. Although little is known of the microbicidal mechanisms of mononuclear phagocytes at present, they do exhibit the metabolic burst and H_2O_2 and $O_2^{\bar{\cdot}}$ generation displayed by PMN's, but to a lesser extent.

The oxygen-independent mechanisms also seem to contribute to the killing capacity of the phagocytic cells, since anaerobiosis does not totally impair their microbicidal activity (Table 2–4). Although there is evidence that lysozyme may be involved directly in the killing of bacteria, the action of this enzyme may also be to function in a digestive manner after the killing of the bacteria. Lactoferrin, an iron-binding protein, leukin, and phagocytin, found in the specific granules of the PMN but not in mononuclear phagocytes, also have been shown to have bacteriostatic properties. The granular cationic proteins also exhibit antimicrobial activity, presumably after binding to the microorganisms, a function that is also lacking in macrophages. Finally, the formation of lactic acid as a result of the respiratory burst reduces the intracellular pH and thus provides conditions favorable for the action of digestive enzymes rather than functioning directly as a microbicidal agent.

Cell Types and Effector Mechanisms Involved in Specific Responses

LYMPHOCYTES AND PLASMA CELLS

The lymphoid cells of the immune system differ from the preceding group of cells by their ability to react specifically with antigen and to elaborate specific cell products. The lymphoid cells include plasma cells and lymphocytes (Figs. 2–10 and 2–11). These cells, once sensitized, become "committed" and are referred to as immunocytes. By definition, an immunocyte is a cell of the lymphoid series that can react with antigen with the production of specific cell products called antibody or a cell-mediated event such as delayed hypersensitivity, e.g., tuberculin reaction (Chapter 9).

The traditional classification of lymphocytes as small, medium, and large was based on the concept that morphologically similar cells had the same functions, life cycles, and metabolic behavior. In recent years, however, it has become apparent that even lymphocytes that appear morphologically identical constitute several cell populations that are extremely heterogeneous in function.

The lymphoid cell line traces its origin to a pluripotential stem cell that in the fetus is found within the yolk sac, bone marrow, and liver and in the adult in the bone marrow. These cells produce two classes of committed stem cells: (1) a committed hematopoietic stem cell that can give rise to the erythroid elements, granulocytes, or megakaryocytes; and (2) a committed lymphoid stem cell precursor that can give rise to cells of the lymphoid series (Table 2–2). The commitment to any of these pathways is dependent upon the microenvironments in which these stem cells develop.

DEVELOPMENT OF THE LYMPHOID TISSUE

Available evidence indicates that the lymphoid system consists of two compartments: (1) a *central* compartment involved in the differentiation of the lymphoid stem cells into lymphocytes capable of reacting with antigen (antigen-reactive cell); and (2) a *peripheral* compartment in which these cells can subsequently react with antigen (Fig. 2–12). The central lymphoid system consists of three components: (1) the *bone marrow,* (2) the *thymus,* and (3) a component whose identity is known with certainty only in birds (the bursa of Fabricius) and that in mammals is designated as the *bursal equivalent tissue.* The peripheral lymphoid system consists of lymph nodes, spleen, and gut-associated lymphoid tissue. In contrast to the differentiation of lymphocytes in the peripheral compartment, which is antigen-dependent, the maturation of lymphoid elements in the central compartment can occur in the absence of antigen (Fig. 2–12).

In higher vertebrates two types of lymphocytes may be found in peripheral lymphoid tissues that are dependent upon their sites of differentiation in the central lymphoid compartment. One type, which develops in the thymus, differentiates into small lymphocytes referred to as T-lymphocytes, which are involved in antigen recognition in cell-mediated immune reactions, including delayed hypersensitivity. The other population of lymphocytes is derived from stem cells, which differentiate in the bursa of Fabricius in birds and in the mammalian (bursal) equivalent and consist mainly of small lymphocytes referred to as B-lymphocytes, the plasma cells, and their progeny. In higher mammals, the location of the bursal equivalent is unknown, and several sites have been postulated, including the bone marrow. Such bursal equivalent– or bone marrow–derived lymphocytes are termed B-lymphocytes. Thus, the bone marrow component of the central lymphoid tissues may serve not only as a site of production of pluripotential lymphoid stem cells but also as a microenvironment for the differentiation of stem cells into antigen-reactive B-lymphocytes as well as a site for mature recirculating lymphocyte populations.

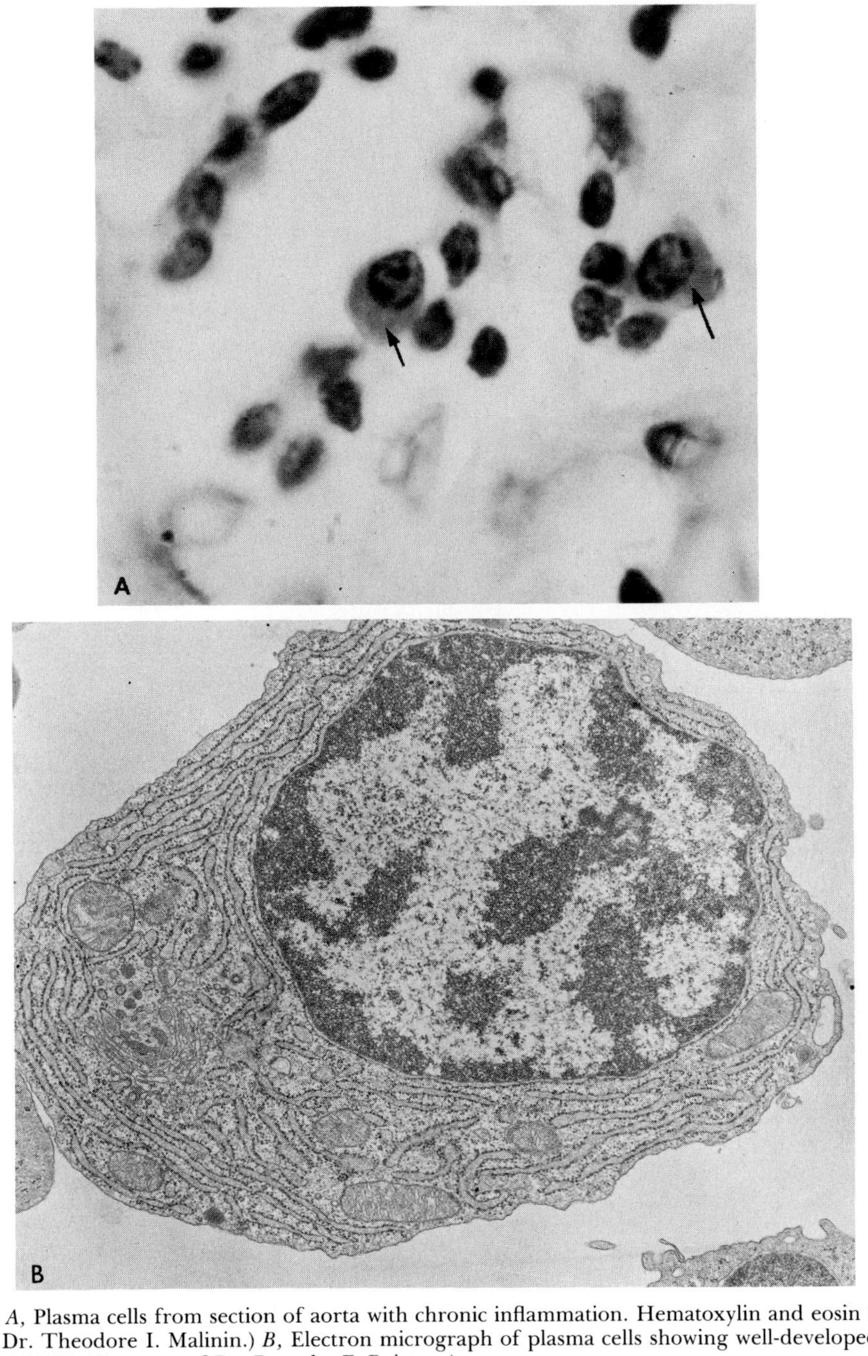

Figure 2–10. *A*, Plasma cells from section of aorta with chronic inflammation. Hematoxylin and eosin stain, × 1000. (Courtesy of Dr. Theodore I. Malinin.) *B*, Electron micrograph of plasma cells showing well-developed endoplasmic reticulum, × 11,000. (Courtesy of Dr. Dorothy F. Bainton.)

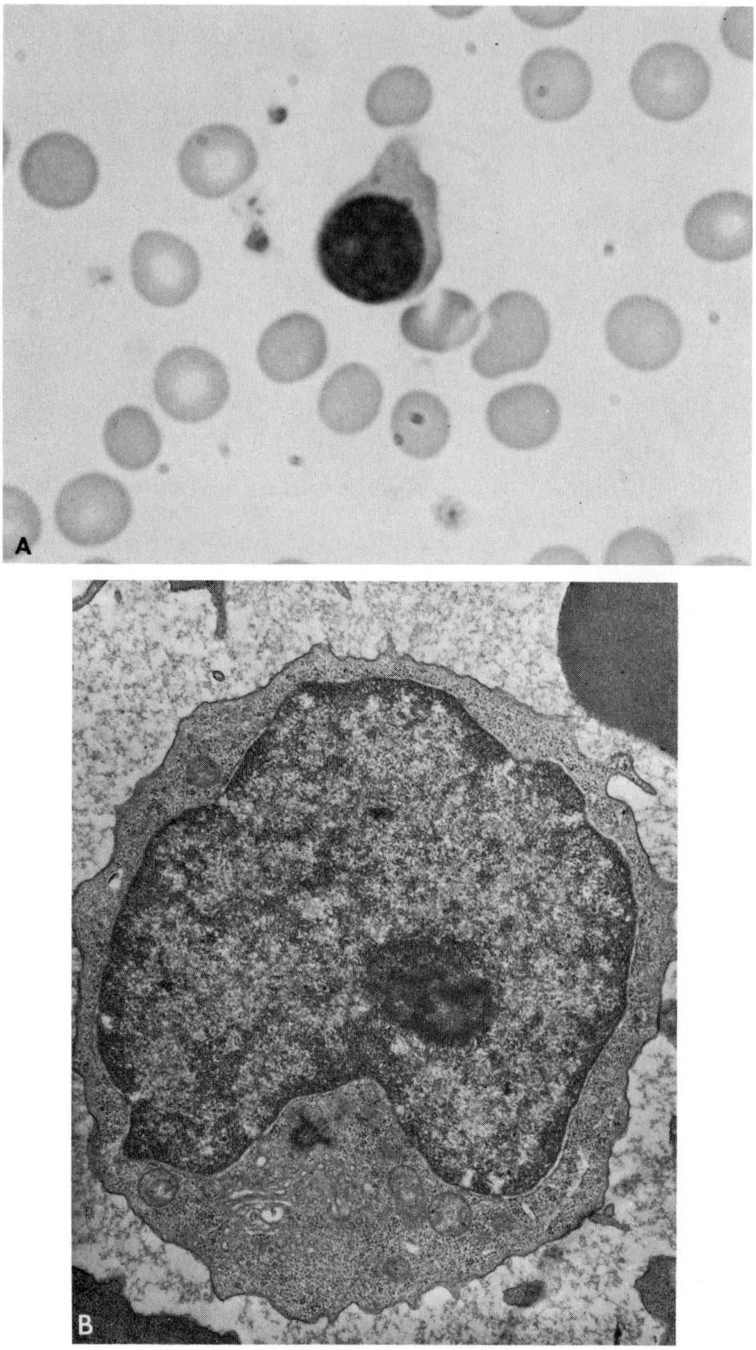

Figure 2–11. *A,* Lymphocytes from peripheral blood. Wright-Giemsa stain, × 1400. *B,* Electron micrograph of a resting lymphocyte, × 11,000. (Courtesy of Dr. Dorothy F. Bainton.)

CELLULAR ELEMENTS

Lymphocytes thus comprise two lines of immunocompetent cells, one concerned with cell-mediated immunity (T-lymphocytes) and the other with humoral immunity (B-lymphocytes) (Fig. 2–12). Ordinarily, in the absence of stimulation the B-lymphocyte does not replicate. Under an appropriate stimulus, such as antigen, it transforms into a large, metabolically more active "blast" cell, which has been termed "an active lymphocyte" or "a large pyroninophyllic" cell (Chapter 7). Plasma cells are characterized by their RNA-rich cytoplasm and eccentrically placed nuclei. Ultrastructurally, the cytoplasm contains

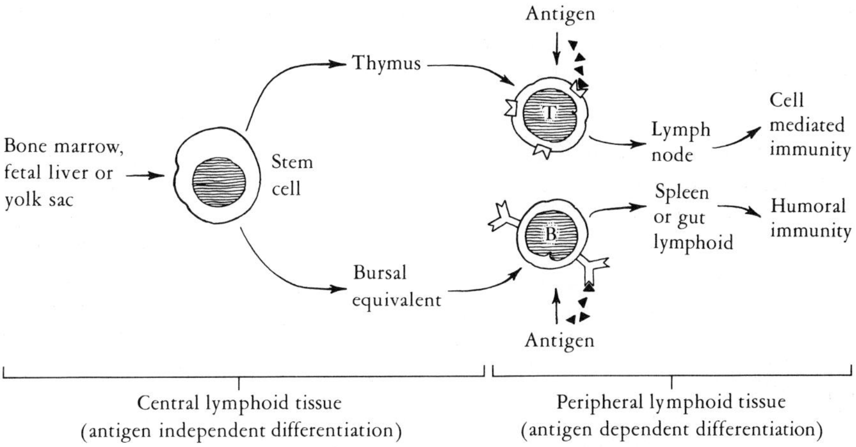

Figure 2–12. Development of the lymphoid system.

an extensive system of endoplasmic reticulum studded with ribosomes (Fig. 2–10). This structure is characteristic of cells active in protein synthesis, and the product of these cells is immunoglobulin.

T-lymphocytes are involved in such cell-mediated immune reactions as graft versus host (GVH), delayed hypersensitivity, and tumor rejection, and develop in an alternative pathway of development. These cells are incapable of differentiating into plasma cells but give rise to a cell capable of producing a variety of factors that trigger inflammatory or cell-mediated damaging reactions leading to cell-mediated events. These factors include migration inhibitory factor (MIF), a substance chemotactic for mononuclear and granulocytic cells, a cytotoxic factor capable of injuring a variety of cell types, interferon, and several other factors whose biologic roles are not yet well defined, e.g., interleukin-2 (Chapters 9 and 13). Some are released upon interaction of sensitized lymphocytes with appropriate antigens; others may remain cell-bound. In either case, they lead to the destruction of foreign target cells or to the damage and destruction of host cells. In addition to the function of releasing these various factors, the T-lymphocyte is now recognized to exist as a family of different T-cell subsets. These are identified by specific surface antigenic markers recognized by monoclonal antibodies or by functional assays of the cells. As described below, two major populations of T-cell subsets include the T-inducer ("helper cells") and the T-cytotoxic/suppressor ("suppressor cells" or "killer cells"). Recently a group of cells have been identified as "natural killer (NK) cells," which are defined by their ability to kill tumor cells without previously being sensitized. The origin of the NK cells is unclear, but they share many of the surface membrane characteristics not only of thymocytes but also of monocytes. Thus, it is apparent that the lymphocytes possess the most diversified function of all cells of the immune system.

Following stimulation of either B- or T-lymphocytes, an alternate pathway of differentiation leads to the production of a subpopulation termed memory cells. Upon reencounter with specific immunogens, these cells have the capacity to proliferate and differentiate into cell lines responsible for either humoral or cell-mediated immunity (Chapter 7).

The conversion of small lymphocytes to blast cells provides the basis for one of the most useful tests employed in clinical immunology, i.e., the test of immunocompetency of patients suspected of having a variety of immune deficiency disorders (Chapter 23). In addition, other tests allow the identification of specific lymphocytes as B- or T-lymphocytes (Chapters 7, 9, and 26). The transformation of the lymphocyte to the activated lymphocyte can be induced by a variety of stimuli including specific antigen, in either a soluble or a cell-associated form, e.g., lymphocytes from a genetically unrelated individual in a mixed lymphocyte response (MLC), or on a graft in graft rejection, or on a tumor cell in tumor rejection; or by antilymphocyte sera or by nonspecific mitogens, some of which selectively stimulate B-lymphocytes, others T-lymphocytes. These reactions take place by virtue of receptors on the surface of lymphocytes, which are described in greater detail in Chapters 3, 7, and 9.

The Structure of Organs That House Immunologic Cells: The Peripheral Lymphoid Tissue

The immune system contains some cells concerned with the initial response to foreign configurations and other cells that function in subsequent encounters. The system is equipped to perform nonspecific events, such as phagocytosis, as well as responses carried out in a specific manner by cells of the lymphoid tissues.

The lymphoreticular cells are strategically located in areas of the body best suited to deal with foreign configurations, which may confront the host *exogenously* or may arise *endogenously* (Fig. 2–1). For example, the foreign configuration may be a microorganism entering the host by such natural portals as the gastrointestinal, respiratory, or genitourinary tract. The lymphoid tissue is arranged in a unique manner in these areas. When the configuration arises *endogenously* within a host, e.g., a worn-out erythrocyte or a tumor cell, elements are mobilized into the lymphatics or the blood stream, where they quickly come into contact with immune effector cells.

The encounter between a configuration and a cellular element involved in immunity appears to be a random event. There are two anatomic features that increase the chance occurrence of these random events. The first feature is that some elements of the system are in constant motion and are recirculating continuously (the phagocytes and lymphoid cells). The second is that certain organs, such as the lymph nodes and spleen, contain a system of conduits through which a continuous recirculation of lymph or blood occurs.

Thus, the system is well organized to carry out its functions in defense, homeostasis, and surveillance. Four types of peripheral lymphatic tissues are important in this regard: (1) the lymph nodules, (2) the lymph nodes, (3) the spleen, and (4) the thymus. Although all four seem to be engaged in lymphopoiesis, only the first three respond actively to antigenic stimulation. The thymus, in contrast, stands autonomous in this regard and appears to be a master central lymphoid organ concerned with embryogenesis and orchestration of the remainder of the peripheral lymphoid tissues.

LYMPH NODULE

Lymph nodules consist of collections of lymphoid elements scattered in the submucous tissues of the respiratory passages, the intestine, and the genitourinary tracts. They are particularly well developed in structures such as the tonsils, which stand guard at the entrance of the gastrointestinal and respiratory tracts, and also in the Peyer's patches, collections of lymph nodules in the gastrointestinal tract. Their structure is demonstrated in Figure 2–13. This type of lymphoid tissue is arranged somewhat differently from that in lymph nodes, insofar as it lacks a connective tissue capsule. These nodules are not well developed in the fetus or in germ-free animals, but develop following exposure to antigens. Their development is believed to be related in some way to exposure of the host to antigens in the environment.

Since lymph nodules contain phagocytic elements as well as lymphoid elements, they are capable of reacting in nonspecific as well as in specific immunity. In the lymphoid cells that line these tracts, there occurs synthesis of the secretory IgA immunoglobulins. This class of immunoglobulin has been shown to be important at mucosal surfaces (Chapter 5). These tracts, contiguous with the exterior, elaborate a secretory form of antibody and provide the host with a cell product well suited to function at body surfaces and to deal with pathogens in the external environment. The IgE globulins have also been shown recently to be synthesized by cells in the same locations. Both IgA and IgE globulins are cell products of the external secretory system (Fig. 2–1).

LYMPH NODES

If a foreign configuration can overcome the initial barriers provided by the skin, mucous membranes, and lymph nodules, it may be handled in three additional ways: (1) It may be attached by wandering macrophages in the connective tissue; (2) it may provoke an inflammatory response with cellular accumulations, e.g., neutrophils; or (3) it may be taken up directly into the lymph or blood. The lymph represents a collection of tissue fluids flowing in lymphatic capillaries into a series of even larger collecting vessels called

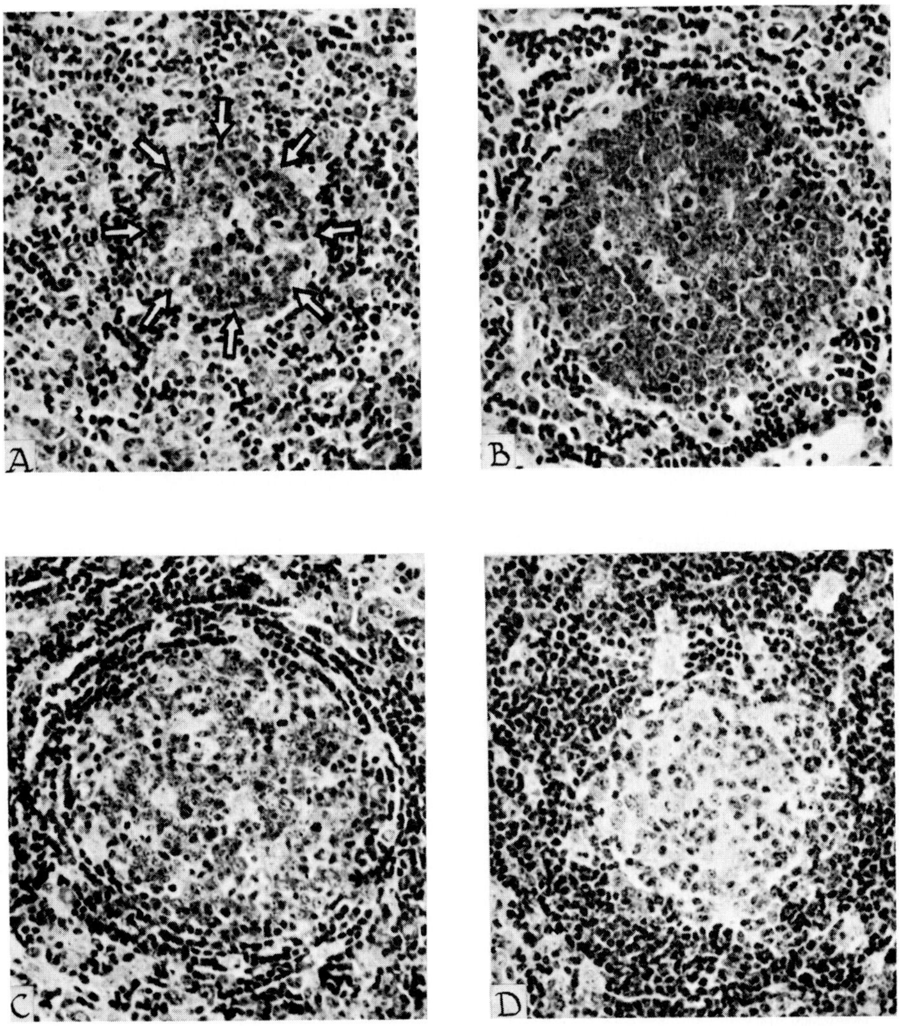

Figure 2–13. Lymphatic nodules of guinea pigs. Note different stages of development following immunization with *Listeria monocytogenes.* Hematoxylin and eosin stain, × 1100. (From Bloom, W., and Fawcett, D. W.: Textbook of Histology. 10th ed. Philadelphia, W. B. Saunders Company, 1975.)

the *lymphatics.* These vessels connect with and pass through a series of structures, the lymph nodes. During this voyage, the lymph becomes progressively enriched with lymphocytes, so that when it finally empties into the blood stream via the thoracic ducts, the fluid is significantly different from the tissue fluids of its origin. Lymphocytes are also added from postcapillary venules and become part of the *recirculating pool.*

The *recirculating pool* consists of a group of lymphocytes found in the circulating blood, lymph, and lymph nodes, which traverse a circumscribed pathway from the blood to the lymph and then back to the blood. The recirculation of lymphocytes from the blood to the lymph occurs through a unique anatomic structure of lymph nodes, the postcapillary venule. These venules, found in the lymph node cortex, are distinguished by their elongated endothelial cell structure. Unlike other interepithelial cell transfers, such as that of the polymorphonuclear neutrophil, the lymphocyte passes from the blood to the lymph by a remarkable process in which the endothelial cell invaginates the lymphocyte and allows it to pass directly through the cell (Fig. 2–14). The recirculating pool of small lymphocytes consists primarily of T-cells that are characterized by their long life spans and are believed to function as memory cells.

Lymph nodes are oval structures distributed throughout the body (Fig. 2–15); through them pass the motile carriers of specific genetic information, the lymphocytes. When enlarged, the lymph nodes be-

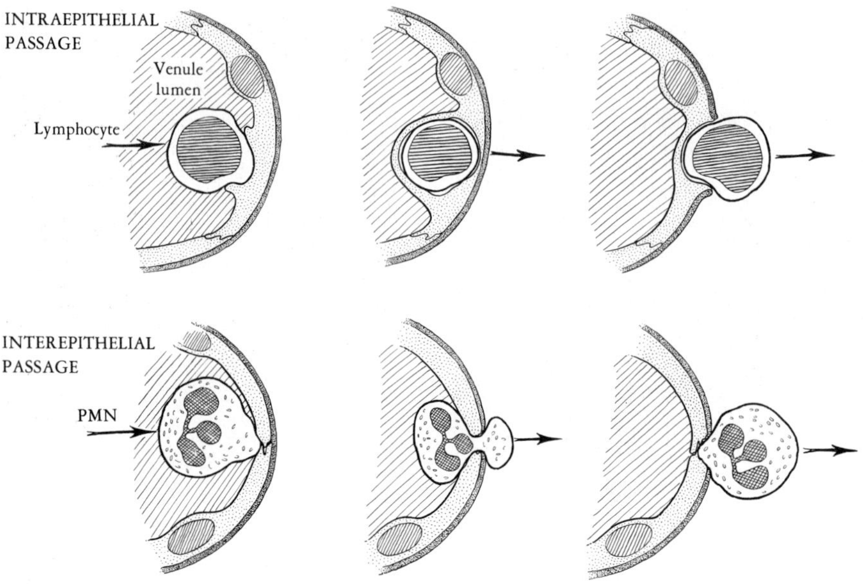

Figure 2–14. Schematic representation of intraepithelial passage of a small lymphocyte and interepithelial passage of a polymorphonuclear leukocyte.

come physically palpable, providing a useful diagnostic sign of infection or malignant disease. The structure of a lymph node is shown in Figure 2–15. It consists of two main portions, an outer portion (cortex) and an inner portion (medulla). The node is surrounded by a connective tissue capsule from which extensions protrude centrally (trabeculae). The capsule provides support and a conduit along which blood vessels run. Weblike structures (reticular fibers) extend from these connective tissue elements into the substance of the node; these contain phagocytic elements of the macrophage system. In the periphery, the node is made up of large numbers of lymphocytes organized into nodules. In the center of the nodules are collections of actively dividing cells termed *germinal centers.* Deeper cortical zones contain the postcapillary venules with their characteristic cuboidal endothelial cells through which passage of lymphocytes from blood lymph occurs (Fig. 2–16). Thus, in the lymph node, lymphocytes enter through both the vascular system and the lymphatics (Fig. 2–16). In mutant strains of mice born without thymuses (nude mice) or following the thymectomy of neonatal animals, there is a depletion of lymphoid elements in these paracortical or subcortical regions; therefore, this region has become known as a *thymic-dependent region* and contains the T-lymphocytes important in cell-mediated immunity. In contrast, upon removal of the bursa of Fabricius (in birds) or the bursal equivalent tissues (in the mammal), there is a failure of formation of the outer cortical regions containing the germinal centers, as well as the deeper medullary region; therefore, these regions have been called the bursal equivalent regions and contain the B-lymphocytes important in antibody synthesis. Following antigen stimulation, antibody synthesis can be noted in both the medullary and the far cortical regions of the node. Although it is tempting to compartmentalize the node according to function, this is undoubtedly an oversimplification of a more complicated process, since elements of each type of tissue may be present in both regions. Nonetheless, the importance of these findings for clinical medicine is illustrated in numerous disease states such as the DiGeorge syndrome, in which T-lymphocytes are absent owing to the congenital absence of the thymus, or X-linked agammaglobulinemia, in which a deficiency of B-lymphocytes occurs as a result of a failure of development of the bursal equivalent tissue (Chapter 22).

There are two basic functions of the lymph nodes. The first function is the filtration of foreign material performed as lymph percolates through the multichanneled structure. This removes particulate matter, and some products of phagocytic degradation become

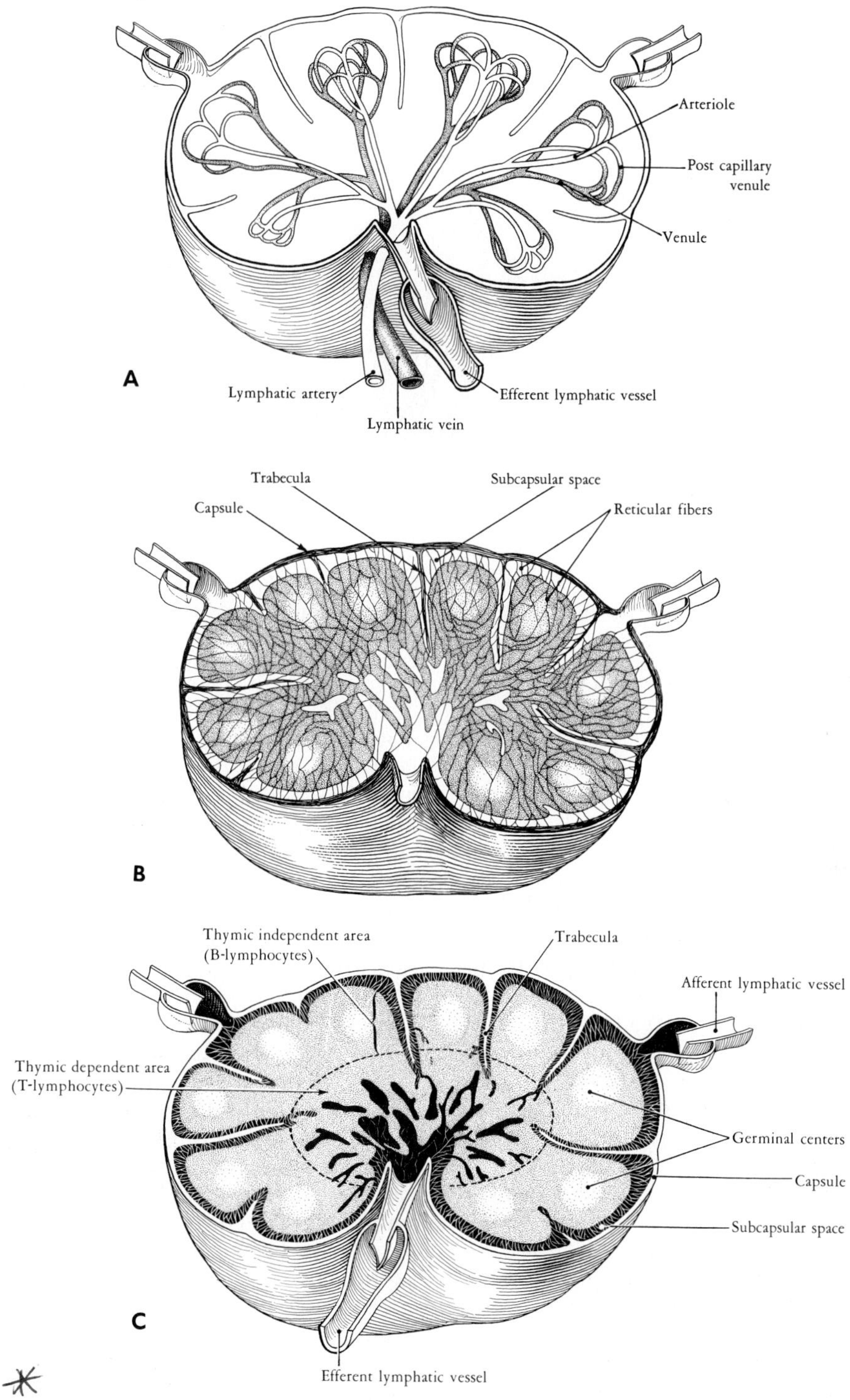

Figure 2–15. Structure of lymph node, schematic. *A,* Circulation; *B,* supporting structures (reticular fibers); and *C,* general areas of thymic-dependent (T-cell) and -independent (B-cell) areas.

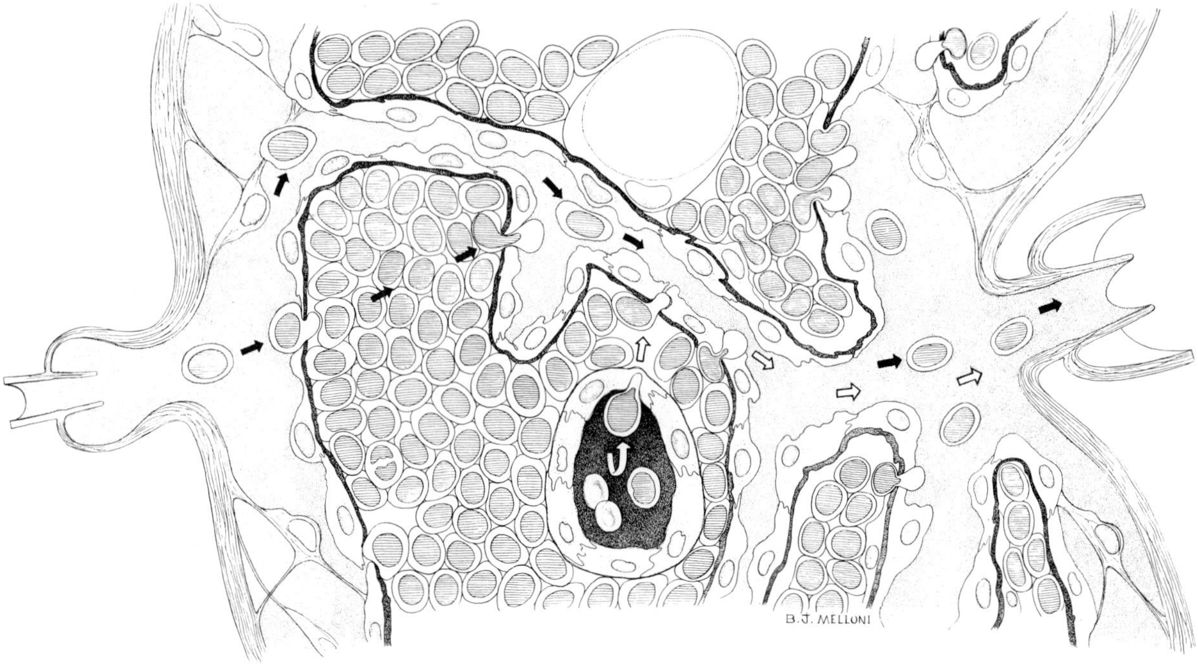

Figure 2–16. Schematic representation of circulation of lymphocytes within a lymph node. Note the dual entry of lymphocytes: from the vascular to lymphatic via postcapillary venule, and from afferent lymphatic vessels.

immunogenic. The second function is the circulation of lymphocytes, which are formed in the central lymphoid pool.

SPLEEN

If these first two barriers are inadequate, foreign constituents may gain access to the blood, either by direct invasion of small vessels (capillaries, venules) or via lymph stream channels emptying into the blood. The spleen is the sole lymphatic tissue specialized to filter blood. This organ has a number of *nonimmunologic* and *immunologic* functions. It removes effete or worn-out cells from the circulatory system (homeostatic function), converts hemoglobin to bilirubin, and releases iron into the circulation for reutilization. Like the lymph nodes, the spleen is a component of the peripheral lymphoid system, produces lymphocytes and plasma cells, and is important in the mediation of specific immunologic events. Yet the organ is important early in life, when other elements of the lymphoreticular system are incompletely developed. Removal of the spleen has been shown to be associated with overwhelming bacterial infections not only in infants and children but also in young adults.

The spleen is surrounded by a connective tissue capsule from which trabeculae extend into its interior (Fig. 2–17). The interior (pulp) is filled with two kinds of tissue: the *white* pulp and the *red* pulp. The white pulp contains lymph nodules and is the chief site of lymphocyte prodution in the spleen. The germinal follicles found in this region contain B-lymphocytes and are considered bursal equivalent tissues. Other lymphocytes surrounding the folicles and periarteriolar sheaths of the white pulp contain T-lymphocytes and are referred to as the thymic-dependent regions. Red pulp, on the other hand, surrounds the white pulp and contains large numbers of erythrocytes consonant with its filtration function. The arterial blood supply enters through the hilus and follows along trabeculae until the smaller arteries become surrounded by sheaths or collars of lymphocytes (white pulp). They then give off capillaries to the lymph nodules. The blood passes through the red pulp, containing elements of the reticuloendothelial system active in phagocytosis. These structures are shown in Figure 2–17. In addition to its phagocytic function, the spleen is capable of responding to antigenic stimulation. Following the intravenous injection of rabbits with antigen, one can demonstrate cells actively engaged in antibody synthesis in the sheaths surrounding arteries and also in lymph nodules.

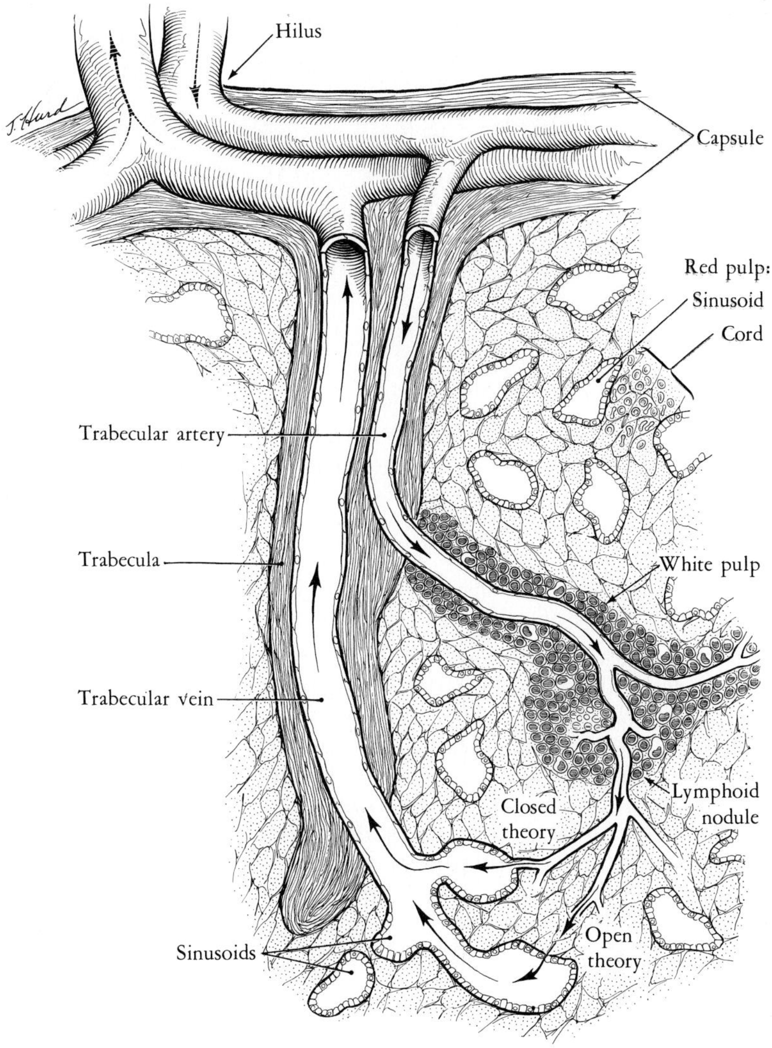

Figure 2–17. Schematic representation of structure of spleen.

THYMUS

The thymus is responsible for the development of lymphocytes involved in cell-mediated immune responses (thymus-derived or T-lymphocytes). The gland appears to be a master organ important in immunogenesis in the young and in orchestrating the total lymphoid system throughout life. This central lymphoid organ differs in a number of respects from other lymphoid tissues. All the lymphoid tissues described thus far are advantageously and strategically positioned for contact with foreign configurations that may enter or arise within the host. The thymus, on the other hand, is protected from rather than exposed to antigen. In addition, the rate of mitotic activity in the thymus is greater than in any other lymphatic tissue, yet the number of cells leaving it is fewer than the number accounted for by this high rate of mitosis. The assumption made from these findings is that a large number of lymphocytes produced within the thymus die within its substance. Although originally considered to be a mechanism for removal of "forbidden" autoreactive lymphocyte clones, this function of the thymus probably represents homeostatic activity involved in the production of T-lymphocytes. The role of the thymus in the development of the immunologic system is described more fully in Chapters 3 and 9.

The thymus consists of two lobes surrounded by a thin capsule of connective tissues (Fig. 2–18). The capsule extends into the substance of the gland, forming septa that partially divide the lobes into lobules. Peripheral portions of the lobule (cortex) are heavily infiltrated with lymphocytes. More

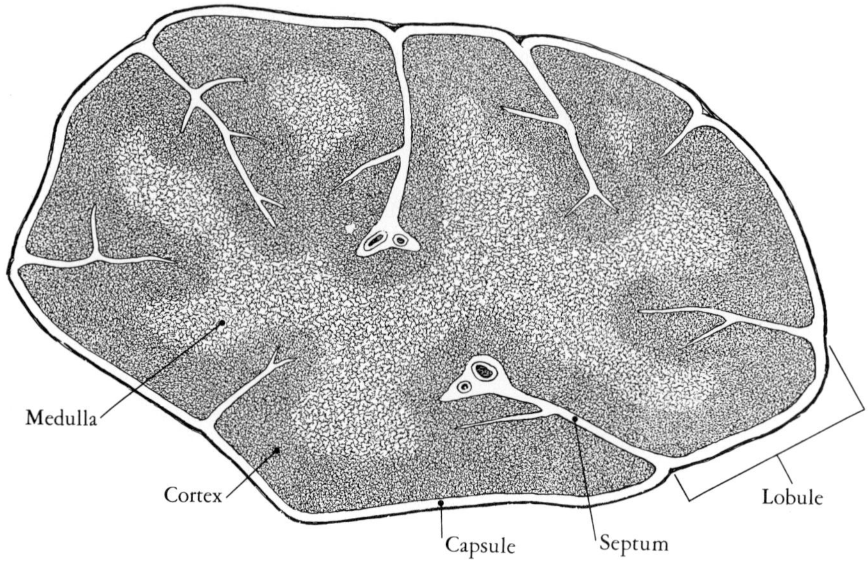

Figure 2–18. Schematic representation of thymus gland, showing division into cortex and medulla.

central portions (medulla) contain fewer lymphocytes but more epithelial elements. Within the substance of the thymus are cystic structures containing keratin (Hassall's corpuscles). The thymus is believed to perform two main functions: the production of lymphocytes within the cortex and the production of a humoral substance(s) by epithelial elements of the gland. These humoral substances (or hormones) may induce differentiation of lymphocytes directly within the thymus or may control their differentiation in the periphery. Although the thymus gland has a cortex and a medulla, neither contains germinal centers or plasma cells in the normal situation. These may appear when the gland is abnormal, e.g., in thymoma or in certain autoimmune diseases (Chapter 20C).

Unlike other lymphoid organs, the thymus is composed of two tissue types: lymphoid and epithelial. The lymphoid cells are of mesenchymal origin, and the epithelial cells

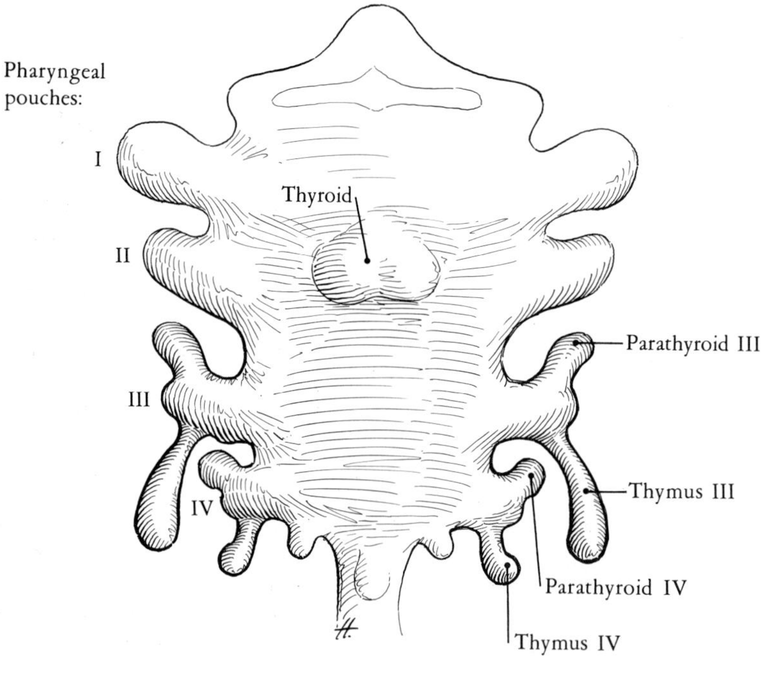

Figure 2–19. Embryology of the thymus gland from III to IV pharyngeal pouches. Note close proximity of site of differentiation of thyroid gland (II–III) and parathyroid glands (III–IV).

are of endodermal origin. The thymus initially develops as a continuous epithelium of cells from the third and fourth pharyngeal pouches Then the mesenchyme-derived lymphoid cells seed this epithelial thymus and convert this structure into a lymphoepithelial organ. The process of differentiation in the human begins as a ventral outpocketing from these pouches about the sixth week of fetal life (Fig. 2–19). It is noteworthy that the parathyroids begin their development about the same time from the same pouches. A caudal migration of epithelium occurs with further differentiation. Failure of this migration is seen in one of the immunologic deficiency disorders—thymic dysplasia (Chapter 22). By the tenth week, the thymic epithelium is differentiated into a compact epithelial structure interlaced with a fibrous reticular network. The epithelial cells are secretory cells with a well-developed Golgi apparatus, a rough endoplasmic reticulum, and a large nucleus with multiple nucleoli (Fig. 2–20). With further development, the thymus is

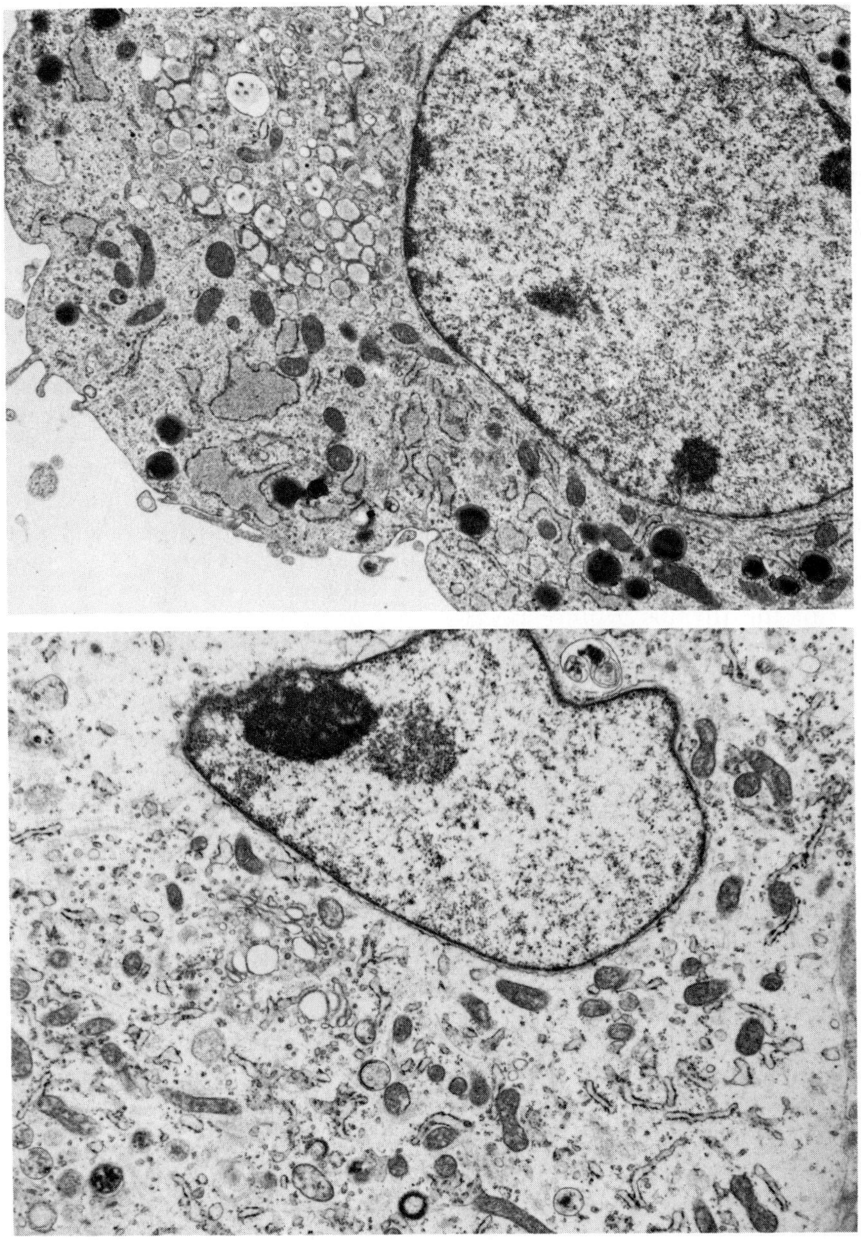

Figure 2–20. Electron micrograph of a thymus epithelial cell in culture, × 11,000. (Courtesy of Sam Waksal.)

infiltrated with precursor cells migrating from the liver and yolk sac during fetal life and bone marrow during adult life. Large lymphoblastoid cells first enter the subcapsular cortex and subsequently undergo further differentiation as they migrate through the different areas of the thymus. The clinical importance of the simultaneous embryogenesis of parathyroid glands and the thymus is seen in another of the immunologic deficiency disorders of man, the DiGeorge syndrome (Chapter 22). Infants with this disorder are born not only lacking in thymic function but also without parathyroid glands. Thus they present with hypocalcemic tetany in the newborn period and with subsequent failure of the development of cell-mediated immunity.

Thymocytes develop within the thymic microenvironment, and autoradiographic studies show that they migrate from cortical areas to medullary areas. This maturation process is characterized by changes in surface (differentiation) antigens as well as functional properties (Table 2–5). In the mouse, one of the more important surface antigens is the Thy-1 (Θ) antigen on thymocytes, which also exists on peripheral T-lymphocytes. Less differentiated thymocytes contain large amounts of Thy-1 and TL (thymus leukemia) antigens and small amounts of H-2 antigen on their surfaces. The more differentiated thymocytes contain large amounts of H-2, small amounts of Thy-1, and no TL antigen. The highly differentiated thymocytes in the medullary regions of the thymus acquire GVH reactivity and cortisone resistance. The thymus may exert its control over the differentiation and maturation of prothymocytes either by direct contact with these cells and the thymus epithelium or via the thymic humoral factors. These factors or thymic hormones are secreted by the epithelial cells of the thymus and may be the control mechanism over peripheral T-lymphocytes.

In man, similar changes in differentiation antigens occur. Following infiltration of the thymus with pluripotential stem cells that have migrated from the yolk sac, fetal liver, or spleen, these cells acquire new surface differentiation antigens and functions. Utilizing monoclonal antibody techniques, three discrete stages of thymic differentiation have been defined (Fig. 2–21). During intrathymic maturation, thymocytes progress through these stages and gradually acquire and then lose or retain various surface markers. The most mature thymocytes eventually differentiate into two separate populations that finally are released into the peripheral blood. These two populations are called (1) T-inducer (T_4) lymphocytes, which facilitate antibody production ("helper cells"); and (2) T-cytotoxic/suppressor (T_5/T_8) lymphocytes, which inhibit antibody production ("suppressor cells") or destroy target cells ("killer or cytotoxic cells"). These events will be more fully described in Chapters 7 and 9.

After birth, the role of the thymus continues to change. The changes in the size of the gland with age are shown in Figure 2–22. Relative to body size it is largest during fetal life and at birth weighs from 10 to 15 gm. The gland continues to increase in size, reaching a maximum of 30 to 40 gm at puberty. This follows the same pattern of change that occurs in all lymphoid tissue during childhood. It is of interest that this pattern of growth parallels the sequential appearance of T- and B-cell function during maturation. Following adolescence, the gland begins to involute. The parallel continues in that lymphoid tissues and immunoglobulins also diminish with increasing age. In addition, the development of autoimmune phenomena and malignant disease increases with advancing age with a loss of T-cell (e.g., suppressor) function. Thus the thymus and its associated lymphoid tissues and their products play a dynamic role from early embryogenesis throughout the life span of the individual.

Table 2–5. **Thymocyte Populations (Mouse)**

	Size		
	Large	Small	Medium
Per cent of thymus	5–7	85–90	5–7
Location	Subcapsular	Deeper cortex	Medulla
Life span	Rapid turnover	Long-lived	Long-lived
Cortisone sensitivity	Yes	Yes	No
Thy 1 (θ)	+ + +	+ +	+
H-2	+	+	+ +
Per cent Fc+	< 1	10	9

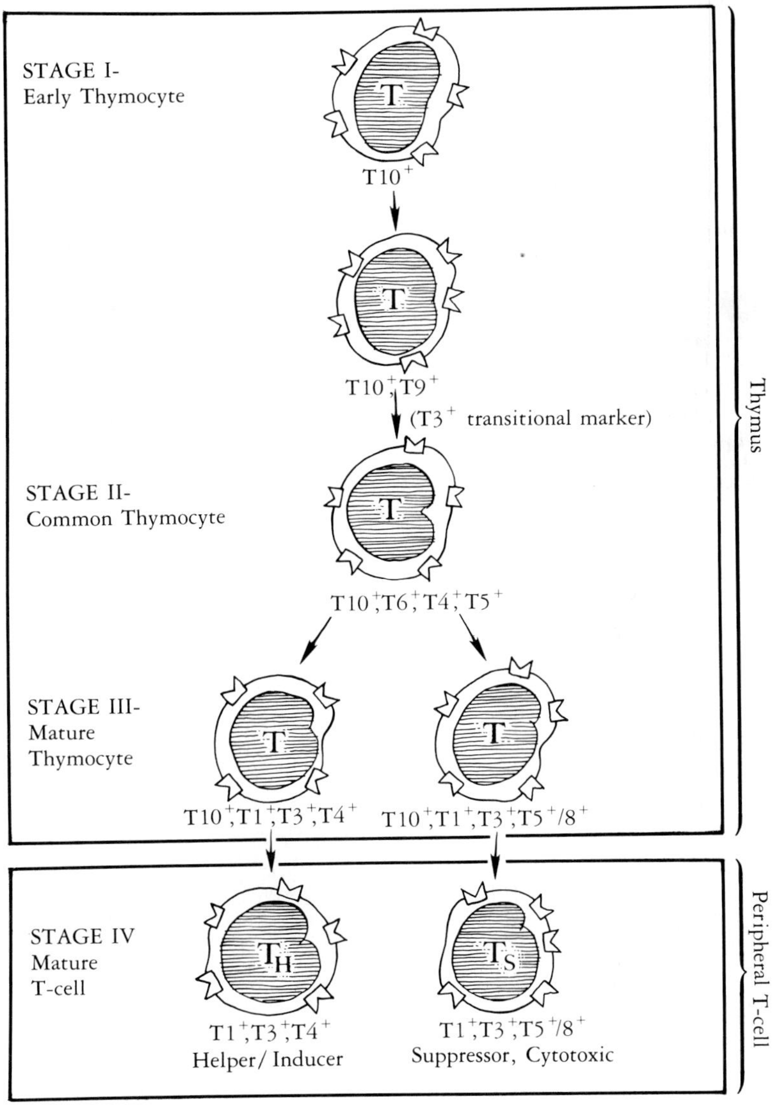

Figure 2–21. Human T-cell maturation as defined by monoclonal antibodies. (After Reinherz and Schlossman.)

The thymus thus appears to be equipped to maintain lymphopoiesis while segreated from antigen. This curious finding may be explained in part by the barrier that is made up of a continuous epithelium surrounding blood vessels in the cortex (Fig. 2–23). This epithelial membrane forms a perivascular space between the capillary endothelium and the epithelial sheath. The barrier might prevent macromolecules in the blood stream from entering the substance of the thymus gland. Although macromolecules may be prevented from entering the epithelial barrier, lymphocytes produced within the cortex are capable of passing freely through this epithelium into the blood system, as in other anatomic sites (e.g., postcapillary venule of the lymph nodes) (Fig. 2–23).

Thus, the thymus may be viewed as a lymphoid organ, anatomically distinct, upon which all other peripheral lymphoid organs are dependent. It is an organ actively engaged in lymphopoiesis but independent of antigenic stimulation. It appears important as a central lymphoid tissue essential for the development and maturation of peripheral lymphoid tissues. Two major functions have been attributed to the thymus: (1) that it acts by the elaboration of a hormone that expands peripheral lymphocyte populations in much the same way as erythropoietin expands erythrocyte populations, and (2) that it acts

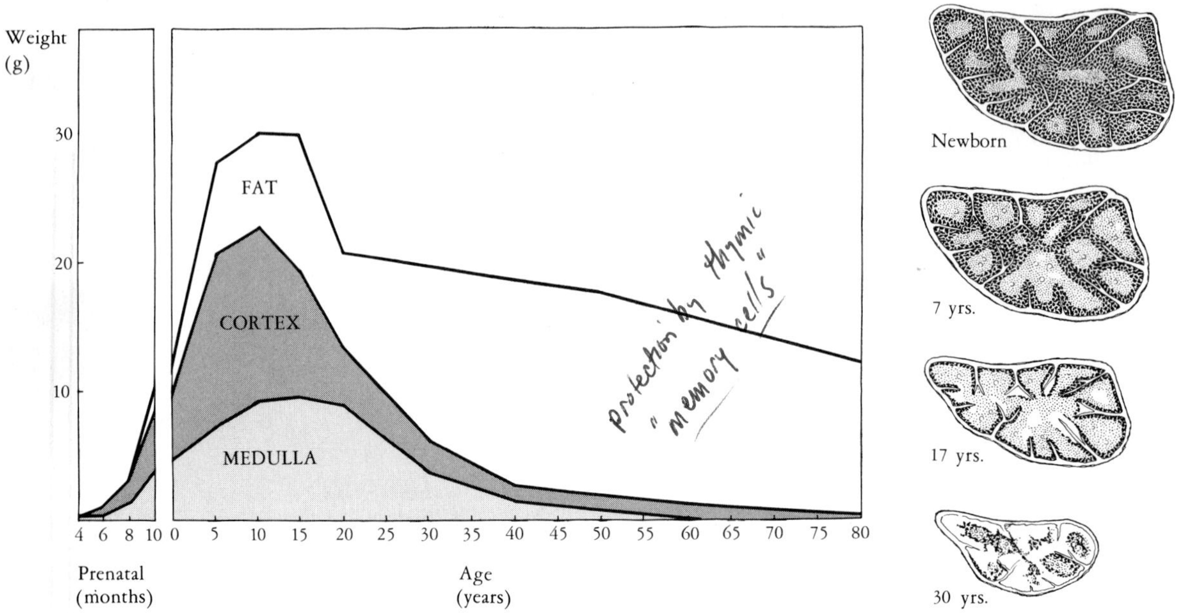

Figure 2–22. Schematic representation of changes in weight and composition of thymus gland with maturation, showing involution of the gland with age. (After Hammar, J. A.: Die normal morphologische Thymusforschung im letzten. Vierteljahrhundert. Leipzig. Barth, 1936.)

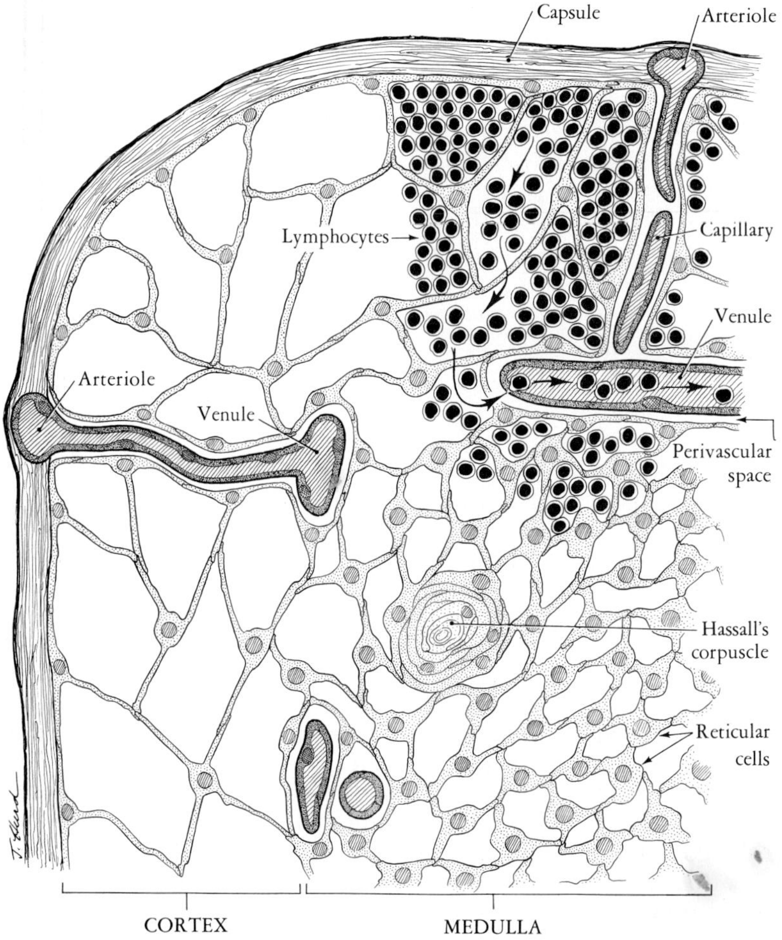

Figure 2–23. Thymus gland. Schematic representation of the perivascular epithelium surrounding blood vessels in the cortex. Note the barrier provided by this sheath and the pathways of lymphocytes formed in the cortex into the blood vessels.

by direct seeding of peripheral lymphoid tissues with lymphocytes. Recent studies have focused upon the role of the thymus as an endocrine gland, and several thymic hormones from the human and animal sources have been described. Some of these, e.g., thymosin(s), are receiving clinical trials in the reconstitution of children with a wide variety of immune deficiencies (Chapter 22). Failure of thymic function has also been implicated in the development of neoplasms and autoimmune disease, e.g., myasthenia gravis.

DEVELOPMENT OF THE IMMUNOLOGIC SYSTEM

The development of the immunologic system may be considered as a series of adaptive cellular responses to a changing and potentially hostile environment (Table 2–6). It may be considered at several levels: *species, individual,* or *cell.*

The effect of the hostile environment ensures by selective pressures the survival of those life forms within the species that are best adapted to that environment. This adaptive process forms the basis for the *phylogeny* of the immune response. The microenvironment in which undifferentiated immunologic progenitor cells exist provides yet another type of inducing stimulus within the developing individual *(ontogeny).* The immunologically mature individual may be considered as the selected form that resulted from this type of development. Finally, when cells find themselves within the molecular milieu of antigen, a series of proliferative and differentiative events occur that are characteristic of the specific immune response. This leads to the synthesis of cell products such as antibody or mediators of cell-mediated immunity. The "memory" cells that are the result of this process may be considered the best adapted forms for the environment initiated by antigen. Moreover, the interaction of macrophages, B- and T-lymphocytes involved in immunologic processes, has genetic requirements (Chapter 7). Thus, the development of immune systems at all levels is the result of selective pressures exerted by a type of environment on either a species, an individual, or a cell, the net effect leading to some survival advantage of the evolving form.

Development of the Immunologic System in Evolving Species: Phylogeny of the Immune Response

PHYLOGENY OF NONSPECIFIC IMMUNITY

The most primitive manifestation of a resistance mechanism is phagocytosis. This event, which is found in the most ancient of the unicellular organisms, served a nutritive function; in higher forms, the process evolved to a *defense* function. This was clearly recorded by Metchnikoff in his writing.

> Immunity is a phenomenon which has existed on this globe from time immemorial. Immunity must be of as ancient date as is disease. The most simple and primitive organisms have constantly to struggle for their existence; they give chase to living organisms in order to obtain food, and they defend themselves against other organisms in order that they may not become their prey. When the aggressor in this struggle is much smaller than its adversary, the result is that the former introduces itself into the body of the latter and destroys it by means of infection. In this case it takes up its abode in its adversary in order to absorb the contents of its host and to produce within it one or more generations. The natural history of unicellular organisms, both vegetable and animal, often presents to us these examples of primitive infection.

From the currently identifiable life forms, there arose an increasingly complex immune system, that ranged from the primitive defense of phagocytosis to the humoral and cell-mediated responses characteristic of specific immunity (Fig. 2–24).

As cellular life differentiated into more complex forms, there developed an increas-

Table 2–6. **Effect of Environment on the Development of the Immune Response**

Target	Inductive Environment	Process	Selected Form
Species	Macroenvironment	Phylogeny	Existing life forms
Individual	Microenvironment (thymus, bursal tissues)	Ontogeny	Immunologically mature individual
Cell	Molecular environment (antigen)	Induction of immune response	"Memory" cells

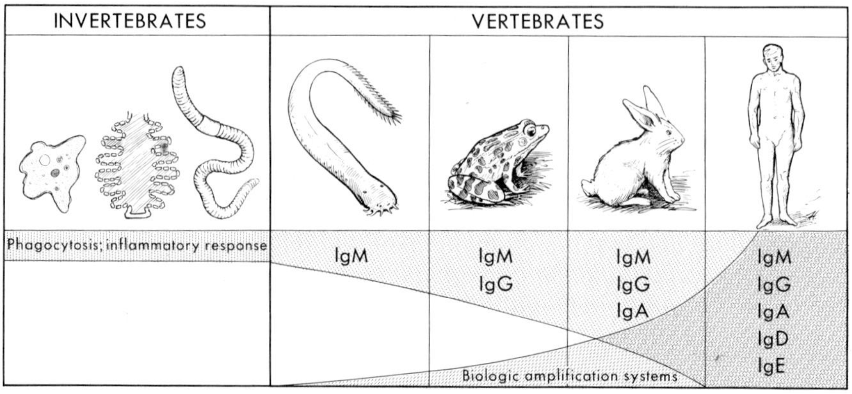

Figure 2–24. Schematic representation of phylogeny of immune response.

ing specialization of the systems concerned with recognition of foreignness. Thus, there evolved ever-increasingly complex immunologic systems. Although phagocytosis was continued as a nutritive function by endodermal cells (sponges, for example), the addition of a newly acquired mesodermal layer added a defense function. *It is the development and specialization of this mesodermal layer in higher life forms, beginning with vertebrates, in which specialization of cells destined for specific immunologic events is seen.*

In higher invertebrates a vascular system developed that allowed phagocytosis to proceed by both *fixed* and *circulating* cells (Fig. 2–24). In man, for example, there are five circulating white cells, three of which are phagocytic (monocytes, polymorphonuclear leukocytes, and eosinophils). Thus, in phylogeny, the two most important nonspecific elements, *phagocytosis* and the *inflammatory response,* were found in primitive life forms. With evolution, these defense mechanisms persisted, and were supplemented and amplified by the addition of new components—*specific immunity* and *biologic amplification systems* (e.g., coagulation system and complement). Thus, these older mechanisms were not replaced with evolution, but rather were continued and reinforced as evolving life forms added new responses.

PHYLOGENY OF SPECIFIC IMMUNITY

The first evidence of a specific immunologic system appeared in primitive vertebrates such as the hagfish (Fig. 2–24). It consisted of a disseminated lymphoid system, rather than the specialized lymphoid structures that occur in higher forms. In these early species there existed a primitive high molecular weight antibody and cells that could manifest cell-mediated immunity. In the elasmobranchs, for example, a tissue transplant consisting of skin or scales would be promptly rejected. Similarly, the introduction of antigens into these species will elicit a high molecular weight antibody analogous to IgM immunoglobulin of higher forms (Chapter 5). During evolution, there occurred specialization of cells and supporting structures to house these tissues—the lymphoreticular tissues. The thymus is the earliest lymphoid organ to appear in phylogeny and is present in the most primitive of vertebrates. There also appeared in birds a separate anatomic structure arising from the primitive gut, the bursa of Fabricius, which is important in the development of cells that elaborate antibody in avian species. The mammalian equivalent of this organ is not known. In the human, it is useful to consider thymic-controlled tissues that elaborate cell-mediated events as *thymic-dependent* tissues and those that elaborate antibody under a separate influence as *thymic-independent* tissues. Both are important to our understanding of the maturation of immune responses and immunologic deficiency states of man (Chapter 22).

The evolutionary order of appearance of immunoglobulin classes in many respects parallels that seen in the maturing individual (ontogeny). It also recapitulates the sequential appearance of immunoglobulin molecular forms that appear following a single antigenic exposure during the immune response (Chapter 7). These are shown in Figure 2–24. In the most primitive of vertebrates, the predominant antibody is a high molecular weight substance, analogous to the IgM globulins of the human. During phylogeny, a second class of antibody with properties similar to the IgG globulins is elaborated. The IgA immunoglobulins appear as rather late evolutionary events and are restricted to mammals. The development of a novel form of IgA immunoglobulin, the secretory IgA globulins, was also elucidated in mammals. This external antibody system has proved to be of immense importance in defense at body surfaces and appears to be a mechanism by which lower forms, such as the ungulates, receive passive antibody via colostrum. The major transfer of antibody in the human occurs primarily via the placenta; however, breast milk still continues to be a source of IgA antibody. This antibody is not absorbed by the infant's gastrointestinal tract but may be important locally within the intestine (coproantibody). Finally, still later additions seen in man are the IgD and the IgE immunoglobulins. The IgE immunoglobulins, seen also in other mammalian forms, are a unique class of antibody involved in immediate-type hypersensitivity.

With evolution there also occurred the development of an elaborate series of substances that could augment and enhance the efficiency of the ancient resistance mechanisms. These are referred to as biologic amplification systems and consist primarily of the coagulation and the complement systems (Chapter 6).

Development of the Immunologic System in the Developing Individual: Ontogeny of the Immune Response

Available evidence suggests that the maturation of the immune response in the human begins *in utero* sometime during the second to third months of gestation. The differentiation of cells destined to perform both nonspecific and specific immunologic functions seems to have a common ancestral origin. Both cell types appear to arise from a population of progenitor cells referred to as *stem cells* or *hemocytoblasts;* these are located within the hematopoietic tissues of the developing embryo (yolk sac, fetal liver, and bone marrow). Depending upon the type of microchemical environment surrounding the cells, development will occur along at least two avenues: the *hematopoietic* and the *lymphopoietic* (Fig. 2–25).

One type of microchemical environment leads to proliferation and differentiation of nonlymphoid stem cell hematopoietic precursors. The products of these cell lines are the hematopoietic elements of the peripheral blood and tissues and include the *erythrocytes, granulocytes, platelets,* and *monocytes.* The second set of progenitor cells are the stem cell lymphoid precursors that can differentiate along two pathways. The first, under the influence of the thymus, perhaps within the substance of the gland itself, includes a population of small lymphocytes that subserve the function of cell-mediated immunity (thymic-dependent or T-lymphocytes). If the lymphoid stem cells come under a second type of microchemical environment, i.e., bursal equivalent, differentiation will occur to produce a population of lymphocytes (B-lymphocytes) and plasma cells concerned with humoral immunity or antibody synthesis (Fig. 2–25).

The functional significance of this *two-compartment system* is important to clinical medicine. It provides a useful basis upon which our understanding of immunologic deficiency disorders rests (Chapter 22). Thus, individuals displaying selective disorders of bursal equivalent tissues, the so-called aggammaglobulinemias or dysgammaglobulinemias, present with recurrent bacterial infections. Selective deficiencies of the thymic-dependent tissues, on the other hand, are also seen in man and are manifested with other types of infections, such as fungal and viral diseases. Still a third type of patient presents with combined deficiencies of both thymic-dependent and thymic-independent tissues. These individuals have profound deficiencies in both cell-mediated and antibody mediated functions and have the most serious sequelae of all the immunologic deficiency syndromes and present with a diversity of infections.

MATERNAL-FETAL RELATIONSHIPS

One of the most significant developments in phylogeny is the appearance of placentation in the species with the ability to bear live young (viviparity). This occurred in higher forms with the development of the multilayered placenta. One of the challenging problems in biology is the question of how a fetus, who inherits one half of its antigens from paternally controlled genes foreign to the mother, can be tolerated successfully during

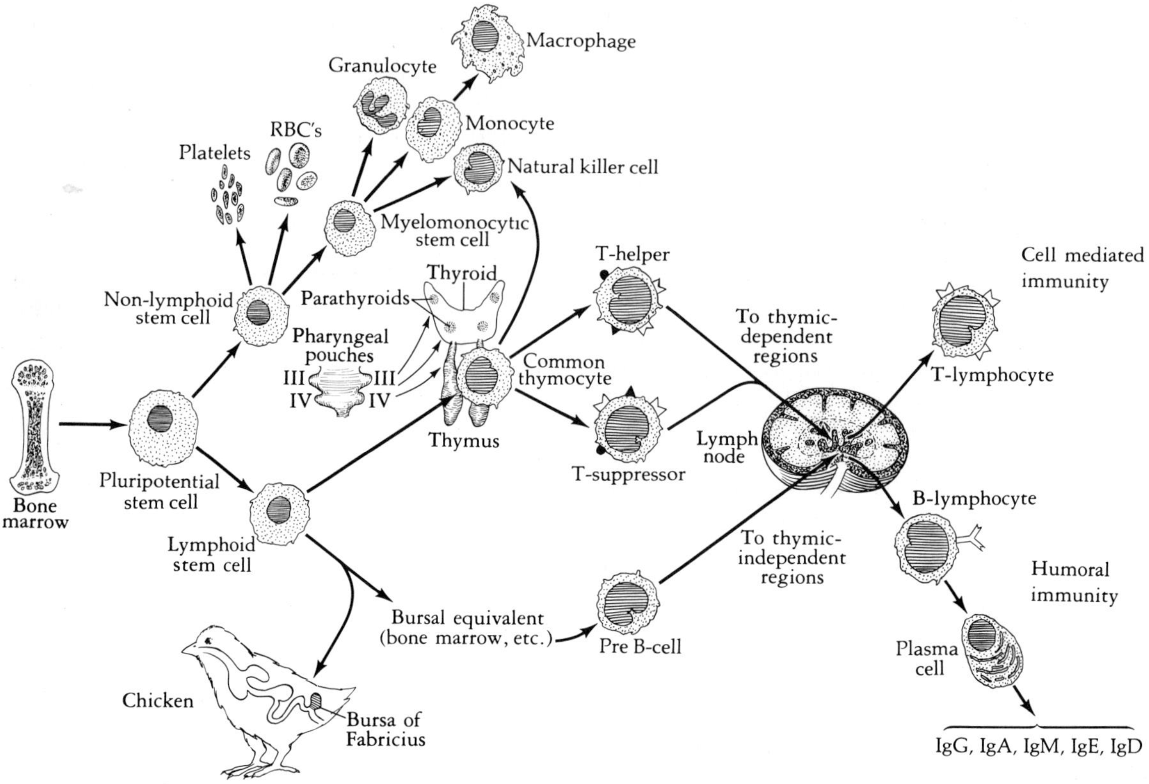

Figure 2–25. Schematic representation of ontogeny of immune response, showing differentiation of progenitor cells into hematopoietic and immunocompetent cells.

pregnancy. This has been attributed largely to the barrier function of the placenta. By acting as a mechanical barrier, the placenta usually effectively separates the formed elements of the blood of the mother from that of the fetus. There are elements, however, that do gain access to the fetus and provide protection—antibodies.

There are different pathways of transmission of maternal antibody to the fetus in different species (Table 2–7). In species with large numbers of membranes intervening between the maternal and fetal circulations, the colostral route seems to be a more important mechanism of transfer. Conversely, as the number of layers of membrane decreases (as in man, for example), the transplacental route seems to assume greater importance. Thus, in man, the prodominant transfer of antibody occurs via the passage of the IgG immunoglobulins from the maternal circulation to that of the fetus. This is accomplished by means of an active transport mechanism of this immunoglobulin by virtue of a receptor located on the Fc fragment of the molecule (Chapter 5). In this manner, the fetus receives a library of preformed antibody from its mother, reflecting most of her ex-

Table 2–7. Relationship of Type of Placentation with Character of Maternal-Fetal Transfer of Antibody in Various Species

Animal	Number of Placental Membranes	Relative Importance of Route	
		Placental	Colostral
Horse	6	0	+ + +
Sheep, cow	5	0	+ + +
Cat, dog	5	+	+ +
Rat, mouse	4	+	+ +
Rabbit, guinea pig	3	+ + +	±
Man, monkey	3	+ + +	0

periences with infectious agents. Occasionally, fetal cells or other proteins may gain access to the maternal circulation and thus actively immunize her to the paternal allotypes (antigen) found on these substances. This process, referred to as isoimmunization, may lead to serious disease in the infant, such as hemolytic disease of the newborn, thrombocytopenia, and leukopenia (Chapter 20B).

The development of serum immunoglobulins during intrauterine life and postnatally is shown in Figure 2–26. If one analyzes the amount and type of gamma globulin found in the blood of the newborn infant at birth, one finds that the levels of immunoglobulin are equivalent to those of the mother and are made up almost exclusively of the IgG immunoglobulins. There is virtually little or no IgA and IgM globulin present in cord sera. This is because the fetus is usually protected *in utero* from antigenic stimuli. If the fetus is challenged *in utero* as a consequence of immunization or infection (e.g., congenital rubella, cytomegalic inclusion disease, toxoplasmosis), it will respond with antibody production largely of the IgM variety. The exclusion of other classes of antibody is beneficial to the fetus in many cases. For example, the exclusion of the IgM isohemagglutinins, leukoagglutinins, or the IgE antibodies of allergy prevents disease that may be produced by these antibodies. However, it also prevents the passage of other maternal antibodies that would be beneficial to the newborn, such as the IgM antibodies important in bacterial defense against gram-negative bacteria (opsonins, agglutinins, and bactericidal antibodies). This may explain, in part, the increased susceptibility of the newborn to infection with gram-negative organisms such as *Escherichia coli.*

Since the IgG immunoglobulins are passively transferred, they have a finite half-life of between 20 and 30 days, and therefore their concentration in serum falls rapidly within the first few months of life, reaching the lowest levels between the second and fourth months. This period is referred to as physiologic hypogammaglobulinemia (Chapter 22). During the course of the first few years, the levels of gamma globulin increase because of exposure of the maturing infant to antigens in the environment. There appears to be a sequential development in gamma globulin at different rates. The IgM globulins attain adult levels by one year of age, the IgG globulins by five to six years of age, and the IgA globulins by ten years of age (Chapter 26). This pattern of appearance of immunoglobulins recapitulates that seen in phylogeny and also appears to parallel that seen following an antigenic exposure during the primary immune response.

It is important to emphasize that the development of immunoglobulin receptors on lymphocytes during fetal life follows the same general pattern as that observed with the appearance of various immunoglobulins in the serum after birth (Table 2–8). It is notable that IgM is present on the surface of cells

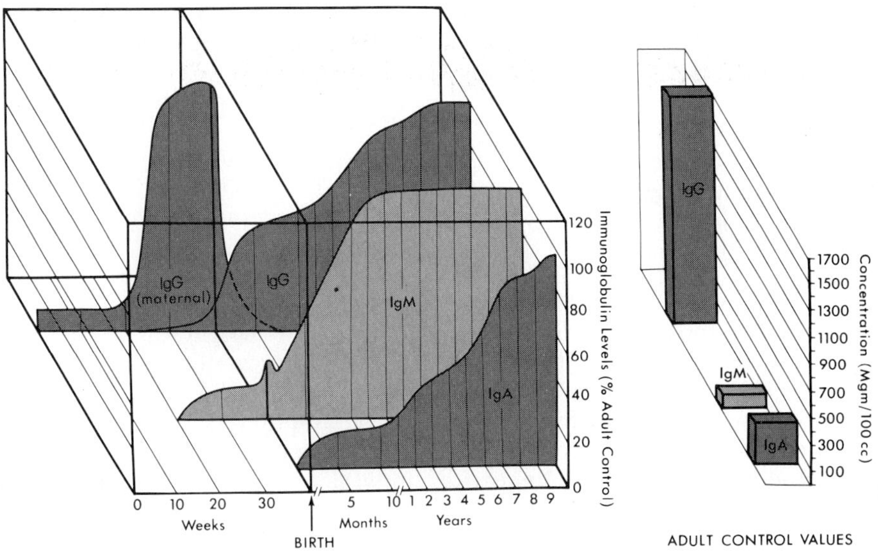

Figure 2–26. Development of serum immunoglobulins in the human during maturation. (After Alford, C. A., Jr.: Immunoglobulin determinations in the diagnosis of fetal infection. Pediatr. Clin. North Am., *18*:99, 1971.)

Table 2–8. **Maturation of Human T- and B-Cells: Surface Markers and Lymphoproliferative Responses**

		Serum Immunoglobulins					Responsiveness				
							Mitogens			Antigens	
	Age	IgM	IgG	IgA	IgD	IgE	PHA	Con-A	PWM	PPD	SK-SD
Fetal	10 weeks	−	−	−	−	−	+	−	−	−	−
	10.5 weeks	+	−	−	−	?	+	?	−	−	−
	12 weeks	+	+	−	−	?	+	+	−	−	−
	20 weeks	+	+	+	±	±	+	+	+	−	−
	Newborn	+	+	+	+	±	+	+	+	−	−
	Adult	+	+	+	+	+	+	+	+	+	+

as early as 10½ weeks. At birth, human immunocompetent cells have become fully responsive to mitogens (Table 2–8). (Mitogens such as phytohemagglutinin [PHA], concanavalin-A [Con-A], and pokeweed [PWM] are substances that will directly stimulate either B-or T-lymphocytes [Chapter 7].) However, the ability of cells to respond to specific antigens, such as tuberculin (PPD) or streptokinase-streptodornase (SK-SD), is limited. Only later do the lymphocytes develop the capability for cell-mediated responses against foreign antigens. Cell-mediated responses can also be measured *in vitro* by the development of lymphotoxin (LT) or macrophage inhibition factor (MIF) (Chapter 9). As can be seen in Table 2–9, at birth, cell-mediated responses are variable; LT can be produced, but MIF cannot.

From the very earliest fetal life, lymphocytes are present that can act both as responders to and stimulators of the mixed lymphocyte reaction (MLR) (Table 2–9). This suggests that the fetus can recognize transplantation antigens even before they can respond to any other foreign antigen, making all the more remarkable the inability of the fetus to react against its mother.

DEVELOPMENT OF THE IMMUNOLOGIC SYSTEM AT THE LEVEL OF THE WHOLE ORGANISM

It is now well established that the ability to respond to certain antigens is determined by the genetic constitution of the host (Chapter 3). Thus, selected strains of guinea pigs and mice fail to respond with antibody formation following immunization with normally immunogenic polypeptide antigens. The precise mechanism of this *nonresponder state* is not yet known, but is believed to be due to the suppression or deletion of genes important in immune responses.

Several studies in the mouse indicate an association between certain histocompatibility antigens and the ability to respond to immunogens (Chapter 3). Histocompatibility typing of mice allows the prediction of immune responsiveness to a wide variety of antigens other than histocompatibility antigens. The association between histocompatibility antigenic composition and immune responsiveness is under intensive study, and various data suggest that the expression of certain antigenic phenotypes may also be an expression of an individual immunologic responsiveness, e.g., association of HLA-B27 antigen with ankylosing spondylitis (Chapters 3 and 20C).

In the human, the precise analog of this nonresponder state is not known. However, in certain of the immunologic deficiency states, such as the Wiskott-Aldrich syndrome (Chapter 22), there is an inability to process certain polysaccharide antigens. It would seem reasonable that with the vast heterogeneity of the human species, variations in responsiveness from individual to individual would exist. Indeed, this appears to be the case and is manifested in clinical practice by the frequent encounter of individuals with susceptibility to infectious disease not expressed by other individuals. The susceptibility to certain autoimmune and malignant diseases is also known to occur in children with immunologic deficiency. A genetic basis may be involved in other hypersensitivity diseases of man. Only in certain individuals does acute glomerulonephritis or rheumatic fever occur following infection with Group A beta-hemolytic streptococci. This may be the human counterpart to the experimental model of serum sickness-type nephritis, which occurs after administration of repeated doses of bovine serum albumin to rabbits (Chapter 13). Such animals could be divided into three groups: good antibody responders,

Table 2–9. **Maturation of Human T- and B-Cells: Mixed Lymphocyte Responsiveness and Mediator Production**

	Age	MLR		Lymphokine	
		Responder	Stimulator	LT	MIF
Fetal	7.5 weeks	+	+	–	–
	10 weeks	+	+	–	–
	12 weeks	+	+	–	–
	20 weeks	+	+	–	–
	Newborn	+	+	+	–
	Adult	+	+	+	+

moderate antibody responders, and poor antibody responders. Limited disease was seen in the good and poor antibody responders; the most progressive and chronic forms of glomerulonephritis were seen in animals with moderate antibody production. This was presumably because of the development of antigen-antibody complexes injurious to their kidneys. This model of immunologic injury will be described in greater detail in Chapter 13.

Development of the Immunologic System at the Cellular Level

Antigen itself may be considered as part of the cellular environment that induces the development of an immune responsiveness (Table 2–6). During the induction of an immune response, antigen comes in contact with an appropriate collection of lymphoid cells, following which a series of proliferative and differentiative steps are initiated (see Fig. 7–2). At the moment of presentation of antigen, at least two, and possibly three, cells are involved. The first is a macrophage, which in some cases is essential for the processing of antigen to a form that can interact with a second series of cells, those of lymphoid type. These latter cells can proliferate and differentiate to become immunocompetent cells, capable of antibody formation or cell-mediated events. Following removal of antigen, there is an involution of this population of immunocompetent cells. However, some cells remain as "memory" cells, capable of carrying out specific immunologic events during any future encounter with the same antigen. These consist of either B- or T-lymphocytes. The whole cellular burst of activity seen in the induction of an immune response may be analogous to genetically controlled differentiation seen in the development of the species or during ontogeny of the individual. The memory cells may be considered as the best adapted forms for this type of environment (Table 2–6).

These processes involve a variety of cell types. As described previously, the lymphoid cell populations that respond to antigens can basically be divided into two populations, the T- and B-lymphocytes, which can act independently as well as in cooperation to produce an immune response (Chapter 7). Specific antigen receptors exist on the surface of both T-cells and B-cells. Certain antigens can directly stimulate the B-cells so that they will subsequently produce plasma cells and antibody; other antigens require the interaction of T-cells, which provide specific and nonspecific helper substances that will allow the B-cell to mature to produce antibody. It is interesting to note that antigen, after processing by macrophages, can lead to the production of activators of helper T-cells. Further, these macrophages must be syngeneic to the T-cells in order for the help to occur. Subsequent to activation, the T-lymphocytes produce factors that can trigger the B-cells (Chapter 9). A separate population of T-lymphocytes can also act to suppress the immune response, i.e., suppressor T-lymphocytes. This appears to involve active processes in the suppression of helper T-cells.

The interaction of T-cells, in both their helper and suppressor functions, is under strict genetic control, which is mediated by genes that are located within the major histocompatibility complex. These immune response (IR) genes are related to histocompatibility identity between the various cell types involved in the immune response (Chapter 3). Immunoregulation and the multiple interactions between specific cell types are only now beginning to be understood.

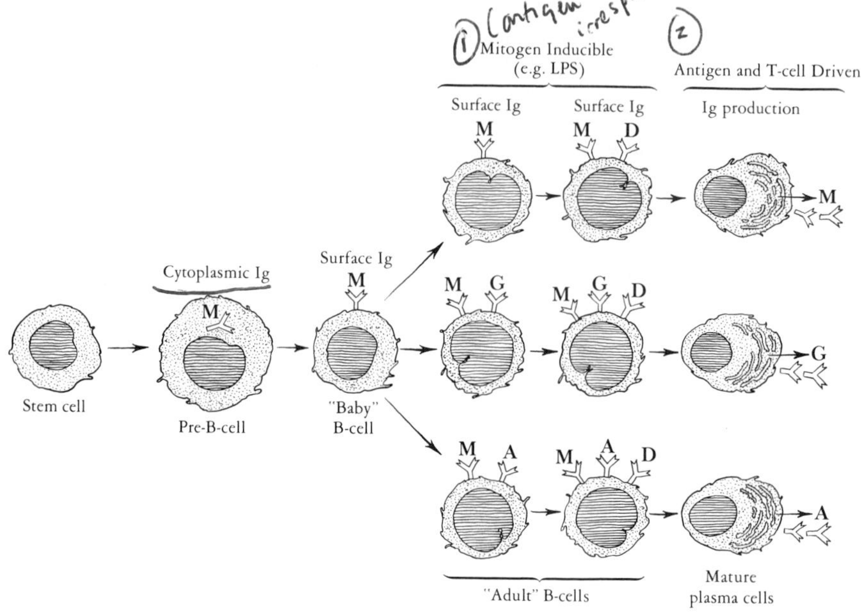

Figure 2–27. Ontogeny of B-lymphocyte system. (Adapted from Cooper, M. D., and Seligmann, M.: B and T lymphocytes in immunodeficiency and lymphoproliferative diseases. *In* Loor, F. and Roelants, G. E. (eds.): B and T Cells in Immune Recognition. West Sussex, England, John Wiley & Sons Ltd., 1977.)

The future directions of clinical immunology will, we hope, provide for the unraveling of these complex events. In the meantime, the clinician must deal with diseases that result from genetic failure to regulate immune response at each level of interaction.

Based upon evidence obtained from the human and experimental animal, Cooper and his coworkers have proposed a model of B-cell differentiation (Fig. 2–27). In this model, B-cells differentiate from a stem cell to a pre–B cell that initially expresses only cytoplasmic IgM. The next stage is represented by a cell expressing surface IgM receptors only. This "Baby B-cell" is a pivotal cell for further differentiation of cells that produce immunoglobulins. After this, two stages of differentiation exist: (1) an antigen-independent stage responsive to mitogen, and (2) an antigen-dependent T-cell driven stage that requires the presence of an IgD surface marker lost after antigenic stimulation.

To summarize, the whole of the immune response appears to be under developmental (genetic) influences. These range from the controls exerted on the evolving species (phylogeny) to those imposed on the maturing individual (ontogeny), the controls exerted within an individual and on the cell and cell products. Both immune responsiveness and unresponsiveness should be considered as genetic processes. This approach to immunology may better enable the physician to appreciate the pathogenesis of many immunologically mediated diseases, their transmissions within families, and their expected reappearances in future offspring.

Suggestions for Further Reading

Anatomic and Functional Organization of the Immune System

Bloom, W., and Fawcett, D. W. (eds.): A Textbook of Histology. 10th ed., Philadelphia, W. B. Saunders Company, 1975.

Cline, M. J. (ed): The White Cell. Cambridge, Harvard University Press, 1975.

Dingle, J. T., and Dean, R. T. (eds.): Lysosomes in Biology and Pathology. New York, American Elsevier Publishing Company, 1976.

Fauci, A. S.: The idiopathic hypereosinophilic syndrome: clinical, pathophysiologic and therapeutic considerations. Ann. Intern. Med., *97*:78, 1982.

Gabrieli, E. R., and Snell, F. M.: Reflection of reticuloendothelial function in studies of blood clearance kinetics. J. Reticuloendothel. Soc., *2*:141, 1965.

Van Furth, R. (ed.): Mononuclear Cells in Immunity, Infection, and Pathology. Oxford, Blackwell Scientific Publications, 1975.

Weiss, L. (ed.): Cells and Tissues of the Immune System: Structure, Functions, Interactions. Englewood Cliff, N.J., Prentice-Hall, Inc., 1972.

Chemotaxis, Phagocytosis, Metabolic Changes, and Antimicrobial Systems of Phagocytic Cells

Bellanti, J. A., and Dayton, D. H. (eds.): The Phagocytic Cell in Host Resistance. New York, Raven Press, 1975.

Cline, M. J. (ed.): The White Cell. Cambridge, Harvard University Press, 1975.

DeChalelet, L. R.: Oxidative bacterial mechanisms of polymorphonuclear leukocytes. J. Infect. Dis., *131*: 295, 1975.

Specific Immune Response

Gell, P. G. H., Coombs, R. R. A., and Lachman, P. T.: Clinical Aspects of Immunology. Oxford, Blackwell Scientific Publications, 1975.

Roitt, I. M.: Essential Immunology. Oxford, Blackwell Scientific Publications, 1974.

Stites, D. P., Stobo, J. D., Fudenberg, H. H., et al.: Basic and Clinical Immunology. 4th ed. Los Altos, Lange Medical Publications, 1982.

Suskind, R. M. (ed.): Malnutrition and the Immune Response. Kroc Foundation Series, Vol. 7. New York, Raven Press, 1977.

Phylogeny and Ontogeny

Cooper, E. L. (ed.): Contemporary Topics in Immunobiology. Vol. 4. Invertebrate Immunology. Plenum Publishing Corp., 1974.

Cooper, M. D., and Dayton, D. H. (eds.): Development of Host Defenses. New York, Raven Press, 1977.

Cooper, M. D., and Seligmann, M.: B and T lymphocytes in immunodeficiency and lymphoproliferative diseases. *In* Loor, F., and Roelants, G. E. (eds.): B and T cells in Immune Recognition. West Sussex, England, John Wiley & Sons Ltd., 1977.

Friedman, H. (ed.): Thymus factors in immunity. Ann. N.Y. Acad. Sci., *249*:1–547, 1975.

Reinherz, E. L., and Schlossman, S. F.: Regulation of the immune response-inducer and suppressor T-lymphocyte subsets in human beings. N. Engl. J. Med., *303*:1153, 1980.

Stites, D. P., Caldwell, J., Carr, M. C., et al.: Ontogeny of immunity in humans. Clin. Immunol. Immunopathol., *4*:519, 1975.

Chapter 3

Immunogenetics

James N. Woody, Capt., M.C., U.S.N., M.D., Ph.D.,
Joseph A. Bellanti, M.D., and Kenneth W. Sell, M.D., Ph.D.

INTRODUCTION

Immunogenetics include all those processes concerned in the immune response that may have a *genetic* basis. In the past, the term has been largely restricted to mean genetic markers on immunoglobulin polypeptide chains. In the light of recent developments, a more contemporary definition of immunogenetics should include *all the factors that control the immunologic responsiveness of the host to foreignness, as well as the transmission of antigenic specificities from generation to generation.*

Immune mechanisms may be viewed from an evolutionary standpoint as a series of genetic adaptations by the evolving species to changing environmental influences exerted upon it (Chapter 2). This has been referred to as *phylogeny* of the immune response. Similarly, the maturation of the immune mechanisms within the developing individual may be considered, and this has been termed *ontogeny* of the immune response. In a narrower sense, the genetic controls can be regarded at a cellular level as the proliferation and differentiation of a variety of cell types in response to antigen (Chapter 7). The action of genes can also be studied at the molecular level in terms of the unlimited variability of immunoglobulin structures that are directly encoded within DNA (Chapter 5). The heritability of antigens themselves, such as the blood group and histocompatibility antigens, is also transmitted within the chromosomes of the germ cells. Finally, of considerable importance are the recent discoveries indicating that the genes that control the expression of certain cellular antigens are nearly identical to those that control immune responsiveness.

The field of immunogenetics can be divided into two broad areas of study. The first major area concerns the genetic regulation and control of the immune system itself. Genes coding for immunoglobulins, the major histocompatibility (MHC) antigens, and the T-cell receptor(s), as well as genes coding for other mediators, interact in regulating and fostering an effective immune response. The second area with the broadest application is the use of antibodies and sensitized immune cells, the products of the immune system, as probes to detect and characterize various antigens that may show genetic variation, i.e., polymorphism. Over the past decade the analytic power of these immunologic probes has increased immensely as they have been used to study the more polymorphic genetic systems, such as the HLA or H-2 histocompatibility systems, blood groups, immunoglobulins, and complement proteins as well as cell surface glycoprotein antigens. The routine availability of exquisitely specific monoclonal antibodies (Chapter 5) and the capacity to prepare T-lymphocyte clones with an equivalent degree of specificity have fostered studies in research disciplines within and outside of immunology. Further, many of these reagents have rapidly found utility as clinical diagnostic reagents, e.g., for the detection of cell surface glycoproteins such as OKT4, which allow the identification of human T-lymphocytes as helper/inducer cells (Chapter 7). Equally important are the monoclonal antibodies capable of recognizing genetic variants of bacteria and viruses, e.g., differentiation between herpes simplex Type I and Type II. The use of sensitized cells as probes is currently limited to the detection of Class II histocompatibility (HLA) antigens with a mixed lymphocyte culture format; however, this will probably expand to include a variety of antigens.

CLINICAL IMPORTANCE OF IMMUNOGENETICS

A knowledge of the tools available, as well as their application, is essential for a thorough understanding of many clinical problems. The major blood group antigens are characterized by antibodies that detect polymorphic determinants; likewise, the human histocompatibility antigens, HLA, are defined by antibodies that detect small changes in these cell surface glycoproteins, which are coded for by the allelic genes at each of the HLA loci. The discovery of the association between HLA types and certain disease states was made possible by the use of antibody detection systems. Similar technologies are being used for diagnosis, treatment, and follow-up of clinical entities in nearly every phase of medicine, ranging from infectious diseases to oncology.

Studies on the development and functioning of the immune system have application to many clinical conditions. The maturation or ontogeny of the immune cells in a given individual is an example of genetic control of cellular proliferation and differentiation. Interruptions or alterations of these developmental sequences lead to immunodeficiency disorders, autoimmune disorders, and perhaps malignancies, as the cells escape the influence of their normal control mechanism(s). The age and maturational level at which the immune cells are of sufficient maturity to react to complex vaccine antigens, such as the polysaccharide vaccine determinants, are a function of the genetic control of this maturational process.

Genetic variability within individuals may determine their ability to respond to a vaccine or a natural infection. Studies in these areas are assuming great importance, especially as recombinant DNA and synthetic vaccines, consisting of small peptides, are being considered as third-generation vaccines (Chapter 23). Interestingly, the histocompatibility-linked immune response genes were discovered in the evaluation of antibody responses to small peptide determinants, and animals were divided into high- and low-responder strains, based on their ability to produce antibodies to synthetic peptides (Chapter 4). The widespread use of small synthetic peptides as vaccines might segregate individuals into high and low responders, based on their genetic backgrounds. This can, of course, be overcome with proper vaccine construction; however, an understanding of the immunogenetic processes involved in generating an effective response is essential.

Genetic variation that yields exaggerated immune responses may lead to harmful consequences, such as anti-platelet antibodies in idiopathic thrombocytopenic purpura (ITP), or autoimmune islet cell destruction during the onset of diabetes in susceptible individuals (Chapter 20C). These hyperresponsive states, some of which are associated with certain HLA phenotypes, as will be described later, point out a need for a clear understanding of immunogenetics.

A knowledge of family genetic susceptibility to allergic rhinitis may aid the pediatrician in arriving at a correct diagnosis of milk allergy in an infant who presents with gastrointestinal colic (Fig. 3–1).

Effective organ and bone marrow transplantation requires a knowledge of the genetic control of histocompatibility antigens and how these antigens are transmitted within families. Many of the current transplant problems, including transplant rejec-

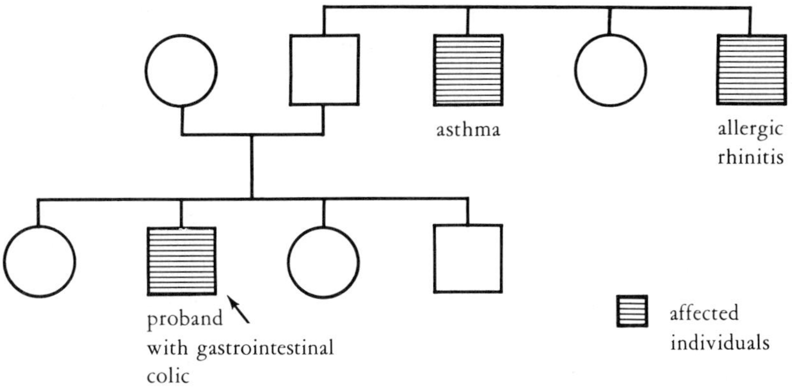

Figure 3–1. Pedigree of an infant who presented with gastrointestinal colic, showing other allergic disorders within the kindred.

tion and graft-versus-host disease, derive from an insufficient understanding of the immune system, its ontogeny, and its immunoregulatory networks. Several novel therapies, such as multiple blood transfusion prior to kidney transplantation, seem to enhance graft survival (Chapter 20C); however, such treatment regimens have poorly understood effects on the immune system, some of which may relate to genetically controlled immune responses. The impact of such drugs as cyclosporine A on graft survival appears promising; however, its impact on the entire immune network has yet to be defined. Studies on the association of HLA antigens and certain diseases suggest that "susceptibility genes" lie nearby. These leads, now strengthened and advanced by the innovative use of c-DNA (complementary DNA) probes to detect unique HLA gene sequences and restriction enzyme fragment length polymorphisms in susceptible individuals, pave the way for identifying immunoregulatory "disease susceptibility genes" at the DNA level, and open the door to understanding important pathophysiologic mechanisms of disease.

GENETICS OF IMMUNE REGULATION

The immune system is a complex network of cells that interact by direct contact and through soluble mediators. The goal of the network is to provide effective immunity for the organism and to prevent harmful internal events. A large number of genes (collectively called immune response or IR genes) exist that code for the regulatory components of the network. It was originally thought that the genes controlling the immune response were located within the genetic segment coding for histocompatibility antigens. Although the histocompatibility-linked IR genes certainly play an important role, they compose only a part of the system. Certain IR genes may code for cellular receptors for antigen as seen with the immunoglobulin molecules, which act as receptors on the surface of B-cells. The genes coding for receptors on T-cells, recently identified, are similar to immunoglobulin genes and compose a third large set of polymorphic genes. Other genes may control mediator secretion or cellular receptors. In this way, a multigenic system controls not only the ability to respond to antigens but also the level and duration of the response.

Disorders of this immunoregulatory network, whether genetic or environmental, can lead to serious consequences ranging from an inability to respond to antigenic exposure (hyporesponsive), as seen in patients with acquired immunodeficiency syndrome (AIDS), to autoimmune disorders such as systemic lupus erythematosus (hyperresponsive). Interestingly, the entire network must be effectively blocked before a foreign kidney, heart, or liver can be successfully engrafted. This iatrogenic intervention must be extremely skillful in order to avoid serious consequences. The future may see the development of innovative schemes to gently perturb this network. Examples might include the short-term blocking of T-cell surface receptors for antigen or interleukin-2, or other mediators using antibodies or receptor-binding drugs.

This chapter will focus on the major histocompatibility systems in mice (H-2) and in man (HLA) as well as on the blood group antigens and will describe their clinical relevance. Immunoglobulin genetics is described in Chapter 5; a discussion of the genetics of the T-cell receptor polymorphisms is, at best, preliminary.

THE MAJOR HISTOCOMPATIBILITY COMPLEX

The major histocompatibility complex (MHC) is a chromosomal region consisting of a series of genes that code for the cell surface expression of strong transplantation antigens. These transplantation antigens are, in general, glycoproteins that are present on the surface of most nucleated cells. The MHC in mammals is also the region where the histocompatibility-linked immune response (IR) genes are located; hence, this chromosomal segment not only controls the synthesis of the transplantation antigens and graft rejection, but also influences immune responses to infectious challenge and susceptibility to the development of immunologically mediated diseases. The two MHC systems that have been most extensively characterized are the H-2 system in the mouse and the HLA (human leukocyte antigen) system in man.

The MHC's of all mammals studied are remarkably similar; in fact, amino acid sequence homology of transplantation antigens between mouse, man, and other species is high, suggesting an evolutionary pressure for conservation of these genetic regions. The genes of the MHC in all animals thus far studied code for two general types of transplantation antigens, Class I and Class II. The complement components (Chapter 6), some of which are coded for by genes in the MHC region, have sometimes been referred to as Class III antigens.

Class I Antigens

The Class I antigen consists of a large transmembrane glycoprotein of about 350 amino acids (44K molecular weight) noncovalently associated with beta-2 microglobulin, a 100–amino acid, 12K molecular weight protein. The beta-2 microglobulin protein is coded for by genes on a separate chromosome from those coding for the Class I heavy chains. The arrangement of these molecules on the cell surface is shown schematically in Figure 3–2.

In humans, three structural genes on chromosome 6 code for the Class I type antigens. The HLA-A, HLA-B, and HLA-C genes code for the 44K heavy-chain portion of the molecule. Each of the HLA-A, -B, or -C genes has multiple alleles (i.e., alternate forms of the gene at each locus). For this reason, the HLA genes have been termed polymorphic, and each of the alleles of a particular locus has been numerically designated; for example, HLA-A1, HLA-A2, HLA-A3, and so forth represent alleles of the HLA-A gene. For a tentative assignment, the prefix "w" (workshop) has been assigned (e.g., HLA-Bw47) to indicate that it is under consideration for acceptance as a formal allele.

In mice there are three genes on chromosome 17 within the mouse H-2 histocompatibility region that code for Class I antigens. These genes have been named K, D, and L; two other genes adjacent to the region, Qa and TLa, also code for Class I–like antigens (Fig. 3–3). The mouse and human Class I antigens are structurally similar, with 60 to 70 per cent of the amino acid sequence showing identity. This similarity has now been confirmed with the DNA sequencing technology.

The allelic Class I products are found on most nucleated cells, exceptions being sperm and trophoblastic cells, and are generally detected by their reactivity with human or mouse alloantisera. Lymphocytes are commonly used for the detection or typing because they are easily obtainable. Since the Class I antigens are similar in the mouse and human systems, the function of the Class I antigens will be described under the murine H-2 genes.

Class II Antigens

The Class II antigens consist of two noncovalently associated glycoproteins (alpha and beta chains) of about 34 and 29K molecular weights, respectively (Fig. 3–2). In humans, at least three genes have been identified that code for Class II antigens, although several more candidates currently exist. The

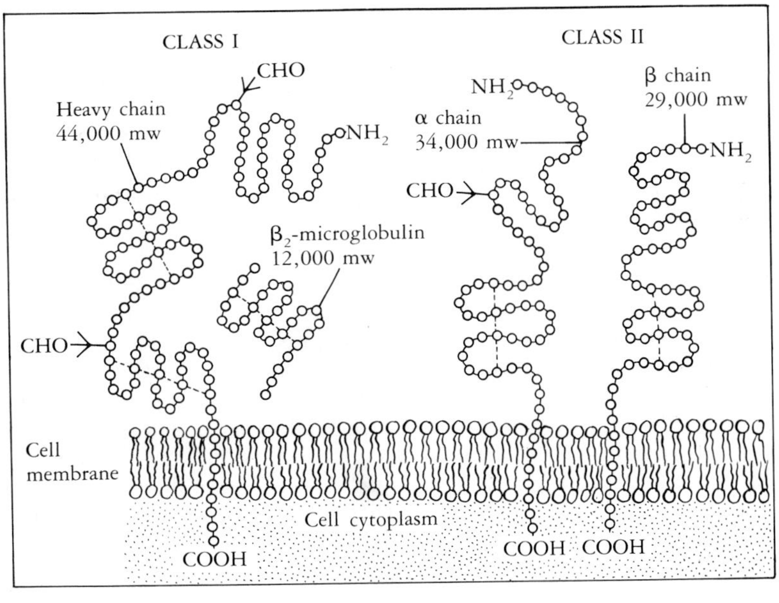

Figure 3–2. Schematic representation of Class I and Class II histocompatibility antigens within the cell membrane. Class I type glycoprotein antigens are coded for by HLA-A, B, and C genes in humans, and by H-2 K, D, L, Qa, and TLa genes in mice. Class II antigens are coded for by HLA-DR, DC, and SB genes in humans, and by IA and IE genes in mice.

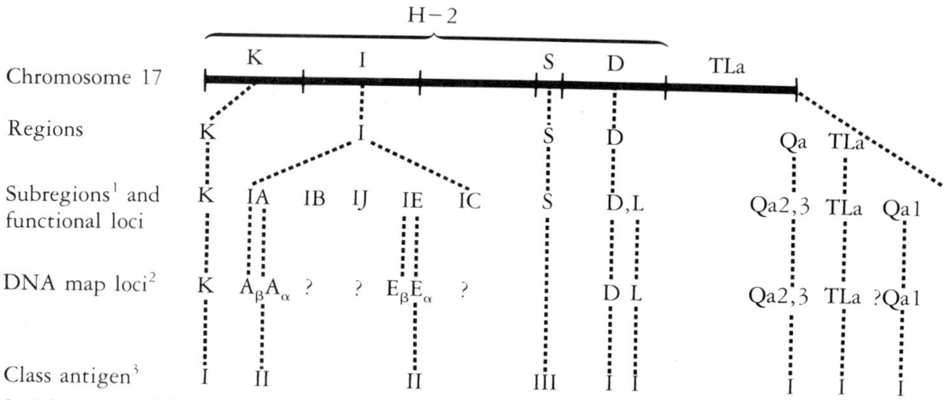

Figure 3–3. Schematic of the mouse H-2 region. (1) Subregions and functional loci were mapped by analysis with recombinant mice and by using functional immune assays such as antibody production, cellular proliferation, or delayed-type hypersensitivity reactions. (2) DNA-mapped loci were determined using DNA sequence analysis to map the position of the genes coding for their respective glycoproteins. (3) It is generally thought that the function of the Class I molecules is to serve as target antigens for immune recognition and killing. The function of the Class II antigen is to serve as restricting molecules for cellular recognition and regulatory events.

three have been designated DR, DC(DS), and SB. In mice, the genes coding for Class II antigens were mapped to a segment in the H-2 MHC called the immune (I) region (Fig. 3–3). Loci that code for the Class II antigens are prefaced by the letter I to designate this region; I-A and I-E represent the structural genes verified by DNA sequence analysis, while IB, IJ, and IC are putative genes, their location having been proposed based on functional assays. These cell surface Class II glycoprotein molecules in mice are collectively termed Ia (immune-associated) antigens, a term often used to refer to either mouse or human Class II antigens. As with the Class I antigens, a high degree of structural similarity exists between mouse and human Class II antigens. In fact, c-DNA probes made to human Class II genes have been used to identify mouse Class II genes. Since the Class II antigens are made up of two chains, alpha and beta, two genes are necessary to code for a single Class II antigen. Gene probes are currently being used to determine the precise location and relationship of the genes. Recent studies suggest that several types of alpha chains may combine with various beta chains to make cell surface "hybrid" molecules.

Using standard tests, some of the Class II antigens can be serologically detected; others are recognized only by T-lymphocytes, which proliferate in response to the foreign Class II determinants. The latter type antigens have been termed lymphocyte-defined or LD antigens, to designate the need for cellular recognition in detection, although in many cases antibodies have been found that bind to the same or similar determinants recognized by the typing cells.

The Class III antigens, or complement components, are discussed in Chapter 6.

MHC of Mice (H-2)

The MHC of mice has been extensively studied and has provided crucial information for our understanding of the human MHC. There are several reasons why the murine MHC has received a great deal of attention.

Some of the early studies on skin graft transplantation survival in mice, for which Sir Peter Medewar was awarded a Nobel Prize, launched the current era of immunogenetics. Transplantation of organs or tissues between nonidentical mouse strains invariably led to rejection of the graft, which was shown to be dependent on the number of genetic differences between animals. It was subsequently learned that certain cell surface antigens, termed histocompatibility antigens, were important in graft rejection. Of the many genetic loci coding for histocompatibility antigens, the H-2 locus was found to be the strongest, although several weaker antigens exist. For several reasons the murine system represented an ideal model for studying the role of these genes, their gene products, and the associated interactions.

1. Inbred strains of mice have been developed and maintained for many years; hence, they are uniform and genetically stable.

2. Because of their rapid breeding cycle,

large numbers of genetically identical animals can be obtained. In studying genetically controlled events, such as graft rejection, it is essential to perform the experiments with a significant number (five to ten animals per experimental group) of genetically identical animals; otherwise, the results would not be statistically valid and it would be impossible to assign functions to specific loci.

3. Inasmuch as the breeding time for mice is very short, one can perform crosses and mapping studies to determine the precise locations of genetic traits.

4. A number of co-isogeneic or congeneic strains have been developed that are genetically identical to a parent strain except for a small section of chromosome. Of particular interest are those with the same parental "background" genes except for the MHC, or H-2 region, and those with small changes within the H-2 region itself. When tested, these strains allow investigators to precisely assign immunologic functions to various loci and provide insight into immune interactions, as demonstrated in Table 3–1. Once defined in the murine system, human counterparts can be sought.

The H-2 region in the mouse is located on chromosome 17 and covers a length of DNA equivalent to 0.5 recombinant units. A schematic representation is shown in Figure 3–3, in which the K, D and L, Qa and TL genes code for Class I antigens, and the I region genes code for Class II antigens.

TERMINOLOGY

Inbred strains of mice are bred to be genetically uniform, their Class I and Class II antigen alleles having been studied and defined using serologic tests such as cytotoxicity and red cell agglutination. The H-2 genes are very polymorphic, with perhaps 50 alleles at each of the H-2K or H-2D loci. These alleles are numbered based on serologic detection. Each inbred strain of mice inherits the MHC genes as a group having a complex but limited group of alleles. It has become standard practice to designate the allelic specificities of the entire H-2 complex by a single, small-script letter; therefore, the CBA strain of mice are designated H-2^k type, which represents a unique sequence of 20 to 30 serologically defined Class I and Class II alleles (antigens). Other strains of mice have a different set of alleles and are designated by different letters, such as the Balb/c strain, which has been designated H-2^d, while the C57 Black 6 is H-2^b. Several of the strains may share a particular set of alleles; hence, the H-2^k strains of mice include not only CBA but also C_3H and AKR. In general, skin grafts may be successfully transplanted between strains of the same H-2 type, although slow rejection may occur owing to weaker histocompatibility antigens not associated with the H-2 complex. Of special interest are the congeneic strains, in which the background genes may derive from an H-2^b or other strains, while the H-2 genes come from an H-2^k or alternate strain. Special strains have been prepared with "isolation" of each of the subregion genes, allowing investigators to assign a specific function for that subregion locus. Such a mapping study, using the H-2 congeneic strains, is demonstrated in Table 3–1.

FUNCTION OF CLASS I ANTIGENS: MICE

What appears to be the major function of the H-2K, D, and L Class I antigens on the

Table 3–1. Mapping of the Murine Genetic Region that Controls Macrophage-T Interactions for Helper Cell Induction Using Congeneic Strains of Mice

Antigen	Macrophage Source	H-2 of Macrophage K	IA	IB	IC	Ss	D	T Cell Source	H-2 of T-cells K	IA	IB	IC	Ss	D	Antibody Response*
KLH	None				—			CBA	k	k	k	k	k	k	73
+	CBA	k	k	k	k	k	k	"							305
+	B10.A	k	k	k	d	d	d	"			"				293
+	B10.A (4R)	k	k	b	b	b	b	"			"				263
+	A.TL	s	k	k	k	k	d	"			"				327
+	AQR	q	k	k	d	d	d	"			"				303
+	B10.D2	d	d	d	d	d	d	"			"				63
+	B10	b	b	b	b	b	b	"			"				70

*Antibody response is measured as antibody-forming cells per culture.

In this experiment, macrophages must cooperate with T-cells to produce T-helper cells, which, in turn, promote an antibody response when mixed with B-cells. Since the B10.A (4R) and AQR macrophages were able to cooperate with the CBA-T cells, the genes controlling or "restricting" this interaction are mapped to the IA region. (From Erb, P., and Feldmann, M. J.: Exp. Med., *142*:460, 1975. Reproduced with permission.)

cell surface was clarified by the work of Zinkernagel and Doherty, who initially showed that these products are necessary for immune T-cell recognition of specific target antigens. They used as their main model the cellular killing of virus-infected targets, demonstrating that vaccinia-specific cytotoxic T-lymphocytes from CBA mice (H-2^{k}) would kill vaccinia-infected targets that exhibited H-2^{k} Class I antigens, but not targets that had H-2^{b} Class I antigens. A similar phenomenon has been observed by Shearer and coworkers using chemicals such as TNP attached to cells. This observation of "genetic restriction" for cytotoxic or killer cells has fostered two hypotheses in explanation, which are schematically outlined in Figure 3–4. The first, termed altered self, assumes that the virus or chemical modifies the Class I molecule so that it presents a new antigenic determinant (neoantigen); i.e., self is altered. This hypothesis uses a single receptor on the cytotoxic cell to recognize the neoantigen, which then initiates killing of the virus-infected target.

The second hypothesis is called dual recognition and postulates that the cytotoxic cell has two separate receptors: one that recognizes the virus or chemical, and a second that is specific for the self–Class I molecules, "restricting determinant," such as H-2K or H-2D, the binding of both receptors being re-

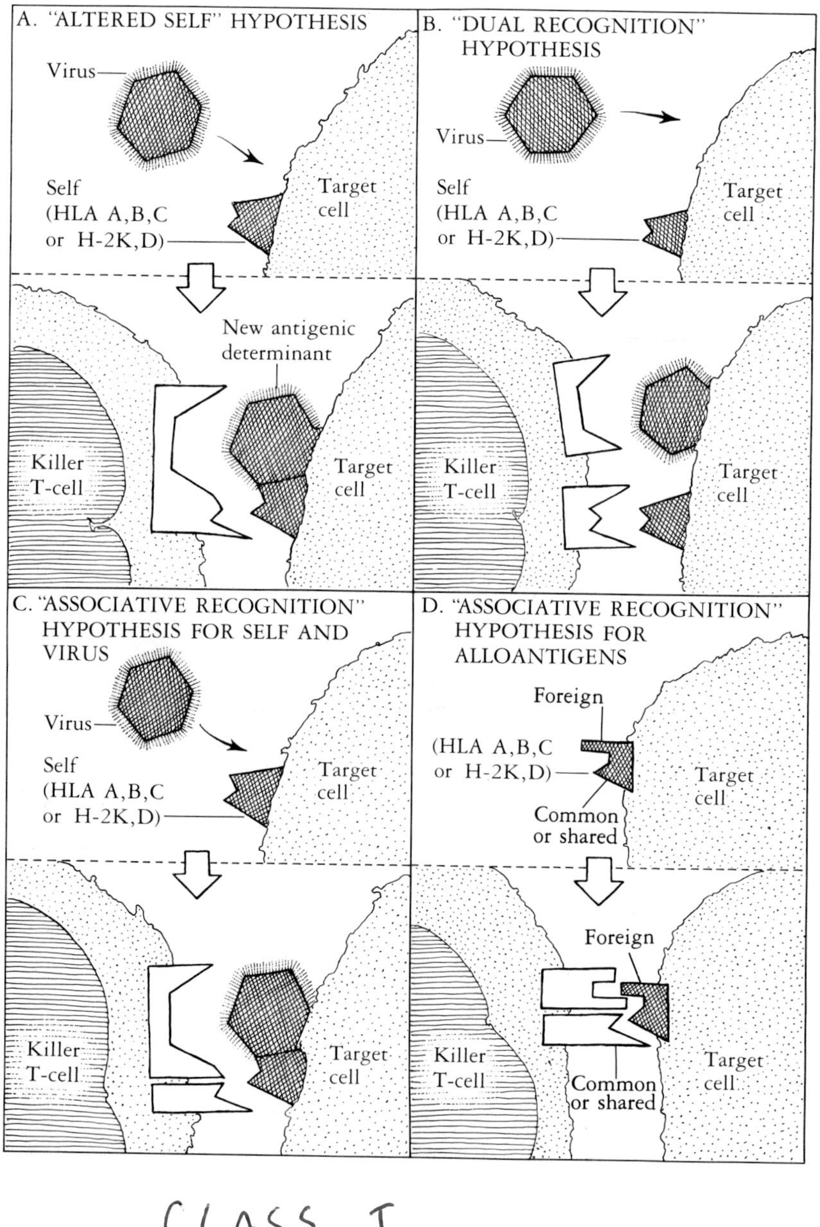

Figure 3–4. Schematic representation of the role played by Class I histocompatibility antigens in T-cell recognition of virally infected cells and allogeneic cells. Two major theories—"altered self" and "dual recognition"—are depicted. A third possibility—"associative recognition"— utilizes portions of both theories. Panel D depicts recognition of "foreign" HLA antigens, as might occur in transplantation rejection, using the "associative recognition" model of receptor interaction.

quired for cell killing. A third "hybrid" hypothesis, recently put forward by Reinherz and Schlossman, using human cytotoxic cells, favors the concept that the antigen-specific receptor displays two major recognition units; one recognizes viral antigen attached to a small, unique portion of self–Class I (altered self), while a second receptor recognizes a "shared" portion of the Class I molecule common to all Class I molecules. This is shown schematically in Figure 3–4, panel D. This associative recognition would account for killing of virus-infected and hapten-modified cells as well as HLA or H-2 incompatible cells, where the target antigen itself may be a Class I alloantigen, as described below.

The Class I antigens were originally defined as strong transplant antigens that serve as targets in graft rejection. Such rejection can be mediated either by antibody, as the foreign Class I antigens evoke a strong antibody response, or by cytotoxic cells that recognize the foreign Class I antigens (Fig. 3–4). Class II antigens can also serve as targets for antibody or cellular recognition and also play a role in graft rejection, as will be discussed later.

FUNCTION OF CLASS II ANTIGENS: MICE

The Class II antigens are coded for by genes located within the I (immune) region of the murine MHC complex (see Fig. 3–3). At one time it was thought that this region contained several sets of genes, some of which coded for products known as immune-associated or Ia antigens, and others that controlled immune responses, the histocompatibility or H-2–linked IR genes. More recently, it has been suggested that the IR genes and the Ia genes are the same, the Class II antigens then representing the IR gene products. The functional activities in which the Class II antigens are involved may be divided into several categories, including immune responsiveness, immune suppression, cellular recognition, and cellular interactions. Dr. Benacerraf, of Harvard University, recently received the Nobel Prize for his work in this field.

The following are Functions of Class II antigens

(A) IMMUNE RESPONSIVENESS

Since the first studies by McDevitt and Tyan 15 years ago, showing linkage of immune responses to the MHC of mice, the number of immune functions ascribed to the H-2 I region genes has been substantial. The early studies, using inbred mouse strains and small synthetic polypeptides, showed clearly that certain autosomal dominant genes controlled the ability of an animal to initiate a cell-mediated or an antibody-mediated response to the peptide antigens. The immune responsiveness was usually relative, and strains were designated as "high" or "low" responders. In general, the responses were functionally measured by capacity to produce antibody, ability of the T-lymphocytes to proliferate, or delayed-type hypersensitivity reactions. A number of excellent reviews, listed at the end of the chapter, detail these studies, which will be briefly outlined here.

The initial step in immune responsiveness, whether measured by antibody production, cellular proliferation, or delayed-type hypersensitivity, requires that antigen be processed and "presented." The cells able to perform this function are those that exhibit surface expression of Class II (Ia) antigens (Chapter 7). In the murine system, presenting cells with Ia antigens include macrophages, dendritic cells, B-cells, and other cell types. The antigen must be "expressed" on the surface either attached to, or nearby, the appropriate Ia molecule. Certain animals that are "nonresponders" are unable to display or effectively "present" certain antigens. Whether the defect is in the type of Class II molecule or in the antigen processing is not clear.

The second step in immune responsiveness appears to be the recognition of the Ia molecule-antigen complex by T-lymphocytes. These T-lymphocytes have been termed helper cells, since they induce B-cells or other cell types into activity. The T-lymphocytes, which in murine systems do not have surface Class II antigens, must have a receptor(s) for the Ia molecule-antigen complex, which triggers proliferation and clone expansion. The structures that the T-cell uses to recognize the processed antigen are schematically shown in Figure 3–5.

The capacity to recognize the various antigens and the critical portions of the Class II molecules, in order to initiate activation, is selected for in the thymus during ontogeny. A nonresponder animal may have T-cells unable to recognize the antigen, the critical Ia antigen, or the complex. This gap in clonal repertoire may be responsible for certain nonresponsive states.

The transmission of information from T-

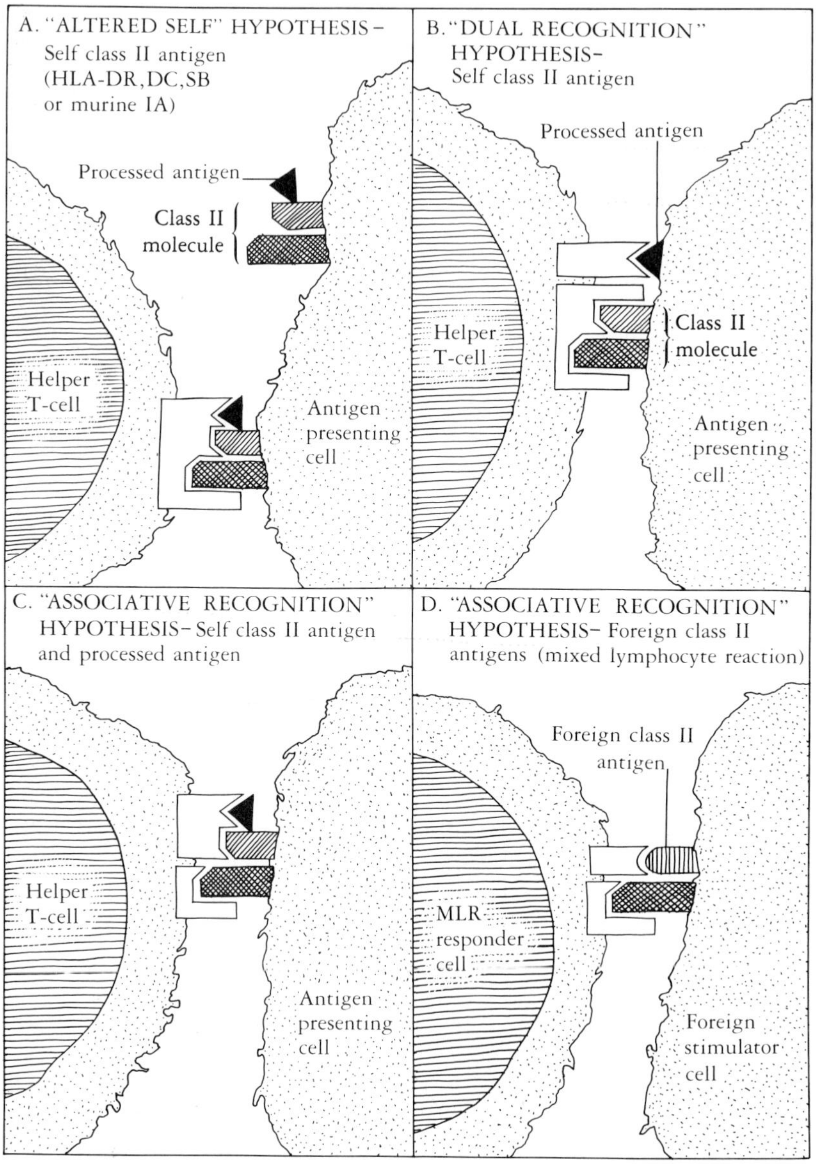

Figure 3–5. Schematic representation of the role of Class II antigen in cellular interactions. The major theories of "altered self" and "dual recognition" as well as "associative recognition" can account for the recognition of antigen on the surface of antigen-presenting cells. The associative recognition concept has one receptor recognizing a public portion of the Class II molecule shared by all such molecules and another receptor that recognizes the antigen that is complexed or adjacent to the Class II molecule. Panel D depicts the model that might occur in recognition of foreign Class II antigens, as is seen in the mixed lymphocyte reaction (MLR).

cells to B-cells can occur by cell-cell contact or via "factors." The various augmenting factors, including "antigen-specific helper" factor and "allogeneic effect" factor, have, in some cases, been shown to contain portions of Class II molecules; others, such as "T-cell replacing factor," do not. How the interaction proceeds is unclear at present; however, it is apparent that the Class II molecules may play a regulatory role in this interaction.

In addition to the macrophage-T and T-B interactions, the early activation of cells that amplify the generation of cytotoxic or killer cells requires macrophages that express the Class II molecules (Chapter 7).

IMMUNE SUPPRESSION

Besides helper T-cells that augment the activities of other cells, there is another class of T-cells that manifest the opposite effect, i.e., the ability to suppress a specific immune response. Several types of T-suppressor cells have been identified and are grouped into those that suppress antibody responses by inhibiting T-helper cells and those that suppress other functional types. The early work with antigen-specific suppressor cells to the synthetic antigens GAT and GT provided information suggesting that the activity of these cells was controlled by genes in the I region. Further studies suggested that both the suppressor cells and the suppressive factors they secreted contained Class II determinants coded for by the functionally defined IJ subregion. The role of these IJ molecules in the suppressive event has not yet been clarified. It is apparent, however, that the generation of suppressor cells requires a complex series of cellular interactions.

Cellular Recognition

In several immunologic systems, cells recognize the presence of Class II antigens on other cells. These may include mixed lymphocyte culture, graft rejection, and graft-versus-host disease.

MIXED LYMPHOCYTE CULTURE

The mixed lymphocyte culture (MLR) represents a reaction in which lymphocytes from strain A are mixed with lymphocytes from strain B, the latter having been irradiated or treated with mitomycin C so that they cannot divide. Under this "one-way" mixed lymphocyte culture condition, strain B cells serve only as "stimulator cells," as they are unable to proliferate. During a five- to seven-day incubation, the strain A "responder cells" undergo blast transformation and cell division that can be measured by the incorporation of tritiated thymidine into new DNA. The stimulator cells in this situation express Class II antigens on their surface that are recognized by the responder cells. The strongest (most stimulatory) Class II antigens are coded for by IA genes, although other I region products and some non–MHC linked gene products (mls) induce significant stimulation. The cells bearing these Class II antigens are generally macrophages, dendritic cells, and B-cells. The recognition of foreign Class II antigens by the MLR responder cell is schematically shown in Figure 3–5*D*; it is discussed in human HLA-D region typing under Figure 3–10.

GRAFT REJECTION

Transplantation of organs or grafts between nonidentical strains of mice result in rejection. The strongest effect (shortest graft survival) is seen when grafts are exchanged between mice nonidentical at the H-2 locus. The use of H-2 recombinant mice has allowed investigators to map the most influential genes to the K, D, and I regions. It is thought that the MLR reaction is the initiator of the rejection process and that the MLR reactive cells amplify or help in the development of cytotoxic effector cells that are targeted for both the H-2K and D Class I antigens and the I region antigens. A similar event has been documented in human kidney transplantation, in which killer cells to Class I (HLA-A,B,C) and to Class II (HLA-DR) antigens have been observed.

GRAFT-VERSUS-HOST DISEASE

It has generally been assumed that the graft-versus-host disease (see Chapter 20C) represents an *in vivo* correlation of the MLR, with donor T-cells recognizing foreign Class II antigens on the macrophages and dendritic cells of the irradiated recipient. In mapping studies, the IA gene products appear to induce the strongest GVHD, although Class I antigens may also participate. As in graft rejection, the *in vivo* cellular events are complex, with the generation of proliferative and cytotoxic cells that may be targeted to cells carrying either Class I or Class II antigens.

Immune Response Genes

In the early 1960's, it was learned that certain autosomal dominant genes controlled the ability of an animal to develop antibodies to certain small synthetic peptide antigens. McDevitt found that the genes controlling the immune response in mice were mapped to the H-2 complex.

Subsequent studies using congeneic mice further mapped the genes to the I region within the H-2 complex. These genes were designated histocompatibility-linked immune response or H-2 IR genes. Sometime later, it was shown that the I region genes coded for Class II antigens, which were termed immune-associated or Ia antigens. Studies of immune responses have used antibody response or T-cell proliferation to characterize further the interactions, with the designation of "responder" or "nonresponder" based on immune reactivity to the particular antigen. How the IR genes function is not clear. At present, much of the cellular-restricting activity is mediated by Class II (I) antigens, as discussed above. The IR genes appear to control fine specificity of responses involving thymic-dependent antigens.

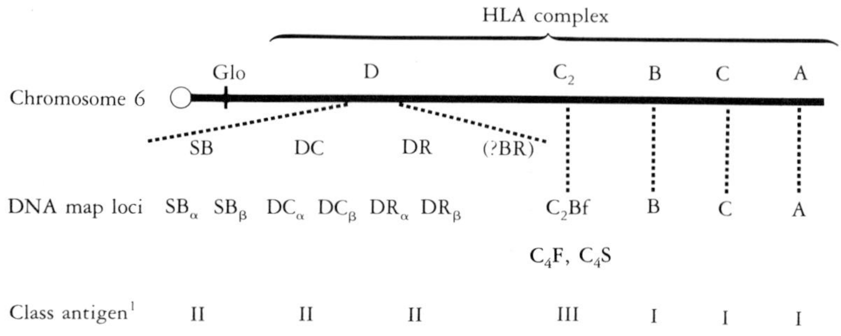

Figure 3–6. Schematic representation of the human HLA complex. The function of Class I molecules is to serve as target antigens for immune recognition and killing, while the function of the Class II antigens is to serve as restricting molecules in cellular regulation.

MHC OF HUMANS (HLA)

The human leukocyte antigen (HLA) system is best known as the typing method used to "match" recipients and donors for organ transplantation, most notably for kidney transplantation, although matching for other organs (heart, liver, pancreas, bone marrow, and so forth) is identical. The HLA typing system has also assumed prominence in paternity testing and is currently utilized to resolve legal questions of heredity. It has recently been shown that certain diseases are closely associated with unique HLA antigens; hence, in some cases the HLA type can be helpful in confirming the clinical diagnosis.

In addition to direct utility in clinical medicine, the HLA genetic system has received much scientific attention, as the genes in the HLA region code for the Classes I, II, and III transplantation antigens and also play a major regulatory role in cell interactions and immune responses, as will be discussed later.

A schematic map of the HLA genes that are located on chromosome 6 is shown in Figure 3–6.

The HLA complex is located on the short arm of chromosome 6, which also carries genes for several enzymes used in blood grouping, such as PGM_3 and GLO. The HLA genes are inherited in a codominant fashion as a group, in accordance with mendelian principles. Individuals receive one set or "haplotype" of the genes from each parent as diagrammatically shown in Figure 3–7 and Table 3–2.

Studies of various populations as well as large families, in which recombinant events can be detected, have made it possible to establish five major genetic loci: A, B, C, DR, and SB. However, several other Class II loci are under consideration as formal loci. The A, B, and C genes code for Class I molecules, whereas DR and SB code for Class II molecules. Each of the five genes has many alleles or alternate forms that represent small variations in the nucleotide sequence of the gene. These small changes result in cell surface glycoproteins with small variations, perhaps a change of one or two amino acids, or a small difference in three-dimensional structure. These variations in HLA antigen structure can be detected using HLA typing antisera, as schematically shown in Figure 3–8, or certain typing cells specific for Class II molecules. Those detected changes are called specificities and are used to assign the numerical alleles for the gene. The HLA-B gene has the largest number of detectable alleles (specificities) with 32, and is said to be the most polymorphic. The HLA-A genes have 17 alleles or specificities detected. The currently accepted list of alleles is shown in Table 3–3. Formal specificities for the SB loci will be determined in late 1984 at the International Workshop for HLA Genetics.

Parent	Haplotype designation	Sib 1 (a/c)	Sib 2 (b/d)	Sib 3 (a/c-d)
Father SB DR B C A				
◆-◆-◆-◆-◆	a	◆·◆·◆·◆·◆		◆·◆·◆·◆·◆
○-○-○-○-○	b		○·○·○·○·○	
Mother SB DR B C A				
△-△-△-△-△	c	△·△·△·△·△		
□-□-□-□-□	d		□·□·□·□·□	△·△·□·□·□

Figure 3–7. Diagrammatic sketch of the mendelian inheritance pattern of HLA antigens within a family. In general, the HLA gene group from either parent is inherited as a set or "haplotype." By convention, the father's haplotypes are designated by the letters a or b, each letter representing the HLA-A, B, C, DR, DC, and SB types on the inherited chromosome. The mother's haplotypes are designated by the letters c, d. The possible haplotypes for the children are then ac, ad, bc, or bd. Sib 3 is a recombinant between the maternal DR and B genes and hence will have the DR and SB type of the c haplotype and the B, C, and A types of the d haplotype.

Table 3–2. **Haplotype Inheritance of HLA Antigens***

	A Series Specificities				B Series Specificities						
	A1	A3	A9	Aw19	B5	B7	B12	B13	Phenotype	Genotype	Haplotype Designation
Father	+		+		+		+		A1, A9; B5, B12	A1, B5; A9, B12	a/b
Mother		+		+		+		+	A3, Aw19, B7, B13	A3, B7; Aw19, B13	c/d
Sib 1	+	+			+	+			A1, A3; B5, B7	A1, B5; A3, B7	a/c
Sib 2			+	+			+	+	A9, Aw19; B12, B13	A9, B12; Aw19, B13	b/d
Sib 3	+	+			+	+			A1, A3; B5, B7	A1, B5; A3, B7	a/c

*In this series, the father's haplotypes are: a = A1, B5 and b = A9, B12; the haplotypes represent the transmission of that HLA gene segment to the offspring. The + signs indicate positive reactions (lysis) of the test lymphocytes with the specific antiserum (see Fig. 3–9).

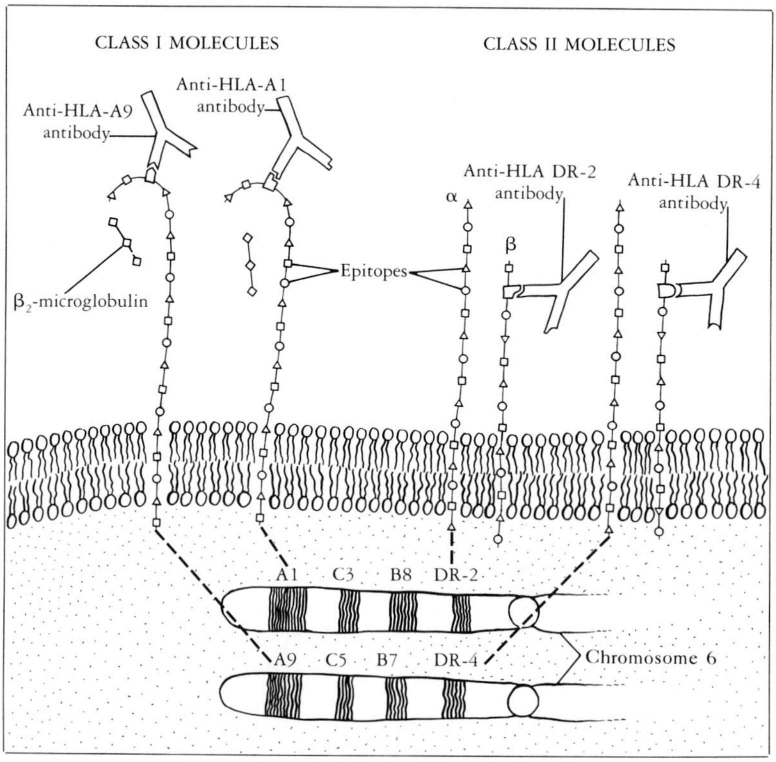

Figure 3–8. Schematic representation of HLA antibodies showing how serologic (allelic) specificities are detected. The small symbols in the schematic molecules represent areas with amino acid variations that can be recognized by specific antibodies. These variations recognized by antibody are known as epitopes.

Table 3–3. **HLA Alleles Identified as Serum Specificities***

A HLA-A	B HLA-B	C HLA-C	D HLA-D	DR HLA-DR
A1	B7	Cw1	Dw1	DR1
A2	B8	Cw2	Dw2	DR2
A3	B13	Cw3	Dw3	DR3
A11	B14	Cw4	Dw4	DR4
Aw23 (A9)	B18	Cw5	Dw5	DR5
Aw24 (A9)	B27	Cw6	Dw6	DRw6
A25 (A10)	Bw35	Cw7	Dw7	DR7
A26 (A10)	B37	Cw8	Dw8	DRw8
A28	Bw38 (B16)		Dw9	DRw9
A29	Bw39 (B16)		Dw10	DRw10
Aw30 (Aw19)	Bw41		Dw11	
Aw31 (Aw19)	Bw42		Dw12	
Aw32 (Aw19)	Bw44 (B12)			
Aw33 (Aw19)	Bw45 (B12)			
Aw34	Bw46			
Aw36	Bw47			
Aw43	Bw48			
	Bw49 (B21)			
	Bw50 (B21)			
	Bw51 (B5)			
	Bw52 (B5)			
	Bw53			
	Bw54 (Bw22)			
	Bw55 (Bw22)			
	Bw56 (Bw22)			
	Bw57 (B17)			
	Bw58 (B17)			
	Bw59			
	Bw60 (Bw40)			
	Bw61 (Bw40)			
	Bw62 (B15)			
	Bw63 (B15)			

*Some of the early antisera contained antibodies that detected several alleles or specificities. In some instances, the original allele was "split" into several. A good example is Bw22, which is now known to contain three alleles: Bw54, Bw55, and Bw56. Alleles in parentheses represent the original allele that has now been split. The letter w indicates a workshop or temporary designation.

Detection of Class I Antigens

Class I molecules, described earlier in this chapter, are coded for by the HLA-A,B, and C genes. They are detected by using antisera that bind to the cell surface molecules bearing the particular specificity determinant.

The Class I antigens are present on all nucleated cells in varying amounts, although red cells and spermatozoa have few molecules on their surface. Antibodies against the HLA-A,B, and C specificities are commonly found in the serum of women who have had several pregnancies, or in individuals receiving an organ transplant or numerous transfusions. Most commonly, serum is collected from multigravida women. It is thought that lymphocytes from the fetus are released into the maternal circulation during the separation of the placenta. These fetal lymphocytes carry paternal HLA antigens that result in the immunization of the mother. Usually, more than one sensitization is necessary to induce a level of circulating antibody that is useful for HLA typing; even then, the antisera are weak. In the case outlined in Table 3–2, the mother may make antibodies to the paternal antigens A1 or B5, with infant 1 and 3, as she does not have those antigens. To prepare an antibody that is monospecific for detecting A1, the maternal antisera must be incubated (absorbed) with cells that have B5 but not A1. The B5 antibody can thereby be removed, leaving an antiserum that detects only A1. Such operationally monospecific serum can then be used for detecting the A1 glycoprotein antigens, as demonstrated in Figure 3–9, which represents the format used for current HLA typing. Using a tray containing two to three antisera for each specificity enables the HLA typing serologist to type most individuals. Certain populations may have HLA antigens that are rare in Americans (of European descent). For example, about 33 per cent of Japanese have the antigen CW-1, which is seen in only 6 per cent of Caucasians. It is important, therefore, to make the serologist aware of the ethnic background prior to HLA typing.

Detection of Class II Antigens

The Class II DR antigens are identified serologically, whereas Dw and SB antigens are generally detected using the one-way mixed lymphocyte culture. In this assay, cells of two nonidentical individuals are mixed together, one cell (the stimulator) being irradiated so that it cannot proliferate. The other cell (the responder) recognizes the foreign Class II antigens on the stimulator cell and begins to proliferate. This proliferation is measured by the uptake of H^3-thymidine into new DNA over a five- to six-day period. The amount of new DNA made (measured as cpm of H^3-thymidine) is an index of the differences in Class II antigens between stimulator and responder. Two basic methods are currently used to type: the homozygous typing cell (HTC) method and the primed lymphocyte typing (PLT) method. These methods are schematically outlined in Figures 3–10 and 3–11, respectively. The recent production of IL-2–dependent populations of PLT cells, which can be continuously maintained, will increase the sensitivity of this assay system.

Using the PLT secondary stimulation type of assay, it is possible to show that primed

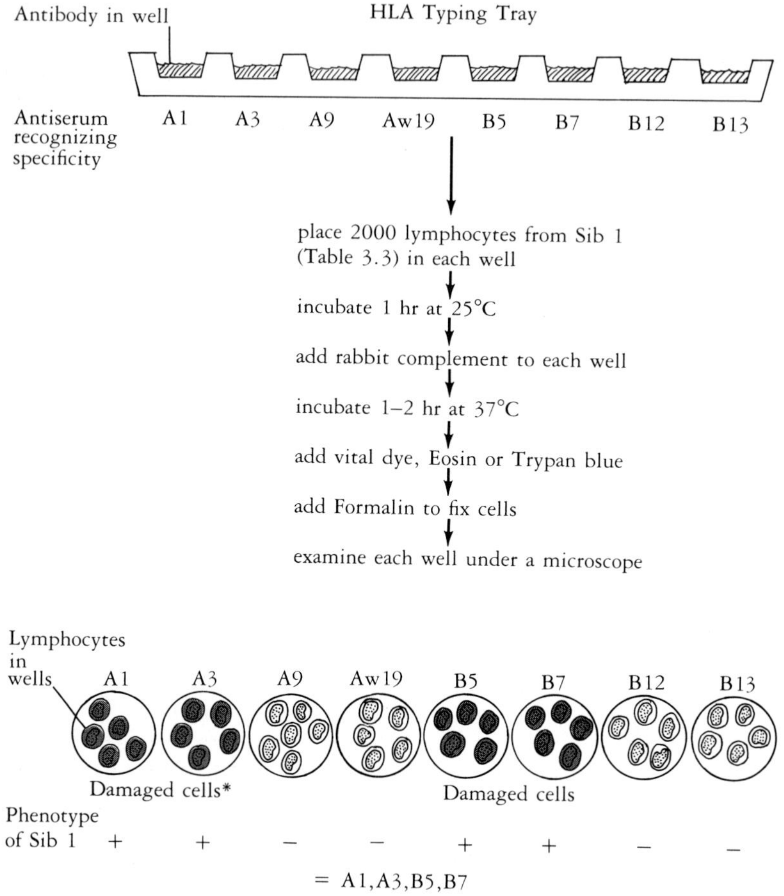

Figure 3–9. Diagram of the HLA serotyping procedures. Damaged or dead lymphocytes allow vital dye to enter the cell and appear dark under phase microscopy.

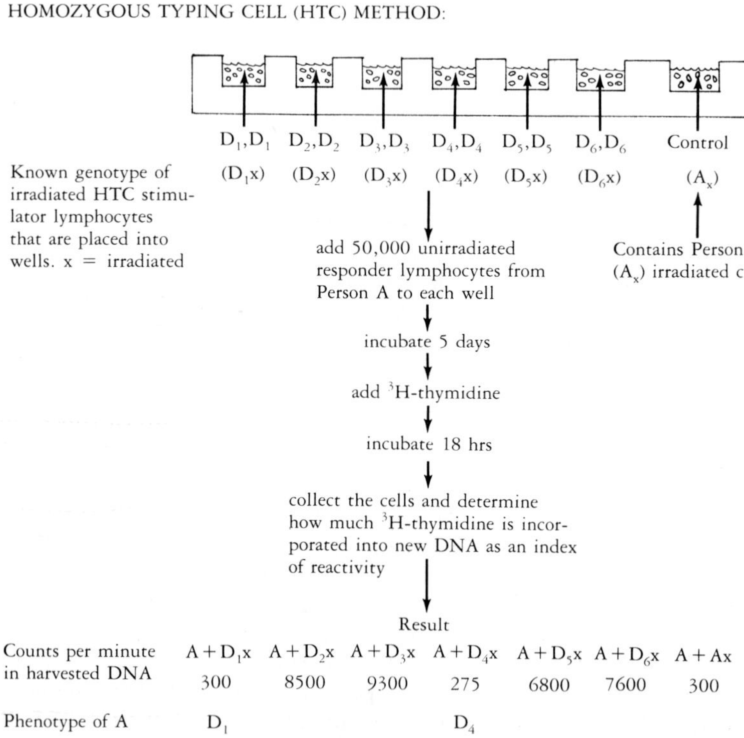

Figure 3–10. Diagram of the procedures for cellular typing of Class II antigens. Since Person A's cells are D_1, D_4, they would respond by proliferation only to the foreign HLA-D types, which are D_2, D_3, D_5, and D_6, and not to D_1 or D_4.

Principles of cellular typing for Class II antigens.
Primed Lymphocyte Typing (PLT) Method:

Responder cell		Stimulator cell (irradiated)
D_1D_1	+	D_2D_2X

↓ wait 10 days ↓

Harvest D_1 cells that are proliferating against the irradiated D_2 cells = primed lymphocyte typing (PLT) cells specific for D_2.

Responder PLT typing cell panel		Stimulator Irradiated cells from Person A		cpm in new DNA
anti-D_1	→ incubated with stimulator cells →	+	After 2–3 days add ^{3}H-thymidine → and harvest cells	9500
anti-D_2		+		300
anti-D_3		+		280
anti-D_4		+		8600
anti-D_5		+		425
anti-D_6		+		318

Figure 3–11. Diagram of the procedures used for cellular typing of Class II antigens using the primed lymphocyte typing (PLT) methodology. The phenotype of Person A is D_1, D_4, as PLT's recognize and proliferate in response to D_1 and D_4 on Person A's lymphocytes.

cells can recognize and react to HLA-DR and HLA-SB molecules, although the latter determinants are just beginning to be studied systematically. The DC(DS) molecules are detected using antisera; however, they are not yet accepted as an allelic Class II gene.

The initial work suggests that the T-cell PLT clones recognize small antigenic determinants (epitopes) similar in size to those recognized by antibodies. It is felt that this technology will lead to a cellular typing system with specificity similar to that of serologic systems.

The detection of the DR antigens is routinely performed using serologic techniques similar to those for the detection of Class I antigens (Fig. 3–9). The serologic specificities generally follow the HTC-determined specificities, although exceptions are becoming more common. Alloantisera specific for DR molecules are somewhat more difficult to use because they are weak, and the DR molecules are normally expressed only on circulating B-cells, which constitute only 10 to 15 per cent of peripheral blood mononuclear cells; hence, B-cells must be separated from the peripheral blood in order to perform an effective typing. This is a time-consuming task and requires 20 to 30 ml of blood; hence, it cannot easily be applied to children. More sensitive techniques, such as two-color fluorescence, do, however, permit DR typing on small samples.

At present, it is thought that the DR antisera, the HTC's, and the PLT's all recognize essentially the same molecules; however, different determinants (epitopes) on the same molecule may be preferentially detected by the different methods. The HTC and PLT technologies can also detect Class II antigens for which only a few antisera exist, for example, the SB antigens. The correlation between serology and cellular typing has proved difficult, as each of the Class II antigens is made up of an alpha and a beta chain, and hybrid molecules may exist, as for the murine system.

Certain of the antisera against Class II antigens are cross reactive, allowing for the detection of "supertypic" groups of DR molecules, or groups that share some common (public) antigenic determinants. The MT1 supertypic group includes DR1, DR2, DRw6, and DRw10, while MT2 includes DR3, DR5, DRw6, DRw8, and MT3 (DR4, DR7, and DRw9). Other recently defined groups include MB1 (DR1, DR2, DRw6) MB2 (DR3, DR7), and MB3 (DR4, DR5). The relationship of these shared determinants with HLA-DR, SB, or DC(DS) loci is currently being worked out.

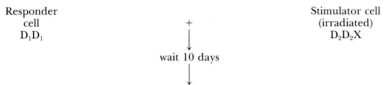

The distribution of Class II antigens in humans is of interest. Under normal circumstances, DR antigens are expressed on the surface of human B-cells, macrophages, and cells of the reticuloendothelial system, including Kupffer cells, Langerhans cells, and endothelial cells. They are also seen on spermatozoa and interstitial cells of the ovary. When activated, T-cells and other cells of the hemopoietic system, including myeloid cells, express the Class II antigens. In this capacity, the Class II antigens may serve as differentiation antigens. It has recently been demonstrated that gamma interferon is a powerful inducer of DR expression, even in some tissues that normally fail to exhibit DR. One theory, proposed by Feldmann and colleagues, suggests that the expression of DR, induced by gamma interferon, may permit and foster the recognition of self-antigens on certain tissues and may be the initiating event in certain types of autoimmunity.

Function of Class I Antigens: Human

The function of the Class I molecules in humans is thought to be similar to that in other mammalian systems. The murine models have provided the greatest insight, as discussed earlier in the chapter. Basically, they serve as determinants necessary for the immune recognition and the elimination of virally infected cells. It is thought that the $T8^+$ killer cell uses the T8 molecule to recognize self–MHC antigen and the T3 associated T-cell "idiotype" region to recognize and bind to antigen. In addition, the Class I antigens may serve as targets in graft rejection, which can be mediated by antibody or sensitized cells.

Function of Class II Antigens: Human

The Class II antigens are involved at many levels in immune interactions. Studies in animal systems, primarily the murine model, have provided us with insights into the various functions of the Class II antigens, as described earlier. Thus far, studies in humans have paralleled the observations in other mammals. This includes the need for sharing of certain Class II (HLA-DR or SB) molecules between macrophages and T-cells in order to obtain effective collaboration for the induction of T-helper cells. The human Class II antigens are detected in the MLC reaction. In some cases of kidney graft rejection, killer cells specific for HLA-D/DR region antigens have been identified. The Class II antigens are thought to play a major role in graft-versus-host disease, seen in bone marrow transplantation; however, the nature of this interaction remains to be resolved. As for the $T8^+$ killer cell, it is thought that the T4 molecules on the $T4^+$ helper cell, with the T3-associated "idiotype" region, form the antigen-specific receptor.

HLA and Paternity Testing

The polymorphism of the HLA system and the reproducibility of the analysis make it ideal for studies of inheritance. One such area is the determination of paternity. The major question to be addressed is, "Can the paternity of the man be excluded?" If the child has none of the HLA haplotypes of the man, which happens in about one quarter of the cases, then paternity can be excluded. In most situations the child may share a few antigens with the putative father, and one must determine, based on haplotype frequencies in the particular ethnic population, the probability of that haplotype's originating from some other male.

HLA and Transplantation

NOMENCLATURE

Transplanted tissues are classified according to the relationship of the donor and recipient. Those terms in common usage are outlined below.

Autograft: A graft taken from one location on the same person and placed elsewhere.

Allograft: A graft taken from one member of a species and given to another member of the same species. There are several types of allografts.

Syngeneic allograft: Grafts between two genetically identical individuals, such as twins or HLA-identical siblings.

Semi-syngeneic allograft or semi-allogeneic allograft: A graft in which half of the HLA genes (one haplotype) are shared and half are different. This usually occurs in a parent-to-child graft, or grafts between siblings who share only one HLA haplotype.

Allogeneic allograft: A graft between two genetically unrelated individuals (non-HLA identical).

Xenograft: A graft taken from one species and placed in a member of another species.

Graft Rejection

It has been clearly shown that the HLA antigens serve as strong transplantation antigens by inducing a powerful immune response. The early events in allograft rejection include the production of T-cells that recognize the foreign HLA antigens. These cells may be of a variety that kill cells bearing foreign Class I or Class II antigens, or they may release mediators (lymphokines) that induce macrophages and neutrophils to enter the graft site, leading to graft destruction. Shortly after the initiation of cellular immunity, antibodies to the Class I and Class II antigens can be detected, which furthers the graft destruction.

Transplantation of organs into an individual with preformed circulating antibodies results in "hyperacute" rejection, as the antibodies immediately destroy the graft (discussed further in Chapter 20C). Recent information has shown that matching of renal allografts for Class II antigens greatly improves graft survival. This matching is performed using DR typing and the mixed lymphocyte culture. Those recipients exhibiting high cellular proliferation to the donor cells are likely to manifest significant rejection reactions.

Linkage Disequilibrium

Assuming that the alleles at the HLA-A and HLA-B loci are independent of each other, one would expect them to occur together in proportion to the gene frequency in the population. Certain combinations occur in much higher frequencies than predicted, such as A1 and B8, and this unusual association is called linkage disequilibrium. The reason for this is unclear, unless it provides some selective advantage.

HLA and Disease Association

One area that has received great attention is the association of certain HLA antigens with various diseases. While the associations are primarily statistical in nature, it is generally agreed that they represent a biologically relevant finding and that the mechanism of this association will eventually be understood.

HLA and disease studies may be initiated in several ways. Most commonly, the HLA types of a group of patients with a particular disease are determined, and the types compared with the HLA types of a random panel of unaffected individuals from the same ethnic group and geographic area.

The most common statistical approach for evaluation is to establish a 2 × 2 contingency table.

		HLA antigen	
		Present	Absent
Disease	Present	a	b
	Absent	c	d

where a, b, c, and d are the number of individuals in each category. The X^2 is determined and the p value calculated. If the result is significant, one may wish to evaluate the strength of this observation. This is done by calculating the relative risk, which is the risk of developing a disease when an antigen is present, relative to the risk when it is lacking. It is calculated using the formula

$$\text{Relative risk} = \frac{ad}{cb}$$

A relative risk of greater than 1 indicates that the antigen is more frequent in patients than in controls.

Several difficulties arise in these types of analysis, one of the major ones being the ability to define clearly a clinical disease that may present as a broad spectrum. A good example is the various forms of arthritis that may vary from mild and nonsymptomatic to severe and disabling. There are, in addition, several statistical pitfalls, one being that associations can occur by chance in 1 of 20 observations (with p of $<.05$). This can be corrected for by multiplying each p value by the number of antigens typed for.

Dr. Arne Svejgaard, in Copenhagen, has established an international registry to evaluate HLA and disease associations. The results are periodically updated and published. A few of the more interesting examples are given in Table 3–4.

While the method described above uses populations with various diseases to develop a statistical association, it is also possible to perform formal linkage analysis between a gene disease and an HLA allele. This requires large families in which several members may have the disease. The information gained, however, is more powerful and may allow investigators to formally map disease-linked genes.

Table 3–4. **HLA and Disease Associations**

Disease Type	HLA Allele	Relative Risk
Rheumatologic Diseases		
Ankylosing spondylitis	B27	88
Reiter's syndrome	B27	37
Acute anterior uveitis	B27	10
Juvenile arthritis	B27, Dw5, or Dw8	4
Rheumatoid arthritis	Dw4(DR4)	4
Autoimmune/Endocrine Diseases		
Chronic hepatitis	Dw3(DR3)	14
" "	B8	9
Celiac disease	Dw3(DR3)	11
Graves' disease	Dw3(DR3)	4
Hashimoto's thyroiditis	Dw5(DR5)	3
Idiopathic Addison's disease	Dw3(DR3)	6
Juvenile-onset diabetes mellitus	Dw4(DR4)	6
" " " "	Dw3(DR3)	3
Congenital adrenal hyperplasia (21-hydroxylase deficiency)	B47	15
" " "	B5	4
Myasthenia gravis	B8	4
" "	Dw3(DR3)	3
Multiple sclerosis	Dw2(DR2)	4
Systemic lupus erythematosus	Dw3(DR3)	6
Malignant Disorders		
Chronic myelocytic leukemia (CML)	A2	39
Chronic lymphocytic leukemia (CLL)	B18	5
Acute lymphoblastic leukemia (ALL)	A2	1
Hodgkin's disease	A1, A11, B8, B15	1–8

Investigators studying the DNA sequence of HLA antigens in individuals with these diseases have found restriction enzyme map patterns (restriction enzyme fragment length polymorphisms) that differ from those of normal individuals. This work would suggest that genes adjacent to the HLA "markers" may be unique in affected individuals, predisposing them to certain illnesses. Assuming that the disease associations are valid and represent a biologically relevant event, what hypothesis can be put forward to explain these observations?

A number of the rheumatologic, autoimmune, and endocrine disorders show an association with HLA alleles of the D/DR region. In many of these disorders, antibodies are found that have specificity for the target organ. One could postulate that the MHC-linked "immune response" alleles in these individuals permit an elevated or exaggerated response status to exogenous or endogenous antigens, which results in the production of autoantibodies (Chapter 20C). To account for some of the observations, one might anticipate that individuals who are homozygous for a particular allele may be more affected than a heterozygote would be; however, this is not the case, and it is necessary to include environmental factors as important in the initiation of the disease process. It was anticipated that strong "susceptibility" associations to infectious diseases would be found; however, this has not been the case, except with tuberculoid leprosy (Rr = 5).

Alternative explanations suggest that the MHC genes influence receptor binding for toxins, oncogenic viruses, bacteria, or other pathogenic materials, thereby opening the way for subsequent disease development and progression; however, this remains to be proved.

It is commonly held that the HLA alleles are not responsible for disease susceptibility but that they are markers in strong linkage disequilibrium with as yet undefined, but responsible, genes. Although these associations are of interest and occasionally are useful to support the clinical impression, the mechanism is poorly understood and awaits future definition.

T-Cell and B-Cell Receptors for Antigen

The cells of the immune system are unique in that the T-cells and B-cells carry surface glycoproteins that must be able to interact with antigen, either alone or complexed with histocompatibility antigens in some specific way.

It has been known for many years that the antigen-binding molecules on the surface of B-cells are immunoglobulin molecules. When the B-cell differentiates to become a plasma cell, the same immunoglobulin molecules that served as receptors for antigen are now secreted. The portion of the immunoglobulin molecule that binds to antigen is called the antigen-binding site or idiotype region (Chapter 5).

It is possible, under certain circumstances, to produce antibodies that recognize and bind to this idiotype region of the immunoglobulin molecule, so-called anti-idiotype antibodies. In several experimental systems it was demonstrated that certain anti-idiotype antibodies could bind to T-cells and T-cell factors; hence, it was suggested that T-cells used the same antigen-recognition system as B-cells, namely, the immunoglobulin variable regions (V_H). This hypothesis seemed reasonable, as the receptor system would then be conserved, and one need not postulate an entire new receptor system, with associated diversity, outside of the well-studied immunoglobulin regions. In a series of recent studies using c-DNA probes to various immunoglobulin regions, it has been demonstrated that antigen-specific T-(suppressor) cells fail to rearrange the immunoglobulin V_H genes, as would be anticipated if they were using those genes to code for receptors, and they fail to make m-RNA with V_H sequences. Furthermore, studies attempting to detect immunoglobulin allotype markers, or other immunoglobulin determinants on cloned T-cells, have been inconsistent. Recent studies by Reinherz, Meuer, and Schlossman, show a 43K and 49K complex associated with T3 that is not immunoglobulin yet appears to be the putative T-cell receptor. It is currently postulated that the T-cell receptor for antigen is coded for by a set of genes unassociated with the immunoglobulin or MHC genes. Such a set of genes might exhibit levels of genetic polymorphism similar to immunoglobulins, within the antigen-binding regions. This is supported by the recently published sequence of portions of the human T-cell receptor by Mak and colleagues as well as similar reports of murine T-cell receptors by Davies and coworkers. The studies indicate that the T-cell receptor has 30 to 60 per cent homology with immunoglobulin, undergoes somatic gene rearrangement during expression, and has "constant" and "variable" regions. The receptors are also likely to have a "hypervariable" region for binding antigen or MHC product. This development implies that, in addition to the immunoglobulin and MHC systems, the T-cell receptor genes form a third polymorphic genetic system that influences immune responsiveness.

GENETICS OF BLOOD GROUPS SYSTEM

One of the genetic traits that have been extensively studied using immunologic methods is the major blood group antigens, including the ABO and Rh systems. The erythrocytes carry a large number of antigenic determinants; however, only a few of them are clinically important, either because of their immunogenicity or because of their frequency in the population.

PRINCIPLES OF BLOOD GROUP DETECTION

The assignment of blood group antigens is made using alloantisera that have been procured from individuals who have been previously immunized by transfusions or pregnancy. In the future, monoclonal antibodies will certainly be utilized to obtain precise definitions of the blood group antigens; however, at present the serum from immunized individuals is rendered operationally monospecific by absorption with red cells of known specificity.

The most common assay used is hemagglutination, whereby the antibodies agglutinate the red cells. IgM antibodies, because they are pentavalent, agglutinate red cells more readily and at lower temperatures (18°C), while IgG antibodies agglutinate best at higher temperatures (37°C).

In saline, IgG antibodies often fail to agglutinate, since the red cell antigens are too distant for cross linking. Under such circumstances, the IgG is an *incomplete antibody*, and because it covers up sites that would permit IgM agglutination, the IgG antibodies are often termed *blocking* antibodies. The standard method to detect IgG antibodies is the indirect antiglobulin test or Coombs' test. This assay utilizes an antibody directed at the IgG bound on the erythrocytes, thereby forming a large lattice that agglutinates and permits detection.

The ABO Blood Group System

For centuries, it was known that recipients of blood transfusions often experienced serious or fatal transfusion reactions. The mechanism for these reactions was not understood until the classic work of Landsteiner, who, in 1900, defined the major isoantigens (alloantigens) of human red cells. He performed a very simple experiment, which is outlined below, using serum and red cells from six members of his laboratory staff, leading to the discovery of blood groups and antigens (Table 3–5).

From this experiment, Landsteiner was able to determine that there were two antigenic determinants present on human red cells, which he called A and B. Some (3 and 4) individuals possessed the A determinant and were A blood group; others (2 and 5) possessed B and were B blood group. A third group (1 and 6) had erythrocytes that failed to agglutinate with any of the sera and were called C. It was subsequently shown that the C group, now known as O, failed to express a unique antigen. Finally, the work of Landsteiner established that individuals have naturally occurring antibodies directed against the antigenic determinants absent from their own erythrocytes. Thus, individuals of blood group A possess anti-B antibodies and vice versa, while individuals with blood group O have both anti-A and anti-B antibodies. Some years later, students of Landsteiner discovered another group that had both A and B antigens and had no antibodies, now known as the AB type (Table 3–6). These original studies formed the foundation of the immunohematology system, for which Landsteiner was awarded the Nobel Prize in 1930.

Table 3–5. Summary of Landsteiner's Original Experiment Leading to the Discovery of Blood Group Antigens

	Erythrocytes						
Sera	**1**	**2**	**3**	**4**	**5**	**6**	**Designated Group**
1	−	+	+	+	+	−	C
2	−	−	+	+	−	−	A
3	−	+	−	−	+	−	B
4	−	+	−	−	+	−	B
5	−	−	+	+	−	−	A
6	−	+	+	+	+	−	C

+ = agglutination

GENETIC GROUP OF ABO ANTIGENS

The erythrocyte expression of the ABO antigens is controlled by a single gene with three alleles—A, B, and O. The alleles A and B are codominant and are dominant over the O allele, which is not expressed. The blood group antigens are known to be glycoprotein and glycolipid in nature, and their antigenic potential relates to the carbohydrate portions. It is now accepted that the A and B alleles code for enzymes that attach carbohydrate molecules to the basic glycoprotein (H substance).

The A allele codes for the enzyme *N*-acetyl galactosaminyl transferase, which adds alpha-D-*N*-acetylgalactosamine to the H stem carbohydrate substance, thereby generating the A antigenic determinant and creating the A antigenic structures. The B allele codes for the enzyme galactosyl transferase, which catalyzes the attachment of an alpha-D-galactose molecule to the H substance, thereby creating the B antigen.

The O allele apparently fails to code for any enzyme and therefore fails to create any unique antigen.

The H Gene and its Alleles. The H gene codes for an enzyme known as fucosyl transferase, which catalyzes the attachment of alpha-L-fucose to the carbohydrate beta-galactosyl-*N*-acetylglucosamine disaccharide (Fig. 3–12). The latter disaccharide is a part of the stem glycoprotein that serves as the backbone structure for the A and B antigens. The addition of alpha-L-fucose to this glycoprotein converts it into H substance, which can then be modified to form the A and B antigens. The majority of the population is H/H or H/h, which enables them to synthesize H substance, as the H allele is dominant. Occasionally, an individual will be h/h and lacks the fucosyl transferase and hence, H substance and A or B antigens. These people phenotypically blood type as O blood group. This phenotype is known as the Bombay phenotype.

ABO SYSTEM AND ITS CLINICAL SIGNIFICANCE

The A, B, and H antigens are examples of substances whose antigenic expressions are influenced by small structural differences in single sugar residues that are under genetic control.

These antigens are of obvious importance in blood transfusions, in which the infusion

Table 3–6. **Summary of Blood Group Typing**

Genotype	Phenotypic	Red Cell Antigen	Antisera Reaction Anti-A	Anti-B	Serum Alloantibody
O/O	O	O	−	−	anti-A, -B
A/O, A/A	A	A	+	−	anti-B
B/O, B/B	B	B	−	+	anti-A
A/B	A/B	A/B	+	+	none

of blood cells carrying A or B antigens into a person with natural anti-A or anti-B antibodies (agglutinins) may result in a life-threatening transfusion reaction. Numerous other blood group antigens may also be involved in such reactions. This possibility has led to the development of a series of tests, called a major crossmatch, that analyzes for the presence of IgM and IgG antibodies in the serum of the recipient for the donor cells.

The presence of anti-A or anti-B antibodies in the serum may induce hemolytic disease of the newborn. In this case, the maternal IgG antibodies cross the placenta and bind to fetal erythrocytes, causing hemolysis. The ABO-induced hemolytic disease is usually milder than that induced by Rh incompatibility.

The ABO antigens are useful in paternity determinations, although testing for more polymorphic antigens, such as the HLA antigens, is usually superior. Forensic pathologists often use ABO antigens to determine the type of blood found at the scene of a crime, as these antigens are very stable. Finally, the ABO antigens, because of their wide distribution on many organs and their binding with natural antibody, are considered to be important in organ transplantation. An ABO-incompatible kidney graft, for example, may be rejected in a hyperacute fashion, if the individual has preformed natural antibodies.

Rh Blood Group Systems

The second red cell antigen system that is of clinical significance is the Rh system.

Levine and Stetson, in 1939, discovered an

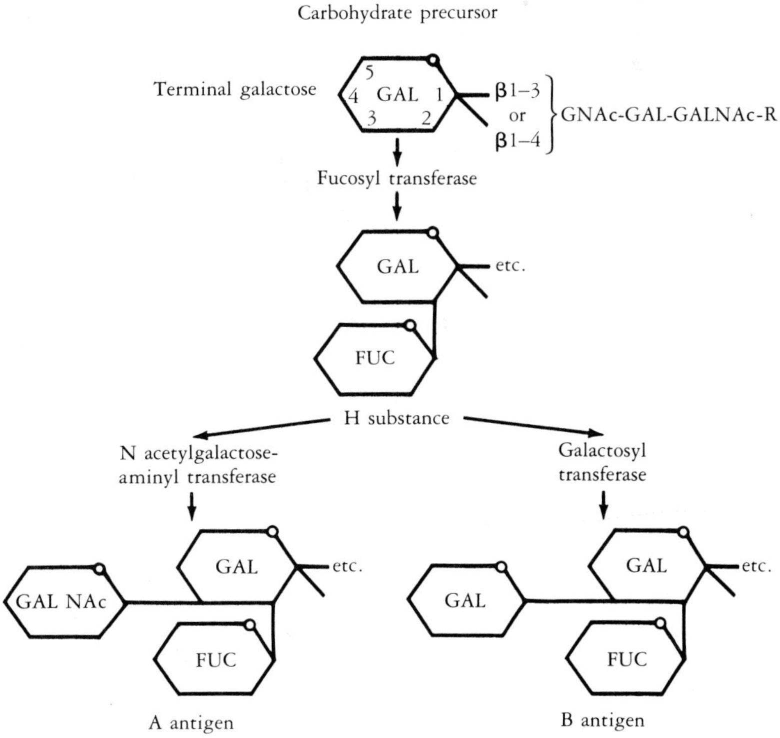

Figure 3–12. Schematic representation of H, A, and B blood group antigens. Shown is a representation of the proposed structure of the A and B blood group antigens. Type A blood cells carry Type A antigens; Type B cells have B antigens, while Type AB has both; and Type O has only H substance. The difference between Types A and B is the N acetylation of the terminal galactose. The sugars are linked to sphingomyelin (R) to form the red cell surface antigen. Linkage of this complex to certain peptides produces "secretory substances." G = glucose, GAL = galactose, FUC = fucose, NAc = acetyl group.

antigen that reacted with serum from a mother who had delivered a child with hemolytic disease of the newborn. This antigen was later shown to be detected by antibodies prepared by injecting rhesus monkey erythrocytes into rabbits or guinea pigs. The later observation, fostered by Landsteiner and Wiener, led to the name "rhesus factor" or Rh antigen.

GENETIC CONTROL OF Rh ANTIGENS

The immense complexity of the Rh system has been revealed over the past 30 years, with the discovery of many additional Rh antigenic types. Approximately 30 types have been identified; however, the original Rh antigen is by far the most important in terms of immunogenicity and clinical significance.

The lengthy interval between the discovery of the ABO and the Rh blood groups was due, in part, to the serologic properties of the anti-Rh antibodies. Unlike those of the ABO system, Rh antibodies do not occur naturally; rather, they are products of frank immunization either through pregnancy or transfusion. The serologic properties of these antibodies are described in Chapter 8.

Two theories have been proposed to explain the inheritance of the Rh antigens. The first of these, suggested by Fisher and Race, proposed that the system consists of three genes, C, D, and E, with paired alleles, coding for five antigenic determinants (D, C, E, c, and e). The three loci are considered to be so closely linked on the chromosome that crossing over is an infrequent event. It is thought that they are inherited, one set from each parent, as depicted in Figure 3–13.

The most important of these loci was called D, which controls the production of the most clinically significant Rh isoantigen, the D antigen. This isoantigen is the strongest immunogen and was responsible for the erythroblastotic infant described by Stetson and Levine, accounting for more than 90 per cent of cases of hemolytic disease of the newborn due to maternal isoimmunization. An alternate allele at this locus was called d (Fig. 3–13). To date, the antigenic product of this hypothetical allele has not been described, and there is considerable doubt that such an antigenic determinant actually exists. The symbol d is used to represent the absence of D, rather than the presence of any known antigenic determinant. A second locus, according to the Fisher-Race scheme, is the position at which one of two alleles, C or c, is located. These genes control the production of either the C or the c antigens. Alleles at a third locus, called E, are responsible for the production of the antigenic determinants E or e. These isoantigens occasionally account for isoimmunization. In order of immunogenicity, the antigens are D > c > C > E > e.

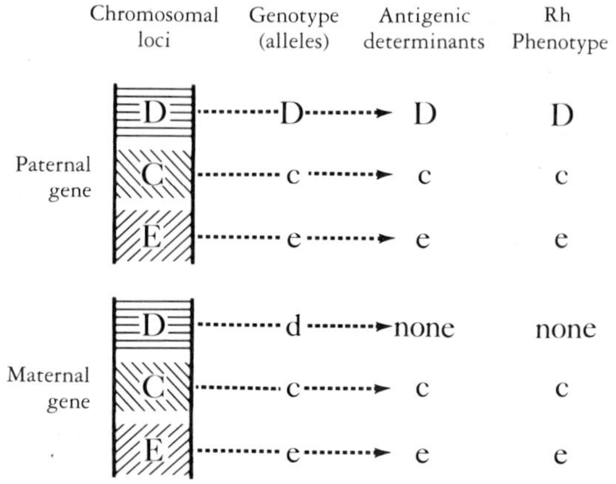

Figure 3–13. Schematic representation of the Fisher-Race Rh phenotype concept with three loci, each having two alleles. The C alleles are C and c, while the E alleles are E and e, these genes being codominant. The D locus has only one allele, D, which is expressed; no antigen for d has been found.

Table 3–7. Notation of Commonly Encountered Rh Isoantigens and Alleles

Genes			Expressed Antigens		
Fisher-Race Rh Haplotypes	Wiener Alleles	Wiener Agglutinogens	Fisher-Race	Wiener	Rh Type
Dce	R^0	Rh_0	D,c,e	Rh_O, hr′, hr″	+
DCe	R^1	Rh_1	D,C,e	Rh_O, rh′, hr″	+
DcE	R^2	Rh_2	D,c,E	Rh_O, hr′, rh″	+
DCE	R^z	Rh_z	D,C,E	Rh_O, rh′, rh″	+
dce	r	rh	– c,e	– hr′, hr″	–
dCe	r′	rh′	– C,e	– rh′, hr″	–
dcE	r″	rh″	– c,E	– hr′, rh″	–
dCE	r^y	rhy	– C,E	– rh′, rh″	–

Table 3–8. Partial List of Proposed Numerical Notation for Rh Antigens

Rosenfield et al.	Fisher-Race	Wiener
Rh1	D	Rh_O
Rh2	C	rh′
Rh3	E	rh″
Rh4	c	hr′
Rh5	e	hr″

If Rh-negative persons are given a unit of Rh-positive blood, over 50 per cent are immunized to D, while less than 5 per cent would form anti-E or e antibodies. In general practice, only compatibility for D is routinely established, except when blood is being transfused into an Rh-negative individual.

A second theory of inheritance, proposed by Wiener, differs to the extent that one locus is responsible for the production of several antigenic determinants. This theory utilizes the concept of "multiple complex alleles," in which a single locus on the chromosome controls the production of the Rh antigenic determinants found on the red cell. At this locus, however, there are a large number of alleles, each being responsible for the production of a single large antigenic structure that encompasses multiple smaller antigenic determinants. The original antigenic determinants were classified as Rh_O, rh′, rh″, hr′ and hr″, which corresponds to D, C, E, c, and e of the Fisher-Race scheme (Tables 3–7 and 3–8). Each allele is given a symbolic designation, such as R^O, to designate the antigenic specificity it controls. For example, Rh^O leads to the production of the

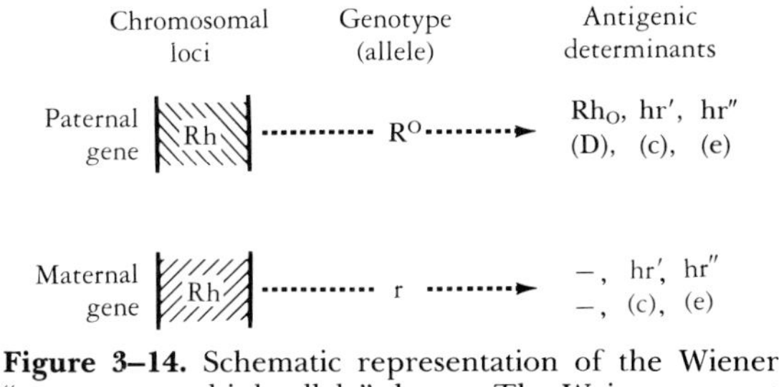

Figure 3–14. Schematic representation of the Wiener "one gene–multiple allele" theory. The Weiner concept suggests that a single "Rh" gene has eight alleles. Each allele codes for a cell surface molecule with two or three antigenic determinants or epitopes, which are recognized by the typing antisera. In this scheme, the Fischer-Race equivalents are in parentheses below the Wiener designations. The allele depicted by R^O code for a molecule with three epitopes, Rh_O, hr′ and hr″, which correspond to the Fisher-Race D, c, and e. The r allele codes for a molecule with only two epitopes hr′ and hr″, which correspond to c and e, as d is not expressed.

antigenic determinants Rh_O, hr′, and hr″ on the red cell. Figure 3–14 depicts the same examples used in Figure 3–13, using the Wiener scheme.

Tables 3–7 and 3–8 present some of the more commonly encountered Rh isoantigens, together with their controlling allelic forms, employing both systems of notation. Table 3–8 shows the newer nomenclature proposed by Rosenfield and colleagues, which simplifies this complex system.

According to the Fisher-Race scheme, the isoantigens are controlled by three linked loci. Since man is diploid, one set of these genetic loci is inherited from each parent. A person is said to be Rh-positive if he inherits D from either parent (DD or Dd). In either case, the father can transmit a D to one of his offspring's chromosomes.

For the physician, therefore, the determination of the genotype of an individual is an important consideration when sensitization due to D has occurred in a D-negative (Rho-negative) mother. For example, a father who is homozygous will transmit D to all the offspring, and each child could suffer from hemolytic disease of the newborn. If, on the other hand, the father is heterozygous, each child has a 50 per cent chance of being negative for D. Thus, by determination of the genotype of the father, the outcome of future pregnancies can be predicted.

Suggestions for Further Reading

Dausset, J., and Svejgaard, A.: HLA and Disease. 1st ed. Baltimore, Williams & Wilkins Company, 1977.

Festenstein, H., and Demant, P.: HLA and H-2, basic immunogenetics, biology and clinical relevance: No. 9. *In* Turk J. (ed.): Current Topics in Immunology. London, Edward Arnold, Ltd., 1978.

Fudenberg, H. H., Pink, J. R. L., Wang, A. C., et al.: Basic Immunogenetics. New York, Oxford University Press, 1978.

Hedrick, S. M., Cohen, D. I., Nielsen, E. A., and Davis, M. M.: Isolation of CDMA clones encoding T cell specific membrane associated proteins. Nature, *308*:149, 1984.

Hedrick, S. M., Nielsen, E. A., Kavaler, J., Cohen, D. I., and Davis, M. M.: Sequence relationships between putative cell receptor polypeptides and immunoglobulins. Nature, *308*:153, 1984.

Hood, L., Steinmetz, M., and Malissen, B.: Genes of the major histocompatibility complex of the mouse. Ann. Rev. Immunol., *1*:529, 1983.

Johnson, R. H., Hartzman, R. J., and Robinson, M. A.: HLA: The major histocompatibility complex. *In* Henry, J. (ed.): Clinical Diagnosis and Management by Laboratory Methods. Philadelphia, W. B. Saunders Company, 1984.

Kindt, T. J., and Robinson, M. A.: MHC antigens in fundamental immunology. *In* Paul, W. E. (ed.): Fundamental Immunology. New York, Raven Press, 1983.
Klein, J., Figueroa, F., and Nagy, Z. A.:Genetics of the major histocompatibility complex, the final act. Ann. Rev. Immunol., *1*:119, 1983.
Melief, C.: Remodelling the H-2 map. Immunol. Today, *4*:57, 1983.
Race, R. R., and Sanger, R.: Blood Groups in Man. 6th ed. Oxford, Blackwell Scientific Publications, 1975.
Reinherz, E. L., Meuer, S. C., and Schlossman, S. F.: The delineation of antigen receptors on human T lymphocytes. Immunol. Today, *4*:5, 1983.
Rosenfield, R. E., Allen, F. H., and Rubinstein, P.: Genetic model for the Rh blood group system. Proc. Natl. Acad. Sci., *70*:1303, 1973.
Schaller, J., and Hansen, J.: HLA relationship to disease. Hosp. Pract., *41*, 1981.
Schwartz, R.: Functional properties of I region gene products and theories of immune response (Ir) gene function. *In* Ia Antigens. Volume 1, Mice. Boca Raton, Fla., CRC Press, 1982, pp. 161–218.
Throwsdale, T., Lee, J., and McMichael, A.: HLA-DR bouillabaisse. Immunol. Today, *4*:33, 1983.
Yanagi, Y., Yoshikai, Y., Leggett, K., Clark, S. P., Aleksander, I., and Mak, T. W.: A human T cell specific cDNA clone encodes a protein having extensive homology to immunoglobulin chains. Nature, *308*:145, 1984.
Zaleski, M. B., Subiski, S., Niles, E. G., et al.: Immunogenetics. Boston, Pitman, 1983.

Chapter 4

Antigens and Immunogenicity

Anne L. Jackson, Ph.D.

DEFINITIONS

Immunogenicity may be defined as that property of a substance (immunogen) that endows it with the capacity to provoke a specific immune response. This consists of the elaboration of antibody, the development of cell-mediated immunity, or both. Antigenicity, on the other hand, is the property of a substance (antigen) that allows it to react with the products of the specific immune response, e.g., antibody or specifically sensitized T-lymphocytes. Substances that are immunogenic are always antigenic, but antigens are not necessarily immunogenic. For example, certain low molecular weight substances, referred to as haptens, e.g., penicillin, are not immunogenic unless coupled to a larger *carrier* molecule. Thus, a hapten functions as an antigen but not as an immunogen. Allergens refer to a specialized class of immunogens that induce hypersensitivity (allergic) reactions (Chapter 20A) and include substances that function as immunogens or haptens.

Portions of the three-dimensional structure of every immunogen contain surface groupings, e.g., amino acids in a globular protein or protruding sugar side chains in polysaccharides. These structures are referred to as antigenic determinants or epitopes and represent exposed active areas of the molecule with which an antibody can combine. Most complex materials, such as red blood cells, tissues, and bacteria, contain numerous antigenic determinants. Because of its small size, an individual antigenic determinant may not be immunogenic and therefore may be considered a hapten. Thus, the immune response to a complex immunogen represents the collective immune responses to a number of antigenic determinants. Of importance to clinical medicine is that new antigenic determinants may appear as a consequence of physical or chemical modifications of that material within the body. The significance of this finding is seen in certain immunologically-mediated diseases of man, such as drug allergies, the autoimmune diseases, and neoplasia (Chapters 19 and 20).

DEFINITIONS OF ANTIGENIC SPECIFICITIES

Broadly speaking, antigens may be classified into two major types: *exogenous* and *endogenous* (Table 4–1). This is an operational classification of antigens, based upon their applications in immunologically mediated diseases of man (Chapter 20).

Exogenous Antigens

Exogenous antigens are those that are presented to the host from the exterior in the form of microorganisms, pollen, drugs, or pollutants (see Table 4–1). These antigens are responsible for a spectrum of human diseases ranging from the infectious diseases to the immunologically mediated diseases of man, such as bronchial asthma (Chapter 20A). There are also genetic mechanisms operating at the level of the exogenous antigens. Influenza virus, for example, which is a major cause of epidemic respiratory disease in man, exists in nature in many antigenic types recognized as A, B, and C. These types represent different mutations of the virus. A

Table 4–1. **Classification of Antigens**

Source	Type	Example	Clinical Significance
Exogenous	Several	Microorganisms, pollen, drugs, pollutants	Susceptibility to infection, immunologically mediated disease (asthma)
Endogenous			
Xenogeneic (Heterologous)	Xenoantigen (Heteroantigen)	Forssman antigen, certain tissue antigens that cross-react with exogenous antigens (e.g., renal and cardiac tissues and beta hemolytic streptococcus)	Pathogenesis of certain diseases, e.g., glomerulonephritis, rheumatic fever
Autologous	Autoantigen	Organ-specific antigens (e.g., thyroid antigen)	Autoimmune diseases, e.g., Hashimoto's thyroiditis
	Idiotype	Immunoglobulin-specific antigens	Switch of immunoglobulin classes
Allogeneic (Homologous)	Alloantigen (Isoantigen)	Blood group, histocompatibility antigens (HL-A)	Hemolytic disease of the newborn, transfusion reactions, transplantation immunity

susceptible population will be infected by a given serotype. Following recovery and establishment of immunity, the virus can no longer propagate, since there are insufficient susceptible individuals to establish continued infection. Owing to selective pressure, however, the virus is known to undergo mutation, following which new variants of influenza emerge. These newly acquired variants, when fully virulent, are responsible for new epidemics. Thus, man survives epidemics, and organisms mutate to re-create epidemics.

Endogenous Antigens

Endogenous antigens are those that are found within an individual and include the following: *xenogeneic* (heterologous), *autologous* and *idiotypic,* or *allogeneic* (homologous) antigens (see Table 4–1).

Xenogeneic antigens are those antigens that are found within a variety of phylogenetically unrelated species. These antigens are also known as *heterogeneic* antigens and are important in clinical medicine, since they give rise to antibody responses associated with or useful in the diagnosis of disease. For example, the cross-reaction of Group A beta-hemolytic streptococcal antigens and human heart tissue is an example of a relationship between the well-known incidence of rheumatic heart disease and infection. It is believed that tissue damage is due to the cross-reaction of antibody with these heterologous antigens. Other types of heterologous responses are helpful in diagnosis. The best known example of this is the Forssman antigen, which is found in the tissue of many species and is closely related to other ubiquitous antigens such as the A blood group antigen. Because the Forssman antigen itself is not found in the tissues of man, it is possible that the great variety of other tissues or cells that contain this antigen could sensitize man. For example, following infectious mononucleosis, an infection caused by the EB virus (Chapter 16), antibody responses develop, some of which are specifically directed against the EB virus and others against this heterogenetic antigen. This latter reaction, referred to as *heterophile antibody response,* is a useful test in diagnosing infectious mononucleosis.

Although generally nonimmunogenic within a species, antigens distinguishing various cell types (e.g., "helper" T-cells) are now being characterized by the use of monoclonal antibodies. Since a monoclonal immunoglobulin recognizes a single epitope, it is now possible to generate an antibody response to previously "weak" or nonimmunogenic antigens by hybridoma technology (Chapter 5).

Autologous body components are constituents of the host and are recognized as self-components. Under ordinary circumstances, they are nonimmunogenic. It is believed that a change in these body components may cause them to become immunogenic under certain circumstances, and the host mounts an immunologic attack against its own tissues. In some instances, human tissues contain antigens that normally can be recognized by the immune system of the host but are separated from the action of antibodies or immune cells by barriers, such as the basement membrane. In these situations, removal of the barrier, for instance, through the effects of inflammation or acute infection, may release the antigens in such a way as to produce an acute secondary immune response, stimulating the host to mount an immunologic attack against its own tissues. In either case, the final condition is referred to as autoimmunity and is described in greater detail in Chapter 20C.

By far the largest group of antigens significant to the clinician are those known as *allogeneic antigens*. Allogeneic antigens are those genetically controlled by antigenic determinants that distinguish one individual of a given species from another. In man, antigenic determinants of this variety are found on red blood cells, white blood cells, platelets, serum proteins, and the surface of cells making up the fixed tissues of the body, including histocompatibility antigens (Table 4–2). These antigens are known to be *polymorphic*. (Polymorphism is the existence of two or more genetically different forms in one interbreeding population due to an array of alleles at one locus of the chromosome. At any one locus, however, an individual has only two alleles of the entire array that exists in the population.) In Table 4–2 are listed some of the important isoantigens of man with their tissue distribution and clinical importance. Immunization with any of these antigens can occur and progress to disease (Chapter 20B). This results when an individual receives an incompatible blood transfusion or a solid graft containing antigenic determinants that are absent in the recipient host. When these specificities are lacking in the recipient, they are perceived as foreign and therefore lead to an immune response. In general, the intensity of the response is proportional to the degree of genetic disparity between immunogen and the host, i.e., the greater the disparity, the more intense the response. These reactions may take the form of a transfusion reaction, as in the case of an incompatible blood transfusion, or the rejection of a solid graft, as in the case of a kidney transplant. Alternatively, immunization can occur during the course of pregnancy when fetal cells (e.g., leukocytes, erythrocytes, platelets) or proteins gain access to the maternal circulation. The maternal production and transplacental transfer of antibody to any of these paternally acquired fetal antigens can lead to severe anemia, leukopenia, thrombocytopenia, or aberrations in gamma globulin production by the fetus (Fig. 4–1).

Within a single given immunoglobulin molecule, additional determinants, unique to that molecule, are found. These are called idiotypic determinants. They are found in all subclasses (isotypes), and antibodies to that epitope are specific for that particular immunoglobulin (anti-idiotype). Anti-idiotypes are thought to be of importance in the regulation of immune responses (Chapter 7).

Structure of an Antigen

A composite picture of an "antigen" may be seen in the case of the Group A streptococcus (Fig. 4–2). The bacterium is composed of several physically and chemically discernible structures, which vary in their immunogenicity. For example, the capsule, which is composed of hyaluronic acid, is relatively nonimmunogenic. This may be accounted for by its close structural similarity to hyaluronates present in animal tissues, and it may not be recognized as foreign by the host. This lack of immunogenicity may also account for the increased virulence of the organism (Chapter 14). The surface antigens, M, T, and R, are found in the cell wall. Of these, the M proteins are the most important biologically since their presence impedes phagocytosis, and they are thought to be the major virulence factor of the Group A beta-hemo-

Table 4–2. Distribution and Clinical Significance of the Alloantigens of Man

Type	Example of Alloantigens	Clinical Significance
Red blood cell	ABO, Rh_O, blood groups (called isoantigens)	Hemolytic disease of newborn, transfusion reactions
White blood cell	Histocompatibility (HL-A) and neutrophil (NA) antigens	Transplantation immunity
Platelets	Platelet (Pl) antigens	Transplantation, thrombocytopenia
Serum proteins	Gamma globulin	Immunologic deficiency
Fixed tissues	Histocompatibility antigens (HL-A)	Transplantation

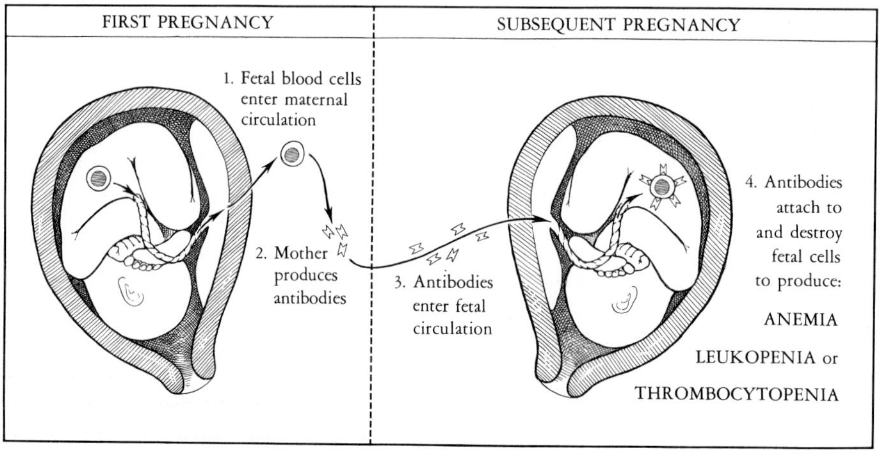

Figure 4–1. Schematic representation of isoimmunization due to feto-maternal incompatibility.

lytic streptococcus. Bacteria that are coated with antibody are more readily taken up and destroyed by phagocytic cells. The M proteins are also important diagnostically because they determine the type specificity of the organism. The group-specific "antigens" (A through N) are carbohydrate in nature and are also found within the cell wall of the streptococcal organism. Antibodies to these carbohydrates are not protective but permit the classification of the streptococci into serologic groups, which were first described by Lancefield. In addition, immunogenic extracellular products are elaborated by the streptococcus. These include the erythrogenic toxins, the streptolysins S and O, and a variety of other toxins. Antibodies to these proteins can serve a protective function (e.g., antierythrogenic toxin in scarlet fever) and may also be of aid in diagnosis of that disease (e.g., antistreptolysin O). When one considers that each of these immunogens has at least one, and probably more, antigenic determinants, the number of antibodies of different specificity that could be produced following immunization or infection becomes quite large. Not all immune responses are protective to the host, however. In assessing vaccines, it is important to determine the degree of protection produced in a patient by these immunogens (Chapter 23).

GENERAL PROPERTIES OF IMMUNOGENS

Foreignness

The first and primary requirement for any molecule to qualify as an immunogen is that

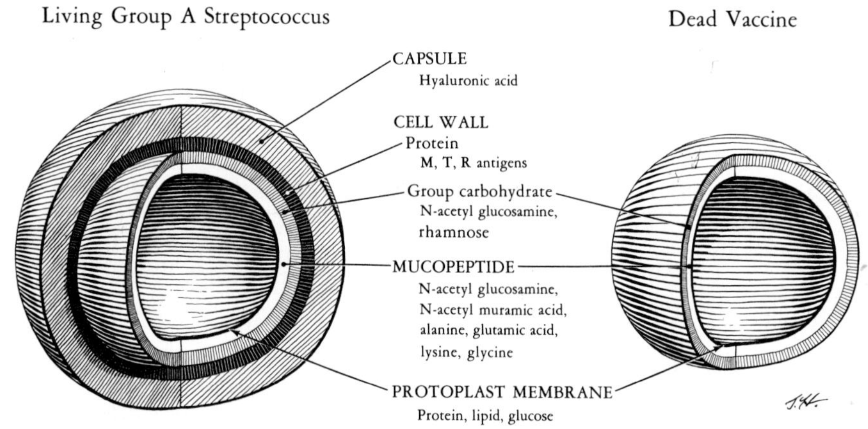

Figure 4–2. Schematic representation of living Group A *Streptococcus* and the dead vaccine prepared from it. (After Krause, R. M.: Factors controlling the occurrence of antibodies with uniform properties. Fed. Proc., *29*:59, 1970.)

the substance be genetically foreign to the host. In nature, an immune response will occur to a component that is not normally present in the body or normally exposed to the host's lymphoreticular system. On occasion, however, body constituents may be recognized as foreign, elicit an immune response, and become the adventitious target of injury, as seen in the autoimmune diseases of man (Chapter 20). Under ordinary circumstances, the immune system discriminates between "self" and "nonself." However, not all foreign substances can induce an immune response. For example, exposure to carbon in the form of coal dust will not induce antibodies to these substances; only the phagocytic response is initiated.

In addition to the requirements for foreignness, there is a large body of evidence showing that the ability to elicit an immune response is under genetic control (Chapter 3). These controls operate both at the level of total immune response, e.g., responders versus nonresponders, and in the control of specific immune products, e.g., IgE antibody. Thus, there exists a genetic requirement with regard to both the immunogen in terms of genetic dissimilarity and the genetic controls of immune responsiveness.

The recognition of a specific immunogen and the commitment to respond to the stimulation by the production of either antibody or cell-mediated immunity or with tolerance also seem to depend on the physical and chemical properties of the immunogen. These responses are mediated by specific receptors on precommitted lymphocytes and will have an influence on the type of cells recruited (Chapter 7). For example, certain immunogens directly stimulate B-lymphocytes with the production of antibody without the requirement for T-cells (T-independent antigens); other types of immunogens require the interaction of T-helper and B-lymphocytes in the full expression of an immune response (T-dependent antigens). Another type of cell cooperation is probably mediated by macrophages (Chapter 7).

PHYSICAL PROPERTIES

Size

In order for a substance to be immunogenic, it must be of a certain minimum size; effective immunogens have molecular weights greater than 10,000. Although some smaller molecules, such as insulin (5000 MW) and glucagon (4600 MW), do function as immunogens, the immune response is minimal in most hosts, and these substances function as haptens after combining with tissue proteins. Haptens can induce a strong immune response if coupled to a carrier protein of appropriate size (greater than 10,000 MW). It should be noted that the response to a hapten-protein complex will be directed to (1) the hapten, (2) the carrier, and (3) an area of overlapping specificity involving the hapten and the adjacent carrier constituents. In the case of humoral immunity, specificity is directed primarily to the hapten; in cell-mediated immunity, reactivity is directed to both the hapten and the carrier protein (Chapter 13).

Much of our understanding concerning the specificity of the immune reactions is derived from Landsteiner's studies of haptens. He was able to successfully distinguish antibody in animals immunized with l-tartaric acid from antibody produced in animals immunized with other isomers of tartaric acid (Table 4–3).

It is becoming increasingly clear that although immunogens are usually large in size, only restricted portions of the molecule are actively involved in the reaction with antibody. Recent studies employing peptide protein complexes have established that molecules of the size of a tetra-peptide participate in the binding of antigen with antibody. The subunits of that antigenic determinant appear to contribute unequally to this binding process. The degree to which these components of an antigen or antigenic determinant induce and are involved in the reaction with antibody is termed *immunodominance.*

Complexity

The factors that determine the complexity of an immunogen include both physical and

Table 4–3. The Reactivity of Sera Prepared Against the Isomers of Tartaric Acid*

	Haptens		
Antisera	l-tartaric acid	d-tartaric acid	m-tartaric acid
Anti-l-tartaric acid	+ + +	±	±
Anti-d-tartaric acid	0	+ + +	±
Anti-m-tartaric acid	±	0	+ + +

*After Landsteiner, K.: The Specificity of Serological Reactions. Cambridge, Harvard University Press, 1956.

chemical properties of the molecule. The state of aggregation of a molecule, for example, influences immunogenicity. A solution of monomeric proteins may actually induce a refractory state or tolerance when present in monomeric form but is highly immunogenic in its polymeric or aggregated state (Chapter 10). Several immunogens that do not induce an immune response when isolated in pure form do so when they are a part of a larger particle. Some artificial particles, or adjuvants, such as bentonite or aluminum hydroxide, may also serve to enhance immunogenicity.

Conformation

There is no one molecular configuration that is immunogenic. Linear or branched polypeptides or carbohydrates, as well as globular proteins, are all capable of inducing an immune response. Nonetheless, antibody that is formed to these different conformational structures is highly specific and can readily discriminate these differences. When the conformation of an antigen has been changed, the antibody induced by the original form no longer combines with it. When a determinant group consists of a sequence of amino acids derived from different portions of a folded polypeptide chain, an antibody directed to it cannot, of course, recognize the extended chains when denaturation-unfolding takes place. Figure 4–3 schematically depicts the relationships of antibody-combining sites for antigenic determinants. It can be seen that antibody to the first antigen (A) will clearly accommodate its own antigen. Determinant B, which has an additional residue, may not be as easily accommodated with antibody to A.

Charge

Immunogenicity is not limited to a particular molecular charge; positive, negative, and neutral substances can be immunogenic. However, the net charge of the immunogen does appear to influence the net charge of the resultant antibody. It has been shown that immunization with some positively charged immunogens results in the production of negatively charged antibodies. These data suggest that the production of antibody may be influenced by the overall charge of an immunogen.

Accessibility

The accessibility of the determinant groups to the recognition system will determine the outcome of an immune response. Recent developments have allowed investigators to prepare synthetic immunogenic polypeptides that contain a limited number of amino acids and in which chemical structure can be defined. In Figure 4–4, three types of multichain branched synthetic polypeptides are shown. In the first example, alanine side chains are attached to the amino groups of polylysine backbone, and on the outside the immunodominant tyrosine and glutamic acid groups are added. An immune response will occur to these immunodominant groupings when this polymer is injected into a rabbit. In the center diagram, the immunodominant tyrosine and glutamic acid determinants are placed next to the polylysine backbone, and the alanine side chains or "whiskers" protrude into the outside milieu. No immune response occurs to this configuration. In the third example, however, the spatial configuration of the side chains has been modified by alternating alanine with lysine residues,

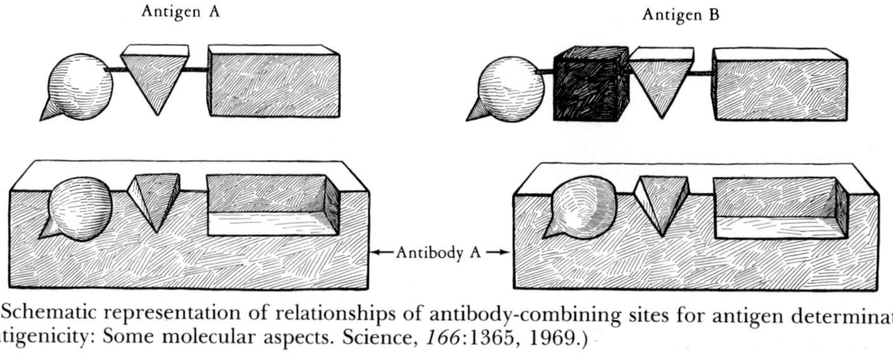

Figure 4–3. Schematic representation of relationships of antibody-combining sites for antigen determinations. (After Sela, M.: Antigenicity: Some molecular aspects. Science, *166*:1365, 1969.)

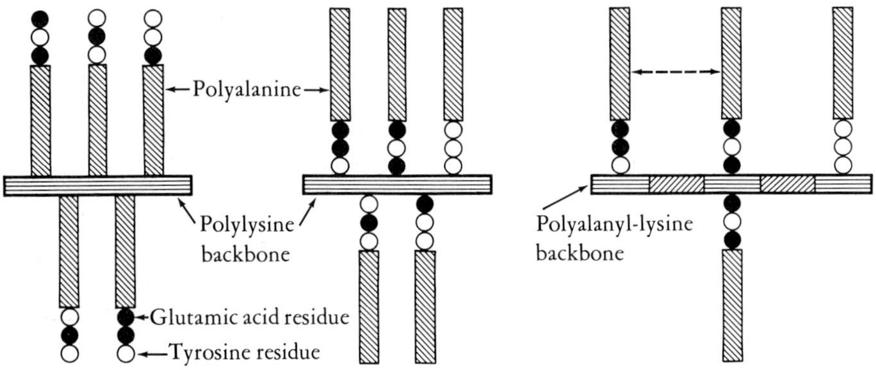

Figure 4–4. Three types of multichain-branched synthetic polypeptides. (After Sela, M.: Studies with synthetic polypeptides. Adv. Immunol., *5*:29, 1966.)

forming a polylysine-polyalanine backbone structure. Since the side chains can be inserted only at the location of the lysine groupings, the space between them is greatly lengthened. When injected into an experimental animal, this polymer will induce an immune response. Thus, the accessibility of determinant groupings on an immunogen will influence whether an immune response will occur.

CHEMICAL PROPERTIES

Most organic chemical groupings, with the exception of pure lipids, can be immunogens. The most effective immunogens are those that display diverse chemical and structural characteristics. However, a single amino acid variation in a protein may give rise to a new antibody specificity owing to a profound change in conformation, which might occur as a result of this single substitution.

There are two kinds of chemical structures that appear to influence immunogenicity: (1) the sequential determinants whose specificity is determined by the sequence of subunits within the determinant, e.g., primary amino acid sequence in the case of a protein, and (2) the conformational determinants that are determined by secondary, tertiary, or quaternary structure.

Digestibility

In general, a potent immunogen is one that is capable of being phagocytosed and degraded within the host. Recent information has shown, however, that nonmetabolized or noncatabolized substances, such as polystyrene, can also be immunogenic in minute quantities. Moreover, it should be noted that the efficiency with which phagocytosis proceeds appears to determine whether an antigen is eliminated or persists. This outcome is of profound biologic significance, since the elimination of antigens will determine whether an immune response will be beneficial or harmful. With successful elimination of antigen, the outcome is beneficial; if antigen persists, the tertiary manifestations of immunity may result in tissue damage by any of the various mechanisms of immunologic injury (Chapters 13 and 20).

Different Chemical Types of Immunogens

The overwhelming majority of immunogens in nature are protein. These may exist as pure proteins or may combine with other substances such as lipids (lipoproteins), nucleic acids (nucleoproteins), or carbohydrates (glycoproteins). Shown in Table 4–4 are some examples of different chemical classes of immunogens.

Some examples of foreign proteins that may be immunogenic include serum and tissue proteins, the structural proteins of viruses, bacteria and other microorganisms, toxins, plant proteins, and enzymes. Antibodies to these substances are sometimes used clinically in immunotherapy (antitoxins) and in the preparation of certain vaccines (Chapters 23 and 24). On the other hand, when they lead to the production of antibodies that are deleterious, they may be responsible for some of the sequelae of the immunologically mediated diseases (Chapter 20). For example, following streptococcal infections, some an-

Table 4–4. Chemical Classes of Immunogens

Type	Source
Protein	Serum proteins, microbial products (toxins), enzymes
Lipoprotein	Serum lipoproteins, cell membranes
Polysaccharides	Capsules of bacteria (pneumococcus)
Lipopolysaccharides	Cell walls of gram-negative bacteria (endotoxins)
Glycoproteins	Blood group substances A and B
Polypeptides	Hormones (insulin, growth hormones), synthetic compounds
Nucleic acids	Nucleoproteins, single-stranded DNA

tibodies that cross-react with cardiac tissue may be associated with some of the disease expressions of rheumatic fever. The lipoproteins are special types of protein immunogens that are found as part of many cell membranes.

Polysaccharides are another class of immunogens. They may occur as pure polysaccharide substances, as in the capsules of bacteria such as the pneumococcus, or they may be lipopolysaccharides occurring within cell walls of gram-negative bacteria (endotoxins). These substances are quite important biologically, since antibodies directed to them may provide protective immunity (antipneumococcal antibody). The lipopolysaccharides account for pathogenicity of certain gram-negative organisms, e.g., cholera endotoxin (Chapter 15).

The best known examples of glycoprotein antigens include the blood group substances A and B and the Rh antigens (Chapter 3). The immunogenicity of these substances has been associated with transfusion reactions and with isoimmunization of pregnancy (Chapter 20). In addition, the histocompatibility antigens (Chapter 3) are also composed of carbohydrate and protein. Polypeptide immunogens have been used experimentally in the form of synthetic polypeptides and have contributed to our understanding of many basic principles underlying immunogenicity. They are also used in clinical medicine, e.g., radioimmunoassay of insulin (Chapter 26). Their immunogenicity is at times undesirable, in which case the production of antibodies is associated with refractoriness to therapy, e.g., insulin antibodies.

The nucleic acids were for many years considered nonimmunogenic; however, under certain conditions they may serve as immunogens, particularly when single-stranded. In patients with the disease systemic lupus erythematosus, circulating antibody to native DNA or other nuclear constituents can be demonstrated. The inflammatory response induced by these antibodies or complexes of DNA–anti-DNA is thought to be responsible for the tissue damage (to blood vessels, glomeruli, and so forth) (Chapter 20) associated with severe forms of the disease.

HOST-RELATED FACTORS

Immunogenicity has profound biologic implications. The response to any given immunogens not only is a function of the physicochemical properties of the substance but also is connected with several host-related factors, including genetic makeup of the host, age, nutritional status, and any of a number of secondary effects that are derived from disease processes (Chapter 1). It should also be clearly understood that the measurement of any immunologic reactant to an immunogen should not necessarily be equated to a protective function in the host (Chapter 23). For example, it is known that the presence of circulating antibody in many types of localized viral infections does not prevent reinfection with these viruses (Chapter 16). Other factors of immunity also appear to be involved with the total host protection, e.g., secretory IgA antibody, as well as cell-mediated immunity.

It is now well established that live attenuated vaccines have greater clinical efficacy in the prevention of disease than do their killed or inactivated counterparts (Chapter 23). Further, serum antibody levels appear to be of longer duration following the use of live replicating vaccines or natural infection. Possibly owing to the continued persistence of immunogen, replicating agents may provide a more sustained stimulation of the immunologic system through the recruitment of additional immunocompetent cells. The methods used in preparation of an antigen may also have an adverse effect on the immunogenicity of a vaccine. Figure 4–2 shows Group A streptococcus from which critical protective immunogens have been removed during processing. As can be seen, the dead vaccine contains neither the capsule nor the M proteins important in inducing protective immunity. The recent development of effective capsular polysaccharide vaccines has been made possible by a knowledge of principles of immunogenicity and has provided effective and safe vaccines for the prevention of serious infections caused by encapsulated bacteria, e.g., *S. pneumoniae, N. meningitides,* and *H. influenzae* Type B (Chapter 23). Obviously, these are important considerations in the preparation of killed microbial vaccines that may lead to products that are more effective in inducing protective immunity.

Immunogenicity varies from species to species and, within a given species, from individual to individual (Chapter 3). For example, although nonimmunogenic in the rabbit, the isolated polysaccharide capsule of the pneumococcus can lead to a full immune response in the mouse. However, if polysaccharide is injected as part of a whole bacterial suspension, the rabbit will produce antibody to these polysaccharides. When all physical and chemical requirements for immunogenicity are fulfilled, the capacity of a given individual or inbred strain of animal to respond to various immunogens is genetically determined. The genes controlling the immune response in the mouse (Ir genes) are found within the same complex as the major histocompatibility (H-2) locus. "Responder" and "nonresponder" strains of mice and guinea pigs have demonstrated the exquisite sensitivity of the immune response to minor variations of immunogen (Chapter 3).

The amount of immunogen injected also influences the response. Studies of immunologic tolerance illustrate that a very low or a very high dose of foreign material can inhibit future responses to the subsequent injection of an otherwise immunogenic dose (Chapter 10). Dose and intervals between injections have also been shown to produce antibody populations of differing titer and avidity.

The route of injection can influence the nature of the immune response. For example, certain immunogens, when injected parenterally, e.g., intravenously, lead to the production primarily of circulating antibody; when given intradermally, the same immunogen may also provoke cell-mediated immunity, in addition to circulating antibody. When assessing the immunogenicity of a preparation, the type of test assay must also be evaluated since false negative reactions may occur when test procedures lack sensitivity or specificity.

Finally, an important biologic property of immunogens is the ability of certain antigens to evoke allergic or hypersensitivity responses (Chapter 20). These reactions, which are expressions of the immune response, may either be cell-mediated or humoral. For example, when certain low molecular weight compounds, such as the catechols from poison ivy, contact the skin, a dermatitis will result that is mediated through sensitized lymphocytes (delayed hypersensitivity). On the other hand, penicillin, when combined with tissue proteins, will evoke an antibody response that may lead to anaphylactic shock or urticarial hives (immediate hypersensitivity). These allergic manifestations are biologic expressions of the immune response that are harmful—the immunologically mediated diseases (Chapter 20).

ADJUVANTS

Certain substances, referred to as adjuvants, enhance the immune response when injected together with an immunogen (Chapter 10). Their function has been considered to increase the surface area of antigen (e.g., alum-precipitated diphtheria toxoid) or to prolong their retention in the body, allowing time for the lymphoid system to have access to the antigen (Freund's adjuvant). Recent evidence suggests that adjuvants may selectively expand T- and B-lymphocyte populations in addition to their classic granuloma-producing effects. The current use of adjuvants in immunotherapy of cancer is described in Chapter 10.

SUMMARY

The term "immunogen" has been proposed to define any substance capable of evoking an immune response. The properties of an immunogen are determined by the physical, chemical, and biologic properties of the substance, which are, in turn, related to its primary structure. Certain chemical groupings on the immunogen that determine specificity of the immunologic reaction are referred to as determinant groups, the most potent of which are termed immunodominant points. Implicit in immunogenicity is the requirement for genetic dissimilarity and recognition of foreignness by the host's surveillance system. Thus, immunogenicity represents the net interplay of the physicochemical properties of the immunogen as well as the response of several host-related factors such as age, genetic makeup, and the general state of the host.

Suggestions for Further Reading

Borek, F. (ed.): Immunogenicity. North-Holland Research Monographs. Vol. 25. Amsterdam, North-Holland, 1972.

Benjamin, E., Scibienski, R. J., and Thompson, K.: The relationship between antigenic structure and immune specificity. *In* F. P. Inman (ed.): Contemporary Topics in Immunochemistry. Vol. I. New York, Plenum Press, 1972, pp. 1–43.

Goodman, J. W.: Immunogenicity and antigenic specificity. *In* Stobo, J. D., Fudenberg, H. H., Wells, J. V., et al. (eds.): Basic and Clinical Immunology. 4th ed. Los Altos, Lange Medical Publications, 1982.

Kabat, E. A.: Structural Concepts in Immunology and Immunochemistry. 2nd ed. New York, Holt, Rinehart and Winston, 1975.

Milstein, C.: Monoclonal antibodies. Sci. Am., *243*:66, 1980.

Sela, M.: Antigenicity, some molecular aspects. Science, *166*:1365, 1969.

Sela, M.: Studies with synthetic polypeptides. Adv. Immunol., *5*:29, 1966.

Williams, R. C., Jr. (ed.): Lymphocytes and Their Interactions. Kroc Foundation Series. Vol. 4. New York, Raven Press, 1977.

Chapter 5

Antibody and Immunoglobulins: Structure and Function

George M. Bernier, M.D.

Immunoglobulins are a remarkable collection of protein molecules, which are the effector molecules of the humoral limb of immunity. These proteins share many antigenic, structural, and biologic similarities, but at the same time significant differences in primary amino acid sequence permit their antibody function and biologic activity to be highly specific for their role in bodily defense. Immunoglobulins are not simply molecules that combine with antigens in a "lock and key" fashion; they are very complex proteins with many highly specialized features in addition to their antigen-combining abilities. For example, to be effective, a human antibody to influenza virus might require several different structural capabilities: (1) a portion of the molecule that could combine specifically with the influenza virus and inhibit it; (2) another portion that could facilitate passage into the respiratory tract at the point of viral replication and permit a high concentration of such molecules in that region; (3) a mechanism to prevent the molecule from being degraded by the proteolytic enzymes that abound in the respiratory tree; and (4) a portion of the molecule that can combine with phagocytic cells. The human immune system has developed the kind of sophisticated specialization that permits this remarkable combination of properties to exist in a single molecular species known as secretory immunoglobulin A. Other equally distinctive features are associated with other kinds of immunoglobulins. As knowledge of the structure of immunoglobulins has developed, as the details of amino acid sequence have been revealed, and, in particular, as the genetic basis of antibody has been unraveled, the chemical basis of these and related phenomena has become more understandable.

HISTORY

The first real chemical information regarding the structure of antibodies was provided by Tiselius and Kabat in the early 1940's. These workers demonstrated that the fraction of serum proteins, the gamma globulins, that migrated most slowly in electrophoresis contained most of the serum antibodies. In the 1950's, Porter treated antibodies with papain, a proteolytic enzyme that split the antibody molecules into three fragments; two retained antibody activity and one possessed most of the antigenic features of gamma globulin. In the early 1960's, Edelman demonstrated that immunoglobulins were multichain structures, and a four-chain model of immunoglobulins was proposed by Porter. Putnam and Titani and Hilschmann and Craig initiated the studies of amino acid sequence of immunoglobulins using Bence Jones proteins, which are excreted in the urine of patients with multiple myeloma (Chapter 21). Determination of the amino acid sequence of the first complete immunoglobulin, an IgG myeloma protein, was completed in 1969 by Edelman and coworkers. In the 1970's, the primary sequence of a great many immunoglobulin molecules, myeloma proteins as well as more normally occurring antibodies, was determined. During the late 1970's and early 1980's the remarkable developments in molecular biology, pioneered by Leder, have unraveled the gene sequences and genetic mechanism of immunoglobulin production and variability.

Just as studies into the chemical nature of immunoglobulins were extremely fruitful, investigations into the complex biology of immunoglobulins clarified the function of the various kinds or classes of immunoglobulins.

In all these studies, the proteins elaborated by plasma cell tumors of man and mouse have proved to be of tremendous value in understanding the biologic, chemical, and genetic features of immunoglobulins.

THE FAMILY OF IMMUNOGLOBULINS

In man, five different classes of immunoglobulins are known to exist, each with a distinct chemical structure and a specific biologic role. These classes are designated by the letters G, A, M, D, and E following the abbreviation Ig (indicating their immunoglobulin function) or, by some writers, following the symbol γ (indicating their electrophoretic mobility as gamma globulins). Table 5–1 lists some of the properties of each class of immunoglobulins.

IgG is the most abundant of the immunoglobulins. These molecules achieve significant concentrations in both the vascular and the extravascular spaces, have a relatively long half-life (23 days), cross the placenta, and are able to activate complement. This class of immunoglobulin is thought to contribute to immunity against many infecting agents that have a blood-borne dissemination, including bacteria, viruses, parasites, and some fungi (Chapters 15 to 18). In addition, it provides antibody activity in tissues. Receptors for IgG exist on human monocytes, on polymorphonuclear leukocytes (polys), on reticuloendothelial cells in spleen and liver, and on some lymphocytes.

Although IgA is the second most abundant serum immunoglobulin, its most important contribution to the immunity of the individual is in the external secretory system. This important secretory immunoglobulin is produced in high concentrations by the lymphoid tissues lining the gastrointestinal, respiratory, and genitourinary tracts. In these secretions (e.g., saliva, tears) IgA is combined with a protein termed *secretory component* that appears to facilitate its transport into secretions and to endow the molecule with some protection against the effects of the proteolytic enzymes normally found in these regions. The IgA molecules do not activate complement by the classic pathway but may do so via the properdin system. IgA does not cross the placenta; however, it contributes to the immunity of the newborn by virtue of its high concentration in colostrum. Receptors for IgA are found on lymphocytes, polys, and monocytes.

IgM is the largest of the immunoglobulin molecules and, because of its large size, is restricted almost entirely to the intravascular space. These macromolecules are highly efficient agglutinators of particulate antigens such as bacteria and red blood cells, and they fix complement with a high degree of efficiency (Chapter 6). This class of immunoglobulin seems to be of greatest importance in the first few days of the primary immune response. When a foreign antigen is introduced into a host for the first time, the synthesis of IgM antibodies precedes that of IgG. However, the level of IgM antibodies peaks within a few days and then declines more rapidly than the level of IgG antibodies (Chapter 7).

The fourth class of immunoglobulins, IgD, was discovered in the mid-1960's by Rowe and Fahey when they encountered a myeloma protein antigenically and chemically different from the then known immunoglobulins. To date, IgD has not been assigned a specific biologic role as a humoral antibody. Antibody activity has been associated with IgD globulin, for example, in cases of penicillin hypersensitivity in the human. This immunoglobulin class is found on the surface of lymphocytes, particularly in neonates, with a frequency that far exceeds its relative serum concentration. A role has been assigned for IgD as a specific surface receptor in the initiation of the immune response (Chapter 7).

The reaginic antibody, IgE, is an immunoglobulin present in only trace amounts in serum. It has the ability to attach to human skin (homocytotropic antibody) and to initiate aspects of the "allergic reaction" (Chapters 8 and 13). IgE was initially isolated by Ishizaka, who purified it from vast quantities of serum containing reaginic antibody. Subsequently, a few myeloma proteins of the IgE class have been identified. Like IgA, IgE is produced chiefly in the linings of the respiratory and intestinal tracts and is part of the external secretory system of antibody (Chapter 2). Deficiency of IgE has been inconstantly associated with deficiency of IgA in individuals

Table 5–1. Some Physical and Biologic Properties of Human Immunoglobulin Classes

Class	Mean Serum Concentration (mg/100 ml)	Molecular Weight	$S_{20\bullet w}$	Mean Survival T/2 (days)	Biologic Function	Receptors on	Heavy Chain Designation	No. of Subclasses
IgG or γG	1240	150,000	7	23	Fix complement Cross placenta Heterocytotropic antibody	Polys, lymphocytes, monocytes	γ	4
IgA or γA	280	170,000	7,10,14	6	Secretory antibody Properdin pathway	Polys, lymphocytes, monocytes	α	2
IgM or γM	120	890,000	19	5	Fix complement	Lymphocytes	μ	1
IgD or γD	3	150,000	7	2.8	Lymphocyte surface receptor	—	δ	2
IgE or γE	0.03	196,000	8	1.5	Reaginic antibody Homocytotropic antibody	Mast cells Lymphocytes	ϵ	1

with impaired immunity who present with undue susceptibility to infection (Chapter 22).

Subclasses

By antigenic analysis, it has been possible to detect relatively minor differences between molecules of a given class of immunoglobulin (Table 5–1). In this way, four different subclasses of IgG have been found and designated IgG1, IgG2, IgG3, and IgG4. In addition, two subclasses each for IgA and IgD globulins have been found and are termed IgA1 and IgA2 and IgD1 and IgD2, respectively. Subsequent chemical analysis has shown that subclass antigenic differences reflect substantial differences in amino acid sequence. As indicated below, important biologic distinctions have been correlated with the various subclasses. For example, IgG4 does not fix complement, whereas the other three IgG subclasses do, and IgG3 globulins have a half-life significantly shorter than that of the other three. A major chemical difference between subclasses is the location and number of interchain disulfide bridges.

Chain Structure of Immunoglobulin

The classification of immunoglobulins, as described above, was made on the basis of antigenic and structural considerations; the real basis for this classification is found in the chemical structure of the molecules. The IgG antibody molecule, for instance, is made up of four polypeptide chains held together by disulfide bonds (Fig. 5–1). Two of the chains are small, with molecular weights of 22,000, and are termed light chains. The other two, with molecular weights of 55,000 are called heavy chains. Each immunoglobulin molecule has two identical heavy chains and two identical light chains. A chemically different kind of heavy chain exists for each of the five classes of immunoglobulin and is responsible for the antigenic differences that have been observed between classes. More important, it is the heavy chain that is responsible for the observed biologic differences between the various classes.

Just as there are five kinds of heavy chains, two different *types* of light chains have been found to exist. The light-chain types are called kappa (κ) and lambda (λ) (for the pair of investigators who originally observed the two types—Korngold and Lipari). Each type of light chain occurs in association with each kind of heavy chain, i.e., in each of the five classes of immunoglobulins. There are ten possible combinations of heavy and light chains, and all ten are normally found in any individual. As indicated in Table 5–1, the five kinds of heavy chains are identified by the Greek-letter equivalent of their class name—γ, α, μ, δ, and ϵ. Any immunoglobulin may therefore be designated by its heavy- and light-chain composition, in a manner analogous to the hemoglobin nomenclature. An IgG molecule, for example, would have a formula $\gamma_2\kappa_2$ or $\gamma_2\lambda_2$.

This basic four-chain structural unit is the form in which IgG, IgD, and IgE exist. A four-chain unit is repeated in the higher molecular weight immunoglobulins; IgM generally exists as a pentamer of basic four-chain subunits with each of five subunits held together by disulfide bonds (Fig. 5–2). A relatively small molecule with high sulfhydryl content, the *J chain,* participates in the polymerization of IgM. The IgM subunits (180,000 daltons) are each made up of two heavy chains (67,000 daltons) and two light chains.

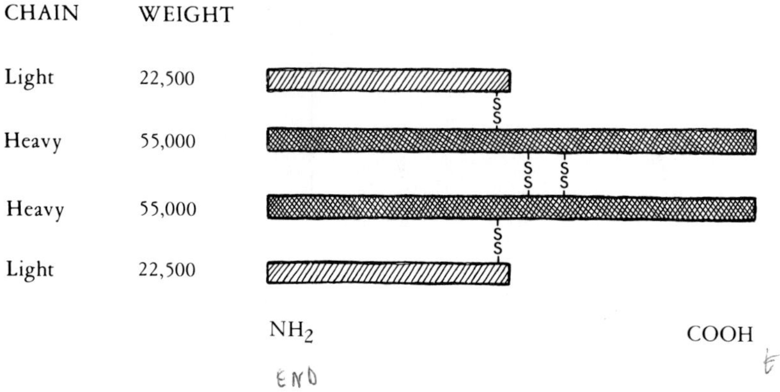

Figure 5–1. Schematic diagram of human IgG1 showing the location of interchain disulfide bonds. The molecule consists of two light chains and two heavy chains. The amino-terminal end is at the left and the carboxyl-terminal end is at the right. The structure depicted here is also applicable to other immunoglobulins with varying heavy-chain composition and polymerization.

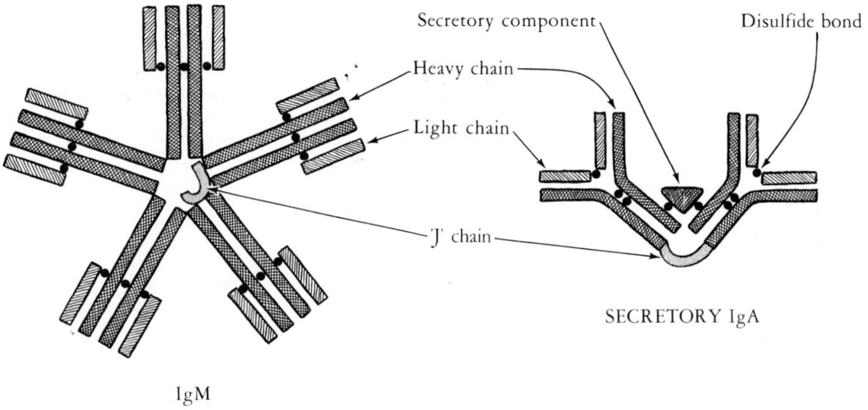

Figure 5–2. Models of IgM and secretory IgA. The former is shown in its usual pentameric form with a J chain involved in the pentamer formation. Secretory IgA is shown as a dimer attached to a secretory component. Note the absence of the light-heavy interchain bonds in the IgA. The IgA predominant in secretions is of the IgA2 subclass, which lacks such bonds.

IgA globulin, and occasionally IgG globulin, may also exist in a polymeric form in serum. Serum IgA, like IgM, may be polymerized through a sufhydryl residue near the carboxyl terminus of the molecule, with the participation of J chain. In secretions, two IgA monomers are linked by J chain and *secretory component* (another non-immunoglobulin) to produce a complex of high molecular weight (Figs. 5–2 and 5–3).

As described before, it has been possible to classify IgA globulins into two subclasses, IgA1 and IgA2, based upon differences in antigenic structure and variation in the arrangement of interchain disulfide bridges. Whereas the IgA2 is a minor component of serum IgA, this subclass is the dominant form in secretions. Curiously, no covalent bonding exists between light and heavy chains in the common genetic variant of this subclass (Fig.

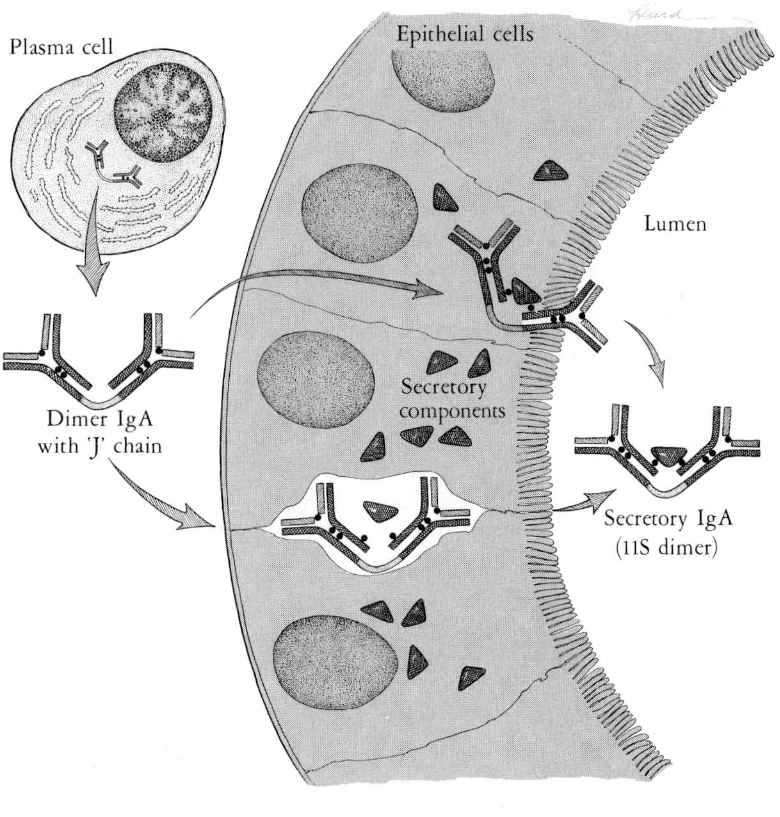

Figure 5–3. Representational drawing depicting the formation of secretory IgA. The IgA globulins are synthesized as monomers but are secreted from the plasma cells as dimers linked by the J chain. As the molecule passes through or in between the epithelial cells, it acquires the secretory component and enters the lumen as the secretory IgA molecule.

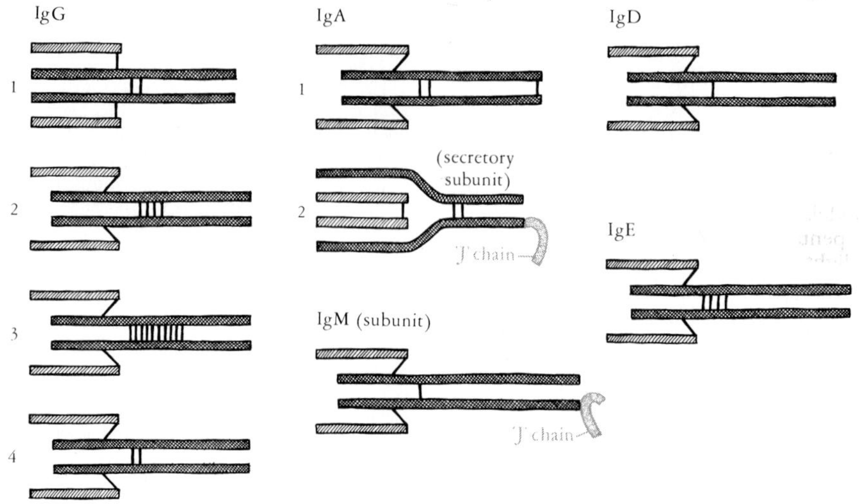

Figure 5–4. Arrangement of peptide chains in various subclasses of immunoglobulins. Disulfide bonds are represented by black bars. In the IgA and IgM subunits, the J chain, in gray, indicates where it would appear in the respective polymeric forms.

5–2). It has been noted that the IgA globulins are synthesized as monomers within plasma cells, which also synthesize J chain and are in contiguity with epithelial cells, containing the secretory component. After passage through the epithelium, IgA is recovered as a dimer, complexed with the secretory component (Fig. 5–3).

Just as the arrangement of interchain disulfide bonds is different in IgA subclasses, so too are there differences in the interchain bonds in the various IgG subclasses (Fig. 5–4). The biologic significance of these differences is not readily apparent, but they may account for some observed differences in such functions as life span or susceptibility to proteolytic degradation. For example, the IgG2 subclass has four heavy-heavy interchain bonds and is quite resistant to papain hydrolysis, as will be described below. Pathologically, the differences may be quite important, too. Myeloma globulins of the IgG3 subclass have an asymmetric structure because of the unusually long hinge region, and the abnormal viscosity this imparts to the blood of individuals with myeloma involving this Ig subclass may create serious problems.

ANTIBODY FUNCTION

An antibody produced in response to one antigen obviously must have structural features that are different from an antibody produced in response to any other antigen. Antibody to tetanus, for example, must differ in some chemically definable way from antibody to diphtheria, since both antibodies can be shown to combine specifically with their homologous antigens. This property, known as *specificity,* is determined by the primary amino acid sequence of the antibody molecule. For example, reduction of disulfide bonds and disruption of all noncovalent forces by dispersing agents such as 8 *M* urea will unfold the polypeptide chains of the molecule, with loss of antibody function. When the molecule is reconstituted by oxidation and removal of the dispersing agent, the antibody will re-form and regain its capacity for combination with its specific antigen.

The "antigen-binding site" or "antibody active site" of the immunoglobulin molecule is the region that combines with a specific antigen. In this region, the antibody specificity is determined by the amino acid sequence that permits its combination with the appropriate antigen. Both heavy and light chains share in this site; specifically, the first 110 amino acids from the amino-terminal end of each polypeptide chain are known to house antibody activity. In Figure 5–5, the IgG molecule is represented in a T-shaped configuration. The amino-terminal regions of variability on both the heavy and the light chains make up the antibody active sites. It is the amino acid sequence in these regions that dictates the specificity of the antibody. In IgG, IgD, and IgE, two antigen-binding sites

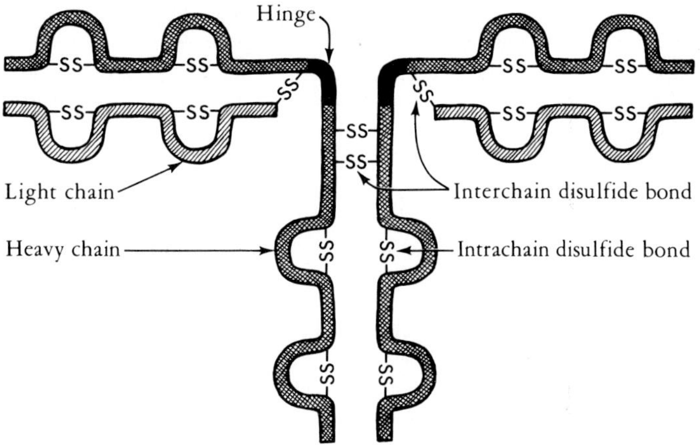

Figure 5–5. Schematic drawing of IgG in T-shaped model. The light chains are shaded by diagonal lines and the heavy chains marked with crosshatching. The hinge region is depicted in black. Disulfide bridges are represented by –SS–. The intrachain disulfide bonds pinch the chains into loops (domains). Extensive overall similarity is apparent in the placement of these loops between light and heavy chains and between the two portions of the heavy chains.

exist per molecule; in IgM, ten such sites exist; in dimeric IgA, such as is found in secretions, four combining sites are present.

A feature critical to the understanding of the overall structure of immunoglobulins is the symmetric arrangement of regions or *domains* for each of approximately 110 amino acids. These domains serve their own functions yet share some sequence homology. An immunoglobulin chain is composed of linked domains—two in light chains; four in the γ, α, and δ chains; and five in the μ and ϵ chains. In heavy chains, a nonhomologous stretch, the hinge region, separates the first two domains of the heavy chain from the other heavy-chain domains (Fig. 5–5).

Fragmentation of Immunoglobulins

Knowledge of the structure of the immunoglobulins has been greatly enhanced by the use of proteolytic enzymes, which degrade the molecule into definable fragments. *Papain* was shown by Porter to split the heavy chains of IgG in the hinge region, the area of the interchain disulfide bonds, yielding three fragments. One fragment, which can be crystallized, contains most of the IgG specific antigenic determinants of the molecule and is designated the Fc fragment; the other two fragments retain the ability to combine with antigen and are designated the Fab fragments (Fig. 5–6). Although of the same approximate size, the fragments differ strikingly in their function. Table 5–2 lists the composition and biologic activities associated with each. An attempt has been made in this table to describe the structure and function of the fragments in a format that is, if not memorable, at least mnemonic.

Another proteolytic enzyme, *pepsin,* acts upon the IgG molecule by degrading the heavy chain, beginning at the carboxyl-terminal end and proceeding to the region of

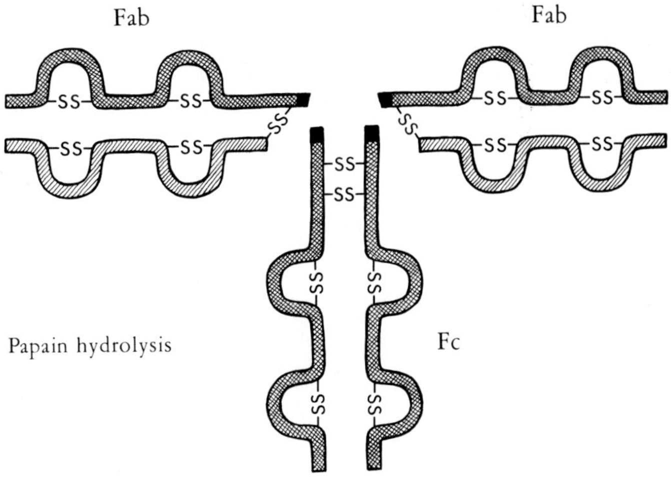

Figure 5–6. Schematic representation of the fragmentation of the IgG molecule by papain, which results in two Fab fragments and one Fc fragment. The Fab fragments possess one antigen-combining site each and can combine with, but may not give a visible reaction with, antigen. The Fc fragment lacks antigen-binding capabilities but retains many antigenic and biologic properties of IgG.

Table 5–2. **Fragments of IgG Produced by Papain Cleavage**

	Fab	Fc
Composition:	1. **A**mino-terminal half of heavy chain and one light chain 2. **A**berrated sequence	1. **C**arboxyl-terminal half of heavy chain dimer 2. **C**arbohydrate 3. **C**rystallizable (in some species) 4. **C**onstant amino acid sequence
Function:	1. **A**ntigen-**b**inding or **a**nti**b**ody active fragment	1. **C**omplement fixation 2. **C**ross placenta 3. **C**ellular attachment through receptors

the interchain disulfide bridge (Fig. 5–7). The splitting with *papain* produces univalent antibody fragments that can combine with antigens but not precipitate them; the *pepsin* treatment leaves a fragment that possesses two antigen-binding sites and can therefore still precipitate antigens. This fragment, termed $F(ab')_2$, has lost most of the specific antigenic determinants of IgG, since most of these are located in the carboxyl-terminal half of the heavy chain (Fc fragment).

In addition to the Fab, $F(ab')_2$, and Fc fragments, the term "Fd" is used to designate the amino-terminal half of the heavy chain, i.e., the half of the heavy chain located in the Fab fragment (Fig. 5–8). This region of the heavy chain is of great biologic importance, since it shares in the antigen-binding site and provides thermodynamically the lion's share of the binding affinity to antigen.

Trypsin has been employed in two different ways in the fragmentation of immunoglobulins. Prolonged digestion with trypsin results in cleavage of the peptide chain next to all arginine and lysine residues and the production of "tryptic peptides." These peptides may be examined by a combination of electrophoresis and chromatography, a technique called "fingerprinting" or "peptide mapping." This method has proved valuable in comparing the structure of two or more proteins, since it provides information about the comparative primary amino acid sequence without requiring exhaustive sequence analysis. The technique has been very useful in studies of variant human hemoglobins and in the study of human and animal immunoglobulins. Shorter periods of digestion of IgG and IgM with trypsin produce fragments similar to those derived by papain hydrolysis.

The other immunoglobulins can also be fragmented by proteolytic enzymes, but the fragments produced are not necessarily comparable to those derived from IgG. For instance, papain digestion of IgA often destroys the Fc portion of the molecule. However, in all immunoglobulin molecules, the regions are named according to the system described for the IgG, i.e., Fab, Fc, and Fd.

Enzymes produced by some bacteria, including the gonococcus and enteric streptococci, have been found to have proteolytic activity specific for the IgA1 subclass. This enzyme cleaves IgA1 molecules in the hinge region and produces fragments quite similar in size to the Fab and Fc fragments of IgG. While at first blush this is a tribute to the evolutionary adaptability of bacteria, in fact, the dominant form of IgA in the human intestinal tract is IgA2, a molecule impervious

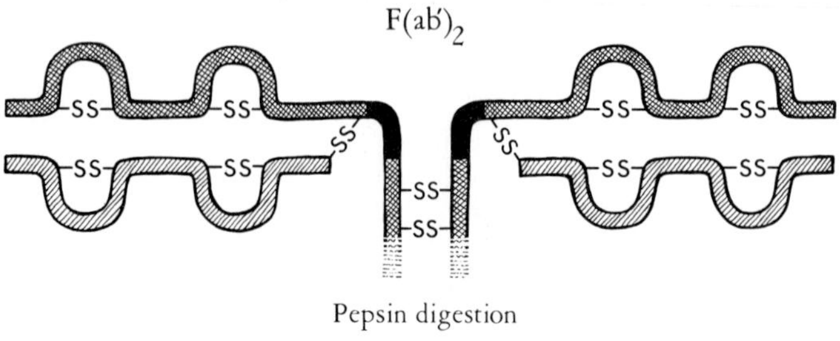

Figure 5–7. Schematic representation of the degradation of IgG by pepsin. The Fc portion is hydrolyzed below the interchain disulfide bonds, leaving a single fragment with two combining sites intact, the $F(ab')_2$.

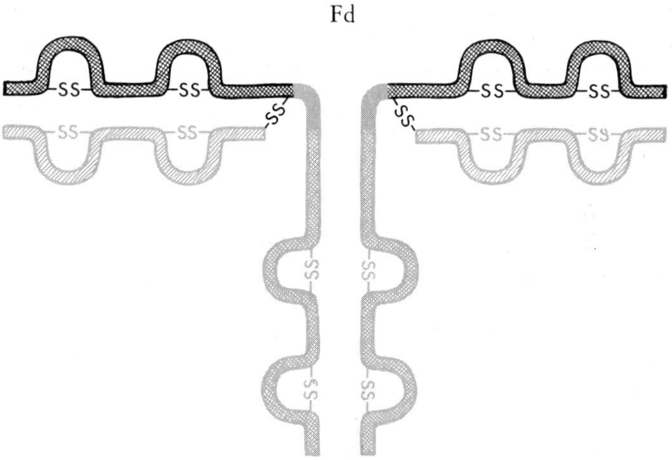

Figure 5–8. Molecular location of the Fd fragment of IgG is indicated in black. The light chains and the Fc portion of the heavy chain are represented in gray.

to the protease. Hence, it would appear that the human intestinal tract has emerged as victor in this particular evolutionary battle.

GENETIC FACTORS ASSOCIATED WITH IMMUNOGLOBULINS: GM, INV, AND AM FACTORS

Genetic markers have been found to be carried on immunoglobulin molecules (Chapter 7). The first two identified were designated Gm and Inv factors (Fig. 5–9) and were detected by the following indirect method.

The sera of some patients with rheumatoid arthritis agglutinate red blood cells coated with human gamma globulin. The anti–gamma globulin antibody contained in the sera of these individuals is called rheumatoid factor (RF) (Chapter 20C). The reaction between the rheumatoid factor from a particular person and gamma globulin–coated red cells was found to be inhibited by preincubation of the rheumatoid serum with serum from some normal persons. Some normal sera inhibited a particular rheumatoid factor reaction; others did not. The ability to inhibit a particular reaction was found to be inherited in a mendelian fashion, and the inhibitory substances in normal serum have been shown to be immunoglobulins. A number of hereditary factors reflecting different loci have been uncovered in this way and are associated with the various IgG heavy chains or with the κ-type light chain. Those factors associated with the heavy chain of IgG are termed Gm (for gamma) and those associated with the light chain are called Inv (the abbreviation of a patient's name) or sometimes Km (analogous to Gm). There are more than 20 recognized Gm factors and 3 Inv factors. As shown more recently (see Table 5–1), four different subclasses of IgG have been detected, and the various Gm factors are asso-

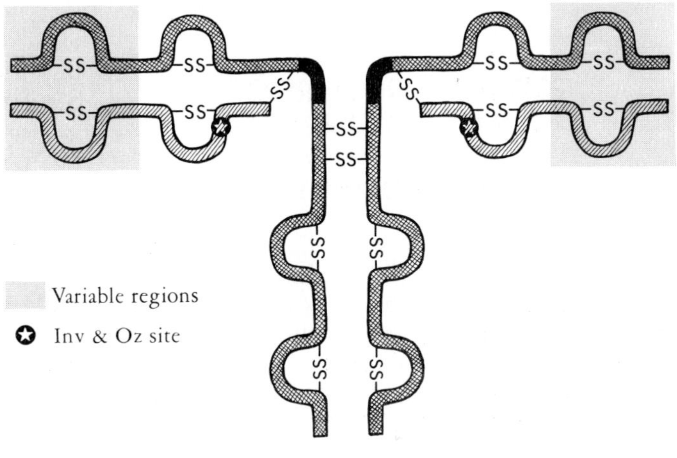

Figure 5–9. In this drawing, the regions of sequence variability are depicted in gray. Note that the variable segment of the light chain is in apposition to the variable segment of the heavy chain—this is the region of antibody specificity. The antigenic markers Inv and Oz are indicated by ⊛. The Gm markers are localized in constant regions of the heavy chains and are the result of minor amino acid sequence variation.

ciated with one of these subclasses. The chemical basis for the Gm and Inv factors will be described later. It is important to point out that the Gm and Inv factors are nonallelic—that is, they are inherited independently of each other.

Another independently inherited group of genetic markers associated with IgA has been described. The reagents for identifying such factors have arisen as a result of transfusion. Some patients have been immunized in this way with an IgA genetically different from their own. Anti-IgA allotypic antibodies have thus been inadvertently produced, and their clinical manifestations have been transfusion reactions ranging from mild to severe. Different genetic factors have been found, and the term "Am" (referring to the IgA equivalent of Gm) has been applied to the system.

In all three systems (Gm, Inv, and Am), the detecting antibody is of human origin. In the first two it is frequently a rheumatoid factor, but, like the third factor, it is sometimes transfusion-induced. Since chemical differences between allotypes are minimal (one amino acid in the case of the Inv factor), detection has required antibodies generated in the same species. Allotypic differences between proteins of other species have been sought and detected immunologically by immunization within the species, under the assumption that the immunized animal's recognition system will detect minor differences between the immunizing antigen and its own proteins.

As might be anticipated, the various Gm factors are associated with specific subclasses of IgG, and the various Am factors are similarly associated with specific subclasses of IgA. To date, in the human system no allotypic markers have been found for the γ light chain or the μ, δ, or ϵ heavy chain.

PRIMARY STRUCTURE OF IMMUNOGLOBULINS

Heterogeneity

An aspect of antibodies that is of paramount interest to the protein biochemist paradoxically proved to be a major impediment to the understanding of immunoglobulins as protein molecules. This aspect is the unique situation of the extreme chemical heterogeneity of the immunoglobulins occurring in the face of a degree of chemical constancy. By way of illustration, albumin, transferrin, and most other serum proteins have a discrete electrophoretic mobility that is a manifestation of chemical homogeneity. Genetic variation in these serum proteins, as in the case of the human hemoglobins, often results in charge differences, which in turn are manifested as different electrophoretic forms. In contrast, the immunoglobulins of all individuals are spread over a very wide electrophoretic range. This electrophoretic variation is most apparent in the case of IgG and is readily illustrated by immunoelectrophoresis, which disperses the IgG molecules from the extreme cathodal end of the electrophoretic field almost all the way to the anode. The extreme electrophoretic heterogeneity of these molecules reflects a degree of variation in primary sequence that is remarkable among protein species. From what has been said before, this heterogeneity is obviously a manifestation of class, subclass, type, and genetic variation. More important, however, it reflects the chemical basis of antibody variability, i.e., of those differences, for instance, that distinguish an anti-tetanus antibody from an anti-diphtheria antibody.

Even when antibodies of a single specificity have been isolated, they too have been electrophoretically heterogeneous. It has been, therefore, most difficult to study the basis of chemical variability by analyzing antibodies themselves, because it is virtually impossible to establish the amino acid sequence in regions of variability. Instead, the problem has been approached by analyzing the homogeneous immunoglobulins produced in some malignant conditions that affect lymphocytes and plasma cells, notably in the human disease states of multiple myeloma and macroglobulinemia and in the mouse plasmacytoma system (Chapter 21).

These disorders are characterized by the elaboration of large amounts of homogeneous immunoglobulins by proliferating cells. Such immunoglobulins are found in the serum or urine of affected individuals. The term "monoclonal" has been applied to the homogeneous immunoglobulin, implying that it is a consequence of the proliferation of a single clone of plasma cells. The proteins elaborated may be complete immunoglobulin molecules of IgG, IgA, IgM, IgD, or IgE class, or free light chains (Bence Jones proteins), or both. In very rare human conditions, such as the heavy-chain diseases, fragments or portions of immunoglobulin chains or molecules are produced.

Because of their homogeneity and their availability in great abundance, the monoclonal immunoglobulins are chemically suitable for amino acid sequence analysis. Much of the information relating to primary amino acid sequence derived from studies of such proteins has been applied to normal immunoglobulins. The rationale for using these abnormal immunoglobulins as models for normal antibody is based upon the following observations and suppositions.

1. Each complete monoclonal immunoglobulin appears to be one of the many normal immunoglobulins. The monoclonal proteins differ from pools of immunoglobulin in terms of restricted electrophoretic mobility, of biologic properties, of chain type, of genetic markers, and of physical properties. However, no unique pathologic features, such as novel amino acids, unusual prosthetic groups, or excessive lengths of peptide chains, have been found in any of the complete monoclonal immunoglobulins.

2. Many monoclonal immunoglobulins have been found to possess antibody activity. Indeed, the frequency of finding monoclonal immunoglobulins with antibody specificity seems proportional to the intensity of the search, and it is likely that all the monoclonal proteins would be *bona fide* antibodies, if only appropriate antigens could be found.

3. Monoclonal mouse and human antibodies have been produced using the hybridoma technology (see below). These antibodies have the characteristics of myeloma globulins: light and heavy chains of only one type and class, electrophoretic homogeneity, and restricted genetic markers.

Each monoclonal immunoglobulin possesses distinctive antigenic and chemical features. To date, complete identity has not been established between the monoclonal immunoglobulins produced by any two individuals. Even in the case of free light chains of one type (κ or λ) that have a molecular weight of only 22,500, no two have been identical. The chemical and antigenic differences are termed idiotypic markers, in contrast to the allotypic markers (Gm, Inv, and Am). If one assumes that one monoclonal immunoglobulin differs from another in the same way and to the same extent that one "normal" antibody molecule differs from another, then detailed examination of relatively few monoclonal immunoglobulins would be expected to provide information about the molecular location of variability, the extent of variability, and the genetic mechanisms responsible for the variability. It should be no surprise that the major antigenic and chemical differences that exist between myeloma proteins occur in that portion of the molecule in which variations between antibodies of different specificities occur.

The sequence of a wide variety of monoclonal immunoglobulins has been determined, and extensive amino acid sequence information is available to aid in the understanding of immunoglobulins. Moreover, the cells that produce these monoclonal Ig's have provided the DNA that has been useful in understanding the genetic basis of antibodies.

Hybridoma Technology as a Source of Monoclonal Antibody

One of the most important recent developments in immunology has been the development of a method for the *in vitro* production of large quantities of homogeneous antibody to a single antigenic specificity, i.e., monoclonal antibody. The source of this antibody is the hybridoma, which is the progeny of fusion between a normal antibody-secreting lymphoid (B) cell and a myeloma cell of animal or human origin. Since normal plasma cells usually die after a few cell divisions, there is a requirement to continue their cell divisions by fusion with a malignant myeloma cell. This technique therefore confers upon the progeny of the fusion the characteristics of both parental cells, namely the antigenic specificity of antibody secreted by the B-cell as well as the perpetuity of monoclonal immunoglobulin production by the myeloma cell.

The technique is schematically shown in Figure 5–10. Spleen cells obtained from mice that have been immunized with the desired antigen are the most commonly used source of antibody-secreting B-lymphocytes. These cells are exposed to an agent that promotes cell fusion, such as polyethylene glycol, while mixed with a suspension of myeloma cells in tissue culture. Following fusion a number of clones of hybrids appear, which are capable of producing various monoclonal antibody to any of the antigenic specificities found on the immunogen. Clones of hybrids of the desired antibody specificity are then selected from the pool and the antibody-producing cell lines are expanded by tissue culture techniques. Clones can be injected back into mice or into tissue culture and the purified

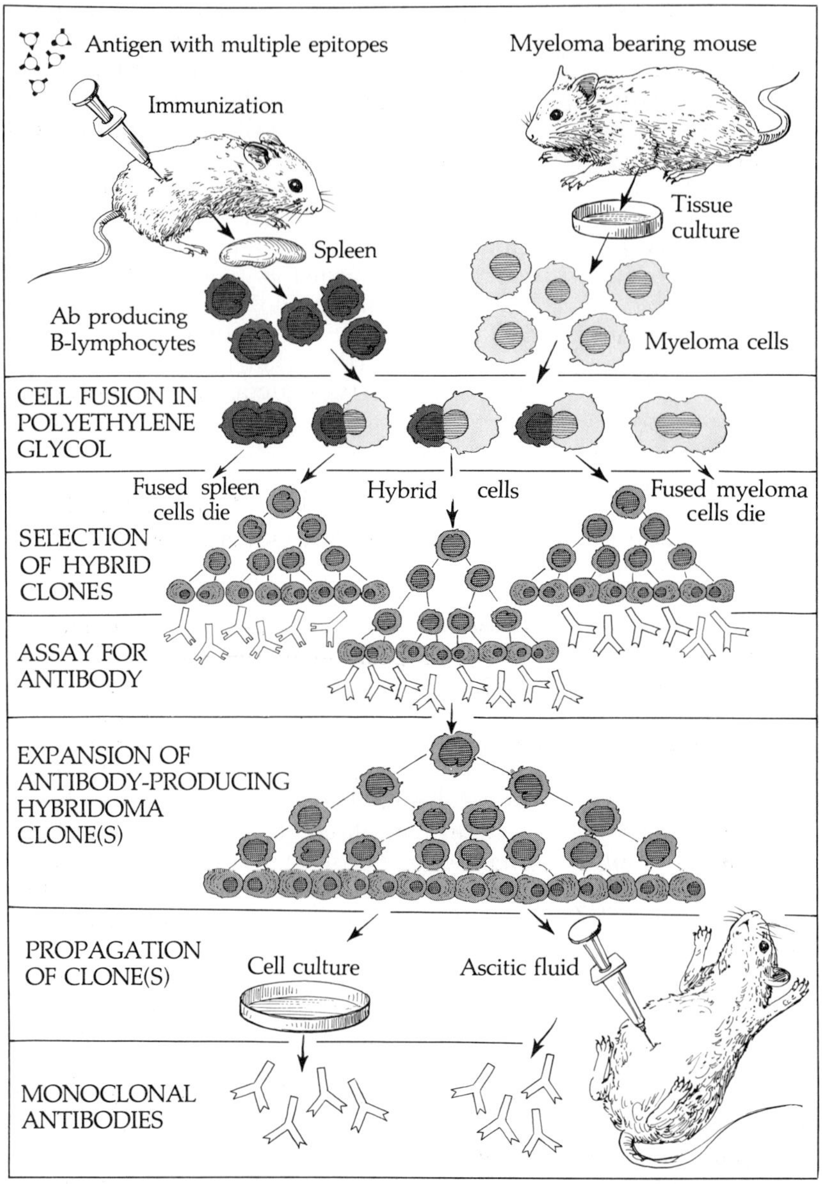

Figure 5–10. Schematic representation of the hybridoma technique for the production of monoclonal antibody.

monoclonal antibody then obtained from ascitic fluid or tissue culture supernatant fluid.

Monoclonal antibody produced by hybridomas is receiving widespread application as a source of diagnostic and therapeutic reagents. These include serologic reagents for identification of infectious agents, tumor antigens, histocompatibility antigens, and functional subpopulations of lymphoid cells, e.g., OKT3, OKT4, and OKT8.

Monoclonal antibodies have been employed in the treatment of lymphomas (Chapter 19), acute and chronic leukemias, and T-cell malignancies and have virtually unlimited potential use in tumor imaging and as vehicles for delivery of cytotoxic agents to tumor cells.

Light Chains

Bence Jones proteins (homogeneous free light chains) from myeloma patients and from mice with plasmacytomas were the first to be studied in appreciable numbers, and the following generalizations can be made. Two types of light chains exist throughout the vertebrate world: κ and λ. In various species one or the other is a predominant form. In man, approximately twice as many molecules have κ light chains as have λ chains. Light chains have been found to possess a region of constancy and a region of variability. The molecular topography of these regions is illustrated in Figure 5–11, and it is apparent that light chains are composed of two approximately equal halves—one constant and the other variable. The sequence of the carboxyl half of the molecule is virtually constant from one λ-type Bence Jones protein to another, or from one κ-type Bence Jones protein to another. Although a degree of homology is present (approximately 40 per cent), the κ chains are very different from the λ chains in this region, i.e., the constant region or domain.

In the amino-terminal half of the molecule, extensive variability is found between Bence Jones proteins of the same antigenic type. The transition from variable to constant region is an abrupt one. When larger numbers of Bence Jones proteins have been examined, it has become apparent that subgrouping of κ and λ chains is possible, based on overall similarity in the amino-terminal half. The variability in this half within a given subgroup is considerably less and is of the kind that would result from changes in single base pairs. Approximately five different subgroups of each light-chain type have been determined on this basis.

There is one notable exception to the pattern of constancy in the carboxyl-terminal half of the light chains. In κ chains, either leucine or valine is found at position 191 and confers one of two genetic factors (Inv1 or Inv3, respectively). The great theoretical importance of this fact is that by inheritance of these markers the carboxyl-terminal half of the light chain can be shown to be transmitted according to mendelian principles. This will be described later as it applies to the genetic basis of antibody variability.

Another factor, called Oz, is found in an analogous position in the λ chain (position 190), where an arginine-lysine interchange

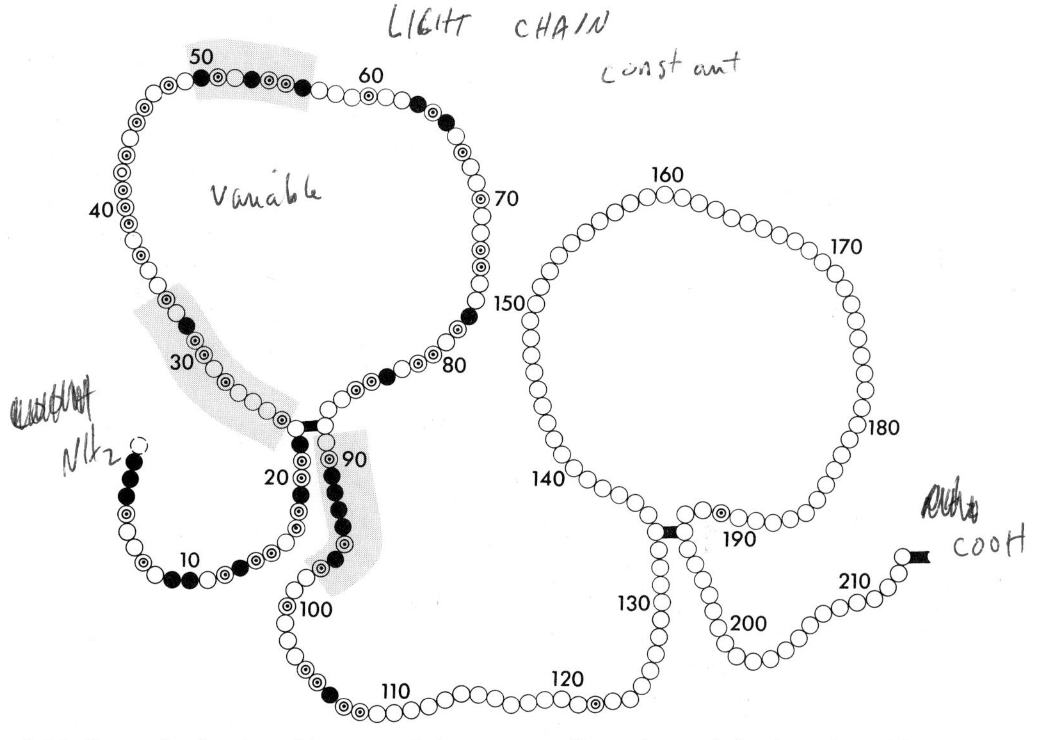

Figure 5–11. Composite drawing of human κ chain sequences illustrating variation in amino acid sequence among several different κ-type Bence Jones proteins. The amino-terminal end of the peptide chain is at the left, the carboxyl terminal at the right. Each circle represents one of the 214 amino acids of the chain. The *white* circles ○ indicate residues where only one amino acid was found. The *shaded* circles ◎ designate positions where two alternate amino acids were detected, and the *black* circles ● indicate positions where three or more different amino acids occurred. Disulfide bonds are indicated by black bars. The variable sequence is confined almost entirely to the amino-terminal half of the molecule. The carboxyl-terminal half is quite constant and the notable variation occurs at position 191, the site of the Inv genetic marker. The gray areas indicate the hypervariable areas that are apparent when sequences of human κ and λ chains and mouse κ chains are compared.

determines the presence or absence of an antigenic determinant. Unlike the Inv determinant, this is not a genetic factor, since all persons produce some λ chains with the Oz determinant and some λ chains without it.

Heavy Chains

The primary sequence of the heavy chains is different for each of the various immunoglobulin classes, but the amino acid sequence variation of the heavy chains is very similar to that observed in light chains. The amino-terminal end, comprising the first 110 or so amino acids, is the area of variable sequence and is termed the *variable domain* of the heavy chain or the V_H domain. The remaining residues represent regions of relative constancy and are termed constant regions or *constant domains* (Fig. 5–12). These are named according to the kind of peptide chain (γ, α, μ, δ, ε) and the relative position in the chain sequence (amino to carboxyl terminus). For example, in an IgG molecule, the domains would be identified in order as $V_H \ldots C\gamma_1 \ldots C\gamma_2 \ldots C\gamma_3$. In the heavy chain of IgM, which is larger by one domain, the order would be $V_H \ldots C\mu_1 \ldots C\mu_2 \ldots C\mu_3 \ldots C\mu_4$.

Each constant domain of each kind of heavy chain has a distinctive amino acid sequence. However, there exists a significant degree of homology from constant domain to constant domain within a peptide chain and between heavy chains of various classes. It is interesting, from an evolutionary viewpoint, that greater similarities exist between a given domain in different heavy chains than between two different domains in the same heavy chain. For example, the $C\alpha_2$ is more like the $C\gamma_2$ than the $C\alpha_3$. This would argue that class divergence occurred after basic immunoglobulin structure was established.

Two important points must be made concerning the V_H regions. These domains appear in every kind of heavy chain and are not distinctive for any class. The V_H of a particular IgG molecule may be more like the V_H of an IgM than that of another IgG. Also, just as subtypes of light-chain variable regions are evident from comparative amino acid sequence, so can the variable regions of heavy chains be subgrouped into V_{HI}, V_{HII}, V_{HIII} . . . . Within a given subgroup, the variation in sequence is much less, as is true of the light chains.

Myeloma globulins have provided the prototype models for analysis in establishing these structural considerations. Although the chemical basis was determined by peptide mapping and amino acid sequence analysis, it has been possible to obtain a significant amount of information from immunologic analysis. It is possible, for instance, to recognize the unique variable region of a given myeloma globulin by immunizing rabbits with the monoclonal protein and absorbing the resultant antiserum with normal immunoglobulins. Antisera so prepared often (but not always) continue to react with the variable domains of the immunizing globulin and can distinguish this monoclonal globulin from all others. The antigens recognized in this way

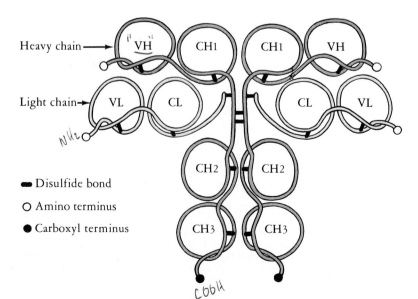

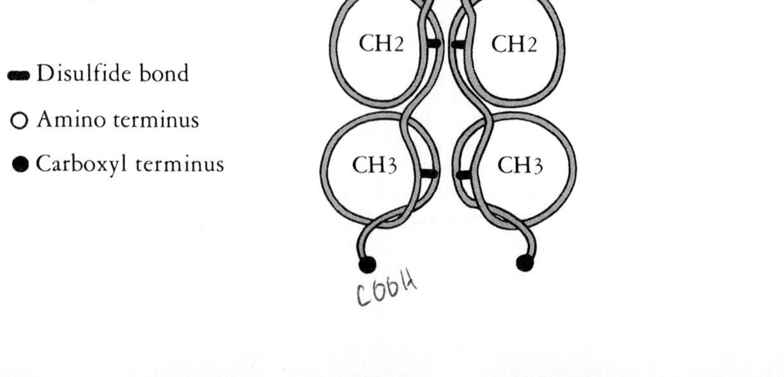

Figure 5–12. Schematic drawing of IgG in a T-shaped model. Each peptide chain is drawn as a continuous line, and attachments between heavy and light chains and between the two heavy chains are indicated by solid bars. Note the two loops in each light chain and the four loops in each heavy chain. These loops are formed by intrachain disulfide bonds and are termed domains. In each chain, one domain (V) has a *variable* amino acid sequence depending on the antibody specificity of the molecule. The other domains (C) have a rather *constant* sequence common among molecules of the same class, subclass, and type. They are numbered in sequence from the amino-terminal end.

are called idiotypic antigens and the antisera are termed anti-idiotype.

By employing antisera made specific for the idiotypic markers of a monoclonal immunoglobulin, it is possible to identify the presence of similar idiotypic markers in cells, on cell surfaces, and in trace amounts in the serum of patients. Anti-idiotypic antibodies have been used to identify antibodies of a common specificity in inbred rabbits. Monoclonal anti-idiotypic antibodies have also been made using the hybridoma technique.

Three-Dimensional Structure

Immunoglobulins have been visualized by the negative staining technique of electron microscopy. X-ray crystallography has also been applied to the study of immunoglobulins, particularly crystallizable monoclonal immunoglobulins, and electron microscopy has been used in the study of sections of such crystalline IgG molecules. By a variety of physical methods, the IgG molecule appears to be composed of three principal units (one Fc and two Fab's). There appears to be a significant amount of flexibility in the hinge region between the Fc and Fab's, with the molecule able to assume a Y or T shape, depending on its association with antigen.

Each of the major fragments has dimensions of approximately 50 × 40 × 70 Å. Hence, the "wing span" of the molecule across the Fab's is approximately 130 to 140 Å (Fig. 5–13).

From hapten-binding studies, as well as physical measurements, the combining site would appear to be a crevice involving the light and heavy chain in the range of 15 Å deep.

Polymeric molecules, such as secretory IgA and pentameric IgM, have been observed by means of electron microscopy. The striking feature of the IgM molecules is their rosette-like structure, similar to that shown schematically in Figure 5–2.

Evolutionary Aspects

A feature common to both heavy and light chains is the location of the intrachain disulfide bonds. As described earlier, these are so situated that the peptide chains are "pinched" into a series of loops of approximately 60 amino acids each. Two loops are found in each light chain, four are found in each IgG, IgA, and IgD heavy chain, and five are found in each IgM and IgE heavy chain. The loops are depicted in highly schematic fashion in Figures 5–11 and 5–12. The recurring periodicity of such loops or domains suggests that the complex immunoglobulin molecule has evolved from a primitive peptide chain approximately 110 amino acids long. A significant degree of homology is found among the various domains of light and heavy chains, and this gives credence to the concept of a common primitive progenitor. It is important to point out that as the particular peptide chains exist today, the differences are more pronounced between classes than between species. For instance, the κ chain of man is closer in sequence to the κ chain of the mouse than it is to the λ chain of man. From a phylogenetic point of view, a low molecular weight IgM class of immunoglobulin appears to be the most primitive of the extant immunoglobulins.

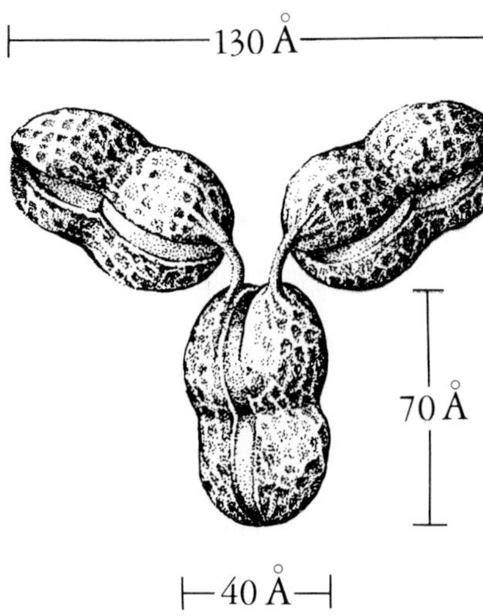

Figure 5–13. Three-dimensional model of IgG showing the close relationship between domains in each of the Fab fragments and in the Fc fragment. The compact areas are linked through the hinge region. This model is based on the studies of x-ray crystallography and electron microscopy.

Of considerable interest along these lines is β_2 microglobulin, an 11,600 dalton cell surface protein associated with the HLA antigen system. This protein, which is also found free in body fluids, has the characteristics of a free domain in that it has a disulfide-bonded loop of 60 amino acids. The β_2 microglobulin has a homology of greater than 20 per cent with virtually every constant domain of every immunoglobulin. It is possible that the earliest forms of immunoglobulins were cell surface–associated protective molecules.

THE GENESIS OF ANTIBODY VARIABILITY

Under appropriate conditions, the introduction of a foreign antigen into a man or an animal results in the production of specific antibody. Two broad mechanisms were invoked to explain the phenomenon of specificity as it occurs in the immune response. The germ line theories held that cells already committed to production of a particular antibody were stimulated by the introduction of antigen to proliferate and elaborate their product. The germ line theories were predicated on the existence of myriad genes, representing all possible antibody specificities. In contrast, the somatic mutation theory postulated few germ line genes that underwent extensive somatic rearrangement and mutation.

In contrast to the "one gene–one polypeptide chain" concept that had been the keystone of molecular biology, new notions had to be invoked to explain the origin of antibody variability. A "two genes–one polypeptide chain" concept was proposed initially to account for the constant and variable portions of the immunoglobulin peptide chain. According to the concept, one gene (a "C" gene) would encode the constant portion of the peptide chain and another gene (a "V" gene) would encode the variable portion. During the selection process, the two genes would link up and the now completed DNA sequence would lead to synthesis of a complete polypeptide chain product. The germ line would contain relatively few "C" genes, one for each type of light chain (κ and the two kinds of λ) and one for each subclass or class of heavy chain (four for IgG, two each for IgA and IgD, and one each for IgM and IgE). A number of "V" genes, however, would have to be present to encode the variable portion of the peptide chain and thereby to confer antibody specificity.

Advances in molecular biology have greatly clarified many of the mechanisms underlying the genesis of antibody variability.

The germ line of an individual can indeed be shown to contain genes that code for the constant regions of immunoglobulins and other genes that encode for the variable segments. As can be shown for many other protein-synthesizing systems, intervening sequences of nonexpressed DNA (introns) separate genes and gene segments from each other. In the mouse the genes that encode for heavy chains are on chromosome 12, those for the κ light chain on chromosome 16, and those for the λ chain on chromosome 6. In each case, those chains responsible for the variable region are on the 5′ side (or "upstream") of the constant-region genes.

On chromosome 12, three distinct gene families that are involved in generating the variable region of heavy chains exist side by side. These three distinct gene families, variable (V_H), diversity (D), and joining (J_H), together generate the unique specificity of an antibody. During differentiation of the B cell, V_H, D, and J_H segments are linked, with a loss of the intervening sequences, to form a V-D-J gene. The process is termed rearrangement. Subsequently, the V-D-J gene and one constant-region gene are transcribed and the messenger RNA derived from this encodes for the complete immunoglobulin heavy chain (Fig. 5–14), deleting the introns.

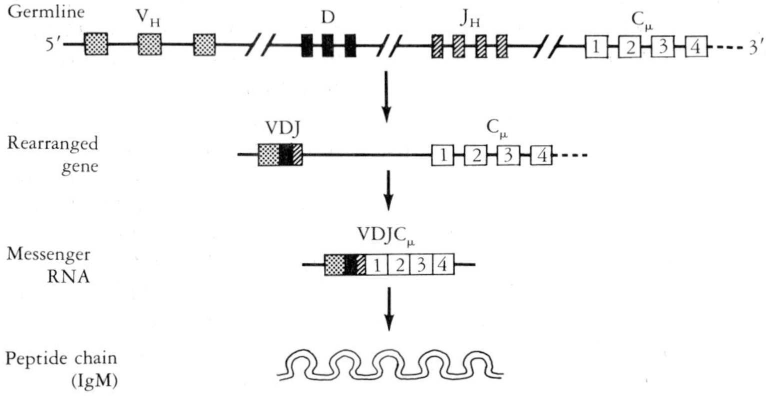

Figure 5–14. Schematic representation of the process whereby gene segments are linked and transcribed. One of many V_H region genes, one of several D genes, and one of several J_H genes are linked through rearrangement with loss of the other V_H, D, and J_H genes. This complex, which now codes the variable region of the antibody is transcribed along with the C region genes of the appropriate class into messenger RNA.

The temporal sequence in which the various immunoglobulins are expressed (μ, δ, γ, ε, α) follows the order of heavy-chain constant-region genes as they exist on chromosome 12. Following gene arrangement, a given heavy-chain constant gene is expressed and is transcribed with the variable-region gene. When a "switch" in Ig classes occurs, the previously expressed constant gene appears to be deleted and a subsequent constant gene is activated and transcribed. In this fashion a single cell can produce sequentially several different classes of immunoglobulin with the same antibody specificity.

A very similar process occurs with the assembly of the messenger for light chains, except that D genes do not exist in the repertoire, only V, J, and constant-region genes. Vλ and Jλ genes are transcribed with the Cλ DNA to produce λ chains, and Vκ, Jκ, and Cκ genes are transcribed for production of that kind of light chain. In the final assembly of antibodies, the heavy and light chains are themselves linked through disulfide bonds and secreted by the antibody-forming cell.

The diversity of the variable regions reflects (a) the V_H gene pool, (b) the D genes that provide frame shifts, (c) the J_H gene pools, and (d) the pairing of the heavy chain with one of many light chains. In addition, during the life of the cell, it appears that a significant degree of somatic mutation occurs, which further defines and refines antibody specificity. Thus, elements of both the germ line and the mutational theories have been shown to be correct.

Suggestions for Further Reading

Edelman, G. M.: The covalent structure of human G-immunoglobulin XI. Functional implications. Biochemistry, *9*:3197, 1970.

Hood, L., and Talmage, D. W.: On the mechanism of antibody diversity: germline basis for variability. Science, *168*:325, 1970.

Ishizaka, T., and Ishizaka, K.: Biology of immunoglobulin E: molecular basis of reaginic hypersensitivity. Prog. Allergy, *19*:60, 1975.

Leder, P., Battey, J., Lenoir, G., et al.: Translocations among antibody genes in human cancer. Science, *222*:765, 1983.

Low, T. L. K., Liu, Y-S. V., and Putnam, F. W.: Structure, function, and evolutionary relationships of Fc domains of human immunoglobulins A, G, M, and E. Science, *191*:390, 1976.

Nisonoff, A., Hopper, J. E., and Spring, S. B. (eds.): The Antibody Molecule. New York, Academic Press, 1975.

Putnam, F. W. (ed.): The Plasma Proteins: Structure, Function and Genetic Control. New York, Academic Press, 1976.

Siebenlist, U., Ravetch, J. V., Korsmeyer, S., et al.: Human immunoglobulin D segments encoded in tandem multigenic families. Nature, *294*:631, 1981.

Teillaud, J. L., Desaymard, C., Guisti, A. M., et al.: Monoclonal antibodies reveal the structural basis of antibody diversity. Science, *222*:721, 1983.

Chapter 6

The Complement System

Steven L. Kunkel, Ph.D., Peter A. Ward, M.D.,
Lynn H. Caporale, Ph.D., and Carl-Wilhelm Vogel, M.D.

INTRODUCTION

The complement system is an integral part of the body's immune system. Although the term "complement" was originally used to describe an auxiliary factor in serum that, acting upon an antibody-coated cell (such as a red blood cell or a bacterium), would cause cell death, the complement system is now known to involve at least 20 proteins that circulate in the plasma in an inactive form. These proteins can be activated by two independent pathways, termed the classical pathway and the alternative pathway.

Activation of the complement system results in a cascade of interactions of these proteins, leading to the generation of products that have important biologic activities and that constitute an important humoral mediator system involved in inflammatory reactions. First, coating of particles, such as bacteria or immune complexes, with certain components of complement facilitates the ingestion of the particle by phagocytic cells (opsonic function of complement). Second, the activation event generates many fission products of complement proteins for which specific receptors exist on a variety of inflammatory cells, such as granulocytes, lymphocytes, and other cells. Binding of these complement-derived products to such receptors results in biologic activities such as chemotaxis and hormone-like activation of cellular functions (inflammatory function of complement). Third, the late-acting proteins of the complement cascade form the macromolecular membrane attack complex, which causes death of target cells. This killing activity may be directed against viruses, bacteria, fungi, parasites, virus-infected cells and tumor cells (cytotoxic function of complement).

An intact complement system is essential to the maintenance of health. Moreover, it has been particularly useful to measure certain components of complement in clinical situations as indicators of disease activity. The importance of complement becomes evident in many patients with congenital defects of a complement protein, who present with recurrent infections or immune complex diseases (Chapters 20C and 22). An understanding of the complement system is therefore important for diagnosis and management of patients who present with recurrent infections, allergic diseases, and autoimmune disorders.

PATHWAYS OF COMPLEMENT ACTIVATION AND THE COMPLEMENT PROTEINS

Activation of complement can occur by two separate pathways: the classical and the alternative pathways. Both pathways lead to a common terminal pathway referred to as the pathway of membrane attack. Twenty plasma proteins, listed in Table 6–1, are now known to be constituents of these pathways. These proteins can be divided into functional proteins, which represent the elements of the various pathways, and regulatory proteins, which exhibit control function. The concentration of the proteins in normal human plasma covers a broad range. They are synthesized in the liver but also by cells of the lymphoreticular system, such as lymphocytes and monocytes.

Both the classical and the alternative complement pathways can be organized into various operational units: initiation, amplification, and membrane attack (Fig. 6–1). Following an initial recognition event, which leads to initiation of the pathway, an ampli-

Table 6–1. **Proteins of the Complement System**

Protein	Molecular Weight	Plasma Concentration
Classical Pathway		
C1q	400,000	65 μg/ml
C1r	190,000	50 μg/ml
C1s	88,000	40 μg/ml
C4	200,000	640 μg/ml
C2	117,000	25 μg/ml
C3	185,000	1400 μg/ml
Alternative Pathway		
Factor B	93,000	200 μg/ml
Factor D	23,000	2 μg/ml
C3	185,000	1400 μg/ml
Membrane Attack Pathway		
C5	200,000	80 μg/ml
C6	128,000	75 μg/ml
C7	121,000	55 μg/ml
C8	154,000	55 μg/ml
C9	79,000	60 μg/ml
Regulatory Proteins		
C1 Inhibitor	85,000	20 μg/ml
C4b Binding protein	570,000	250 μg/ml
Carboxypeptidase N	310,000	50 μg/ml
Factor H	150,000	500 μg/ml
Factor I	80,000	35 μg/ml
Properdin	180,000 (heterogeneous)	25 μg/ml
S-Protein	71,000	600 μg/ml

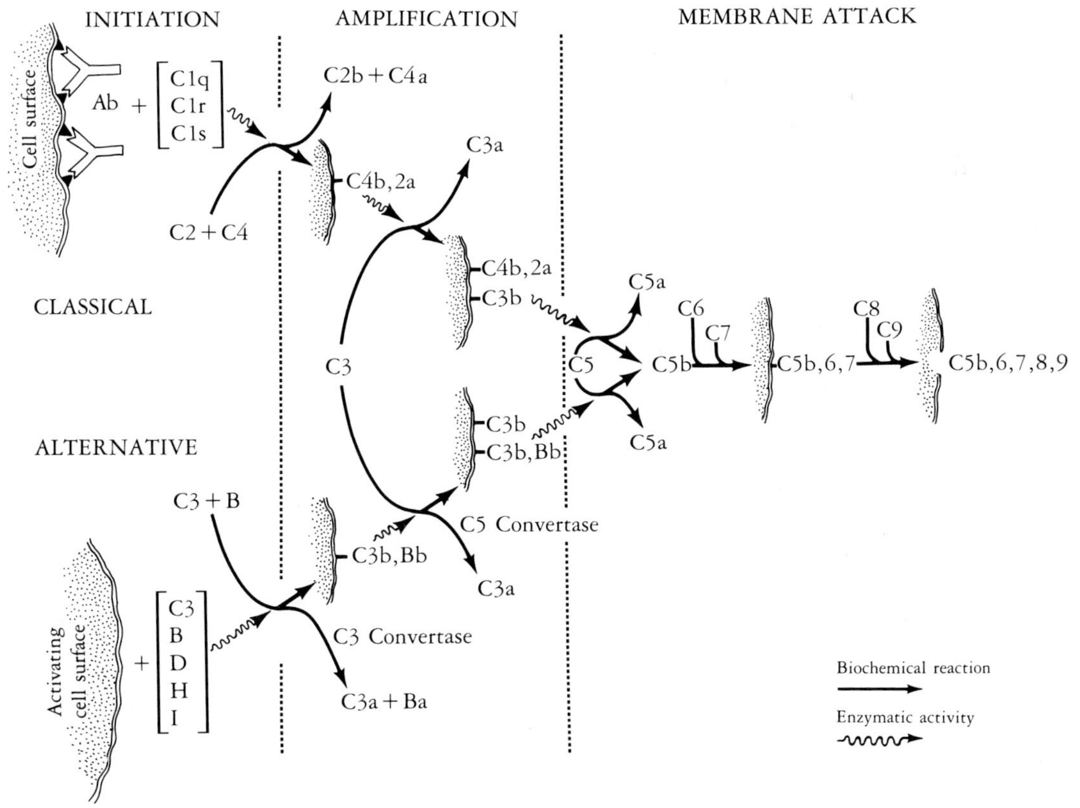

Figure 6–1. Schematic representation of the two pathways of complement activation.

fication phase takes place that involves the action of proteases and the recruitment of additional molecules; this is followed by a terminal phase of membrane attack during which the cell dies.

The recognition unit for the classical pathway, C1, is composed of three separate proteins, C1q, C1r, and C1s. The initiation of this pathway of complement typically involves the reaction of antibody with antigen, which may be soluble or on the surface of a target cell. This antigen-antibody reaction allows the binding of C1q to two or more Fc regions of certain IgG subclasses (IgG_1, IgG_2, IgG_3) or IgM. Activators of the classical pathway are listed in Table 6–2. The ultrastructure of C1q has been demonstrated by electron microscopy to consist of six subunits similar to a bouquet of six flowers. The central stalks of C1q resemble collagen in primary and secondary structure. Upon binding of one C1q molecule to the Fc regions of two or more antigen-bound antibody molecules, C1r proenzymes are activated. The chemical basis of this activation is the cleavage of a peptide bond by an autocatalytic mechanism, leading to the formation of activated C1r, a protease that subsequently cleaves the proenzyme C1s. Thus, the binding of C1q to an immunoglobulin in complex with the antigen represents the recognition event of the classical pathway, resulting in the activation of C1r and C1s. The final result is the generation of an enzymatically active component, C1s, which will cleave and thereby activate the next proteins in the cascade, leading to amplification of the recognition event.

The enzyme C1s has two physiologic substrates, C4 and C2. C4 is cleaved by C1s into C4a, one of the three anaphylatoxins (molecules that promote increased vascular permeability and smooth muscle contraction), and C4b, which binds to the target cell surface. C1s also cleaves C2 when C2 is in complex with C4b. Cleavage of C2 generates C2b, which is released, and C2a, which remains bound to C4b. The bimolecular complex C4b,2a is a protease that cleaves C3 and therefore is called C3 convertase. Cleavage of C3 by the C3 convertase generates two important biologically active peptides, C3a (another anaphylatoxin) and C3b, which attaches to target cell surfaces and can bind to C5. C5, when in complex with C3b, can be cleaved by the C3 convertase (then referred to as C5 convertase). The C5 convertase hydrolyzes C5, which generates the C5a anaphylatoxin and C5b. C5b is the nucleus for the formation of the membrane attack complex.

Table 6–2. Activators of the Classical Pathway

Immunoglobulins	
	IgG (human subclasses 1, 2, and 3)
	IgM
Nonimmunoglobulin Activators	
	Bacterial lipopolysaccharide (lipid A portion)
	C-reactive protein bound to pneumococci
	Retroviruses
	Heart mitochondrial membranes
	Polyanions (e.g., polynucleotides)
	Urate crystals

Immediately following their generation, C3b and C4b exhibit a unique transient ability to covalently bind to target cells ("metastable binding site"). This property has recently been shown to be due to an intramolecular thioester bond that is present between the sulfhydryl group of a cysteine residue and the gamma carbonyl group of a glutamine residue on C3 and C4 (Fig. 6–2). Upon activation of C3 or C4, this thioester becomes highly reactive and can react with a cell

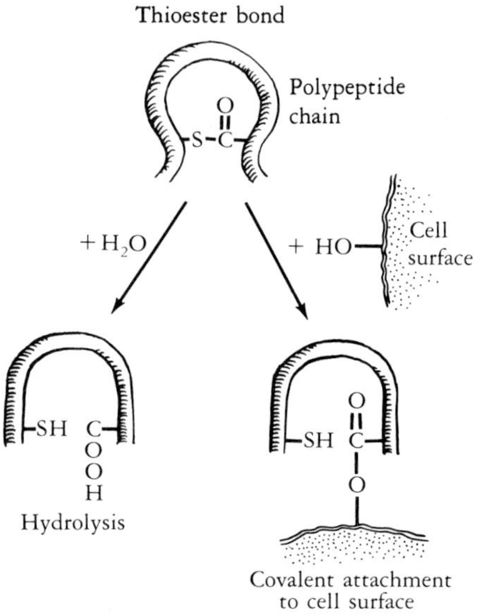

Figure 6–2. Schematic representation of the intramolecular thioester bond in C3 and C4, which upon cleavage to C3b or C4b, respectively, becomes highly reactive. Subsequent opening of this reactive bond by cell surface hydroxyl groups leads to covalent attachment of C3b or C4b to the cell surface. Prior opening of the bond by water (i.e., hydrolysis) prevents covalent attachment. In addition, slow hydrolysis of the thioester in native C3 is responsible for the activation of the alternative pathway (see text).

surface hydroxyl or amino group. This results in the covalent attachment of C3b or C4b to the target cell (Fig. 6–2). An additional function of the thioester bond is its hydrolysis by water, occurring during activation of the alternative pathway as described below.

The alternative pathway can be activated when a molecule of C3b is bound to a target cell. This C3b molecule combines with the plasma protein Factor B, which is a zymogen, and which, when bound to C3b, can be activated by the plasma protein Factor D by cleavage into two fragments, Ba and Bb. The Bb fragment, which contains the active enzymatic site, remains bound to C3b, as C3b,Bb. This complex, like C4b,2a in the classical pathway, is a C3 convertase (C3b,Bb); it is stabilized by the binding of another plasma protein, properdin. Thus, the alternative pathway used to be called the properdin pathway.

The presence of a single molecule of C3b generates many molecules of C3b,Bb, resulting in a tremendous amplification. The C3 convertase (C3b,Bb) cleaves C3, thereby generating more molecules of C3b, which can combine with other molecules of Factor B to give more molecules of C3b,Bb, which can, in turn, cleave more molecules of C3. Therefore, the central feature of the alternative pathway is a positive feedback loop that amplifies the original recognition event (Fig. 6–3). As in the classical pathway, attachment of many C3b molecules to the target cell will allow binding of C5 and its cleavage into C5a and C5b by the enzyme C3b,Bb, now referred to as C5 convertase.

Owing to the potential of this positive feedback loop to rapidly use up Factor B and C3, the positive feedback must be carefully regulated. There are two important regulatory proteins in plasma. The first protein, Factor H (formerly referred to as β1H), competes with Factor B for binding to C3b and also dissociates C3b,Bb into C3b and Bb. The second control protein, Factor I (formerly referred to as C3b inactivator), cleaves C3b that is bound to Factor H or to a similar protein found on the surface of the host cell. The resulting cleaved C3b, termed iC3b, can no longer form a C3 convertase. The action of these two control proteins prevents the consumption of Factor B and C3 in plasma; in addition, these two proteins inactivate C3b,Bb on host cell surfaces. In contrast, surfaces of many target cells, such as bacteria and other microorganisms, protect C3b,Bb

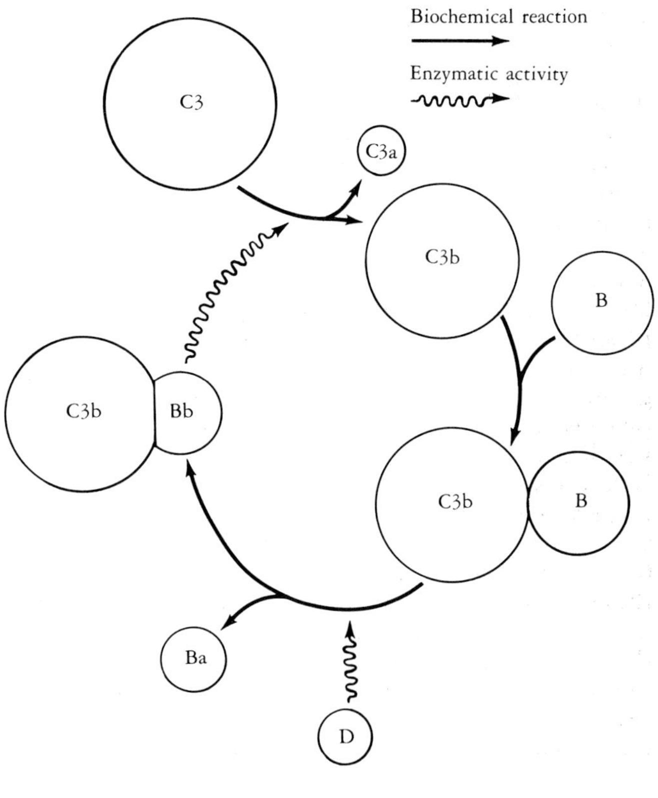

Figure 6–3. Schematic representation of the positive feedback loop of the alternative pathway.

Table 6–3. Activators of the Alternative Pathway

Polysaccharides (e.g., inulin)
Yeast cell walls (zymosan)
Bacterial cell wall components (lipopolysaccharide, peptidoglycan)
Influenza and other viruses
Schistosoma and other parasites
Cryptococci and other fungi
Certain tumor cells
Cobra venom factor
Nephritic factor (autoantibody that stabilizes C3b,Bb)
X-ray contrast media
Dialysis membranes

from inactivation by Factors H and I. This protection allows the positive feedback loop to proceed on the surface of the target cell, leading to the activation of the pathway and subsequent cell death. In other words, the alternative pathway is activated by those substances that prevent the inactivation of the positive feedback loop enzyme C3b,Bb. A substance is therefore treated as "foreign" if it restricts the action of Factors H and I and allows the positive feedback loop to continue. The chemical structures on surfaces of particles and cells responsible for activation or nonactivation of the alternative pathway have not been identified. There is some evidence that carbohydrate moieties are involved, particularly sialic acid. The alternative pathway protein(s) responsible for the recognition of these structures also remains to be determined. Table 6–3 lists known activators of the alternative pathway.

As pointed out earlier, the activation of the alternative pathway requires a C3b molecule bound to the surface of a target cell. An intriguing question is, "Where does the critical first C3b molecule come from?" Although it can be provided by the C3 convertase of the classical pathway or by cleavage of C3 by plasmin and certain bacterial and other cellular proteases, the alternative pathway can generate this first C3b molecule without these proteases. The intramolecular thioester, which is highly reactive in nascent C3b and is responsible for the covalent attachment to targets (see above), is also accessible in native C3 to water molecules (Fig. 6–2). Thus, spontaneous hydrolysis of the thioester bond occurs constantly in plasma at a low rate. The C3 molecules in which the thioester bond has been hydrolyzed behave like C3b, although the C3a domain has not been removed. C3 with a hydrolyzed thioester is called C3(H_2O) or C3b-like C3. It can bind Factor B and allow Factor D to activate Factor B, which results in formation of a fluid-phase C3 convertase, C3(H_2O),Bb. This enzyme is continuously formed and produces C3b molecules that can randomly attach to cells. Although these C3b molecules will be rapidly inactivated on host cells by Factors H and I, they will start the positive feedback loop on foreign surfaces, as outlined previously. In other words, the alternative pathway is constantly activated at a low rate, but amplification with subsequent cell death occurs only on foreign particles.

PRODUCTS OF COMPLEMENT ACTIVATION POSSESSING BIOLOGIC ACTIVITY

Activation of either the alternative or the classical pathway results in the generation of many important peptides involved in inflammatory responses (Table 6–4). The anaphy-

Table 6–4. Biologic Effects of Complement Activation Products

Substance	Biologic Activity
C3a	Smooth muscle contraction Increase of vascular permeability Degranulation of mast cells and basophils with release of histamine Degranulation of eosinophils Aggregation of platelets
C3b	Opsonization of particles and solubilization of immune complexes with subsequent facilitation of phagocytosis
C3e	Release of neutrophils from bone marrow resulting in leukocytosis
C4a	Smooth muscle contraction Increase of vascular permeability
C5a	Smooth muscle contraction Increase of vascular permeability Degranulation of mast cells and basophils with release of histamine Degranulation of eosinophils Aggregation of platelets Chemotaxis of basophils, eosinophils, neutrophils, and monocytes Release of hydrolytic enzymes from neutrophils
C5a-des-arg	Chemotaxis of neutrophils Release of hydrolytic enzymes from neutrophils
Bb	Inhibition of migration and induction of spreading of monocytes and macrophages

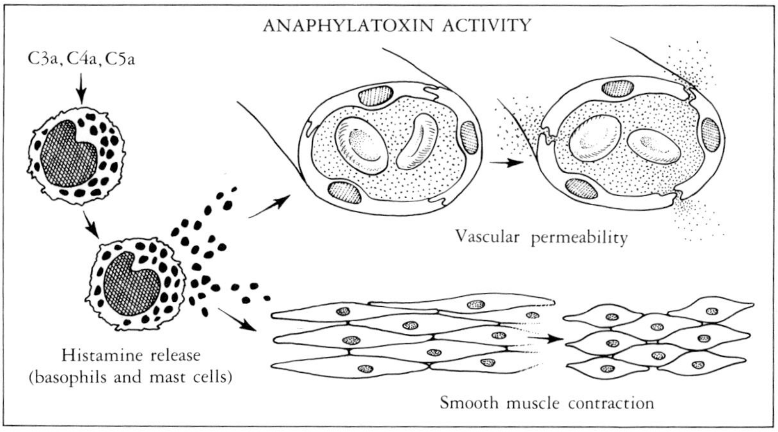

Figure 6–4. Anaphylatoxin activity of C3a, C4a, and C5a causing mediator release, e.g., histamine, from basophils and mast cells with subsequent smooth muscle contraction and alterations in vascular permeability.

latoxins C3a, C4a, and C5a are derived from the enzymatic cleavage of C3, C4, and C5 respectively. Historically, C3a and C5a were defined as factors derived from activated serum possessing spasmogenic activity. The anaphylatoxins are now recognized as having many additional biologic functions. Both C3a and C5a are known to induce the release of histamine from mast cells and basophils (Chapter 20A). As shown in Figure 6–4, both anaphylatoxins cause smooth muscle contraction and induce the release of vasoactive amines, which cause an increase in vascular permeability.

The effect of C5a anaphylatoxin on neutrophils is of considerable importance in the inflammatory response (Chapters 12 and 13). Not only can C5a induce neutrophil aggregation, but this anaphylatoxin appears to be the main chemotactic peptide generated by activation of either complement pathway (Fig. 6–5). *In vitro,* nanomolar concentrations of C5a will induce the unidirectional movement of neutrophils. Other inflammatory cells, such as monocytes, eosinophils, basophils, and macrophages, have also been shown to exhibit a chemotactic response to C5a. The removal of the carboxy-terminal arginine from C5a by serum carboxypeptidase N, generating C5a-des-arg, inactivates the spasmogen, yet restoration of full chemotactic activity of C5a-des-arg may occur in the presence of serum. Therefore, C5a-des-arg may also be responsible for *in vivo* neutrophil chemotactic activity.

As described earlier, the cleavage of C3 by either the alternative or the classical C3 convertases results in the production of two major split products, the C3a anaphylatoxin and C3b. The larger C3b fragment can serve as an opsonin (promoter of phagocytosis) by binding to a target through the thioester

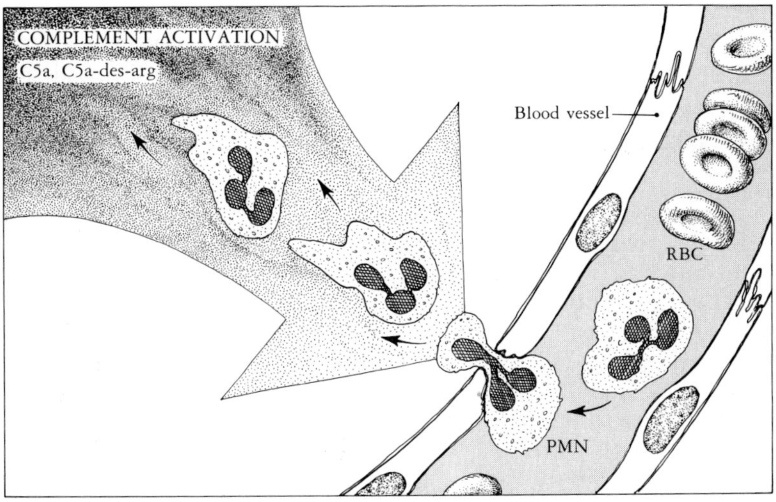

Figure 6–5. Schematic representation of unidirectional movement of neutrophils (chemotactic response) to C5a and C5a-des-arg generated by complement activation.

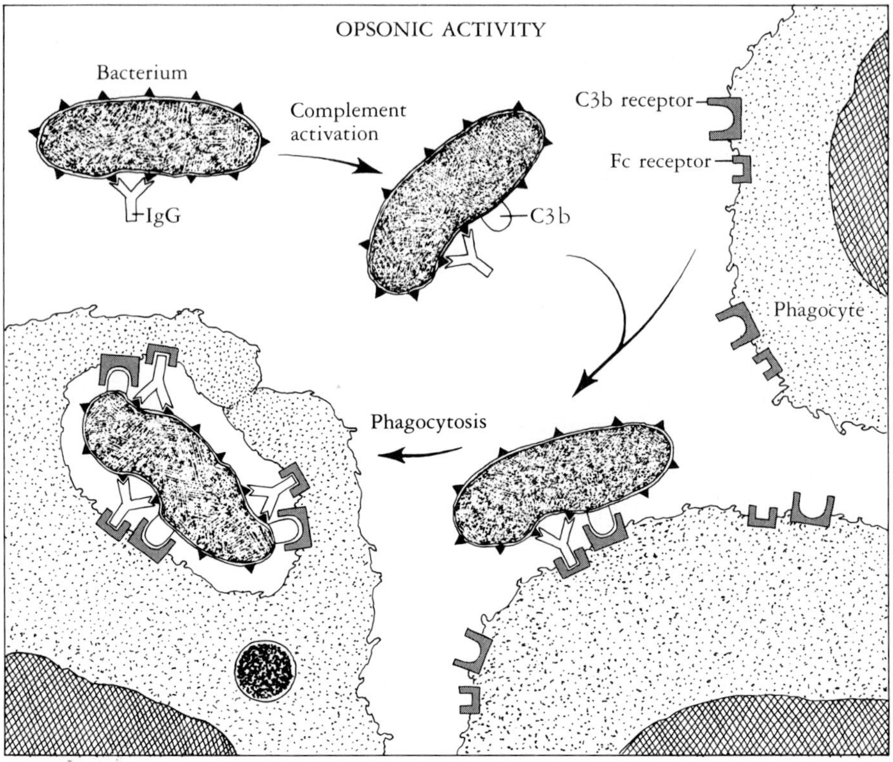

Figure 6–6. Schematic representation of the phagocytic-promoting activity (opsonin function) of complement, associated with the binding of C3b to cell surfaces.

mechanism. This renders the particle or cell immediately susceptible to ingestion by a variety of phagocytic cells that carry specific receptors for C3b (Fig. 6–6).

Many recent observations point to additional roles for complement fragments in regulating the activity of cells of the immune system. These observations include the presence of receptors on lymphocytes for various complement proteins, including C3 split products and Factor H, affecting B- and T-cell function. This is an important area for future research.

THE PATHWAY OF MEMBRANE ATTACK

The formation of C5b by the classical or alternative C5 convertase marks the initiation of the membrane attack pathway. Nascent C5b can bind to C6, resulting in the formation of the stable C5b,6 complex. Subsequently, C5b,6 reacts with C7 to form the trimolecular complex C5b,6,7, which exhibits a metastable binding site through which the complex can bind itself to the target cell membrane. Although the exact biochemical nature of this metastable binding site is unknown, it is believed that binding occurs through hydrophobic interactions with membrane lipids. Next, binding of C8 to the C5b,6,7 complex occurs on the cell membrane, which causes the transposition of C9 from the plasma into the target cell membrane by inducing a polymerization of C9. The polymerization of C9 in the membrane occurs typically in a circular fashion, inserting poly C9 cylinders consisting of about 12 to 16 C9 molecules. The poly C9 cylinders are responsible for the characteristic ring-like appearance of the complement lesions seen by electron microscopy (Fig. 6–7). The poly C9 with the attached C5b,6,7,8 complex is usually referred to as the membrane attack complex (MAC).

It has been established that the membranolytic action of the MAC is due entirely to physical interactions. The MAC is a hollow structure with an inner diameter of 100 Å; therefore, its insertion into the membrane results in transmembrane channels that are large enough to allow molecules the size of proteins to pass through. In addition, the

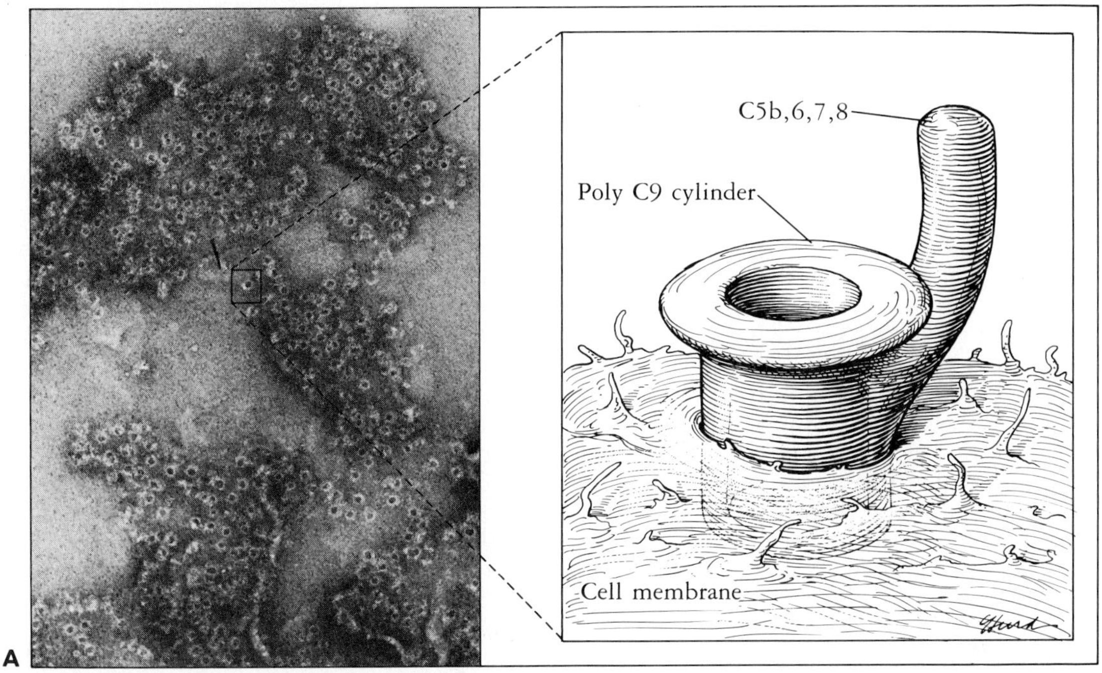

Figure 6–7. *A,* Electron micrograph of a membrane lysed by many membrane attack complexes (magnification approximately 130,000 ×). *B,* Schematic drawing of a MAC.

strong lipid-binding capability of the MAC results in disorganization of the phospholipid bilayer, causing impairment of membrane function. In the case of gram-negative bacteria, the peptidoglycan layer prevents MAC-mediated lysis. However, these bacteria are killed by the insertion of the MAC into the outer membrane. Lysis of these bacteria requires the presence of lysozyme, which can cleave the peptidoglycan.

REGULATORY MECHANISMS OF THE COMPLEMENT CASCADE

Activation of the complement cascade results in a complex series of molecular events with potent biologic consequences. Accordingly, modulating mechanisms are necessary to regulate complement activation and to control the production of biologically active split products.

The first mechanism by which the activity of many activated complement components is modulated is spontaneous decay. Examples of this mechanism are the transient stability of the activated thioester bond in C3b and C4b, and the short half-life of the enzymatically active complexes C4b,2a and C3b,Bb.

The second type of regulatory mechanism is the inactivation of certain components by proteolytic enzymes. For example, the plasma protease Factor I can, in the presence of certain cofactors (see below), inactivate C3b and C4b. A major mechanism for controlling the biologic activity of C3a and C5a anaphylatoxins is serum carboxypeptidase N, as described earlier. Another control protein that may exert a regulatory effect on the C5a anaphylatoxin is the chemotactic factor inactivator. Although the chemical basis of the inactivation is not known, this serum-derived factor appears to irreversibly inactivate many of the biologic activities of C5a.

A third mechanism of regulation involves specific binding proteins that modulate the activity of certain complement components. Examples are Factor H and C4b-binding-protein, which, when bound to C3b and C4b, respectively, make them susceptible to cleavage by Factor I. Another example is S-protein, which binds to the MAC if the MAC is assembling in plasma rather than on a target cell. Binding of the S-protein to the MAC abrogates its ability to attach to a cell membrane, thus limiting attachment of MAC to cells at the site of complement activation. Another important binding protein is C1 esterase inhibitor (C1 INA), which regulates activation of the classical pathway by forming irreversible complexes with C1r and C1s. Patients who lack C1 INA or who possess it in a nonfunctional form suffer from hereditary angioedema (Chapter 20A). They present with episodes of angioedema, which are life-threatening if they involve the larynx. Because C1 INA also inactivates activated kallikrein and Hageman factor, it is difficult to determine which of these enzymes causes the release of mediators most relevant in clinical episodes of angioedema in patients with deficiency of C1 INA.

Modulation of the activity of complement is also achieved by regulation of its synthesis. Cells that can synthesize these components are present at sites of inflammation, thereby helping to prevent complement depletion at the site of complement activation. The importance of complement in inflammation is further evidenced by the finding that certain complement proteins (e.g., C3 and C9) are acute-phase reactants; that is, their synthesis is increased during inflammation, resulting in higher plasma concentrations.

COMPLEMENT-DEPENDENT REACTIONS RESULTING IN TISSUE INJURY

Complement activation is responsible for tissue injury in the pathogenesis of certain diseases. Two major causes of complement-mediated pathogenesis are activation by autoantibodies and activation by immune complexes (Chapter 20A).

Autoantibodies may arise secondary to tissue damage or infection or by mechanisms that are not understood. The binding of an autoantibody will direct complement activation against the host's target tissue. This is the mechanism of tissue injury in Goodpasture's syndrome, in which autoantibodies to glomerular, tubular, and alveolar basement membranes are present. Autoantibodies to the acetylcholine receptor in the postsynaptic membrane of the motor end plate cause myasthenia gravis. Autoimmune hemolytic anemias and thrombocytopenias are caused by autoantibodies to erythrocytes and platelets. Autoantibodies to streptococcal antigens cross reacting with antigens of host tissues seem to be involved in the pathogenesis of rheumatic myocarditis and endocarditis.

Activation of complement in the walls of the small vessels and capillaries by immune complexes, either locally formed or deposited from the circulation, leads to tissue injury and inflammation causing vasculitis. This immunopathologic mechanism is known as the Arthus reaction (Chapter 13) and has been shown to be the pathogenesis of serum sickness and hypersensitivity pneumonitis. Circulating immune complexes are found in a variety of diseases, including infections, neoplasms, and autoimmune disorders. In rheumatoid arthritis, immune complex deposition in the synovial membranes causes polyarthritis. In patients with systemic lupus erythematosus, skin lesions, polyarthritis, myocarditis, polyserositis, and glomerulonephritis are the clinical manifestations of immune complex deposition. The renal glomeruli are the most common site of immune complex deposition causing glomerulonephritis. This is the mechanism of renal injury in Schönlein-Henoch purpura, in poststreptococcal glomerulonephritis, and in other acute glomerulonephritides.

In a form of membranoproliferative glomerulonephritis associated with low levels of C3, the nephrotoxic effects seem to be due to an autoantibody, called nephritic factor, which stabilizes C3b,Bb, resulting in chronic activation of the alternative pathway, which leads to tissue injury.

In paroxysmal nocturnal hemoglobinuria, an acquired alteration in the erythrocyte membrane leads to a slower decay of C3b,Bb on the surface of these cells. The erythrocytes therefore exhibit an increased susceptibility to complement-mediated lysis.

Among substances that have been found to provide activating surfaces for complement are nylon fibers and membranes used in hemodialysis and cardiopulmonary bypass. The released anaphylatoxins are thought to contribute to adverse reactions frequently seen in patients after extracorporeal circulation.

Finally, cobra venom contains a protein called cobra venom factor (CVF), which activates the alternative pathway by a unique mechanism. CVF is an analog of C3b. Like C3b, it forms a C3 convertase, CVF,Bb. This C3 convertase is resistant to inactivation by Factors H and I. Consequently, the enzyme will continuously activate C3 and thereby consume complement.

COMPLEMENT AND INFECTION

The bactericidal power of the complement system was demonstrated by the killing of laboratory strains of *E. coli* by a mixture of the purified complement proteins of the alternative and membrane attack pathways. The ability to destroy such organisms, without waiting for the synthesis of specific antibody, provides an immediate mechanism of defense. However, bacteria have evolved ways to protect themselves against the complement system. For example, most clinical isolates of *E. coli* (e.g., from neonatal coliform meningitis) are not killed by the alternative pathway. The resistance of these bacteria is due to the fact that their lipopolysaccharide coat, which would otherwise activate the alternative pathway, is hidden under a capsular polysaccharide. This capsular polysaccharide does not provide an activating surface. Thus, the classical pathway, activated by antibody that binds to the capsular polysaccharide, is needed to kill these organisms.

Similarly, viruses can activate, and be inactivated by, complement in the presence or absence of antibody. For many viruses, inactivation requires only the early complement components C1, C4, and C2, whereas other viruses are inactivated by MAC-mediated lysis.

Parasites, such as schistosomes, can activate complement by the alternative pathway in the absence of antibody. The resultant coating of these organisms by C3b has been found to greatly stimulate their killing by eosinophils.

Tumor cells have been shown to be susceptible to killing initiated through the alternative and classical complement pathways. C3b can be demonstrated on tumor cells *in vivo.*

All microorganisms can activate complement through the classical pathway once specific antibody of the appropriate class is available. A representative list of non–antibody-dependent methods of activation by a variety of organisms is given in Tables 6–2 and 6–3.

COMPLEMENT DEFICIENCIES

Deficiencies of complement components can be divided into congenital and acquired deficiencies of complement components and their inhibitors. Acquired multicomponent deficiencies are associated with circulating immune complexes, such as in systemic lupus erythematosus (Chapter 20C). This disease is characterized by low C1, C4, C2, and C3 levels in the early stages, with a return toward normal levels as the disease activity diminishes. As described earlier, low levels of C3 are seen in hypocomplementemic membranoproliferative glomerulonephritis. Genetic deficiencies of most complement components have also been described. The most common defect found in humans is a deficiency in C2. Although rare, deficiency states of other complement components have been reported (Table 6–5). Patients with a deficiency of an early component of the classical pathway often possess symptoms associated with connective tissue disease. Patients with a genetic deficiency in one of the terminal components (e.g., C8) have an increased susceptibility to *Neisseria* infections, while patients deficient in C3 or C5 present mainly with pyogenic infections. This points to different mechanisms of complement-depend-

Table 6–5. **Genetic Complement Deficiencies**

Component	Clinical Appearance
C1q	Systemic lupus erythematosus–like syndrome
C1r	Systemic lupus erythematosus–like syndrome
C1s	Systemic lupus erythematosus–like syndrome
C4	Systemic lupus erythematosus–like syndrome
C2	Systemic lupus erythematosus–like syndrome
C3	Severe recurrent pyogenic infections
C5	Recurrent infections (pyogenic, neisserial, and others), Leiner's disease, systemic lupus erythematosus–like syndrome
C6	Recurrent neisserial infections
C7	Recurrent neisserial infections
C8	Recurrent neisserial infections
C9	Apparently healthy
Factor H	Hemolytic uremic syndrome, infections
Factor I	Recurrent infections
Properdin	Recurrent neisserial infections
C1 Inhibitor	Hereditary angioedema
Carboxypeptidase N	Recurrent angioedema

ent control of these organisms. As described previously, a genetic deficiency of C1 esterase inhibitor manifests itself as the syndrome called hereditary angioedema. During an episode of angioedema, activated C1 is found in serum accompanied by a decrease in C4 and C2, while serum levels of C3 and the terminal complement components remain in the normal range.

AN OVERVIEW

The complement system has evolved essentially for protective functions. The complement system fulfills three major roles in host defense: first, coating of pathogenic organisms or immune complexes with opsonins, resulting in their removal by phagocytes; second, activation of inflammatory cells; third, killing of target cells. Activation of these biologic functions can occur by the classical or the alternative pathway. Both pathways exhibit a similar molecular organization: An initial recognition event is amplified, resulting in the generation of many effector molecules. Owing to the potentially destructive consequences to the host of uncontrolled complement action, this system is tightly regulated. Regulatory mechanisms include the inherently transient stability of certain activated complement components (generation of metastable binding sites, rapid decay of the convertases) and modulation of activities by regulatory proteins (binding to or limited proteolysis of activated components). All regulatory mechanisms are directed toward a common goal: to confine the effects of complement to the site of activation, thereby preventing generalized activation with potentially harmful effects on host cells. Just as the coagulation system may suddenly proceed through its activation sequence in an unchecked manner, resulting in the serious consequences of intravascular coagulation, the complement system, although tightly regulated, is involved in the pathogenesis of disease. Complement activation due to recognition of autoantibodies or tissue deposits of immune complexes will direct the response against the host's own tissues. Both acquired and inherited deficiencies of complement have been described. Common clinical manifestations of inherited complement deficiencies are recurrent infections and immune complex diseases; this demonstrates the importance of complement in the control of pathogenic organisms and in the removal of immune complexes.

Thus, complement can be considered as an array of proteins composing a tightly regulated system that is centrally involved in the initiation and coordination of the molecular and cellular response of a host to invasive foreign substances.

Suggestions for Further Reading

Esser, A. F.: Interactions between complement proteins and biological and model membranes. *In* Chapman, D. (ed.): Biological Membranes. Vol. 4. New York, Academic Press, 1982, pp. 277–325.

Fearon, D. T., and Austen, K. F.: The alternative pathway of complement—a system for host resistance to microbial infection. N. Engl. J. Med., *303*:259, 1980.

Hugli, T. E.: The structural basis for anaphylatoxin and chemotactic functions of C3a, C4a, and C5a. CRC Crit. Rev. Immunol., *1*:321, 1981.

Müller-Eberhard, H. J., and Schreiber, R. D.: Molecular biology and chemistry of the alternative pathway of complement. Adv. Immunol., *29*:1, 1980.

Porter, R. R.: Interactions of complement components with antibody-antigen aggregates and cell surfaces. Immunol. Today, *2*:143, 1981.

Reid, K. B. M., and Porter, R. R.: The proteolytic activation systems of complement. Annu. Rev. Biochem., *50*:433, 1981.

Ward, P. A.: Leukotaxis and leukotactic disorders. Am. J. Pathol., *77*:519, 1974.

Chapter 7

Immunophysiology: Cell Function and Cellular Interactions in Antibody Formation

Herbert B. Herscowitz, Ph.D.

INITIATION OF THE SPECIFIC IMMUNE RESPONSE

Individuals may acquire specific immunity either (1) through natural exposure by infection or immunization with specific agents or their products (*active immunity*); or (2) by the passive acquisition of preformed antibody, specifically sensitized lymphocytes, or their products, e.g., transfer factor (*passive immunity*). The fundamental differences between active and passive immunity are shown in Table 7–1.

Active Immunity

The acquisition of active immunity depends upon the participation of host tissues and cells after an encounter with the immunogen. It involves differentiation and proliferation of immunocompetent cells in lymphoreticular tissues, which lead to synthesis of antibody or the development of cell-mediated reactivity, or both. This type of immunity appears only after a specified time lapse subsequent to exposure to the immunogen. The duration of active immunity is relatively long and can be measured in terms of months or years, in some cases. This type of immunity results from natural exposure to immunogens by infection or through the use of vaccines (Chapter 23).

Passive Immunity

Passive immunity may result from the transfer of serum-containing antibodies or products from specifically sensitized cells obtained from an immunized host to a nonimmune individual. Since this type of immunity

Table 7–1. Comparison of Active and Passive Immunity

	Active	Passive
Genesis:	Active host participation after exposure to immunogen either naturally (subclinical or clinical disease) or by immunization (vaccine)	No host participation; transfer of preformed substances (antibody, transfer factor, thymic graft, interleukin-2) from an actively immunized host to a nonimmune host
Components:	Humoral and cell-mediated immunity	Humoral and cell-mediated immunity
Onset of action:	Only after a latent period	Immediate
Duration:	Long-lived	Transitory
Application:	Vaccination	Immune deficiency, prophylaxis

involves the transfer of preformed substances, the onset of its action is immediate; however, because there may be no stimulus for continued production, its effect is usually of short duration. The passive transfer of immunity (specific IgG antibodies) from mother to fetus and the use of transfer factor in immunotherapy are examples of passive immunity. Prior to antibiotic therapy it was common practice to transfer pooled serum from individuals containing specific antibodies to certain infectious agents to susceptible hosts. Although this is generally no longer practiced, passive transfer of preformed antibodies against venoms and toxins is still used in some situations.

RESPONSE OF THE HOST: THE FATE OF IMMUNOGEN

Foreign substances either may enter the body naturally or may be introduced artificially. Most frequently, they gain entrance through the respiratory or gastrointestinal tract, although they may enter naturally through any body surface, including the mucous membranes and skin, or by transplacental passage. Artificial introduction of foreignness occurs by injection (e.g., vaccination) or by surgical intervention (e.g., transplantation).

An interesting and potentially clinically important observation has been made in animals given large amounts of protein antigen by the oral route. Animals treated this way do not produce specific antibodies after systemic challenge with the same antigen. This induced lack of ability to respond, called *tolerance* (Chapter 10), is thought to be due to the appearance of antigen-specific suppressor T-cells in the Peyer's patches. The suppressor cells or soluble suppressor factors exert their influence in peripheral lymphoid tissue (e.g., spleen), where they inhibit the production of IgM and IgG antibodies without affecting the secretory IgA response. These cells also appear to inhibit the development of delayed-type hypersensitivity to the same antigen. These observations served as the basis for the design of a protocol to treat severely Rh-immunized pregnant women in an attempt to save their fetuses. A group of women were given daily oral administration of extracts of Rh+ erythrocyte membranes. In all cases, the anti-Rh antibody titers of the women did not increase during gestation and all of them delivered live-born infants, whereas each had previously experienced stillbirth or intrauterine fetal death secondary to Rh sensitization. Thus, a potentially clinically useful modality can be achieved by manipulating the mode of antigen administration.

Metabolic Fate

The *in vivo* fate of an immunogen can be followed by the use of radioactively labeled materials. Following intravenous injection of the foreign substance (e.g., human serum albumin) into a rabbit, three phases of antigen disappearance are distinguishable (Fig. 7–1). The first phase involves the *equilibration* of the foreign material between the intravascular and the extravascular space by a process of diffusion. This phase is relatively rapid for a diffusible substance and is of similar duration whether the injected material is autologous or foreign. Particulate immunogens (e.g., bacteria or erythrocytes), when injected into animals, are ingested by phagocytic cells and do not diffuse into the extravascular space. Thus, there is no initial equilibration phase.

The second stage of antigen clearance, referred to as *catabolism*, occurs over a period of several days and involves the gradual degradation and digestion of the material. The actual duration of this phase is determined

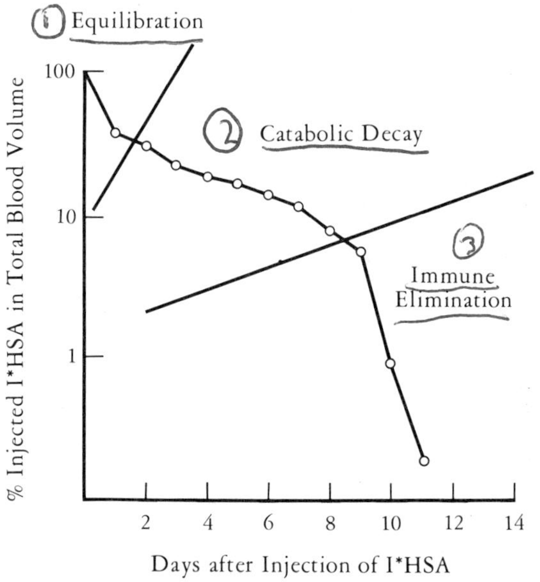

Figure 7–1. Rate of elimination of radiolabeled immunogen from blood.

by both the biologic half-life of the material and the enzymatic capabilities of the host for the particular type of substance. Certain substances will remain in the circulation for fairly long periods of time if the host is deficient in the metabolic machinery required for their degradation (e.g., poly D-amino acids, polysaccharide).

In the third phase of clearance, there is a further rapid removal of the antigen, referred to as *immune elimination*. This stage results from the appearance of newly synthesized antibody that combines with the circulating antigen, leading to the formation of antigen-antibody complexes that are phagocytized and degraded. These antigen-antibody complexes, particularly when formed in antigen excess, have clinical significance, since they may induce tissue injury (Chapter 13). Following the third phase, free antibody appears in the serum. Although the curve shown in Figure 7–1 reflects almost complete elimination of the immunogen, absolute removal may take weeks, months, or years, if it ever occurs. Thus, persistence of a portion of the immunogen may provide continued stimulus to the cells involved in the immune response.

Organ Distribution of Immunogen

When injected intravenously, the immunogen is initially found at sites where fixed phagocytic cells are numerous, e.g., liver, spleen, bone marrow, kidney, and lung. When injected by other routes (e.g., intradermally), the major portion of the material either remains at the site of administration or is localized in the draining lymph node. The physicochemical properties of the injected material determine the degree of localization in the lymph node. For example, particulate materials (e.g., viruses) are more effectively retained in the lymph node than are soluble substances (e.g., human serum albumin).

Foreign substances most frequently enter the body via the gastrointestinal and respiratory tracts, where they become localized in lymphoid tissue, resulting primarily in the production of IgE and secretory IgA antibodies.

Cellular Distribution of Immunogen

Most immunogens are readily taken up by the endocytic processes (*phagocytosis* or *pinocytosis*) of the cells of the *mononuclear phagocyte system* within the body. Macrophages in the medullary cords of lymph nodes and in the red pulp of the spleen remove much of the injected material in animals that have not previously been exposed to the foreign substance. In previously immunized animals, the immunogen can be found associated with dendritic cells located in the follicles of the lymph node cortex. The immunogen appears to be retained, to a large extent, extracellularly between the membranes of dendritic cells. The ability of these cells to retain the immunogen appears to be dependent upon the presence of antibody.

There is conflicting information regarding the precise cellular location of endocytosed material because of the breakdown of internally labeled proteins used in these studies and the reutilization of the radiolabeled amino acids into new cellular components. Immunogenic material has been reported to be localized within the cytoplasm in small or large lysosomal granules, on the cell membrane, and in association with ribonucleic acid. It should be pointed out that there is still some controversy about the phagocytic function of macrophages in the immune response. While some investigators feel that the major function of the macrophage is to degrade and eliminate the foreign configuration, there is compelling evidence to indicate that this cell is necessary for the "processing" of foreign substances for presentation to lymphocytes in a form that will initiate the immune response.

ANTIBODY FORMATION IN THE INDIVIDUAL

Primary Response

The injection of a single dose of a foreign substance into an immunocompetent animal will cause specific antibody to appear in the serum after a definite time lapse. First exposure to an immunogen evokes the *primary response* (Fig. 7–2). Immediately after introduction of the immunogen, little or no anti-

primary- antigen comes in contact with an immunocompetent cell.

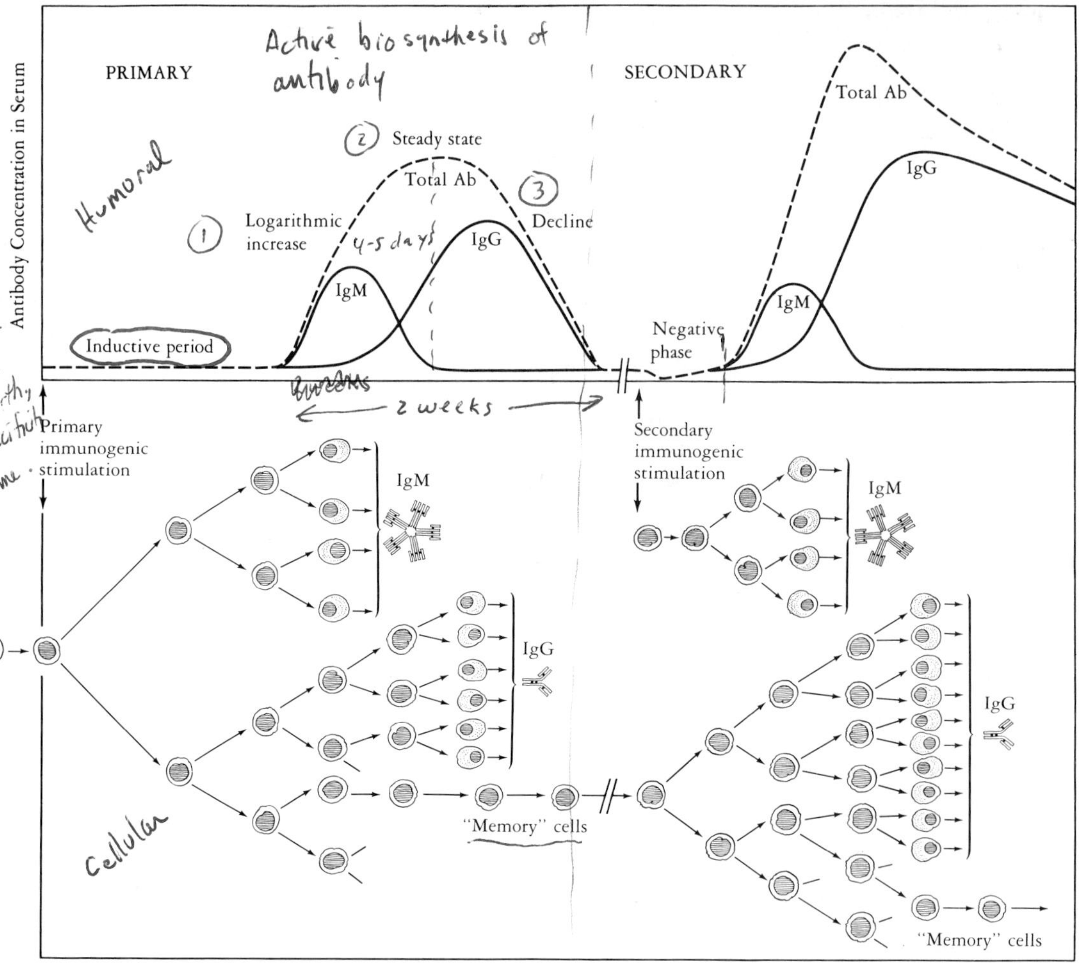

Figure 7–2. Schematic representation of humoral and cellular events in the primary and secondary (anamnestic) antibody responses.

body is detected in the serum. This period is referred to as the *inductive* or *latent* period. It is during this time that the immunogen is recognized as foreign and is processed, and an unknown signal is transferred to the appropriate cells destined to make antibody. This period is characterized by cellular proliferation and differentiation. The duration of this period is variable and depends upon (1) the immunogenicity, quantity, form, and solubility of the stimulant; (2) the animal species into which it is injected; (3) the route of immunization; and (4) the sensitivity of the assay used to detect the newly formed antibody. For example, antibodies can be detected three to four days after the injection of foreign erythrocytes (e.g., transfusion reaction), five to seven days after soluble proteins, and 10 to 14 days after bacterial cells.

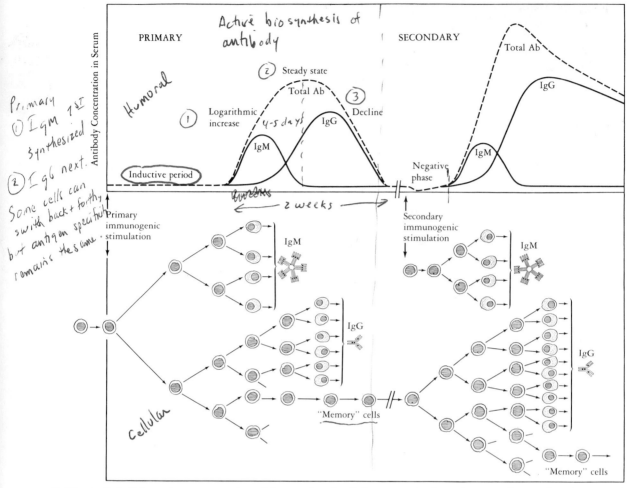

Following the appearance of the first antibody at the end of the induction period, there is a time of active biosynthesis of antibody that can be further subdivided into three phases. In the first, the *logarithmic* phase, the antibody concentration increases logarithmically for four to ten days, again depending upon the nature of the immunogen, until it reaches a peak. During this phase the doubling time (that time required to achieve a twofold increase in serum antibody concentration) has been reported to be as short as five to eight hours. Peak antibody titers against heterologous erythrocytes are usually attained in four to five days; against soluble proteins, in 8 to 12 days; and against toxoids prepared from toxins of gram-positive bacilli (e.g., *Corynebacterium diphtheriae*), in as long as two to three months. On a cellular basis, the number of differentiated plasma cells increases soon after immunization, while peak cellular synthesis of antibody precedes the peak serum antibody response by several days.

The level of circulating antibody attained after primary immunization is a reflection of the difference between the antibody's rates of synthesis and catabolism. When these rates are the same the serum antibody concentration is constant, as shown in Figure 7–2 as a *plateau* or *steady state*. This phase of the response is highly transitory and in some cases almost nonexistent. The rate of antibody synthesis is dependent upon the number of antibody-forming cells, which can be influenced by the conditions of immunization. The rate of antibody catabolism, however, is a reflection of the half-life of the class of immunoglobulin (Chapter 5).

Finally, a *decline* phase is observed, in which the rate of antibody catabolism is greater than that of its synthesis. The duration of this phase is also variable, since there may be varying degrees of difference between rates of synthesis and catabolism.

The early primary response to most immunogens is characterized by the predominance of IgM antibody; the IgG class of antibody appears somewhat later. IgM antibody production is usually transient, and within two weeks after the initiation of the immune response, IgG antibody predominates. Whether or not IgM antibodies are always produced in greater quantity before their corresponding IgG counterparts is subject to question. The basis for this controversy is the fact that the IgM antibody is more readily detectable because of the greater sensitivity of the IgM assay methods. Administration of the immunogen in adjuvant (Chapter 10) usually results in the continued synthesis of both IgM and IgG antibodies for several months.

The antibodies formed early in the immune response usually have a low *affinity* (the attractive force between complementary conformational sites on the antibody and antigen that causes them to combine); the affinity of late antibodies is usually greatly increased. Differences in affinity are readily observed with IgG antibodies since such changes can be a thousand fold. In addition to increases in affinity with the passage of time, there is also an increase in *avidity* (the strength of the binding of antibody to antigen); in other words, antigen-antibody complexes formed with late antisera are less dissociable. These changes are related to the diverse antigenic determinants on the immunogen that give rise to a variety of antibody specificities, which appear after different latent periods. As a consequence of these changes, the *cross reactivity* of a given antiserum also increases with time, probably owing to the fact that high-affinity antibodies can react with closely related antigenic determinants more readily than their low-affinity counterparts can. The compilation of all of these changes exemplifies the fact that the humoral immune response is *heterogeneous*, the manifestation of a population of antibodies with differences in Ig class, affinity, avidity, and specificity.

Secondary Response

Upon a second exposure to the same immunogen, weeks, months, or even years later, there is a markedly enhanced response that is characterized by the accelerated appearance of immunocompetent cells and antibody (Fig. 7–2). If antibody is still present in the serum at the time of the second injection of immunogen, it disappears at a faster rate than in the decline phase of the primary response. This *negative phase* is due to the immediate reaction of pre-existing antibody with newly injected immunogen, resulting in the formation of antigen-antibody complexes. If the second dose of immunogen is very small, an enhanced immune response may not occur, possibly because all of the newly injected immunogen is consumed in antigen-antibody complexes, phagocytized, and effectively removed, so that the antibody-forming cells are deprived of a stimulus. However, if the dose of immunogen is sufficient to allow the material that remains after complex formation to stimulate the immune system, then a typical *secondary* (*anamnestic* or *recall*) response is initiated. This enhanced response serves as the principle for giving booster doses of vaccines (Chapter 23).

The differences between the primary and secondary responses are summarized in Table 7–2. In contrast to the primary response, the secondary response is characterized by a shorter latent period, a more rapid rate of antibody synthesis, and a higher peak titer of antibody that persists for a longer period of time. The shorter latent period and more rapid rate of antibody synthesis, in spite of the fact that doubling times are similar in primary and secondary responses, are related to the number of antigen-sensitive cells,

affinity - attractive force
avidity - strength of binding

Table 7–2. **Relative Differences Between Primary and Secondary Response**

	Primary	Secondary
Latent period	Long	Short
Rate of antibody synthesis	Low	High
Peak antibody titer	Low	High
Persistence of antibody titer	Short	Long
Affinity of antibody	Low	High
Crossreactivity of antibody	Low	High
Presence of memory cells	Few (?)	Many
Predominating Ig class	IgM	IgG
Dose of immunogen to elicit	High	Low

called *memory cells,* present at the time of secondary stimulation. The scheme presented in Figure 7–2 shows that upon primary stimulation the precursor cell divides and differentiates into a number of antibody-forming cells producing either IgM or IgG immunoglobulins. During this process, a small number of memory cells are also produced. Following secondary challenge the proliferative events appear qualitatively similar, but the number of antigen-sensitive cells is greatly increased over that present in the primary response; the result is a greater pool of antibody-forming cells, and thus an increased amount of antibody is synthesized. Serum antibody formed in the secondary response may reach levels as high as 10 to 12 mg per ml and is predominantly of the IgG class, although some IgM is also expressed.

The dose of immunogen required to elicit a secondary response is far less than that required for the initiation of the primary response. Again, this is related to the number of antigen-sensitive cells bearing high-avidity receptors available for secondary stimulation and to the presence of circulating antibody remaining from the primary response. This circulating antibody will form complexes with the newly introduced material; antigen-antibody complexes formed in antigen excess are extremely immunogenic. The magnitude of the secondary response depends on other factors, including the interval between stimuli. Both short and long intervals result in decreased responses, the former because of the complete removal of immunogen and the latter possibly as a result of cell senescence. Immunologic memory may persist for many years and thereby provide long-lasting immunity against infection. Indeed, in the case of some bacterial and viral infections, immunity to reinfection may be lifelong. It is postulated that this immunity is related to the restimulation of long-lived memory cells by persisting antigen or newly introduced antigen. As in the primary response, antibody produced late in the secondary response has higher avidity and affinity for antigen than does that synthesized earlier. Late antibodies also appear to exhibit broad specificity. This may be attributed to the appearance of antibodies against certain antigenic determinants that do not stimulate antibodies early in the response (e.g., minor antigenic determinants). Therefore, the apparently broader specificity occurs because late antibodies exhibit a greater degree of *cross reactivity* with structurally related substances than do early antibodies.

A secondary response can be initiated by an immunogen that is closely related to the primary stimulating agent. In this case, the major portion of the antibodies produced will react more effectively with the first than with the second immunogen. This phenomenon, referred to as *the doctrine of original antigenic sin,* was first noted in studies of the response to influenza virus. It was observed that booster immunization with influenza vaccines induced antibodies that were directed mainly against strains of the virus that the individual had previously experienced, and the immune response to the booster vaccine was weaker. A possible explanation for this phenomenon is that the high-affinity antibody-forming cells are selectively stimulated in a population consisting of both low- and high-affinity antibody-producing cells.

Immunologic Memory

It appears that both B- and T-cells display immunologic memory. This finding was obtained from studies of cell cooperation in the immune response to hapten-carrier complexes. Although the hapten-carrier conjugates used in these studies may be considered unnatural immunogens, they are, in fact, true analogs of antigens that occur in nature, since the latter are also composed of multiple antigenic determinants, each of which can be considered a hapten. Under ordinary circumstances, when an animal is given a primary immunization with a hapten-protein conjugate, e.g., dinitrophenyl coupled to bovine serum albumin (DNP-BSA), and then is given a second injection of the same immunogen at a later time, antibodies against the hapten

(DNP) are formed at a rate typical of the secondary response (Fig. 7–3*A*). If the second injection is given with DNP coupled to a non–cross-reacting protein carrier, e.g., ovalbumin (OA), a secondary anti-DNP response is not usually manifested (Fig. 7–3*B*). However, if the animal that receives the second injection of DNP-OA has been previously primed with OA itself, then a substantial anti-DNP response will be elicited (Fig. 7–3*C*). This phenomenon, referred to as the *carrier effect,* suggests that recognition of both hapten and carrier is required for the secondary response. Further experiments have shown that T-cells recognize the carrier determinant and B-cells are responsible for recognition of the hapten.

The carrier effect is not always operative in secondary anti-hapten responses. In some cases, up to two years after animals have been given a primary injection with DNP-BSA, a potent secondary anti-DNP response can be induced with DNP coupled to a non–cross-reacting carrier, such as hemocyanin. This suggests that memory resides in B-cells. Evidence for T-cell memory comes from the inability of the so-called T-independent antigens (e.g., lipopolysaccharide, pneumococcal polysaccharide) to induce a secondary IgG response. Further, data obtained from studies with the congenitally athymic mouse strain (nude, nu/nu) suggest that T-cells regulate secondary responses of the IgG class.

Secondary stimulation of the immune response is not entirely without untoward effects, especially when soluble immunogens or haptens capable of binding to autologous substances are used. A portion of the anti-

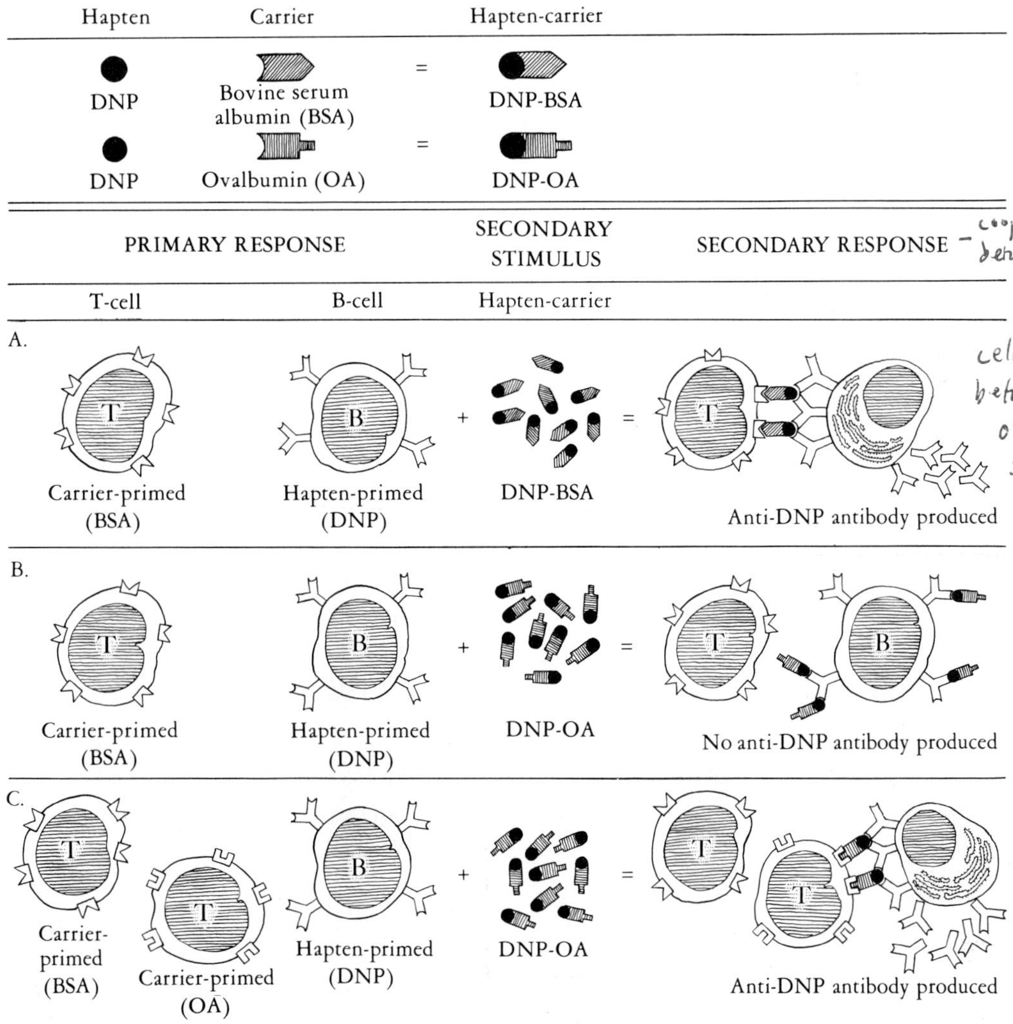

Figure 7–3. Schematic representation of carrier effect in the secondary antihapten antibody response.

body produced, as well as certain classes of antibody (e.g., IgE) made following primary stimulation, has the ability to fix to tissue cells. These cell-associated antibodies can bind the secondarily injected antigen, and, in some instances, this event can initiate a series of reactions that may be injurious or lethal to the individual. This antibody-mediated tissue injury is based on a secondary response and is further described in Chapters 13 and 20.

CELLULAR EVENTS INVOLVED IN THE SPECIFIC IMMUNE RESPONSE

Functional Cells

Much of our current information regarding the nature of cells and cellular interactions involved in the immune response has been obtained from studies of the "experiments of nature" that take the form of human immune deficiency diseases (Chapter 22). The results of these studies have shown that there is a functional division of the immune system involving two lines of immunocompetent cells, one concerned with humoral immunity and the other with cell-mediated immunity. Although the early events occurring in the *afferent* arm of both divisions are essentially similar, as depicted in Figure 7–4, the products of the *efferent* arm are different; specific antibody is the product of *humoral immunity,* and specifically sensitized lymphocytes and their lymphokines are the products of *cell-mediated immunity* (Chapter 9).

According to our current knowledge, both lymphocytes and macrophages are involved in the immune response. There are two major types of lymphocytes that are morphologically indistinguishable. These antigen-specific cells, which act upon stimulation of surface membrane receptors, have been classified on the basis of their site of differentiation into *thymus-derived* (*T-cells*) and *bursa- or bone marrow–derived* (*B-cells*) (Chapter 3). In addition to there being differences in functional capabilities between the two major classes of lymphocytes, there is also functional diversity among lymphocytes of the same class. For example, T-cells in both humans and mice can be further classified into *helper* and *suppressor* or *regulatory* and *effector* subpopulations. Similarly, B-cells exhibit functional diversity based on the different classes of immunoglobulin that they synthesize.

Macrophages have a wide variety of functions in the immune response that are also thought to be associated with distinct functional subpopulations. These cells, which function as *accessory cells (A-cells),* are not specific for a given immunogen. In addition to their function as "antigen-presenting cells," macrophages secrete a variety of biologically active mediators (*monokines*), which regulate the response of both B- and T-cells either by augmenting or by suppressing cell division and/or differentiation. Tables 7–3 and 7–4 summarize some of the major properties of these cell types.

Lymphocytes

Lymphocyte precursors arise in the bone marrow from pleuripotent stem cells, pass through the blood stream, and enter the central lymphoid organs where further development takes place (Chapter 2). Those cells that enter the thymus (thymocytes) may be modified therein or may pass through the organ and be eliminated. It has been suggested that maturation of T-lymphocytes in the thymus may be influenced by one of several soluble hormones elaborated by the epithelial cells of the thymus, e.g., *thymosin.* It has also been suggested that macrophages or their soluble products have an influence on lymphocyte differentiation in the thymus. Evidence for a thymic humoral factor is derived from experiments in which animals made immunologically deficient by removal of the thymus were rendered immunologically competent after transplantation of fetal thymus tissue contained within a cell-impermeable chamber. Attempts have been made to use thymic factors to reconstitute immunologic competence to humans having congenital T-cell defects, with some reported success (Chapter 22).

Precursors of B-lymphocytes, which are also of bone marrow origin, may go directly to the peripheral lymphoid tissue or may first pass through or be influenced by the liver, bone marrow, appendix, intestines, or tonsils in order to develop into functional B-cells. Evidence for the existence of an organ analogous to the bursa of Fabricius of birds is missing in mammalian species (Chapter 2).

In spite of their different maturation pathways, only in recent years, through the de-

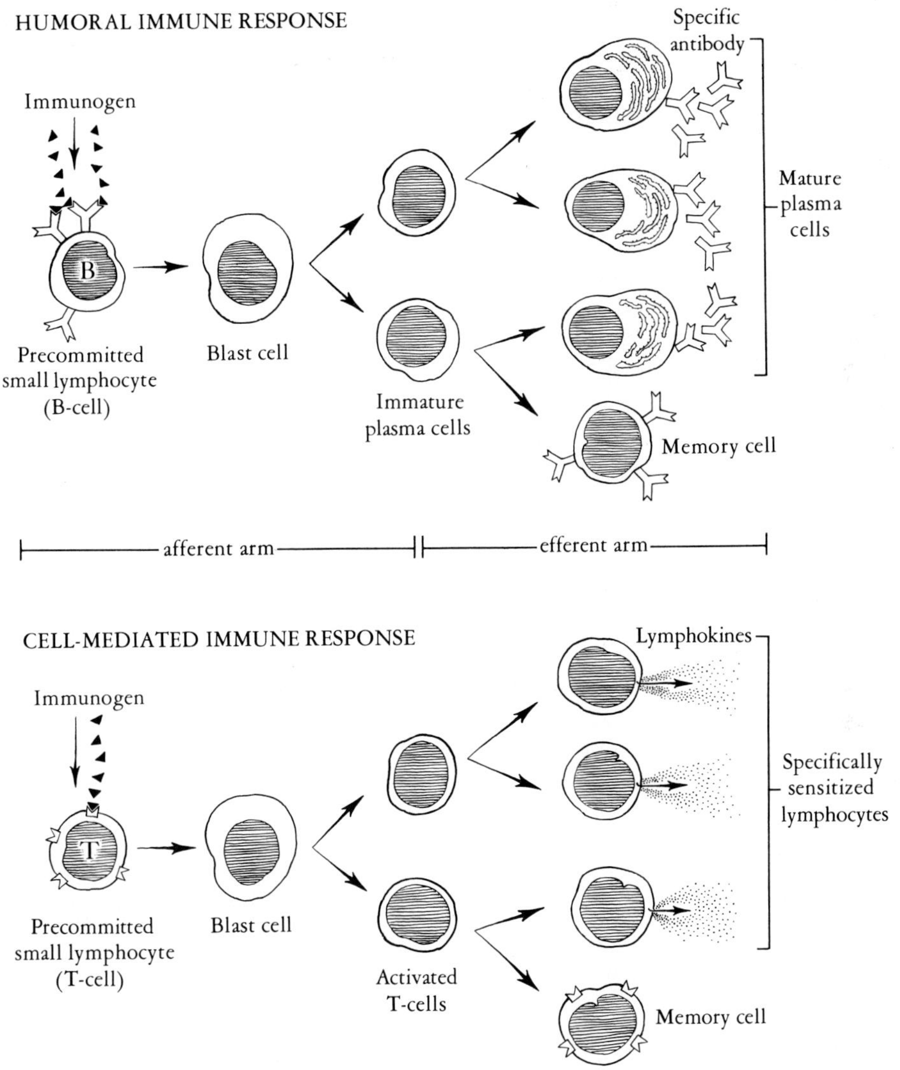

Figure 7–4. Schematic representation of the activation of immunocompetent cells by immunogen for humoral and cell-mediated immune responses.

Table 7–3. **Characteristics of Human Lymphocytes and Macrophages**

	T-Cells	B-Cells	Macrophages
Site of Differentiation	Thymus	Bone Marrow	Bone Marrow
Surface markers			
Specific surface antigen	OKT and Leu series*	HBLA (?)	OKM1
Antigen-binding receptor	V region idiotype	Immunoglobulin	–
Receptors for:			
SRBC (E-rosette)	+	–	–
IgG Fc (EA-rosette)	+ (Suppressor)	+	+
IgM Fc (EA-rosette)	+ (Helper)	–	–
C3b (EAC-rosette)	–	+	+
Measles virus	+	–	–
Epstein-Barr virus	–	+	–
HLA alloantigens: A,B,C,	+	+	+
HLA alloantigens: D/DR	±	+	+
Location: per cent lymphocytes			
Peripheral blood	55–75	15–30	2–12
Thoracic duct	<75	<25	<10
Lymph node	75	20	5
Spleen	35–45	50–60	5–10
Bone marrow	<10	<75	10–15
Thymus	<75	<10	<10
Tissue location	Cortex	Germinal center	Sinuses
Life span	Both long- and short-lived	Most are short-lived	Long-lived
Traffic	Recirculate	Little recirculation	Little, if any, recirculation
Blast transformation induced by:			
Phytohemagglutinin (PHA)			
soluble	+	–	–
insoluble	+	+	–
Concanavalin-A (Con-A)			
soluble	+	–	–
insoluble	+	+	–
Lipopolysaccharide (LPS)	–	– (?)	–
Pokeweed mitogen (PWM)	+	+	–
Anti-immunoglobulin	–	+	–
Specific antigen	+	+	–
Susceptible to inactivation by:			
Corticosteroids	+	+ +	–
X-irradiation	+ +	+ + +	–
Anti-lymphocyte serum (ALS)	+ + +	(+)	–
Immunosuppressive drugs:			
Cyclophosphamide	+ (Suppressor)	+ + +	+
Azathioprine	+ + +	+	+

*The Leu series of monoclonal antibodies is a trademark of Becton Dickinson Company, Sunnyvale, California. The OK series of monoclonal antibodies is a trademark of Ortho Pharmaceutical Corporation, Raritan, New Jersey.

Table 7–4. Immunologic Functions of T-Cells, B-Cells, and Macrophages

	T-Cell	B-Cell	Macrophage
Humoral response	Helper Suppressor Regulator	Differentiate into antibody-secreting cells	Accessory cell for induction
Cell-mediated response	Helper Suppressor Regulator	?	Accessory cell for induction Effector cell
Specificity	Clonally restricted	Clonally restricted	Nonspecific
Products elaborated	Lymphokines Helper factors Suppressor factors	Immunoglobulins	Monokines (e.g., interleukin-1) Regulatory factors
Memory	Antigen-specific	Antigen-specific	None
Can be made tolerant?	Yes	Yes	No

velopment of sensitive immunologic techniques (e.g., immunofluorescence, rosette analysis), has it become possible to describe characteristic markers useful for the identification of morphologically indistinguishable B- and T-cells.

* A cells activity can be predicted by what is on its surface.

SURFACE MARKERS

In murine systems, some of the lymphocytes that enter the thymus acquire a surface alloantigen formerly called *theta* (θ) that occurs in two allelic forms now referred to as *Thy 1.1 and Thy 1.2*. This antigen is found on lymphocytes that leave the thymus (thymus-derived or T-cells), on brain cells, and on skin and fibroblast cells in very small amounts, but it is absent from B-cells. The presence of the Thy 1 antigen is detected by an antiserum prepared by immunizing mice not carrying the specific antigen with thymus cells from mice that do. This antiserum, in the presence of complement, can be used to deplete lymphocyte populations of Thy 1–bearing cells. T-cells express different concentrations of the Thy 1 alloantigen on their surface at different stages of their maturation. In the cortex of the thymus, thymocytes express the greatest amount of Thy 1. The more mature thymus medullary lymphocyte expresses a lesser amount of the Thy 1 antigen, and even less is expressed on circulating (peripheral) T-cells. An analogous thymus alloantigen in humans, called *human thymus lymphocyte antigen* (HTLA), has been used for the preparation of a cytotoxic antiserum that has immunosuppressive capabilities. This reagent has been used clinically to prevent the immunologic rejection of organ or tissue transplants (Chapters 20 and 24).

Other alloantigens have been detected primarily on the surface of T-cells. Among these is the *TL alloantigen,* which is expressed on the surface of lymphocytes within the thymus of genetically TL^+ mouse strains and is lost as the cells mature into T-cells. The TL antigen also appears on T-cells of leukemic mice in TL^- strains, suggesting that derepression of a previously existing gene occurs. In humans, alloantibodies against T-cells are found in the sera of patients with infectious mononucleosis and systemic lupus erythematosus, which suggests antigenic modulation of the cell surface or derepression of genetic information for expression of the given antigen.

The *Ly antigens* constitute a group of cell surface markers that are differentially expressed on murine T-cells (Lyt) and B-cells (Lyb). Further differential expression of Lyt antigens delineates functionally distinct subpopulations of T-cells (to be described later in this chapter). Functional subsets of murine T-cells can also be identified by the presence of Qa and Ia antigens (described later).

The development of flow fluorocytometry technology and hybridoma methodology for the production of monoclonal antibodies has led to the analysis of human lymphocyte subpopulations. Monoclonal antibodies that define various functional subsets of human T-cells have been developed. These monoclonal antibodies also react with human T-cells at different stages of maturation (see Chapter 2, Fig. 2–21). The earliest thymocytes bear the T10 marker alone or in combination with T9. During maturation, the cells acquire a unique thymocyte antigen, defined as T6. These cells also express the T4 and T5/T8 markers, which are also found on peripheral T-cells. Anti-T6, anti-T9, and anti-T10 monoclonal antibodies react almost exclusively with thymocytes and not with peripheral T-cells. Cells bearing the T10, T6,

T4, and T5/T8 markers account for 70 to 75 per cent of total thymocytes. As the cells undergo further maturation within the thymus, they lose T6, acquire T1 and T3 markers, and segregate into the T4 and T5/T8 subsets. Upon leaving the thymus to populate the peripheral T-cell compartment, the cells lose the T10 marker. Monoclonal anti-T1 and anti-T3 antibodies react with virtually 100 per cent of peripheral T-cells but with only about 10 per cent of mature thymocytes. Anti-T4 reacts with 75 per cent of thymocytes and 60 per cent of peripheral T-cells, identifying the *helper or inducer* subset of human T-cells. Anti-T5 and anti-T8 react with 80 per cent of thymocytes and 20 to 30 per cent of peripheral T-cells, identifying the *suppressor or cytotoxic* subset of human T-cells. Table 7–5 summarizes the functional properties of these cells. Monoclonal antibodies with specificities similar to those described above are commercially available and are readily applicable to quantitating lymphocyte subpopulations in clinical disease states in hospital laboratories.

Alloantigens on B-cells with a relationship similar to that which Thy-1 (theta) has for T-cells have not yet been described. In murine species, a *mouse B-lymphocyte antigen* (MBLA) has been used for the preparation of a heterologous anti-B cell antiserum. This reagent was used in studies of B-cell function only after it had been absorbed extensively with mouse tissue to remove cytotoxic activity against thymus cells. Another murine alloantigen, referred to as *PC.1*, is present on the surface of plasma cells, the terminally differentiated product of the antigen-stimulated B-cell, and on certain mouse myeloma cells. This surface marker is thought to be a differentiation antigen. Although several attempts have been made to generate antisera against human B-cells, they have been unsuccessful for the most part because of the lack of identification of a unique B-cell alloantigen. The most useful marker to aid in the identification of B-cells to date is the presence of immunoglobulin on the cell surface. It is highly likely that in the not too distant future a collection of antibodies that define B-cells at various stages of maturation will also be available, as is the case for T-cells.

Immunoglobulins are present on B-cells.

Macrophages, which also arise from bone marrow progenitor cells, find their way into the blood stream as monocytes (Chapter 2). The monocytes wander through tissues and, together with their fixed-form counterparts, serve both phagocytic and immunoregulatory functions. In recent years, monoclonal antibodies that react with surface antigens on both rodent and human mononuclear phagocytes have been described. At present there are more than 15 reagents that appear to be specific for antigens on human monocytes/macrophages. While none of these monoclonal antibodies, as yet, defines a molecule of known function (e.g., Fc receptors), some of the marker-bearing cells have distinct immunologic function (e.g., antigen-presentation). Several mouse anti-human monoclonal antibodies define antigens shared among monocytes and other blood cells. For example, monoclonal antibodies designated OKM1, Mo1, and MY4 are expressed on monocytes and granulocytes, while TA-1 and Mo4 are found on T-cells and platelets, re-

Table 7–5. Immunologic Function of Human T-Cell Subsets Recognized by Monoclonal Antibodies

Function	T-Helper T-Inducer ($T\ 4^+$)	T-Cytotoxic T-Suppressor ($T\ 5/8^+$)
Proliferation induced by		
Soluble antigen	+	–
I-region (D/DR) products	+	+
Concanavalin-A	+	+
Phytohemagglutinin	+	–
Helper induction in		
T-Mϕ interactions	+	–
T-T interactions	+	–
T-B interactions	+	–
Suppressor effector in		
Antibody production	–	+
Cell-mediated reactions	–	+
Cytotoxic effector cell	–	+

spectively. Anti-OKM1 and anti-Mo1 also have reactivity against null cells. Deletion of OKM1-positive cells abrogates antibody-dependent cellular cytotoxicity (ADCC) and natural killer (NK) activity by human mononuclear cells. There are several rat anti-mouse monoclonal antibodies that define antigens expressed on macrophages alone as well as a number of reagents that detect antigens that are shared among myeloid cells. For example, anti–Mac-1 reacts with mouse macrophages, granulocytes, and some mouse cell lines as well as with human peripheral blood monocytes, granulocytes, and null cells. Of clinical significance is the observation that many of the mouse anti-human monoclonal antibodies are reactive with myeloid leukemia cells but not with malignant lymphoid cells. These reagents may prove useful not only for the diagnosis of myeloid leukemia when conventional methods are questionable, but also as specific immunotherapeutic agents for treatment of disorders of the reticuloendothelial system. Very recently, a series of monoclonal antibodies that are reactive with distinct stages of monocyte/macrophage differentiation have been developed. Similarly, monoclonal antibodies that are capable of defining functional macrophage subsets are now beginning to appear.

In addition to the above-described surface markers, nonlymphoid cells as well as B-cells, T-cells, and macrophages express on their surface, to varying degrees, antigens representing the gene products of the *major histocompatibility complex* (MHC) of the species. A detailed description of these alloantigens is found in Chapter 3, while their role in cellular interactions is discussed later in this chapter.

SURFACE RECEPTORS

Specific *receptors* with binding affinity for a variety of ligands are found on the surface of cells that participate in the immune response. Methods that have been developed for the detection of these receptors can also serve as a means of evaluating the quantity or quality of a particular cell type. One such method involves the formation of *rosettes* consisting of either a lymphocyte or a macrophage surrounded by an appropriate indicator cell. In humans, three types of rosettes can be distinguished that correspond to different cell surface receptors (Fig. 7–5). T-lymphocytes from normal humans, when mixed with sheep erythrocytes (E), form spontaneous rosettes (Fig. 7–5*A*). While there is no specific immunologic basis for the formation of these *E-rosettes* (also called T-rosettes), the presence of E-receptors on the surface of mature T-cells has proved to be extremely useful for quantitating these cells in peripheral blood. A second type of receptor that is involved in rosette formation binds antigen-antibody complexes or aggregated immunoglobulin through the Fc portion of the IgG molecule (Fig. 7–5*B*). These *Fc receptors* are normally readily detectable on the surface of B-cells and macrophages and form *EA-rosettes* with sheep erythrocytes that have been coated with specific anti-sheep erythrocyte antibody (A). In addition to finding receptors for the Fc portion of IgG on B-cells and macrophages, the subset of human T-cells (called T_γ cells) that function as *cytotoxic and suppressor cells* (analogous to the $T1^+$, $T3^+$, $T5^+/T8^+$ cells) also possess Fc receptors, which can be detected using an IgG antibody prepared against ox erythrocytes. Receptors for the Fc portion of monomeric IgM are differentially expressed on macrophages and the subset of human T-cells (called T_μ cells) that function as *helper and inducer cells* (analogous to the $T1^+$, $T3^+$, $T4^+$ cell). Recently, lymphocytes and macrophages expressing Fc receptors for IgE and IgA have been described. These cells appear to have class-specific regulatory function on IgE and IgA antibody production. Finally, Fc receptors have been demonstrated on natural killer and K-cells (Chapter 9) involved in antibody-dependent cellular cytotoxicity (ADCC). The third type of receptor, found on some B-cells, some macrophages, and a limited number of other cell types, recognizes the third component of complement (C3b). These *EAC-rosettes* are formed with sheep erythrocytes coated with specific antibody and complement. The complement receptor does not appear to be a single molecular species. Recent studies indicate that there are unique membrane-binding sites for at least C3b, C3d, and C4. Lymphocytes bearing this receptor are referred to as *complement receptor (CR^+) lymphocytes.* This receptor is useful in distinguishing immature B-cells (CR^-) from mature B-cells (CR^+) by rosette analysis.

Microscopically you can distinguish rosette type.

ANTIGEN-BINDING RECEPTORS

The initiation of the immune response is dependent upon recognition of a foreign

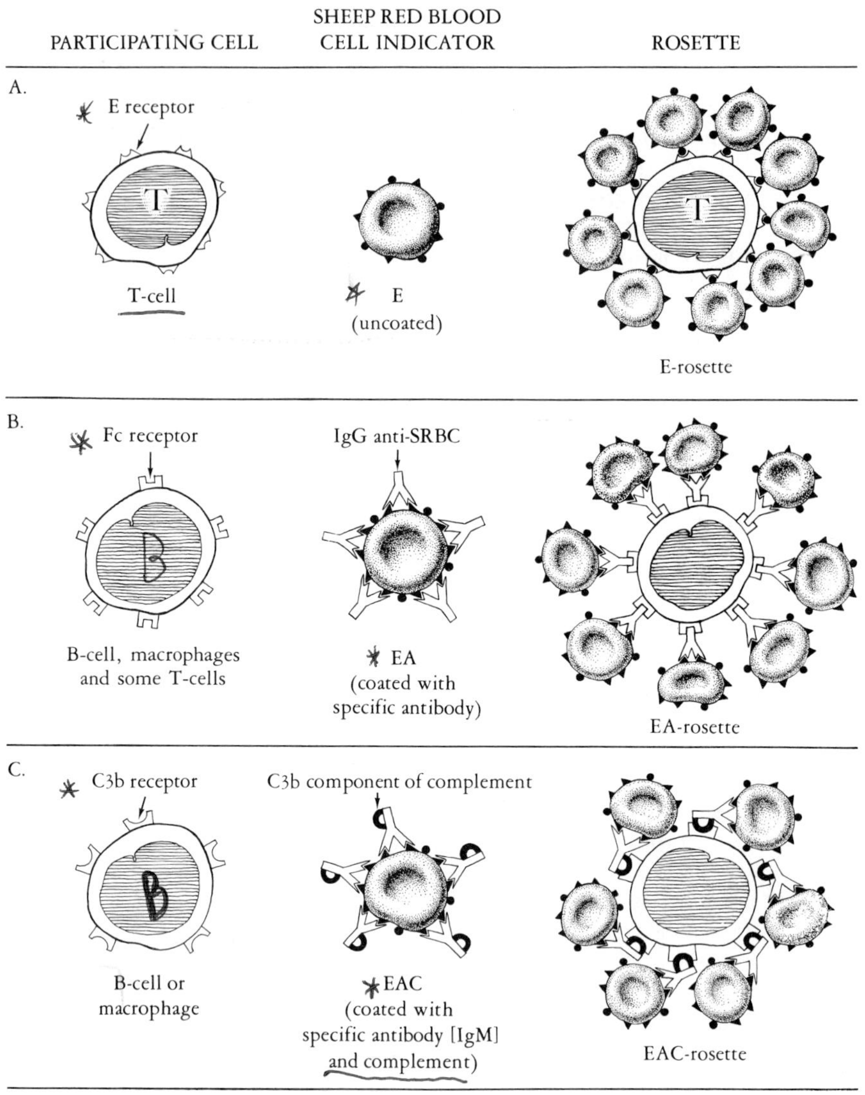

Figure 7–5. Schematic representation of different types of rosettes.

configuration (antigen) by specific receptors on B- and T-cells.

Receptors for Antigen on B-Cells. Immunoglobulin (Ig) can be readily detected on the surface of B-cells from human and most mammalian species through the use of fluorescent-labeled antisera prepared against various immunoglobulin classes. These surface Ig's are capable of binding specific antigens and function as antigen receptors that are likely to be involved in the differentiation events culminating in antibody synthesis. B-cells contain about 100,000 randomly distributed Ig molecules per cell. While it was originally thought that the Ig receptor on the B-cell was identical to the antibody product ultimately synthesized by the antigen-stimulated cell, current evidence indicates that surface-bound and secreted Ig differ somewhat in their C_H domains.

Specific Ig classes can be associated with B-cells. In humans and mice, IgM-bearing cells are more common than those bearing IgG. The relative proportion of κ and λ light chains on the surface of B-cells corresponds to that expressed on serum immunoglobulins. However, whereas the major serum Ig expresses the γ heavy chain, the major Ig expressed on B-cells bears the μ heavy chain. The cell surface IgM appears to exist predominantly in the monomeric form as IgM_S (8S), containing more carboxy-terminal hydrophobic amino acids and fewer carbohydrate moieties than are found in the pentameric serum IgM. In addition to expressing surface IgM, many B-cells also simultaneously express IgD on their surface. The immunoglobulin molecules on cells that simultaneously express IgM and IgD appear to be limited to the same type of light chain and idiotype. There is also evidence that the surface and secreted Ig have the same specificity and affinity for their specific antigen, which suggests that they possess the same V_L and V_H domains and the same idiotype.

The surface immunoglobulins are neither rigidly held in fixed position nor loosely bound; in fact, there is fluidity and movement of these molecules. For example, when a radiolabeled or fluorescein-labeled anti-immunoglobulin serum is reacted with living B-cells, changes can be observed at the cell surface (Fig. 7–6). If the reaction is carried out at low temperature (4°C), the labeled material can be seen in a *diffuse* arrangement over the entire cell surface, indicating that the surface immunoglobulin is randomly distributed. As the temperature is raised, the labeled material assumes a distribution of spots or patches over the surface. *Patch formation* is independent of cell metabolism but is dependent upon the bivalence of antibody (e.g., $F(ab')_2$. This reaction is thought to depend upon cross-linking of the receptors. After a short time the label coalesces into a cap over one pole of the cell. *Cap formation* is an energy-dependent process. Following this the cap is either released or internalized within the cell, where the material is seen in vesicles. The cell surface remains devoid of immunoglobulin for a period of time before newly synthesized receptors can be detected. The same phenomenon can be demonstrated when B-cells expressing specific receptors bind a multivalent antigen. It has been suggested by some that these events are crucial to the triggering of cell differentiation and proliferation required for the initiation of the immune response. Others suggest that the above events function solely to remove excess antigen from the cell surface.

Receptors for Antigen on T-Cells. Based upon our understanding of the specificity of the antigen-antibody reaction, it would be

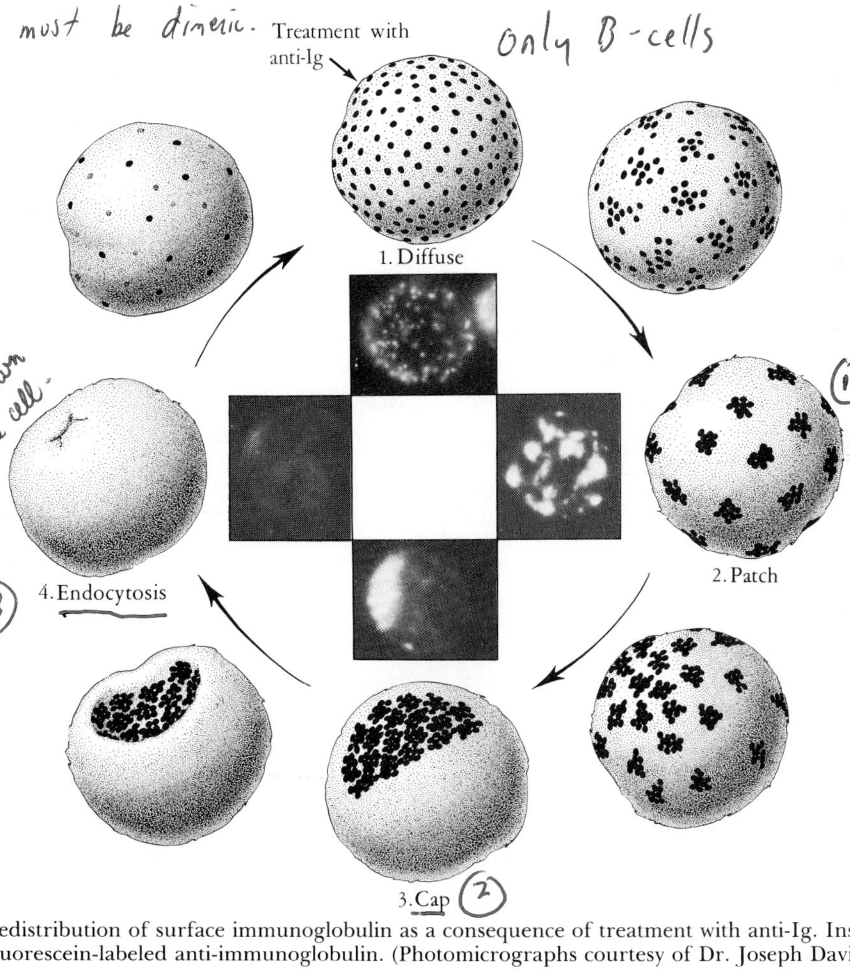

Figure 7–6. Redistribution of surface immunoglobulin as a consequence of treatment with anti-Ig. Inserts show cells treated with fluorescein-labeled anti-immunoglobulin. (Photomicrographs courtesy of Dr. Joseph Davie.)

logical to conclude that the T-cell receptor must also be represented by immunoglobulin. However, the nature of the T-cell receptor is controversial and, at present, uncertain. Immunoglobulin can be detected on the surface of T-cells, but only in trace amounts, and it is uncertain whether this is passively acquired from B-cells or made by the T-cell. The fact that anti-immunoglobulin antisera do not readily block the immunologic functions of these cells argues against the receptor's being an immunoglobulin. Those who favor the immunoglobulin nature of the T-cell receptor suggest that it is located deeper in the cell membrane than that of B-cells; that it is sterically hindered by other surface components; or that it belongs to a class of hitherto unidentified immunoglobulins that lack a conventional constant (C) region domain, since antisera to such domains react poorly, if at all, with T-cells. Studies on the genetic control of antibody formation have shown that antigen recognition by T-cells is regulated by genes closely associated with the major histocompatibility complex (MHC), called Ir genes (Chapter 3). It is currently believed that T-cell receptors for antigen are represented by variable (V) region domains, since their antigen-recognition units express idiotypes in response to activation by antigen, which are the same as those of antibody molecules stimulated by the same antigen. It is likely that these V-region domains on the T-cell are associated with MHC gene products rather than with conventional C-region domains.

In the human, an additional substance is associated with the cell surface. The material is a low molecular weight protein fragment found in association with the histocompatibility antigens (HLA). This β_2 *microglobulin* in many ways resembles the homology regions of immunoglobulins; its amino acid sequence is very similar to the homology regions in the constant portion of the light chain (C_L) and the heavy chain (CH_3) of IgG. It has been suggested, although this is no longer believed, that the β_2 microglobulin functions as the T-cell receptor by serving as the recognition site for B- and T-cell interactions or some regulatory substance. Its similarity in structure to immunoglobulin and its close association with HLA suggests an important evolutionary interaction between the products of the immune system and the histocompatibility system.

Blast Transformation. The recognition of an immunogen by specific receptors on B- and T-cells leads to the initiation of a series of events in which the cells increase in size, the nucleolus enlarges, rough endoplasmic reticulum and microtubules become prominent, the rate of DNA synthesis increases, and mitosis ensues. Figure 7–7 shows a typical blast cell. This process of *blast transformation* can also be induced by the addition of bivalent $F(ab')_2$, but not of monovalent Fab fragments of anti-immunoglobulin or anti-allotype antisera, to cultures of immunoglobulin-bearing lymphocytes. The addition of other agents, including certain plant proteins and endotoxin, called *mitogens*, to cultures of nonsensitized lymphocytes may also initiate blast transformation. These observations suggest that some membrane perturbation induced by the cross-linking of certain surface macromolecules stimulates the lymphocyte to divide.

Plant mitogens have the potential to activate large numbers of lymphocytes without regard to the antigenic reactivity of the responding cells. The different mitogens bind to and have specificity for diverse sugar moieties of glycoproteins on the lymphocyte membrane (e.g., concanavalin A [Con-A] binds to glycoproteins containing α-mannosyl moie-

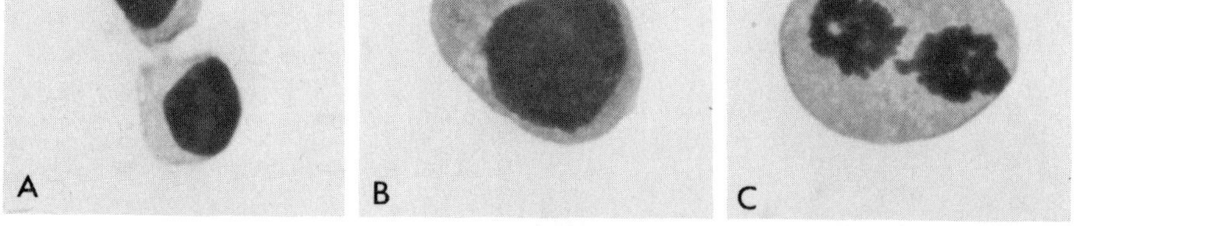

Figure 7–7. Photomicrographs of lymphocytes in the process of blast transformation. Giemsa stain, ×900. *A,* Unstimulated small lymphocytes; *B,* PHA-stimulated blast cell; *C,* PHA-stimuated lymphocyte in mitosis. (Courtesy of B. Zeligs.)

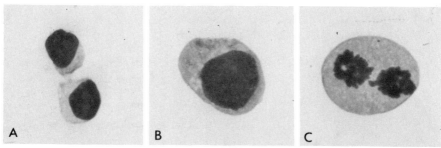

ties). Some of the mitogens have the ability to activate T-cells, others to activate B-cells, and some induce changes in both. It is important to note that a given mitogen will have diverse effects on lymphocytes obtained from different species. For example, whereas the lipopolysaccharide (LPS) of gram-negative bacteria is a potent mitogen for murine B-cells (but not for T-cells), it does not induce blast transformation in rabbit B-cells. Currently, there is question as to the mitogenic effect of LPS on human B-cells. Some believe that LPS induces a clonally restricted response in human B-cells (i.e., similar to that induced by any specific immunogen), but one report suggests that after an initial culture period in the absence of LPS, human B-cells will respond to the addition of LPS in a polyclonal manner. It is thought that the initial culture period is necessary to remove the influence of suppressor T-cells. Pokeweed mitogen (PWM) stimulates both B- and T-cell subpopulations of mouse and human lymphocytes. It has been suggested that stimulation of human B-cells by PWM depends on the presence of T-cells. Both phytohemagglutinin (PHA) and Con-A, in their soluble forms, selectively stimulate murine T-cells to synthesize DNA, divide, and produce a nonspecific factor that can replace the T-cell helper function in some immune responses. When rendered insoluble by attachment to large particles, Con-A and PHA induce blast transformation in both B- and T-cell subpopulations. In this case, B-cell stimulation could be indirect, since nonspecific products elaborated by PHA-stimulated T-cells initiate the activation of B-cells.

In addition to stimulating DNA synthesis in both T- and B-cells, certain mitogens, such as PWM, will initiate synthesis and secretion of IgM in cultures of B-cells, and others, such as PHA, will induce lymphokine production (Chapter 9) in cultures of T-cells and are called *polyclonal activators.* The reaction of lymphocyte populations to the various mitogens (Table 7–3) may, with caution, be used by the clinician to identify the type of cell (T- or B-cell) and to reveal developmental or functional deficiencies (Chapter 22).

Macrophages

Although the involvement of macrophages in both *in vivo* and *in vitro* immune responses has been known for many years, their precise function still remains unclear. The basic functional property of a macrophage is its ability to engulf and remove foreign and effete materials. The endocytic processes of macrophages appear to be initiated by the interaction of the foreign material with the cell membrane. Phagocytosis can be facilitated by the presence of antigen coated with antibody, a process called *opsonization.* In addition, antibodies of a variety of specificities can be attached to the macrophage surface through its Fc receptor. This *cytophilic* antibody endows macrophages with enhanced abilities to recognize, engulf, and destroy antigenic substances. The receptors for complement components, which are independent of Fc receptors, also aid the macrophages in removing antigens from their environment.

Evidence for the role of the macrophage in humoral responses has been provided by numerous *in vivo* studies using irradiated animals, reticuloendothelial blockade, and anti-macrophage serum. The essentiality of macrophage participation in the *in vitro* immune response has been shown by experiments in which mouse spleen populations were separated into adherent (macrophage-rich) and nonadherent (lymphocyte-rich) populations. Neither of these populations by themselves can respond to antigen; however, when they are combined, an antibody response equivalent to that of the unseparated spleen cell population is obtained.

Numerous functional roles have been ascribed to macrophages participating in the immune response. In early experiments, it was thought that macrophages "*processed*" antigens into an immunogenic form that was recognized by a particular lymphocyte subclass. Processing appears to be an important event associated with the initial steps of the immune response to particulate materials; it is thought that this event may expose determinants otherwise unavailable to react with lymphocytes or may change pre-existing determinants into a recognizable form. In support of this concept, it has been shown that aggregation of soluble antigens leads to more efficient phagocytosis, which also results in enhanced immunogenicity.

It has also been suggested by some that processing of antigen by macrophages results in the production of a new class of macrophage-derived RNA that carries genetic information. Two fractions of macrophage-derived RNA have been described; however, one of these contains a portion of the original antigen. This antigen-RNA complex is more efficient in stimulating an immune response than the original antigen and has been referred to as a *superantigen*. In this case, the enhanced immunogenicity has been attributed to the adjuvant properties of the component nucleic acid.

The second class of RNA has been shown to be free of antigen fragments and is thought to have messenger RNA activity. It is referred to as *informational* RNA (i-RNA). This RNA has a molecular weight between 400,000 and 750,000 and selectively induces the formation of IgM antibody. Support for an informational role of macrophage-derived RNA was obtained from the following type of experiment. If, after incubation with antigen, macrophage RNA is prepared from cells of a strain of animal that produces antibody with a unique allotype marker (b^4b^4) and is added to lymphoid cells obtained from another animal that produces antibody of a different allotype (b^5b^5), the antibody molecules formed will be of the allotype of the macrophage donor animal (b^4b^4). Recent evidence has also shown that this i-RNA can direct the synthesis of 19S protein of a particular allotype in cell-free extracts, suggesting that the i-RNA functions as messenger RNA.

A second function attributed to the macrophage is *antigen presentation*. It has been amply demonstrated that after incubation of antigen with macrophages, a portion of the antigen remains associated with the macrophage surface. This macrophage-bound antigen is more immunogenic than an equivalent amount of free antigen. It is not clear whether the surface-bound antigen is derived from material taken up by the macrophage, processed, and subsequently exocytosed or whether it is a result of direct interaction of the material with components (e.g., antibody affixed to Fc receptors) on the macrophage membrane. This surface-associated antigen appears to be tightly bound and can be recovered in macromolecular form after limited treatment of the cell surface with proteolytic enzymes.

It is now clear that antigen presentation is mediated by a subset of macrophages bearing surface Ia molecules that are encoded by genes of the major histocompatibility complex (Chapter 3). Since anti-Ia antibody interferes with the presenting function of macrophages possessing membrane-bound antigen, it has been suggested that Ia and specific antigen molecules "interact" on the macrophage surface. It is thought that it is the "Ia–antigen complex" on the *antigen-presenting cell* that is recognized by the responding lymphocyte subset. In spite of the current belief in this hypothesis, it must be considered with caution, since it has been difficult to demonstrate that antibody against the specific antigen can interfere with antigen presentation as has been shown to be the case with anti-Ia antibody.

An additional function attributed to macrophages is the production and secretion of a wide variety of biologically active factors that influence the activity of lymphocytes. Macrophage extracts or supernatant fluids from macrophage cultures can substitute for the function of intact macrophages in *in vitro* systems measuring antibody formation. However, it has also been shown that macrophage function can be replaced by 2-mercaptoethanol (2-ME) during the induction of the *in vitro* immune response to sheep red blood cells (SRBC) by mouse spleen cells. It has been suggested that in this system, 2-ME substitutes for macrophage function by acting in combination with a serum component of the tissue culture medium, leading to the activation of T-cells. An additional factor produced by macrophages that has a positive effect on lymphocyte function is *interleukin-1* (IL-1), formerly called lymphocyte activating factor. This material, which has been purified to homogeneity, stimulates maturation and proliferation in T-cells. In addition, IL-1 appears to stimulate the production of a second interleukin, IL-2, by T-cells, which acts together with the signals initiated by antigen and Ia such that T-cell activation is achieved. The production of IL-2 by helper T-cells has also been reported to be important for the stimulation of B-cells to proliferate and differentiate into immunoglobulin-secreting cells. Alternatively, macrophages may also suppress the activities of lymphocytes nonspecifically through the elaboration of other biologically active substances. These include: arginase, thymidine, complement-cleavage products, prostaglandins, interferon, and oxygen intermediates.

Although all of the above postulated functions of macrophages are worthy of further consideration, attention has been directed toward the surface membrane of the macrophage. Macrophage-bound antigen is highly immunogenic for T-cells. The fact that maximal stimulation is achieved when the macrophage and lymphocyte possess common histocompatibility molecules (Ia determinants) suggests that something more than antigen is required. Indeed, in several systems direct contact between macrophages and lymphocytes has been observed and suggests the necessity of cell surface interaction or the transfer of information from one cell to the other (Fig. 7–8) via soluble factors.

Null Cells

A relatively small proportion of lymphocytes can be detected that bear neither the Thy-l antigen nor the surface immunoglobulin that are characteristic of T- and B-cells, respectively. These *null cells,* originally recognized for their ability to lyse tumor cells either spontaneously or through an ADCC mechanism (Chapter 9), have characteristics distinct from other types of lymphoid cells. This population, representing 5 to 15 per cent of the cells in peripheral blood, consists of hemopoietic stem cells, which are thought to include precursors of T- and B-cells, myeloid, erythroid, and thrombocytic series. Two types of cells are considered in this category.

KILLER CELLS (K CELLS)

This is a heterogeneous group of cells that, when taken from normal individuals, can lyse diverse target cells *in vitro* if incubated in the

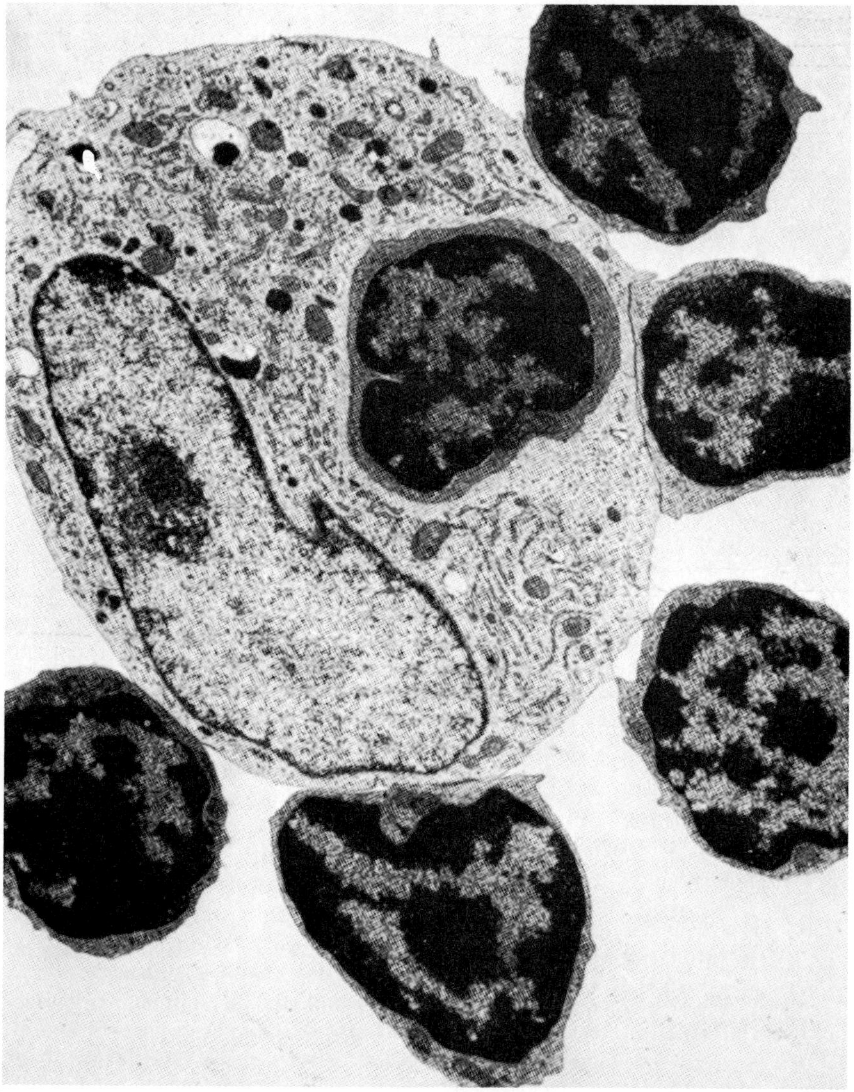

Figure 7–8. Photomicrograph of macrophage-lymphocyte interaction. (Reproduced from Lipsky, P. E., and Rosenthal, A. S.: Macrophage-lymphocyte interaction. I. Characteristics of the antigen-independent-binding of guinea pig thymocytes and lymphocytes to syngeneic macrophages. J. Exp. Med., *138*:900, 1973.)

presence of specific antibodies against surface antigens on the latter. Fc receptors for IgG on these cells can bind monomeric IgG, aggregated IgG, or IgG that has already reacted with antigen, e.g., on the surface of target cells. About 40 per cent of K cells possess receptors for SRBC, a typical T-cell marker, in addition to the Fc receptor for IgG. Another 40 per cent lack the T-cell marker as well as surface-bound immunoglobulin, a marker of B-cells, but possess receptors for complement components. The remaining 20 per cent of K cells do not possess any of the above-mentioned markers.

NATURAL KILLER CELLS (NK CELLS)

NK cells are nonphagocytic and nonadherent cells found in normal individuals of most mammalian species. They resemble large granular lymphocytes and compose about 5 per cent of peripheral blood and splenic leukocytes. They express surface receptors for the Fc portion of IgG and can function as K cells that mediate ADCC. Although these cells do not appear to be thymus-dependent, with significant levels of NK activity detected in athymic nude or neonatally thymectomized mice, these cells share T-cell–associated markers. About 50 per cent of human NK cells have receptors for SRBC, and the majority react with monoclonal antibodies against T-cell markers (e.g., $T10^+$) as well as monocyte/macrophage markers (e.g., OKM1). NK cells can react against a wide variety of target cells. Not only are tumor cells susceptible to lysis by NK cells but also fetal cells, virus-infected cells, and some subsets of thymus cells, bone marrow cells, and macrophages. Unlike the case with antigen recognition by T-cells, recognition by NK cells does not appear to require the sharing of histocompatibility antigens. The activity of NK cells can be augmented by interferon as well as other stimuli (e.g., retinoic acid). There is increasing evidence that these cells may play an important role in immune surveillance.

CELL INTERACTIONS IN THE INITIATION OF ANTIBODY FORMATION

The clonal selection theory of antibody formation proposed by Burnet states that an immunologically responsive cell (small lymphocyte) contains within its genome the genetic information to respond to a single immunogen (or a few related ones) even before the cell encounters the foreign configuration. Thus, the lymphocyte population of an individual is preprogrammed to contain a diverse library of cells, some of which respond to one antigen, others to a second, and so forth. The encounter between the immunogen and the precommitted cell results in the proliferation of the latter and the generation of a clone of differentiated antibody-forming cells (Fig. 7–9). This hypothesis implies that an antiserum prepared against a complex immunogen (e.g., bacterium) consists of a population of different antibodies, each produced by separate clones preprogrammed to respond to a particular antigenic determinant on the complex microorganism. In order to provide experimental evidence to support this hypothesis, attempts were made to determine the number of antibodies produced by single cells. It was found that a single plasma cell produces antibodies with a single antigen-binding specificity. The uniformity in primary structure of a given class of antibody produced by a single cell is similar to that of the myeloma protein produced in multiple myeloma and suggests that the immunoglobulin molecule is subject to *allelic exclusion;* that is, the cell expresses only one of its several alleles for the different polypeptide chains of the immunoglobulin molecule at any one time. However, in view of the fact that a single cell can be shown to produce more than one class of immunoglobulin (e.g., IgM and IgD) at one time, what was once referred to as the *one cell–one antibody* rule has now been modified to the *one cell–one idiotype* rule. Since the early immune response is characterized by the predominance of IgM antibody followed later by IgG, it has been suggested that cells can undergo an *IgM→IgG switch* during the course of the response. Immunologic evidence to support such a switch mechanism is based on the observation of patients with biclonal myelomas. One such patient produced both homogeneous IgM and IgG paraproteins. Analysis of these proteins revealed identity in primary amino acid sequence in all regions of the immunoglobulins except for the C_H region, which was μ in one protein and γ in the other. This switch can be explained on a genetic basis, whereby in making IgM the cell expresses genes for V_L, C_L, V_H, and $C\mu$ regions (Fig. 7–10). The

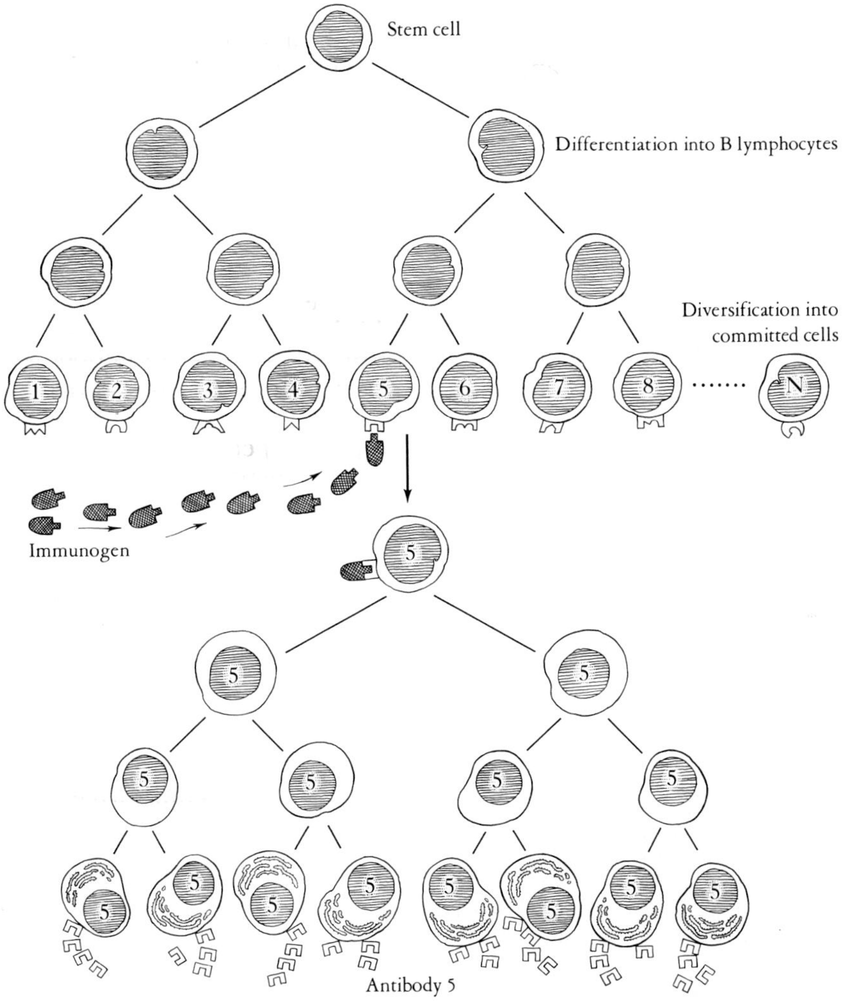

(Bursa or Bursal equivalent)

Figure 7–9. Schematic representation of clonal expansion of committed lymphocytes as a consequence of subsequent encounter with immunogen.

Clonal selection theory, Burnet

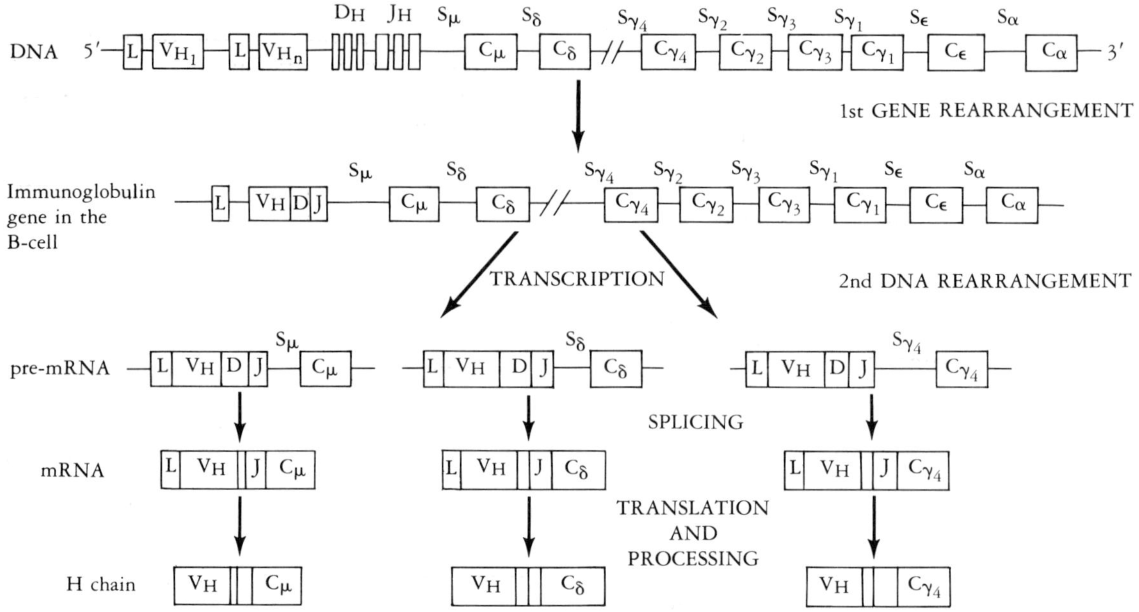

Figure 7–10. Schematic diagram of a proposed human heavy-chain locus demonstrating possible gene rearrangement involved in the dual expression of IgM and IgD as well as the IgM → IgG shift. L, leader sequences; V_H, variable region; J_H, joining segments; D_H, diversity segments; C, family of constant regions; and S, family of switch sites that precede each of the C-region genes. (After Rabbits, R. H., et al., 1981.)

switch to IgG synthesis preserves the expression of V_L, C_L, and V_H but involves a DNA rearrangement event in which Cγ gene can now be expressed. As indicated in Figure 7–10, the coding sequences for all C_H classes are found on the same chromosome separated at various lengths by intervening DNA segments containing specific switch sites (S). The Cμ gene is closest to the joining segment (J), and the Cα is farthest. A change in immunoglobulin class could occur when a switching site in the J-Cμ intervening DNA segment becomes joined to a switching site (S) between Cμ and any other C_H gene (e.g., $C\gamma_4$). As a consequence of looping out and excision of the Cμ gene, the V_HJ sequence previously adjacent to Cμ will now be adjacent to $C\gamma_4$. In a similar manner, the expression of IgD or other immunoglobulin heavy chains can be understood.

Compartmentalization of the Immune Response

Studies concerning the number of cells required for antibody formation have generated a vast amount of literature in the past decade. It was found that removal of the bursa of Fabricius from neonatal chickens, by either surgical or hormonal methods, resulted in an impairment of the ability of these animals to synthesize antibodies. Similarly, injection of neonatal mice with anti-μ chain antiserum resulted in animals with severe deficiencies of the humoral immune response, as manifested by their inability to produce not only IgM antibodies but also IgG and IgA antibodies later in life. The clinical diseases observed in such animals are virtually identical to those seen in children suffering from a congenital sex-linked disease called Bruton's agammaglobulinemia (Chapter 22). In none of the above situations is there impairment of cell-mediated immunity. On the other hand, removal of the thymus gland from neonatal animals resulted in a severely impaired cell-mediated response concomitant with variable deficiencies in the humoral response. Congenitally athymic (nude) mice display similar immunologic deficiencies of the cell-mediated response, although they respond normally to some immunogens and poorly, if at all, to others. In humans, a congenital developmental anomaly called the DiGeorge syndrome (Chapter 22) results in the birth of children lacking a thymus and displaying severe defects in cell-mediated immunity, along with variable defects in humoral immunity. Integration of these laboratory and clinical findings, which showed both a division of the immune response into humoral and cell-mediated immunity and combined immunodeficiencies related to the absence of the thymus, suggested, even before the nature of B- and T-cells was known, that cooperation between the cells of the two *central lymphoid organs* (bursa and thymus) was required for full expression of humoral immunity.

The current information regarding the mechanisms of cell cooperation involving macrophages, B-cells, and T-cells has been obtained from both *in vivo* and *in vitro* experiments. In 1966, it was first shown that thymus-derived and bone marrow–derived cells act synergistically in the restoration of the immune response of immunodeficient animals, and that if either population was omitted, a response did not take place. Subsequently, it was shown that depletion of spleen cell populations of adherent cells (macrophages) resulted in marked suppression of the immune response to SRBC and that this response could be restored by the addition of macrophages. Elegantly designed experiments showed that B-cells are the specific precursors of the antibody-forming cells and that T-cells, even though they do not differentiate into antibody-producing cells, can be stimulated to divide in response to antigen, can be specifically *educated* (have the ability to be primed by antigen and recognize it at a later time), and can provide a specific *helper* function for the initiation of the humoral response. Further understanding of the functions of B- and T-cells was obtained from studies of the carrier effect, in which it was shown that two receptors were involved in the elicitation of a secondary anti-hapten response, one hapten-specific, the other carrier-specific, and that B-cells carried the former, while T-cells carried the latter.

Cell Cooperation

In discussing potential mechanisms of antibody formation, two points should be addressed: The first is the mechanism by which the antigen-sensitive cell recognizes the immunogen, and the second is the nature of the signal required to trigger the B-cell to produce antibody. Regarding the first point, evidence has been presented that B-cells express clonally restricted immunoglobulin on their surface capable of reacting with a specific immunogen, and that this reaction leads to changes in the surface membrane, possibly initiating proliferation and differentiation into an antibody-forming cell. While the precise nature of the T-cell receptor has not been defined, there is evidence to indicate that T-cells also express clonally restricted receptors for antigen on their surface, possibly in the form of idiotypic determinants. It is believed that interaction of the immunogen with these receptors contributes, in part, to the activation process in T-cells.

Influence of the Thymus on Immunogenicity

There is a growing body of evidence to suggest that the triggering of B-cells requires either one complex signal or two separate signals. Bacterial lipopolysaccharide, which has been shown to be mitogenic for murine B-cells, has the ability to activate B-cells nonspecifically. Such activation results in a *polyclonal* response, in which many clones of B-cells are activated in the absence of a specific antigen to make small amounts of their predetermined antibodies. Thus, a B-cell mitogen can provide a *nonspecific* signal to trigger B-cell activation. It is thought that the antigenic determinant carries a *specific second signal* that activates specific clones to produce large amounts of antibody. Thus, the triggering of B-cells appears to require two signals, a *specific signal* represented by the antigenic determinant that is recognized by the Ig receptor and influences the differentiation and proliferation of the clone. The specific signal is referred to as *immunogenicity* and the nonspecific signal as *mitogenicity* or *adjuvanticity*.

In recent years, by means of *in vitro* systems, some interesting observations have been made concerning the idea that the nature of the immunogen may influence the types of cells that interact in the immune response. A small number of immunogens appear to elicit B-cell responses in the absence of T-cell help. These so-called *T-independent antigens* have been characterized as polymeric substances having a large number of repeating identical determinants that are relatively resistant to degradation and include such substances as dextran, levan, ficoll, polyvinylpyrrolidone, lipopolysaccharide, polymerized flagellin, and pneumococcal polysaccharide (Fig. 7–11*A*). The immune response to these materials is characterized by the almost exclusive production of IgM

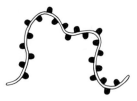

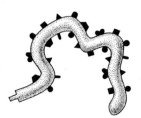

A. T-independent antigen - contains many copies of identical antigenic determinants (e.g., levan, pneumococcal polysaccharide, lipopolysaccharide)

B. T-dependent antigen - few copies of many different antigenic determinants (e.g., RBC, bacterium, protein)

Figure 7–11. Schematic representation of T-independent and T-dependent antigens.

with little or no IgG production and no production of immunologic memory. In addition to the lack of a requirement for T-cell help, the immune response to these materials was also thought to be independent of macrophage function. However, experiments using highly selective methods for the depletion of macrophages have suggested that these cells are required, albeit in small numbers, for responses to certain T-independent antigens. Interestingly, it has been found that T-cells may even play a suppressive role in the response to certain T-independent antigens (e.g., pneumococcal polysaccharide S-III), since removal of these cells by thymectomy or by treatment with anti-lymphocyte serum results in enhanced antibody production. Therefore, although these antigens appear to be independent of T-cell helper function, they may not be totally T-independent, in that T-cells may still play a regulatory role. To explain the triggering of B-cells it has been postulated, although not without controversy, that T-independent antigens carry both the specific and the nonspecific signal on the same molecule. The specific signal is represented by the ability of the multiple copies of the repeating antigenic determinant to cross link specific immunoglobulin receptors on the surface of B-cells. The nonspecific signal is represented by the ability of these substances, when introduced at high doses, to function as polyclonal B-cell activators, in that they stimulate multiple B-cell clones to proliferate and secrete immunoglobulin without regard to specific recognition by B-cell surface receptors. For example, LPS of *E. coli* is a polyclonal activator of mouse B-cells when given at high doses. However, while it also reacts with B-cells when given at low doses, it activates only those B-cells that are precommitted to make an anti-LPS antibody response. These results suggest that T-independent antigens possess separate antigenic and mitogenic sites and that these bind to separate receptors on B-cells (Fig. 7–12).

Almost all of the immunogens encountered in nature are not polymers of repeated similar antigenic determinants. Indeed, they are usually made up of a single copy or a few copies of diverse antigenic determinants (Fig. 7–11*B*). These substances induce immune responses, potentially involving all of the immunoglobulin classes and immunologic memory, and require T-cell help. Cells, proteins, glycoproteins, and hapten-carrier combinations are but a few examples of substances that make up the class of *T-dependent antigens.* It has been shown that the immune response to these antigens in T-cell–deficient animals is greatly suppressed and is limited, for the most part, to the IgM class of antibody, suggesting that T-cells are involved in the transition from IgM to IgG antibody synthesis.

T-Cell Subpopulations

It is now well accepted that there are three major subsets of murine T-cells that influence the activity of other T-cells as well as that of B-cells. These T-cell subpopulations, referred to as inducers, regulators, and effectors, have been defined through the use of antisera prepared against alloantigens described earlier in this chapter. Three T-cell subsets have been defined by cytotoxic antisera prepared against the murine Lyt alloantigens, which are coded for by two unlinked genetic loci (Lyt-1 on chromosome 19, and Lyt-2 and Lyt-3, which are closely linked on chromosome 6). These subsets have been designated as Lyt-1,2,3$^+$, Lyt-1$^+$, and Lyt-2,3$^+$. Of the T-cells found in peripheral lymphoid tissue, about 60 to 65 per cent are Lyt-1,2,3$^+$, 30 to 35 per cent are Lyt-1$^+$, and 5 to 10 per cent are Lyt-2,3$^+$.

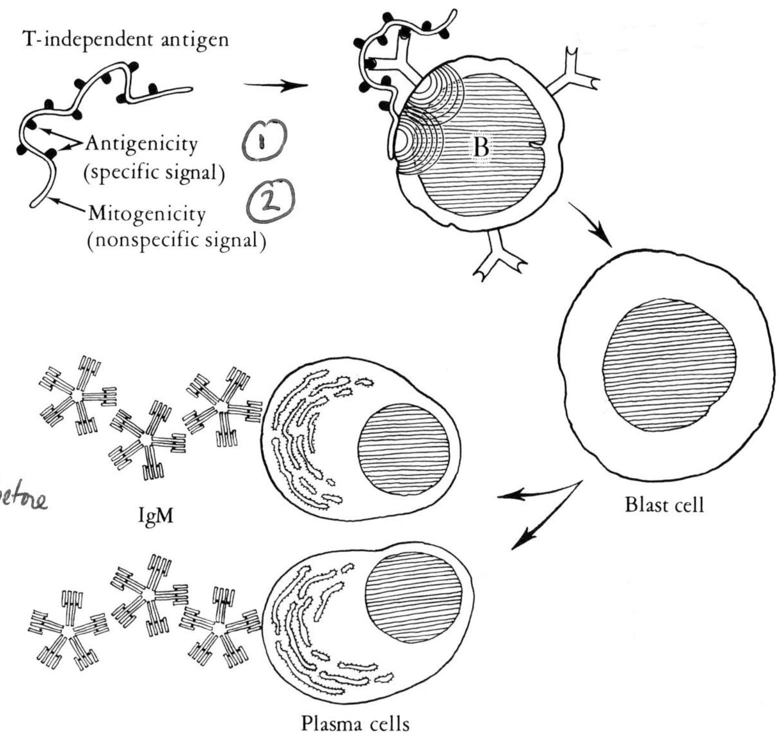

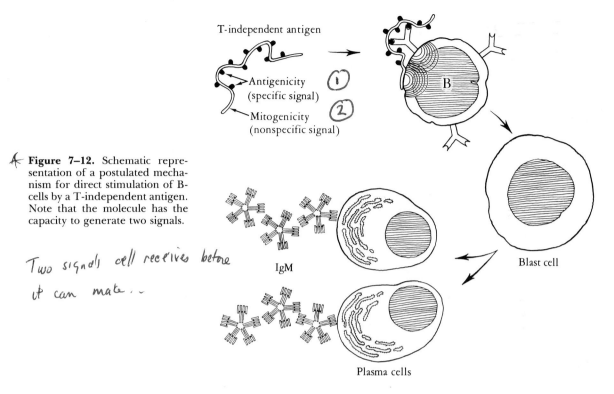

Figure 7–12. Schematic representation of a postulated mechanism for direct stimulation of B-cells by a T-independent antigen. Note that the molecule has the capacity to generate two signals.

Two signals cell receives before it can mate..

The Lyt-1,2,3$^+$ cells are the earliest to appear in T-cell ontogeny and are greatly reduced in numbers in peripheral lymphoid tissue shortly after adult thymectomy. The Lyt-1$^+$ and Lyt-2,3$^+$ subsets appear in peripheral lymphoid tissue later, and their numbers are relatively unaffected by adult thymectomy. It is believed that the precursor of these T-cell subsets, designated as the TL$^+$ Lyt-1,2,3$^+$ cell, directly differentiates into the Lyt-1,2,3$^+$ cell with the loss of the TL antigen. It is also thought that the Lyt-1$^+$ and Lyt-2,3$^+$ cells arise from the Lyt-1,2,3$^+$ cell as two separate lines of differentiation rather than from sequential stages with one maturing into the other (Fig. 7–13).

Cytotoxic antisera have been used to selectively deplete lymphoid cell populations of specific Lyt-bearing cells in an attempt to define unique immunologic functions associated with these subpopulations. These studies revealed that the T-cell subsets were precommitted to serve a particular immunologic function during a process of thymus-dependent differentiation, which occurs before the cells encounter specific antigens. In other words, maturation of these cells is independent of antigen stimulation.

The Lyt-1$^+$ cell responds to immunogenic stimulation by proliferating and elaborating various factors (specific and nonspecific) that stimulate B-cells to differentiate into antibody-producing cells. Thus, the Lyt-1$^+$ cell is the carrier-specific T-cell in the hapten-carrier response and is the cell responsible for *T-cell helper function* (T_H). In addition, this T-cell subset also contains cells that help in the development of cytotoxic T-cells, which normally display the Lyt-2,3$^+$ phenotype as well as cells that function as effectors in delayed-type hypersensitivity responses. Thus, there is synergy between Lyt-1$^+$ and Lyt-2,3$^+$ T-cells in immune responses. The Lyt-2,3$^+$ population contains cells that manifest *T-cell suppressor function* (T_S) as well as cells that function as cytotoxic effectors involved in the destruction of tumor cells and transplanted allogeneic cells. Recent studies using the fluorescence-activated cell sorter have indicated that some Lyt-2,3$^+$ cells also bear the Lyt-1$^+$ marker, which could not be detected by conventional assays. The significance of this finding remains to be elucidated. The Lyt-1,2,3$^+$ cell appears to function as a precursor of

Lyt-1$^+$

TL$^+$, Lyt-1,2,3$^+$ → Lyt-1,2,3$^+$

Lyt-2,3$^+$

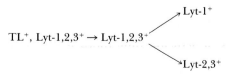

Figure 7–13. A proposed model of T-cell subset differentiation in the mouse.

both Lyt-1$^+$ and Lyt-2,3$^+$ cells as well as a cell that regulates the development of both T_H and T_S functional cell populations. This population functions as a precusor of killer cells that destroy virus-infected cells having altered self-antigens (Chapter 16). In addition, these cells appear to interact with the Lyt-2,3$^+$ cells for other killer functions.

Further subdivision of the Lyt-1$^+$ and Lyt-2,3$^+$ subsets can be made on the basis of expression of MHC determinants. Some Lyt-1$^+$ cells also express markers coded by the Qa-1 region, while others lack these antigens. Similarly, some Lyt-2,3$^+$ T-cells also express I-J encoded markers, while others do not. The function of these cells will be discussed later in this chapter in the section on regulation of immune responses. Table 7–6 summarizes the properties of these murine T-cell subsets. As indicated previously, functional subpopulations of human T-cells have been defined by monoclonal antibodies. Table 7–7 outlines the similarities between human and mouse T-cell subsets with respect to their functional capabilities.

Genetic Control of Cell Cooperation

As indicated in Chapter 3, the immune response is subject to genetic influence at various levels, including that which encompasses cellular interactions. Such control can exist at the level of antigen presentation (macrophage), antigen recognition (T- and B-cells), and cell cooperation.

Advances in our understanding of the genetic control of cell cooperation were made possible by studies of the immune response of inbred animals, mainly mice and guinea pigs (Chapter 3). Specific responses to many antigens have been shown to be under the influence of autosomal dominant genes that are linked to the *major histocompatibility complex* (MHC), a multigenic system determining the structure and expression of a number of cell-surface glycoproteins. In the mouse, the H-2 is the major histocompatibility complex. Within the H-2 complex are two regions, *K and D,* which are approximately 0.5 centimorgan apart, a distance sufficient to include the genetic information for up to 2000 structural genes. The products of the K and D regions (called *Class I determinants*) are ubiquitously distributed cell-surface glycoproteins that appear to be in close association with β_2 microglobulin. These gene products are serologically defined antigens that elicit antibodies involved in graft rejection. The K and D gene products also appear to interact with cytopathogenic viruses, a process that has been shown to be necessary for recognition of virus-infected cells by cytotoxic T-cells. A new locus of undetermined function, called H-2L, has recently been described. This

Table 7–6. Characteristics of Lyt$^+$ Subsets of Mouse T-cells

Property	Lyt-1,2,3$^+$	Lyt-1$^+$	Lyt-2,3$^+$
Ontogeny	Early	Later	Later
Percent of T-cells in			
Periphery	60–65	30–35	5–10
Thymus	90	10	10
Helper activity for			
Antibody production	±	+	–
Generation of killer cells	±	+	–
DTH effector cell	±	+	–
Suppressor activity in			
Antibody production	±	–	+
Mixed-leukocyte reaction (MLC)	±	–	+
Regulator function			
Precursor	+	–	–
Amplifier	+	–	–
MHC reactivity			
I-region determinants	–	+	+
K/D region determinants	–	–	+
Killer potential	±	–	+
Cytotoxic effector	–	–	+

Table 7–7. T-Cell Subsets of Mice and Humans*

Human Marker	Mouse Marker	Function of Subsets
OKT 10,6,4,5† Leu-1	Lyt-1,2,3	$T_{regulator}$ $T_{precursor}$
OKT 4 Leu-3a,3b	Lyt-1	T_{helper} T_{DTH}
OKT 5/8 Leu-2a,2b	Lyt-2,3	$T_{suppressor}$ $T_{cytotoxic}$

*The Leu series of monoclonal antibodies is a trademark of Becton Dickinson Company, Sunnyvale, California. The OK series of monoclonal antibodies is the trademark of Ortho Pharmaceutical Corporation, Raritan, New Jersey.

†To date, no monoclonal antibody has been produced that is specific for this population of cells. However, the OKT 10,6,4,5 cell represents a cell that is found in the thymus but not in the peripheral lymphoid compartment, whereas the Leu-1 and Lyt-1,2,3 cells are found in the periphery as well as in the thymus.

locus lies close to, but is independent of, the H-2D locus. The murine K and D loci are equivalent to human B, C, and A loci (see Figs. 3–3 and 3–6).

Genetic markers have been identified between the K and D regions. The *S locus* contains structural genes coding for the synthesis of complement components (C3 and C4). An analogous region, coding for the second and fourth components of complement and the properdin factor B (BF) of the alternative pathway (Chapter 6) has been described in the human MHC.

Located between the K and S regions of the mouse MHC is the *I-region,* which controls immune responses to a large number of antigens and codes for cell surface glycoproteins (called *Class II determinants*) important in mediating cellular interactions. The I-region has been further divided into several subregions: I-A, I-B, I-J, I-E, and I-C. There are some questions about the existence of some of these regions. For example, it has been shown that some I-region functions can be explained by cooperation between I-A and I-E products on interacting cells. Whether I-B, I-C, and even I-J, which has been reported to be associated with certain T-cell subsets, actually exist is currently being evaluated. As with the K, D, and S regions, the human MHC possesses a region analogous to the murine I-region. This region is found close to the HLA-D locus and is referred to as the *D-related* (DR) locus. In addition to D and DR, several other yet incompletely defined loci have been detected in this region of the human MHC. These include DC, MB, and SB. The products of the DR and SB loci appear to be analogous to the products of the murine I-E subregion, while the product of the human MB locus resembles that of the mouse I-A subregion.

The gene product of the I-region, referred to as *I-region–associated* or *Ia determinant (antigen),* plays an important role in antigen recognition by T-cells and in the interactions among macrophages, T-cells, and B-cells. These determinants have been defined by antibodies obtained by cross immunization between recombinant mice that differ in the I-region. Of the more than 20 Ia specificities currently recognized, the majority have been localized in the I-A subregion, with others having been identified in the I-E subregion. Some Ia specificities have also been described in the I-B and I-J subregions; the latter are thought to code for determinants present on suppressor T-cells. In contrast to K and D determinants, Ia determinants have a restricted distribution. They are found on B-cells, on some macrophages, and on certain T-cell subsets as well as on spermatozoa and epidermal Langerhans cells. It is now well documented that Ia determinants participate in the presentation of antigen by macrophages, since anti-Ia antibodies block the generation of T-helper cell activity. Ia determinants have been detected on both antigen-specific and nonspecific factors released by T-cells and macrophages. Ia determinants can be detected on killer T-cells, mitogen-responsive T-cells, MLR-stimulator T-cells, helper T-cells, and suppressor T-cells. It is likely that the Ia determinant represents the product of the postulated *cell interaction (CI) genes* located within the MHC that mediates cellular interactions.

The murine I-region also contains the so-called immune response genes (*Ir genes*) that appear to control the ability of an individual to respond to a specific antigen as well as the magnitude of the response to that antigen. These genes have been mapped primarily in the I-A subregion. A small number of Ir genes that appear to require complementation are found in both the I-A and the I-E subregions; their presence in the I-B subregion is not definitively established. Specific Ir genes have been delineated by measuring immune responses to structurally defined immunogens (Chapter 3). For example, the immune response to the synthetic branched copolymer of tyrosine, glutamic acid, alanine, and lysine, called (T,G)-A-L, has been shown to be under genetic control. Mice of the

C57Bl strain (responder) produce high titers of both IgM and IgG antibody to this T-dependent antigen. Mice of the CBA strain (nonresponder) produce a normal IgM primary response but do not produce IgG antibodies in the primary or secondary response. Thymectomized mice of responder strains react like nonresponders, suggesting that the product of the Ir gene is associated with the T-cell, since these cells appear to be needed for IgG production.

Additional information has been obtained from studies of the immune response of guinea pigs to poly-L-lysine (PLL). Inbred strain 2 guinea pigs (responder) respond well to DNP-PLL, giving high antibody titers to the haptenic (DNP) portion with cell-mediated hypersensitivity and helper activity to the PLL portion. Strain 13 animals (nonresponder) do not give the aforementioned responses. As with F_1 generations of responder × nonresponder mice, F_1 hybrids of strain 2 × strain 13 guinea pigs are all responders, as are about 50 per cent of the progeny of the backcross of hybrids to low-responder strains. Both nonresponder mouse and guinea pig strains will make anti-hapten responses like that of responder strains if the hapten is administered as a complex with an immunogenic carrier such as BSA (e.g., DNP-PLL-BSA or (T,G)-A-L-BSA). These findings suggest that the Ir gene product is concerned with the recognition of the carrier portion of the immunogen, a function normally ascribed to T-cells.

Although there are some studies that suggest that Ir gene control is also expressed at the level of the B-cell, the most convincing evidence points to the macrophage as the cell most intimately involved in I-region regulation of immune responsiveness. In an elegant series of experiments, Rosenthal and Shevach demonstrated that it was the I-region determinants on the macrophage, not the T-cell, that controlled the ability of lymphocytes to proliferate in response to *in vitro* stimulation by antigen. They immunized (2 × 13) F_1 guinea pigs simultaneously with DNP-GL (to which strain 2 responds, but strain 13 does not) and GT (to which strain 13 responds, but strain 2 does not). These antigens were then presented to lymphocytes from immunized guinea pigs either in their soluble form or in association with macrophages from strains 2,13 or (2 × 13) F_1 of normal animals (Table 7–8). Lymphocytes from (2 × 13) F_1 animals responded to both DNP-GL and GT when presented alone or by (2 × 13) F_1 macrophages. In a similar manner, strain 2 lymphocytes (responder to DNP-GL) or strain 13 lymphocytes (responder to GT) proliferated only when the antigen to which they normally respond was presented on strain 2 or strain 13 macrophages, respectively. No response was observed when DNP-GL was presented to (2 × 13) F_1 lymphocytes by strain 13 macrophages (nonresponder to DNP-GL) or when GT was presented by strain 2 macrophages (nonresponder to GT). On the other hand, proliferation of (2 × 13) F_1 lymphocytes occurred when DNP-GL was presented on strain 2 macrophages (responder for DNP-GL) and GT was presented on strain 13 macrophages (responder for GT). These results demonstrate that macrophages that present antigens to T-cells must share the same I-region determinants expressed by T-cells. In a manner similar to that described

Table 7–8. Regulation of T-Lymphocyte Proliferation by I-Region Determinants on Macrophages

Source of Sensitized T-Lymphocytes*	Antigen Used for In Vitro Challenge	Source of Macrophage for Antigen Presentation	Proliferative Response (DNA Synthesis)
Strain 2 (Responder)	DNP-GL	Strain 2 (Responder)	+ + +
		Strain 13 (Nonresponder)	–
Strain 13 (Responder)	GT	Strain 2 (Nonresponder)	–
		Strain 13 (Responder)	+ + +
(2 × 13) F_1	DNP-GL	(2 × 13) F_1	+ + +
		Strain 2	+ + +
		Strain 13	–
(2 × 13) F_1	GT	(2 × 13) F_1	+ + +
		Strain 2	–
		Strain 13	+ + +

*Animals were immunized simultaneously with DNP-GL and GT. (After Rosenthal and Shevach.)

for antigen-induced activation of helper T-cells described above, shared MHC determinants on macrophages are also required for the activation of killer T-cells involved in removal of virus-infected cells as well as allogeneic and tumor target cells and effector T-cells involved in delayed-type hypersensitivity responses. Whereas H-2K and H-2D determinants are involved in the activation of killer T-cells (Chapters 3 and 9), I-region determinants in the form of the Ia antigen participate in activation of helper T-cells and effector T-cells of DTH. Two models have been proposed in an attempt to explain the complex nature of the T-cell recognition unit (see Fig. 3–4). The *dual receptor* model suggests that T-cells either have two separate receptors or that the receptor consists of two distinct regions—one that recognizes antigen and the other that recognizes self-MHC determinants (either H2-K and H-2D or I-region). The second model, referred to as *altered-self*, suggests that the T-cell receptor is a single unit that recognizes a complex determinant generated by an interaction between antigen and MHC molecules. Both of these models indicate that T-cells cannot be activated by interacting with either antigen or self-MHC determinants alone. The ability of T-cells to recognize self-MHC determinants is acquired in the thymus during differentiation rather than being determined by the cell's own H-2 haplotype.

START HERE:

MODELS OF ANTIBODY FORMATION

The immune response to T-dependent antigens requires the activity of Ia-bearing accessory cells (represented by macrophages, dendritic cells, and epidermal Langerhans cells). Figure 7–14 depicts the postulated cellular events involved in T-cell activation. As indicated in the previous section, the initial stage of T-cell activation occurs as a consequence of the recognition of processed antigen in association with self-MHC (Ia) determinants. Possibly, as a result of surface changes due to ligand binding, the macrophages are stimulated to synthesize and secrete interleukin-1 (IL-1). This soluble mediator appears to provide a second signal that exerts its effect both by stimulating an increase in the number of receptors on the T-cell for a second distinct interleukin, called IL-2, and also by inducing the synthesis of IL-2 by the T-cells. Whether the T-cells that synthesize IL-2 are the same as those that react with it is not clear at this time. As a consequence of IL-2 stimulation, full activation of T-cells is achieved. In addition to their ability to cooperate with other cell types for further expression of the immune response, activated T-cells release products that increase the reactivity of macrophages. Soluble materials released by activated T-cells appear to augment the density of Ia determinants expressed on the surface of macrophages, thereby augmenting the antigen-presenting capabilities of these cells.

In addition to the activation of T-cells resulting from direct cellular contact between histocompatible macrophages and T-cells, helper cells can be generated by soluble factors produced by macrophages. Two of these factors, designated genetically related factor (GRF) and nonspecific macrophage factor (NMF), have been described. GRF is released from macrophages only after they have been incubated with soluble antigen. The macrophages that release this factor share I-region determinants (I-A) with responding lymphocytes. GRF is a heat-labile protein with a molecular weight of 55,000 to 60,000 whose biologic activity cannot be absorbed with anti-immunoglobulin, but can be with anti-Ia antibody. This factor was shown to contain Ia determinants linked to a small antigenic fragment. The nonspecific factor, NMF, was shown to be released from normal macrophages. It activated T-helper cells only when the T-cells were obtained from animals immunized with particulate antigens. This factor is not I-region–restricted. Thus, T-cell activation has a twofold requirement: (1) the recognition of antigen in association with Ia determinants on the surface of accessory cells, and (2) the release of biologically active factors from accessory cells, which then act on T-cells.

Just as two signals seem to be needed for the activation of T-cells, two signals have been shown to be required for triggering of the B-cell differentiation process that leads to antibody synthesis. As indicated previously, one of these signals involves the recognition of antigen by immunoglobulin receptors on B-cells. The second signal, which is incompletely defined, appears to be mediated by helper T-cells, which induce proliferation in B-cells, probably through a soluble factor (e.g., B-cell activating factor). Several models have been proposed to explain the

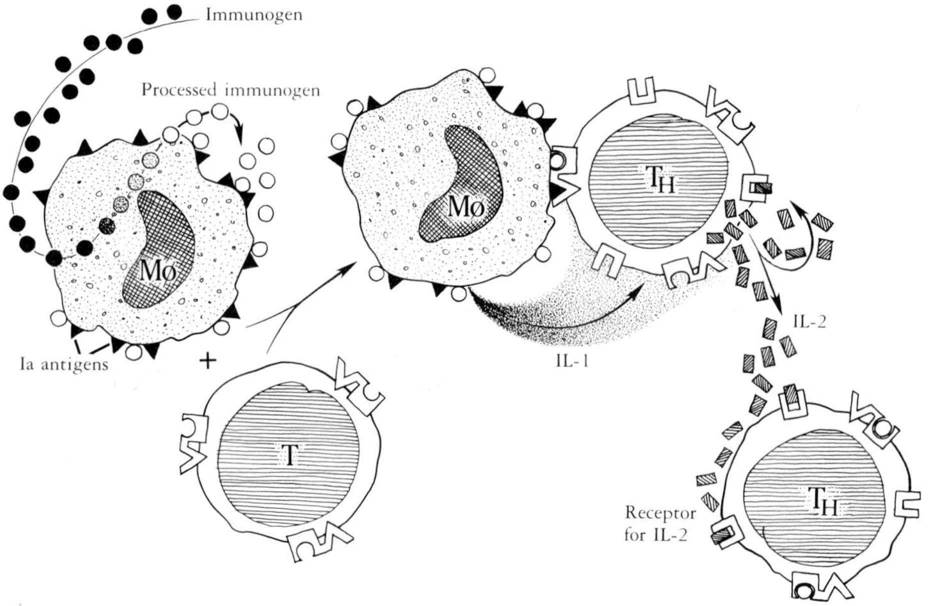

Figure 7–14. Schematic representation of the cellular events involved in T-cell activation.

interactions between helper T-cells and B-cells.

The *antigen-focusing hypothesis,* based on the carrier effect (see p. 123), suggests that there is simultaneous binding of complex antigens by T- and B-cells. In this model, the T-cell presents a polyvalent pattern of haptenic determinants whose critical function is the cross-linking of hapten-specific Ig receptors on the surface of B-cells. Evidence derived from *in vitro* experiments involving cellular interactions has cast doubt on the foregoing hypothesis, which relegates the T-cell to an essentially passive role. These experiments have demonstrated that cooperation between B- and T-cells can occur even when the two cell populations are separated by a membrane that is impermeable to the cells, and suggest that helper T-cells operate through soluble factors.

Two classes of soluble factors produced by T-cells have been shown to influence the activity of B-cells. The first of these factors is nonspecific (produced by T-cells in response to nonspecific stimuli) and can be generated in several ways. These factors have been used to replace the requirement for a carrier in anti-hapten secondary responses. One such factor has been produced by injection of allogeneic lymphoid cells into an animal primed with a hapten-carrier complex. For example, if animals primed with DNP-BSA are injected with allogeneic lymphoid cells from a donor whose cells will attack the host's cells in a graft-versus-host reaction, and if at a later time they receive a second injection of DNP coupled to a non–cross-reacting carrier such as OA, then a secondary anti-DNP response can be elicited in the absence of OA-primed T-cells. The factor responsible for this so-called *allogeneic effect* is referred to as the *allogeneic effect factor* (AEF). The active factor appears to be a bimolecular complex consisting of 35,000 and 12,000 dalton subunits. The AEF contains determinants coded for by genes of the major histocompatibility complex of the mouse, since its activity can be removed by absorption with antisera prepared against the product of these genes, specifically anti-Ia. Similar nonspecific factors can be prepared from supernatant fluids of short-term cultures of histoincompatible mouse spleen cells that have participated in an *in vitro* mixed leukocyte reaction or from supernatant fluids of cells stimulated *in vitro* with T-cell mitogens such as Con-A or PHA. Together with the hapten-specific signal, these nonspecific factors are thought to function as a second signal in triggering the activation of B-cells.

T-cells have also been shown to elaborate antigen-specific factors, which cooperate with B-cells in immune responses. One such factor, produced by T-cells, was called "IgT" because it was initially thought to be a monomeric (8S) IgM molecule. This factor has the capacity to bind the specific antigen used to activate the T-cells and also has the ability to bind to the membrane of macrophages, probably through an Fc receptor. Using *in vitro* systems in which B- and T-cells were separated by a membrane permeable only by molecules, it was shown that upon stimulation with antigen, the T-cells release a factor that is complexed with antigen that can diffuse across the membrane and become associated with macrophages. The macrophage-bound antigen-"IgT" complex induces B-cells to respond specifically to the hapten determinants present on the molecule. Subsequent studies have shown that this factor, as well as other antigen-specific factors, are produced by Lyt-1^+ T-cells and that such factors carry Ia determinants coded for by the I-A subregion.

It has also been shown that (T,G)-A-L–activated spleen cells release an antigen-specific factor after *in vitro* challenge with the same material. This factor replaces the specific T-cell helper function and reacts with antisera prepared against molecules specified by genes located on the left side of the H-2 complex, specifically the I-A region. It has been demonstrated that both responder and nonresponder T-cells produce this "antigen recognition" factor. On the other hand, this factor, whether derived from responder or nonresponder animals, will cooperate effectively only with B-cells from responder animals. It has been suggested that B-cells carry an "acceptor" site for T-cell factors. Thus, a genetic defect that gives rise to a nonresponder animal may also be found at the level of the "acceptor" site (B-cell). In examining several strains for their ability to produce the "antigen-recognition" factor (T-cell) or the "acceptor" site (B-cell), investigators have found strains that are defective in T-cell factor, B-cell "acceptor," or both. These results suggest that two I-region genes are involved in the control of the response to (T,G)-A-L. One, expressed in T-cells, codes for an "antigen recognition" factor and is coupled to an "interaction" factor; the other, expressed in B-cells, codes for the "acceptor" site. It is the "interaction" factor that reacts with the B-cell "acceptor" site and thus facilitates cell cooperation.

Utilizing the foregoing information, it is possible to present a hypothetical model of antibody formation that illustrates potential interactions among T-cells, B-cells, and macrophages (Fig. 7–15). While it is clear that the immunogen plays an important role in selecting the specific receptor (idiotype)-bearing B- and T-cells that cooperate for antibody production, it is also well accepted that these cellular interactions are under the control of genes coded for by the MHC. This model is based on *in vitro* events and may be subject to complete revision as new information arises and ideas and concepts change in this rapidly moving area of immunobiology.

In this model, the initial event most likely involves the interaction of the immunogen with an accessory cell (e.g., macrophage) in a nonspecific manner, leading to the processing of this material into an immunogenic form that is expressed on the macrophage surface. In the case of T-dependent antigens, the first specific recognition event involving carrier determinants occurs at the level of the T-cell and is mediated by the incompletely defined T-cell receptor, which recognizes the antigen in the context of self-MHC determinants on the macrophage surface. Full activation of T-cells in some systems involves the activity of a soluble factor produced by the accessory cell (interleukin-1), which stimulates the production and release of a second factor, interleukin-2 (also called T-cell growth factor [TCGF]), by the T-cell (Fig. 7–14). Additional antigen-specific factors that carry Ia determinants (e.g., GRF, described above) and are produced by macrophages have also been shown to be involved in T-cell activation. Alternatively, there is also some experimental evidence that helper T-cells can be activated as a consequence of the direct interaction of antigen with T-cell receptors. However, this appears to be unlikely, since current thinking suggests that those antigens that bypass the initial event of interacting with an accessory cell and react directly with the T-cell induce a population of suppressor T-cells rather than helper T-cells (see discussion on regulation later in this chapter).

Once activated, helper T-cells or their factors can cooperate with B-cells by one or more of several possible mechanisms. According to one mechanism, B-cell triggering involves the direct interaction of activated T-cells with B-cells possessing specific Ig receptors. In this case, there is some evidence to indicate that the cooperating cells must also share MHC-coded surface determinants in order for optimal interaction to occur. For reasons indicated earlier in this chapter, this does not appear to be the favored mechanism. The remainder of the mechanisms to be described involve soluble factors produced by activated helper T-cells. In the first of these, the activated T-cell has been reported

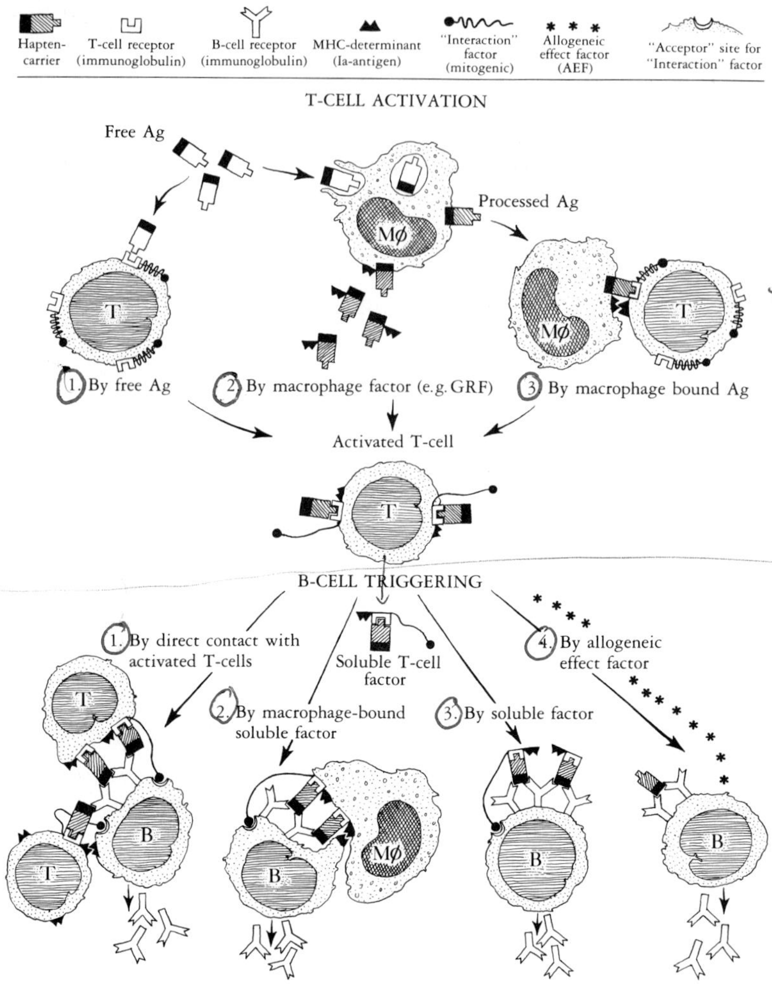

Figure 7–15. Schematic representation of cellular interactions involved in the generation of the humoral immune responses. Note that T-cells can be activated in three ways: (1) by free antigen (Ag); (2) by macrophage-processed antigen; or (3) by macrophage-associated antigen. In turn, B-cells may be triggered to produce antibody in four ways: (1) by direct contact with Ag-bearing activated T-cells; (2) by macrophage-bound factor; (3) by a soluble Ag-specific T-cell factor; or (4) by a nonspecific (allogeneic effect) factor produced by T-cells.

to release its receptor ("IgT")-containing antigen, which then becomes associated with the surface of a macrophage, possibly through Fc receptors. As a consequence of this binding, a lattice of repeating similar antigenic determinants, resembling that found on T-independent antigens, is thought to be created. Thus, both types of antigens can be visualized as being presented to B-cells in an analogous manner. While this hypothesis is attractive, it remains unproved.

An additional antigen-specific factor has been shown to contain MHC-coded determinants, specifically Ia. At present, it is not clear whether the B-cell and macrophage must share I-region determinants for efficient cooperation to occur. This mechanism of cell communication is also not favored in view of the fact that it requires a direct interaction between antigen and T-cell as the initial event, instead of the more widely held view that antigen first interacts with macrophages. An additional mechanism suggests that the activated helper T-cell can release an immunologically active substance containing an "interaction" factor that bears I-region determinants (Ia) and represents the mitogenic signal provided by the T-cell. This soluble material can react with a B-cell that carries both an antigen-specific Ig receptor and an "acceptor" site (which also may be coded for by an I-region gene) for the T-cell "interaction" factor. Since there is no direct contact between T- and B-cells, there may not be a requirement for the sharing of common MHC gene products. Indeed, efficient cooperation between soluble T-cell factors and B-cells has been achieved with various combinations of allogeneic cells. For example, the *allogeneic effect factor* described earlier is capable of providing the second signal to antigen-stimulated B-cells in certain experimental systems.

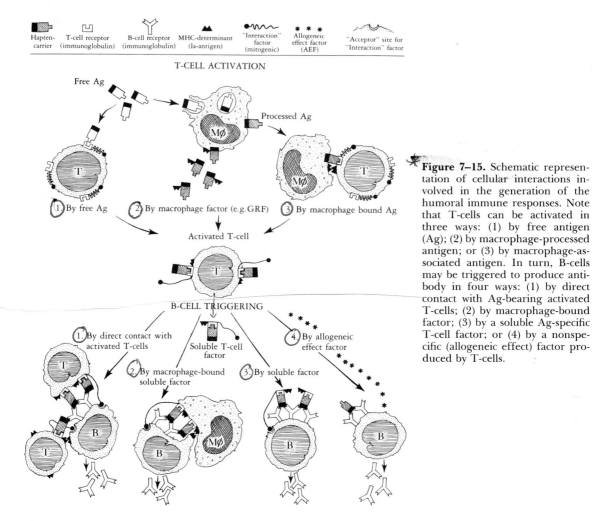

In each of the mechanisms described

above, the precommitted B-cell recognizes the appropriate antigenic determinants (hapten) through its surface Ig receptors, providing the antigen-specific signal. The non–antigenic-specific or mitogenic signal is provided by the activated helper T-cell or its product(s). The activated B-cell then goes through a series of events involving its differentiation into a plasma cell, accompanied by the proliferation of a clone of antibody-secreting cells. Our understanding of Ir genes, their control of complex cellular interactions in the immune response, and their relationship to the antigenic makeup of the individual is in a very early stage. This area of immunology is destined to have a strong impact on our understanding of disease processes.

REGULATION OF ANTIBODY FORMATION

It soon becomes apparent that there must be some regulatory mechanism(s) operating to control antibody formation. If this did not occur, antigen stimulation might lead to proliferation of antibody-forming cells comparable to that seen in neoplasia. Several potential mechanisms are described below.

Antigenic Competition

Simultaneous or close administration of two unrelated immunogens in some cases results in the transient and nonspecific suppression of the immune response to one of the antigens and a normal response to the other. This phenomenon, called *antigenic competition,* is defined as the inhibition of the immune response to one antigen or determinant as a consequence of the administration of another antigen or determinant. Competition between two separate antigens is called *intermolecular* antigenic competition, while that which occurs between antigenic determinants on the same molecule is called *intramolecular* antigenic competition. The maximum suppressive effect is observed when the second antigen is administered a few days after the first one. If the second antigen is given after a booster injection of the first one, competition is more apparent. The mechanism involved in antigenic competition is not known. Several possible explanations have been advanced, including (1) activation of suppressor T-cells; (2) interference with the ability of macrophages to present antigen to lymphocytes owing to saturation of essential cooperating sites on the macrophage surface; (3) competition for nutrients; or (4) release of soluble suppressor factors.

Antigenic competition is of both theoretical and practical importance. For the immunologist, it is important to understand the mechanism by which two unrelated immunogens interfere with each other. This is difficult to understand if we accept the premise of the clonal selection theory, which states that antigen-sensitive cells are precommitted to produce antibody of one specificity. This phenomenon has been used as a major argument for multipotentiality of antigen-sensitive cells. For the clinician, antigenic competition has practical significance when vaccination programs are considered (Chapter 23). For example, if appropriate dose adjustments of diphtheria and tetanus toxoids are not made in the DPT vaccine given to children, antigenic competition might occur. The clinician must also consider the immunosuppressive effects of this phenomenon in relation to disease processes. For example, in murine systems it has been shown that infection with leukemia viruses results in an immunosuppressed animal. Similarly, certain virus infections in humans (e.g., measles) can result in an immunosuppressed host.

Passive Antibody

It has been shown that the administration of preformed antibody can interfere with the host's ability to produce its own antibody in response to immunogenic stimulation. This suppressive effect can be achieved by injection of antibodies directed against different targets. For example, administration of anti-SRBC antibody (anti-immunogen) at the same time or soon after injection of SRBC results in suppression of anti-SRBC antibody formation in mice. This suppression is antigen-specific and most pronounced when the anti-immunogen antibody is given in relative excess. Antibodies of the IgG class are more effective at inducing suppression than are IgM antibodies, as are high-affinity antibodies compared with low-affinity antibodies. This phenomenon does not occur when passive antibody is given to previously immunized animals; thus, it does not appear to affect immunologic memory.

The clinician has made use of this phenomenon in the prevention of severe hemolytic disease of the newborn due to Rh incompatibility. Preformed antibody prepared against Rh^+ red blood cells is injected into Rh^- mothers at the time of delivery of Rh^+ babies. This antibody binds to and enhances the elimination of Rh^+ red blood cells that enter the maternal circulation as the placenta separates. This procedure prevents the immunization of the mother, who, if untreated, would produce a secondary IgG response to Rh^+ red blood cells in a subsequent Rh-incompatible pregnancy. These IgG antibodies are capable of crossing the placenta and could result in the destruction of fetal red blood cells (Chapter 24). In addition to the desirable immunosuppressive effect of passive antibody described above, the clinician must be aware of undesirable effects that may occur naturally. For example, the placental transfer of maternal antibody against certain viruses (e.g., polio and measles) could interfere with the initiation of an active immune response against these agents in the young child. Therefore, the clinician must adjust the immunization timetable to allow for the disappearance of maternal antibody if successful active immunization is to be achieved. Although the mechanism of action of this feedback effect is not clear, it has been suggested that passive antibody acts by blocking antigenic determinants so that the appropriate antigen-sensitive cells cannot be stimulated.

As with passive administration of anti-immunogen antibody, injection of antibodies against the antigen-binding surface receptors on B- or T-cells also results in suppression of antibody formation. This type of suppression can be achieved using anti-receptor antibodies of various specificities. For example, injection of newborn animals with antibodies against the μ chain of IgM results in the loss of ability of the maturing animal to synthesize not only IgM but also IgG and IgA immunoglobulins. Passive transfer of anti-γ or anti-α antibodies interferes with the production of only IgG or IgA, respectively. This phenomenon, called *isotype suppression*, does not occur in adults and lends credence to the hypothesis that B-cells expressing IgM on their surface are precursors of cells that secrete other classes of immunoglobulin later in life.

Injection of newborn animals with antibody prepared against allotypic markers on paternal immunoglobulin molecules results in suppression of the appearance of Ig molecules bearing the paternal allotype. Normal Ig levels are maintained because of an overproduction of molecules bearing the maternal allotype. This phenomenon, called *allotype suppression*, usually lasts for several months even after the natural catabolic decay of the passively transferred Ig has occurred. This suggests that suppression is due to an active process. T-cells have been implicated in this phenomenon, since the cells responsible for suppression can be eliminated by treatment with anti-Thy-1 plus complement. Although the mechanism remains unclear, it has been suggested that suppressor T-cells exert their effect on helper T-cells rather than directly on the antibody-forming B-cell.

A third type of anti-receptor antibody can also suppress antibody formation. In this case, administration of antibodies against idiotypic determinants can suppress the production of immunoglobulins that bear that particular idiotype. This inhibition, referred to as *idiotype suppression*, can be of two types. One results from administration of high doses of anti-idiotypic antibody, causing immediate but transient suppression. A second type, resulting from low doses of anti-idiotypic antibody is characterized by delayed but chronic suppression. This type of suppression appears to play a major role in the regulation of antibody formation.

In 1974, Jerne proposed his *network hypothesis* in an attempt to explain the complex interactions that regulate antibody formation. He suggested that the immune system is self-regulating and is composed of a network of idiotypes and anti-idiotypic antibodies. According to this hypothesis, an antigen elicits the production of an antibody (Ab_1) that possesses a unique sequence of amino acids, called the idiotype (Id_1), in its antigen-binding region, which distinguishes it from other antibodies. The unique sequence displayed by Id_1 can also function as an immunogen in the same host (since this new array of amino acids is not recognized as self) and stimulates the production of another antibody (Ab_2) that has anti-idiotypic specificity for Ab_1 and at the same time displays its unique idiotype (Id_2). In a similar manner, Ab_2 will stimulate the production of Ab_3, which has its unique sequence (Id_3) and which displays anti–anti-idiotypic antibody activity against Ab_2, and so on, such that each idiotype that is expressed will stimulate the production of a corresponding anti-idiotypic antibody. From previous discussion it should be recalled that both B- and T-cells, as well as their soluble products (e.g., antibody, T-cell suppressor and helper factors) display idiotypic determinants. Further, inherent in the clonal selection theory is the fact that the idiotype of the Ig secreted by a B-cell is the same as its surface Ig receptor for antigen. In other words, each clone of B- or T-cells possesses a receptor capable of recognizing not only a specific antigenic determinant but also an idiotype expressed by the receptor on another clone of B- or T-cells. Figure 7–16

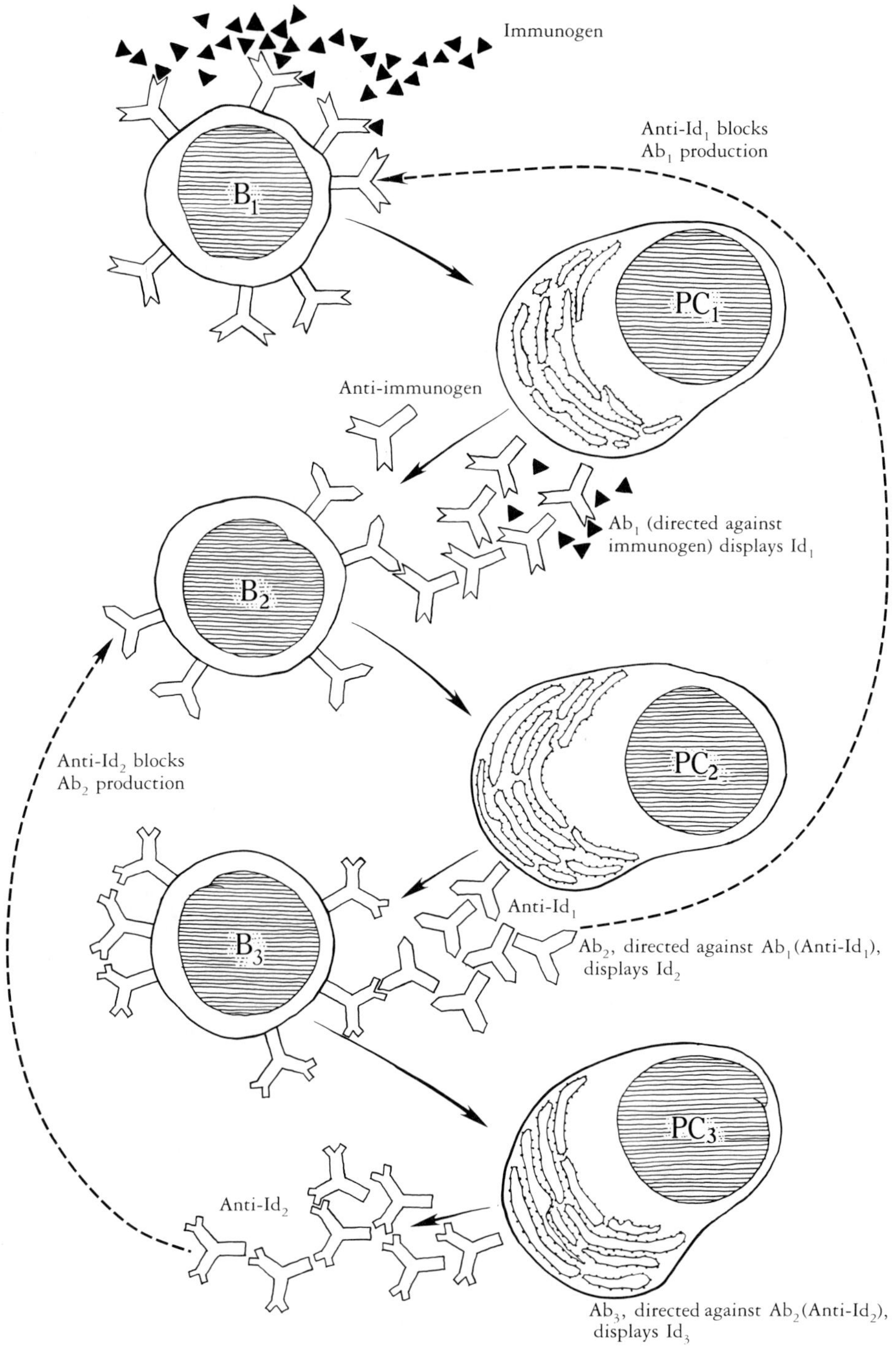

Figure 7–16. Schematic representation of idiotype–anti-idiotype regulation of antibody formation.

schematically presents the idiotype–anti-idiotype network operative in B-cells. In this scheme, the immunogen stimulates the first cell to produce its antibody (Ab_1). This antibody then stimulates another clone of B-cells, which has specific receptors for Id_1 of Ab_1, to make large amounts of Ab_2, which can suppress production of Ab_1 by a mechanism involving *idiotypic suppression*. The presence of Ab_2 can lead to the formation of Ab_3, which recognizes Id_2 and suppresses the formation of Ab_2, thereby terminating the suppression of Ab_2 on Ab_1 production. It should be noted that the network can also involve T-cells, whereby helper or suppressor T-cells can express idiotypes identical to those displayed on antibody molecules. Perturbation of this network, initiated by exposure to antigen, results in interaction between idiotypes, anti-idiotypes, and anti–anti-idiotypes that either turn on or turn off antibody formation through the activities of the various subsets of immunoregulatory T-cells.

Regulatory T-Cells

It has been amply demonstrated that in addition to the helper function provided by T-cells, the presence of this class of lymphocytes can also result in a reduction in the magnitude of the normal immune response or the level of immunoglobulin synthesis. The concept of a suppressor T-cell population was intially derived from studies involving the transfer of normal or immune cells to tolerant (Chapter 10) hosts and of tolerant cells to normal irradiated hosts. It was found that, as a result of the encounter of antigen with T-cells during the induction of tolerance, B-cells were "turned off" and could no longer cooperate with normal syngeneic T-cells to induce an immune response. This phenomenon is termed *infectious tolerance* and suggests a role for *suppressor T-cells* in the induction of tolerance.

Additional support for the presence of a population of suppressor T-cells can be summarized as follows: (1) In the immune response to T-independent antigens, removal of the thymus or treatment with anti-lymphocyte serum results in enhanced antibody formation; (2) T-cells from animals displaying chronic allotype suppression will cause allotype suppression by normal cells either *in vitro* or when passively transferred *in vivo*; (3) T-cells stimulated nonspecifically by mitogens (e.g., Con-A) suppress *in vitro* immune responses; (4) on the basis of studies of the hapten-specific IgE response, it appears that T-cells determine the class of immunoglobulin produced following antigenic stimulation; and (5) genetically defined nonresponder strains of animals appear to possess this characteristic owing to the presence of cells capable of suppressing immune responses to specific antigens.

It has been shown that suppression can be mediated by soluble factors that are either extracted from or released by T-cells. One such suppressor factor is involved in the regulation of the response to KLH in mice. This factor displays carrier-specific suppressor activity for IgG antibody production and appears to be under genetic control of the I-J subregion of the MHC. The target of this factor appears to be the carrier-primed helper T-cell rather than the hapten-primed B-cell. This observation indicates that interaction among T-cell subsets is responsible for the suppression of antibody formation. Further information regarding the nature of soluble regulatory factors produced by T-cells is expected in the near future in view of the development of techniques that enable T-cells to be immortalized as hybridomas in much the same way as B-cells have been for the production of monoclonal antibodies.

As indicated earlier in this chapter, it has been possible to further differentiate Lyt-bearing subsets of T-cells on the basis of their expression of MHC-associated determinants. For example, it has been shown that while interaction between both Lyt-1^+, Qa-1^+ and Lyt-1^+, Qa-1^- T-cells is required for generation of helper activity for antibody production by B-cells, the Lyt-1^+, Qa-1^+ subset is also involved in a *feedback regulatory loop* that generates active suppression by the Lyt-2,3^+ subset of T-cells. Mobilization of the Lyt-2,3^+ suppressor subset occurs as a consequence of a signal transmitted by the Lyt-1^+, Qa-1^+ *inducer T-cell* to the Lyt-1,2,3^+ *regulator T-cell*, which, in turn, generates suppressor function in the Lyt-2,3^+ cells. Thus, two subsets of Lyt-1^+–bearing T-cells can be identified, one that is Qa-1^- and is called a *helper-effector*, and a second that is Qa-1^+ and is called a *helper/suppressor-inducer*. Subpopulations of the Lyt-2,3^+ T-cell subset have also been delineated on the basis of their expression of I-J subregion products. While Lyt-2,3^+, I-J^- cells function as *suppressor-effectors*, the Lyt-2,3^+, I-J^+ T-cells appear to transmit a signal, also through the Lyt-1,2,3⁺ regulator T-cell, for a second feedback regulatory loop that turns off suppressor activity mediated by the Lyt-2,3⁺, I-J⁻ effector cells. This regulatory loop has been called *contrasuppression,* and the Lyt-2,3⁺, I-J⁺ T-cell that stimulates this loop is referred to as a *contrasuppressor-inducer.*

Figure 7–17 is a schematic representation of the proposed cellular interactions that might occur among the already recognized subsets of regulatory T-cells. Presentation of the immunogen on macrophages results in the activation of Lyt-1⁺, Qa-1⁻, I-J⁻ (helper-effector T-cell) and Lyt-1⁺, Qa-1⁺, I-J⁺ (inducer T-cell), which cooperate with B-cells to initiate antibody formation (Pathway 1). At the same time, the Lyt-1⁺, Qa-1⁺, I-J⁺ (helper/suppressor-inducer T-cell) population is activated to stimulate Lyt-1,2,3⁺, Qa-1⁺, I-J⁺ (regulator) T-cells, which influence the Lyt-2,3⁺, Qa-1⁻, I-J⁻ (suppressor-effector) T-cells to exert their regulatory effect (Pathway 2). As mentioned previously, it is currently thought that the suppressive effects mediated by the Lyt-2,3⁺, Qa-1⁻, I-J⁻ T-cells are manifest at the level of the helper-effector T-cells (Lyt-1⁺, Qa-1⁻, I-J⁻), rather than by direct action on B-cells. In situations in which the immunogen appears to bypass interaction with macrophages (e.g., high antigen dose), Lyt-2,3⁺, Qa-1⁻, I-J⁻ (suppressor-effector T-cells) can be directly activated by antigen (Pathway 3). These cells also exert their suppressive effects at the level of the helper-effector T-cell. Finally, the contrasuppression circuit (Pathway 4), initiated by the activation of Lyt-2,3⁺, Qa-1⁺, I-J⁺ T-cells, has a dual regulatory effect in that it appears to interfere with the suppressive activities of the Lyt-2,3⁺, Qa-1⁻, I-J⁻ (suppressor-effectors) as well as to render the Lyt-1⁺, Qa-1⁻, I-J⁻ (helper-effector) resistant to the activity of the suppressor-effector (Lyt-2,3⁺, Qa-1⁻, I-J⁻) cells. This pathway also is thought to occur through the Lyt-1,2,3⁺ regulator cell. Recently, it was demonstrated that similar T-T interactions are required for the generation of human suppressor-cell activity. In this system, cooperation between OKT4⁺ and OKT5/8⁺ T-cells was required for suppression to be exerted in an antigen-specific primary immune response.

The importance of regulatory T-cells is being recognized in clinical medicine. It has been shown that certain patients with common variable immunodeficiency (CVI) appear to have an increase in suppressor cell activity. This has been shown by the inhibition of immunoglobulin synthesis by normal cultured cells after the addition of lympho-

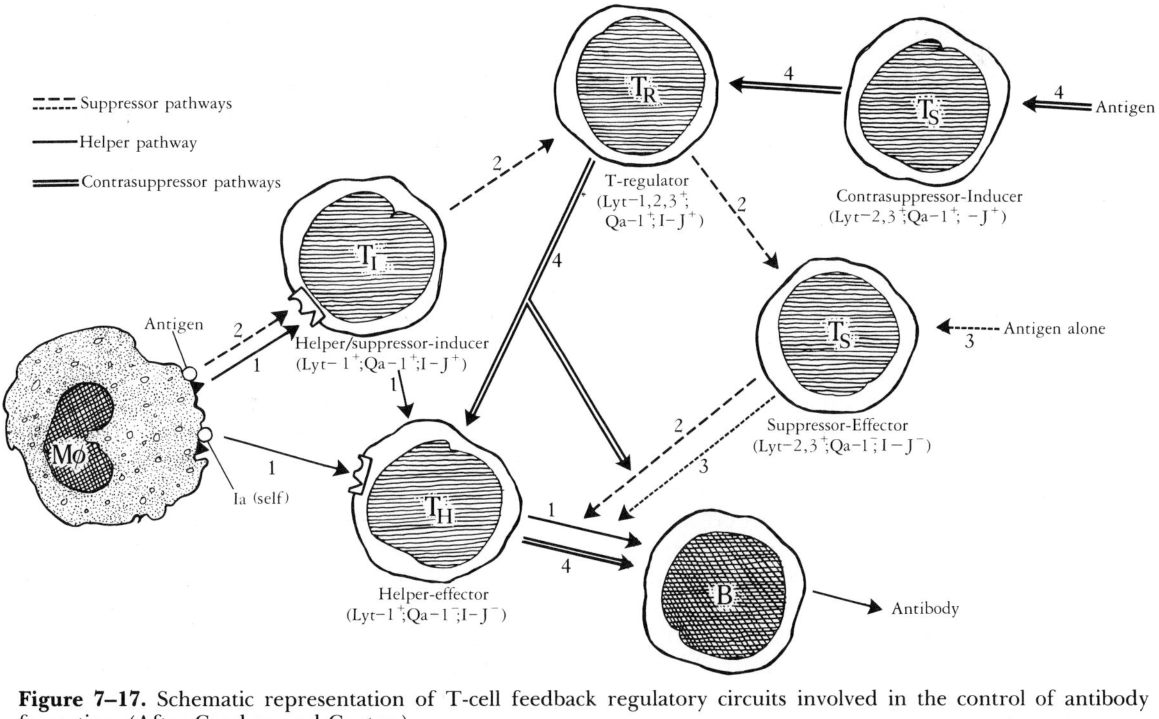

Figure 7–17. Schematic representation of T-cell feedback regulatory circuits involved in the control of antibody formation. (After Gershon and Cantor.)

cytes from CVI patients. Recently, a great deal of attention has been focused on gaining an understanding of the pathogenesis of acquired immunodeficiency syndrome (AIDS). Immunologic studies of several patients reveal a primary T-cell defect as indicated by a reduction in the absolute number of T-helper cells and depressed T-helper/T-suppressor cell ratios. Whether these immunologic aberrations are the cause or the effect of this newly described disease remains to be determined.

It has also been suggested that there is an enhancement of suppressor cell function in patients with multiple myeloma. The normal polyclonal response of the myeloma patient may be suppressed by these cells, resulting in an increased susceptibility to infection. Further, there is evidence to indicate that suppressor cells are closely involved in the control of autoimmune disease. It is thought that with advancing age there is a decrease in number or function of suppressor T-cells that allows for the expression of autoimmune disease. A similar argument has been advanced to explain the higher incidence of cancer in aging patients.

Thus, the reader can appreciate that a delicate balance exists between help and suppression, which serves to regulate the immune response.

THEORIES OF ANTIBODY FORMATION

The observation that an animal can produce antibody molecules not only against pathogenic microorganisms but also against foreign proteins and synthetic configurations has led to many speculations regarding the mechanism of antibody formation. The theories proposed fall into two categories that are based on the action of the immunogen, which can be either *selective* or *instructive* in the process of antibody formation.

In 1900, in what we would consider the Dark Ages of immunology, before the nature of the antibody molecule was known, before the nature of the reactions between antigen and antibody was known, before the nature of the cells that made antibody was known, Ehrlich proposed a theory of antibody formation that was remarkably similar to currently accepted ideas (see Fig. 1–11). He proposed that all cells of the body possess side chains on their surface, termed haptophores (antibody), that function as receptors for metabolites, termed toxophores (antigens). As a result of the reaction between the metabolite and the receptor, the receptor is consumed and the cell compensates by synthesizing new side chains in excess, some of which are released into the circulation. Ehrlich's concept of selection of cells with preexisting receptors for antigen was challenged in the 1930's by the work of Landsteiner, who showed that an animal could respond, by producing antibody, to a large number of synthetic haptens that it would never be expected to meet in nature.

At about the same time, *instructive,* or *template,* theories became popular. One of these theories proposed that antigen directs the formation of antibodies from its precursor molecules. Breinl and Haurowitz suggested that under the influence of antigen, the subunits of the antibody molecule (subunit structure was unknown at that time) combine with each other in an anomalous manner so that a specific antibody is formed. This modification was due to the presence of antigen within the antibody-forming cell, and thus the antigen served as a direct template. This view was expanded by Linus Pauling, who suggested that all antibody molecules have identical primary structure and differ from each other only in the conformation of their peptide chains. He proposed that antigen within the cell at the time of antibody synthesis serves as a template to stabilize a specific complementary conformation on the antibody molecule. These theories implied that antibody-forming cells are multipotent, that is, they can make all types of antibody specificities. They also predicted that antibody activity would be recovered from denatured antibody by renaturation only in the presence of specific antigen. When it was shown that antibody specificity resides in the primary sequence of amino acids in the antibody molecule, that antibody-forming cells have restricted potentiality, and that renaturation, in the absence of antigen, restores antibody activity, the direct template theory was modified.

An indirect template theory was put forth, in which it was suggested that antibody specificity is influenced directly though the action of antigen on DNA. This implies an alteration in the sequence of events in protein synthesis from the usual DNA → RNA → protein. It also implies that the antigen can function as a mutagen. These theories are untenable in view of our current knowledge of molecular biology.

In 1955, Jerne proposed a modern view of the selective theory, in which he suggested that the population of antibody-forming cells is endowed with a finite number of randomly distributed specific receptor molecules that arise spontaneously in the absence of antigens. These specific receptor molecules (natural antibodies) are released from individual cells, and antigen selects these specific receptors, thereby initiating antibody formation (natural selection). This hypothesis suggested that there are separate genes coding for each antibody molecule and that the entire library of genes required for all antibodies is present in each potential antibody-forming cell. This idea served as the basis of *germ-line* theories.

Burnet evolved the basic principles of the above-stated theory into the modern *clonal selection theory*. This theory suggested that there are a large number of previously programmed clones in the adult, each one carrying specific receptors on its surface capable of reacting with a specific immunogen. The outcome of the reaction between receptor and immunogen is either antibody formation or suppression (death of the clone if stimulated during fetal development or tolerance, Chapter 12). Burnet suggested that the progenitor cells of the immune response are highly mutable omnipotent cells. He postulated that the diversity of specificities formed is the result of *somatic mutation*. Somatic development results in the differentiation of a population of individual antigen-sensitive cells, each of which has the capacity to respond to one or to a limited number of antigenic configurations. The antigen selects a specific precursor cell, which then proliferates into a clone of cells producing specific antibody. Although this theory, in its present form, leaves the explanation of certain immunologic phenomena unanswered, it is the most widely accepted among immunologists.

ANTIBODY FORMATION AT THE MOLECULAR LEVEL

The IgG molecule is a multichain protein that, upon partial reduction, yields two heavy chains and two light chains (Chapter 5). In addition, each chain is composed of a variable sequence of amino acids (V_H and V_L) associated with its antigen-binding activities, and a constant sequence of amino acids (C_H and C_L) reflective of that particular class of polypeptide chain. The observation that immunoglobulin polypeptide chains of the same type have identical sequences in the constant region but different sequences in the variable region seems difficult to reconcile with the dogma of molecular biology that states: "one gene, one polypeptide." Based on work done with the inheritance of allotypic markers, it was concluded that each constant region sequence is coded for by a single structural gene. In order to account for the great diversity of antibody specificities, it was postulated that there were multiple V region genes and that each V subgroup must be specified by at least one gene. It is now believed that one of many V region genes can become associated with a single C region gene for the synthesis of a single immunoglobulin chain (Chapter 5). Therefore, a departure from dogma exists and we now speak of *"two genes, one polypeptide."* The potential mechanism by which two genes recombine to direct the synthesis of a single polypeptide chain has been discussed (Fig. 7–10 and Chapter 5).

The early molecular events preparatory to the formation of antibody follow established patterns of protein synthesis. Following stimulation of the antigen-sensitive cell, there is a period of cellular proliferation accompanied by differentiation. The cells begin to synthesize DNA in as little as three hours after stimulation, and peak synthesis occurs three to four hours thereafter. Increases in RNA synthesis parallel those of DNA, with both mRNA and ribosomal RNA synthesis occurring. The use of inhibitors of nucleic acid synthesis during this time results in marked suppression of the immune response. Morphologic changes become apparent, with the cell displaying a well-developed endoplasmic reticulum and Golgi apparatus.

In the same manner that myeloma proteins have aided our understanding of the structure of immunoglobulins, studies of their synthesis have also aided our understanding of the molecular events of antibody formation. With the use of cell-free systems, it has been shown that only one mRNA molecule is involved in the synthesis of a single heavy or light polypeptide chain, rather than two mRNAs, where one codes for the variable and the other codes for the constant portion of the given chain. The base sequences and structure of several Ig mRNAs are now known. It has been shown that the precursor of mRNA, found in the nucleus, is of very high molecular weight and is processed into a smaller unit before it reaches the cytoplasm. Cytoplasmic mRNAs for both heavy and light chains contain a larger number of bases than can be accounted for in the translated polypeptide chains. The function of these extra bases is unclear at present.

After transcription and processing in the nucleus, the mRNA is transported into the cytoplasm, where it becomes associated with membrane-bound ribosomes to form the rought endoplasmic reticulum (Fig. 7–18). The individual polypeptide chains of the immunoglobulin molecule are made on separate polyribosome units. The immunoglobulin heavy chain is synthesized as a complete unit on heavy polysomes (16 to 18 ribosomes) having a sedimentation coefficient of 270S. Similarly, the light chains are synthesized as complete units on light polysomes (seven or eight ribosomes) having a sedimentation coefficient of 190S. It appears that both heavy and light chains are synthesized as larger precursors, containing an additional 20 *N*-terminal amino acid residues. This leader sequence of relatively hydrophobic amino acids, which appears to be involved in membrane interactions with the Ig molecule, is cleaved as the chains enter the lumen of the endoplasmic reticulum. The newly formed L-chains are released from the polysomes and enter an intracellular pool of free L-chains. Although there is thought to be some assembly of L- to H-chain at the level of the heavy polysomes, most of it occurs postribosomally as the individual chains pass through the cisternae of the endoplasmic reticulum. Assembly into the full molecule containing two identical heavy chains and two identical light chains (H_2L_2) occurs by means of two major pathways with a variety of convalently linked intermediates. In the first pathway, two H-chains form an H_2 dimer followed by the addition of each of the L-chains to give H_2L, then the H_2L_2 molecule. In the second pathway, the H- and L-chains combine to form a half-molecule (HL), which then combines with another half-molecule (HL) through inter–H-chain disulfide bridges to give the complete molecule. While there is some preferential assembly by one of these pathways within a given species and Ig subclass, both have been shown to function.

Synthesis of H- and L-chains occurs at a

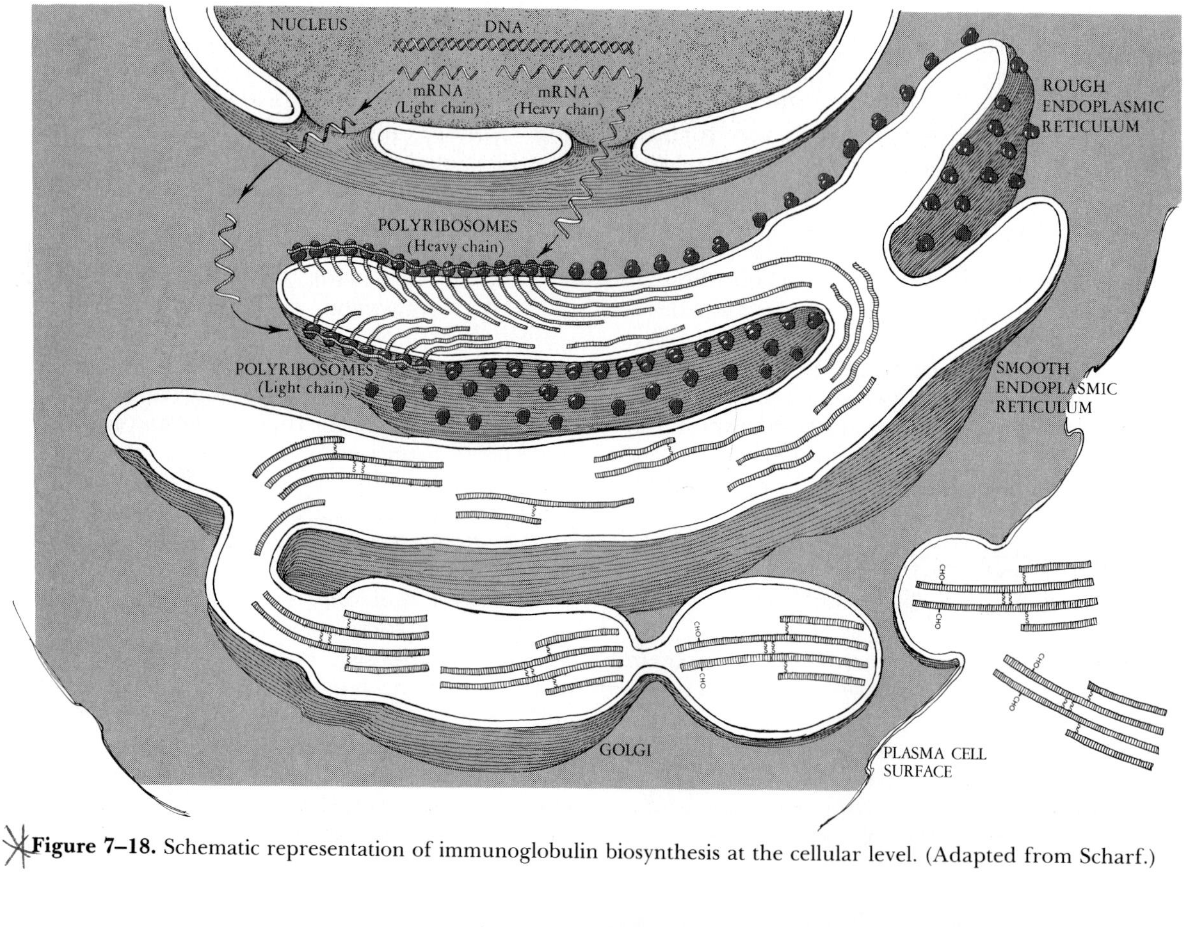

Figure 7–18. Schematic representation of immunoglobulin biosynthesis at the cellular level. (Adapted from Scharf.)

rapid rate, 60 seconds and 30 seconds, respectively. In spite of this, secretion of the newly synthesized molecule does not occur until after a lag of about 20 to 30 minutes. It is during this time that carbohydrate is added and the molecule is transported to the membrane. The H-chains, and in some cases the L-chains, are glycosylated in both the rough and the smooth endoplasmic reticulum. The assembled molecules traverse the Golgi apparatus and then move toward the cell surface. As they are transported to the cell surface in secretory vesicles, interchain disulfide bonds are formed and sugars are added successively to form oligosaccharide groups of the complete molecule. Most of the immunoglobulin molecules are secreted into the membrane and remain there for a period of time before being released.

In the case of IgM and IgA, polymerization occurs with the addition of the J-chain either shortly before or simultaneously with secretion of these molecules from the plasma cell. Finally, the mechanisms that control both the synthesis and the secretion of Ig molecules are not yet well understood, but should be of importance for the design of potential therapeutic modalities to be used in treatment of immunoproliferative diseases such as multiple myeloma.

Suggestions for Further Reading

The Fate of Immunogen

Ada, G. L., Nossal, G. J. V., and Pye, J.: Antigens in immunity. II. Distribution of iodinated antigens following injection into rats via the hind foot pads. Aust. J. Exp. Biol. Med. Sci., *42*:295, 1964.

Bellanti, J. A., and Herscowitz, H. B. (eds.): The Reticuloendothelial System—A Comprehensive Treatise, Vol. 6: Immunology. New York, Plenum Press, 1984.

Bierme, S. J., Blanc, M., Abbal, M., et al.: Oral Rh treatment for severely immunised mothers. Lancet, *1*:604, 1979.

Campbell, D. H., and Garvey, J. S.: Nature of retained antigen and its role in immune mechanisms. Adv. Immunol., *3*:261, 1963.

Dixon, F. J.: The metabolism of antigen and antibody. J. Allergy, *25*:487, 1954.

Mattingly, J. A., and Waksman, B. H.: Immunologic suppression after oral administration of antigen. I. Specific suppressor cells formed in rat Peyer's patches after oral administration of sheep erythrocytes and their systemic migration. J. Immunol., *121*:1878, 1978.

Antibody Formation in the Animal

Abramoff, P., and Brien, N. B.: Studies of the chicken immune response. I. Correlation of cellular and humoral immune response. J. Immunol., *100*:1204, 1968.

Eisen, H. N., and Siskind, G. W.: Variations in affinities of antibodies during the immune response. Biochemistry, *3*:996, 1964.

Fazekas de St. Groth, S., and Webster, R. G.: Disquisitions on original antigenic sin. I. Evidence in man. J. Exp. Med., *124*:331, 1966.

Mitchison, N. A.: The carrier effect in the secondary response to hapten-protein conjugates. II. Cellular cooperation. Eur. J. Immunol., *1*:18, 1971.

Uhr, J. W., and Finkelstein, M. S.: The kinetics of antibody formation. Prog. Allergy, *10*:37, 1967.

Cells of the Specific Immune Response

Bach, J. F.: Evaluation of T cells and thymic serum factors in man using the rosette technique. Transplant. Rev., *16*:196, 1973.

Binz, H., and Wigzell, H.: Antigen binding, idiotypic receptors from T lymphocytes: An analysis of their biochemistry, genetics, and use as immunogens to produce specific immune tolerance. Cold Spring Harbor Symp. Quant. Biol., *41*:275, 1976.

Cantor, H., and Boyce, E.: Regulation of the immune response by T-cell subclasses. Contemp. Top. Immunobiol., *7*:47, 1977.

Cooper, M. D., and Buckley, R. H.: Developmental immunology and the immunodeficiency diseases. JAMA, *248*:2658, 1982.

Cowing, C., Schwartz, B. D., and Dickler, H. B.: Macrophage Ia antigens. I. Macrophage populations differ in their expression of Ia antigens. J. Immunol., *120*:378, 1978.

Cramer, M., and Krawinkel, U.: Immunochemical properties of isolated hapten specific T-cell receptor molecules. *In* Pernis, B., and Vogel, H. J. (eds.): Regulatory T-Lymphocytes. New York, Academic Press, 1980.

Fishman, M., Adler, F. L., and Rice, S. G.: Macrophage RNA in the *in vitro* immune response to phage. Ann. N.Y. Acad. Sci., *207*:73, 1973.

Förster, O., and Landy, M. (eds.): Heterogeniety of Mononuclear Phagocytes. New York, Academic Press, 1981.

Greaves, M., and Janossy, G.: Elicitation of selective T and B lymphocyte responses by cell surface binding ligands. Transplant. Rev., *11*:87, 1973.

Herberman, R. B., and Ortaldo, J. R.: Natural killer cells: Their role in defenses against disease. Science, *214*:24, 1981.

Herscowitz, H. B., Holden, H. T., Bellanti, J. A., et al. (eds.): Manual of Macrophage Methodology: Collection, Characterization and Function. New York, Marcel Dekker, 1981.

Klinman, N., Mosier, D. E., Scher, I., et al. (eds.): B Lymphocytes in the Immune Response: Functional, Development and Interactive Properties. New York, Elsevier/North Holland, 1981.

Mishell, B. B., and Shiigi, S. M. (eds.): Selected Methods in Cellular Immunology. San Francisco, W. H. Freeman, 1980.

Moretta, L., Webb, S. R., Grossi, C. E., et al.: Functional analysis of two human T cell subpopulations: Help and suppression of B cell responses by T cells bearing receptors for IgM (T_M) and IgG (T_G). J. Exp. Med., *146*:184, 1977.

Nelson, D. S. (ed.): Immunobiology of the Macrophage. New York, Academic Press, 1976.

Pernis, B., and Vogel, H. J. (eds.): Regulatory T Lymphocytes. New York, Academic Press, 1980.

Pernis, B., Forni, L., and Amante, L.: Immunoglobulin

spots on the surface of rabbit lymphocytes. J. Exp. Med., *132*:1001, 1970.
Raff, M. C.: Surface antigenic markers for distinguishing T and B lymphocytes in mice. Transplant. Rev., *6*:52, 1971.
Reif, A. E., and Allen, M. J. V.: The AKR thymic antigen and its distribution in leukemias and nervous tissue. J. Exp. Med., *120*:413, 1964.
Reinharz, E. L., and Schlossman, S. F.: The differentiation and function of human T lymphocytes. Cell, *19*:821, 1980.
Taylor, R. B., Duffus, W. P. H., Raff, M. C., et al.: Redistribution and pinocytosis of lymphocyte surface Ig molecules by anti-Ig antibody. Nature [New Biol.], *233*:225, 1971.
Unanue, E. R., and Rosenthal, A. S. (eds.): Macrophage Regulation of Immunity. New York, Academic Press, 1980.
Vitetta, E. S., and Uhr, J. W.: Immunoglobulin-receptors revisited. Science, *189*:964, 1975.
Warner, N. L.: Membrane immunoglobulins and antigen receptors on B and T lymphocytes. Adv. Immunol., *19*:67, 1974.

Cellular Interactions in the Initiation of Antibody Formation

Bona, C. (ed.): Idiotypes and Lymphocytes. New York, Academic Press, 1981.
Claman, H. N., Chaperon, E. A., and Triplett, R. F.: Thymus-marrow combinations: Synergism in antibody production. Proc. Soc. Exp. Biol. Med., *122*:1167, 1966.
Early, P., Rogers, J., Davis, M., et al.: Two mRNAs can be produced from a single immunoglobulin μ gene by alternative RNA processing pathways. Cell, *20*:313, 1980.
Feldmann, M.: Cell interactions in the immune response *in vitro*. V. Specific collaboration via complexes of antigen and thymus-derived cell immunoglobulin. J. Exp. Med., *136*:737, 1972.
Feldmann, M., Rosenthal, A. S., and Erb, P.: Macrophage-lymphocyte interactions in immune induction. Int. Rev. Cytol., *60*:149, 1979.
Gillis, S., and Watson, J.: Biochemical and biological characterization of lymphocyte regulatory molecules. V. Identification of an interleukin-2–producing human leukemia T cell line. J. Exp. Med., *152*:1707, 1980.
Katz, D. H.: Adaptive differentiation of lymphocytes: Theoretical implications for mechanisms of cell-cell recognition and regulation of immune responses. Adv. Immunol., *29*:138, 1980.
Katz, D. H., Paul, W. E., Goidl, E. A., et al.: Carrier function in antihapten responses. III. Stimulation of antibody synthesis and facilitation of hapten-specific secondary antibody responses by graft-versus-host reactions. J. Exp. Med., *133*:169, 1971.
Lawton, A. R., III, and Cooper, M. D.: Modification of B lymphocyte differentiation by anti-immunoglobulins. Contemp. Top. Immunobiol., *3*:193, 1974.
Lee, K-C.: Regulation of T cell activation by macrophage subsets. Lymphokines, *6*:1, 1982.
McDevitt, H. O. (ed.): Ir Genes and Ia Antigens. New York, Academic Press, 1978.
Miller, J. F. A. P.: Influence of the major histocompatibility complex on T-cell activation. Adv. Cancer Res., *29*:1, 1979.
Miller, J. F. A. P., Basten, A., Sprent, J., et al.: Interactions between lymphocytes in immune responses. Cell. Immunol., *2*:469, 1971.
Mishell, R. I., and Dutton, R. W.: Immunization of dissociated spleen cell cultures from normal mice. J. Exp. Med., *126*:423, 1967.
Mizel, S. B., and Mizel, D.: Purification to apparent homogeneity of murine interleukin-1. J. Immunol., *126*:834, 1981.
Moore, K. W., Rogers, J., Hunkapiller, T., et al.: Expression of IgD may use both DNA rearrangement and RNA splicing mechanisms. Proc. Natl. Acad. Sci. U.S.A., *78*:1800, 1981.
Mosier, D. E.: A requirement for two cell types for antibody formation *in vitro*. Science, *158*:1573, 1967.
Rabbits, T. H., Bentley, D. L., Dunnick, W., et al.: Immunoglobulin genes undergo multiple sequence rearrangements during differentiation. Cold Spring Harbor Symp. Quant. Biol., *45*:867, 1981.
Rajewsky, K. V., Schirrmacher, V., Nase, S., et al.: The requirement for more than one antigenic determinant for immunogenicity. J. Exp. Med., *129*:1131, 1969.
Rosenthal, A. S., and Shevach, E. M.: Function of macrophages in antigen recognition by guinea pig T-lymphocytes. I. Requirement of histocompatible macrophages and lymphocytes. J. Exp. Med., *138*:1194, 1974.
Shimpl, A., and Wecker, E.: Replacement of T cell function by a T cell product. Nature [New Biol.], *237*:15, 1972.
Smith, K. A., and Ruscetti, F. W.: T-cell growth factor and the culture of cloned functional T-cells. Adv. Immunol., *31*:137, 1981.
Tada, T., and Okumura, K.: The role of antigen-specific T-cell factors in the immune response. Adv. Immunol., *28*:1, 1979.
Waldmann, H., and Munro, A. J.: The interrelationships of antigenic structure, thymus independence and adjuvanticity. Immunology, *28*:509, 1975.
Watson, J., Frank, M. B., Mochizuki, D., et al.: The biochemistry and biology of interleukin-2. Lymphokines, *6*:95, 1982.
Zinkernagel, R. M., and Doherty, P. C.: MHC-restricted cytotoxic T-cells: Studies on the biological role of polymorphic major transplantation antigens during T-cell restriction-specificity, function and responsiveness. Adv. Immunol., *27*:52, 1979.

Regulation of Antibody Formation

Aune, T. A., and Pierce, C. W.: Preparation of a soluble immune response suppressor and macrophage-derived suppressor factor. J. Immunol. Methods, *53*:1, 1982.
Baker, P. J., Stashak, P. W., Amsbaugh, D. F., et al.: Evidence for the existence of two functionally distinct types of cells which regulate the antibody response to type III pneumococcal polysaccharide. J. Immunol., *105*:1581, 1970.
Beller, D. I., and Unanue, E. R.: Reciprocal regulation of macrophage and T-cell functions by way of soluble mediators. Lymphokines, *6*:25, 1982.
Benacerraf, B.: Genetic control of the specificity of T-lymphocytes and their regulatory products. *In* Fougereau, M., and Dausset, J. (eds.): Immunology 80. New York, Academic Press, 1980.
Bona, C., and Paul, W. E.: Cellular basis of regulation of expression of idiotype. I. T-suppressor cells specific for MOPC 460 idiotype regulate the expression of

cells secreting anti-TNP antibodies bearing 460 idiotype. J. Exp. Med., *149*:592, 1979.

Cantor, H.: Control of the immune system by inhibitor and inducer T lymphocytes. Ann. Rev. Med., *30*:269, 1979.

Eichmann, K.: Expression and function of idiotypes on lymphocytes. Adv. Immunol., *26*:195, 1978.

Gershon, R. K.: T cell control of antibody production. Contemp. Top. Immunobiol., *3*:1, 1974.

Gershon, R. K.: Suppressor T-cells: miniposition paper celebrating a new decade. *In* Fougereau, M., and Dausset, J. (eds.): Immunology 80. New York, Academic Press, 1980.

Gershon, R. K., Eardley, D. D., Durum, S., et al.: Contrasuppression: a novel immunoregulatory activity. J. Exp. Med., *153*:1533, 1981.

Herzenberg, L. A., and Herzenberg, L. A.: Short-term and chronic allotype suppression in mice. Contemp. Top. Immunobiol., *3*:41, 1974.

Jerne, N. K.: Towards a network theory of the immune system. Ann. Immunol., *125C*:373, 1974.

Kohler, H.: Idiotypic network interactions. Immunol. Today, *1*:18, 1980.

Liacopoulous, P., and Ben-Efriam, S.: Antigenic competition. Prog. Allergy, *18*:97, 1974.

McDevitt, H. O.: The evolution of genes in the major histocompatibility complex. Fed. Proc., *33*:2168, 1976.

Moller, G., and Wigzell, H.: Antibody synthesis at the cellular level. Antibody-induced suppression of 19S and 7S antibody responses. J. Exp. Med., *121*:969, 1965.

Pross, H. F., and Eidinger, D.: Antigenic competition. A review of nonspecific antigen-induced suppression. Adv. Immunol., *18*:133, 1974.

Taussig, M. J., Munro, A. J., Campbell, R., et al.: Antigen specific T-cell factor in cell cooperation. J. Exp. Med., *142*:694, 1975.

Uhr, J. W., and Moller, G.: Regulatory effects of antibody on the immune response. Adv. Immunol., *8*:81, 1968.

Unanue, E. R.: The regulatory role of macrophages in antigen stimulation. Adv. Immunol., *31*:1, 1981.

Yamauchi, K., Murphy, D., Cantor, H., et al.: Analysis of antigen-specific, H-2–restricted cell-free product(s) made by "I-J$^-$" Ly-2 cells (Ly-2TsF) that suppress Ly-2 cell–depleted spleen cell activity. Eur. J. Immunol. *11*:913, 1981.

Theories of Antibody Formation

Burnet, F. M.: The Clonal Selection Theory of Acquired Immunity. Nashville, Vanderbilt University Press, 1959.

Ehrlich, P.: On immunity with special reference to cell life. Proc. R. Soc. Lond. (Biol)., *66*:424, 1900.

Haurowitz, F.: The problem of antibody diversity. Immunodifferentiation versus somatic mutation. Immunochemistry, *10*:775, 1973.

Jerne, N. K.: The somatic generation of immune recognition. Eur. J. Immunol., *1*:1, 1971.

Pauling, L.: A theory of the structure and process of formation of antibodies. J. Am. Chem. Soc., *62*:2643, 1940.

Antibody Formation at the Molecular Level

Buxbaum, J. N.: The biosynthesis, assembly and secretion of immunoglobulins. Semin. Hematol., *10*:33, 1973.

Parkhouse, R. M. E.: Biosynthesis of polymeric immunoglobulins. Prog. Immunol. II, *1*:119, 1974.

Scharff, M. D., and Laskov, P.: Synthesis and assembly of immunoglobulin polypeptide chains. Prog. Allergy, *14*:37, 1970.

Scharff, M. D., Birshtein, B., Dharmgrongartama, B., et al.: The use of mutant myeloma cells to explore the production of immunoglobulins. *In* Smith, E. E., and Ribbons, D. W. (eds.): Molecular Approaches to Immunology. New York, Academic Press, 1975.

Sherr, C. J., Schenkein, I., and Uhr, J. W.: Synthesis and intracellular transport of immunoglobulin in secretory and nonsecretory cells. Ann. N.Y. Acad. Sci., *190*:250, 1971.

Stevens, R. H.: Distribution of immunoglobulin mRNA in mouse lymphocytes. Prog. Immunol. II, *1*:119, 1974.

Williamson, A. R.: Biosynthesis of immunoglobulins. *In* Porter, R. R. (ed.): Defense and Recognition. London, Butterworth, 1973.

Chapter 8

Antigen-Antibody Interactions

Chester M. Zmijewski, Ph.D., and Joseph A. Bellanti, M.D.

The reactants of the specific immune response are either antibody, a product of the B-lymphocytes, or specifically sensitized T-lymphocytes. This chapter will deal with the reactions of antigen with antibody—the antigen-antibody interaction. Manifestations of the reaction of antigen with specifically sensitized T-lymphocytes and other cellular reactions, i.e., cell-mediated reactions, will be described in Chapter 9.

DEFINITIONS

Antigen-antibody interactions can be divided into three categories: (1) the *primary*, (2) the *secondary*, and (3) the *tertiary* (Fig. 8–1). The *primary* or initial interaction of antigen with antibody is the basic event and consists of the binding of antigen with an antibody molecule (Fig. 8–2). Since this interaction is rarely visible, its detection is usually accomplished by *secondary* reactions, which provide auxilliary means to visualize the reaction, e.g., precipitation. Tertiary reactions are biologic expressions of the antigen-antibody interaction that may be either beneficial or deleterious.

The measurement of *primary* antigen-antibody interactions can be accomplished by several techniques, including the ammonium sulfate precipitation method (Farr technique), equilibrium dialysis or visualization by immunofluorescence, ferritin labeling, or by a series of immunoassays, including radioimmunoassay (RIA), enzyme immunoassay (EIA), and fluoroimmunoassay (FIA) (Fig. 8–1). These methods are assuming clinical value in the measurement of antibodies important in disease processes, e.g., anti-DNA antibody in lupus erythematosus determined by fluorescent technique, and hepatitis virus B antigen (HB_sAg) or HB_sAg antibody by radioimmunoassay.

The *secondary* manifestations of the antigen-antibody reaction include *precipitation, agglutination, complement-dependent reactions, neutralization,* and *cytotropic effects.* These reactions are of practical importance to the physician, since they form the basis of a number of laboratory tests used in the detection and identification of antigens, antibodies, or antigen-antibody complexes involved in disease processes.

The antigen-antibody interactions are sometimes expressed as *tertiary* manifestations (Fig. 8–1). Such reactions are by definition biologic expressions of the antigen-antibody interaction and at times may be helpful to the patient but at other times may lead to disease through immunologic injury. Since the *in vivo* tertiary manifestations of the immune response that are harmful will be described in Chapters 13 and 20, this chapter will be concerned only with the *in vitro* manifestations of the interaction of antigen with antibody. An interesting trend has been observed in recent years in which the earlier first-order immunoassays, e.g., RIA, are being replaced by second-order immunoassays, e.g., EIA (ELISA). It is likely that these too, in time, will be supplanted by third-order immunoassays, e.g., FIA (immunofluorescent techniques).

PRIMARY MANIFESTATIONS OF THE ANTIGEN-ANTIBODY INTERACTION

The primary interaction of antigen with antibody consists of the initial binding of

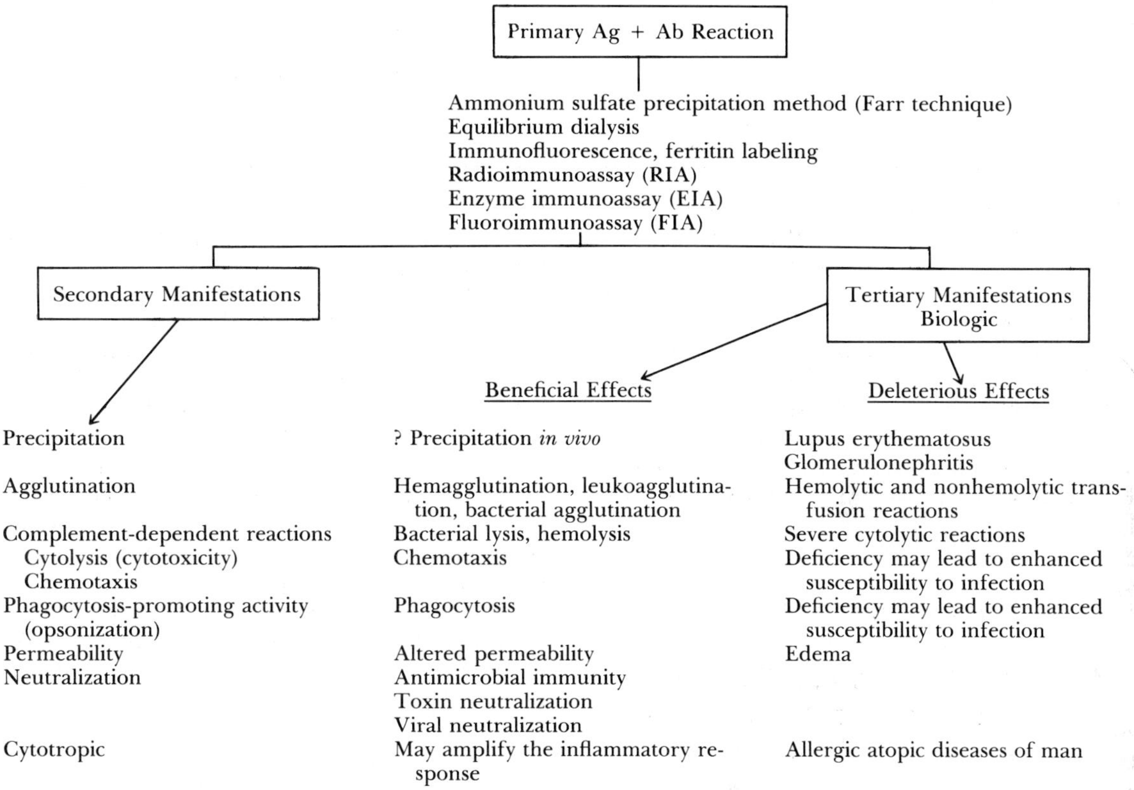

Figure 8–1. Schematic representation of antigen-antibody reactions.

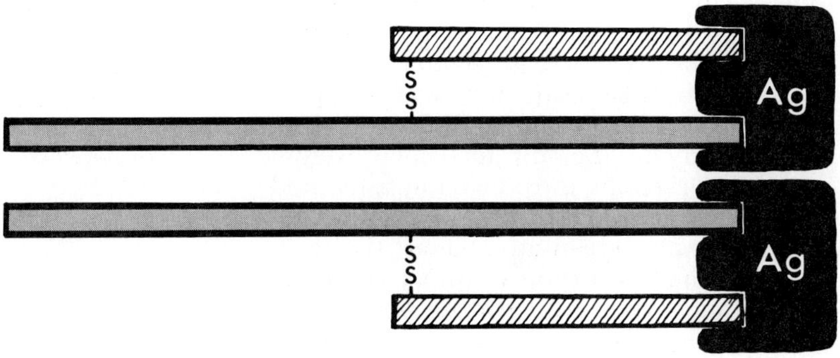

Figure 8–2. Schematic representation of the binding of antigen to antibody sites.

Table 8–1. **Clinical Applications of Primary Antigen-Antibody Interactions**

Label	Type of Assay: Quantitative Methods	Type of Assay: Immunohistochemical Methods
Fluorescent	Fluoroimmunoassay (FIA)	Fluorescent antibody method
Radioactive	Radioimmunoassay (RIA)	Autoradiography
Electron-dense		Ferritin labeling
Enzyme	Enzyme immunoassay (EIA), e.g., enzyme-linked immunosorbent (ELISA)	Immunoperoxidase labeling

antigen with the two or more available antigen-binding sites on any given antibody molecule. This is shown schematically in Figure 8–2. The primary interaction of antigen with antibody is rarely directly visible, and visualization is usually accomplished by labeling antibody or antigen with fluorescent, radioactive, electron-dense, or enzymatic markers. These methods include both *quantitative* assays performed on sera and *immunohistochemical* techniques performed on tissues (Table 8–1).

Quantitative Methods for the Measurement of Antigen or Antibody Based on Primary Manifestations of the Antigen-Antibody Interaction

At present, the classic quantitative assay for the measurement of antigen-antibody reactions is the *radioimmunoassay* (RIA), in which a radioactively labeled substance (radioligand) is employed either directly or indirectly for the quantitative measurement of the unlabeled substance by a binding reaction to a specific antibody or other receptor system. Even substances that are not immunogenic by themselves (e.g., haptens) can be measured in these assays if they are coupled to larger carrier substances capable of inducing antibody to the low molecular weight material. Originally introduced as a method for the measurement of plasma insulin concentrations by Berson and Yalow, the technique has had an explosive impact upon all areas of medicine and has made possible the accurate measurement of small concentrations of a wide range of biologic substances, some of which could not be accurately measured previously, e.g., digoxin (Table 8–2). Although the vast majority of these assays employ an antigen-antibody reaction, some substances, e.g., hormones, may be assayed by virtue of their binding to hormone receptors on cells or receptor proteins in the serum, e.g., thyroxin-binding protein (radioreceptor assay). These latter assays differ only in that receptors rather than antibody are used to bind the radioactive ligand. Radioimmunoassays are carried out either in solution, e.g., *liquid- or soluble-phase radioimmunoassays,* or on a supporting matrix to which the antigen (ligand) or antibody is adsorbed or covalently linked, e.g., *solid-phase radioimmunoassay* (Table 8–3). In contrast to the liquid-phase RIA, which depends upon a competitive binding principle and in which reactants are added together, the solid-phase RIA involves a two-step reaction, the first being the antigen-antibody binding and the second, the detection step.

LIQUID-PHASE RIA

The basic principle of the liquid-phase RIA is that the ligand to be measured (Ag) is assayed indirectly through its competition with a labeled derivative (Ag*) for binding a

Table 8–2. **Examples of Substances Measurable by Radioimmunoassay**

Serum proteins	Angiotensin
IgE (PRIST)	Bradykinin
IgE antibody (RAST)	Calcitonin
Anti-DNA	Glucagon
Carcinoembryonic antigen (CEA)	Kinins
	Drugs
Microbial agents and antibodies	Digoxin
HB_sAg or HB_sAb	Morphine
Hormones	*Metabolites*
Insulin	Cyclic AMP
ACTH	Cyclic GMP
Growth hormone	Folic acid
Steroid	Vitamin B_{12}
Estrogen	Intrinsic factors
Testosterone	
Thyroid hormones	

Table 8–3. Quantitative Radioimmunoassay Procedures

Type	Principle	Example
Liquid or soluble phase	Radioimmunoprecipitation	Ammonium sulfate method (Farr technique)
	Double-antibody method	
Solid phase	Competitive binding	Radioimmunosorbent test (RIST)
	Noncompetitive binding (sandwich)	Radioallergosorbent test (RAST) Paper radioimmunosorbent test (PRIST) HB_sAg, Clq, DNA
	Competitive inhibition of binding	RAST inhibition assay

limited amount of antibody (Ab). This is shown schematically in Figure 8–3.

The assay is performed by reacting a standard quantity of Ag* with Ab in the presence of varying concentrations of unlabeled Ag in order to establish a standard curve (Fig. 8–4). In a similar fashion, the Ag containing the unknown is reacted with a standard quantity of Ag* plus Ab in a separate reaction mixture. When the reaction comes to equilibrium it is necessary to remove the Ag*Ab from the free Ag* in order to estimate the amount of unlabeled Ag present in the unknown. In the soluble phase, radioimmunoassay can be accomplished by the selective precipitation of the Ag*Ab complex from the solution by physicochemical techniques, e.g., ammonium sulfate method (Farr technique), or by the specific-antibody (double-antibody) method in which a second antibody is directed at the first. The amount of Ag in the unknown is then determined indirectly by the degree of binding of Ag* in the Ag*Ab complex from the standard curve.

SOLID-PHASE RIA

In addition to being performed in solution, the RIA assays have been modified so that the Ag or Ab can be immobilized or attached to a supporting medium (solid-phase RIA) (Table 8–3). The main advantage of this technique over the liquid phase is the simplicity of performance and the ease with which the Ag*Ab can be separated from the unreacted Ag*, either by washing or by centrifugation. One example of the competitive binding technique is the radioimmunosorbent test (RIST) for the quantitative measurement of IgE, which is represented schematically in Figure 8–5.

Other types of solid-phase RIA are the noncompetitive binding techniques for the measurement of Ag or Ab (Table 8–3). In this technique, represented schematically in Figure 8–6, either antigen or antibody is attached to a supporting matrix, and then the unknown specimen is added. When antibody is being analyzed, the antibody-containing specimen is added to the antigen-coated matrix, following which a second radiolabeled anti–gamma globulin reagent is added. When antigen is to be determined, antibody is immobilized on the matrix, the antigen-containing specimen is added, and a radiolabeled antibody to the antigen is added (Fig. 8–6). By means of this sandwich technique, which is a noncompetitive direct binding technique, specific antibody or antigen can be detected in a patient's serum. Examples of this technique include the radioallergosorbent test (RAST) for the measurement of specific IgE antibody to a variety of allergens, the PRIST test for the direct measure-

Labeled antigen (ligand)		Specific Antibody or Binding Receptor		Labeled antigen-(ligand-) antibody complex
Ag*	+	Ab + Ag ⇅ Ag-Ab unlabeled antigen-antibody complex	⇌ unlabeled antigen	Ag*Ab (in standard or unknown)

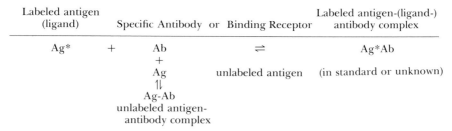

Figure 8–3. Schematic representation of the competitive binding radioimmunoassay.

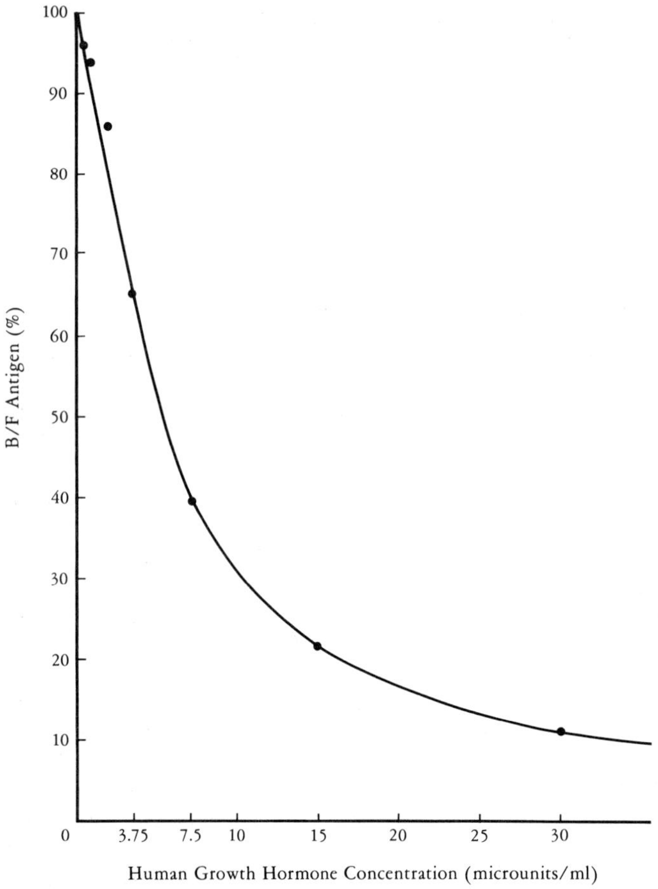

Figure 8–4. Standard curve for use in the radioimmunoassay of human growth hormone. (Courtesy of Dr. Malcolm M. Martin.)

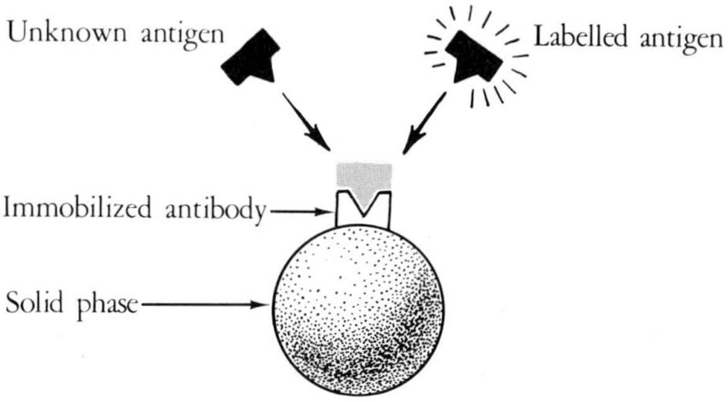

Figure 8–5. Schematic representation of the competitive binding RIA technique, e.g., RIST.

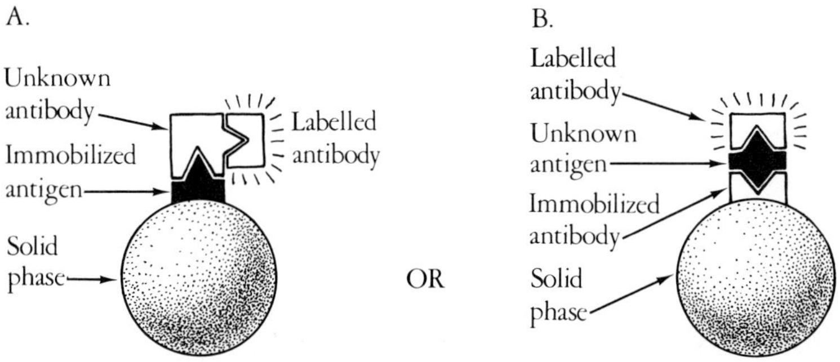

Figure 8–6. Schematic representation of the noncompetitive (direct) RIA-binding technique illustrating the use of the test (*A*) in detecting unknown antibody, e.g., RAST and HB_sAb, in which case antigen is immobilized, or (*B*) in detecting unknown antigen, e.g., PRIST and HB_sAg, in which case antibody is immobilized onto the solid phase.

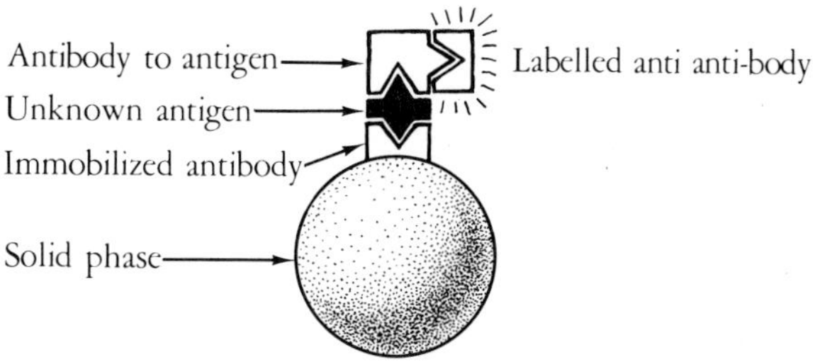

Figure 8–7. Schematic representation of the noncompetitive (indirect) RIA binding ("sandwich") technique.

ment of IgE globulin, and the measurement of hepatitis B antigen (HB_sAg) or specific HB_sAg antibody in the sera of patients with hepatitis (Chapter 20). In some cases, the sandwich may be expanded to include an additional layer(s) (noncompetitive indirect binding technique) to increase the sensitivity of the assay or to allow the detection of antibody to antigens that cannot be readily attached to solid surfaces, e.g., penicillin RAST (Fig. 8–7).

Another modification of the solid RIA has been developed for the standardization of biologically active substances. This technique is illustrated in Figure 8–8 and consists of a two-step reaction: A solid-phase antigen is reacted with a known amount of Ab and radiolabeled anti-human gamma globulin, as in the direct sandwich technique described above; and (2) the unlabeled antigen to be assayed is added in a separate reaction mixture. The degree of inhibition of the reaction is used to quantitate the substance. The RAST inhibition assay is an example of this technique, which is currently being utilized for the standardization of allergenic extracts for use in immunotherapy of allergic disease in the human (Chapter 20).

Another radioimmunoassay technique, the immunoradiometric assay, has been developed, in which purified antibody is radiolabeled and employed either in a liquid- or in a solid-phase radioimmunoassay. The primary advantage of this technique is its improved sensitivity and specificity; its main disadvantage is the complexity of the sophisticated technique required for antibody purification.

ENZYME IMMUNOASSAYS (EIA) AND FLUOROIMMUNOASSAYS (FIA)

Following the widespread use of radioimmunoassays during the past two decades, other markers have been introduced for the quantitative measurement of primary antigen-antibody interactions (see Table 8–1). One of these methods utilizes an enzyme as a label and is referred to as enzyme immunoassay (EIA) or enzyme-linked immunosorbent assay (ELISA). These assays have gained increasing popularity in recent years not only for their simplicity but also for a variety of factors both technical and regulatory (e.g., availability, elimination of the problem of disposal of radioactive wastes). The method utilizes an enzyme-linked antibody, e.g., alkaline phosphatase, and the end point of

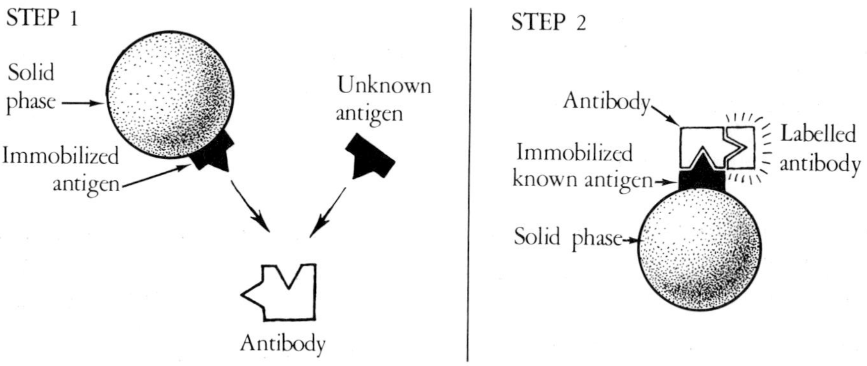

Figure 8–8. Schematic representation of competitive inhibition of binding, e.g., RAST inhibition assay. The assay is performed in two steps: (1) A known quantity of antibody is allowed to react in a competitive reaction between antigen immobilized on a solid phase and the unknown antigen to be measured, and (2) the bound antibody is measured, in a standard noncompetitive (direct) RIA assay, allowing the quantitation of the unknown antigen.

measurement is the enzymatic generation of a product from its substrate that can be measured colorimetrically or by the naked eye. This method has wide clinical application in the serodiagnosis of many diseases, including infectious diseases and particularly viral infections, for the detection of either antigen, e.g., hepatitis B antigen or antibody, e.g., rubella.

Another method for the detection of antigen and antibody is the fluoroimmunoassay (FIA), which utilizes a fluorescent label as a marker, e.g., fluorescein. Although the method can detect either antigen or antibody, thus far it has been used predominantly for the detection of antibody only.

Immunohistochemical Techniques

In addition to quantitative methods for the detection of antigen-antibody reactions, the manifestations of primary antigen-antibody interactions also form the basis of a wide variety of immunohistochemical techniques (see Table 8–1). These include the use of fluorescent-labeled antibody (e.g., immunofluorescence), enzymes (e.g., immunoperoxidase), electron-dense markers (e.g., immunoferritin labels), and radioactive markers (e.g., autoradiography).

Detection of Immune Complexes

Recent evidence indicates that antigen-antibody complexes play a major role in the pathogenesis of certain autoimmune diseases, in the modulation of graft and tumor rejection, and in several chronic infectious diseases, including the slow virus infections of man (Chapters 16, 19, and 20). Several techniques are now available for the detection of these immune complexes and are listed in Table 8–4. The clinical usefulness of these techniques has been rather limited, since several of them are research tools and are not readily demonstrated. However, newer techniques, e.g., the measurement of Clq, or monoclonal 19S anti-IgG, or the binding of immune complexes to surface receptors on cultured lymphoblasts (RAJI cells), have been developed that may allow new approaches to the elucidation of obscure diseases, which heretofore have been diagnostic and therapeutic orphans.

Table 8–4. Techniques for the Detection of Immune Complexes

Physicochemical methods (ultracentrifugation; gel filtration)
Precipitin reaction with Clq or monoclonal anti-IgG
Platelet aggregation
Binding to surface receptors of cultured RAJI cells
Clq binding test
Radioimmunoassays with monoclonal RF (MRF) or polyclonal RF (PRF)

USE OF MONOCLONAL ANTIBODIES IN IMMUNOASSAYS

The principles of monoclonal antibody production from hybridomas has been described in Chapter 5. These monoclonal antibodies are finding application in a variety of immunoassays because they offer a number of distinct advantages over reagents prepared by more classic immunization techniques. These include a high degree of specificity, relative ease of *in vitro* production, great sensitivity, and almost limitless supply. The high degree of specificity may present potential pitfalls, however, because if monoclonal antibody is directed at the wrong antigenic specificity, an assay based on this reagent could give misleading results.

SECONDARY OR *IN VITRO* MANIFESTATIONS OF THE ANTIGEN-ANTIBODY INTERACTION

The humoral immune response to an immunogenic stimulus results in the production of circulating antibody belonging to one or more of the five major immunoglobulin classes: IgM, IgG, IgA, IgD, and IgE. Evidence for the presence of this type of response may be obtained from any of several serologic assay systems, listed in Figure 8–1, that are based upon secondary manifestations of the antigen-antibody interaction.

Precipitation, Agglutination, Phagocytosis, Cytotoxicity, and Toxin Neutralization

The type of assay system used to detect antibody depends not so much on the antibody produced as on the physical and chemical form of the antigen in question. Soluble antigens, when combined with their specific antibody, will lead to precipitation, in which the antigen-antibody complexes form large isoluble aggregates. The same antigens, if naturally or artifically attached to particulate matter, e.g., bacterial cells, red cells, latex particles, or bentonite particles, will form agglutinates or clumps. This process is referred to as agglutination. If living phagocytic cells, such as polymorphonuclear leukocytes, are added to the assay system, engulfment or phagocytosis of the antigen-sensitized particles may occur. Complement may or may not participate in this reaction; however, should antibody interact with cell-bound antigen to initiate the entire complement cascade, then cytotoxicity (cell death with lysis) may take place.

Toxin neutralization, the ability of specific antibody to neutralize toxin, forms one of the oldest of serologic reactions. It may be demonstrated *in vitro* or *in vivo*. The serum to be tested is first added to a potent toxin *in vitro* and then injected into a living animal or tissue culture system. The survival of the animal or the tissue culture is used as an index of toxin neutralization (LD_{50}) and will occur when antibody (antitoxin) is present in the test serum. On certain occasions, when a toxin is mixed *in vitro* with its specific antiserum, visible precipitation or flocculation will occur because of toxin-antitoxin formation. The Schick test for the detection of antibody to diphtheria toxin and the Dick test for the detection of antibody to scarlatinal toxin are examples of *in vivo* toxin neutralization.

To some degree, precipitation and agglutination may be considered as manifestations of the same antigen-antibody interaction, the only difference being the physical form of the test antigen. In both, a two-stage reversible chemical union takes place. In the first stage, antibodies present in the immune serum react with specific antigenic determinants present on the ligand. The ease of combination depends on several factors, notably pH, ionic strength, and temperature. For this reason, *in vitro* antigen-antibody reactions are carried out at specific temperatures in buffered media containing electrolytes. The union between antigen and antibody is accomplished by means of noncovalent binding, e.g., van der Waals forces. When the primary coupling reaction has reached equilibrium, the second stage, or *lattice formation,* takes place. During this phase, the unbound receptor sites on the antibody molecules attache to suitable receptors or additional antigen molecules, forming a lattice. This is represented schematically in Figure 8–9.

As in the first stage of the reaction, the

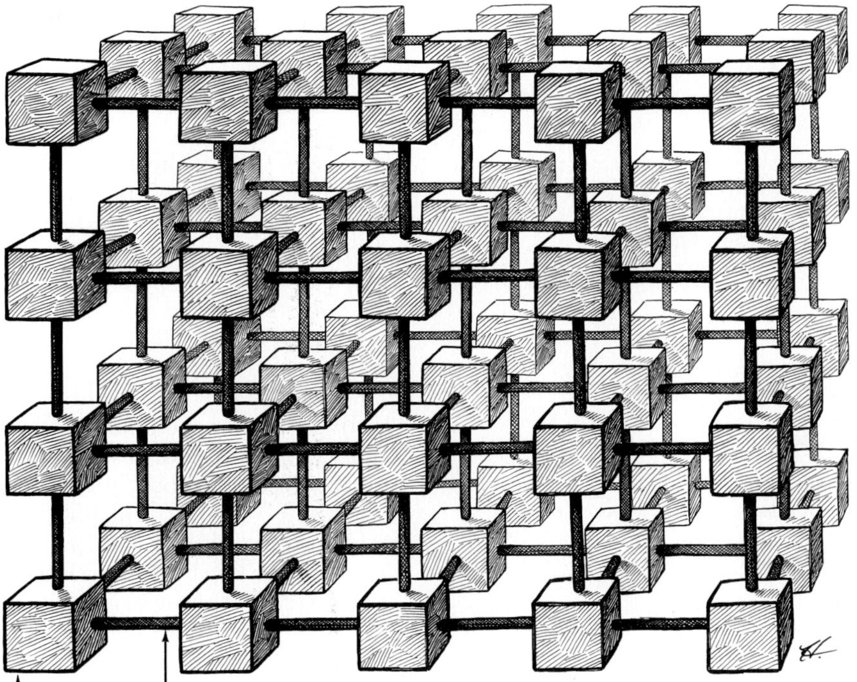

Figure 8–9. Schematic representation of antigen-antibody lattice formation.

second stage is also specific. Since two antigenic receptor sites of divalent antibody molecules are identical, an antibody with one specificity can link only identical antigens or antigenic determinants on the same molecule, never dissimilar ones. An illustration of this specificity can be noted in the following example:

When red blood cells from individuals belonging to blood groups A and B are mixed and then exposed to an immune serum containing only anti-A, the aggregates will be composed only of A cells. The B cells remain free in suspension.

In precipitation, the antigen is a soluble molecule. Therefore, a fairly large lattice must be formed before a visible aggregate is seen. In order to build a lattice of sufficient magnitude, a larger number of antibody molecules are required and the reactants must be present in optimal proportion. In agglutination, on the other hand, the antigen is part of a large insoluble particle, such as a red cell or a bacterial cell, and relatively fewer molecules are required for visible aggregation. Consequently, agglutination is a more sensitive serologic assay for antibody detection than is precipitation. This is an important consideration when choosing and interpreting serologic assay systems such as hemagglutination and bacterial agglutination. Sometimes it may become necessary to convert an ordinary precipitating system to an agglutinating system in order to increase the sensitivity of the assay. Shown in Table 8–5 are relative sensitivities of various antigen-antibody tests. In addition to the physical properties of the antigen, the nature of the antibody is important. On a molar basis, the IgM antibodies are more efficient agglutinators than are the IgG antibodies because of the greater number of antibody-combining sites on the IgM molecule; the IgG, on the other hand, are better precipitins than are the IgM.

Table 8–5. Sensitivity of Quantitative Tests Measuring Antibody Nitrogen of High-Avidity Antibody

Test	mg Ab N/ml or Test
Precipitin reactions	3–20
Immunoelectrophoresis	3–20
Double diffusion in agar gel	0.2–1.0
Complement fixation	0.01–0.1
Radial immunodiffusion	0.008–0.025
Bacterial agglutination	0.01
Hemolysis	0.001–0.03
Passive hemagglutination	0.005
Passive cutaneous anaphylaxis	0.003
Antitoxin neutralization	0.003
Antigen-combining globulin technique (Farr)	0.0001–0.001
Radioimmunoassay	0.0001–0.001
Enzyme-linked assays	0.0001–0.001
Virus neutralization	0.00001–0.0001
Bactericidal test	0.00001–0.0001

Quantitative Precipitin Reaction

If increasing amounts of soluble antigen are mixed with a constant amount of antibody and the resultant precipitate is measured quantitatively, a dose-response relationship will be seen similar to that shown in Figure 8–10.

Initially, no precipitate will be formed. As the amount of antigen increases, small amounts of precipitate will result and gradually increase until the amount of precipitate is maximal. With continued addition of antigen, the amount of precipitate slowly diminishes until none is observed. This curve can be divided into the three zones shown in Figure 8–10.

In the first zone of the reaction, there is relative *antibody excess* (Fig. 8–10). Each of the two antigen-combining sites of an antibody molecule can react with a molecule of antigen, resulting in the formation of complexes composed of one antibody holding two antigens. No antigen is available for further union with the excess antibody, and therefore continued lattice formation with subsequent precipitation ceases. If the supernatant fluids are examined, it becomes evident that no free antigen exists. The composition of the supernatant fluids is shown in the accompanying inset of Figure 8–10.

In the middle, or equivalence, zone the concentrations of antigen reach optimal proportions (Fig. 8–10). Here the relative concentrations of antigen and antibody are such that maximal precipitation can occur. If, after removing the precipitates, the supernatant fluids are examined, it becomes evident that neither free antibody nor free antigen remains (Fig. 8–10). The multivalent antigen molecules are tightly held in a three-dimensional lattice by divalent antibody molecules.

The area to the right is known as the *region of antigen excess* (Fig. 8–10). Here, little precipitate is formed, although free antigen can be found in the supernatant. At this point, there is too little antibody to combine with

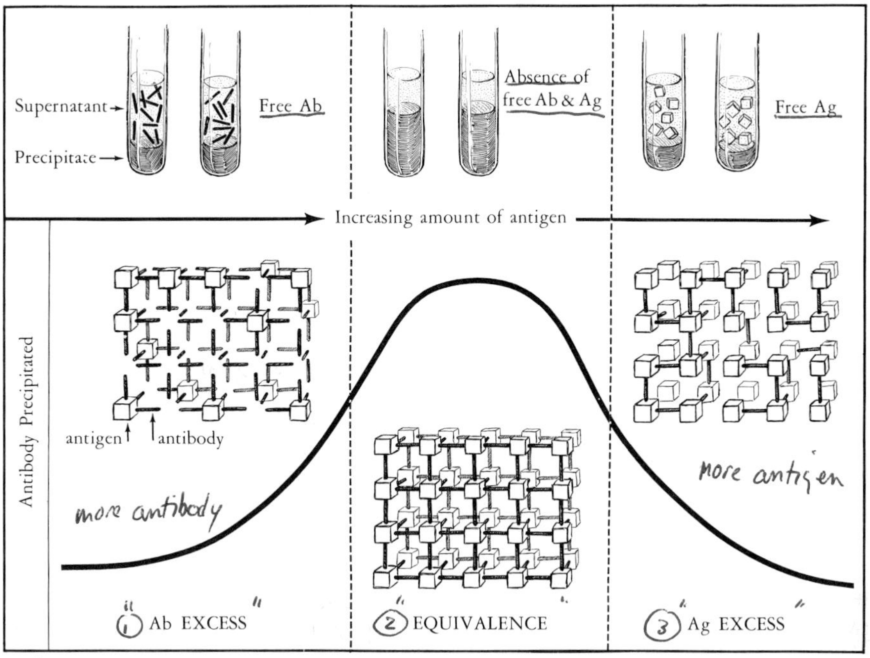

Figure 8–10. Schematic representation of the quantitative precipitation curve.

Three zones in these rxns.

all the antigenic receptor sites. Examination of the supernatant fluid will reveal that free antigen is present in excess.

These relationships of antigen and antibody in precipitin reactions are most relevant to clinical medicine. Phagocytosis is efficient in the removal of aggregates that are formed in the region of optimal proportions. Antigen-antibody complexes formed in relative antigen excess, however, have the capability of initiating a sequence of destructive inflammatory damage, characteristic of the serum sickness type of disease (Chapter 13). These complexes are small enough to remain soluble in the circulation but large enough to produce immunologic injury of tissues through complement activation.

Precipitation assays, apart from being performed in liquid media, are also carried out in semisolid media, e.g., agar, in which one or both constituents are allowed to diffuse into or toward the other. A solution of agar is placed in a Petri dish; wells are cut into the gel; and antigen and antibody are placed in them. During incubation, both antigen and antibody diffuse toward each other from the wells and interact to form precipitates in the agar. A schematic representation of this reaction is shown in Figure 8–11. It can be seen that as diffusion progresses, concentration gradients of both antigen and antibody are established. When optimal concentrations are attained, a precipitate will form that is visible through the agar as a distinct band or line (Fig. 8–11). If the reaction is allowed to continue, the precipitin line may decrease in intensity or actually disappear owing to an excess of antigen or antibody.

The precipitin reaction is a useful analytic tool for the identification of unknown antibodies or antigens. If two different antigens, A and B, are each allowed to diffuse in agar from adjacent wells toward their specific antibody (anti-A or anti-B) in different plates,

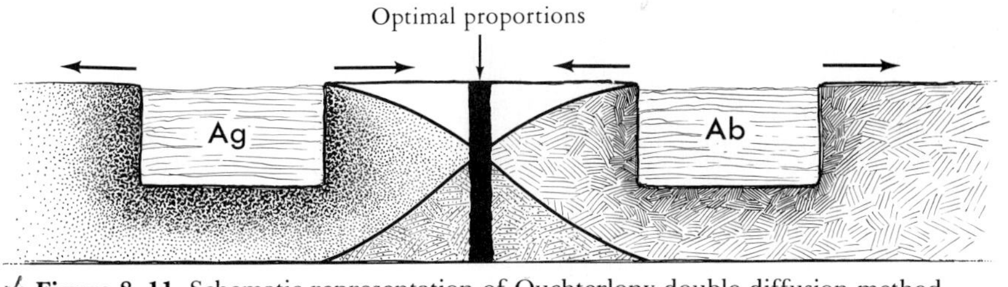

Figure 8–11. Schematic representation of Ouchterlony double diffusion method.

The test can be used to quantify immunoglobulins.

lines of precipitation will be obtained for each antigen-antibody system. The region of optimal proportion for the A–anti-A reaction may differ from that of the B–anti-B reaction. This may be due to differences in molecular weight or concentration, both of which can influence the rate of diffusion. With this technique, however, it is possible to determine whether two antigens are *identical, similar,* or *different* (Fig. 8–12) by juxtaposing the reactions between adjacent wells. For example, an antiserum reactive with both antigens is placed in a central well surrounded by wells containing the two suspected antigens. Diffusion is allowed to take place and bands of precipitate are formed. If the two antigens are identical, they will diffuse at the same rate and the zone of optimal proportions will be reached in the same location. Therefore, the two bands will coalesce, as shown in Figure 8–12, in the *reaction of identity.* With further diffusion of antigen or

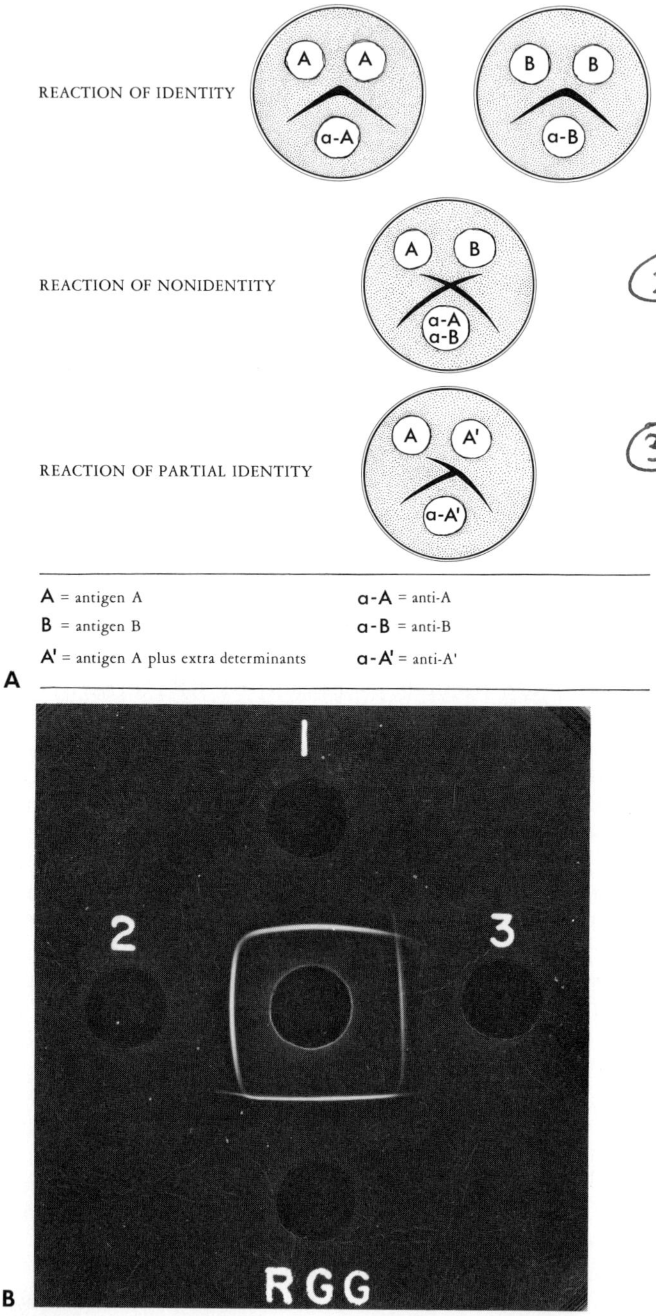

Figure 8–12. *A,* Schematic representation of three types of Ouchterlony double diffusion reactions. *B,* Ouchterlony double diffusion plate showing the reaction of identity between fractions 1 and 2, the reaction of partial identity between whole rabbit gamma globulin (RGG) and fractions 2 and 3 and the reaction of nonidentity between fractions 1 and 3. (From Putnam, F. W., et al.: The cleavage of rabbit γ-globulin by papain. J. Biol. Chem., *237*:717, 1962; courtesy of Dr. Shunsuke Migita.)

antibody, the formation of soluble complexes will occur. Coalescence will be maintained, however, since the bands continue to form and dissolve at the same rate. If, on the other hand, the two antigens are completely different, the bands will cross in the *reaction of nonidentity*, as shown in Figure 8–12. In this case, the concentration of one antigen has little influence on the behavior of the other, and the two bands that form will cross over each other. Sometimes two antigens may be similar and share a common determinant; this results in spur formation—the reaction of partial identity (Fig. 8–12).

Precipitation in agar gels is widely used in diagnostic immunology. It is most useful in the quantification of immunoglobulin concentrations and in immunoelectrophoresis (Chapter 21). In immunoquantification, the agar is impregnated by the antiserum and the material to be tested is placed in wells. The diameters of the concentric rings that form are directly proportional to the concentration of the antigen in question (Chapter 26). In recent years, the method of detection of antigen-antibody precipitin reactions has been improved by nephelometric or light-scattering techniques, which have been used for the quantification of a wide variety of serum proteins and other body fluid proteins (Chapter 26). These techniques are useful in the quantification of immunoglobulins in many disease states such as the immunoproliferative diseases (Chapter 21) and the immunologic deficiency states (Chapter 22).

Agglutination Reactions

The same principles governing the antigen-antibody relationships seen in precipitin reactions also apply to agglutination reactions. The notable difference is that soluble complexes are not formed by the latter. Instead, in the region where antibody is in excess, visible agglutination may be inhibited. This is referred to as a *prozone phenomenon*. Owing to the particle size, electrostatic surface charge density, or immunochemical nature of the antibody, certain physicochemical conditions occur that affect agglutination reactions.

Any large particle, such as a red blood cell, suspended in solution contains a net surface electrostatic charge. This is due, in part, to cell surface chemical groupings that may be completely or partially ionized. Since red blood cell particles in any given reaction are similar, they carry an identical charge and therefore tend to repel each other. The strength of the effective electrostatic charge (zeta potential), as described below, tends to keep the particles at a given distance.

In agglutination, the first stage of the initial antigen-antibody union takes place as in precipitation and is dependent upon ionic strength, pH, and temperature. The second stage, lattice formation, is dependent upon overcoming the electrostatic repulsion forces of the particles. In the agglutination of red blood cells, for example, in which antigenic receptor sites may be located in deep valleys on the cell surface, antibody is firmly bound to receptor sites on one cell. Lattice formation cannot occur until its free receptor valence attaches to antigen between adjacent cells. If the cells are held apart by repulsive forces, the free end of the antibody molecule will not approach the antigen closely enough to make a firm bond. The repulsive forces may be overcome by physical methods that force the cells into closer proximity, e.g., centrifugation or sedimentation. With some antigen-antibody systems, however, such measures have no effect and agglutination cannot occur.

Those antibodies capable of reacting with antigen in saline solution have been termed *saline* or *complete* antibodies and, for the most part, consist of IgM antibody. Those incapable of reacting in saline have been termed *incomplete* or *blocking* antibodies and include the IgG antibodies. *It should be pointed out, however, that the terms "complete" and "incomplete" are misnomers, since all antibodies are functionally complete.* Certain types of 7S IgG antibodies cannot agglutinate red cells in saline suspension even though firmly attached to antigens. In these cases, the size of the antibody molecule and its wide spatial arrangement prevent agglutination. Even high centrifugal forces cannot overcome these electrostatic repulsion effects and allow lattice formation to occur. Nevertheless, if these same antibodies are mixed with red blood cells in a colloidal medium such as albumin, agglutination will occur. This principle becomes important in the interpretation of various types of antibody associated with alloimmunization, e.g., hemolytic disease of the newborn or transfusion reactions (Chapter 20).

ZETA POTENTIAL

The distance between two particles in suspension is not solely dependent upon their net surface charge density. Ions in solution orient themselves around a particle so as to form a diffuse double layer or cloud. The difference in charge density between the inside and the outside of the ionic cloud creates an electrostatic potential known as the zeta potential. The zeta potential is the essential determining factor of the repulsion effects of two adjacent particles. By controlling this potential, it is possible to control the minimal distance two particles may achieve in suspension.

The zeta potential may be reduced by two methods: (1) pretreatment with enzymes, such as trypsin or neuraminidase, that alter chemical groupings on cell surfaces; and (2) the use of various colloidal diluents, e.g., serum albumin or Ficoll, that lower the zeta potential by changing the dielectric constant of the aqueous electrolyte solution. The net result is that the electrostatic repulsion effects are overcome and the cells or particles can approximate each other, permitting the firm coupling of antigen with antibody necessary for agglutination.

The Antiglobulin (Coombs) Reaction

In some cases, a short antibody molecule directed against a deeply located antigenic determinant cannot agglutinate, even when these various manipulations are employed. In such situations, a third type of serologic technique, such as the antiglobulin (Coombs) reaction, must be employed in order to demonstrate that antibody is present. The antiglobulin test consists of the addition of an antibody directed against gamma globulin, which provides a bridge between two antibody-coated cells (Fig. 8–13). Most commercially available Coombs reagents used in the clinical laboratory contain anti-human IgG in combination with some anti-human "non-gamma" antibody to detect bound complement components. These are the so-called broad-spectrum Coombs sera and contain broadly reactive antiglobulin activity. Additional sera are available to detect class-specific antibody, e.g., IgG-, IgM-, IgA-associated antibody.

The Coombs test is performed in two ways: (1) the *direct* antiglobulin test, consisting of the detection of cell-bound antibody by the addition of the antiglobulin reagent directly to the cell suspension; and (2) the *indirect* antiglobulin test, detecting the presence of circulating antibody that is first adsorbed to the test red cells to which is added the antiglobulin reagent. For example, the direct Coombs test would be useful for the detection of IgG-sensitized red cells in an infant suspected of having hemolytic disease of the newborn; the indirect Coombs test would be useful for the detection of IgG-associated antibody in the serum of a mother suspected of being sensitized to the Rh antigen (Chapter 20).

Passive Agglutination

Since agglutination tests are more sensitive indicators of antibody, it is sometimes desir-

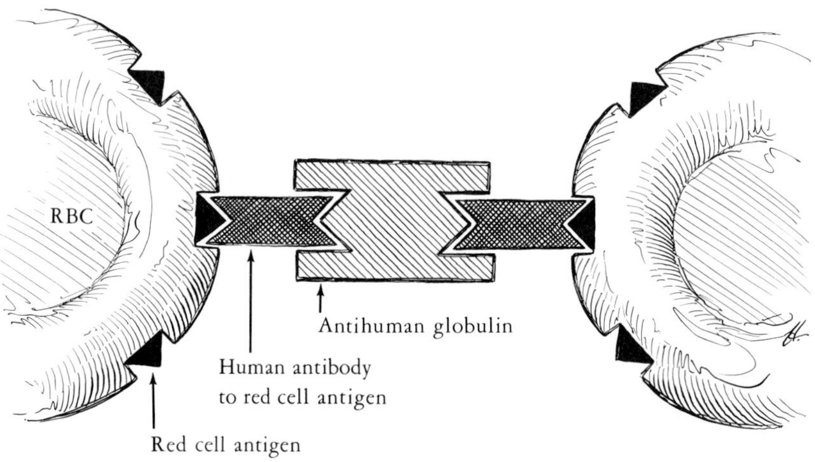

Figure 8–13. Schematic representation of the antiglobulin (Coombs) reaction.

able to convert systems that precipitate to those that agglutinate. This is referred to as *passive agglutination* and can be accomplished by coating a small soluble antigen onto a larger insoluble particle, such as polystyrene, latex, bentonite, or red blood cells. Diagnostic tests employing this technique are in widespread use for the detection of a variety of antibodies, such as the rheumatoid factor (an IgM antibody directed against partially denatured IgG globulin) (Chapter 20).

Antigens may be coupled to erythrocytes by various techniques. Polysaccharide antigens readily adhere to the surface of unaltered red blood cells. Thus, specific polysaccharide antigens of certain bacteria adhere to erythrocytes and are used as test antigens for the detection of antibody. Protein substances may be attached to red cells that have been treated with tannic acid. The tanned-cell hemagglutination technique is valuable in detecting antibody to thyroglobulin in Hashimoto's disease (Chapter 20). Finally, certain antigens may be attached to red cells by means of a chemical linkage such as the bis-diazotized benzidine (BDB) coupling reaction. Thus, both precipitation and agglutination provide very specific and sensitive tests in current use in diagnostic immunology (Chapter 26).

COMPLEMENT-DEPENDENT REACTIONS

Complement has been described in detail in Chapter 6. Those complement-dependent effects useful in identifying antigen-antibody reactions include *lysis, phagocytosis, chemotaxis, opsonization, immune adherence, complement fixation,* and *altered permeability* (see Fig. 8–1).

Lysis

Lysis represents destruction of the cell membrane through the action of the late-acting complement components (C8, C9) that are activated by the reaction of specific antibody to a surface antigen and mediated through the activation of the complete complement sequence. These reactions usually result in the destruction of red blood cells (hemolysis), white blood cells (lymphocytotoxicity), or certain gram-negative bacteria (bacteriolysis).

Chemotaxis, Opsonization, Immune Adherence, Phagocytosis, and Altered Permeability

The interaction of antigen with antibody together with complement can also affect the inflammatory response through chemotaxis, opsonization, immune adherence, phagocytosis, and altered permeability. This involves a multiphasic act including the generation of chemotactic factor (C3a, C5a, C567), the activation of the phagocytosis-promoting factor (C3b), and the presence of complement receptors (C3b) and Fc receptors on the surface of phagocytic cells. The chemotactic and phagocytic factors can be initiated through the activation of either the classic or alternative complement pathway (Chapter 6). The antigen-antibody reaction usually leads to the activation of the classic pathway. Once initiated, these principles lead to the accumulation of phagocytic cells and to the enhancement of phagocytosis.

The activation of the complement cascade by the antigen-antibody interaction can also lead to the production of factors that alter the permeability of blood vessels. The action of these split products (C3a, C5a) is indirect and occurs through the release of vasoactive amines from mediator cells (Chapters 2 and 13).

Complement Fixation

The sera of all animal species contain varying quantities of complement. For many years, normal guinea pig serum was used as the primary source of complement in most serologic systems, since this species of animal contains high levels of complement having very efficient lytic properties. Different sources of complement are used in various *in vitro* tests; for example, in cytotoxicity tests used in transplantation, rabbit complement is the ideal source.

Lytic antibodies are rarely used directly in *in vitro* tests. The reasons for this are the low sensitivity of the method and the unavailability of antigen in proper form. For example, although it is possible to detect lytic antibodies against *Bordetella pertussis,* it takes at least one molecule of IgM antibody or two molecules of IgG antibody to initiate the complement sequence for the lysis of a single cell.

In order to produce a perceptible change by direct lysis, a huge number of bacterial cells would be required. The second limiting factor may be the type of antigen itself. There are certain organisms such as viruses, rickettsiae, fungi, and some spirochetes that are not susceptible to direct lysis.

For these reasons, the complement-fixation test capable of detecting the same antibody represents one of the most sensitive and frequently employed serologic tests in clinical medicine. The assay is based upon a two-stage reaction in which complement is consumed in the first stage of the antigen-antibody reaction. The binding of complement is assayed indirectly by a detection system consisting of antibody-coated erythrocytes that detect residual complement activity. In the first stage, the test antigen and the patient's heated serum (complement-inactivated) are incubated in the presence of a measured quantity of guinea pig complement. The amount of complement used is critical and represents a slight excess of that amount required to lyse a standard suspension of sheep red cells sensitized with rabbit anti–sheep red cell antibody (hemolysin or amboceptor). At the end of the primary incubation, the sensitized sheep red cells are added. If the patient's serum contains antibody directed against the test antigen, an antigen-antibody reaction occurs that consumes the complement. Therefore, little or no complement is available to lyse the sensitized sheep red cells. This is termed *complement fixation* and represents the presence of antibody. If, on the other hand, the patient's serum is devoid of antibody, no antigen-antibody reaction takes place in the first stage, and complement remains in the system and is available for the lysis of the added sensitized sheep cells. This represents the lack of complement-fixation and implies the absence of the complement-fixing antibody. This technique is much more sensitive than is the direct lysis of bacteria and provides a simple and quantitative method of antibody detection.

A special case of complement-dependent lysis is the *cytotoxicity test.* This assay employs a system in which the living cells are mixed with antibody and complement. When antibody to a cell-bound antigen is present, cell death will occur in the presence of complement. The end point or cell death can be ascertained by any of a number of methods, including supravital staining, gross appearance of cells, or enzymatic function. This assay has wide application in histocompatibility testing for organ transplantation and is also assuming importance in tests of cell-mediated immunity to viruses (Chapter 9 and 16) and tumor antigens (Chapter 19). A specialized example of the use of lytic techniques *in vitro* is the Jerne plaque technique. In this method, a suspension of presensitized immunocompetent lymphoid cells is incubated in agar in which red cells, antigen, and complement are also present. The *in vitro* production of antibody by these cells is detected by clear areas of lysis surrounding each of the antibody-producing cells.

Cytotropic Effects

Cytotropic effects are a property of some classes of antibody that can bind to a limited number of mediator cells of the body, such as mast cells and basophils, and in most mammalian species, including man, appear to be primarily associated with the IgE class of immunoglobulin. When involved in antigen-antibody interactions, this class of immunoglobulin has the capacity to release from mediator cells a number of vasoactive amines important in localized and generalized forms of anaphylaxis (Chapter 13). This class of antibody can be detected *in vitro* by means of the release of vasoactive amines from sensitized mediator cells (e.g., leukocyte histamine release) or by assays involving their effect on isolated target tissue (e.g., Schultz-Dale). In addition, these antibodies can be detected by radioimmunoassay tests (e.g., RAST).

SUMMARY

The manifestations of antigen-antibody interactions can be divided into three categories: the primary, the secondary, and the tertiary. The primary interaction of antigen with antibody is the basic event and may be demonstrated directly or through secondary manifestations, which include precipitation, agglutination, complement-dependent reactions, neutralization, and cytotropic effects. The secondary manifestations of antigen-antibody reactions encompass a number of physical and chemical interactions between antibody, antigen, complement, and the suspending medium in which the antigen-antibody reaction occurs. The tertiary manifestations of the antigen-antibody interaction are biologic expressions, which may be either beneficial or harmful to the host.

Suggestions for Further Reading

Haber, E., and Krause, R. M. (eds.): Antibodies in Human Diagnosis and Therapy. New York, Raven Press, 1977.

Henriksen, S. D. (ed.): Immunology. Baltimore, Williams & Wilkins Company, 1970.

Kabat, E. A. (ed.): Structural Concepts in Immunology and Immunochemistry. 2nd ed. New York, Holt, Rinehart and Winston, 1975.

Rose, N. R., and Friedman, H. (eds.): Manual of Clinical Immunology. 2nd ed. Washington, D. C., American Society for Microbiology, 1980.

Stites, D. P., Stobo, J. D., Fudenberg, H. H., et al.: Basic and Clinical Immunology. 4th ed. Los Altos, Lange Medical Publications, 1982.

Voller, A., Bidwell, D. E., and Bartlett, A.: Enzyme immunoassays in diagnostic medicine. Bull. WHO, *52*:55, 1976.

Chapter 9

Cell-Mediated Immune Reactions

Joseph A. Bellanti, M.D., and Ross E. Rocklin, M.D.

The previous chapter describes those manifestations of the specific immune response concerned with the reactions of antibody with antigen—the *antigen-antibody interactions.* This chapter is concerned with those expressions of the immune response that involve the interaction of cells of the immune system with antigen and are termed *cell-mediated immune* (CMI) reactions. Until recently, these reactions were considered to be mediated only by T-lymphocytes independent of antibody; it is becoming increasingly clear, however, that they may also be carried out by a variety of cell types, humoral substances, or combinations of both.

Although the term "delayed hypersensitivity" has been used previously to include both normal and pathologic expressions of cell-mediated immunity, its use here will be restricted to include only those *in vivo* manifestations of the cellular immune response that lead to tissue injury (Chapter 13). The more inclusive term "cell-mediated" or "cellular immunity" will be used to encompass both *normal* and *pathologic* events and will include both *in vitro* and *in vivo* expressions of specifically sensitized T-lymphocytes as well as those activities carried out by other cellular and humoral components of the immune response.

The series of reactions involved in this type of immunity seem to be characteristically associated with effector–target cell interactions involved in (1) acquired microbial resistance, particularly that associated with intracellular parasitism (Chapters 14 through 18); (2) transplantation immunity (Chapter 20B); and (3) tumor rejection (Chapter 19). In each of these situations, antigen is either intracellular or architecturally inaccessible, and antigen-antibody reactions appear to be relatively inefficient. Cellular reactions, on the other hand, appear to be more effective in the elimination of such sterically inaccessible antigens.

HISTORICAL ASPECTS

The phenomenon of delayed hypersensitivity was first discovered by Edward Jenner in 1798, during the course of his studies with cowpox virus immunization, when he observed that an inflammatory lesion occurred within 24 to 48 hours at the site of revaccination of a previously immunized individual. In the nineteenth century, during attempts at developing a vaccine for tuberculosis, Robert Koch observed a similar phenomenon. Following inoculation of culture broth of the tubercle bacillus into the skin of tuberculous guinea pigs, he observed a localized red lesion within 24 to 48 hours that occasionally became necrotic.

The characteristics and mechanisms of various types of tissue injury resulting from immunologic mechanisms, including delayed hypersensitivity reactions, will be described more fully in Chapter 13. The following biologic characteristics of the delayed hypersensitivity reaction in skin are presented briefly to illustrate the basic immunobiologic principles underlying these effects.

Following the intradermal injection of antigen into a sensitized host, a reaction occurs at the localized skin site within 24 to 48 hours, reaching a maximum at 72 hours. The lesion consists of a firm indurated "red bump," whose intensity is directly related to the degree of sensitization of the host. For years, this *in vivo* method of testing for cell-mediated responses was the only procedure available and by its nature was difficult to quantify.

It was subsequently shown that this dermal reactivity could be passively transferred from a sensitized individual to a normal host by the use of living lymphoid cells, e.g., blood lymphocytes, but not by serum. Cell extracts of human leukocytes (transfer factor) were also shown to have the capacity to transfer this reactivity from sensitized donors to normal recipients.

The histology of the dermal skin site reveals the presence of mononuclear cells, basophils, and few neutrophils, in contrast to cellular reactions mediated by antibodies, in which neutrophilic infiltration and edema predominate (Chapter 13). The early histologists were noncommital in their descriptions of these cells and used the term "round-cell infiltration." Recently, the predominant type of leukocyte in cell-mediated reactions has been shown to be the macrophage. In experimental studies in guinea pigs in which radioactively labeled macrophages were employed to determine the source of these cells, it was demonstrated that the macrophages present in the reaction site were those of the recipient and not the donor. Furthermore, most of the cells in the cell-mediated lesion appeared to be derived from rapidly dividing populations of macrophages originating in the bone marrow. These cells arrive at the test site via the motile form of the macrophage, the monocyte (Chapter 2).

CELL TYPES AND EFFECTOR MECHANISMS

There are a variety of cell types and cellular mechanisms involved in the expressions or regulation of cell-mediated reactions. Shown in Table 9–1 are the cell types with their sites of origin, surface characteristics, and mechanisms of action. These cell types include (1) T-lymphocytes, (2) macrophages, (3) killer or K-cells, and (4) natural killer or NK-cells.

T-Lymphocytes

The first cell type to be described is the T-lymphocyte (Table 9–1). In addition to its collaborative role with B-lymphocytes in either a "helper" or a "suppressor" function (Chapters 7 and 10), it is now recognized that the T-lymphocyte, either alone or in concert with other subsets of T-lymphocytes, is important in the expressions of cell-mediated immunity. The clinically important reactions include the rejection of allografts, the rejection of tumors, and antimicrobial immunity.

The T-lymphocytes arise in the bone marrow and differentiate in the thymus; the mature forms contain characteristic markers (Table 9–1). Upon further differentiation these cells give rise to a population of cytotoxic T-cells that can destroy appropriate target cells either directly or through the elaboration of specific cell products, e.g., lymphokines. These cytotoxic lymphocytes can be generated *in vitro* in a mixed lymphocyte (MLC) reaction, *in vivo* during a graft-versus-host (GVH) reaction, or during the rejection of an allograft, tumor cell, or virally transformed or chemically modified target cell. Such cytotoxic cells can be demonstrated *in vitro* by the lysis of appropriate target cells.

Recently, cytotoxicity experiments in the murine system have suggested that certain genetic restrictions are involved in the recognition and destruction of virally infected or chemically modified target cells by T-lymphocytes. A requirement for identity at the H-2K or D locus has been demonstrated for both the sensitized T-lymphocyte and the target cell (Chapter 3). Although a similar relationship has not yet been demonstrated for the human, the biologic implications of these findings are very important with respect to antiviral immunity, autoimmunity, and malignancy. Furthermore, based upon these findings, the ability to differentiate between "self" and nonself" appears to be intimately related to histocompatibility and immune responsiveness. From an evolutionary standpoint, it has been suggested that minor alterations of these strong immuno-

Table 9–1. **Effector Cell Types Involved in Cell-Mediated Reactions**

Cell Type	Precursor Cell or Site of Differentiation	Surface Markers or Receptors: mIg	Fc	C3b	T Antigen	Mechanisms of Action
T-lymphocytes	Thymus	–	–	–	+	Direct or elaboration of lymphokines
Macrophages	Monocyte precursor	±	+	+	–	Direct or armed with antibody; enhanced by MIF
K-cells	?	–	+	–	–	Armed with antibody (ADCC)
NK-cells	?	–	–	–	–	Direct

genic histocompatibility antigens by viruses or chemicals will immediately stimulate the immunologic system. Very recently, a genetic requirement for T-helper function in antibody synthesis by B-cells has also been demonstrated (Chapter 7).

Mononuclear Phagocytes

The mononuclear phagocytes make up a second set of cell types active in cellular immunity. These cells not only are important in the "processing" or "presentation" of antigen for the initiating events of T cell activation and antibody production by B-cells but also may perform an accessory function in the expressions of cell-mediated immunity by T-lymphocytes. Their actions are mediated in part through the elaboration of monokines such as interleukin-1, which is involved in the activation of T-cells, and colony-stimulating factor, neutral proteinases (plasminogen activator, elastase, and collagenase), and complement proteins, which are involved in various effector functions. Moreover, they may take part directly in the destruction of foreign substances by *phagocytosis* or by direct cytotoxic effect on target cells. In addition, some of the products of T-lymphocytes, e.g., migration inhibitory factor (MIF), may influence macrophage function by affecting cell movement or cellular metabolism. The enhancement of these macrophage functions by agents, e.g., immunopotentiators, is receiving widespread attention in cancer immunotherapy (Chapter 10).

The presence of an Fc receptor and a receptor for C3b may facilitate the uptake of complexes of antigen and antibody or antigen-antibody and complement, respectively. In addition, the presence of the Fc receptor may allow the cell type to participate in antibody-dependent cellular cytotoxic (ADCC) reactions, as described for the killer (K) cell.

Killer Cells

Another cellular type important in cell-mediated reactions is the killer or K-cells (see Table 9–1). Although their precise identity and site of origin are unknown, these cells are morphologically indistinguishable from small lymphocytes and Fc receptor–positive, surface immunoglobulin–negative (mIG—), and C3b receptor–negative (i.e., null cells). These cells have been shown to have cytotoxic activity with target cells coated with specific IgG antibody in an antibody-dependent cellular cytotoxic (ADCC) reaction, in which an antibody molecule appears to form a bridge between the target cell and the effector cell. This presumably occurs through a binding of the Fab region of the immunoglobulin molecule with the antigenic determinants on the target cell and the Fc portion of the antibody with the Fc receptor on the surface of the lymphocyte. Complement does not appear to participate in these reactions, and unlike the situation with T-lymphocytes, these reactions can occur with nonsensitized K-cells.

Natural Killer Cells

A fourth cell type has very recently been described that appears to be a natural killer or NK-cell. The identity of these cells is also unknown; they contain no known T- or B-cell markers and do not require prior sensitization for their generation. These cells occur naturally and are found in increased quantity in mice lacking thymuses (nude mice). This finding may explain the apparent discrepancy in the immune surveillance theory, which would predict an increased incidence of tumors in such animals. The apparent increase in NK-cells may offer an explanation for the absence of increased tumorigenicity in these animals. These cells are thought to be involved in nonspecific killing of virally transformed target cells, allografts, resistance to some infections, and tumor rejection. Although their role in man is as yet undefined, these cells may be of profound biologic significance in immune surveillance of malignant diseases in the human.

Effect of Antibody on Cell-Mediated Reactions

In addition to its role in facilitating cell-mediated immunity through an ADCC mechanism, antibody may also exert a direct cytotoxic effect on a target cell through a complement-dependent reaction (Table 9–1) (Chapter 6). Alternatively, antibody directed against a target cell can "block" the cytotoxic effect of T-lymphocytes, macrophages, K-cells, or NK-cells, presumably by binding with antigenic determinants on the target cell surface. This interference by antibody or antigen-antibody complexes may have relevance for host immunologic reactions against certain tumors, and such "blocking antibody" may result in intensified tumor growth, a phenomenon referred to as *enhancement.* Other species of antibody formed in the tumor-bearing host can "unblock" this blocking antibody and lead to the destruction of the tumor. Whether this unblocking effect is related to direct complement-dependent effects of antibody or is favored by an ADCC effect is unknown.

COMPONENTS OF THE CELL-MEDIATED REACTION

Like the antigen-antibody reactions, the T-lymphocyte–antigen reactions may be divided into three stages: the *primary* stage, the *secondary* stage, and the *tertiary* stage (Fig. 9–1).

The Primary Stage: Combination of Antigen with Specifically Sensitized T-Lymphocytes

The cell-mediated reaction is initiated by the binding of antigen with an antigen receptor on the surface of a sensitized T-lymphocyte (Chapter 7). This may occur directly or, more likely, may be mediated by macrophage-bound antigen in association with "self" determinants. There are a number of other substances that can attach to the surface of the T-lymphocyte and either activate it, e.g., mitogens, or provide a basis for its identification, e.g., sheep erythrocyte binding in an E-rosette reaction (Chapter 7). Following the reaction of antigen with a sensitized T-lymphocyte, a sequence of morphologic and biochemical events occurs that forms the secondary stage.

The Secondary Stage: Morphologic and Biochemical Reactions

The second stage of the antigen–T-lymphocyte interaction is made up of the *in vitro* manifestations of cell-mediated immunity that presumably result from the membrane perturbations established following the primary interaction of the T-lymphocyte with antigen or mitogen, and are detected indirectly through morphologic or biochemical events. The morphologic changes of lymphocytes in tissue culture consist of blast cell transformation with subsequent mitosis. Many investigators suggest that the macrophage is essential for this reaction to proceed and that cell populations depleted of these cells may be deficient in lymphoproliferative activity. The biochemical events that occur during the secondary stage are revealed by *de novo* DNA, RNA, or protein synthesis, detected by use of radiolabeled precursors. Collectively, these morphologic and biochemical changes have proved to be of considerable clinical importance, since they are used in *in vitro* measurements to assess the functional reactivity of blood lymphocytes in patients suspected of having impaired thymic-dependent immunity (Chapters 22 and 26).

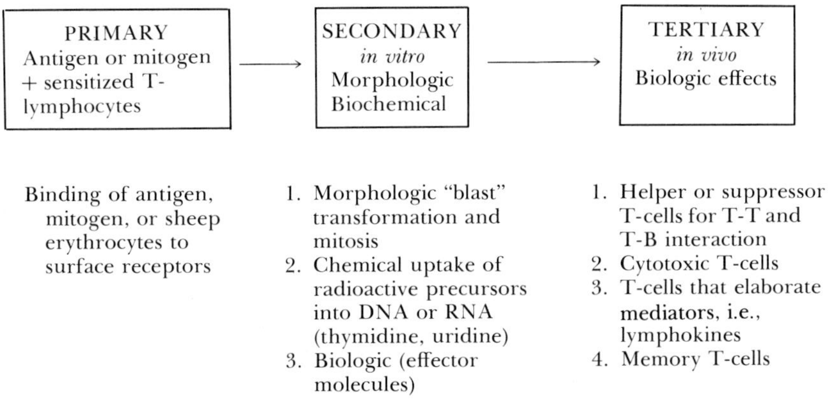

Figure 9–1. Schematic representation of cell-mediated events.

The Tertiary Stage: Biologic Expressions

The tertiary effects of cell-mediated immunity are the biologic expressions of these earlier events (Fig. 9–1). They consist of the following steps: (1) the generation of helper or suppressor T-cells for T-T and T-B interactions, including the role of macrophages; (2) the generation of cytotoxic T-cells; (3) the generation of T-cells that elaborate the effector molecules (mediators) of CMI; and (4) the generation of memory T-cells.

Thymocytes and thymus-derived lymphocytes (T-cells) are a heterogeneous population of cells. This heterogeneity is reflected in differences in organ localization, surface antigen properties, recirculation potential, and function.

T-lymphocyte development depends on the presence of a thymus. Immunocompetent cells migrate from the thymus to T-dependent areas in peripheral lymphoid tissue—the periarteriolar areas of the spleen and the deep cortical areas of the lymph nodes.

The genetic controls and immunoregulatory aspects of T-cell function in the mouse system have been described in Chapters 3 and 7, respectively. This section will focus primarily on the human T-cell–mediated immune responses.

Cell-mediated immune reactions are found to involve the sequential interactions of at least two types of thymus-derived lymphocytes (T-lymphocytes). T-lymphocytes in the mouse have been characterized by both Thy-1 (θ) antigen and a series of alloantigens termed Ly. One T-lymphocyte subpopulation bearing the Ly-1 marker responds to antigenic stimulation by proliferation and is responsible for T-lymphocyte proliferation in a mixed lymphocyte culture. A factor may then be elaborated (putatively Ia, see Chapter 3) that triggers a population of Ly-2,3-bearing T-lymphocytes. These cells mediate what has been termed cell-mediated lympholysis (CML) through a number of proposed mechanisms (lymphotoxin, for example). T-lymphocytes bearing Ly-1 markers may also produce factors such as MIF, which allows macrophages to provide additional help during an immune response against a tumor or tissue graft.

For ease of discussion, the cellular events that make up the tertiary stage of CMI in the human following interaction of antigen with T-lymphocytes are shown in Figure 9–2. T-helper/inducer (T_H) cells play a central role along with macrophages in providing positive signals for a number of cells that are involved in the expression of cell-mediated immune reactions. Initiation of cell-mediated immune reactions requires an antigen-presenting (processing) cell such as the macrophage. Other specialized cells, such as dendritic cells or cutaneous Langerhans cells, that are part of or related to the monocyte-macrophage lineage may also subserve this function. Initially, macrophages activate the small number of T-helper lymphocytes ($T4^+$) that possess receptors for the antigen in question by presenting the antigen to the T-cells in conjunction with "self-recognition" molecules (Ia). Activated T-helper cells elaborate lymphokines, some of which activate macrophages and also recruit other lymphocytes and monocytes-macrophages to participate in the reaction. Activated macrophages produce monokines, some of which are necessary for T-cell activation and induction of inflammation. Thus, a reaction that initially involves a small number of sensitized cells can be amplified and expanded to include a large number of cells that are not sensitized to the antigen that initiated the reaction.

Macrophages liberate interleukin-1, a monokine that seems identical to leukocyte pyrogen (the cause of febrile reactions) and is required for activation of T-helper lymphocytes. The later cells elaborate IL-2 and, together with IL-1, bring about the differentiation of the TDTH ($T4^+$) cells. The T_{DTA} cell activated by antigen and IL-1 then releases a series of molecules that can enhance the function of macrophages. One such factor(s) is macrophage activation factor (MAF); this may in fact be an activity due to multiple molecules, one of which seems to be γ interferon. When the macrophages are activated, they secreted not only interleukin-1 but also a series of enzymes (neutral proteases, e.g., colagenase and elastase) that can digest connective tissue, procoagulant molecules (tissue factor and factor VII) that can cause local coagulation via the extrinsic coagulation pathway, and a plasminogen activator. This last enzyme converts plasminogen to plasmin, and plasmin will digest fibrin and thereby slowly reverse clot formation. Fibrin is deposited at sites of DTH and an intermediate degradaton produce, "fibrinoid," is found in increased amounts in connective tissue diseases. Release of other lymphokines, such as

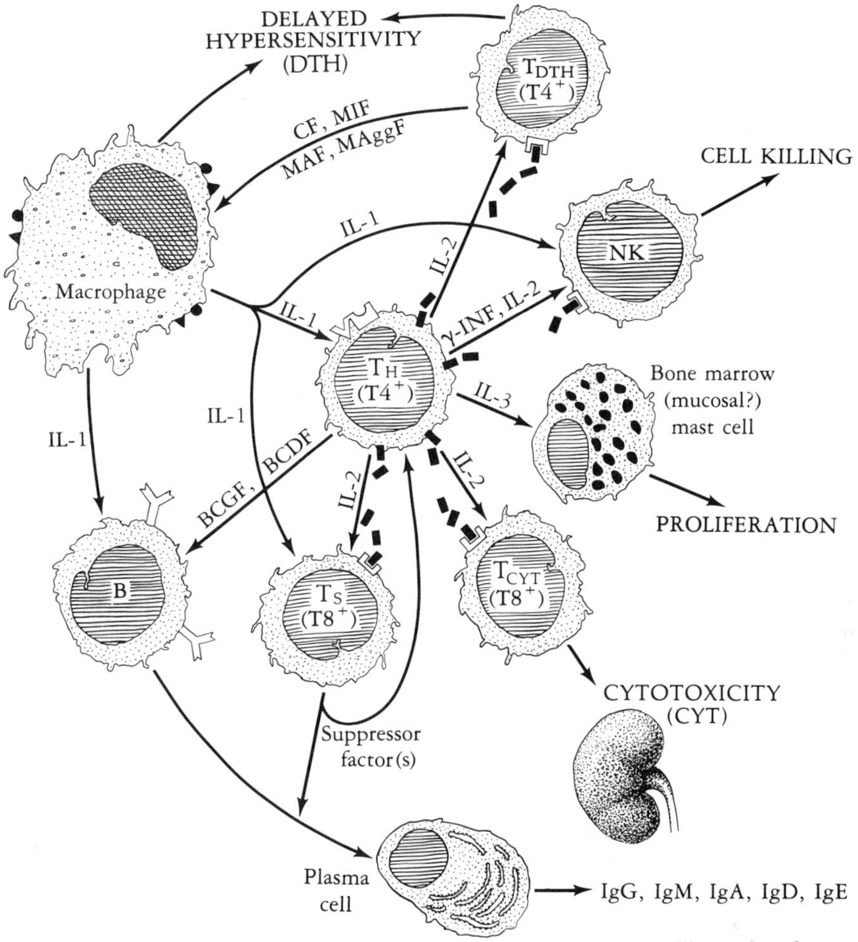

Figure 9–2. Cellular events that make up the tertiary stage of CMI in the human, illustrating the central role of the T-cell in the immunoregulatory network.

macrophage chemotactic factor (CF), recruits the cells to the site of reaction, while migration inhibition factor (MIF) immobilizes macrophages and tends to localize them in the vicinity of the immune reaction. Release of another factor, a macrophage aggregation factor (MAggF), facilitates their adherence to each other. The latter factor appears to be fibronectin or fragments derived therefrom. Interleukin-2 (IL-2) is required for the proliferation of certain subpopulations of lymphocytes. IL-2 released by the T-helper cell interacts with an IL-2 receptor on T-suppressor cells ($T8^+$) and, in conjunction with IL-1, activates them. The T_S cell regulates both T- and B-cells functions, usually by means of suppressor factors that block the activity of T-helper cells and the differentiation of B-cells into plasma cells. Also contained within the $T8^+$ subpopulation is a cytotoxic T-cell (T_{CYT}), whose function in cell-mediated immune reactions is that of transplant rejection and destruction of tumor cells.

The names "helper" and "suppressor" for these lymphocyte subpopulations refer in part to their role in the maturation and proliferation of B-cells to form antibody-secreting plasma cells (Chapter 7). The helper cell elaborates factors (B-cell growth factor [BCGF] and B-cell differentiation factor [BCDF], which facilitate differentiation of B-cells and secretion of antibody, while the suppressor cell produces factors that inhibit antibody formation. A proper balance between help and suppression appears necessary for regulation of all the immunoglobulin isotypes (IgG, IgM, IgA, IgD, and IgE). In some systems, IL-1 may also be required for B-cell activation. Once differentiation into a plasma cell has occurred, immunoglobulin synthesis proceeds.

Certain other lymphocyte functions have recently been shown to be mediated by lymphokines. For example, natural killer cells are lymphocytes that can kill target tissues, such as tumor cells, in the absence of antibody (killer function). Gamma interferon has been shown to promote the activity of these cells. There is also a third interleukin, IL-3, whose function in lymphocyte proliferation is as yet unclear. However, this molecule appears to stimulate the proliferation of bone marrow mast cells. The latter group of cells appears to populate mucosal lining tissue and represents a subpopulation of mast cells that differs from those usually identified within tissue.

EFFECTOR MOLECULES OF CELL-MEDIATED REACTIONS

Following the interaction of a sensitized lymphocyte with antigen, the lymphocyte is capable of elaborating an array of diverse substances. These factors have recently been shown to possess a variety of biologic activities that are thought to be the *in vitro* correlates of cell-mediated immunity. The physical and biologic activities of these effector molecules are shown in Tables 9–2 and 9–3. The knowledge of these effector molecules "has liberated immunologists from the firm, red bump" and allowed a better understanding of the dynamics of the *in vivo* reaction.

Table 9–2. **Products of Activated Lymphocytes**

I. Mediators Affecting Macrophages
- (a) migration inhibitory factor (MIF)
- (b) macrophage activating factor
- (c) macrophage aggregation factor (? same as MIF)
- (d) factor causing disappearance of macrophage from perioneum (? same as MIF)
- (e) chemotactic factor for macrophages
- (f) antigen-dependent MIF

II. Mediators Affecting Neutrophil Leukocytes
- (a) chemotactic factor
- (b) leukocyte inhibitory factor (LIF)

III. Mediators Affecting Lymphocytes
- (a) mitogenic factors (Interleukin-2)
- (b) antibody enhancing factors
- (c) antibody suppressing factors
- (d) chemotactic factor

IV. Mediators Affecting Eosinophils
- (a) chemotactic factor*
- (b) migration stimulation factor

V. Mediators Affecting Basophils (mast cells)
- (a) chemotactic augmentation factor
- (b) histamine releasing factor
- (c) interleukin-3

VI. Other Cells
- (a) cytotoxic factors—lymphotoxin
- (b) growth inhibitory factors
  - (1) clonal inhibitory factor
  - (2) proliferation inhibitory factor
- (c) osteoclast activating factor (OAF)

VII. Immunoglobulin Binding Factor

VIII. Procoagulant Activity

IX. Skin Reactive Factor

X. Interferon

XI. Immunoglobulin

*Requires antigen-antibody complexes.

Transfer Factor

Following the *in vitro* interaction of the sensitized lymphocyte with its specific antigen, a substance is released that has the capacity to transfer delayed hypersensitivity to another nonreactive individual. This substance is referred to as transfer factor and has been described in the human and in primates. Lysates containing transfer factor are produced by freezing and thawing blood leukocytes. Both a dialyzable and a nondialyzable transfer factor have been identified. The dialyzable transfer factor has a molecular weight of less than 10,000, is stable at 37°C, and is resistant to treatment with DNase, RNase, and trypsin. The nondialyzable factor has not been well characterized. Transfer factor is immunologically specific; i.e., it will confer reactivity only toward the antigen that caused the factor to be generated initially. For example, transfer factor produced from the interaction of tuberculin with tuberculin-positive cells will confer the ability to react only with tuberculin, not with any other antigen. Transfer factor also has been shown to be capable of mediating homograft (skin) immunity.

Migration Inhibitory Factor

Migration inhibitory factor (MIF) inhibits the migration of normal macrophages *in vitro*. When cells from a peritoneal exudate of animals are put into a capillary tube, the macrophages migrate peripherally from the end of the tube. If one adds to the medium small quantities of antigen to which the animal exhibits CMI, the macrophages fail to migrate from the tube. This phenomenon, referred to as migration inhibition, is the *in vitro* assay for the substance migration inhibitory factor. This phenomenon has also been observed in humans; it is not species-specific and can be produced by antigen or mitogen stimulation of lymphocytes. The MIF generated by human lymphocytes, for example, can inhibit the migration of guinea pig macrophages (Fig. 9–3). MIF has a molecular

Table 9–3. Physical and Biologic Properties of Effector Molecules of Cell-Mediated Immunity*

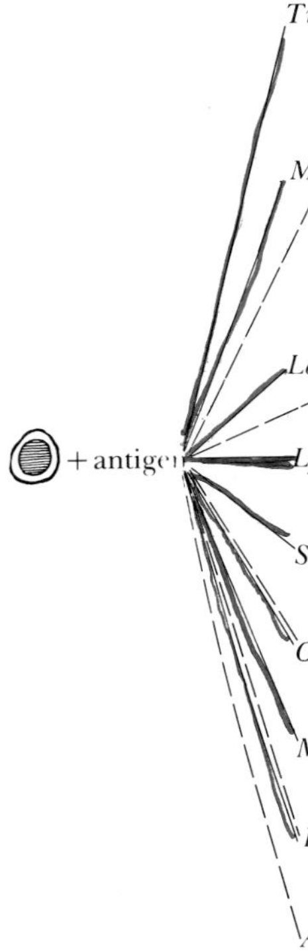

	Molecular Weight	Physical Properties	Activities: In vitro	Activities: In vivo
Transfer factor(s)	<10,000 ?	Heat labile; (a) dialyzable polypeptide (b) nondialyzable	Mediator production Lymphocyte transformation	Transfer of reactivity to uncommitted lymphocytes
MIF (macrophage activating factor)	25,000–55,000	Heat stable; nondialyzable protein	Prevents random migration of macrophages; may activate macrophages	May lead to accumulation of macrophages; may increase phagocytosis and killing
Leukocyte inhibitory factor	68,000	Protein	Prevents migration of PMN's	Untested
Lymphotoxin(s)	25,000–150,000	Heat labile; nondialyzable protein	Target cell injury	May destroy target cells
Skin-reactive factor(s)	70,000			Localized cutaneous reaction
Chemotactic factors	12,000–60,000	Heat stable; nondialyzable protein	Attracts macrophages; attracts PMN's	Untested
Mitogenic factors	25,000	Heat stable; nondialyzable protein	Nonspecific lymphocyte transformation	Untested
Interferons	25,000–100,000	Heat stable; nondialyzable	Inhibits viral replication	Inhibits viral replication
Antibody	160,000	Heat stable; nondialyzable	Reactive with antigen	Varied

——— Involving thymic-dependent (T) lymphocytes.
– – – Involving thymic-independent (B) lymphocytes.
*Additional factors with undefined physical-chemical properties are listed in Table 9–2.

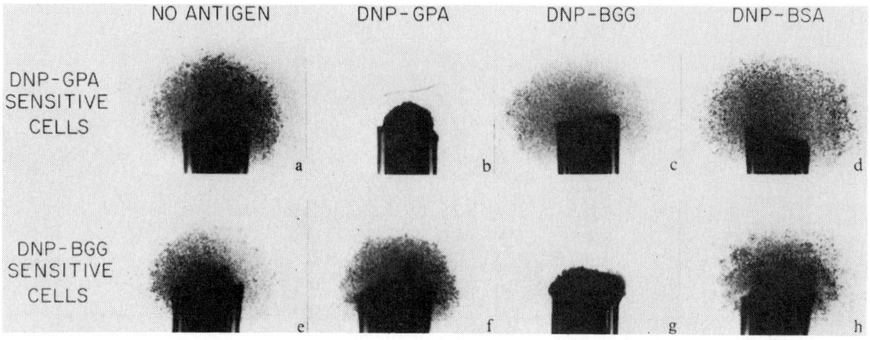

Figure 9–3. Inhibition of macrophage migration. *a–d,* Peritoneal exudate cells (macrophages and lymphocytes) from a guinea pig exhibiting delayed hypersensitivity to DNP coupled to guinea pig albumin (DNP-GPA). Migration of macrophages from the capillary tube has been inhibited (*b*) only by the immunizing antigen, not by DNP coupled to BSA (bovine serum albumin) or BGG (bovine gamma globulin). *e–h,* Cells from an animal exhibiting delayed hypersensitivity to DNP coupled to BGG. Again, this is the only antigen that inhibits migration. The experiment demonstrates the role of the carrier protein in determining the specificity of this *in vitro* correlate of delayed hypersensitivity. (From David, J. R., Lawrence, H. S., and Thomas, L.: J. Immunol., *93*:280, 1964.)

weight estimated to range from 25,000 to 55,000; is destroyed by trypsin and neuraminidase, but not by DNase or RNase; and is stable when heated to 56°C for 30 minutes. Guinea pig and human MIF have properties of an acidic glycoprotein.

MIF may be important *in vivo* as a substance that contains macrophages to the area of injury. It might also be involved in the formation of granulomatous lesions and those infectious diseases in which cell-mediated immunity and mononuclear infiltration are prominent features, e.g., the tuberculoma or tubercle granuloma. There is also evidence that MIF-rich fluids may alter morphology of macrophages, increase their ability to stick to glass surfaces, and augment their capacity to kill certain bacteria (Chapter 15). Therefore, MIF, or some similar factor, may profoundly alter the functional capacity of macrophages, the net outcome of which has been termed "macrophage activation."

Lymphotoxin

Lymphotoxin (LT) is the term for a series of molecules (alpha, beta, gamma) liberated from specifically sensitized lymphocytes or nonspecific stimulants such as phytohemagglutinin (PHA). Lymphotoxin seems to be associated with target-cell injury and inhibits the capacity of cells to divide (Fig. 9–4). They have a molecular weight range between 25,000 and 150,000; are heat stable; and resist RNase, DNase, and trypsin but are destroyed by chymotrypsin. The biologic role of this mediator is unknown, but the obvious possibility exists that it destroys cells directly.

Skin-Reactive Factor

This material is also produced by the interaction of specifically sensitized lymphocytes with antigen and mitogens. When introduced into the skin of normal guinea pigs, skin-reactive factor or factors produce an indurated and erythematous lesion within three hours. The lesion reaches its peak at 10 hours and disappears by 30 hours. The histologic picture of the lesion is similar to that produced in the delayed-type cutaneous lesion. Its biologic activity may well be the sum of the factors described above.

Chemotactic Factors

Several chemotactic factors have been described that are released from the reaction of specific antigen with sensitized lymphocytes and can also be generated by nonspecific mitogens. One factor induces chemotactic migration of macrophages or monocytes; other factors are selectively chemotactic for neutrophils, eosinophils, and basophils. These substances have molecular weights ranging from 12,000 to 60,000.

Mitogenic Factor (Blastogenic Factor)

When sensitized lymphocytes are stimulated with specific antigen, a substance is released with the capacity to cause non-specific blast cell transformation and increase tritiated thymidine uptake. This factor has a molecular weight of 25,000 and, together with transfer factor, may be important in

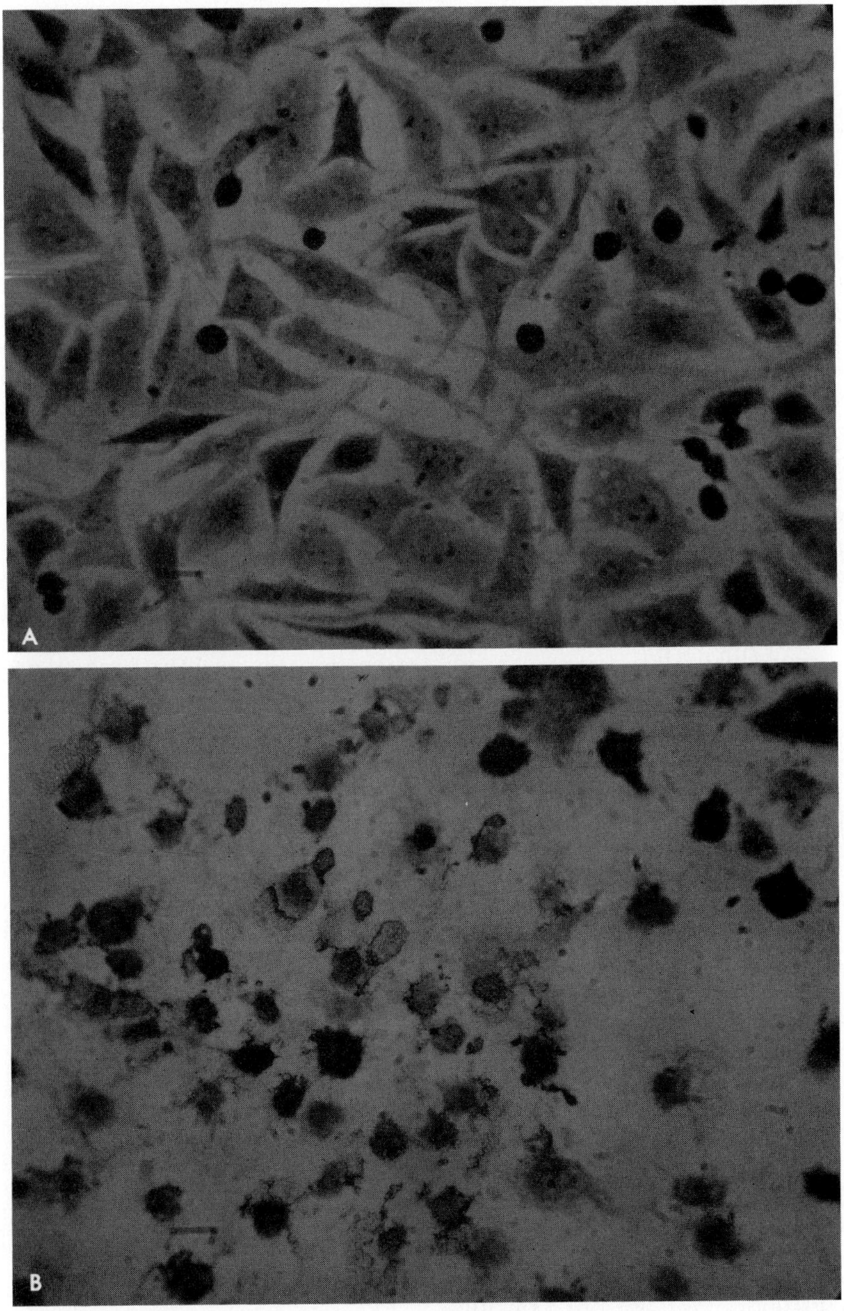

Figure 9–4. The effect of lymphotoxin on target cells. *A*, Control monolayer of L-strain fibroblasts. *B*, A similar monolayer after 24 hours of reaction with the supernatant from activated human lymphocytes that contained lymphotoxin. Extensive cell death is apparent. (Courtesy of Dr. G. A. Granger.)

augmenting or amplifying the cell-mediated response by recruiting uncommitted lymphocytes. This factor may be identical to the recently described interleukin-2, which causes proliferation of T-cells.

Interferons

The interferons are a group of substances whose approximate molecular weight ranges from 25,000 to 100,000. They are produced in cells following viral infection (nonimmune or α- and β-interferon) (Chapter 16). They are also released from sensitized lymphocytes (immune or γ-interferon) upon interaction with specific antigens and nonspecific stimulators such as PHA. These factors are known to be important effector molecules, significant not only in the recovery mechanisms of viral infections (Chapter 16) but also involved in immunoregulatory processes, including the activation of natural killer (NK) cells. The substances are particularly well suited to cell-mediated responses involving viral interactions *in vivo*.

Antibody

Antibody may also be released following interaction of antigen with specifically sensitized B-lymphocytes; however, it is not known whether antibody is produced by the same cells that elaborate MIF and other mediators. The role of antibody has been presented in previous chapters. Its function may be to augment the cell-mediated responses in a variety of ways, e.g., ADCC reactions.

Cell Types Elaborating Mediators

Studies in animals indicate that thymus-derived (T) lymphocytes are responsible for producing soluble mediators. The recent availability of methods to purify lymphocyte subpopulations with almost complete recovery of cells has permitted further investigation into the basis for antigen-induced lymphocyte activation. By use of purified populations, it has been shown that both T- and B-cells proliferate in response to mitogens such as PHA, Con-A, and pokeweed, but only T-cells proliferate directly in response to antigen. Both T- and B-cells produce MIF, chemotactic factor, and interferon in response to specific antigen or mitogens. However, only T-cells produce lymphocyte mitogenic factor or interleukin-2.

Although the production of lymphocyte mediators may correlate with the presence of cell-mediated immunity, it is clear that these factors are not solely products of activated T-cells.

Lymphocyte-Macrophage Interactions

A surprising number of lymphocyte functions appear to be based upon low molecular weight substances. A small number of sensitized lymphocytes (effector cells) could amplify the total response by the recruitment of larger numbers of uncommitted cells (transfer factor, mitogenic factor). The elaboration of lymphotoxin could destroy unwanted foreign cells; the attraction of macrophages and polymorphonuclear leukocytes could be accomplished through the action of chemotactic factors; and interferon could be of particular value in inhibiting the replication of viruses. Finally, the role of antibody could participate in several of the antigen-antibody reactions or in ADCC reactions.

SUMMARY

Cell-mediated immunity includes those manifestations of the specific immune response expressed by a variety of cells and cell products. The hallmarks of these reactions, which differentiate them from humoral antigen-antibody reactions, are their delayed onset, the requirement for living lymphocytes or their products to elicit the response, and the recently discovered effector molecules with relatively low molecular weights, which appear to be the *in vitro* correlates of the *in vivo* response. This type of immunologic mechanism appears to be particularly well suited to antigens that are cell-bound or in other ways inaccessible to the antibody mechanism.

IN VIVO EXPRESSIONS

The *in vivo* manifestations of the immune response are a continuum consisting of the interactions of the host with all foreign macromolecular substances (immunogens) and include all the possible expressions of the immune response appropriate for the type of stimulus. The separation of these responses into "harmful" and "helpful" expressions of the immune response is artificial, since the total spectrum of the immune response is available for the disposal of a foreign substance. The types of *in vivo* expressions that are available are shown in Figure 9–5. They consist of phagocytosis, the inflammatory response, and those responses mediated by products of the specific immune response, antibody and cell-mediated immunity. The host response depends on whether the encounter is *initial* or a *repeat.*

The Body's First Encounter with Antigen

If a material is a particulate substance, such as a bacterium or a virus, the body will attempt to eliminate it by phagocytosis. Since this is the first encounter, there is no preexisting antibody (opsonins) to facilitate engulfment. The fate of the disposal is decided by the efficiency of the unenhanced phagocytic process. If processing is successful, the material is eliminated and disease symptoms are not seen or are minimal. This is represented schematically in Figure 9–5. The specific immune response is induced to elaborate cells capable of antibody production or cell-mediated events (Fig. 9–5). Subsequent encounter with the same material will result in an enhanced efficiency of this process (see below). This is shown schematically in Figure 9–5 and represents the elimination of all exogenous antigens (bacterial organisms, viruses, and particulate matter) as well as altered or dead self components (effete red blood cells).

Phagocytosis may be unsuccessful because of the quantity or physical characteristics of the material or the general condition (health) of the host. For example, many encapsulated bacterial organisms (pneumococcus) escape engulfment because of the smoothness of the capsule. Other organisms may be engulfed but survive within the phagocyte (e.g., tubercle bacillus). In either event, active disease or death can occur (Fig. 9–5). The outcome of the disease is then determined by the effi-

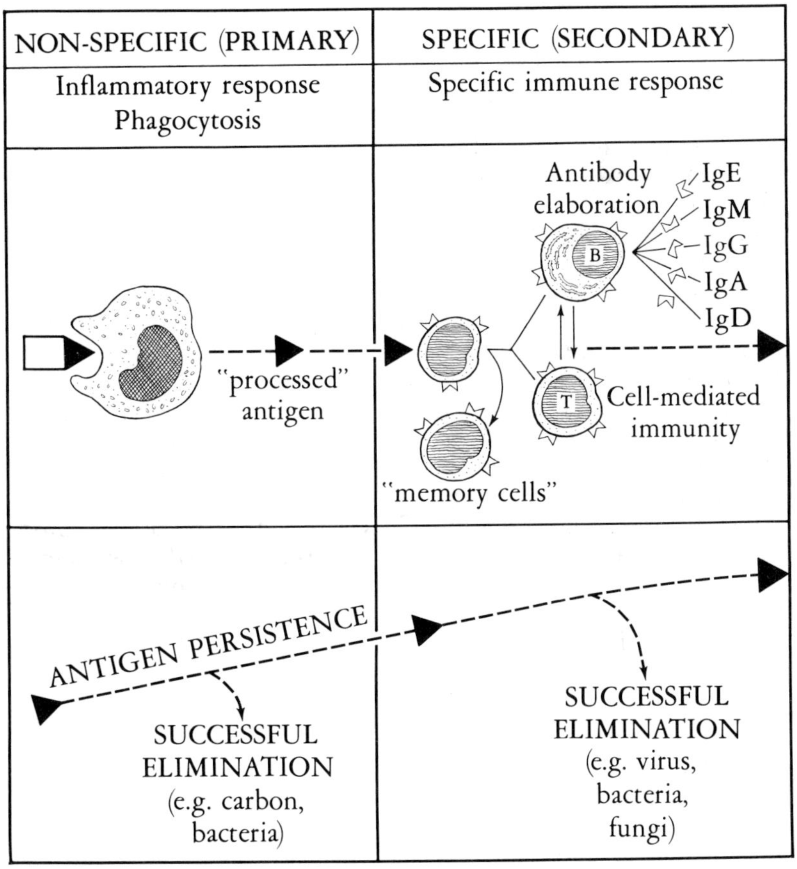

Figure 9–5. Schematic representation of the *in vivo* expressions of the immune responses.

ciency of the specific immune response, both antibody production and cell-mediated immunity. After the appearance of antibody, which with complement facilitates the uptake of an encapsulated organism, the phagocytes successfully destroy the disease-producing organism. Further, with the appearance of cell-mediated immunity and the elaboration of the effector molecules (MIF, mitogenic factor, and so on), phagocytosis by macrophages is enhanced, with elimination of organisms in this fashion. These events are described more fully in Chapter 15.

Subsequent Encounters

All subsequent encounters of the host with a foreign substance lead to the same events described previously, except that the responses are greatly enhanced. Because of rapid recall, there is an increased number of cells involved in antibody production or in cell-mediated events resulting in products of the specific immune response. These processes, either alone or in concert with phagocytosis, expedite the elimination of the unwanted material (Fig. 9–5). However, even a subsequent encounter may be unsuccessful because of the general condition of the host, e.g., underlying disease, immunosuppressive therapy, or an overwhelming dose of challenge inoculum. The efficiency with which the immune response can dispose of foreign antigens determines whether the outcome will be beneficial or harmful. If antigen is successfully removed or eliminated by the more primitive responses of phagocytosis and inflammatory response, with or without enhancement by the specific immune response, then the outcome will be beneficial. If antigen cannot be eliminated, the more deleterious, devastating effects of the immune response (tertiary immune response) occur, manifested as the immunologically mediated diseases of man (Chapter 20).

Summary

The *in vivo* manifestations of the immune response may be viewed as the total capacity of the host recognition system to dispose of foreign substances (antigens). These include the primitive responses of phagocytosis and inflammatory responses, which can dispose of most foreign substances. In the case of pathogens that have assumed virulent characteristics to evade these responses, a more sophisticated secondary system, the specific immune response, can lead to products that facilitate or enhance these primitive responses. The products include the elaboration of antibody or cell-mediated events that can effect disposal of the antigen, either alone or in concert with the more primitive responses. The outcome of this encounter of the host with a foreign configuration will be either beneficial or harmful, depending upon the efficiency with which the foreign substance can be eliminated.

Suggestions for Further Reading

Bloom, B. R., and Glade, P. R. (eds.): In Vitro Methods in Cell-Mediated Immunity. New York, Academic Press, 1971.

David, J. R., and David, R. R.: Cellular hypersensitivity and immunity: inhibition of macrophage migration and the lymphocyte mediators. Progr. Allergy, *16*:300, 1972.

Edelman, G. M. (ed.): Cellular Selection and Regulation in the Immune Response. New York, Raven Press, 1974.

Lawrence, H. S.: Transfer factor. Adv. Immunol., *11*:195, 1969.

Rocklin, R. E.: Clinical applications of in-vitro lymphocyte tests. Progr. Clin. Immunol., *2*:21, 1974.

Rose, N. R., and Friedman, H. (eds.): Manual of Clinical Immunology. Washington, D.C. American Society for Microbiology, 1980.

Williams, R. C., Jr., (ed.): Lymphocytes and Their Interactions. Kroc Foundation Series. Vol. 4. New York, Raven Press, 1975.

Chapter 10

Immunomodulation: Immunopotentiation, Tolerance, and Immunosuppression

Paul Katz, M.D.

The immune network in man involves a complex series of interrelated and mutually regulatory events. Under optimal conditions, that is, in the absence of certain diseases or pharmacologic agents, this scheme functions efficiently to rid the host of "foreign" configurations (e.g., microorganisms, tumors) while sparing native antigen-bearing tissues (i.e., "self"-antigens). In instances of disordered immunoregulation, the host may be unable to mount an immune response sufficient to eliminate detrimental antigens, resulting in widespread infection or malignancy, for example (Chapter 19). Conversely, host responses may become aberrant and tissues bearing "self"-antigens may be incorrectly perceived as being foreign. Such circumstances would favor the development of the so-called autoimmune diseases (Chapter 20C).

Either intentionally or unintentionally, normal homeostatic responses may be modified by intrinsic alterations in the immune network or by exogenous influences. As noted previously, potentiation or suppression of immune responses may be either detrimental or beneficial. In some cases, immunomodulation is a desirable and often obtainable goal, while in other situations it must be combated in order to prevent undesirable and potentially life-threatening effects.

For ease of discussion, immunomodulation may be broadly defined as the overall regulation of immune responsiveness, which includes both *immunopotentiation* ("up-regulation") and *immunosuppression* ("down-regulation"). Further, we will examine tolerance, that is, the state of immunologic unresponsiveness. The principles to be discussed will find application in those chapters devoted to the host response to infectious agents (Chapters 14 to 18), tumors (Chapters 19 and 21), immunologically mediated diseases (Chapters 20 and 22), and immunoregulatory agents (Chapter 25).

IMMUNOPOTENTIATION

Immunopotentiation refers to the specific or nonspecific enhancement of immune responsiveness. This augmentation can be intrinsic, that is, arising from within the host, or extrinsic and secondary to exogenous influences. The overall potentiation of the immune response may occur by an alteration in any one of the many steps involved in the host's immunologic reactions. Thus, a given potentiator may increase an immunologic event by (1) shortening the "latent" time for the response to become manifest; (2) augmenting the overall "level" or "height" of a given response; (3) lengthening the duration of the response; (4) delaying the cessation of the response; or (5) developing a new response to a previously nonstimulatory antigen.

Immunopotentiation can occur in both the classic humoral and the cell-mediated immune systems. It is noteworthy, however, that a substance capable of enhancing a response in one system may be suppressive in the other system. Therefore, the overall biologic effects of a given response-modifying factor must be

Table 10–1. Nonspecific Immune Potentiators

Water and oil emulsions (e.g., Freund's adjuvant)
Microorganisms (e.g., BCG)
Microorganism components (e.g., lipopolysaccharides, endotoxin)
Synthetic polynucleotides (e.g., polyinosinic-polycytidylic acid)
Lymphokines (e.g., migration inhibitory factor, interferon)
Pharmacologic agent (e.g., levamisole)

viewed as the sum total of potentially divergent reactions.

The concept of immunopotentiation has become increasingly important in recent years, particularly in regard to enhancing responses against tumors and infectious agents above that which could be expected by exposure to the tumor or the infectious agent alone.

Compounds capable of augmenting immunologic reactivity may be divided into two classes: (1) *nonspecific* or *general* immune enhancers, which increase humoral and cell-mediated responses to a multitude of widely differing antigens; and (2) *specific* potentiators, which increase a restricted group of immune responses to an equally restricted group of antigens. Both of these classes will be examined.

Table 10–1 lists some of the nonspecific immune potentiators. These substances, often referred to as adjuvants, probably differ in their modes of action, yet their net responses are often comparable. Although the means by which these nonspecific stimulators exert their biologic effects remain elusive, one can postulate several potential mechanisms. The biologic half-life of a given antigen could be prolonged. Such is the case with the classic adjuvant, Freund's adjuvant, a mixture of oil and killed mycobacteria. Although prohibited for human use owing to the induction of granulomas, complete Freund's adjuvant, when administered with antigen, can markedly enhance the immune responses of animals to that antigen, in part secondary to a prolonged release of the antigen. Substances such as aluminum hydroxide and alum have shown comparable results, presumably related to the increased antigenic half-life.

These agents could also induce their biologic effects by attracting or activating immunocompetent cells at the site of the antigen. Such is probably the case for the lymphokines, the collective term applied to that group of antigen-induced, soluble, mononuclear cell–derived substances reviewed in Chapter 9. Likewise, complete Freund's adjuvant, as evidenced by its propensity to induce granulomas, can recruit immunoreactive cells.

Immune potentiators could induce the proliferation, differentiation, and activation of immunoregulatory cells. Such is clearly the case with nonspecific mitogenic substances such as lipopolysaccharide, endotoxin, and many of the lymphokines.

These substances could also exert a variety of effects on the metabolic pathways of cells involved in the immune response. Many of these agents, for example, are known to alter the intracellular concentrations of the cyclic nucleotides, cyclic adenosine monophosphate (cAMP) and cyclic guanosine monophosphate (cGMP). Considerable data have accrued indicating that cAMP or its intracellular inducers are capable of inactivating suppressor T-lymphocytes, with a resultant boost in antibody formation. Additionally, the increased intracellular cGMP:cAMP ratio noted after *in vitro* interferon treatment may account for the enhanced natural killer (NK) cell activity (Chapter 19) induced by this agent by increasing the release of lysosomal enzymes. These potential mechanisms of nonspecific induction and augmentation of immune responses are listed in Table 10–2.

Of the nonspecific immune potentiators, perhaps the best studied has been the attenuated strain of *Mycobacterium bovis*, bacille Calmette-Guérin (BCG). After the observation that tuberculous patients appeared to be relatively resistant to the development of certain other types of infections, a possible role as adjuvant was ascribed to the mycobacteria. Early animal studies suggested that BCG administration could induce the regression of transplanted tumors if the host were immunocompetent. Subsequent studies in man and continued studies in animal models have suggested numerous possible mechanisms by which immunopotentiation could occur. Included among these are: (1) activation of the reticuloendothelial system; (2) induction of

Table 10–2. Potential Mechanisms of Action of Nonspecific Immunopotentiators

Prolongation of antigenic half-life
Attraction and/or activation of immunocompetent cells
Proliferation and/or differentiation of immunocompetent cells
Modulation of intrinsic metabolic pathways of immunocompetent cells

lymphokine production by mononuclear cells, resulting in the attraction and activation of immunocompetent lymphoid cells; (3) stimulation of NK-cells; (4) cross-reactivity between tumor antigens and BCG, inducing an immune response against common antigenic determinants; and (5) increased susceptibility of tumor cells to destruction.

BCG has found some usefulness in the treatment of human malignancies, most notably malignant melanoma (Chapter 19). Although not without risk, BCG therapy may be valuable in certain clinical situations, particularly those in which other forms of therapy are also utilized.

Corynebacterium parvum is an anaerobic gram-positive bacillary organism that also has immunopotentiating capabilities. Used as a heat-killed suspension, *C. parvum* increases tumor resistance in animals, prevents the growth of established tumors, and diminishes the frequency of metastatic disease. As with BCG, the precise mechanism by which this organism augments immune responses is unclear; however, the ability of macrophages to phagocytose and kill is markedly enhanced. Paradoxically, some T-cell responses are depressed, including mitogen-induced proliferation and other blastogenesis-dependent processes, while B-cell activity is either normal or increased. Conceivably, *C. parvum* may act on various effector limbs of the immune response with an overall enhancement of immune reactivity favoring antitumor effects.

The synthetic polynucleotides, such as polyinosinic-polycytidylic acid (poly I:C) and polyadenylic-polyuridylic acid (poly A:U) have also demonstrated nonspecific immunoenhancing capabilities. Werner Braun very elegantly demonstrated that these agents could augment multiple aspects of the immune response. In particular, they increase antigen-specific antibody formation to a variety of antigens. Other effects have been demonstrated on helper T cell–mediated stimulation of B-cell responses and delayed-type hypersensitivity reactions. A direct B-cell effect has been reported, most likely mediated by changes in cyclic nucleotide concentrations. A considerable body of accumulated evidence has demonstrated that these agents can boost NK responses through their ability to induce interferon production by NK-cells.

As noted earlier, the lymphokines can potentiate immune reactivity. These compounds and their capabilities are reviewed in Chapters 9 and 19.

Of the pharmacologic agents with immunoenhancing capabilities, perhaps levamisole is the most exciting. This anthelmintic agent has been demonstrated to increase tumor resistance in certain animal models, perhaps through stimulatory action on macrophages and T-cells. Interestingly, this agent has shown promise in the treatment of diseases characterized by excessive immunologic activity, such as rheumatoid arthritis and systemic lupus erythematosus. It is quite possible that this agent eventually will be found to affect multiple limbs of the immune network.

Although agents that nonspecifically augment the immune response form the bulk of the immunopotentiators, there are some antigen-specific immunoenhancing compounds. Included in this group are the immunogenic RNAs and tranfer factor.

RNA obtained from murine or rabbit mononuclear cells has been shown to transfer specific antigenic responsiveness to an animal not exposed to that antigen. Subsequent studies have yielded considerable conflicting data, and it is not yet clear what the role of immune RNA is as an immune potentiator. RNA extracted from mononuclear cells of tumor-bearing animals reduced the tumor load in other tumor-bearing animals. Further work is clearly indicated in this area.

Transfer factor is a less than 10,000 molecular weight, dialyzable, cell-free extract of immune lymphocytes that can transfer cell-mediated immune responses from antigen-responsive to antigen-nonresponsive individuals. The activity transferred is antigen-specific, and a generalized immunoenhancement is usually reported. The original experiments using transfer factor demonstrated transfer of cutaneous reactivity to purified protein derivative (PPD) from a PPD-positive donor to a PPD-negative one.

Transfer factor is probably a heterogeneous group of compounds of T-cell origin that act on multiple different populations of T-cells. The factor is DNAase-resistant, dialyzable, and heat-sensitive. Although its mechanism(s) of action is unclear, transfer factor may induce lymphocyte proliferation, soluble mediator production and release, and the recruitment of immunocompetent cells. Conceivably, part of the effects of this agent could be secondary to adjuvant-like characteristics. Most clinical studies to date have employed transfer factor in the therapy of immunodeficient states, malignancies, and certain infectious diseases. These trials have met with varying degrees of success and failure, but, unfortunately, it is unlikely that transfer factor will be the hoped-for panacea to convey antigen-specific cell-mediated immunity.

SUPPRESSION OF IMMUNE RESPONSIVENESS

Just as it is necessary to potentiate the immune response in some instances, it becomes necessary at other times to benefit the host by manipulating the immunologic system in a negative way so that it cannot respond to the presence of a foreign configuration or, at best, will have a diminished response to it. As in the case of immunopotentiation, negative manipulation can affect both specific and nonspecific responses and collectively comes under the general heading of *unresponsiveness. Immunologic tolerance* is a form of specific unresponsiveness and may be defined as the inability to respond to a specific antigenic stimulation, based upon an immature or incompetent immunologic system, the genetic constitution of the host, or the properties of the antigen. *Immunosuppression* comes under the heading of nonspecific unresponsiveness, refers to the artificial prevention or diminution of expression of immune response, and involves a more generalized form of unresponsiveness (Chapter 25).

Immunologic Tolerance: Historical Aspects

Implicit in all previous discussions of immunity is the fundamental ability of the immunologic system to differentiate "self" from "nonself." The idea that the body should never react with its own tissues was clearly enunciated by Ehrlich in his dogma "horror autotoxicus." One of the first challenges to this dogma came from the brilliant observations of Owen, who in 1945 demonstrated that each of nonidentical twin calves derived from two separate ova frequently shared two sets of red cells in their circulation, one set of its own, the other from its twin. This state is referred to as *mosaicism* or *chimerism*. Owen correctly assumed that this state of chimerism resulted from the well-known finding in such twin cattle of a common placental circulation that allowed the exchange of hematopoietic elements from one twin to the other early in fetal life. Paradoxically, if these same cells were introduced into the calf at a later time, they would lead to an immunologic response and their prompt rejection and destruction.

The second set of observations that challenged the classic dogmas of immunology were made in the late 1940s by Medawar, who used specifically inbred strains of mice. If, for example, one obtains two strains of mice, A and B (A with white skin, B with black), A will accept skin grafts from another A mouse but not from a mouse of the B strain; similarly, a B mouse will accept a graft from another B mouse but not from a mouse of the A strain (Fig. 10–1). However, when lymphoreticular cells of strain B were introduced into mice of strain A, the recipients treated were capable of accepting skin grafts from mice of strain B (Fig. 10–1). Medawar termed this effect "specific immune tolerance."

Once these observations were connected, further studies showed other ways to induce tolerance. The inoculation of embryos or young animals with antigens, for example, failed to elicit an immune response. Additional experiments showed that these animals actually became tolerant to the antigen with which the immature immune system had come in contact. In older animals, moreover, repeated high doses of certain antigens appeared to have a similar effect.

IMMUNOLOGIC TOLERANCE

Immunologic tolerance, a state of immunologic unresponsiveness, may, in many respects, be viewed as a form of immunosuppression. Strictly speaking, tolerance has been the term applied to that state in which exposure to an *immunogen* (an antigen capable of normally inducing immune reactivity) does not result in an immune response and appears to be secondary to a loss of immunoresponsive cell clones prior to their interaction with antigen. Under these circumstances, a "foreign" antigen is perceived in the same manner as a "self"-antigen and no response against that *specific* antigen is mounted. Tolerance should be viewed as antigen-specific, that is, tolerance to one antigen does not imply tolerance to all others.

Pseudotolerance or *immunologic paralysis* refers to that state in which antigen-responsive cells are present, but antigenic concentration is high enough that the binding to and neutralization of the antibodies formed occur. In this state, it seems reasonable to assume that persistent synthesis and elimination of antibody would also result in dissipation of the inciting antigen and a reduction in the pseudotolerant state. This situation is obviously quite distinct from true tolerance, in which the cells and their products needed to participate in the immunologic reaction are not available.

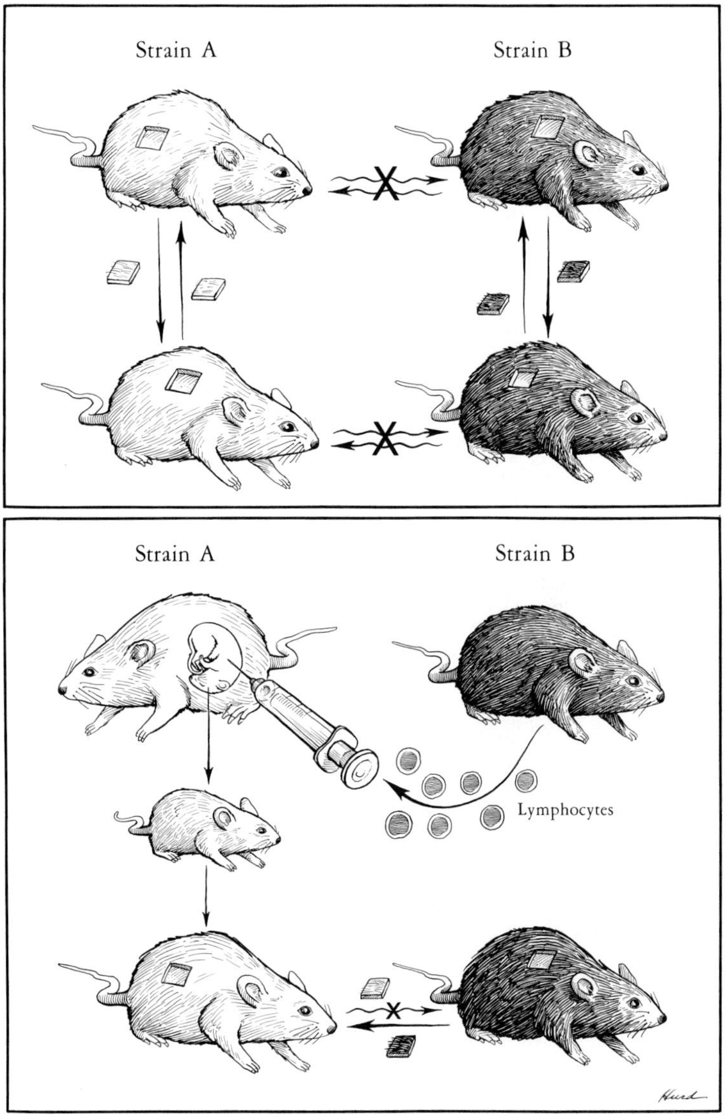

Figure 10–1. Representation of Medawar's experiment illustrating the fetal induction of tolerance in the mouse.

The induction of immunologic tolerance is dependent upon a variety of host and antigenic factors (Table 10–3). Immunologic immaturity greatly favors the development of tolerance, particularly in animal models, as described previously. Once an antigen-specific response has started, tolerance induction becomes progressively more difficult. In these circumstances, tolerance can be achieved by depleting the animal of antigen-reactive cells (e.g., with irradiation or antilymphocyte serum) and then reintroducing the antigen. Following the depletion of immunoreactive cells, the animal once again becomes immunologically naive and tolerance can be established. The ease of tolerance induction in the immature host may be, in fact, beneficial, as it enables the host to gradually accumulate self-antigens; the development of the tolerant state toward these antigens might then preclude autoimmune disease later in life.

Certain antigenic characteristics influence tolerance. For example, the physical state of gamma globulins in part determines their tolerogenicity. Aggregation of molecules favors immunogenicity, whereas monomers

Table 10–3. Factors Affecting the Development of Tolerance

Immunologic immaturity
Characteristics of antigen—physical state, complexity, persistence, distribution, etc.
Dose of antigen
Route of antigen administration
Genetic factors

more frequently evoke tolerance. Figure 10–2 shows how aggregated human gamma globulin (HGG) induces antibody formation by mouse spleen cells, whereas disaggregated HGG does not elicit an antibody response.

The complexity of antigenic structure also affects tolerogenicity. Substances of simple configuration equilibrate well between intra- and extravascular spaces and persist for some time. This is particularly true for simple antigens borne on replicating cells, where antigen persistence is readily achieved.

The dose of the antigen can likewise alter immunogenicity. As depicted in Figure 10–3, there is a certain dose of an antigen that will elicit a maximal antibody response. *Low-dose tolerance* is induced by antigens below the concentration for optimal responses. These low antigen concentrations may induce tolerance by an effect primarily on T-cells. Few antigens appear to be capable of producing low-zone tolerance. *High-dose tolerance* occurs when the dose of antigen is greater than optimal. This may be mediated by both a T- and a B-cell effect.

The route of administration also appears to be critical in determining immunogenicity and tolerogenicity. Soluble antigens administered intradermally with adjuvants induce antibody formation and cell-mediated immune responses. Conversely, intravenous inoculation favors tolerance, perhaps because of the high concentration of antigen achieved by this route.

Genetic factors may impair or enhance immune responsiveness. Studies in animal models have demonstrated that certain strains can be more easily tolerized than other strains.

It is apparent that T- and B-cell tolerance are separate and distinct. Induction of tolerance occurs more rapidly, persists longer, and requires less antigen in T-cells than in B-cells. It should be noted that apparent B-cell tolerance can be elicited by T-dependent antigens. Such antigens require T-cell help to provide the appropriate "signal" to B-cells to induce antibody formation. Tolerance to such antigens, then, may really be T-cell tolerance rather than B-cell tolerance, with a resultant net failure of antibody production. It is probably such T-cell tolerance that protects us from most self-antigens.

Tolerance does not necessarily imply an indefinite state of immunologic unresponsiveness. Elimination of the antigen by normal catabolism will reduce the concentration to a level at which the tolerant state can no longer be perpetuated. Tolerance can likewise end by the introduction of the inciting antigen in an altered form or by the use of a cross-reactive antigen. The precise mechanism by which tolerance is halted in these cases is not entirely clear.

IMMUNOSUPPRESSION

Suppression of naturally occurring immunologic responses can be either beneficial or detrimental to the host. Immunosuppression can occur in one of several ways: (1) secondary to normal immunoregulatory mechanisms; (2) secondary to an underlying disease or as a result of disordered immunoregulation; and/or (3) secondary to exogenous factors such as pharmacologic agents.

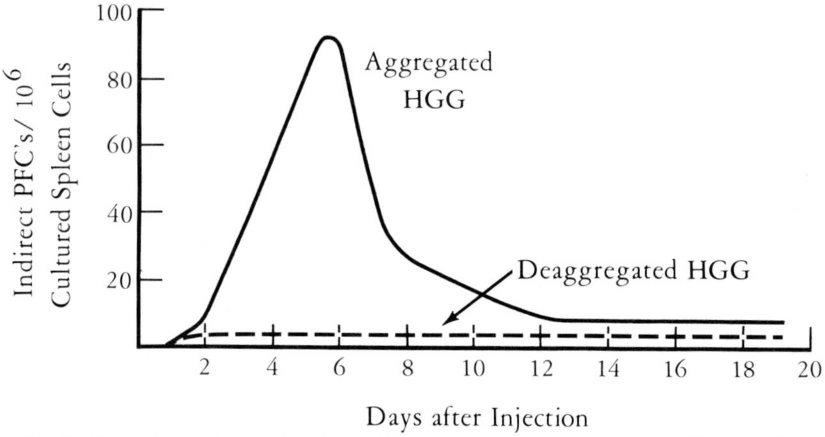

Figure 10–2. Antibody formation (plaque-forming cells, PFCs) by murine spleen cells after injection with either aggregated or deaggregated human gamma globulin (HGG). Aggregated HGG induces antibody formation, whereas deaggregated HGG is tolerogenic.

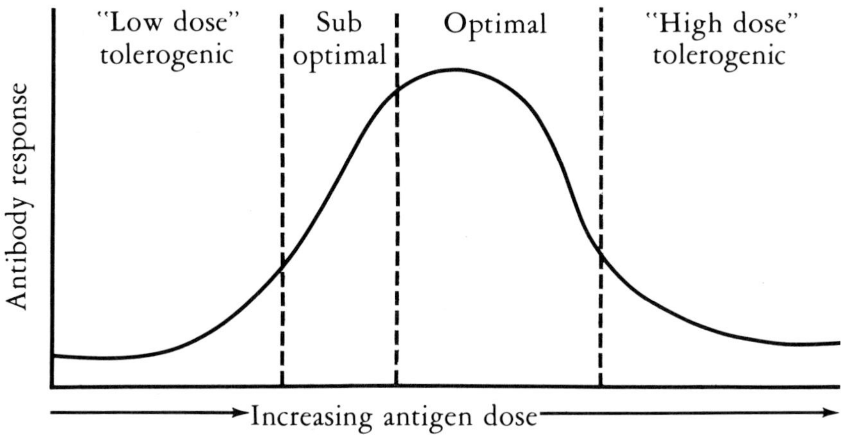

Figure 10–3. Relationship of antigen concentration to antibody formation. Low or high antigen concentrations prevent optimal antibody formation.

As discussed in the preceding sections, normal immunoregulatory mechanisms in combination with certain antigenic characteristics may induce specific immunologic unresponsiveness. This is quite obviously desirable in circumstances that prevent the immunogenicity of self-antigens. A breakdown in normal mechanisms of tolerogenicity could conceivably favor the development of autoimmune disease. It is also possible that immunosuppressive activities mediated by immunocompetent cells assist in the termination of a given immune reaction. This concept has been buoyed by the finding of naturally occurring suppressor cells in animals and man that may serve to down-regulate or modify ongoing immunologic activity. Such activities have been ascribed to various subpopulations of T-cells as well as cells of the monocyte-macrophage series, which are described more fully in Chapters 7 and 11.

It is not difficult to imagine how an overzealous suppressor network could result in or contribute to the pathogenesis of immunologic disease. In such circumstances, an overdampening of normal immune activities prevents the host from responding appropriately to specific or nonspecific signals. In 1974, Waldmann and coworkers reported a pioneering group of experiments involving the mitogen-induced B-cell responses of patients with common variable hypogammaglobulinemia (CVH). These investigators demonstrated that lymphocytes from these patients were unable to normally produce antibody *in vitro* in response to stimulation with the polyclonal B-cell activator pokeweed mitogen. Coculture of CVH lymphocytes with normal lymphocytes suppressed normal B-cell activity, indicative of excessive suppressor cell function. It was determined that excessive suppressor T-cell activity was responsible for these abnormalities and that removal or inactivation of CVH suppressor T-cells abrogated these responses. Subsequently, numerous cases of excessive suppressor cell activity have been reported in a variety of immunologically mediated immunodeficiency states, infectious diseases, autoimmune disorders, and malignant states. One must be wary of extrapolating too much from the situation *in vitro* to the situation *in vivo*. Furthermore, it is often unclear whether the *in vitro* phenomenon antedates the development of the disease or merely reflects subsequent nonspecific immunologic aberrancies.

Excessive suppressor cell activity can be mediated by a specific subpopulation of T-cells. These cells have been phenotypically characterized in a number of systems as bearing Fc receptors for IgG (T-gamma cells), or as bearing antigens recognized by the OKT8 monoclonal antibody, or both. An alteration in the frequency of these cells does not necessarily imply a relative or absolute alteration in suppressive capabilities, however. Cells of the monocyte-macrophage series have also shown excessive suppressor function in such diverse diseases as multiple myeloma, sarcoidosis, Hodgkin's disease, and tuberculosis. It is quite likely that the mechanisms of T-cell suppression and monocyte suppression are distinct. Studies to better characterize these activities are currently in progress in a number of laboratories. In some instances, it has been possible to abrogate excessive immunosuppressive activity by pharmacologic agents. Such abrogation has been demonstrated with corticosteroids in sarcoidosis and with indomethacin in Hodgkin's disease. Whether the elimination of excessive suppressor influences alters immune reactivity is not defined at present. The reader is referred to Chapters 14 to 22 for in-depth reviews of suppressor cell activities in clinical disease.

Perhaps the greatest degree of immunosuppression that is clinically observed is that which occurs as a direct result of the treatment of an underlying condition, usually a malignant or autoimmune disorder. It should be noted that in many cases it may be difficult to distinguish between immunosuppression secondary to drug treatment and immunosuppression resulting from the primary disease.

The agents most commonly reponsible for immunosuppression today are the corticosteroids and the cytotoxic drugs. These drugs, their mechanisms of actions, and their roles in immunosuppression are discussed in detail in Chapter 25.

Corticosteroids alter the immune response by their effects on leukocyte function or circulatory kinetics or both. A variety of *in vitro* studies have shown myriad effects on immunologic activity. Many of these studies, however, have employed drug concentrations that are unobtainable *in vivo*, and therefore these results are uninterpretable. Furthermore, corticosteroids can transiently induce changes in the composition of leukocytes in the intravascular space by redistributing certain cell types to extravascular compartments while limiting the egress of other cells. It should be noted that the degree of immunosuppression induced by these drugs will vary depending on the corticosteroid preparation, the dosage, and the dosage schedule.

Cytotoxic drugs have been increasingly utilized in the therapy not only of tumors but also of immunologically mediated diseases. Both by intent and by happenstance, these agents can powerfully dampen selected aspects of the immune response. In most cases, the suppression of aberrant immune responses cannot be separated from the suppression of desirable immune responses, rendering patients so treated susceptible to a variety of infectious complications.

The two agents most widely utilized to achieve immunosuppression are cyclophosphamide and azathioprine (Chapter 25).

Other immunosuppressive agents that have been used clinically include antilymphocyte serum (ALS) and antithymocyte globulin (ATG). These antisera have been employed primarily in transplantation in the hope of preventing allograft rejection. Radiation therapy has long been used in tumor therapy and has recently been used experimentally in rheumatoid arthritis. It is probable that ionizing radiation destroys replicating cells nonspecifically and prevents the further propagation of an abnormal immune response. Cyclosporin A is a fungal metabolite recently employed in bone marrow transplantation. This agent somewhat selectively permits engraftment while preventing graft-versus-host reactions.

SUMMARY

The complicated array of interconnecting immunologic networks is obviously susceptible to augmentation and suppression. A variety of seemingly diverse innate factors, exogenous agents, and diseases can induce relative and absolute immunopotentiation or immunosuppression. This alteration in immune reactivity either may be harmful to the host or may, in fact, be a sought-after goal.

Suggestions for Further Reading

Immunopotentiation. Ciba Foundation Symposium 18. Amesterdam, Associated Scientific Publishers, 1973.

Katz, D. H., and Benacerraf, B.: The regulatory influence of activated T cells on B cell responses to antigen. Adv. Immunol., *15*:1, 1972.

Steinberg, A. D.: Immunoregulatory agents. *In* Kelley, W. N., Harris, E. D., Jr., Ruddy, S., et al. (eds.): Textbook of Rheumatology. Philadelphia, W. B. Saunders Company, 1981.

Waldmann, T. A., and Broder, S.: Suppressor cells in the regulation of the immune responses. Progr. Clin. Immunol., *3*:155, 1977.

Chapter 11

A Unifying Model for Immunologic Processes

Joseph A. Bellanti, M.D.

It may now be possible to construct a unifying model for immunologic processes based upon the various principles of the immunologic system described in Section One. The model, which is an adaptation of one suggested by Talmage, will also serve as a framework for further descriptions of immunologic mechanisms (Section Two) and the clinical applications of immunology (Section Three). For ease of discussion, we may speak of five components of the host's encounter with foreignness: (1) *the environment,* (2) *the target cell,* (3) *the phagocytic cells,* (4) *the mediator cells* and mediator products, and (5) *the specific antigen-recognition cells* (B-lymphocytes and T-lymphocytes) and their products.

THE ENVIRONMENT

Since most substances that confront, and ultimately activate, the host's immunologic system arise from the exterior world, the place to begin in any discussion of the immunologic system is with the external environment (Fig. 11–1). Included within the external environment are the myriad foreign substances that range from the simplest of low molecular weight chemicals to the most complex microbial agents. It should also be emphasized that the immunologic system may be activated not only by foreign substances that arise from the external environment, but also by those that present from the internal environment, e.g., transplanted cells or altered self-components (virally or chemically altered or malignant cells). Those substances that have the capacity to evoke immunologic responses are referred to as *immunogens* or *antigens,* and all share the common characteristic of being recognized as *foreign* by the host (Chapter 4). Occasionally, the encounter with a foreign configuration may lead to an inability to respond, a state that is referred to as *immunologic tolerance;* such configurations are referred to as *tolerogens* (Chapter 10). Allergens are a specialized class of immunogen and take part in hypersensitivity (allergic) reactions (Chapter 20A). Antigens may be complete and lead to an immune response *per se* (immunogens), or they may be incomplete (haptens) and require prior attachment to a carrier protein to become fully immunogenic (e.g., penicillin). As our environment becomes more complex, not only does the number of antigens increase but also the potential number of allergens to which we are exposed (Fig. 11–1). In addition to those diseases that are triggered by the effects of the immune response to an environmental agent, e.g., allergy, recent evidence suggests that a number of diseases may result from the direct toxic effects of environmental agents, e.g., heavy metals, on the immunologic system. Collectively, these adverse effects fall under the heading of *immunotoxicology* and are becoming increasingly important as our environment becomes more polluted and complex. Thus, the physician must be constantly aware of the many types and varied routes of exposure to immunogens and allergens and toxins that compose our complex environment, not only to prevent and treat certain diseases (e.g., vaccines), but also to be able to recognize the possibility of immunologically mediated diseases that may take unexpected forms or masquerade as other entities.

TARGET CELLS

The introduction of an environmental agent into a host may have an adverse effect

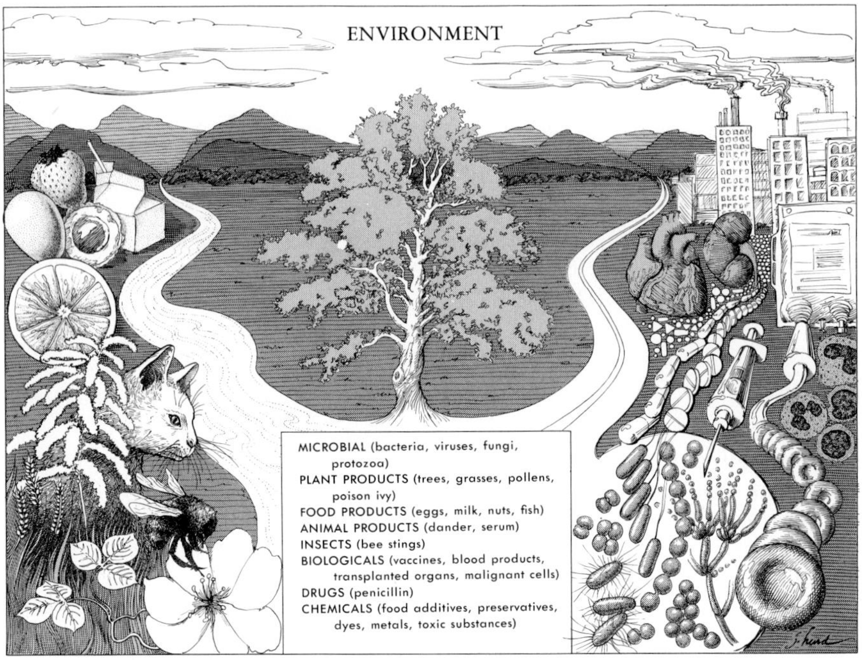

Figure 11–1. Examples of environmental agents.

on a target cell (Fig. 11–2, Table 11–1). There are a variety of target cells upon which an environmental agent may impact. They vary according to their type and location as well as the portal of entry of the foreign substance. It is important to emphasize that the target cells may be normal host cells that become the adventitious targets of injury by the environmental agents or immunologic processes, or they may represent altered host cells that have become modified through the interaction with the environmental substance (e.g., chemical), by infection (e.g., virus), or by malignant transformation (e.g., tumor cells); alternatively, the target cell may be a foreign cell introduced by transplantation (Chapter 20). The target cell may thus sustain direct injury from the environmental agent or indirect injury through immunologic processes (Chapter 20). The net effect leads to disruption of cell function or cell death. Some of the more common target cells are shown in Table 11–1. Included are cells of the skin, gastrointestinal tract, respiratory tract, and circulatory system. For example, disruption of epidermal cells following contact with an environmental agent, e.g., poison ivy, could lead to dermatitis; destruction of mucosal cells of the gastrointestinal tract secondary to ingestion of an environmental agent, e.g., an offending food substance, may result in gastrointestinal bleeding. If the target cells are smooth muscle and glandular cells of the respiratory tract, the impact of the environmental agent may lead to increased contractility with bronchospasm and increased secretion of mucus characteristic of bronchial asthma. Alternatively, endothelial target cells

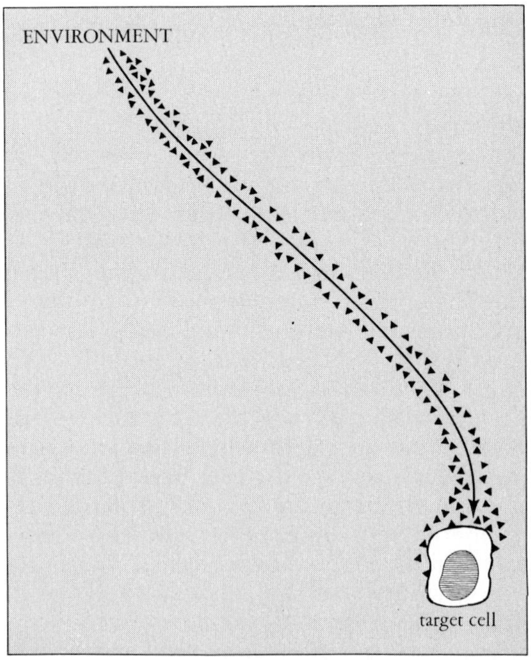

Figure 11–2. Effects of environmental agents on target cells.

Table 11–1. **Effects of the Environment on Target Cells**

Location of Target Cell	Example of Effect	Result
Skin	Disruption of epidermal cells	Dermatitis
Gastrointestinal tract		
Mucosal cell	Destruction	Gastrointestinal bleeding
Smooth muscle	Increased contractility	Diarrhea, vomiting
Glandular cell	Increased secretion	Increased mucus production
Respiratory tract		
Smooth muscle	Increased contraction	Bronchospasm
Glandular cell	Increased secretion	Increased mucus production
Circulatory system		
Endothelial cell	Increased intercellular pore size	Edema
Formed elements	Destruction of erythrocytes	Anemia

of blood vessels might respond by showing an increase in intercellular pore size with resultant loss of fluids and the production of edema. The impact of the foreign substance on the formed elements of the blood, such as red cells, might lead to their destruction and the development of anemia.

During the course of evolution, a number of *nonspecific* and *specific* immunologic mechanisms have appeared within the vertebrates (Chapters 1 and 2). This collection of cellular elements, referred to as the lymphoreticular system, is distributed strategically throughout the body and lines the lymphatic and vascular channels. Its function may be considered the protection of the target cell from injury. *Phagocytosis* and the *inflammatory response* are the body's first line of defense and represent the most primitive of the nonspecific immune responses (Chapters 2, 12, and 13).

THE PHAGOCYTIC CELLS

The phagocytic cells are those elements that are involved in the process of engulfment and uptake of particles from the external environment; subsequent digestion of these substances may lead to their elimination (Chapter 2). The phagocyte may be considered, then, as a barrier between the environment and the target cell, protecting the target cell from subsequent injury (Fig. 11–3, Table 11–2). In the human, phagocytosis is carried out primarily by mononuclear phagocytes (macrophages), neutrophils, and eosinophils (Chapter 2). These phagocytic cells, together with the effector mechanisms triggered by or involved in their mobilization, are shown in Table 11–2. There are a variety of chemotactic factors—generated from the complement system (Chapter 6) or derived from specific lymphocytes, e.g., the lymphokines (Chapter 9) or from the phagocytic cells themselves—that can lead to the accumulation of phagocytic cells in an area of inflammation. The net effect of these processes is the mobilization of phagocytic cells into areas in which their action is required for the protection of target cells from injury. However, on occasion the phagocytic cells themselves may contribute to tissue injury by the release of intracellular products, e.g., lysosomal enzymes, as seen in the autoimmune diseases (Chapter 20C).

MEDIATOR CELLS

Certain cells of the body contain macromolecular and low molecular weight sub-

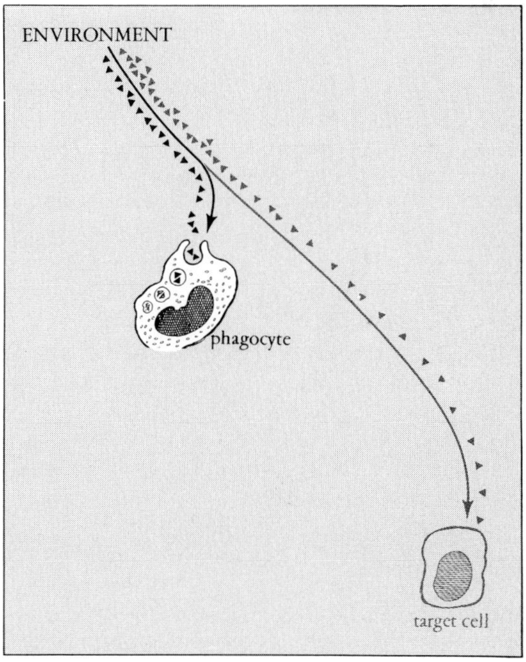

Figure 11–3. Phagocytic cells: mobilization factors and functions.

Table 11–2. Mobilization Factors and Functions of Phagocytic Cells

Phagocytic Cell	Agents Responsible for Mobilization of Cells	Cell Product or Function
Macrophages (monocytes)	Chemotactic factors, e.g., migration inhibitory factor (MIF), lymphokines	Processed immunogen, removal of environmental agent, prostaglandins
Neutrophils	Chemotactic factors (complement-associated and bacterial factors), lymphokines	Kallikreins (producing kinins), basic peptides, prostaglandins
Eosinophils	Identical with neutrophils, specific chemotactic factors, lymphokines	Ingestion of immune complexes, antagonize effects of mediators, e.g., leukotrienes (formerly SRS-A)

stances with biologic properties that can amplify the effects of the phagocytic cells or that may have a direct effect on the target cells. These cells are referred to as mediator cells. Following their interaction with the environmental agent, they perform their function by the release of chemical substances having a variety of biologic activities, e.g., the increase of vascular permeability or the enhancement of the inflammatory response (Fig. 11–4, Table 11–3). The mediator cells, like the target cells, represent a heterogeneous collection of morphologic types that includes mast cells, basophils, platelets, enterochromaffin cells, and neutrophils (Table 11–3). The best studied of these are the mast cells and basophils, which are important in certain immediate hypersensitivity diseases of man (Chapter 20A).

The term "mediators" encompasses a group of substances that are formed and released by mediator cells in response to an environmental agent (Fig. 11–5, Table 11–4). The best studied of these substances include histamine, serotonin, kinins, and, recently, the products of metabolism of arachidonic acid (eicosanoid system), including prostaglandins, thromboxanes, and leukotrienes, slow reactive substance of anaphylaxis (SRS-A) (which has now been identified as leukotrienes C_4, D_4, and E_4), eosinophilic chemotactic factors of anaphylaxis (ECF-A), and platelet-activating factor (PAF) (Chapter 13). Other macromolecular substances are derived from the phagocytic cells, e.g., lysosomal enzymes. Although most of these substances are synthesized in the mediator cells, some mediators, e.g., the complement and coagulation components, are synthesized in other cells and are found predominantly as serum components (Chapter 6).

Once they are released or generated, the

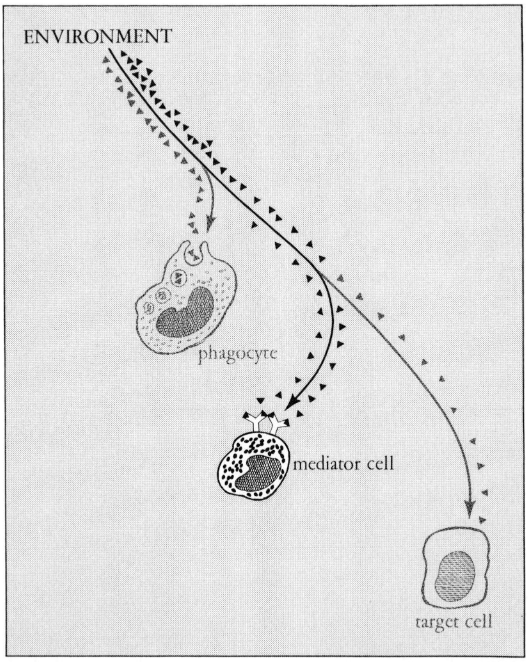

Figure 11–4. Mediator cells: products (mediators) and functions.

Table 11–3. **Products and Functions of Mediator Cells**

Mediator Cell	Product	Action
Mast cells	Histamine, leukotrienes C_4, D_4, E_4 (formerly SRS-A), prostaglandins, ECF-A	Increased vascular permeability, bronchoconstriction, eosinophilotaxis
Basophils, platelets	Vasoactive amines (histamine, serotonin)	Increased vascular permeability, smooth muscle constriction
Enterochromaffin cells	Serotonin	Vasodilation
Neutrophils	SRS, ECF	Contractility of smooth muscle, eosinophilotaxis

mediators have a twofold effect on the nonspecific immunologic responses and act with (1) the target cell, e.g., allergy, or (2) the phagocytic cells, e.g., promotion of chemotaxis (Fig. 11–5, Table 11–4).

CELLS OF THE SPECIFIC IMMUNOLOGIC SYSTEM: THE SPECIFIC ANTIGEN-RECOGNITION CELLS

These cells, in contrast to those of the nonspecific immunologic system, interact with the environmental agent in a highly specific way. The responses display *specificity, memory,* and *heterogeneity* and are basically carried out by two universes of lymphocytes: (1) the bone marrow or bursal-dependent B-lymphocytes, which provide humoral immunity; and (2) the thymus-dependent or T-lymphocytes, which participate in cell-mediated immunity (Chapter 2).

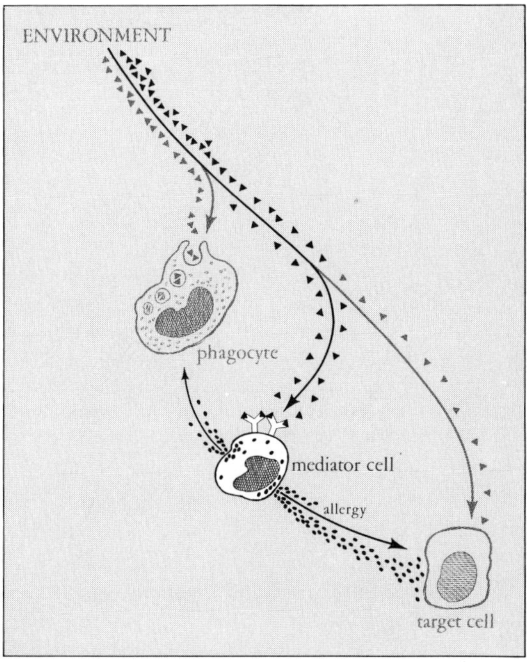

Figure 11–5. Mediator products and their effects on target cells (e.g., allergy) or phagocytic cells.

The B-lymphocytes are those cells that ultimately respond to the environmental agent, through either immunization or infection (Fig. 11–6). The exquisite specificity for the recognition of antigen by the B-cell is a function of immunoglobulin on the surface of these cells. As a consequence of the binding of antigen with the surface receptor, the cell differentiates into clones of antibody-secreting plasma cells, each of which secretes a single class of immunoglobulin that is specific for the antigen. There are five classes (isotypes) of immunoglobulins, IgG, IgM, IgA, IgD, and IgE, each differing in physical, chemical, and biologic properties (Chapter 5). The primary effect of antibody is its direct binding with the environmental agent (Fig. 11–6). In addition, antibody may interact with the phagocytic cells, the mediator cells, or the target cells. The effect of antibody on phagocytic cells is shown in Figure 11–7. Three types of interactions are seen: (1) the direct binding of antibody to the surface of the phagocytic cells (cytophilic antibody), (2) the uptake of antigen-antibody (Ag-Ab) complexes through the Fc receptor, and (3) the

Table 11–4. **Mediators Released in Response to Environmental Agents**

Low molecular weight mediators (< 1000)
Histamine
Serotonin
Kinins
Slow reactive substance of anaphylaxis (SRS-A) (now leukotrienes C_4, D_4, E_4)
Prostaglandins
Eosinophilic chemotactic factors of anaphylaxis (ECF-A)
Platelet-activating factor (PAF)
Macromolecular mediators (> 1000)
Lysosomal enzymes
Cationic proteins of polymorphonuclear leukocytes
Complement and coagulation components

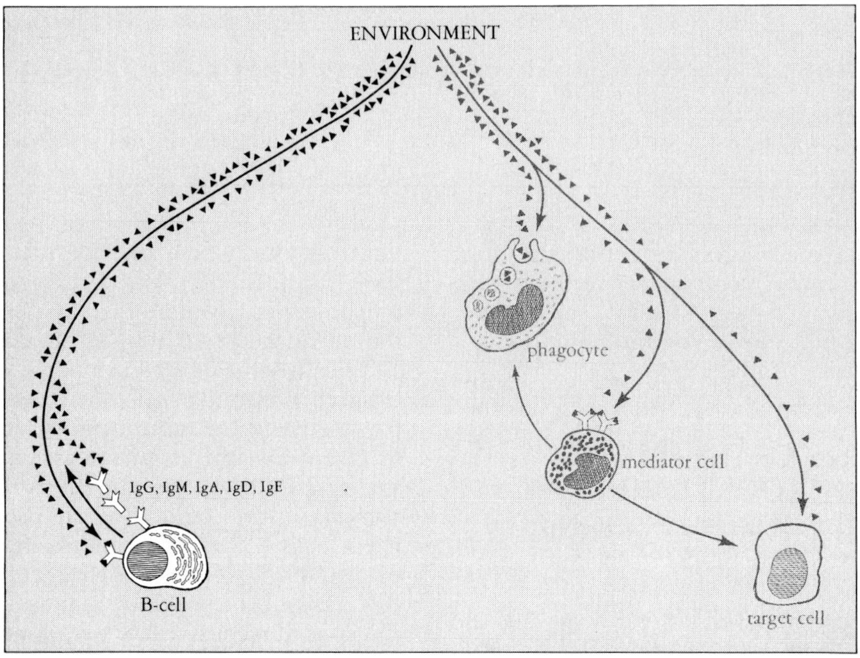

Figure 11–6. Reaction of B-lymphocyte to environmental agent through its surface receptor, with resultant antibody production.

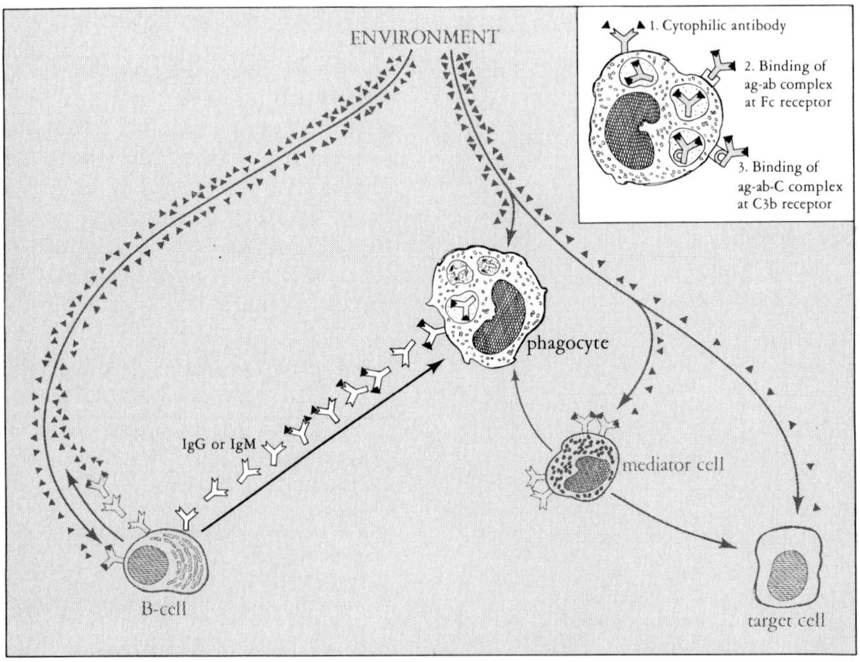

Figure 11–7. Responses of antibody with phagocytic cells.

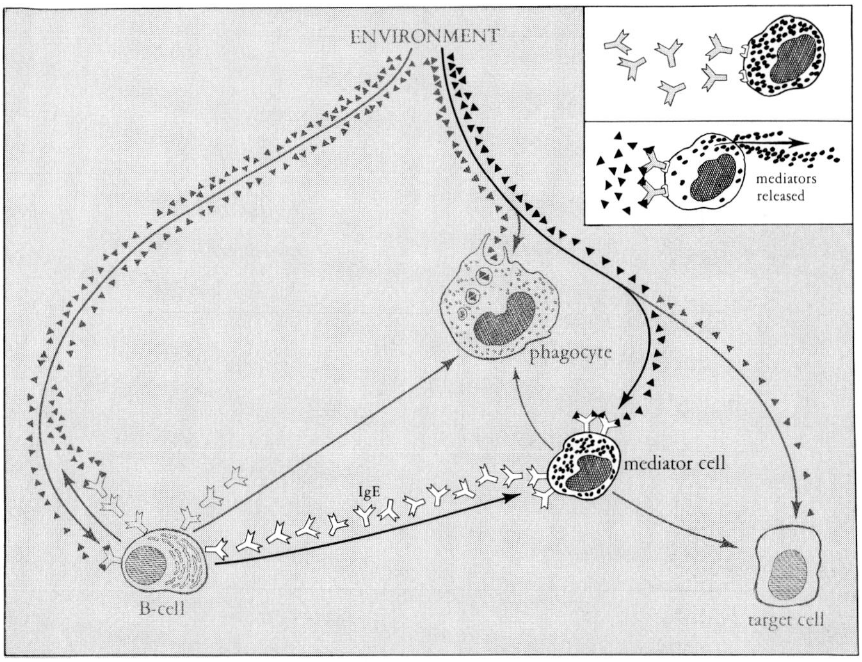

Figure 11–8. Responses of antibody with mediator cells with resultant release of mediators (insert).

uptake of antigen-antibody-complement (Ag-Ab-C) complexes through the C3b receptor (Fig. 11–7 inset). The coating of certain encapsulated bacterial organisms by immunoglobulins (IgG, IgM) or by certain complement components (e.g., C3b) facilitates their uptake by phaogcytic cells; collectively these substances are referred to as opsonins. The effect of antibody on mediator cells is shown in Figure 11–8. Certain classes of gamma globulin, e.g., IgE, can attach to the mediator cells by virtue of their Fc fragments. Following the interaction of at least two of these membrane-bound molecules with antigen, the release of mediators occurs (Fig. 11–8 inset). Occasionally, under abnormal circum-

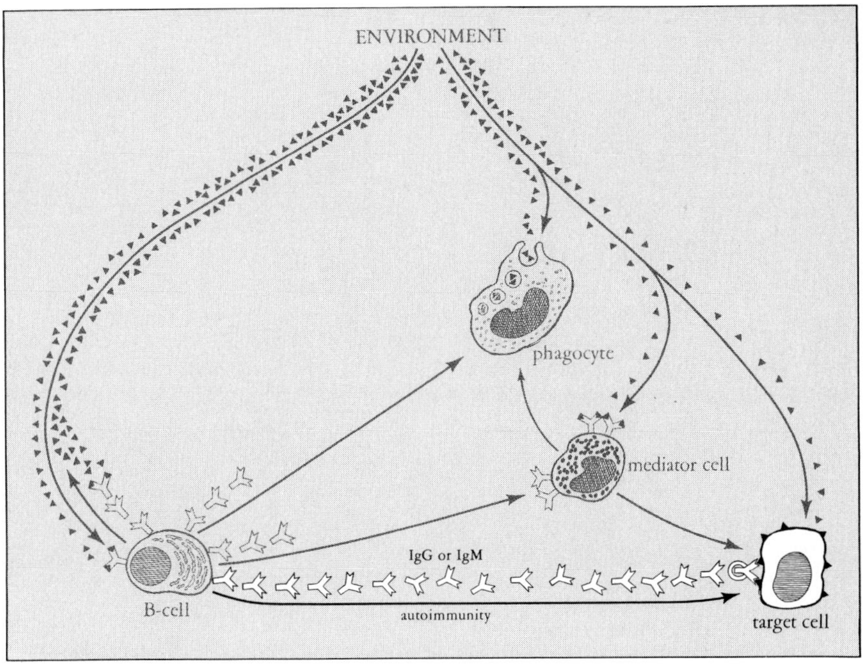

Figure 11–9. Effects of antibody on target cells with resultant autoimmunity.

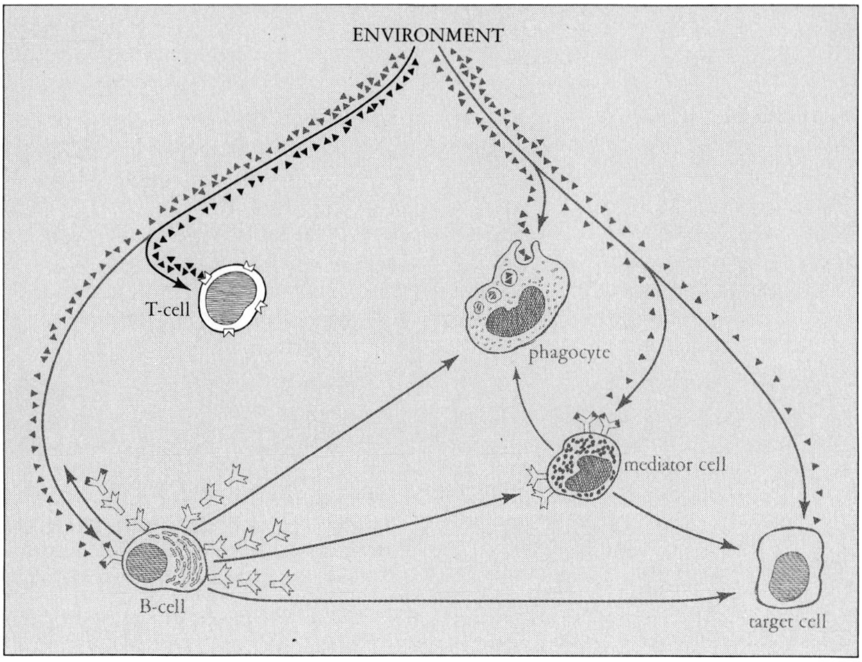

Figure 11–10. Reaction of T-lymphocyte to environmental agent through its surface receptor.

stances, antibody may be directed against the target cells (Fig. 11–9). This is a totally anomalous situation but is seen in some of the immunologically mediated diseases of man—the autoimmune diseases (Chapter 20C).

The T-lymphocytes are those cells responsible for cell-mediated immunity (Chapter 9). These cells respond to the environmental agent through surface receptors (Fig. 11–10). Although not intact immunoglobulin, these receptors are analogous to the antigen-binding receptors (the V-region determinants) on the B-cells (Chapters 5 and 7).

Following the interaction of the environ-

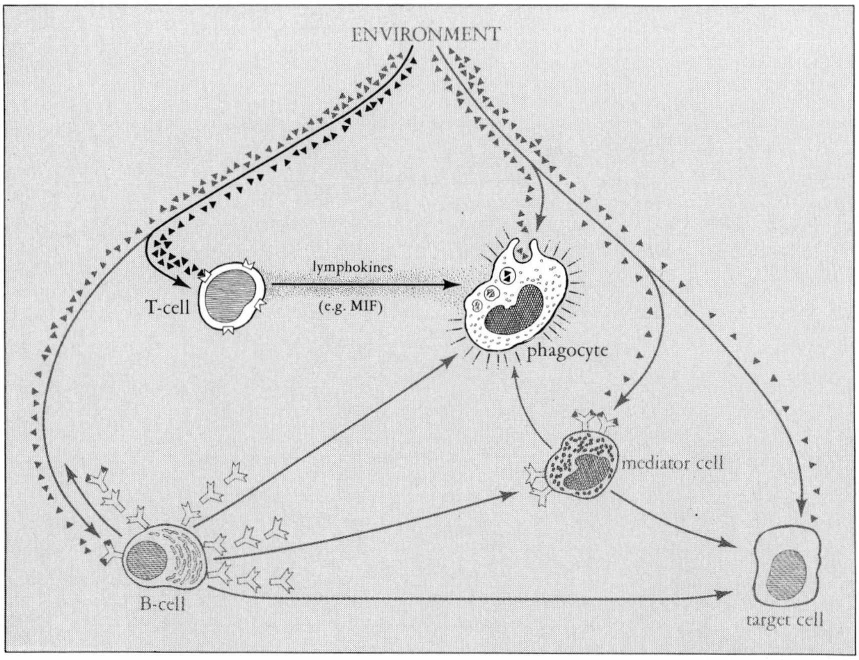

Figure 11–11. Responses of lymphokines (e.g., elaborated from T-lymphocytes) on phagocytic cells (e.g., macrophages).

mental agent with the T-cell, a series of morphologic, biologic, and biochemical events occur, in which the cell may function either directly or through the elaboration of certain products, the lymphokines (Chapter 9). The best studied of the lymphokines is migration inhibitory factor (MIF), which not only inhibits the migration of macrophages but also can activate the cell metabolically (Fig. 11–11). In addition, the T-lymphocyte can participate in the recognition of antigen on the surface of foreign target cells in any of three ways (Fig. 11–12). The cell may participate in direct lymphocyte-dependent cytotoxicity; or the elaboration of cytotoxin may lead to target-cell destruction; or certain subsets of lymphocytes, the killer or K cells, may lead to target-cell destruction through antibody-dependent cytotoxicity (ADCC) reactions (Fig. 11–12 inset).

An additional pathway of target cell destruction is mediated by a group of cells (natural killer or NK cells), which does not require prior sensitization by antigen, whose lineage is of uncertain origin (monocytic or T-cell), but which can directly destroy target cells. These cells appear to be enhanced by the action of interferon(s) and are importantly involved in transplant and tumor rejection (Chapters 19 and 20B).

The T-lymphocytes may also interact with the B-cells in two ways: (1) A subset of T-cells (the helper [T4] cells) can interact with B-cells to facilitate the production of antibody, and (2) another subset of T-cells (the suppressor/cytotoxic [T5/T8] cells) can inhibit the production of antibody by B-cells (Fig. 11–13).

The macrophage has been shown to be an essential cell that interacts with the T- and B-lymphocytes and is necessary for the induction of T-cell responses as well as T cell–dependent B-cell responses to antigen. Moreover, these cellular interactions of macrophages, T-cells, and B-cells appear to be genetically restricted by products (Class I and Class II molecules) of the major histocompatibility complex (MHC) locus, which are located on the surface of these cells (Figure 11–14) (Chapter 3). A number of cell prod-

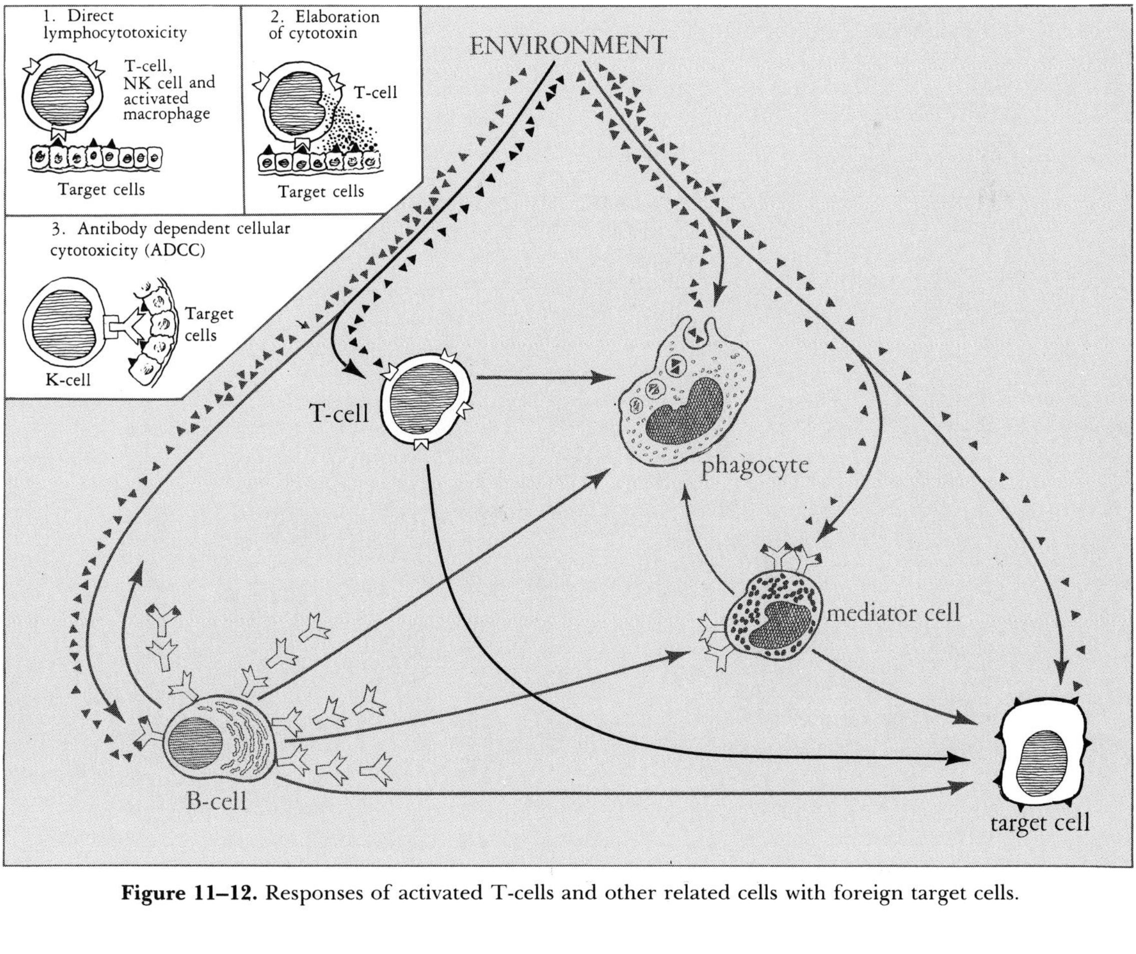

Figure 11–12. Responses of activated T-cells and other related cells with foreign target cells.

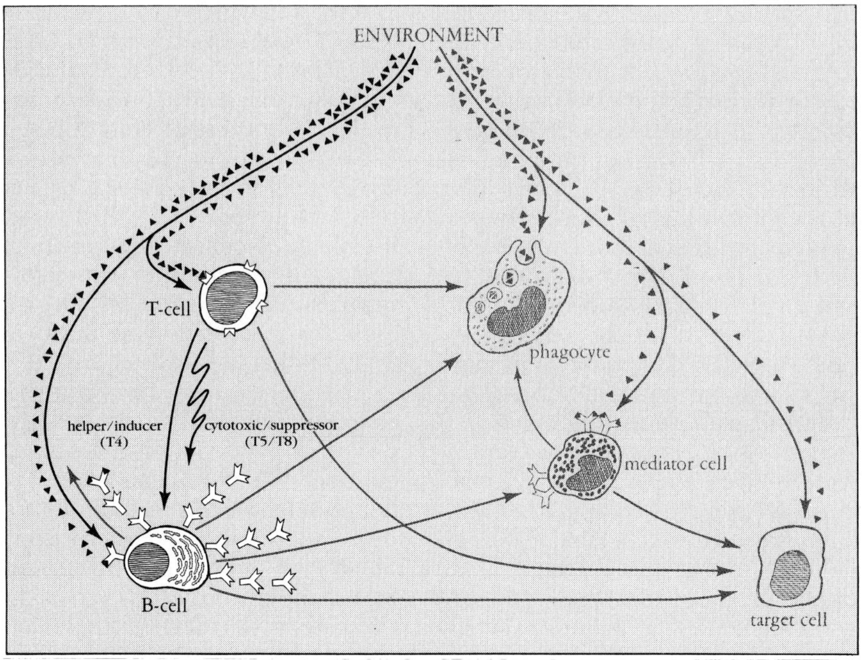

Figure 11–13. Helper and suppressor effects of T-lymphocytes on B-lymphocytes.

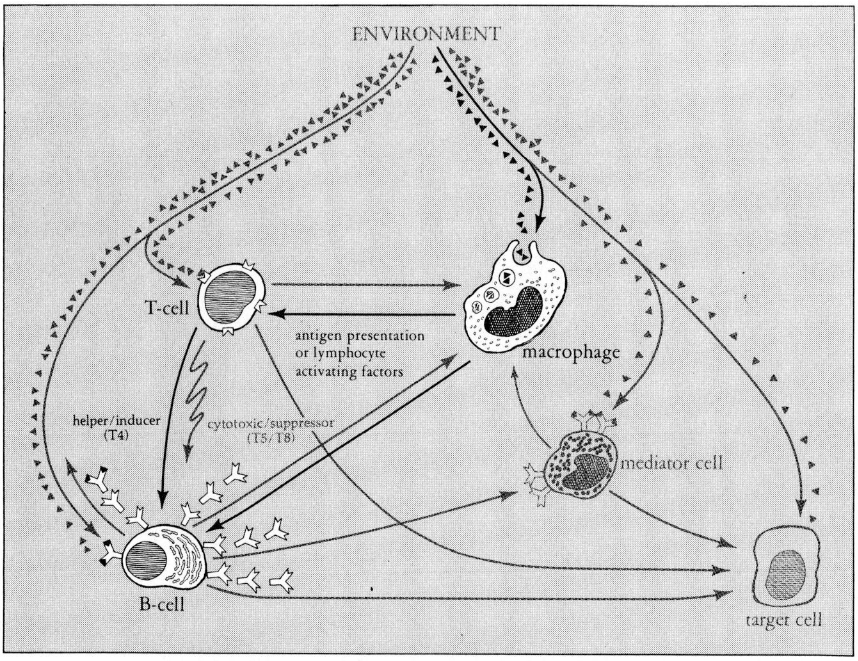

Figure 11–14. Responses of macrophages with T- and B-lymphocytes.

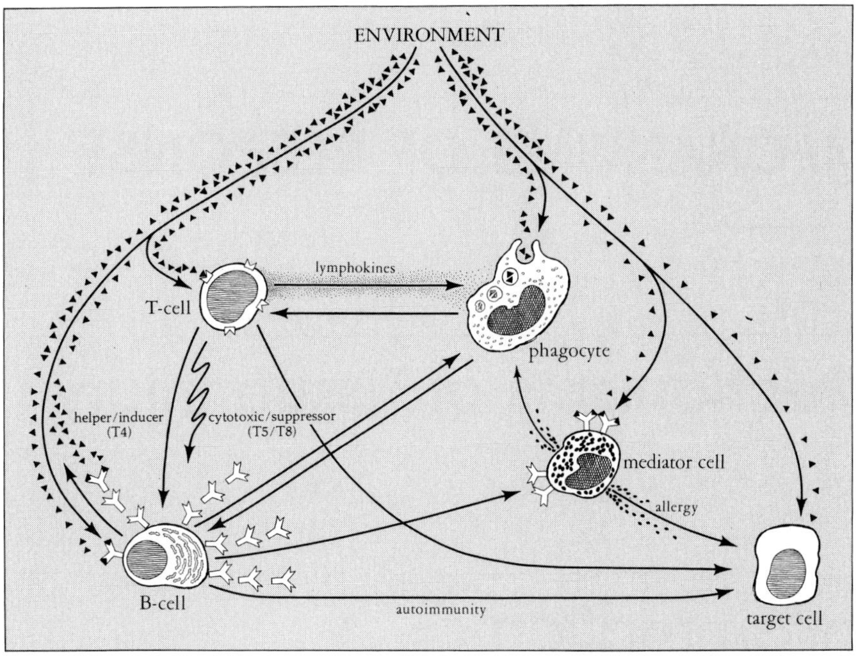

Figure 11–15. Total array of immunologic responses to the environment.

ucts (e.g., monokines and lymphokines), produced respectively by both macrophages (e.g., interleukin-1) and lymphocytes (e.g., interleukin-2), play an important role in the intercellular communication (Chapters 7 and 9).

Thus, the immunologic system may be viewed as a multicellular system involving the interaction of foreign substances with a wide variety of cell types (Fig. 11–15). The immunologic responses concerned with the recognition and disposal of foreignness are termed immunity when they lead to a beneficial response; when the interaction of the immunologic components and the environmental agent leads to injury of target cells, the responses are referred to as hypersensitivity or allergy; when the target cells of the host are injured directly by immunologic mechanisms, these responses are referred to as autoimmunity (Chapter 20). Occasionally, when the immunologic surveillance of a foreign target cell, e.g., tumor cell, is evaded, the manifestations of malignant disease may be manifested (Chapter 19). The total array of these responses is shown in Figure 11–15.

Suggestions for Further Reading

Bellanti, J. A., Balter, N. J., and Gray, I.: A unifying model for immunotoxicology: A summation presentation. *In* Dean, J. H., and Podarthsingh, M. (eds.): Biologic Relevance of Immune Suppression as Induced by Genetic, Therapeutic and Environmental Factors. New York, Van Nostrand Reinhold Company, 1981.

Fauci, A. S., et al.: Activation and regulation of human immune responses: implications in normal and disease states. Ann. Intern. Med., *99*:61, 1983.

Section Two

MECHANISMS OF RESPONSE

Part I

Mechanisms of Tissue Injury

Chapter 12

Inflammation

Peter A. Ward, M.D.

Inflammation can be considered as that complex series of events that develop when the body is injured either by mechanical or chemical agents or by self-destructive (autoimmune) processes. Although there is a tendency in clinical medicine to consider the inflammatory response in terms of reactions harmful to the body, a more balanced view is that inflammation is essentially a *protective* response in which the body attempts either to return to the preinjury condition or to repair itself after inflicted injury. The inflammatory response sets apart living bodies from machines, since, in the latter case, there is no intrinsic capacity for restoration of a damaged or broken part. Thus, the inflammatory response is an essentially protective and restorative reaction of the body since it attempts to maintain homeostasis under adverse environmental influences.

The classic signs of inflammation are well known. They include *swelling, redness, heat, pain,* and *altered function.* The inflammatory response is critically dependent upon both intact blood vessels and the circulating cells and fluids within these channels. Generally, three states of inflammation are recognized: *acute, subacute,* and *chronic,* each being defined by typical histologic criteria. The *acute inflammatory* response is heralded by dilatation of blood vessels and the outpouring of leukocytes and fluids. Grossly, the results is *redness* (erythema) due to blood vessel dilatation, *swelling* (edema) due to escape of fluids into soft tissues, and *firmness* (induration) due to accumulation of fluids and cells. The result of these processes leads to a loss of the normal capacity of blood vessels to retain fluids and cells within the vasculature; however, such changes do not necessarily reflect structural impairment of the vessel. Leukocytes may be responding to chemical attractants that are diffusing toward the vessel from an extravascular site. Moreover, it is known that the release of certain factors, e.g., histamine from tissue mast cells, may subsequently render the vessel more permeable to plasma fluids (Chapter 13). In most cases, the acute inflammatory response reflects the effects of mediators acting on the blood vessel, rather than a nonspecific injury to the vessel, resulting in the selective release of fluids and cells. Following mechanical trauma or thermal injury, vasopermeability changes may appear early in the acute inflammatory response. In fact, histamine-dependent permeability appears within minutes after thermal injury, probably owing to the release of granular contents of tissue mast cells. This phase of permeability is brief, however, lasting only a few minutes. Within 30 minutes, a more prolonged phase of permeability begins. The mediators responsible for this delayed phase of increased permeability are not known but are believed to consist of several factors, including complement products, kinins, and prostaglandins.

Within 30 to 60 minutes of injury, neutrophilic granulocytes make their appearance. They are first seen clustering along endothelial cells of vessels in the injured area. This remarkable accumulation of neutrophils, still within lumens of vessels, is referred to as *margination*. Soon thereafter, the leukocytes thread their way out of the vessel by squeezing through junctions between endothelial cells (see Fig. 12–1). Within minutes, the granulocytes are extravascular and begin

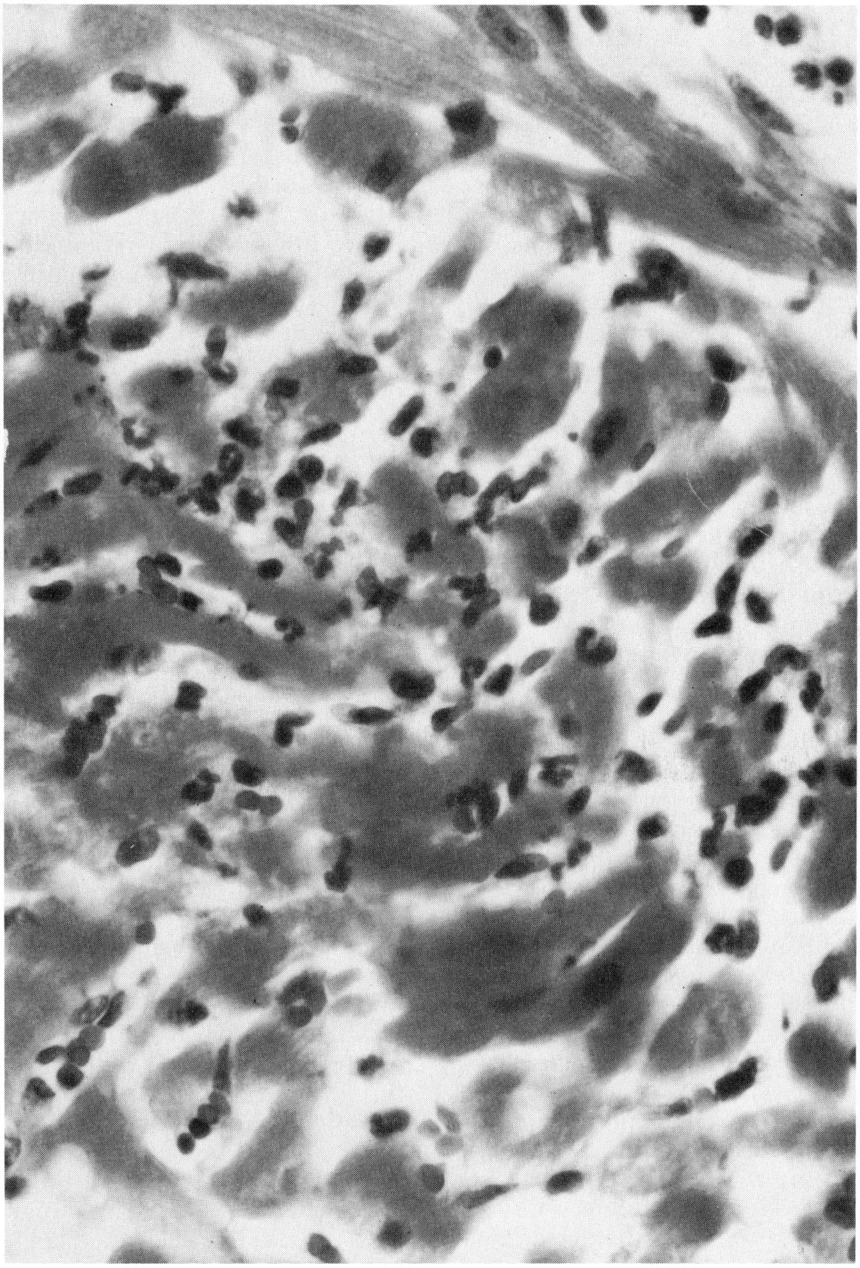

Figure 12–1. Accumulation of neutrophilic granulocytes in myocardium five hours after damage or destruction of tissue to anoxia. Hematoxylin and eosin stain, ×530. (Armed Forces Institute of Pathology photograph.)

to accumulate in the area of injury (Fig. 12–1). Once out of the confines of vessels, neutrophils represent the first line of defense against invading microorganisms. The prime function of neutrophils is to ingest (phagocytose) and destroy potentially dangerous agents, such as bacteria. Within four to five hours, if the acute inflammatory response progresses, mononuclear cells (including lymphocytes and monocytes) will appear at the inflammatory site, after leaving the vessels through mechanisms similar to those of the neutrophils. The arrival of these cells augments the protective barrier between foreign agents and the lymphatic channels, blood vessels, and neighboring tissues. Monocytes augment the defense by adding their own phagocytic function to the area, while lymphocytes convey the immunologic capacity to respond to foreign agents by specific *humoral* and *cell-mediated* phenomena, described in Chapter 2.

The description so far has stressed the protective function of the inflammatory process. It should be understood, however, that if the inflammatory response is aberrant, serious consequences may occur. The outpouring of too much fluid from the vasculature into an area such as the brain may lead to a serious rise in intracranial pressure. The accumulation of fluid due to inflammation in the pleural or pericardial cavities may seriously compromise organ function. Likewise, the arrival of excessive numbers of neutrophils and the subsequent discharge of their enzymatic contents may result in serious structural damage. This is well illustrated in cases of immunologic vasculitis or nephritis, in which dissolution of basement membrane occurs as a consequence of enzymatic hydrolysis, sometimes with catastrophic results (Chapters 13 and 20). Many diseases confronting the clinician are due to an uncontrolled inflammatory response. The joint damage in rheumatoid arthritis, the functional and structural damage in glomerulonephritis, and the demyelinating diseases of the central nervous system are examples of excessive or uncontrolled inflammatory responses. The treatment of these entities (since we lack information about the causative agents) is anti-inflammatory therapy (Chapters 10 and 25). Some of the most active areas under investigation at the present time concern the identification and characterization of mediators of the acute inflammatory response and the mechanisms by which homeostasis or immunologic balance can be maintained (Chapter 2).

Mediators of the acute inflammatory response may be separated into those that carry out either *vasopermeability* or *chemotactic* (leukotactic) functions. The vasopermeability factors achieve their effects by causing a reversible opening of endothelial junctions, perhaps as the result of activation of contractile elements within endothelial cells. The open junctions permit the flow of solutes (electrolytes, water, and proteins) until closure of these junctions occurs, at which time the permeability changes diminish. The *permeability factors* (described more fully in Chapter 13) include vasoactive amines (histamine from mast cells and basophils, serotonin from platelets), peptides, and lipids. Peptides with vasopermeability activity include the kinins (the most well known being bradykinin, which is generated after activation of plasma kallikrein) and the anaphylatoxins (C3a and C5a) generated from the complement system. In human skin, C3a in a concentration of 10^{-12}M causes pronounced permeability increases.

One of the most significant recent advances in immunology is the discovery that the lipid-related vasopermeability factors include some of the products of polyunsaturated fatty acids (eicosanoids), of which arachidonic acid appears to play a pivotal role (Fig. 12–2). Following activation of leukocytes by a variety of agents (chemotactic factors, phagocytic stimuli, and so forth), a membrane-associated phospholipase is activated, resulting in liberation of arachidonic acid. From this point, arachidonate metabolism proceeds via two pathways: One results in generation of a series of leukotriene (LT) compounds designated as LTA_4 to LTF_4; the second (cyclooxygenase) pathway results in generation of a variety of metabolites, including the prostaglandins (with prostacyclins) and thromboxane. The factor that determines the products that will be generated is the cell type under consideration (e.g., endothelial cells produce large amounts of prostacyclin, whereas the chief product of platelets is thromboxane).

Biologic Functions of Arachidonic Acid Metabolites: Leukotrienes, Prostaglandins (Including Prostacyclins), and Thromboxanes. The most important immune functions of the arachidonic acid metabolites are shown in Table 12–1. Biologic functions of the leukotrienes include chemotactic activity associ-

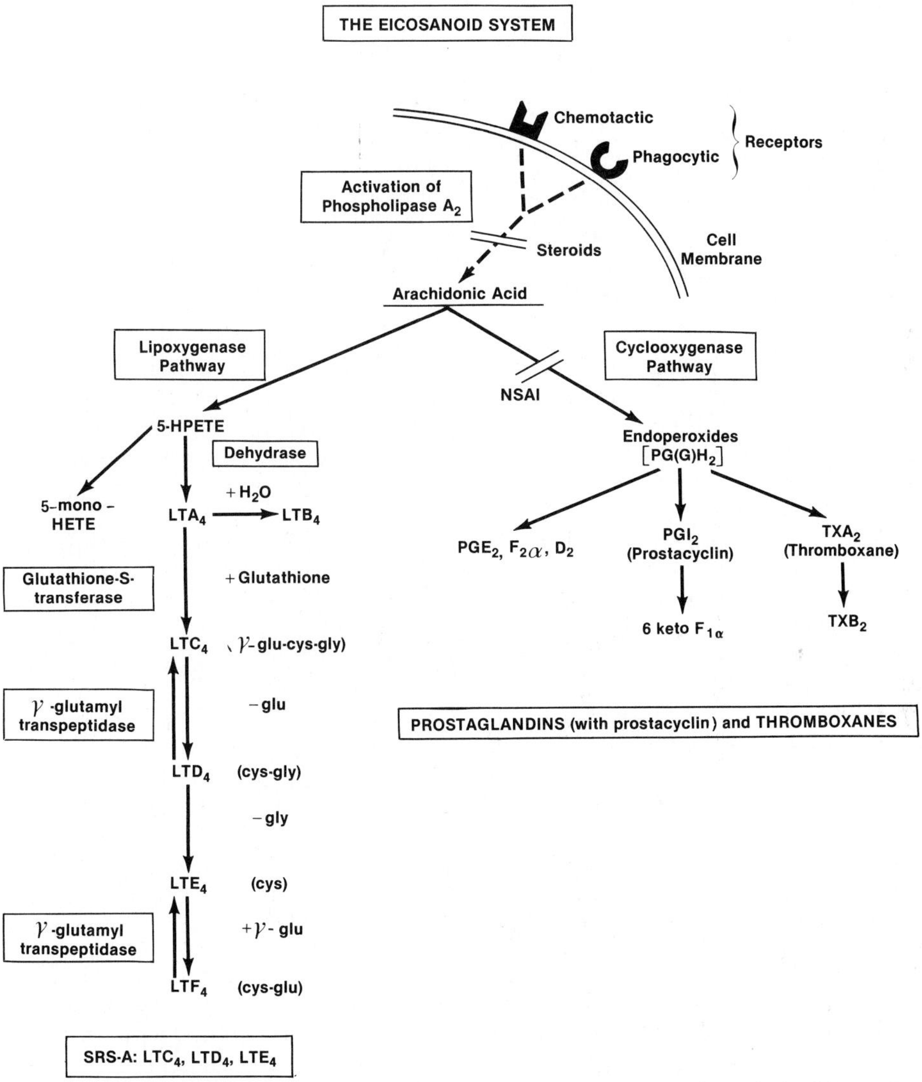

Figure 12–2. Schematic representation of the generation of biologically active products derived from the metabolism of polyunsaturated fatty acids (the eicosanoids), illustrating the pivotal role of arachidonic acid.

Table 12–1. Biologic Functions of Arachidonic Acid Metabolites: Leukotrienes, Prostaglandins (Including Prostacyclins), and Thromboxanes

Metabolite	Biologic Function(s)
LTC_4, LTD_4, LTE_4 (SRS-A)	Bronchoconstriction; Increased vascular permeability; Enhanced mucus secretion
LTB_4	Adhesion and chemotaxis of leukocytes; Stimulates neutrophils: aggregation, enzyme release, and generation of superoxides
Thromboxane A_2	Platelet aggregation; Smooth muscle constriction and vasoconstriction
PGE_2	Vasodilation and edema
PGI_2 (prostacyclin)	Antiaggregation effects on platelets
$PGF_{2\alpha}$	Bronchoconstriction; Vasoconstriction

ated with LTB_4 (and, to a lesser extent, 5-HETE) and smooth muscle contractile activity for LTC_4, LTD_4, and LTE_4. In the latter regard, the spasmogenic activity is equivalent to what was originally described as slow-reacting substance of anaphylaxis (SRS-A). The leukotriene compounds LTC_4–LTE_4 also cause enhanced mucus secretion and have limited effects in increasing vasopermeability changes. The cyclo-oxygenase products involve vasoconstrictive and platelet-aggregating activities (thromboxane A_2), vasodilating activity and antiaggregating effects on platelets (prostacyclin), and some spasmogenic and vasopermeability activities (PGE_2). The E_2 and I_2 prostaglandins also affect functional responses of a variety of leukocytes by increasing intracellular levels of cyclic AMP (Chapter 20A). In general, the whole arachidonate acid metabolite system includes a complex area of biologically active lipids with numerous proinflammatory activities.

Chemotactic factors represent an important class of inflammatory mediators. Their effects are brought about by interaction with surface receptors on leukocytes. The receptor chemotactic ligand interaction results in cation (Na^+, K^+, Ca^{++}) fluxes across the cell membrane, causing a depolarization and hyperpolarization. At the same time, phospholipase activation occurs, resulting in stimulation of arachidonate metabolism. It appears that activation of the lipoxygenase pathway results in generation of some critical lipid that facilitates the cell response to the chemotactic signal (LTB_4). Included in the response of the leukocyte to a chemotactic stimulus is a focal area on the cell membrane of increased adherence, which probably permits the cell to gain a foothold on a surface so that contractile events resulting in cell movement can take place. With actin filament condensation in the vicinity of the chemotactic receptor–ligand complexes, the cell assembles the contractile apparatus that facilitates cell movement.

Although motility responses of leukocytes are the most obvious outcome of chemotactic factor–receptor interaction, other functional and biochemical responses also occur. These include increased glycolysis, hexose monophosphate pathway activation, production of toxic oxygen products (e.g., superoxide anion O_2^-, H_2O_2, hydroxyl radical $OH^\cdot$, singlet oxygen $^1O_2$), and secretion to the cell's exterior of lysosomal granule contents (proteases, glycosidases, and so forth). The ability of chemotactic stimulation of leukocytes to cause multifunctional responses is of considerable interest, since the toxic oxygen derivatives produced and the proteases released have the ability to injure tissues (see further on).

Chemotactic factors fall into three structural categories: peptides, proteins, and lipids. Of the peptides, *N*-formyl oligopeptides produced by bacteria are an important class. The chief activation product of the complement system in C5a is a *glycopeptide* with a molecular weight of 12,500 (Chapter 6). Receptors for C5a have been found on neutrophils, monocytes, and macrophages. There is reason to believe that eosinophils and basophils also contain these receptors. Endothelial cells may also contain receptors for C5a, accounting for their ability, following contact with C5a, to become adhesive to leukocytes. Proteins with chemotactic activity for leukocytes are not structurally defined but are present in the repertoire of activities in lymphokine fluids. Lipids with chemotactic activity for leukocytes have been referred to earlier and include arachidonate metabolites such as leukotriene (LTB_4) and HETE compounds. Based on these data, it is obvious that chemotactic factors can be generated in several ways: following activation of the complement system; by proteases (such as leukocytic elastase and cathepsin G) that will cleave C5; by leukocyte stimulation resulting in release of arachidonate (lipoxygenase) metabolites; and by activation of T-cells. There is also evidence that lymphocytes themselves are under chemotactic control, although the nature of the factors affecting T- and B-cells has not been well defined.

Defects in chemotactic responsiveness of human leukocytes are seen with surprising frequency (Chapter 22). The abnormalities may be unassociated with any clinical problem, or they may be accompanied by serious, life-threatening, recurrent bacterial infections. Curiously, susceptibility to viral infections is not associated with defects in leukocyte chemotaxis. The defects seen in humans are *cellular* and *humoral* in nature. Cellular defects are usually acquired and are reversible, such as those found in association with metabolic disorders. Only rarely are the cellular defects of a genetic nature, as in the Chédiak-Higashi syndrome. Humoral defects involving the chemotactic system occur in conditions of deficiency of plasma factors (such as in genetic deficiency of C5). In addition, abnormal levels of regulatory factors in the plasma for the chemotactic system may be associated with defects of chemotaxis.

The *subacute inflammatory response* is, by definition, a somewhat delayed phase of the acute inflammatory response and is characterized by the accumulation of lymphocytes and monocytes and the formation of *granulation tissue.* For example, one to three days following a skin laceration, there occurs a dramatic proliferation of endothelial cells and fibroblasts. Collectively, these cells form a lush forest of fine capillaries that grow into the area of injury (Figs. 12–3 and 12–4). The capillaries deliver a greatly increased supply of blood to the area and provide nutrients for the accelerated metabolic requirements of inflamed tissues. Fibroblasts are actively synthesizing proteins and mucopolysaccharides, and their main function seems to be the deposition of collagen in the injured area. There is now evidence that proliferation of endothelial cells is induced by factors generated from activated T-lymphoid cells or activated macrophages. Plasma and platelet factors have also been found to have growth-inducing activity for endothelial cells. Fibroblasts growth factors, which cause proliferation of cells as well as increased synthesis of collagen, are also found in supernatant fluids of activated T-cells or macrophages. As fibroblasts secrete tropocollagen that ultimately becomes cross-linked, tensile strength of the tissue gradually increases and reaches its maximum within five days, at which time there is a bridge of connective tissue across a previously open and exposed area. For the wound to heal properly, there must be adequate nutrition following surgery. Concomitant with the appearance of granulation tissue is the proliferation of epithelial cells, which provide a protective structure for the exposed and injured area.

If the inflammatory response is not completely successful in restoring the injured tissue to its original state (e.g., failure of elimination of foreign substance) or if repair of tissue cannot be accomplished, events may progress to a state of *chronic inflammation.* This is characterized by the continued presence of lymphocytes, monocytes, and plasma cells. The explanation for progression of events to this stage may be persistence of foreign material, either living or dead, that mobilizes immunologic reactions. For example, in viral hepatitis, replicating virus may persist within the liver. Plasma cells and lymphocytes accumulate in large numbers, probably conveying immunologic defenses to the local area in the form of specific antibody-synthesizing B-cells or sensitized T-lymphocytes. The persistence of these inflammatory cells could result in functional impairment of the tissue, either because of the direct action of mediators elaborated by lymphoid cells, e.g., lymphotoxin (Chapter 9), or because of unremitting deposition of collagen by fibroblasts. If this happens in the liver, dense fibrous scar tissue results in cirrhosis. In the heart, the outcome may be a fibrous scar that replaces muscle.

It should be stressed that although a given inflammatory response may follow the progression of events as described, this is not always the case. In pneumococcal pneumonia, an acute inflammatory response may be seen with massive exudate of neutrophils and fibrin deposition in an entire lobe of lung (lobar pneumonia). Yet, if the outcome is favorable, particularly with antibiotic therapy, the entire exudate disappears dramatically within 48 hours. Under unusual circumstances, the inflammatory response progresses to the subacute stage, and the individual is under duress as the exudate is invaded by granulation tissue. In this case, the only result can be massive fibrosis with functional loss of a large area of lung. In other situations, such as rejection of a solid homograft, chronic inflammatory (lymphoid) cells are seen in the inflammatory reaction. Very little is known about factors that govern the initiation of the inflammatory response

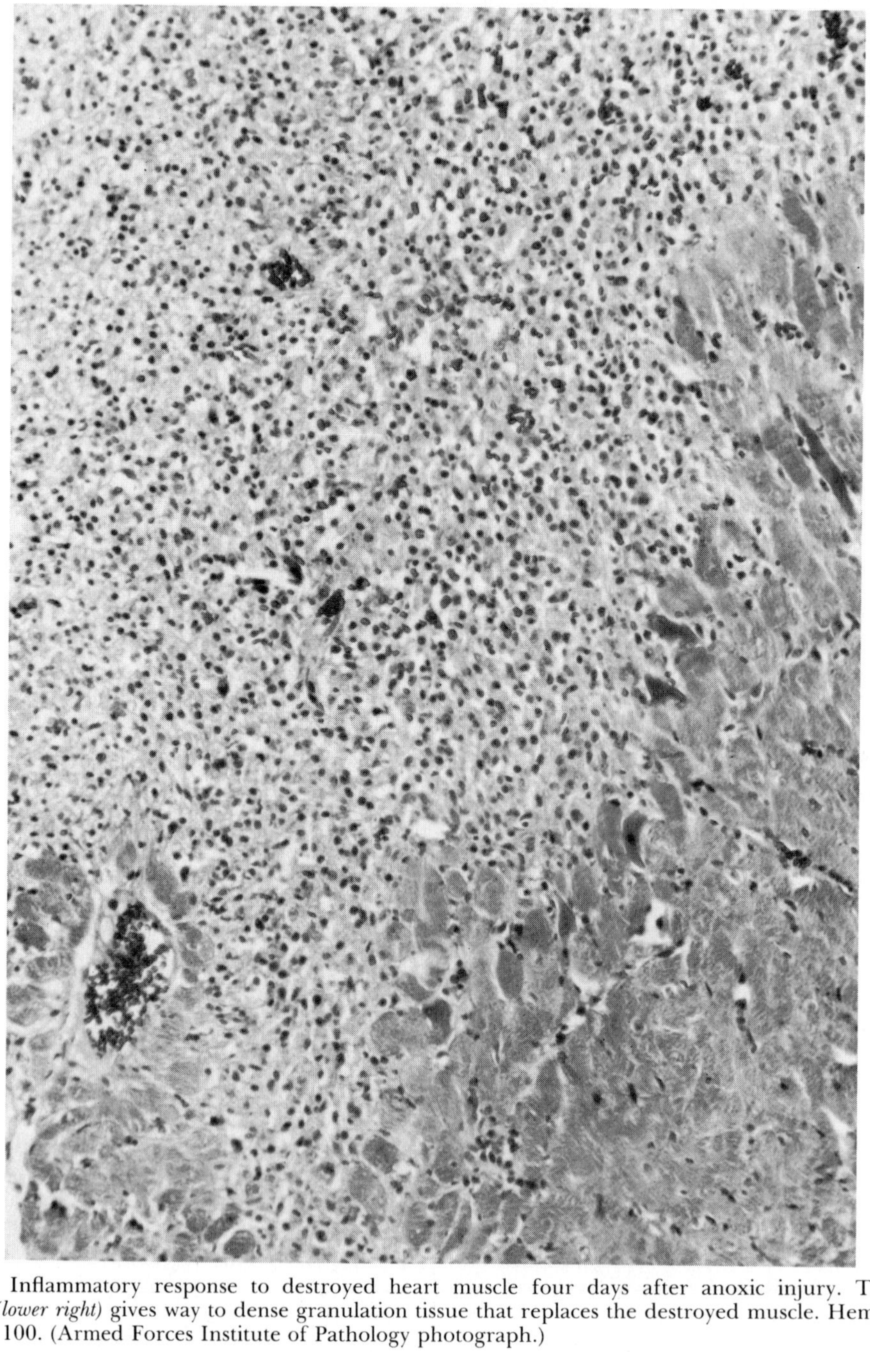

Figure 12–3. Inflammatory response to destroyed heart muscle four days after anoxic injury. The surviving myocardium *(lower right)* gives way to dense granulation tissue that replaces the destroyed muscle. Hematoxylin and eosin stain, ×100. (Armed Forces Institute of Pathology photograph.)

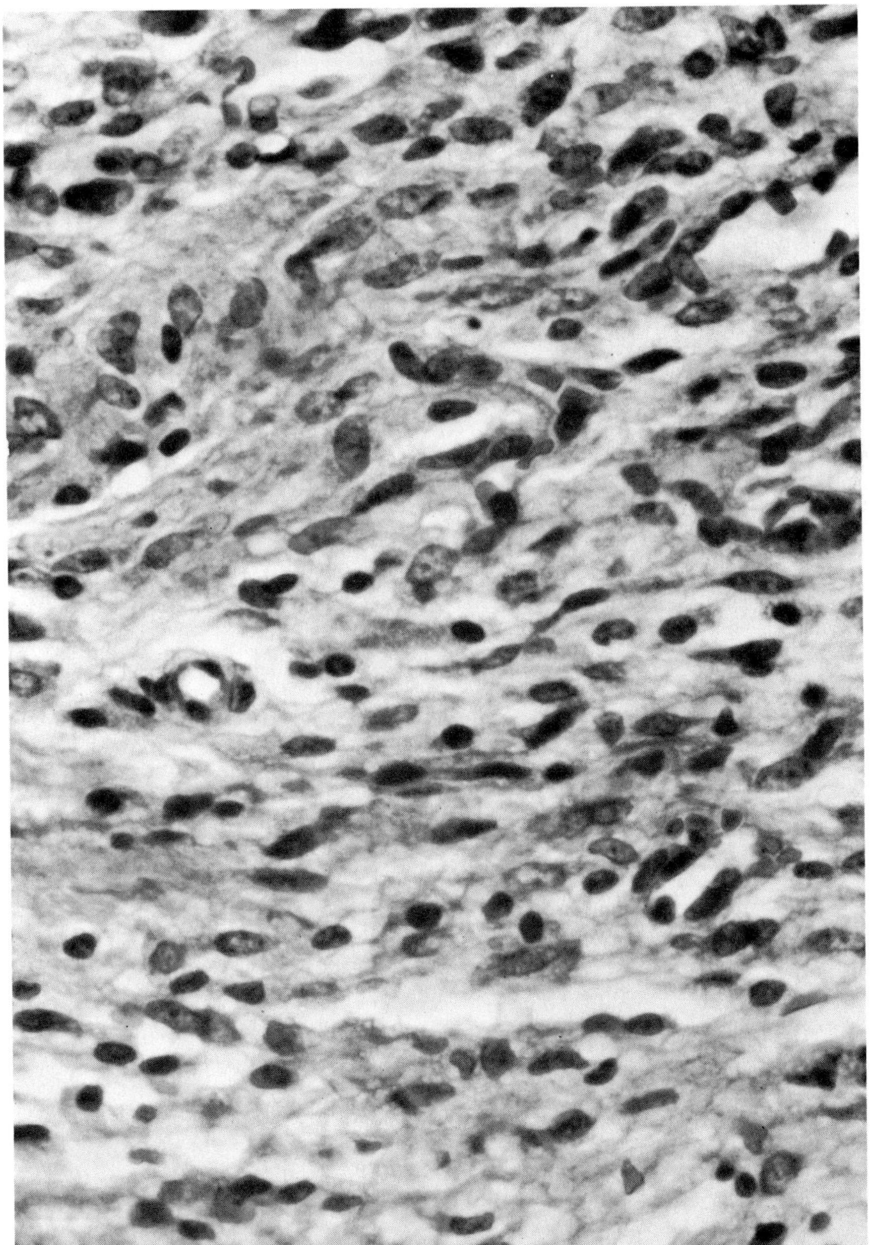

Figure 12–4. Higher magnification of granulation tissue in Figure 12–3. A lush network of fibroblastic and angioblastic elements is present. Between elongated nuclei, collagen fibrils are being laid down. Eventually these will form a dense collagenous scar. This is one outcome of the inflammatory response. Hematoxylin and eosin stain, ×530. (Armed Forces Institute of Pathology photograph.)

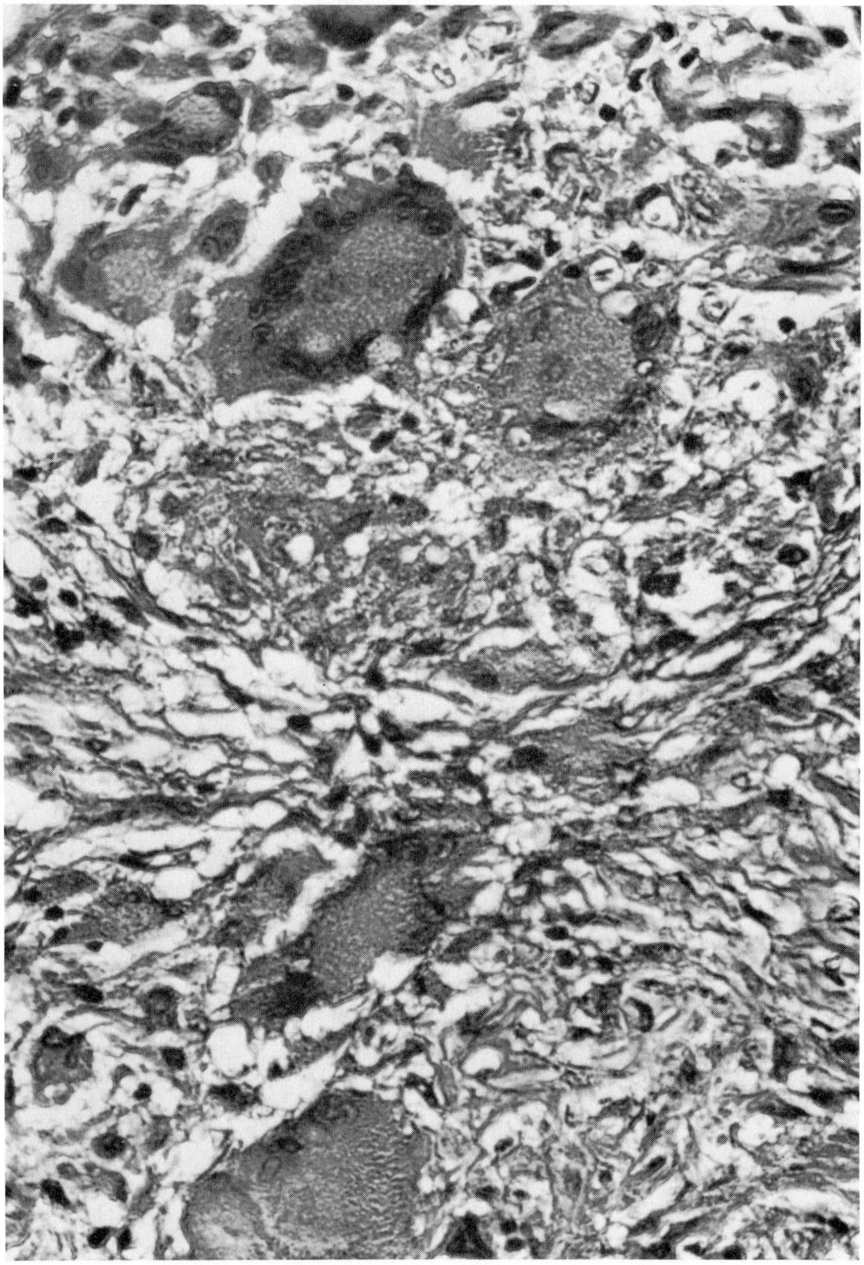

Figure 12–5. Granulomatous inflammation with elliptical macrophages ("epithelioid cells") and giant cells. From a patient with pulmonary sarcoidosis. Hematoxylin and eosin stain, ×350. (Armed Forces Institute of Pathology photograph.)

or the manner in which it is modulated or controlled. The lack of such an understanding represents one of the deficient areas of knowledge in medicine. Successful treatment for a large number of diseases awaits the accumulation of this knowledge.

A special type of chronic inflammation is *granulomatous inflammation.* This condition was first appreciated in tuberculosis, when it was noted that in certain patients dying of the disease there were peculiar white granules (granulomas) scattered throughout the body. It was found that these small bodies, also referred to as tubercles, consisted of characteristic spheric accumulations of large phagocytic or histiocytic cells (unfortunately termed epithelioid cells). A prominent feature of the granuloma is the formation of giant cells (Fig. 12–5) containing a peripheral zone of lymphocytes, with or without plasma cells. Granulomatous inflammation is now known to occur in other disease states in which there is presistence of foreign agents, either infectious (e.g., fungal infections) or noninfectious (e.g., silica). Generally speaking, granulomatous inflammation is an undersirable outcome of the inflammatory response, since, as in syphilis, tuberculosis, or helminthic infections, there may be extensive destruction of tissue with cavitation (necrosis) or scarring (fibrosis).

It is now known that granulomatous inflammation may reflect either *immunologic* or *nonimmunologic* mechanisms. The pioneering studies of Warren indicate that in experimental schistosomiasis, intact immunologic responsiveness is a prerequisite to the formation of granulomas. In that disease, a variety of immunosuppressive measures preclude granuloma formation and the extensive pulmonary scarring is prevented. On the other hand, Warren has also shown that another system of granuloma formation, induced by the injection of talc (a trisilicate), is unaffected by immunosuppressive therapv but significantly retarded by drugs that interfere with activation of the kinin-generating (kallikrein) system (Chapters 2 and 13). It thus appears that granulomatous inflammation may result from two separate mechanisms: (1) an immunologically determined pathway (as in granulomatous inflammation of tuberculosis, with extensive tissue destruction due perhaps to the release of factors from lymphocytes [see Chapter 9], and (2) a nonimmunologic pathway requiring an intact kinin-forming system.

Tissue injury due to immunologic reactions has its origin in the inflammatory response, which is initiated by the reactions to antigen in tissues (Chapter 13). The initiating event may be either a mediator such as a leukotactic factor generated from the complement system or a factor produced by bacteria. Once the leukocyte has arrived from the blood stream, the inflammatory process is initiated and the tissue will recover if adequate leukocyte defense is marshaled. Conversely, if too many leukocytes arrive, or if control mechanisms fail to function adequately, the tissue may become the adventitious target of damage. When the factors that determine these differences are understood, therapeutic measures may be more effectively applied in the prevention of these aberrancies rather than in the symptomatic treatment of disease manifestations.

Suggestions for Further Reading

Boros, D. L.: Granulomatous inflammations. Prog. Allergy, *24:*183, 1967.

Casale, T. B., and Marom, Z.: Mast cells and asthma. The role of mast cell mediators in the pathogenesis of allergic asthma. Ann. Allergy, *51*:2, 1983.

Fantone, J. C., and Ward, P. A.: Role of oxygen-derived free radicals and metabolites in leukocyte-dependent inflammatory reactions. Am. J. Pathol., *107*:397, 1982.

Goetzl, E.: Mediators of immediate hypersensitivity derived from arachidonic acid. N. Engl. J. Med., *303*:822, 1980.

Houck, J. C.: Chemical Messengers of the Inflammatory Process. Vol. 1. Amsterdam, Elsevier/North Holland, 1979.

Marom, Z., and Casale, T. B.: Mast cells and their mediators. Ann. Allergy, *50*:367, 1983.

Samuelsson, B.: Leukotrienes: mediators of immediate hypersensitivy reactions and inflammation. Science, *220*:568, 1983.

Ward, P. A.: Immunology of Inflammation. Vol. 4. Amsterdam, Elsevier/North Holland, 1983.

Weissmann, G.: The Cell Biology of Inflammation. Vol. 2. Amsterdam, Elsevier/North Holland, 1979.

Chapter 13

Mechanisms of Tissue Injury Produced by Immunologic Reactions

Peter M. Henson, Ph.D., B.V.M.&S., M.R.C.V.S.

The encounter between a foreign substance and a host is followed by the induction of an immune response; the host is then in an immunologically primed state. Upon subsequent contact with the same antigen, the immune response will occur more rapidly and with greater vigor (secondary or anamnestic response) (Chapter 7). This subsequent reaction, which has exquisite immunologic specificity, can have either a *protective* function, forming the basis of host resistance to infectious diseases (Chapters 14 to 18) and malignant diseases (Chapter 19), or a *deleterious* function, the outcome causing *tissue injury* (Chapter 20). These protective or injurious responses that follow the recognition of an antigen as foreign are intimately associated with the process of inflammation (Chapter 12). Inflammation itself, which predates the immune system in evolution, is a nonspecific response of tissues to a stimulus or insult. Many of these inflammatory mechanisms have become closely interwoven with the effector arm of the immune system. This chapter is concerned primarily with the mechanisms of tissue injury due to immunologic responses and secondarily with those due to the inflammatory process.

The term "allergy" was originally coined by von Pirquet to include both facets of the altered state: the beneficial was termed *immunity* and the harmful, *hypersensitivity*. Today, however, despite the advantages of this nomenclature, the term "allergy" has become synonymous with the deleterious effects of hypersensitivity, and the broader responses to antigens are encompassed by the term "immunity" (Chapter 2). Allergy, or hypersensitivity, may therefore be defined as the altered reactivity to an antigen that can result in pathologic reactions upon the exposure of a sensitized host to that particular antigen (Chapter 20A).

Originally, the pathologic effects of immunologic processes were separated into two hypersensitivity reactions, *immediate* and *delayed,* which referred to the time required for the reaction to appear after challenge with antigen. With the increase of knowledge in many areas of immunobiology, Gell and Coombs further classified these reactions as Types I, II, III, and IV allergic reactions. These included immediate hypersensitivity reactions (Type I), toxic effects of anticell and antitissue antibodies (Type II), toxic effects of complexes between antibody and antigen (Type III), and delayed hypersensitivity (cell-mediated) reactions (Type IV), which are listed in Table 13–1. More recently, as we have come to understand the underlying mechanisms that produce these reactions, it has become apparent that Types II and III injury are very closely related. In effect, we can consider these responses as due to antigen-antibody complexes, whether they form upon a cell surface, with the cell membrane constituent as the antigen, or whether they form free in the blood or tissues with an exogenous or endogenous antigen in solution or suspension.

It is important at the outset to emphasize that any given pathologic process (e.g., the production of an autoimmune disease) may comprise mechanisms belonging to several or

Table 13–1. **Immunologic Mechanisms of Tissue Injury**

Type	Manifestations	Mechanism
I	Immediate hypersensitivity reactions	IgE and other immunoglobulins
II	Antibody directed against cells	IgG and IgM
III	Antigen-antibody complexes	IgG mainly
IV	Delayed hypersensitivity (cell-mediated)	Sensitized T-lymphocytes

all of these groups of reactions. The clinical applications of these overlapping reactions will be described more fully in Chapter 20.

PATHOGENESIS OF IMMUNOLOGIC INJURY

Immediate Hypersensitivity

Administration of a soluble antigen to a previously sensitized host can, under appropriate conditions, produce a reaction within minutes of the challenge. This reaction has been termed immediate in order to distinguish it from those of slower onset, which are called delayed. The most rapid hypersensitivity reaction of the immediate type is known as *anaphylaxis*. It is characterized by an explosive response that occurs within minutes of the challenging dose, and it can be either *systemic* (generalized) or *localized* (cutaneous). In immediate-type reactions, a variety of immunologic mechanisms may be operative but most have a mediation pathway that involves the release of pharmacologically active substances from mediator cells. The primary effect of these mediators is interaction with target cells, producing a functional alteration, e.g., contraction of smooth muscle, increase of vascular permeability, or increased secretion. These reactions are all characteristic features of Type I immediate hypersensitivity reactions.

GENERALIZED ANAPHYLAXIS

In the laboratory, generalized anaphylaxis is usually produced by injecting a small dose of antigen (sensitizing dose) into an animal, followed within several days by an intravenous dose of antigen (challenging dose). The manifestations of generalized anaphylaxis vary with different species, in which different shock organs may be affected. The guinea pig, a few minutes after challenge with antigen, will scratch, sneeze, and cough, may convulse, and can collapse and die. This is primarily the result of respiratory impairment due to constriction of smooth muscle in the bronchioles and to bronchial edema. A sharp drop in blood pressure and a generalized increase in vascular permeability may also accompany the reaction. The lungs at post-mortem examination are characteristically overinflated. In the rabbit, both cardiovascular and pulmonary functions are severely impaired with a drop in systemic blood pressure, a rise in pulmonary arterial pressure, and constriction of airways. In the human, generalized anaphylaxis presents with itching, erythema, vomiting, abdominal cramps, diarrhea, and respiratory distress. In severe cases, laryngeal edema and vascular collapse may result in death.

Passive Transfer of Anaphylaxis. Since the reaction is antibody-mediated, anaphylactic sensitivity can be transferred to a normal recipient by means of serum. The source of antibody may be the same species, e.g., the human, in which case the predominant immunoglobulin involved is of the IgE class, or a different species, as described below. For example, a guinea pig sensitized by an intravenous injection of rabbit antibody to ovalbumin and challenged with ovalbumin 48 hours later will suffer a fatal anaphylactic shock. A similar reaction can occur following the use of homologous (i.e., guinea pig) antiserum.

TYPES OF ANAPHYLAXIS

The rapid severe generalized response that comprises the syndrome of anaphylaxis may be caused by a number of different etiologic processes: (1) *cytotropic,* (2) *aggregate,* and (3) *cytotoxic*. The intravascular injection of large amounts of the complement fragments C5a or C3a also can produce similar responses (Chapter 6).

Cytotropic Anaphylaxis. In cytotropic anaphylaxis, the antibodies become fixed to mediator cells (e.g., mast cells) in the tissues of the recipient after a two-day latent period between injection of antiserum and antigen challenge. These antibodies with the property of binding are called cytotropic; those derived from the same species are call *homocytotropic,* and those from a different species are called *heterocytotropic.* Challenge with small amounts of antigen can then produce anaphylaxis. The antigen combines with antibody bound to the mast cells, which then release an array of mediator substances, including both preformed materials such as histamine as well as newly synthesized mediators such as leukotrienes (see below).

Aggregate Anaphylaxis. A second type of anaphylactic reaction occurs following the release of the same type of mediators that is triggered by antigen-antibody complexes. In this type, referred to as aggregate anaphylaxis, a latent period is not required. Antigen may be injected immediately after the injection of antiserum. After the antigen-antibody interaction in the blood, a secondary effect may be exerted on target cells through the release of mediators. The injection of soluble immune complexes may be used to induce a similar anaphylactic response, although not strictly caused by "aggregates." Aggregate anaphylaxis, therefore, is an example of tissue injury mediated through antigen-antibody complexes (Type III reaction) and is considered here because the final common pathway is similar to that of cytotropic anaphylaxis.

Cytotropic and aggregate anaphylactic reactions can occur simultaneously. For example, if antigen is rapidly injected into a sensitized animal containing both tissue-bound and circulating antibody, a massive release of mediators will result in anaphylaxis. Anaphylaxis can be avoided by injecting the antigen *slowly* or in divided doses, or by employing the subcutaneous or intraperitoneal routes. These observations assume clinical importance in the administration of antigen in the human. Intravenous routes, in contrast to other routes, are generally more likely to be associated with severe anaphylactic reactions.

Cytotoxic Anaphylaxis. Cytotoxic anaphylaxis is caused by the injection of antibodies directed against antigens present on cells and represents a Type II reaction. For example, the intravenous injection of rabbit anti-Forssman antiserum into a guinea pig will produce anaphylaxis. Since all guinea pigs have this heterophil antigen on their cell surfaces, extensive cytotoxic damage can lead to an anaphylactic reaction in the presence of complement. In man, some transfusion reactions may be of this type (Chapter 20B). Cytotoxic anaphylaxis is therefore due to antitissue antibodies. These effects are described in greater detail below.

It is apparent that generalized anaphylaxis may be induced by different immunologic reactions, including Type I, II, and III mechanisms. However, the pathogenesis in each involves a common final pathway—the release of pharmacologically active substances (mediators) from mediator cells.

CUTANEOUS ANAPHYLAXIS

Active Cutaneous Anaphylaxis. Upon injection of antigen into the skin of a sensitized animal, a local anaphylactic reaction will occur within a few minutes. It consists of localized swelling and redness—a wheal and flare reaction. Skin tests in man for allergy to a wide variety of antigens (allergens) are characteristic of this phenomenon (Chapter 20A).

In animals, the cutaneous reaction is similar to that in man but is less readily visible. The local increase in vascular permeability that is characteristic of this reaction may be demonstrated by the use of tracer dyes such as Evans blue dye. This binds to albumin in the blood, and when the blood vessels exhibit increased permeability, the albumin that leaks out is dyed blue and stains the tissues. The anaphylactic reactions are mediated by substances such as histamine and serotonin, which have only a transient effect, since they are quickly inactivated by tissue and plasma enzymes, e.g., histaminases. Consequently, the true immediate hypersensitivity reaction is short-lived and recovery occurs within hours.

Passive Cutaneous Anaphylaxis. Localized anaphylaxis can also be passively transferred by specific types of antibody, most importantly, in the human, of the IgE class. In animals, this type of transferred reaction in the skin was described by Ovary and called *passive cutaneous anaphylaxis (PCA).* Sensitizing antibody is injected intradermally, and, after an obligatory latent period (usually 24 to 72 hours), antigen is given intravenously with Evans blue dye. The local permeability reaction, as evidenced by bluing of the skin, appears within minutes (Fig. 13–1). The requirement for a latent period in the skin is not fully understood but presumably represents the time required for cytotropic antibodies to diffuse and become fixed to mediator cells in the tissues, particularly the mast cells.

The PCA reaction is especially useful for

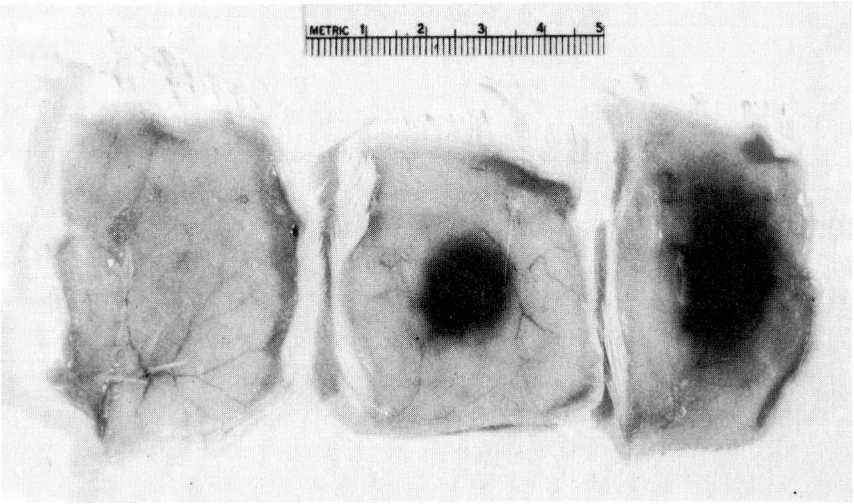

Figure 13–1. Passive cutaneous anaphylaxis (PCA) in guinea pigs. The two skins on the right come from animals injected intradermally with cytotropic antibody and, after a latent period, intravenously with antigen and Evans blue dye. The skin on the left is a control, injected with saline only. The leakage of the dye out of vessels with increased permeability is apparent.

study, since when carried out with IgE antibody it provides a model for a purely cytotropic reaction. Although initial histologic examination of the skin usually reveals minimal cell infiltration in most species, including man, a leukocytic infiltration is noted 2 to 24 hours after a challenge with antigen. In *active cutaneous anaphylaxis,* on the other hand, the animal has formed circulating antibodies, and the reaction evoked by intradermal antigen is often complex, with an Arthus lesion (see below) superimposed on the anaphylaxis.

Human Atopy and the Prausnitz-Küstner (P-K) Reaction. A significant proportion of humans are susceptible to natural sensitization by a variety of environmental antigens, including pollens, spores, animal danders, house dusts, and foods. These individuals appear to be genetically predisposed or susceptible (Chapters 3 and 20). This susceptibility is known as *atopy* (from *atopia:* Gr., strange disease); however, the term "allergy" is often used synonymously. Subsequent contact of these individuals with the antigens by inhalation or ingestion produces such conditions as allergic rhinitis, asthma, and allergic urticaria (Chapter 20A).

These hyperactivities in man can also be passively transferred to unreactive subjects by the injection of serum antibodies. In order to avoid generalized reactions and sensitization, a completely localized transfer may be performed. This procedure is referred to as the Prausnitz-Küstner, or P-K, reaction. Serum from a sensitized individual is injected intradermally into a normal recipient. After a latent period of one or more days, antigen is injected into the same site and a localized wheal and flare reaction occurs within minutes. The P-K test, the human counterpart of the PCA reaction, although of importance in the study of immediate hypersensitivity in man in the past, has now been largely replaced by *in vitro* tests (Chapters 20A and 26).

ANTIBODIES RESPONSIBLE FOR IMMEDIATE HYPERSENSITIVITY

In man, the term *reagin* or skin-sensitizing antibody was formerly used interchangeably with cytotropic antibody. In recent years, however, the bulk of antibodies responsible for immediate hypersensitivity in man has been shown to belong to the IgE class of immunoglobulin. Purified normal IgE, injected with reaginic antibody, can inhibit the P-K or PCA reaction by competing for receptor sites on mediator cells, e.g., mast cells. Moreover, as an indication that IgE is present in the skin of atopic as well as nonatopic individuals, intradermal injection of a specific rabbit antibody to IgE will induce a typical wheal and flare reaction. The salient properties of IgE globulins are shown in Table 13–2. IgE antibody is slightly larger than IgG and does not fix complement through the classic pathway. There is no evidence, however, for complement requirement in immediate hypersensitivity reactions mediated by

Table 13–2. **Comparison of Properties of IgE and IgG Antibodies**

IgE Antibody	IgG Antibody
200 kilodalton	150 kilodalton
Non–complement fixing	Complement requirement in many reactions
Heat-labile	Heat-stable
Present in trace amounts in serum	Highest concentrations in serum
Biologic activity seen in both atopic and nonatopic individuals; higher in atopic	Biologic activity seen in both atopic and nonatopic individuals

IgE antibody. Another property of the antibody that has been used for characterization is its heat lability. Heating antibody at 56°C for two to four hours results in alteration of the Fc fragment of the IgE molecule and loss of its ability to fix to receptors on mediator cells. IgE is present in only nanogram quantities in human serum and is also present in individuals who show no evidence of atopy, suggesting that other factors in addition to the mere ability to synthesize IgE are involved in the induction of the atopic state.

Other Homocytotropic Antibodies. In the guinea pig, PCA reactions are produced by antibodies of the IgG1a and IgG1b, as well as IgE. These IgG1 antibodies exhibit some clear differences from the IgE antibodies. They are less heat labile and persist in the skin for relatively shorter periods of time. In addition, shorter latent periods are required for detection of the IgG1 than for the IgE homocytotropic antibody by the PCA reaction.

In the rat, IgG_{2a} has cytotropic properties, i.e., it can mediate a local anaphylactic reaction. Rabbit IgG antibody has also been shown to induce, under special circumstances, a PCA-like reaction. In addition, there are suggestions that cytotropic IgG antibodies, e.g., IgG_4, may occur in man. However, despite these indications, the predominant antibody involved in immediate hypersensitivity reactions in man is IgE.

"Late-Phase Responses." Challenge of sensitized animals and man by the intradermal or airways route sometimes elicits a delayed response (permeability or bronchial constriction, respectively) after four to six hours (Chapter 20A). Recent evidence suggests that IgE antibody is responsible for this process in rats, rabbits, and probably man. The phenomenon may result from a delayed attraction of leukocytes as a result of the IgE-induced release of mediators from mast cells (see below).

Stimulation of Homocytotropic Antibodies

Synthesis of IgE Antibodies. A variety of circumstances may be associated with higher levels of total IgE in the plasma and/or larger amounts of specific IgE antibody (Chapter 20A). These include atopic disease, bronchopulmonary aspergillosis, parasitic disease, certain deficiencies of T-cell function, and the hyperimmunoglobulinemia E syndrome with recurrent staphylococcal infection. Moreover, the control of IgE synthesis appears now to be strongly influenced by genetic factors that are thought to predispose to the atopic state. Deficiency of IgE-specific suppressor cells as well as the presence of suppressor factors has been described in the atopic individual as well as in the experimental animal model.

Of particular interest is the observation that infestation with fungi, such as *Aspergillus,* or parasites, especially helminths, leads to the production of homocytotropic antibody (Chapter 17). It is not known what properties of helminthic antigens predispose the host toward synthesis of these antibodies; however, the phenomenon has been observed in a variety of species. For example, humans infected with ascaris have elevated levels of IgE globulins, and their serum can be used to induce PCA reactions in baboons, with ascaris antigens. (PCA activity in primates is a known property of human IgE antibody.) The possibility that a homocytotropic, antibody-mediated, local anaphylactic reaction in the gut of rats is involved in the ridding of infestation by the intestinal worm *Nippostrongylus braziliensis* is of some interest. Furthermore, this reaction may be dependent on the presence of eosinophilic leukocytes.

Fixation to Tissues. One of the most common properties of IgE antibodies is their ability to become attached to mediator cells in the tissues, e.g., mast cells. The skin-fixing properties of the antibody molecule reside in the Fc fragment, since its removal by enzymatic digestion or its alteration by heating leads to a loss of its biologic activity, e.g., cutaneous anaphylaxis. Once antibody is fixed to mediator cells, a combination of antibody with the antigen-binding sites on the Fab fragments can occur. This leads to cross linking of the antibody molecules and thus of the receptors on the cell surface and then to the release of mediators from these cells. Intradermal injection of preformed complexes of antigen with IgE antibody will also cause a wheal and flare reaction. The fixation of homocytotropic antibody to mediator cells appears to be due to a particularly firm, but not irreversible, bond. IgE antibody will remain at the site of intradermal injection in man for up to two months and will still be capable of reacting with a subsequent injection of antigen. Such antibody fixed to mast cells has been demonstrated in humans, monkeys, and guinea pigs by the use of a wide variety of immunohistochemical techniques, e.g., immunofluorescent, autoradiographic, and ferritin-labeled antibody techniques. In addition to their skin-fixing ability *in vivo,* IgE antibodies will bind to isolated mast cells and basophils *in vitro.*

The receptor on basophils or mast cells for the Fc fragment of homocytotropic antibody seems to be quite specific, since passive sensitization of cells can be performed by incubation with whole serum from a sensitive animal. The low levels of homocytotropic antibody compete successfully with large amounts of other immunoglobulins present in the serum. After a suitable incubation with antibody, the cells may be washed and will release contained histamine upon incubation with specific antigen. This forms the basis of an *in vitro* measurement of IgE antibody in the human through the release of histamine—the leukocyte histamine release assay (Chapter 26). The fact that IgE immunoglobulin binds avidly to mast cell receptors means that *in vivo,* the levels of IgE detected in the plasma are those that are *left over* after the tissue binding has occurred. In other words, they may represent only a proportion of the total IgE in the body, and low serum levels can coexist with at least some *in vivo* reactivity to inhaled or injected antigen.

Nonhomocytotropic Antibodies. Release of mediators from cell reservoirs can also be induced by immune complexes of antigen combined with antibody that is not homocytotropic, as described previously. Thus, aggregate anaphylaxis in rabbits can result from rabbit IgG antibody reacting with antigen, but the pathogenesis is more closely related to that of the Arthus reaction than that of immediate hypersensitivity. The reaction involves many cell types, including platelets and neutrophils. *Heterocytotropic antibodies* are another example of cytotropic antibodies that are usually IgG in nature. Rabbit IgG antibodies, injected into the skin of guinea pigs, will allow the induction of a strong PCA reaction after intravenous challenge with antigen. Whether or not binding sites for these heterologous antibodies are the same as those for homologous antibody, however, is at present unknown.

Blocking Antibodies and Desensitization (Immunotherapy). Immediate hypersensitivity reactions do not occur in the presence of large amounts of so-called *blocking antibodies.* A blocking antibody presumably competes locally or in the circulation for the antigen and prevents the reaction with homocytotropic antibody fixed to mediator cells. In serum, these antibodies are predominantly IgG and may be induced in man by repeated injections of antigen.

This observation forms the basis for an approach to desensitization or hyposensitization (immunotherapy) of allergic individuals (Chapter 20A). Minute quantities of the allergen to which the patient is sensitive are injected in increasing doses over a prolonged period. There seems to be a therapeutic benefit from this procedure in some individuals, but it is not certain whether the production of blocking antibodies is the sole mechanism involved.

Pharmacologically Active Mediators of Immediate Hypersensitivity

Early in the study of anaphylaxis, it was found that histamine injected into normal guinea pigs could mimic the immediate reaction. Since that time, many pharmacologically active substances have been implicated in immediate hypersensitivity reactions, including histamine, serotonin, kinins, prostaglandins, prostaglandin intermediates, platelet-activating factor (PAF), and slow-reacting substances (SRS-A), now known as leukotrienes (LTC_4, LTD_4, and LTE_4). The structures of many of these molecules are known (Fig. 13–2). However, there are still "mediators" whose structures are unknown and which have been described on the basis of activity alone, for example, a variety of chemotactic factors that may contribute to some of the slower phases of immediate hypersensitivity reactions. There is no direct evidence

Histamine

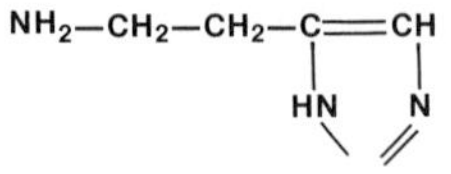

Serotonin
(5 Hydroxytryptamine)

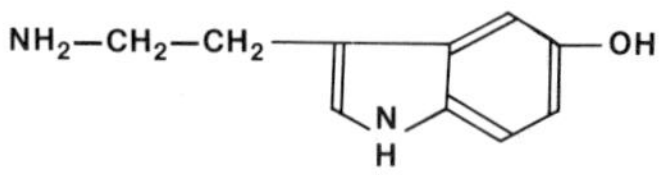

Bradykinin — Arg. pro pro. gly. phe. ser. pro. phe. arg.

Lysylbradykinin — Lys. arg. pro. pro. gly. phe. ser. pro. phe. arg.

PAF (platelet activating factor)

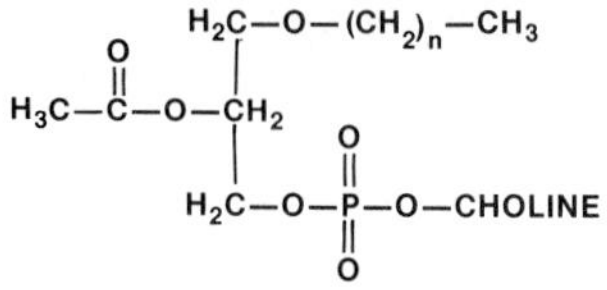

n = 15 or 17

(acetyl glyceryl ether phosphorylcholine)

ECF-A (eosinophil chemotactic factor of anaphylaxis) — mixture of two tetrapeptides (<500 MW) Ala-gly-ser-glu-and Val-gly-ser-glu and higher molecular weight factors.

Thromboxane A_2, Prostacyclin, PGE_2 (and other prostanoids)

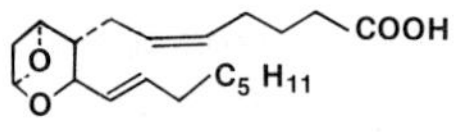

TXA_2

PGI_2 (Prostacyclin)

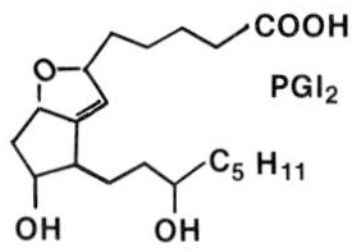

PGI_2

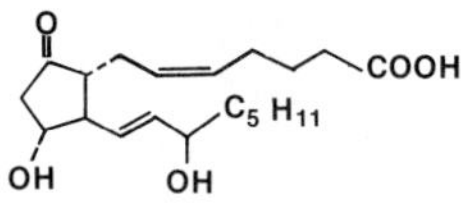

PGE_2

Leukotriene C_4 (SRS-A) — (glu—cys—gly)

Leukotriene D_4 (SRS-A) — (cys—gly)

Leukotriene E_4 (SRS-A) — (cys)

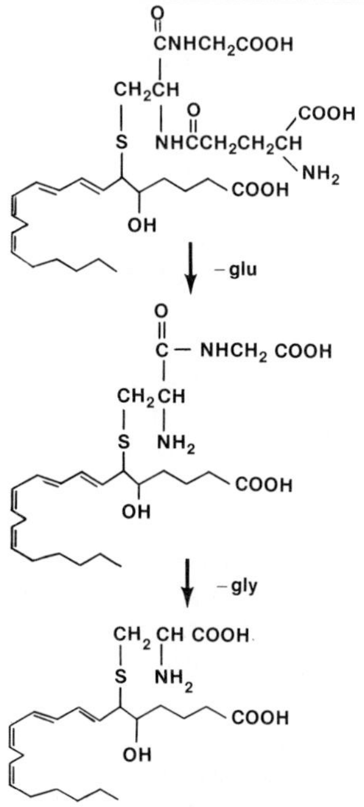

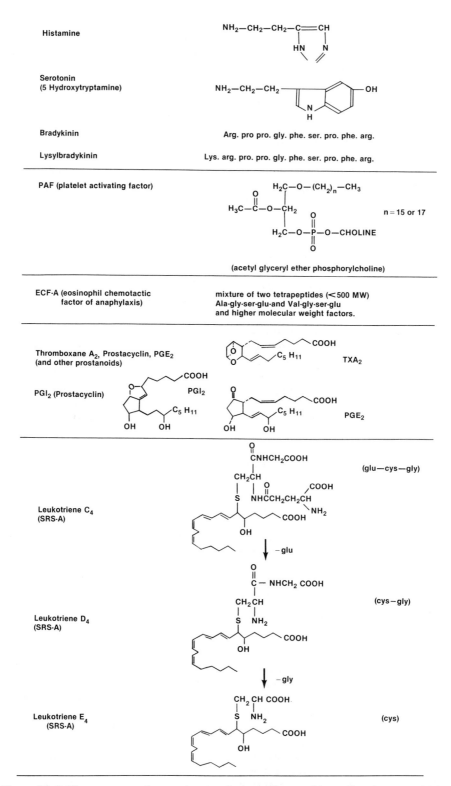

Figure 13–2. The structure of some pharmacologic mediators of immediate hypersensitivity.

that any one of these agents actually causes anaphylaxis. The presence of some mediators during an anaphylactic reaction *in vivo* or *in vitro* is the only available information. Specific antagonists of mediators, such as histamine and serotonin, prevent some manifestations of the hypersensitivity reactions. However, specific inhibitors for some of the other mediators are not yet available. Additional evidence for the involvement of such mediators comes from the reproduction of actual hypersensitivity reactions when a substance such as histamine is injected in pure form.

Much of the information concerning mediators has been obtained from *in vitro* studies using isolated perfused organs or suspensions of organs, such as the lung and skin, as well as suspensions of mast cells and basophilic leukocytes. Antigen added to chopped lung tissue from a guinea pig sensitized to that antigen will induce the release of up to 30 per cent of the total histamine in the tissue. In addition, other mediators, including leukotrienes, PAF, and eosinophil chemotactic factor of anaphylaxis (ECF-A), may be detected in the supernatant after the reaction. Lung tissue can also be passively sensitized when incubated with serum containing homocytotropic antibody, and it has provided a useful tool for the study of the anaphylactic reaction. Today, however, studies are concentrated upon individual cells that cause the release of these mediators.

Histamine. Histamine is found in many tissues and is particularly localized in the granules of mast cells and basophils. Some species (e.g., the rabbit) also store large quantities of histamine in granules within platelets. Mast cell and basophil granules also contain heparin, which gives them their characteristic metachromatic staining with toluidine blue, but there is little evidence that this plays a direct role in anaphylaxis. Recent studies suggest a possible role for mast-cell heparin in vascular repair and regeneration processes. The reaction of antigen with mast cells from sensitized animals results in extrusion of the granules (degranulation) and the release of histamine. Degranulation of mast cells may be seen *in vivo*, as well as *in vitro*, in tissue sections that have undergone anaphylactic reaction. It is noteworthy that degranulation of mass cells and basophils is now suspected to play a role in immune complex–induced injury and also in delayed hypersensitivity (see below). This represents another example of the difficulties inherent in attempts to classify complex networks of interacting mechanisms.

Histamine is formed by decarboxylation of histidine, which is stored in the mast cell granules. Once released, histamine can exert its many pharmacologic effects, including smooth muscle contraction, increased vascular permeability, and increased mucus secretion. The effects of histamine are transient, however, since the amine is rapidly broken down in the plasma and tissues by histaminases. The bioassay for histamine makes use of its effect on smooth muscle and measures the contraction of the guinea pig ileum by the Schultz-Dale reaction. Histamine can also be assayed by chemical, enzymatic, and radioactive techniques (Chapter 26).

There are two types of histamine receptors: the H1 receptors, inhibited by standard antihistamines, and the H2 receptors, affected only by specific antihistamines such as burimamide and metiamide. Acting through H1 receptors, histamine contracts smooth muscles, increases vascular permeability, and increases mucus secretion of goblet cells. Interaction of histamine with H2-type receptors results in increased gastric secretion and a decrease of mediator release from anaphylactically reacting mediator cells (e.g., mast cells and basophils). This action of histamine through H_2 receptors suggests an important negative feedback loop in which the released histamine inhibits further release of this mediator. Moreover, there is evidence for a greater complexity of the feedback loop that includes the H_2 receptor on T-suppressor lymphocytes. Another important biologic action of histamine that relates to immediate hypersensitivity reactions is its chemotactic potential for eosinophilic leukocytes. Not only can histamine attract eosinophils into sites of allergic reactions, but it can also deactivate and arrest these cells from further outward migration.

Just as histamine can mimic some of the effects of anaphylaxis in the guinea pig, so can antagonists of histamine, the antihistamines, prevent anaphylactic reactions. This indicates that histamine is an important mediator of immediate hypersensitivity in both man and animals. However, the inability of these useful therapeutic substances to completely abolish the reactions *in vivo* indicates that other mediators participate. In rats and in mice, mast cells contain serotonin as well as histamine, and both mediators may participate in these species.

Serotonin (5-Hydroxytryptamine). This vasoactive amine is found in mast cells in rats and mice and in the platelets of most species. It is also present in the brain and the gastric mucosa. The role of serotonin in human anaphylaxis is questionable, but it may be important in other species. Although it does not directly induce increased vascular permeability in rabbit skin, as it does in rats and mice, it may participate in immune complex disease in the rabbit. The amine produces increased vascular permeability, capillary dilatation, and contraction of smooth muscle. It is a neurotransmitter, and recently it has been suggested as a possible stimulus for some inflammatory cells as well as of neuronal and smooth muscle cells.

Kinins. Kinins are basic peptides with vasoactive properties that are produced in plasma and in tissues. They are split by kallikreins from certain precursor plasma proteins, the kininogens. Kallikreins may be activated in the plasma but are also present in organs such as the pancreas. The kinins produced include bradykinin, a nonopeptide, and lysylbradykinin, a decapeptide (Fig. 13–2). These peptides increase vascular permeability and cause a lowering of blood pressure and a contraction of smooth muscle. They are bioassayed by their ability to contract the uterus from a rat in estrus. Although kinin levels in the blood do increase slightly in some species during anaphylaxis, there is little evidence that they play a major role in the reaction. However, recent experiments have suggested that some of the effects of kinins may have been overlooked because of a great enhancement of these actions by prostaglandins (PGE_2). A similar synergism occurs between PGE_2 and some of the actions of C5a and leukotriene B_4 (see below). As with other mediators, they are rapidly degraded by enzymes in the plasma (kininases).

Leukotrienes C_4, D_4, and E_4 (Slow-reacting Substance of Anaphylaxis, SRS-A). The molecules are now identified as products of lipoxygenation of arachidonic acid (Chapter 12; Fig. 12–2; Fig. 13–2). The addition of glutathione to an unstable precursor molecule, leukotriene A_4, leads to production of leukotriene C_4(LTC_4). This has SRS activity. In fact, SRS-A appears to be a mixture of LTC_4 and its derivatives LTD_4 and LTE_4, the relative amounts of which may vary from cell source to cell source. The leukotrienes are synthesized and secreted by a number of cell types, including macrophages, and by mast cells and basophils. However, the exact range of cells that secrete these molecules, and the relative amounts they produce, remain to be determined. Substances that can produce a relatively slow contraction of an isolated smooth muscle preparation were termed slow-reactive substances (SRS). Slow-reactive substance of anaphylaxis (SRS-A) was found in the perfusate from sensitized guinea pig lungs perfused with antigens and was released from chopped sensitized human lung fragment by antigen. Its action on smooth muscle is not inhibited by antihistamines. In the human, leukotrienes C_4, D_4 and E_4 may be partly responsible for the prolonged bronchospasm seen in asthma and may account for the inability of antihistamines to completely alleviate the reaction.

Leukotriene B_4. By contrast with the slow-reacting substances, leukotriene B_4 is a dihydroxyeicosatetraenoic acid. It is also derived from LTA_4 but does not usually contract smooth muscle. Its biologic activity seems directed toward leukocytes, particularly perhaps as a chemoattractant. *In vivo,* when injected into the rabbit skin it induces an increase in vascular permeability but only when PGE_2 is also injected and neutrophils are present. However, LTB_4, or some other related product of arachidonate lipoxygenation may be involved in the release of mediators from basophils (and neutrophils). These complex events are not yet completely worked out, but this probably represents another example of feedback regulation of cell function, in this case a positive feedback loop.

Eosinophil Chemotactic Factor of Anaphylaxis (ECF-A). Following the reaction of antigen with cell-bound IgE, there also is the release of mediators that are selectively chemotactic for eosinophils, ECF-A. Stored as a preformed moiety in mast cells and basophils, the mediators may represent a mixture of at least two tetrapeptides that have an overall molecular weight of less than 500 (see Fig. 13–2). A higher molecular ECF weight may also be liberated, and, in addition, histamine itself has been reported to have eosinophil chemotactic activity. It is noteworthy that eosinophilic leukocytes are commonly found at sites of allergic reactions, although their function is at present unknown.

Platelet-Activating Factor. PAF is a low molecular weight lipid whose structure is shown in Figure 13–2. This glycerol ether has potent activating effects on platelets from some species but may be even more important as a general allergic and inflammatory mediator. It induces a rapid wheal and flare in human skin, and in rabbits it mimics completely the IgE-induced anaphylactic reaction. Small amounts injected into rats, rabbits, dogs, goats, and primates are lethal, although the exact modes of action of this mediator are not yet fully elucidated.

Prostaglandins. A variety of C_{20} unsaturated hydroxy aliphatic acids with potent biologic properties have been termed prostaglandins. They are derived from arachidonic acid via the cyclooxygenase pathway. They are widely distributed in tissues and, depending on their nature, can contract (e.g., thromboxane A_2 [TxA_2] or PGF_2) or relax (e.g., prostacyclin [PGI_2] or PGE_2) smooth muscle. Prostaglandins are released from tissues undergoing anaphylaxis. As indicated above, certain prostaglandins may have potentiating action on some allergic and inflammatory processes. Possibly this will explain the anti-inflammatory action of the nonsteroidal anti-inflammatory agents, such as aspirin, indomethacin, ibuprofen, and the like, which inhibit the cyclooxygenase pathway. An additional area in which prostaglandins may contribute to the pathogenesis of immunologic reactions is in enhancing the painful effects of some of the mediators, e.g., in sunburn.

Reaction of Antibody and Antigen (Types II and III Injury)

ANTITISSUE ANTIBODIES

Injury may be produced by the reaction of antibodies with antigens on cells. This has been referred to as a *cytotoxic or Type II reaction.* Previously, antitissue antibodies were considered important contributors to immunologic disease. Now their role appears more limited compared with injury mediated by antigen-antibody complexes. Nevertheless, such antibodies are involved in human disease and have been shown to induce experimental tissue damage in animals.

There are a number of related mechanisms for such injury. The first is the reaction of antibody with tissue cells. The antibody can induce direct cytolysis and killing by activation of all nine components of complement (Chapter 6). The cytotoxic anaphylaxis described earlier may be the result of this type of process. In the human, certain hemolytic reactions may be of this type. The second mechanism of injury by cytotoxic antibody involves the participation of cells, such as the neutrophil and macrophage. When the antitissue antibody reacts with its antigen, whether on a tissue cell or basement membrane, the antigen-antibody complex so formed can interact with phagocytic cells. These cells adhere to the bound immunoglobulin itself, but the adherence is greatly enhanced by the fixation of complement through C3b and iC3b, a split product of the third component of complement, C3 (Chapter 6). Reaction of antibody with circulating cells such as the erythrocyte, therefore, can cause not only cytolysis but also phagocytosis by cells of the reticuloendothelial system. In tissues, the fixation of antibody and complement can cause accumulation of cells, such as neutrophils, that release injurious constituents when they react with antibody or complement. This process is identical with that for immune complexes, the only difference being that antigen is itself part of the target tissue. In addition to these effects, antibody can also facilitate the cytotoxic action of lymphocytes and perhaps macrophages, e.g., killer (K) cells, in the so-called antibody-dependent cellular cytotoxic (ADCC) reactions (Chapters 9 and 11) described below. These processes may occur together, as in autoimmune hemolytic anemia in which both hemolysis and increased clearance contribute to the destruction of erythrocytes. Another example of the damage produced by antitissue antibody is *nephrotoxic nephritis,* produced experimentally by the injection of heterologous antiglomerular basement membrane (a-GBM) antiserum. The response that generally ensues involves the activation of complement and accumulation of inflammatory cells with subsequent tissue injury (Figs. 13–3 and 13–4). This is a similar response to the deposition or formation of immune complexes in most sites in the body (Type III reaction). Later the animal mounts its own immune response against the foreign antibody that was injected. Here both humoral and cellular immune responses may contribute to this later (or autologous) phase of nephrotoxic nephritis. Glomerulonephritis in man is sometimes associated with synthesis of anti-GBM antibodies. Some evidence of binding of immunoglobulins to human glomeruli *in vivo* has been obtained, for example, in patients with Goodpasture's syndrome and chronic glomerulonephritis (Chapter 20C).

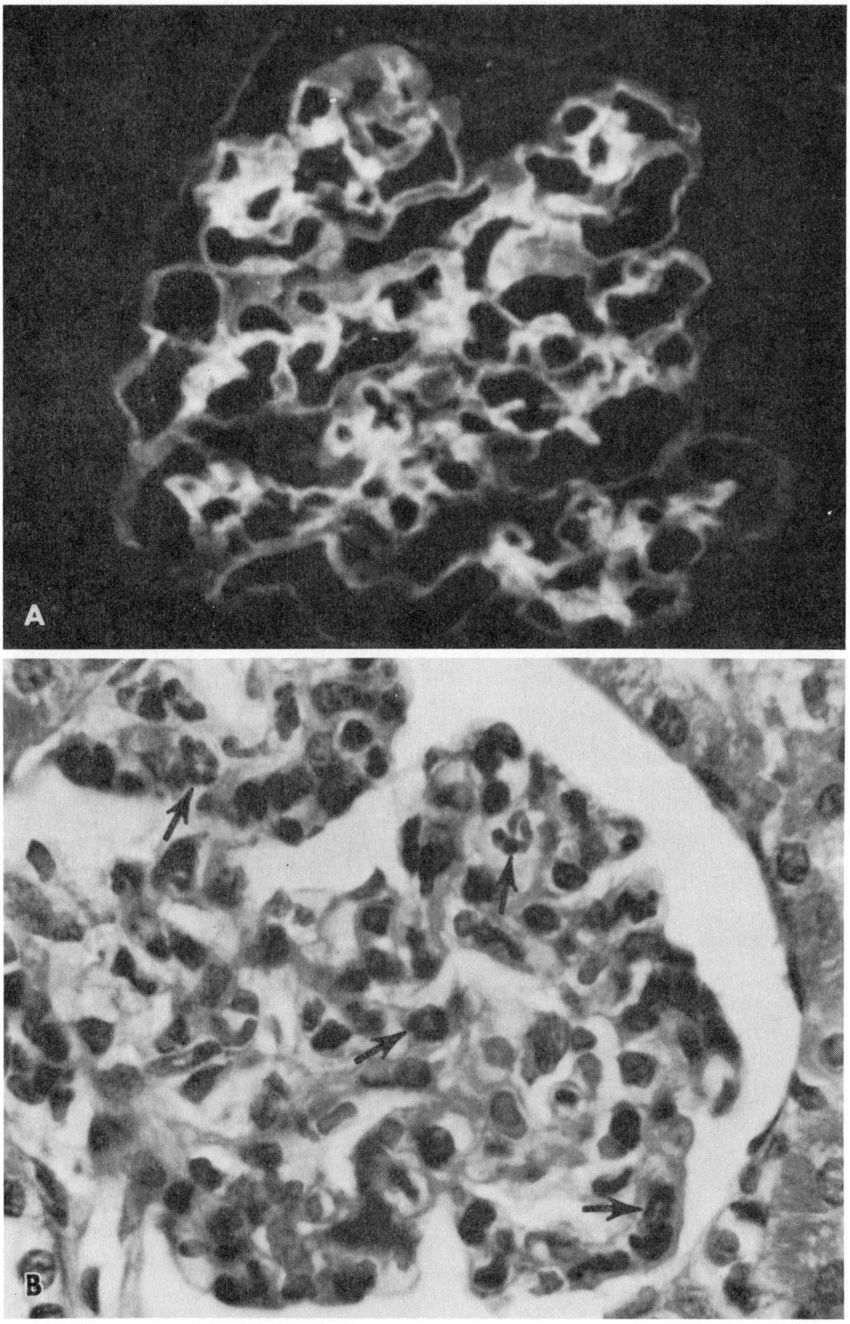

Figure 13–3. Nephrotoxic glomerulonephritis in the rat. The sections were taken two hours after injection of rabbit antirat glomerular basement membrane antiserum. *A,* Section stained for the presence of rabbit IgG with fluorescent antibody. The IgG can be seen lying in a *linear* fashion along the glomerular basement membrane. Staining for rat C3 revealed a similar pattern of fluorescence. ×850. *B,* Section stained with hematoxylin and eosin. Neutrophils are filling the capillary loops *(arrows).* ×1000.

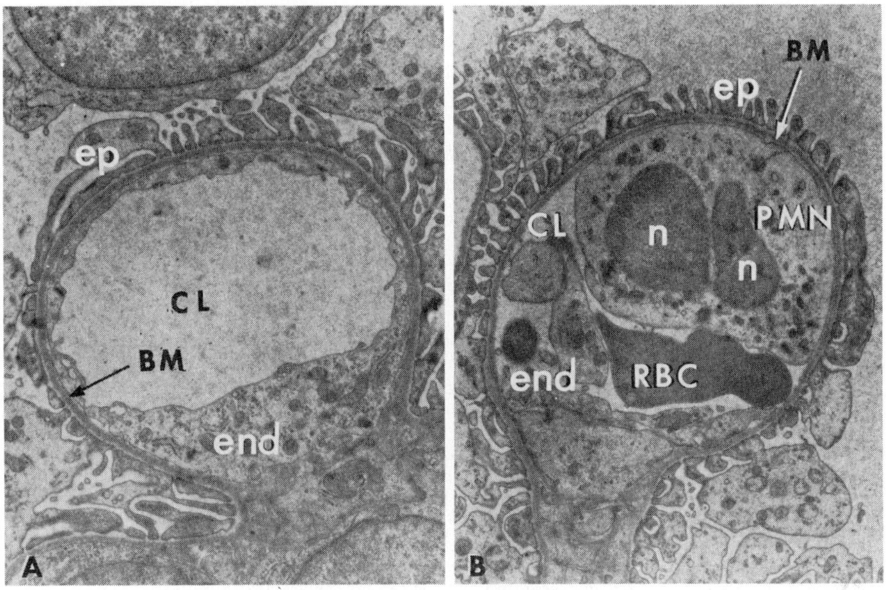

Figure 13–4. Electron photomicrograph of glomerular capillary loops in nephrotoxic nephritis. *A*, Neutrophil infiltration has not occurred and the endothelial cell (end) is spread normally over the basement membrane (BM). *B*, A neutrophil has pushed aside the endothelial cell and is closely adherent to the denuded basement membrane. CL: Capillary lumen; ep: epithelial cell. ×7000. (From Cochrane, C. G., Unanue, E. L., and Dixon, F. J.: A role of polymorphonuclear leukocytes and complement in nephrotoxic nephritis. J. Exp. Med., *122*:99, 1965.)

Sections of kidneys from patients with these diseases often show a linear fluorescence along the basement membrane. Moreover, the fact that antihuman GBM can be eluted from such kidneys and can induce nephritis if transferred to monkeys suggests that this antibody may have a possible pathogenetic role. Patients with this type of antibody in their glomeruli who are given kidney homografts often develop glomerulonephritis in the transplanted kidney as well.

AUTOIMMUNE ANTITISSUE ANTIBODIES

Antibodies against various tissues have been described in human autoimmune diseases (Chapter 20C). Indeed, their detection by immunofluorescence has generally been the only indication that the disease is related to autoimmunity. Unfortunately, there is little evidence available in man to determine whether the antibodies actually cause the damage or are the result of it. Where complement-fixing antibodies that can react with the surface of cells in the body are present, destruction of cells can occur. This may be most clearly seen in autoimmune hemolytic anemia. Activation of the entire cytolytic sequence of complement components results in lysis of the erythrocytes, and in addition, they may be engulfed by phagocytes reacting with the C3b fixed to their surfaces. In a similar way, idiopathic thrombocytopenic purpura may result from the presence of antiplatelet antibodies. The possible nature of the abnormality that leads to the production of these antibodies is described in Chapter 20C.

ANTIRECEPTOR ANTIBODIES

A third mechanism by which antibodies can affect cells directly is by reaction against specific receptors on the cell. A number of human diseases may result from this type of process. The classic example is myasthenia gravis, in which autoantibodies develop against the acetylcholine receptor and interfere with its function. However, even here it seems likely that the mechanism of interference, as often as not, involves complement and perhaps other effector mechanisms. That is, they too represent another example of the potentially injurious effects of the formation of immune complexes in tissues.

Injury Produced by Antigen-Antibody Complexes

After antibody has combined with antigen within the body, certain effector mechanisms, such as phagocytosis, eventually result in the elimination of the immune complexes. In some cases, however, the process is accompanied by a variety of inflammatory reactions, known collectively as the *Type III reaction*. Since these pathogenic effects of immune complexes are important contributors to a number of human disease conditions, a considerable amount of experimentation has been directed toward elucidation of the mechanisms involved.

In general, the pathogenesis of injury produced by immune complexes can be divided into four phases: (1) the combination of antibody with antigen to produce the complexes; (2) the localization of these complexes at particular sites in the body (if the complexes were formed in, or liberated into, the blood stream); (3) the accumulation of humoral and cellular factors; and (4) the production of tissue injury. The process can be best understood by first considering the local effects of immune complexes in the skin, the Arthus reaction, and then considering a more complicated systemic immune-complex disease such as serum sickness.

THE ARTHUS REACTION—A TYPICAL IMMUNE COMPLEX–INDUCED INFLAMMATORY REACTION

Injection of antigen into the skin of a sensitized animal results in an edematous, hemorrhagic, and eventually, necrotic lesion, which was first described by Maurice Arthus in 1903. This reaction, known as the Arthus phenomenon, is produced by the combination of precipitating antibody with antigen in the skin and may be elicited in four ways. The *active Arthus reaction* is that originally described, whereby antigen is injected into a previously immunized animal possessing circulating antibodies. The *direct passive Arthus reaction* is identical, except that circulating antibody is supplied passively to a normal recipient by an intravenous injection of antiserum. If the administration is reversed so that antiserum is injected intradermally and antigen intravenously, a *reversed passive Arthus reaction* is produced. Finally, both antibody and antigen can be injected at the same site and, in fact, may even be combined together *in vitro* prior to injection.

Specificity and Type of Antibody. Since the reaction is produced by antigen-antibody combination, its specificity is that of the antibodies produced (active) or administered (passive). A wide variety of antigens and species of animal exhibit the reaction. From 50 to 100 μg of antibody nitrogen is generally required for the reversed passive lesion, and similarly large amounts of circulating antibody are necessary for the direct reaction. The process thus requires an appreciable quantity of immune complexes. The antibodies must also be of a precipitating, complement-fixing type, but for the passive reaction they need not come from the same species of animal.

Morphology. The typical lesion develops rapidly. Local swelling, erythema, and edema appear within an hour, and the lesions become hemorrhagic and increase in intensity over the next few hours (Fig. 13–5). The severity is dependent upon the quantity of antigen and antibody available, and, with large amounts of antigen-antibody complex, necrosis may result. Over the next two days, the reaction gradually diminishes and eventually disappears. The response to a tetanus toxoid injection into the skin of an individual who is already immunized against tetanus is largely of this type.

Microscopically, an acute inflammatory reaction is seen. Retarded blood flow in small vessels is accompanied by leukocyte clumping and diapedesis, with occasional microaggregates of platelets and leukocytes. The strikingly characteristic feature of this lesion,

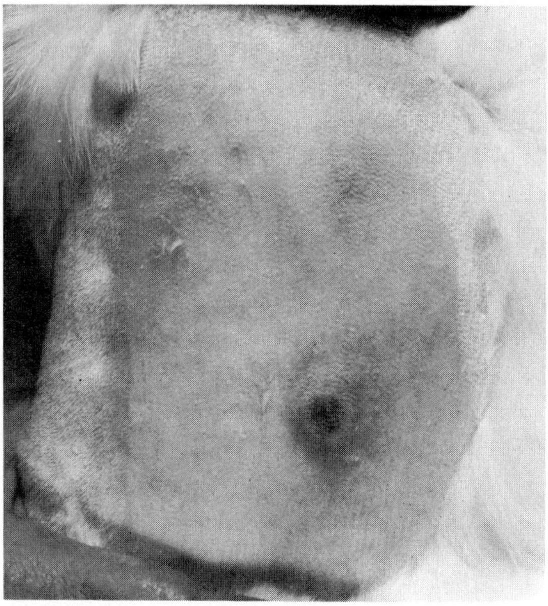

Figure 13–5. Active Arthus reaction in an immunized rabbit eight hours after the intradermal injection of antigen (60 μg N and bovine serum albumin). The edema and central hemorrhagic area are apparent. A control site injected with saline is above the lesion. No reaction can be seen.

however, is the marked accumulation of neutrophils within capillary and venule walls (Fig. 13–6*A*). After about eight hours, there is a gradual infiltration of mononuclear cells, such as lymphocytes, macrophages, endothelial cells, and fibroblasts. By 24 hours, mononuclear elements predominate, and after three to six days plasma cells are seen in islands of lymphoid cells in the perivascular spaces. This transition from acute inflammatory cells (neutrophils, eosinophils) to mononuclear phagocytes is typical of the acute inflammatory reaction, and the same sequence of events can be initiated by bacteria, trauma, and other nonimmunologic triggers.

Pathogenesis. In the active Arthus reaction, antigen such as bovine serum albumin (BSA) is injected into the skin. Circulating antibody meets this antigen at the local blood vessel wall and precipitates with it. In the reversed passive reaction, the process is sim-

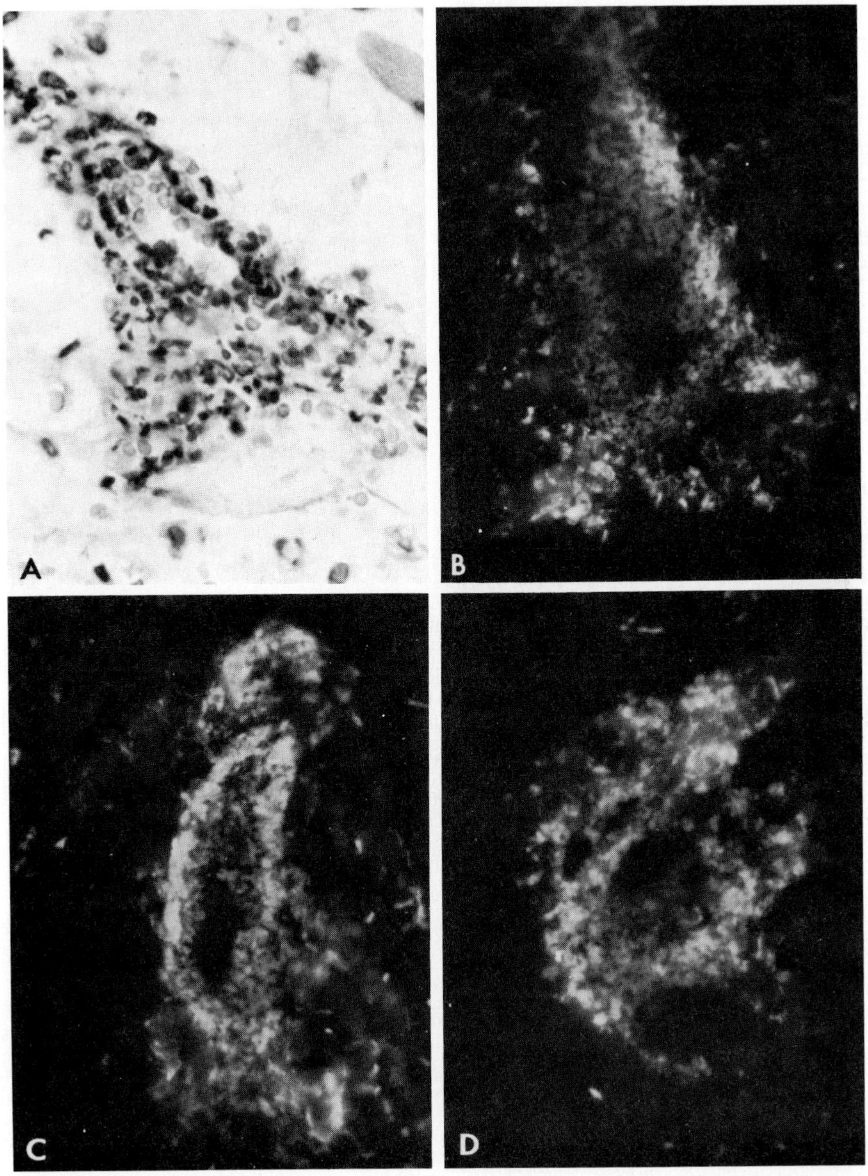

Figure 13–6. Reversed passive Arthus reaction. *A,* Section of a venule taken three hours after the injection of antigen (bovine serum albumin [BSA]) intravenously and antibody (rabbit anti-BSA) intradermally. Large numbers of neutrophils have accumulated in the vessel wall. Edema and extravasated red cells may also be seen. ×250. A section of a similar venule was stained with fluorescent anti-BSA *(B),* antirabbit IgG *(C),* and antirabbit C3 *(D).* Antigen, antibody, and complement may be seen in the vessel walls.

ilar, except that it is the antigen that is circulating. The antigen-antibody complexes have ample opportunity to fix complement, and immunofluorescent techniques show that BSA, antibody (gamma globulin), and complement (C3) are localized within the blood vessel wall at the site of antigen injection (Fig. 13–6*B*, *C*, and *D*).

The formation and localization of the immune complexes do not themselves induce tissue damage. From the characteristic observation of neutrophil infiltration it might be expected that these cells are also involved in the reaction, and indeed, this seems to be the case. Thus, if the reaction is performed in rabbits depleted of circulating neutrophils, immune complexes can be seen within blood vessel walls, but no inflammatory reaction ensues.

The process whereby neutrophils accumulate at the site of immune-complex deposition requires activation of the complement sequence. This conclusion follows the observation that the Arthus reaction may be largely prevented or reduced by depletion of circulating complement components or performing the reaction in mice genetically unable to make C5 (see Fig. 13–7). A likely mechanism for the action of complement in the induction of neutrophil accumulation is the release of chemotactic factors C5a and C5a des arg (C5a from which the C-terminal arginine has been cleaved by tissue and plasma carboxypeptidases) during complement fixation by the immune complexes (Chapter 6). Neutrophils are induced by these C5 fragments to bind to the endothelial cells of the blood vessel and then are presumed to migrate toward the source (highest concentration) of these fragments, i.e., the immune complexes. This process is known as chemotaxis (see below). This process would be augmented by local hemostasis, since the factors would not be carried away by blood flow. Injection of purified C5 fragments into various sites in the body in fact induces exactly the sequence of events observed in the immune complex–induced reaction (Fig. 13–8). This occurs even in the animals deficient in C5 (the precursor for the C5 fragments), which cannot themselves respond to the immune complexes. However, despite the evidence implicating C5 fragments in early leukocyte accumulation in immune-complex reactions, this

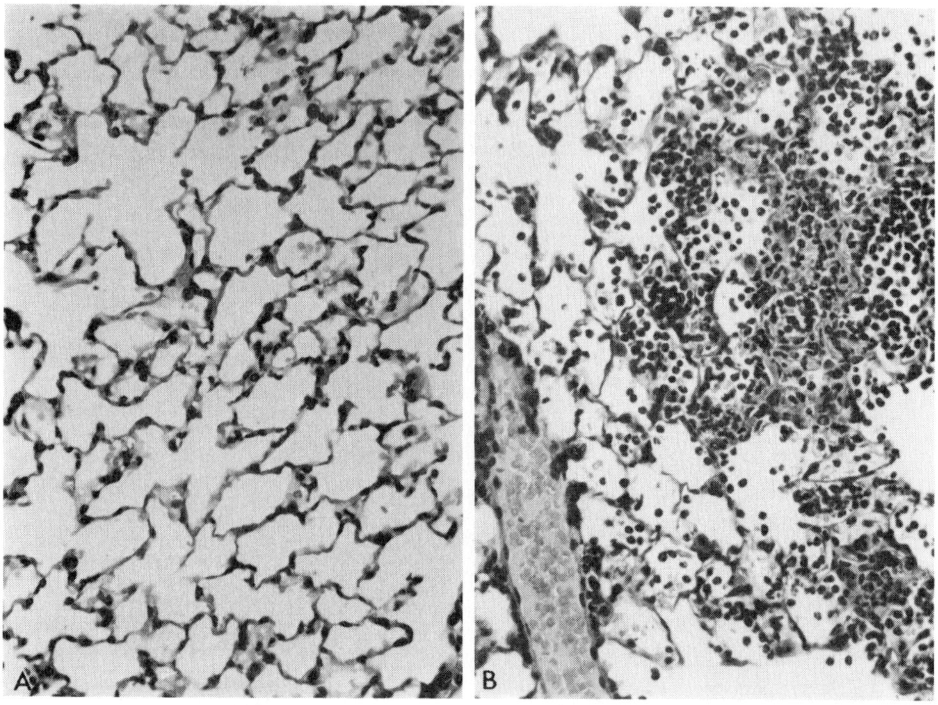

Figure 13–7. The inflammatory effects of immune complexes in the lung are mediated in part by fragments derived from C5. *A*, Lung from a mouse genetically deficient in C5 in which preformed immune complexes were instilled via the airways six hours previously. No inflammation is seen. *B*, Lung from a similarly treated mouse which had normal levels of C5. A severe reaction may be seen, with leukocyte infiltration, edema, and damage to alveolar walls. A dilated blood vessel is also apparent (see text). (Photomicrographs courtesy of Dr. G. Larsen.)

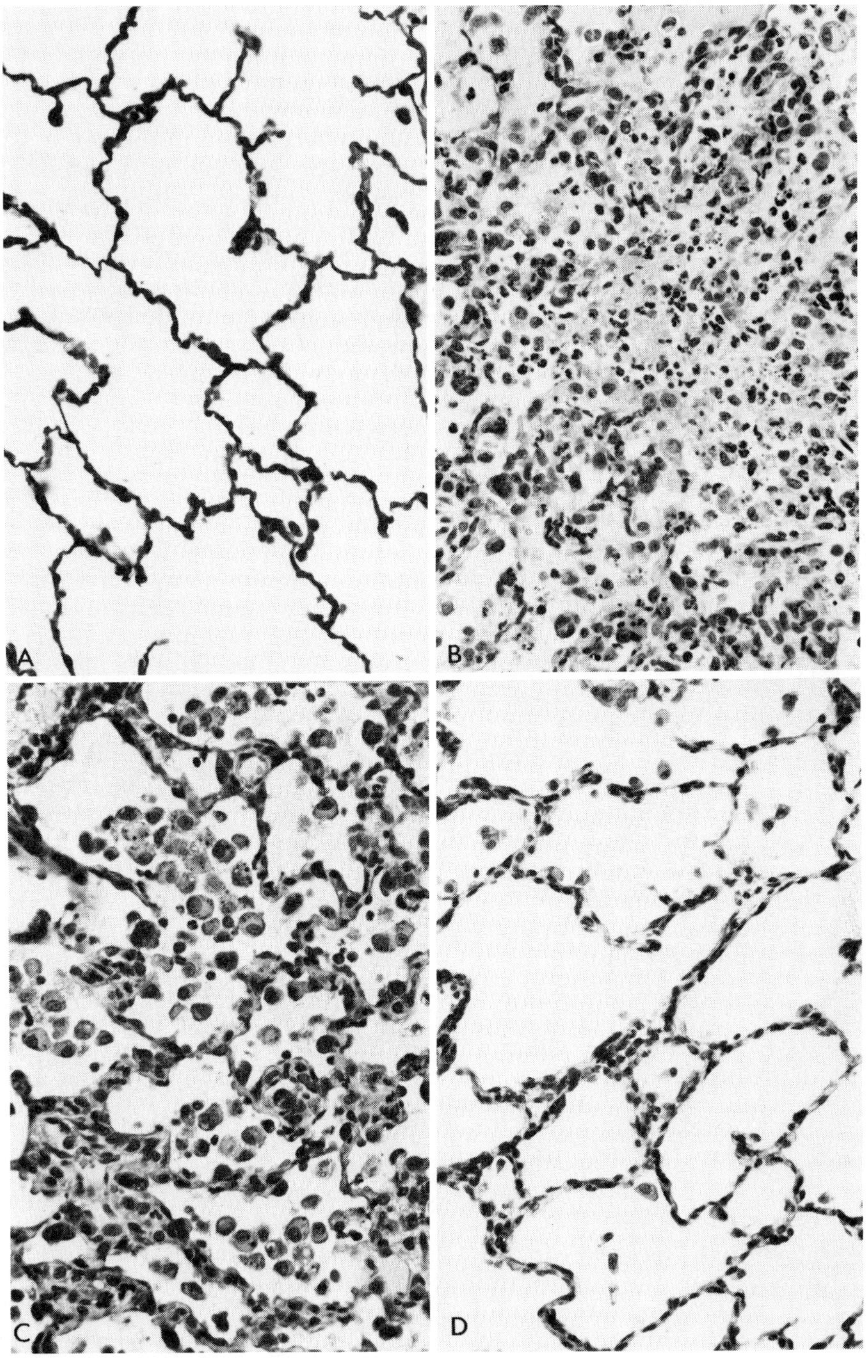

Figure 13–8. Stages in the inflammatory reaction induced in the lung by C5a des-arg. A similar sequence occurs when immune complexes are instilled into the lung, and it is suggested that C5 fragments generated as a result of the immune complexes are responsible in part for the tissue injury seen. *A,* Control lung in which saline was instilled (equivalent to zero time). *B,* Twenty-four hours after instillation of 10 μg C5a des-arg. This is the time at which the granulocyte infiltration is switching to monocyte accumulation. Granulocytes, mononuclear phagocytes (macrophages), and severe edema (increased vascular permeability) may be seen. *C,* After 48 hours the predominant cell type is the macrophage. Some neutrophil debris is still present, and neutrophils have been phagocytosed by the macrophages. *D,* By five days the lung has almost returned to normal histologically and is also functionally normal. (Photomicrographs courtesy of Dr. G. Larsen.)

is certainly not the only mechanism involved. Inflammation is a highly redundant process and alternative (collateral) mechanisms (i.e., different chemotactic factors) can often be operative, though perhaps less efficiently.

Another property of neutrophils, which may be of importance in their accumulation at sites where antigen-antibody complexes are localized, is their ability to adhere to immune reactants. Neutrophils will adhere both to antibody that has combined with antigen and to complement fixed to antigen-antibody complexes. The name "immune adherence" has been given to the latter reaction (Chapter 6), and it is the third component of complement (C3) that is primarily involved (C3 immune adherence). The immune adherence bond is a strong one, and there are many available sites for adherence on the neutrophil. When such cells pass immune complexes in or on a blood vessel wall, they may become adherent and thus localized at this site. Moreover, adherence would be the end result of chemotaxis after the cell has reached the immune complex that is generating the chemotactic factor. Adherence of neutrophils is generally followed by phagocytosis of the immune complexes, and, in the lesions of the Arthus reaction, the neutrophils have engulfed the immune complexes they encounter (Fig. 13–9).

The process described so far has still not accounted for the tissue damage that ensues. However, neutrophils contain a variety of hydrolytic enzymes and other active materials that, if released, could produce the observed effects. Studies of these cells *in vitro* have revealed that they do release some of these materials into the extracellular environment during the process of phagocytosis. Within the neutrophil may be found proteolytic enzymes capable of hydrolyzing collagen, elastic tissue, and cartilage (see below); thus they are capable of destroying basement membrane and other supporting structures. At least some of these enzymes are known to be released and may be implicated in the damage to blood vessel walls, hemorrhage, and necrosis of the immune complex–induced lesions.

Another feature of the lesion is the increased vascular permeability and edema. This may be clearly demonstrated by intravenous injection of Evans blue dye with the antigen or antibody. The increased permeability is also mainly dependent upon the neutrophil accumulation, since depletion of these cells largely prevents it. In the search for the mediators of this effect, neutrophils were found to contain a variety of permeability-increasing factors, in addition to the proteolytic enzymes. Four small basic proteins have been described that are released from neutrophil granules and induce vascular permeability when injected into the skin. In addition, the release of oxygen radicals (see below) from neutrophils (and other inflammatory cells) can cause changes in endothelial cells that permit the passage of plasma proteins. Whether this necessarily represents *damage* to the endothelial cells is a subject of debate. Certainly, oxygen radicals can kill these (and other) cells. However, permeability increases are often transient and may be considered to be an important physiologic component of the protective aspects of inflammatory reactions. They allow the influx of a battery of inhibitors of the injurious processes. Release of vasoactive amines from mast cells may play a supportive role in the initiation of some immune complex–induced reactions, as in some delayed hypersensitivity reactions also. However, the major component of the permeability increase is not due to vasoactive amines.

An influx of neutrophils in the Arthus reaction is thus the primary factor responsible for the observed tissue damage. However, not all the results of the accumulation are harmful. The cells phagocytose and digest the immune complexes that induced the reaction. Later, there is a change in cell population from granulocytes to mononuclear cells (monocytes) in the lesion (Fig. 13–10). In immune complex–induced inflammatory reactions in the lung the prior accumulation of neutrophils is apparently necessary for the emigration of monocytes, although the nature of the monocyte-directed chemotactic factors is not yet known. An attractive possibility is that degradative fragments of connective tissue proteins (including fibronectin) are specifically attractive for monocytes. This would explain the neutrophil requirement (tissue destruction by neutrophil proteases) and would provide a general mechanism for the attraction of monocytes to the site of injury.

The monocytes mature in the tissues into macrophages (Fig. 13–10). In a self-limiting inflammatory reaction such as the Arthus reaction, these cells act to clean up the mess. They phagocytize remaining neutrophils and tissue debris, and can also take up by pinocytosis many of the degradative enzymes that have been released at the site of injury. Of

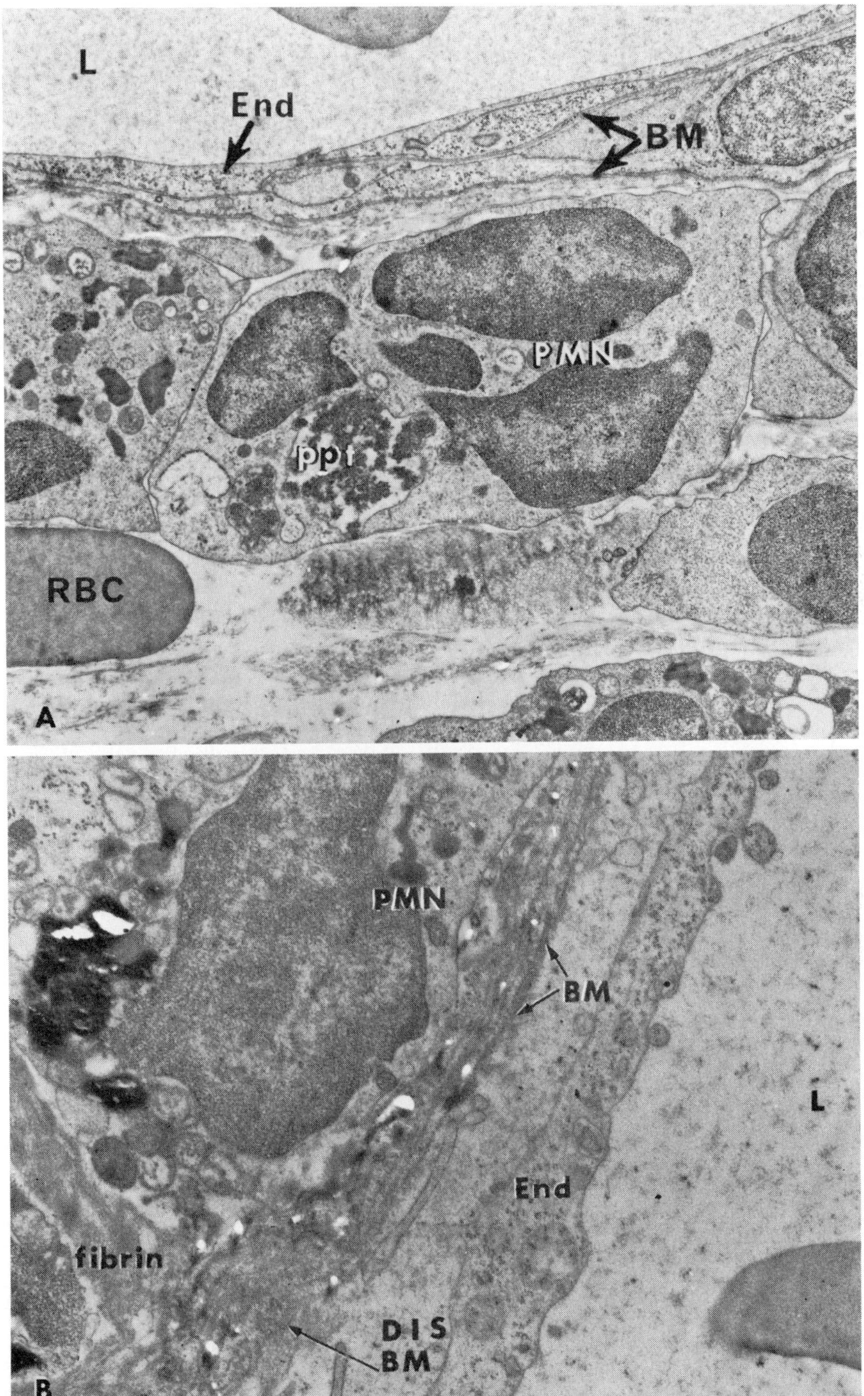

Figure 13–9. Electron photomicrograph of Arthus reactions in the rabbit bladder wall. *A,* Ferritin was used as the antigen. Immune complexes of this electron-opaque material and antibody (ppt) may be seen in the vessel wall and within phagocytic vacuoles of neutrophils that have accumulated at this site. This is an early lesion and little basement membrane damage is apparent, although an extravasated red cell is present. *B,* At a slightly later stage, dissolution of the basement membrane (dis BM) can be seen and fibrin has been deposited. PMN: neutrophil; BM: basement membrane; L: vessel lumen; End: endothelial cell. ×10,500.

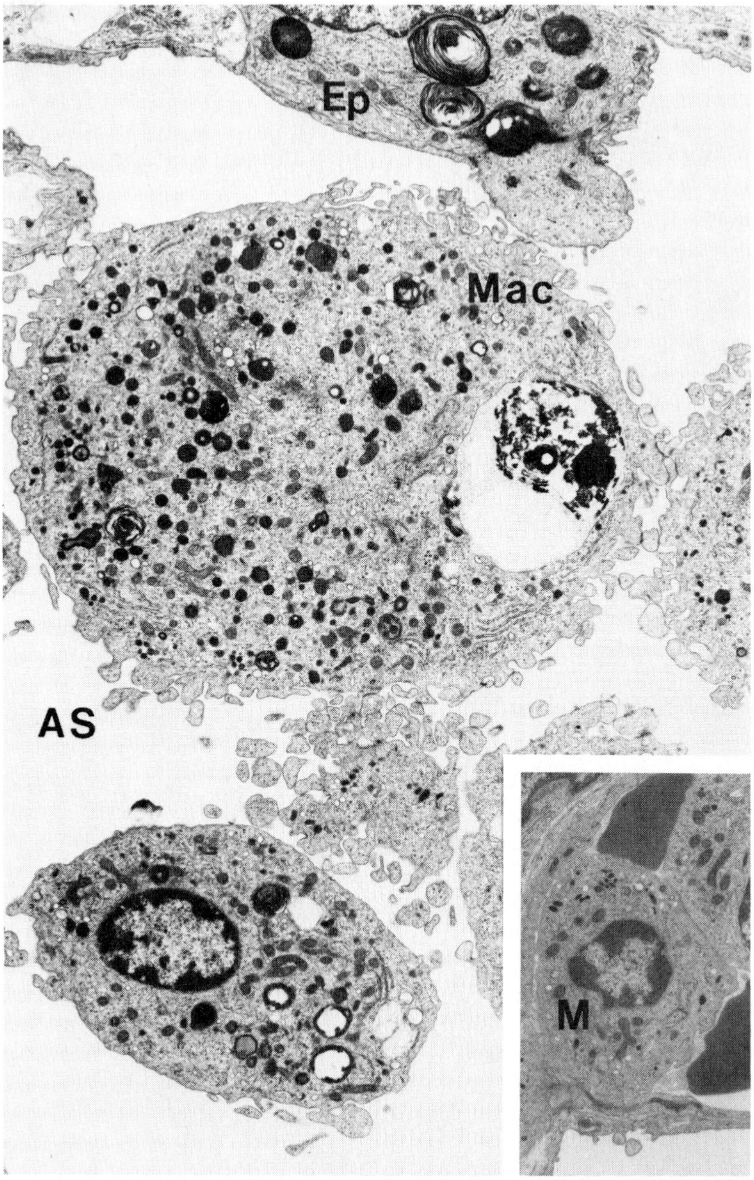

Figure 13–10. Maturation of monocytes into macrophages in inflammatory sites. *Insert,* Electron micrograph of monocytes in the alveolar wall of a rabbit lung 24 hours after the initiation of an inflammatory reaction. These cells are in the capillary lumen and interstitium and may be presumed to be migrating out of the vessels. They have a high nucleus-to-cytoplasm ratio and contain only a few primary lysosomes. ×5700. *Main photomicrograph,* Mature macrophages in an alveolus from a similar animal, taken 48 hours after initiation of the lesion. These cells have abundant cytoplasm with many secondary lysosomes and phagocytosed debris. M: Monocyte in a capillary; Mac: macrophages in alveloar air space; Ep: epithelial cell; AS: air space. ×5700.

great importance is the recent recognition of the reparative properties of these cells. They secrete growth factors for a number of cells, including fibroblasts and endothelial cells. (The fibroblast-stimulating factor may be related to interleukin; see Chapter 9.) Such factors may promote repair, although it should be noted that whereas fibrotic reactions in the skin may be important in healing by "first intention," in many other sites in the body they severely and permanently impair tissue function.

The implication that macrophages are involved only in removal and repair is, however, to seriously underplay the potential for these cells to participate in all aspects of immunologic injury. Thus, phagocytosis of immune complexes by macrophages stimulates the release of potent chemotactic factors for neutrophils and can *initiate* the whole inflammatory sequence. This may be particularly important in the case of surveillance macrophages found normally, for example, in the lung. Macrophages can also cause extensive tissue damage (remodeling) themselves, being possessed of the capability of secreting their own battery of proteases. These Jekyll and Hyde properties seem to be related to the environment (and stimuli) the cell is exposed to in the inflammatory lesion.

This relatively simple immune complex–induced injury, which is largely dependent on neutrophils, may, at times, be confused with superimposed processes of different pathogeneses. Thus, the presence of homocytotropic antibody in the skin may contribute to an immediate histamine-mediated increase in vascular permeability. Such antibody usually requires a latent period in the skin for maximal activity when given passively, but may be present in an actively immunized animal. The characteristic feature of this immediate hypersensitivity reaction is its onset within minutes of intravenous antigen administration, as compared with the Arthus reaction, which develops more slowly. After the Arthus reaction has occurred in suitably sensitized animals, a delayed hypersensitivity lesion may follow. This reaction is characterized by its delay in onset and by the type of cells (mononuclear) involved.

SERUM SICKNESS (ACUTE GENERALIZED IMMUNE COMPLEX DISEASE)

Following the injection of foreign serum to humans, a number of unpleasant side effects are known to occur. The disease, which came to be known as serum sickness, can result in vascular, cardiac, renal, cutaneous, and joint lesions. Evidence has accumulated that the immune complexes formed when antibodies are produced against the foreign serum proteins are the cause of the tissue damage. Other antigens may induce disease by a similar process, i.e., following combination with specific antibody in the blood stream. Such antigens include bacterial, viral, and even autologous materials, which may for a variety of reasons be recognized as foreign.

The Arthus reaction follows the formation of antigen-antibody complexes locally. Immune complexes formed in the blood stream produce a more generalized effect and can induce tissue injury in a variety of target organs, depending upon where they become localized. The pathogenesis of these lesions therefore includes mechanisms of deposition of immune complexes, as well as their subsequent effect on the tissues.

A description of the pathogenesis of experimentally induced acute serum sickness in rabbits will serve to indicate some of the factors and mechanisms involved in the production of tissue injury by circulating immune complexes. An antigen, bovine serum albumin (BSA), is given as a single large intravenous injection (250 mg per kilogram). Following an initial equilibration with the extravascular space, the BSA is for a time catabolized at the same rate as rabbit albumin. Production of antibody to the BSA then causes an increased clearance rate and, at this time, complexes between antigen and antibody can be detected in the blood.

Concurrent with the formation and circulation of the immune complexes is the appearance of the characteristic lesions, such as glomerulonephritis and arteritis. (In fact, immune complexes may deposit at many sites in the vasculature and there cause injury.) Sections of the kidney (Fig. 13–11) reveal that the capillaries in the glomeruli have been almost completely occluded, mainly because of proliferation of the endothelial cells (proliferative glomerulonephritis). Neutrophil accumulation is not a characteristic feature of this acute immune-complex disease nephritis. Figure 13–12 shows a section of a coronary artery, which is a common site for this lesion. Endothelial proliferation or accumulation of mononuclear cells, or both, is apparent. In addition, and in contrast to the glomerular lesions, neutrophil accumulation is marked. Damage to the internal elastic lamina, penetration of neutrophils into the media, and medial necrosis are seen.

Pathogenesis. The immune complexes are deposited in the blood vessels at the site of the lesions. Immunofluorescent techniques demonstrate this clearly in the kidney, where, by use of suitable antisera, BSA, rabbit immunoglobulin, and rabbit complement can be detected in a characteristically granular pattern (Fig. 13–11*A*). Deposited complexes have also been demonstrated in the arteries, although the presence of neutrophils soon results in their phagocytosis and digestion.

Deposition of Circulating Immune Complexes in Blood Vessel Walls. The deposition of circulating immune complexes in blood vessel walls is an intricate process. Earlier studies with inhibitors of vasopermeability-inducing agents, such as antihistamines and antiserotonins, suggested that local increases in vascular permeability caused trapping of circulating complexes of appropriate sizes at the filtering basal laminae of the vessels. IgE antibody and the mediators of acute allergic vasopermeability (see above) were apparently involved in this deposition process. More recently, a series of additional factors have been suggested, particularly in the case of chronic immune complex diseases (see below). Of great interest is the possibility that a positive charge on the immune com-

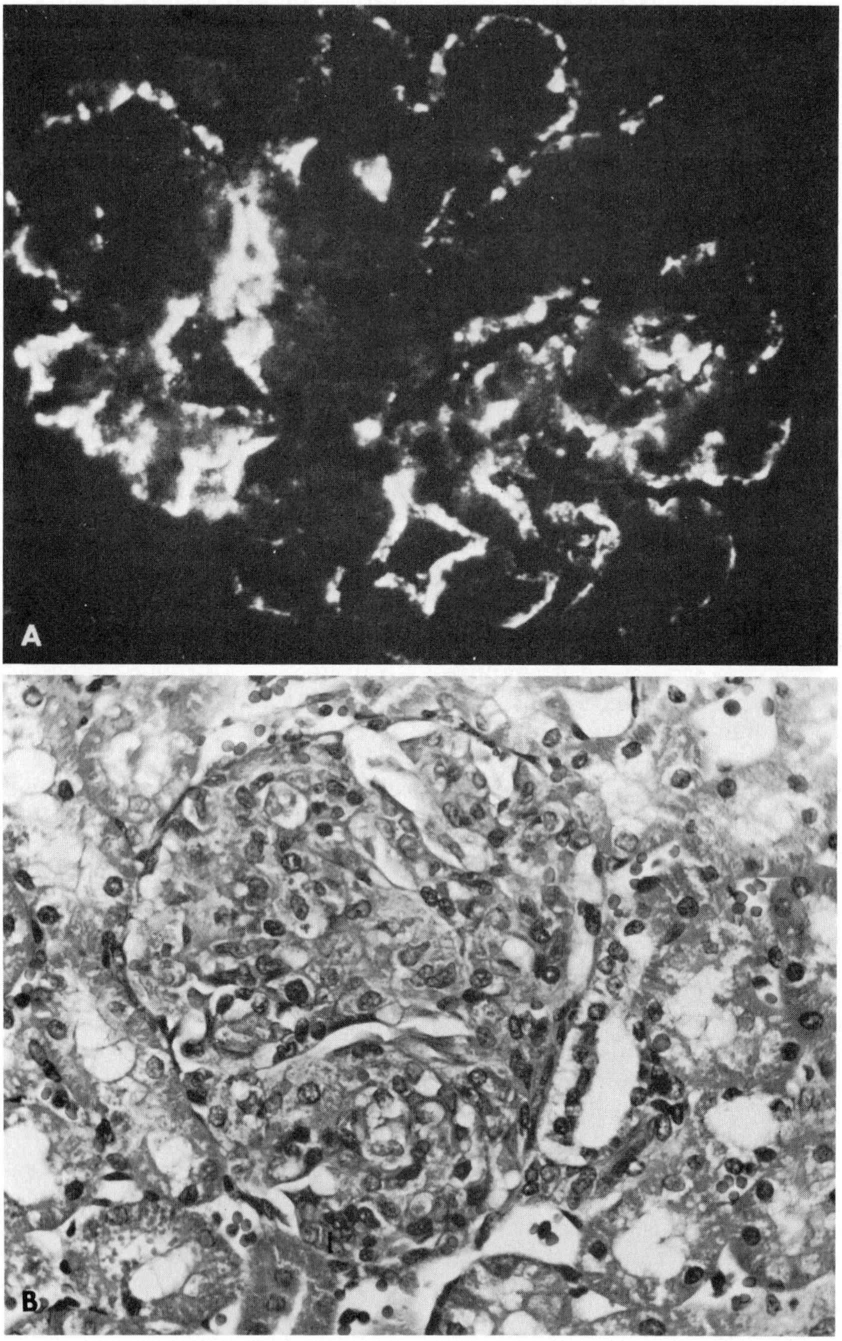

Figure 13–11. Kidney sections from a rabbit with acute immune-complex disease. *A,* Glomerulus showing staining with fluorescent antirabbit IgG in *granular* deposits along the basement membrane. Fluorescent antisera against the antigen (BSA) and rabbit C3 give a similar pattern of fluorescence. *B,* Hematoxylin and eosin–stained section. There is great proliferation of cells in the glomerulus, and the capillary lumens have been occluded. Neutrophils cannot be seen. ×300.

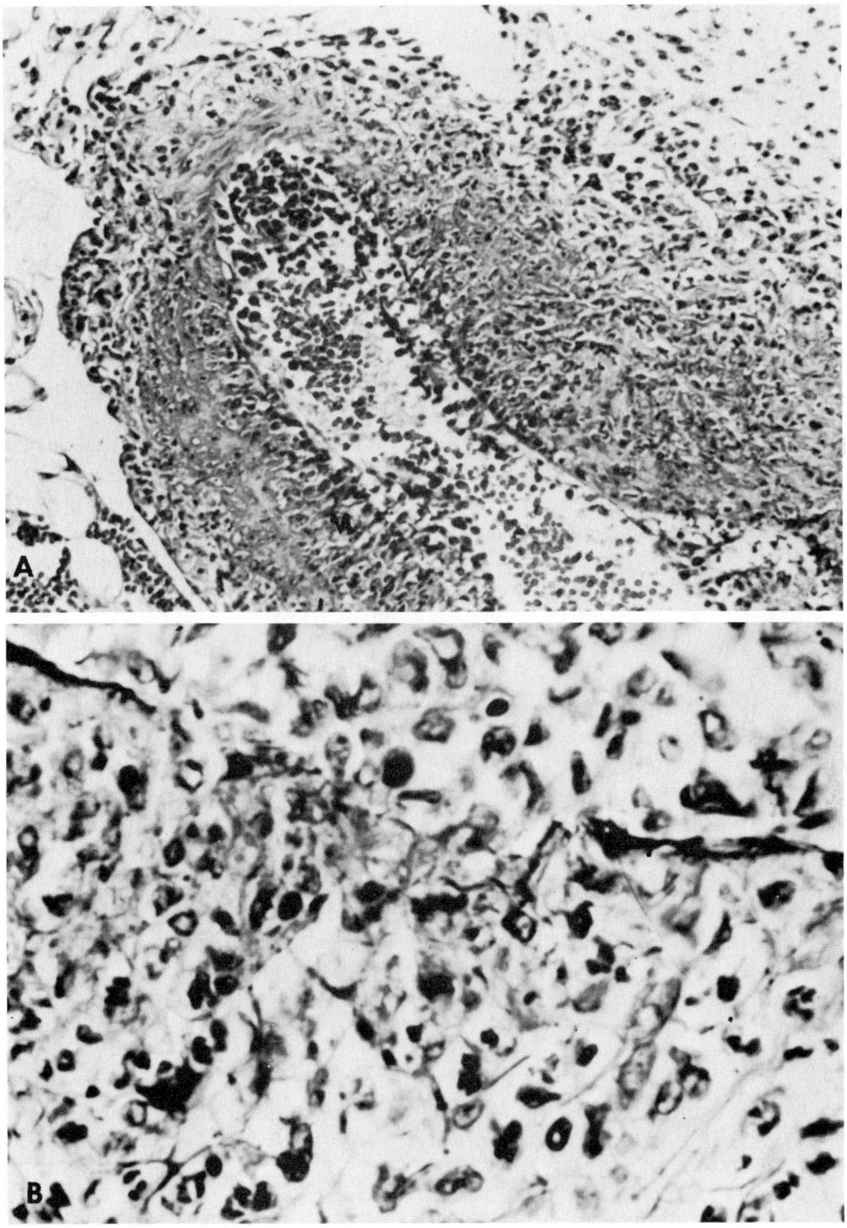

Figure 13–12. Arteritis in acute immune-complex disease in rabbits. *A*, Neutrophil accumulation, intimal proliferation, and early medial necrosis are present. ×200. *B*, Higher power showing breaks in the internal elastic lamina and penetration of neutrophils into the media. The lumen is toward the top.

plexes may contribute to trapping or negatively charge vessel wall components.

Production of Tissue Injury. For reasons that are not clear, the glomerular lesions in acute immune-complex disease are relatively free of neutrophils. Unlike the case in nephrotoxic nephritis, depletion of neutrophils or complement does not prevent the glomerulonephritis. The mechanism by which deposited immune complexes induce endothelial cell proliferation, increased glomerular permeability, and subsequent proteinuria is unknown.

The arteritis lesions, on the other hand, appear to be neutrophil-mediated. As with the Arthus reaction, neutrophil or C3 depletion prevents neutrophil accumulation and tissue damage, although complexes are still deposited and some endothelial changes occur. Following neutrophil accumulation, damage to the internal elastic lamina occurs, probably the result of released neutrophil elastase. The cells may then penetrate into the media and perpetuate their injurious action there. Similarities to the Arthus reaction are apparent. The lesions generally heal within a few days after disappearance of the immune complexes. Table 13–3 compares glomerulonephritis induced by antiglomerular basement membrane antiserum with that caused by circulating immune complexes.

Systemic Immune-Complex Disease (Serum Sickness) in Man. Administration of large amounts of foreign serum to humans results in a disease process identical to that in rabbits. At the time when antibodies are first formed, they complex with circulating antigen and produce the serum sickness syndrome. Manifestations of this immune-complex disease include fever, enlarged lymph nodes, erythematous rashes, painful joints, and vascular inflammatory reactions. The clinical details of serum sickness in man are described in Chapter 20A. Evidence for a similar pathogenesis of deposition of immune complexes in blood vessels in man comes from studies of leukocytoclastic angiitis. Injection of histamine into normal areas of skin in an individual with an attack of this disease results in localization of gamma globulin and complement and the development of tissue injury (Chapter 20).

Chronic Immune-Complex Disease. The acute immune-complex disease is transient and disappears when no more complexes circulate. However, some diseases of man that may be mediated by immune complexes are chronic and persistent, including lupus erythematosus.

Daily injections of antigen to experimental animals (e.g., rabbit) can result in a chronic immune-complex disease model. Glomerulonephritis develops after 1 to 14 weeks of continued insult by the circulating complexes. Histologically, the appearance is one of membranous glomerulonephritis (Fig. 13–13*B*). Basement membranes are thickened, but there is less endothelial cell swelling and proliferation found in the glomeruli in chronic serum sickness. After more prolonged insult, proliferation, crescent formation, adhesions, and scarring may occur.

Antigen, antibody, and complement may be detected by fluorescence in these glomeruli and are distributed in a lumpy, irregular fashion, indicating that immune complexes are again deposited in the kidney (Fig. 13–13*A*). Electron microscopic examination of sections of glomeruli reveals electron-dense masses (immune complexes) on the epithelial side of the basement membrane.

Pathogenesis. The deposition of immunologic reactants in the glomerulus in this type of lesion (and thus presumably in man) seems

Table 13–3. A Comparison of the Glomerulonephritis in Immune-Complex Disease and Nephrotoxic Nephritis

	Glomerulonephritis	
	Nephrotoxic Nephritis	Acute Immune-Complex Disease
Antibodies	Directed against the glomerular basement membrane	Directed against circulating antigens (immune complexes are deposited in glomeruli secondarily)
Fluorescence	Linear (IgG, complement)	Granular (antigen, IgG, complement)
Histology	Neutrophil accumulation	Proliferative glomerulonephritis
Complement and neutrophils	Generally required for injury	Not required for injury (in contrast to the vasculitis of this disease)

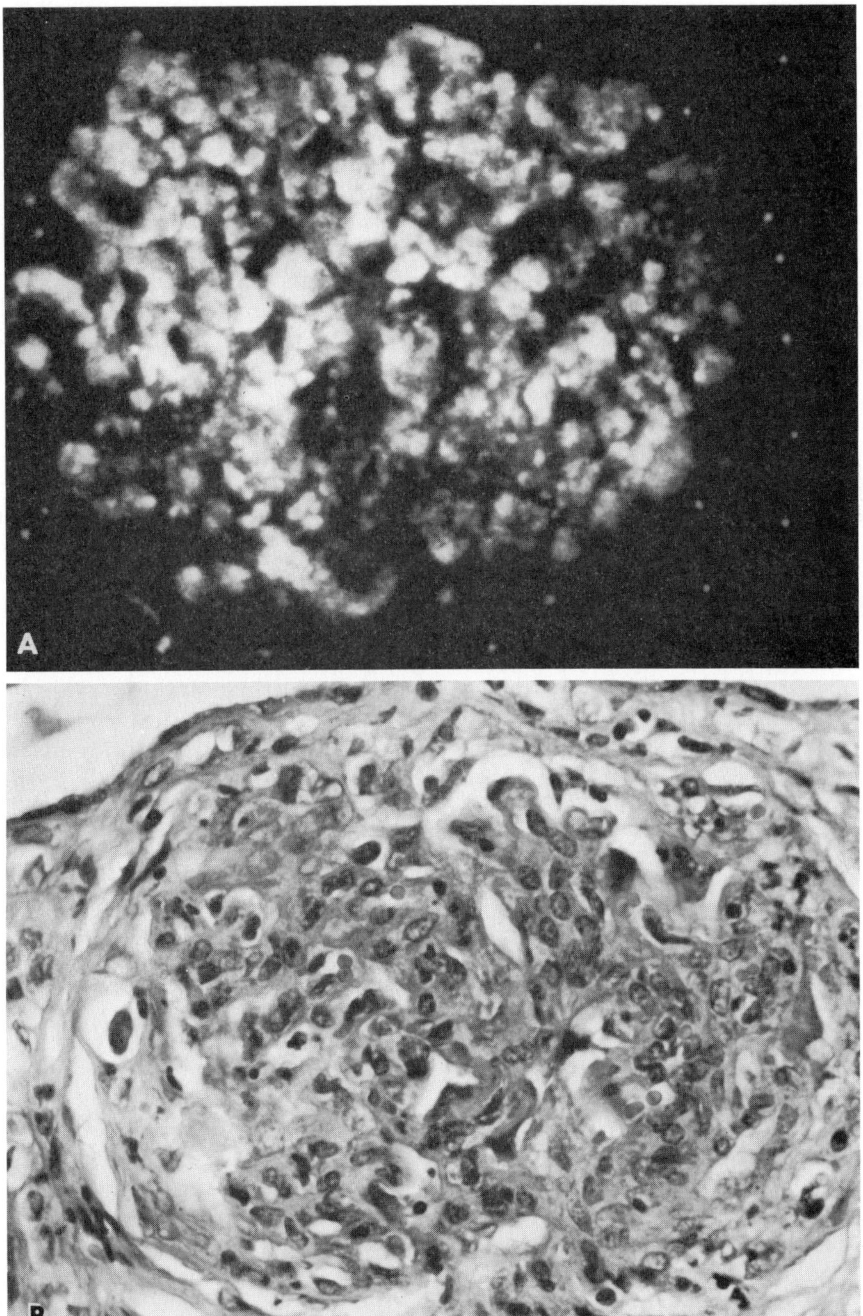

Figure 13–13. Kidney sections from a rabbit having immune complexes circulating for several months as a result of daily injections of antigen (chronic immune-complex disease). *A*, Coarsely granular fluorescent staining of the glomerulus due to deposited antigen (or rabbit IgG or C3) demonstrated with fluorescent anti-BSA antiserum. *B*, The glomerulus shows proliferation of cells, obliteration of capillaries with crescent, and adhesion formation.

to involve a different process from that outlined above. Although circulating immune complexes can be detected, the accumulation process probably involves a formation *in situ.* Antigen (for example, DNA in systemic lupus erythematosus) may become fixed to the basement membrane, and then antibody, or immune complexes, gradually become bound to this antigen and then to the growing immune complex. Whether the same types of processes are involved in formation of complexes in other sites (e.g., the lung) in SLE is not known. The pathogenesis of chronic immune-complex disease is less well understood than that of the acute form. Complex localization may initially follow processes similar to those seen in the acute disease, but once initial deposition has occurred it is self-perpetuating. For reasons that are not clear, vascular and joint lesions are an uncommon finding. The high rate of blood flow through the glomerulus and its filtering action may predispose this structure to injury by continuously ciculating complexes.

Glomerulonephritis Produced by Immune Complexes in Man and in Animals. Considerable emphasis has recently been placed on immune complexes as being involved in a large number of immunologically mediated diseases in man (Chapter 20). However, it should be noted that a causative role for these immune complexes in the pathogenesis of the disease has not been demonstrated. In few cases is the antigen within the complex known. Nevertheless, when the characteristic granular deposits of immunoglobulin and complement are found in sections of glomeruli of patients, an etiology involving immune complexes is suggested. In some cases, however, a knowledge of the antigen is available. A number of groups of possible antigens involved in these processes are listed below.

Autoantigens. In systemic lupus erythematosus in man and in the autoimmune disease of New Zealand black (NZB) and New Zealand white (NZW) hybrid mice, antinuclear antibodies are found in the serum. Glomerulonephritis in these conditions has been shown to be related to immune complexes of DNA and anti-DNA. Immunoglobulin and complement can be detected in the glomeruli by immunofluorescent techniques. Moreover, elution of the kidneys or lungs reveals the presence of nuclear antigens and antibody in the eluates.

Viral Antigens. Chronic infection with certain viruses results in a situation in which virus persists in an animal for a long period of time. Antibodies to the virus that are produced can thus precipitate with it and induce a chronic glomerulonephritis. Examples in animal systems include lymphocytic choriomeningitis (LCM) virus in mice and Aleutian disease in mink. There have been preliminary reports of virus-like particles observed in the kidney biopsies of patients with lupus erythematosus.

Bacterial Antigens. Poststreptococcal glomerulonephritis in man may be an example of deposition of complexes with bacterial antigens inducing immune complex nephritis (Fig. 13–14).

Cross-Reacting Antigens. Body constituents that normally circulate in small amounts in the blood may be involved in immune-complex nephritis. Experimentally, rats injected with rat-kidney homogenates produce an antibody that cross-reacts with normal kidney tubular antigens circulating in low levels. The immune complexes thus formed become deposited in the kidneys and induce a glomerulonephritis that is due to the complexes and is quite unrelated to the source of the antigen. It is possible that exposure to environmental (e.g., bacterial) antigens cross reacting with antigens within the body may produce a similar type of disease.

MEDIATORS OF IMMUNE COMPLEX–INDUCED INFLAMMATORY REACTIONS

The mediators of the tissue injury that is caused by antigen-antibody complexes probably include all those listed earlier as being involved in immediate hypersensitivity reactions (Fig. 13–2). However, the relative contributions of each molecule are different in these slower and more prolonged reactions. For example, antihistamines do not block the Arthus reaction even though a number of lines of evidence have suggested that for optimal reactions, a component of immediate-type hypersensitivity is involved. In addition, however, we need to invoke a number of other molecules, including the C5 fragments mentioned above. Unfortunately, these are generally not as well characterized as the mediators described in Figure 13–2.

C5a and C5a des arg. The origin of these fragments of C5 is described in Chapter 6. *In vitro,* C5a is the more potent molecule,

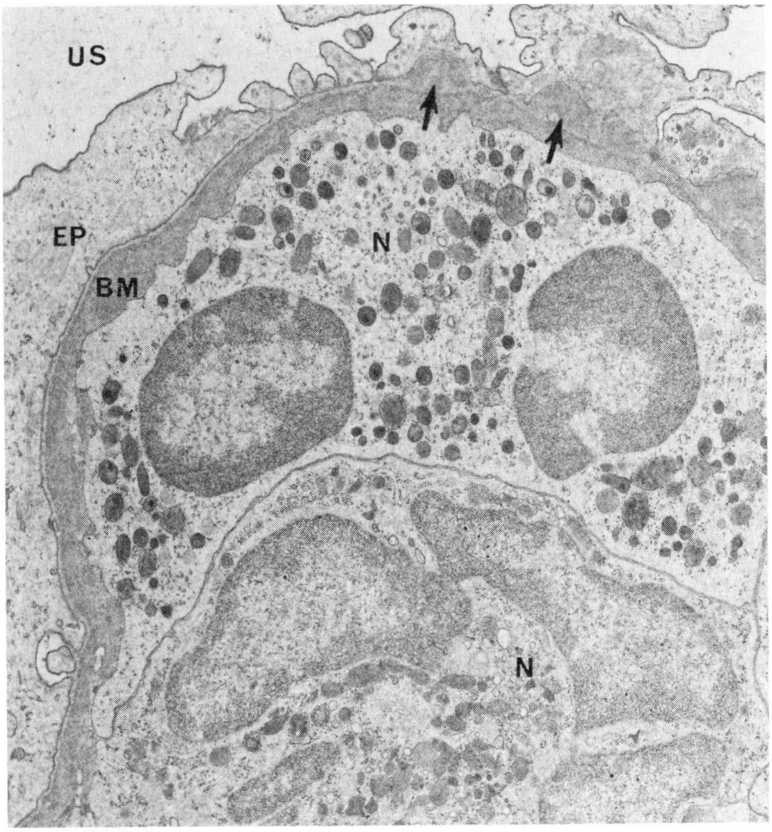

Figure 13–14. Electron photomicrograph of a glomerulus from a case of poststreptococcal glomerulonephritis in man. Neutrophils (N) fill the capillary lumen and push the endothelial cell away from the basement membrane (BM). Deposits *(arrows)* can be seen along the basement membrane and human IgG and C3 could be detected in a granular distribution along the basement membrane with fluorescent antisera. EP: epithelial cell; US: urinary space. (Courtesy of Dr. J. D. Feldman.)

inducing contraction of smooth muscle and stimulation of neutrophil functions such as chemotaxis, secretion, and production of oxygen radicals (see below). *In vivo,* however, C5a des arg (i.e., C5a with the C-terminal argine removed) appears more potent at inducing inflammation (see Fig. 13–9). These molecules also induce increased vascular permeability in the skin (and lung), apparently by mechanisms involving neutrophils and vasodilator prostaglandins (see Fig. 13–2).

In the case of molecules such as C5a, the possibility that the observed effects *in vivo* are in fact mediated indirectly must always be considered. C5a causes release of histamine from mast cells, and the smooth muscle contraction may depend in part on release from mast cells within the muscle. Part of the contractile effect also appears to be mediated by release of leukotrienes C and D (Fig. 13–2), and finally, there may also be a direct effect of C5a on smooth muscle cells. C5 fragments can also stimulate macrophages—providing another indirect pathway into the inflammatory response.

Prostaglandins. These have been mentioned earlier. At high concentrations, PGE_2 and PGI_2 (and the nonmammalian prostaglandin PGE_1) are inhibitory to various cells involved in the inflammatory response. Such molecules are thought to modulate the functions of a number of cells *in vivo*—for example, PGI_2 is produced by normal endothelial cells and renders the blood vessel surface nonthrombogenic by inhibiting platelet activation. By contrast, these same prostaglandins (at lower concentrations and in different circumstances) enhance the emigration of neutrophils and the induction of vascular permeability. A delicate balance is implied, which can be tipped one way or another to *induce* or perhaps also to *suppress* the injurious consequences of immune-complex formation.

Oxygen Radicals. These are discussed in more detail below. While not considered strictly as "mediators" in the same class with those mentioned above, they are of key importance in tissue damage due to immune complexes.

Vasopermeability Factors. An understanding of the exact mechanisms by which increased vascular permeability occurs in immune complex–induced inflammation is still elusive. Granulocyte-derived oxygen radicals and cationic proteins represent prime candidates at present, but a number of other molecules have been suggested to participate, including the vasoactive peptide angiotensin II and PAF.

Chemotactic Factors. A number of these have already been mentioned. The attraction of cells to the sites of immune-complex formation is a key component of the injurious process. A vast array of molecules have been shown to exert chemotactic influence *in vitro* on neutrophils, and the number described for eosinophils and monocytes is steadily growing. *In vivo,* however, the clear-cut demonstration of involvement of these factors in a real-life inflammatory response is usually lacking. From the point of view of potency, availability, and likelihood to be generated as a result of immune-complex formation, the following may be considered of key interest at present: for neutrophils—C5 fragments, leukotriene B_4, a macrophage-derived 10,000 molecular weight peptide, a specific lymphokine, and a high molecular weight protein from mast cells (neutrophil chemotactic factor or NCF); for eosinophils—ECFs and a specific lymphokine; for monocytes—C5 fragments, aspecific lymphokine, and products of connective tissue degradation. Final characterization of many of these molecules remains to be carried out.

Delayed Hypersensitivity

Delayed hypersensitivity is a manifestation of what has come to be called cellular or cell-mediated immunity. The principles underlying this phenomenon have been described in a previous chapter (Chapter 9). Delayed hypersensitivity may be defined as an increased reactivity to specific antigens mediated not by antibodies but by T-cells. This phenomenon was first observed in 1801 by Jenner in connection with cowpox reinoculation and was later developed by Koch and von Pirquet into a test for tuberculosis. The reaction in the skin that follows intradermal injection of antigen into a suitably sensitized animal was called "delayed" hypersensitivity because of its slow onset, taking 24 hours to reach maximal intensity. The phenomenon, which is exemplified by the tuberculin reaction, was thus distinguished from immediate hypersensitivity and the Arthus reaction. Differences underlying the pathogenesis of these immunologic reactions became apparent later.

Cell-mediated immunity is more difficult to define or quantify than humoral immunity (Chapter 9). The reaction of antibody with its antigen can be detected directly or indirectly in a number of ways. Until recently, the reaction of a specifically sensitized lymphocyte with its antigen could be ascertained only by *in vivo* reactions of the delayed type (Chapter 9). One of the characteristics of the delayed response is that it can be transferred to an unreactive recipient by cells but not by serum. This procedure was first described by Landsteiner and Chase in the 1940's and has assisted considerably the study of the phenomenon. Even now, however, despite a vast quantity of accumulated literature, our understanding of delayed hypersensitivity is relatively superficial.

Interest in this phenomenon lies in its involvement in such problems as graft rejection, tumor rejection, autoimmune disease, and contact sensitivity and its role in antimicrobial immunity. The benefit to the animal from the presence of a cellular reactivity to antigens has long been debated and may be related not only to resistance to bacterial and viral infection but also to recognition of abnormalities of self, as in autoimmune disease and neoplasia. Unfortunately, as with humoral immunity, the manifestation of the cellular response to antigen sometimes involves tissue damage and disease.

A discussion of the cutaneous delayed reaction will serve to illustrate some characteristics of the phenomenon. Its involvement in graft rejection and autoimmunity are considered in Chapter 20.

INDUCTION OF DELAYED HYPERSENSITIVITY

Classically, delayed hypersensitivity was found after infection with bacteria such as *Mycobacterium tuberculosis.* In addition, it may be produced experimentally by the injection of a variety of protein antigens, usually in low doses and accompanied by killed tubercle bacilli. Antigen incorporated into an oil-in-water emulsion containing tubercle bacilli (Freund's complete adjuvant) is generally used to induce delayed hypersensitivity. The component of the bacteria responsible for the increased sensitizing effect is a lipopolysaccharide—Wax D. The route of sensitization is important, the intradermal route being the most efficacious (Chapter 10).

Although they may be produced in all animals, including man, delayed hypersensitivity reactions have been studied most productively in the guinea pig. The sensitivity generally appears early, e.g., four to seven days after antigen injection. In some situations, delayed hypersensitivity is the only immunologic reaction evoked by the sensitization. However, since complete Freund's adjuvant also increases antibody production, the early onset of delayed hypersensitivity is often followed by a humoral immune response. Testing an animal at this time for delayed reactivity may be complicated by superimposed immediate hypersensitivity and Arthus reactions. Since larger quantities of antigen induce antibody formation, small sensitizing doses (1 to 50 μg) are generally more effective.

THE CUTANEOUS REACTION

The tuberculin test in man is an example of this process. To test for delayed hypersensitivity *in vivo,* a small quantity of antigen (often less than 1 μg) is injected intradermally. In detecting sensitivity to *Mycobacterium tuberculosis,* the antigen employed for skin testing is tuberculin, a purified protein derivative (PPD) of the organism. Characteristically, the onset of the skin reaction is slow, and nothing may be seen for 6 to 12 hours. Erythema and nonedematous, indurated swelling gradually develop, reach maximal intensity after 24 to 72 hours, and then slowly regress. In severe reactions, hemorrhage and necrosis may be seen. With protein antigens, a milder but similar reaction occurs. The reaction is sometimes considered qualitatively different and is called a Jones-Mote reaction.

HISTOLOGY

The delayed hypersensitivity lesion is characterized by mononuclear cell infiltration, although some neutrophils may appear in the early (six hour) lesion. Nests of macrophages and lymphocytes may be seen around blood vessels and nerves (Fig. 13–15). Macrophages are found invading tissues such as the dermis. A previously ignored cell, the basophil, has recently been found to accumulate quite commonly in these lesions, and although its effect

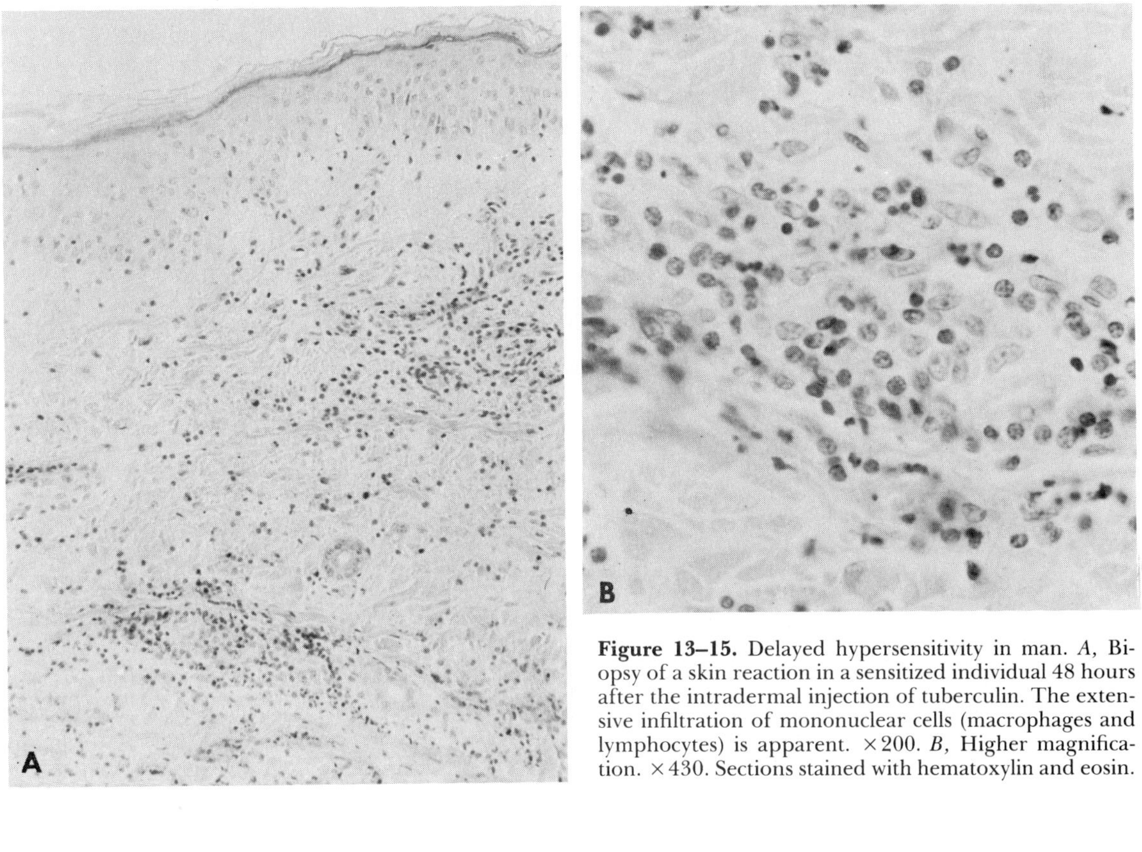

Figure 13–15. Delayed hypersensitivity in man. *A,* Biopsy of a skin reaction in a sensitized individual 48 hours after the intradermal injection of tuberculin. The extensive infiltration of mononuclear cells (macrophages and lymphocytes) is apparent. ×200. *B,* Higher magnification. ×430. Sections stained with hematoxylin and eosin.

is unknown, it is seen in the Jones-Mote reaction. Occasionally in tuberculin sensitivity, a lesion is seen with fibrin, neutrophils, and central necrosis. In addition, where antibody production has begun, a superimposed Arthus reaction may contribute to the overall picture. With protein antigens the mononuclear cell invasion is characteristic and is usually accompanied by some disruption in the surrounding tissues. This type of lesion is also found in all the reactions involving delayed activity, such as graft rejection, and in many of the autoimmune diseases.

OTHER FORMS OF DELAYED HYPERSENSITIVITY

A systemic reaction can be elicited in a hypersensitive animal following intravenous administration of antigen, e.g., tuberculin. The generalized reaction is initially a febrile one, and tuberculin has been shown to release endogenous pyrogen in sensitive animals (Chapter 14). This tuberculin shock reaction can result in lymphocytopenia, shock, and even death. In animals with tuberculosis, absorption of tuberculin into the blood stream can result in reactions around the tuberculous lesions anywhere in the body.

CONTACT HYPERSENSITIVITY

A delayed inflammatory reaction can be produced by application of certain low molecular weight materials to the skin. The response has been best studied in the human and in the guinea pig. Sensitization follows the same general pattern as the usual delayed hypersensitivity reaction. A week after the percutaneous application of a low molecular weight sensitizer, such as picric acid or dinitrochlorobenzene (DNCB), a delayed skin reaction may be elicited by a second application of a challenging dose of antigen to the skin. In man, this is sometimes applied as a patch test (a piece of filter paper soaked in a solution of the substance applied to the skin).

The cutaneous inflammation is similar to that described for classic delayed hypersensitivity lesions. The onset is slow and erythema and swelling are observed. Histologically, there is a mononuclear cell infiltration more closely concentrated in the upper layers of the skin and around hair follicles because of the route of antigen administration (Fig. 13–16).

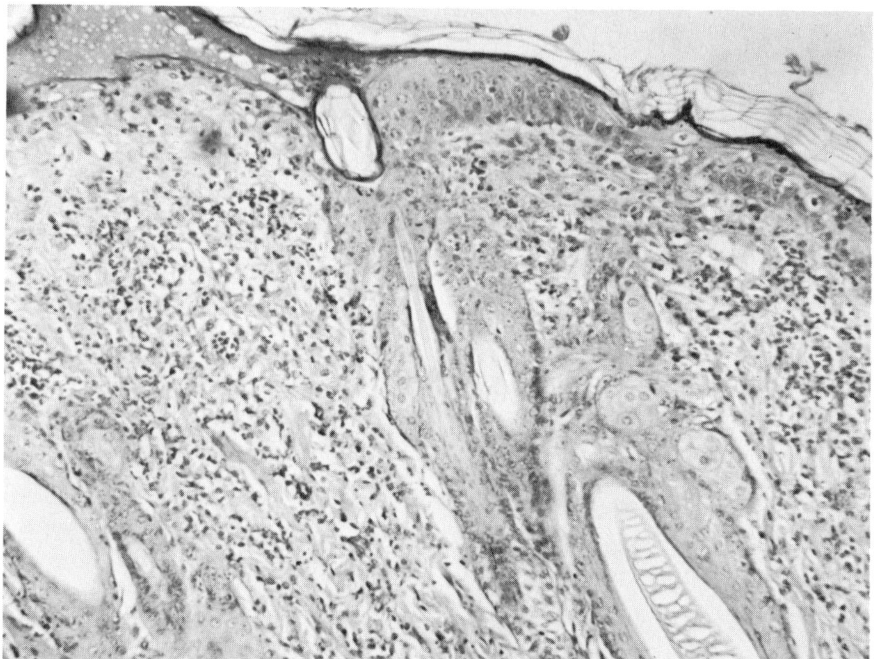

Figure 13–16. Contact sensitivity in a guinea pig. Section of a skin reaction in a sensitized animal 24 hours after the percutaneous application of dinitrofluorobenzene (DNFB). The mononuclear cell infiltration is similar to that in Figure 13–15 but is more superficial and is seen surrounding the hair follicles (reflecting the route of administration of antigen). (Courtesy of Dr. J. D. Feldman.)

The unique feature of this reaction is the size of the antigen employed (less than 1000 molecular weight). Such materials are not usually immunogenic and act only as haptens, i.e., require a carrier protein (Chapter 4). In contact sensitivity, the low molecular weight sensitizer is bound to protein in the skin itself. To induce the sensitivity, it has been shown that the antigen (hapten) must be able to bind covalently to proteins. Thus, 2,4 dinitrobenzene requires a Cl, F, Br, or SO_3H group for activity; H, CH_3, or NH_2 groups, which do not bind to proteins, are incapable of causing this hypersensitivity.

Interestingly, administration of preformed hapten-protein complexes (e.g., picrylated bovine gamma globulin) will elicit only weak contact sensitivity skin reactions when the guinea pig is later tested with the hapten itself. This is due to the nature of the specificity of the reaction, which is directed not only to the hapten but also to the carrier protein (Chapters 4 and 7). In the skin test, when the hapten enters the skin it combines with proteins different from those to which it was bound in the initial inoculum, and no reaction ensues. In support of this conclusion is the observation that testing with the original hapten-protein conjugate will produce a delayed hypersensitivity reaction. Moreover, if the initial sensitization was performed with hapten bound to homologous skin proteins, later skin testing with hapten alone will result in positive reactions.

CONTACT SENSITIVITY IN MAN

One of the best known examples of contact sensitization is the allergic contact dermatitis resulting from exposure to poison ivy. The sensitizer in this instance is a plant catechol, urushiol, that acts in the same way as the synthetic chemicals described earlier. Skin reactions to industrial chemicals, cosmetics, and drugs (such as penicillin) are often manifestations of contact hypersensitivity. Sensitization requires penetration of the chemical into the skin, which is generally easier for hydrophobic materials; however, the sweat glands in humans do provide a penetration route for hydrophilic substances. Sensitization of an individual persists, and, even though the reaction is weaker, a skin test can elicit a response after many years. In man, the histologic picture is similar to that in animals and that of classic delayed hypersensitivity; however, damage to the epidermis often results in vesicle and blister formation.

TRANSFER OF DELAYED HYPERSENSITIVITY

Characteristically, delayed hypersensitivity is a cellular phenomenon and the reactivity to a given antigen can be transferred passively to a normal recipient by sensitized T-lymphocytes from a sensitized donor. Serum is ineffective. Delayed hypersensitivity is thus clearly differentiated from immediate hypersensitivity, which is transferred by serum. However, it must be noted that transfer of antibody-forming cells (B-cells) will also elaborate antibody in the host, perhaps resulting in cellular transfer of immediate hypersensitivity and Arthus reactions. In spite of the requirement for transfer by cells, however, one mechanism of delayed hypersensitivity has postulated the presence of minute amounts of high-affinity antibody in the circulation. This possibility does not seem likely, since passive transfer of large amounts of high-affinity antibody has not been effective, but it cannot be completely excluded until the true mechanism is known.

Cells from the spleen, lymph nodes, or peritoneal exudates have usually been used for transfer. The lymphocyte responsible is the T-cell or thymus-derived lymphocyte, and there is increasing evidence that this cell belongs to a different population from that responsible for "helper" function in antibody synthesis (Chapter 7). The cells in species other than man must be viable. It has also been shown that active metabolism of the transferred cells is required. Twenty-four hours after transfer of cells from a sensitized donor to a normal guinea pig, for example, delayed reactions may be detected in the recipient. In inbred strains, the sensitivity persists. Where the donor cells are incompatible with the recipient, reactivity will disappear after a week, when the host mounts an immune attack against the foreign cells. The transient nature of the transfer in outbred animals suggests that the sensitized cell itself is involved in the reaction and is not merely passing "information" to host cells.

Cell transfer has been an important tool in the study of delayed hypersensitivity and its possible involvement in experimental diseases. By using this technique, it has been possible to show that labeled donor cells (i.e., sensitized cells) constitute only a small proportion of the cells in a lesion; the majority are of host origin. A more difficult problem has been whether there is a specific accumulation of sensitized T-cells at a site of antigen injection as compared with a control site. Experiments from different laboratories have yielded conflicting results. What specific accumulation there is seems to be small. The cells that do make up the cell infiltrate (i.e., predominantly unsensitized host cells) are dividing cells. Of interest is that transfer of cells to irradiated recipients fails to support delayed hypersensitivity, again showing the importance of dividing host cells.

TRANSFER FACTOR IN MAN

In man, the situation is somewhat different. Delayed hypersensitivity can be transferred with cells such as peripheral leukocytes. What is unique, however, is that extracts of the leukocytes will also transfer the specific sensitivity. The material responsible has been called transfer factor, is dialyzable, and appears to have a molecular weight below 10,000 (Chapter 9). It is resistant to trypsin, ribonuclease, and heat. Its character and mechanism of action remain unknown, and it is possible that more than one factor is involved. The factor is released from sensitized leukocytes upon incubation with antigen *in vitro;* and, upon injection into a human recipient, it can sensitize him within a matter of hours. Following the injection of transfer factor into skin test–negative recipients, the previously negative skin sites become positive within six hours, but "conversion" can last for years. This short latent period provides evidence that the phenomenon is not due to antigen transfer resulting in sensitization of the host. Moreover, transfer has been achieved with sensitization to synthetic antigens that the recipient could not have experienced, so that stimulus by transferred antigen of a pre-existing sensitivity cannot be the explanation. Attempts to detect antibody in the transfer factor have always been negative, and since its small molecular weight became known, this possibility has been excluded. The nature of this factor is an important question and its answer may help to elucidate the mechanisms of delayed hypersensitivity. Recently, transfer factor prepared from normal donors has been used in the immunologic reconstitution of individuals with impaired cellular immunity, e.g., Wiskott-Aldrich syndrome, and chronic mucocutaneous candidiasis. The uses of transfer factor will be described more fully in Chapter 22.

SPECIFICITY OF DELAYED HYPERSENSITIVITY

Cellular immunity, like humoral immunity, is exquisitely specific. There are, however, some clear and interesting differences between the two responses. Antiserum to a hapten-carrier complex will usually contain antibodies to the hapten itself, which will react with it free in solution or attached to another carrier. Delayed hypersensitivity, on the other hand, tends to be directed toward the carrier proteins as well as to the hapten. Guinea pigs sensitized to dinitrophenol–guinea pig albumin (DNP-GPA) conjugates will give delayed reactions to DNP-GPA but not to DNP or GPA separately or to dinitrophenol–bovine gamma globulin (DNP-BGG). An *in vitro* model for delayed hypersensitivity, the inhibition of macrophage migration, exhibits exactly the same type of specificity. As we have seen earlier, contact sensitivity involving haptenic groups also exhibits this carrier specificity. In this case, the carriers are proteins in the skin to which the chemical (e.g., DNCB) is administered topically or intradermally. It appears, therefore, that delayed hypersensitivity requires a larger antigenic determinant, i.e., the hapten and a portion of the carrier.

An indication of the necessity for the antigen to be degraded in the animal prior to the induction of delayed hypersensitivity has been obtained by the use of polymers of the nondegradable D-amino acids as carriers. In this case, delayed hypersensitivity could not be produced, in contrast with the effectiveness of haptens coupled to L-amino acid polymers. It is also extremely difficult to induce delayed hypersensitivity to polysaccharides, which are known to be difficult to degrade; however, since polysaccharides can induce humoral antibody, degradation does not appear to be the only explanation.

DESENSITIZATION AND TOLERANCE

Administration of large doses of antigen can specifically desensitize animals that had previously exhibited delayed hypersensitivity, so that a subsequent skin test with antigen is negative. Desensitization is considerably easier for proteins than for bacterial antigens such as tuberculin. Thus, 1 to 2 mg of ovalbumin given intravenously or intradermally can effectively prevent a delayed reaction, even if the desensitizing injection is given up to two hours after the intradermal challenge.

This emphasizes that the interaction of antigen and cells in the skin is relatively slow, probably because of the reduced rate of accumulation of specific cells. Flooding the system with excess antigen can prevent the local lesion, even though the initial reaction has already started.

Animals may be made tolerant or unresponsive to specific antigens so that it is not possible to stimulate an antibody response to that antigen (Chapter 10). In the same way, tolerance usually results in the inability to induce delayed hypersensitivity. Injections of large quantities of antigens to neonates appear to be the most effective method of induction of unresponsiveness. Tolerance to homografts can also be produced in this way. The feeding of contact allergens, such as DNCB, to guinea pigs can cause a state of unresponsiveness to a subsequent application of the chemical to the skin. However, these animals are not tolerant to the hapten if it is conjugated to a non–guinea pig protein, such as egg albumin. Such experiments indicate once again the critical role of the carrier in delayed hypersensitivity and show that immunologic unresponsiveness in this type of reaction has similar specificity.

PATHOGENESIS OF TISSUE DAMAGE IN DELAYED HYPERSENSITIVITY

It is generally thought that the specifically sensitized T-lymphocyte is responsible for recognition of the antigen in lesions of delayed hypersensitivity. When the antigen is injected there are two possibilities for contact with lymphocytes—either antigen leaks out into the blood stream to react with passing lymphocytes, or lymphocytes that are constantly migrating through tissues by chance encounter the locally deposited antigen. Lymphocytes have been observed to accumulate and migrate out of blood vessels in the lesions; however, the mechanisms involved in the accumulation are still to be determined.

The sensitized lymphocyte, after encounter with antigen, becomes a metabolically activated cell and may release a variety of factors. These have been described in Chapter 9. The release of these factors has been observed *in vitro* but is only surmised *in vivo*. One of these substances is chemotactic for macrophages. Macrophages are known to accumulate with lymphocytes at the delayed hypersensitivity site. The migration inhibition factor (MIF) capable of inhibiting the macrophages' migration *in vitro* may possibly be involved in keeping the macrophages in the lesion once they have arrived. Other factors may "activate" the macrophage, inducing increased metabolism and increased synthesis and perhaps secretion of its constituents. Some of these constituents may be injurious to the tissues, e.g., elastase. The reciprocal reaction, macrophage-mediated or catalyzed activation of lymphocytes, may also be operative in this phenomenon through lymphocyte-activating factors (Chapters 7 and 11). In addition, nonsensitized lymphocytes make up most of the accumulated cell population, and their localization may be related to a mitogenic factor (Chapter 9).

The most likely cause of the actual tissue damage would be soluble agents released from the participating cells. Candidates for these are lysosomal enzymes and cytotoxic factors from macrophages and toxic factors (lymphotoxin liberated from lymphocytes). Macrophage lysosomes contain the usual array of hydrolytic enzymes, and some of these can be released to the external environment during phagocytosis. Cytotoxic factors are released from lymphocytes *in vitro* when they react with antigen. The release from lymphocytes is fairly slow, taking 24 hours to yield appreciable levels. Moreover, injection of these supernatants into the skin produces a reaction that, to some extent, mimics the delayed hypersensitivity reaction (skin-reactive factor). The characteristic mononuclear cell infiltrate is, in this case, greatly enhanced and the reaction becomes intense within four to six hours. These recent observations support the idea that lymphocyte factors play some role in the lesion, although the actual tissue damage could still result from macrophage infiltration with release of harmful factors.

It will be clear from this brief consideration that the pathogenesis of delayed hypersensitivity is not fully understood and only now are techniques becoming available that may eventually answer this vitally important question.

CELL REACTIONS INVOLVED IN IMMUNOLOGIC INJURY

Damage to tissues by immunologic reactions *in vivo* involves a variety of cellular and humoral interactions. Study of these cells and their activities *in vitro* has increased our knowledge of their *in vivo* function and may ultimately yield the means to control the injurious processes while retaining those that are beneficial. In this section, reactions of the immunologically important cells will be described, together with their interaction with plasma mediation systems, such as the complement, coagulation, and kinin systems (biologic amplification systems). Some *in vitro* models of the delayed hypersensitivity phenomena that have gained prominence will also be considered.

Mast Cells and Basophils

The main cell reservoirs of the vasoactive amines, particularly histamine, have been extensively studied because of their importance in immediate hypersensitivity reactions. In most species, histamine resides primarily in mast cells and basophils, but in the rabbit high levels are also found in platelets (Chapter 2). Many earlier experimental studies of anaphylaxis involved perfused or chopped sensitized lungs and measured the release of histamine and other pharmacologic mediators following challenges with antigen. More recently, histamine release from preparations of peritoneal mast cells (rat, mouse) or pulmonary mast cells (human) or blood leukocytes containing basophils (man, rabbit, guinea pig) have provided a more defined system. However, the possibility of other sources of histamine and the relative importance of other mediators, such as serotonin, leukotrienes, kinins, and prostaglandins, must be taken into account.

MAST CELLS

Some of the triggers that result in release of histamine from mast cells are indicated in Figure 13–17. Probably the most important mechanism is that mediated by homocytotropic antibody, the analog in the rat of human IgE globulin. Mast cells may be actively sensitized with this type of antibody if they are taken from an animal producing the antibody *in vivo*. Alternatively, passive sensitization can be achieved by incubating the normal mast cells with homocytotropic antibody *in vitro*. Upon subsequent reaction of specific antigen with at least two IgE antibodies on the mast cell surface, the cell is stimulated to release its contained chemical mediators (Chapter 20).

Factors produced by immunologic reactions unrelated to mast cells may also induce release of histamine. Fixation of complement to antigen-antibody complexes results in the liberation of C3a and C5a and will cause isolated rat peritoneal mast cells to release histamine. A basic protein contained in neutrophil granules can act in a similar manner and cause degranulation of mast cells. Since this protein is liberated from neutrophils during their interaction with immune complexes, its participation in the increase of vascular permeability seen in neutrophil-mediated reactions must be considered. A syn-

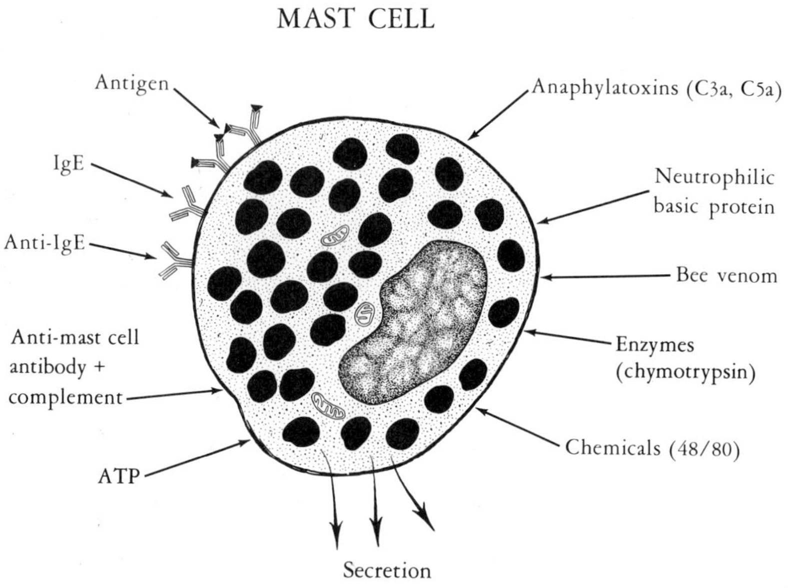

Figure 13–17. Stimuli that can induce release of vasoactive amines and other materials from mast cells.

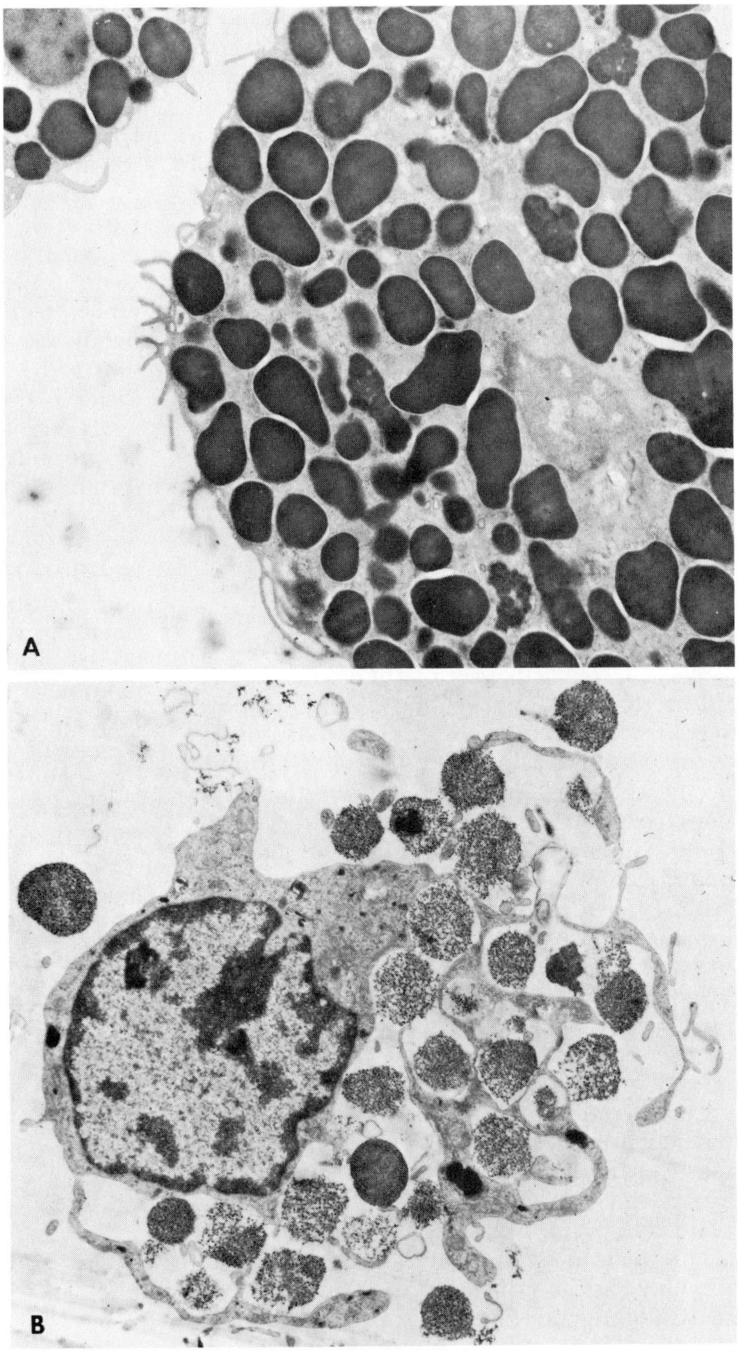

Figure 13–18. Degranulation of rat peritoneal mast cells. *A*, Electron photomicrograph of a control mast cell. Note dense granules filling the cytoplasm. ×9200. *B*, Cell treated with C3a anaphylatoxin (Chapter 6). The granules are being extruded from the cell and are apparently disintegrating. The cell itself is not lysed by this process. ×7500. (Courtesy of Dr. C. G. Cochrane.)

thetic material, compound 48/80, and certain bee and snake venoms have also been used in studies of mast cell reactions. They, too, induce release of histamine.

The complete mechanism of release is not yet understood. Stimulation of the mast cell membranes by these various agents activates cell enzymes (esterases), and, by a process that requires mast cell energy metabolism, histamine is released into the extracellular environment. Additional changes accompanying histamine release include alterations in intracellular cAMP (Chapter 20A). The histamine is contained in characteristic mast cell granules, and, in some of these reactions, there is an overt extrusion of granules to the outside (Fig. 13–18). Importantly, the cells are not killed and do not release potassium or the cytoplasmic enzyme lactic dehydrogenase. In fact, guinea pig basophils, for example, can resynthesize their granules after a release reaction. A completely different mechanism of release follows the reaction of anti–mast cell antibodies with mast cells in the presence of complement. This is a cytotoxic reaction and involves a breakdown of the cell with liberation of all its constituents.

BLOOD LEUKOCYTES AND BASOPHILS

Blood leukocytes enriched in basophil content release histamine by reactions similar to those described for mast cells. These cells have been shown to contain IgE on their surfaces (approximately 20,000 to 80,000 molecules per cell) and will release their histamine if reacted with an antigen to which the individual is sensitive, e.g., ragweed. In addition, the reaction of anti-IgE with leukocytes from an atopic individual will release histamine. The stimulus to the cell membrane in both cases is probably the same and involves the participation of the cyclic nucleotide system (Chapters 7 and 20A) and more recently products of the lipoxygenase transformation of arachidonate as well. Basophils are morphologically different from the tissue mast cells but are also stimulated to secrete their content of vasoactive amines by C5a anaphylatoxin. Other mediators released from or made in basophils (and mast cells) include leukotrienes, ECF-A, a basophil kallikrein of anaphylaxis, and PAF. Recent studies have also concentrated on the control mechanisms that are operative on the secretion process, and a number of therapeutically effective drugs (e.g., isoproterenol, disodium cromoglycate) have been shown to inhibit particular steps in the secretory processes of mast cells and basophils. More precisely, beta-adrenergic agents, e.g., isoproterenol, stimulate adenylate cyclase for increased cAMP accumulation; methylxanthines, e.g., theophylline, lead to an accumulation of cAMP by inhibiting the enzyme phosphodiesterase (Chapter 20A).

EOSINOPHILS

Eosinophilia is considered to be the "hallmark of the allergic disease," but the exact function of eosinophils in allergic reactions is yet to be fully understood. Tissue eosinophilia is marked at the sites where immunologic reactions involving reaginic antibodies occur. The initial blood eosinopenia accompanying acute anaphylaxis results from the migration of these cells to the tissue sites involved in the allergic inflammation, where at least two chemotactic factors are released from reacting cells. These events are shown schematically in Figure 13–19. The first factor, ECF-A, generated from mediator cells, e.g., mast cells, during the allergic reaction, is involved in the unidirectional migration of eosinophils against a concentration gradient. Once at the reaction sites, ECF-A may deactivate and arrest the eosinophils from further outward migration. The second chemotactic factor is histamine, which has been shown to exert a selective chemotactic action on the eosinophils. The chemotactic activity of the histamine is concentration-dependent. At concentrations between 3×10^{-7} and 1.25×10^{-6} molar, for example, histamine is selectively chemotactic for eosinophils. Higher concentrations inactivate and inhibit eosinophil migration, effects similar to those observed for ECF-A. That the chemotactic activation of histamine is not inhibited by either H-1 or H-2-type antagonists suggests the existence of a different histamine receptor on the eosinophils.

The role of eosinophils in allergic reactions (or inflammation in general) is still unclear. An earlier theory was that the cells served to inactivate many of the mediators of acute allergic responses and therefore to "switch off" the reactions. Although this may be part of the story, recent data do not suggest this as a major role for the eosinophil. An alternative suggestion (also somewhat controversial) is that the eosinophil may be particularly important in the defense against helminth parasites. The enhanced ability of such organisms to stimulate IgE synthesis is of additional interest in this regard.

Platelets

The importance of the circulating platelets in hemostasis is well known; however, platelets also contain pharmacologic mediators that are involved in immunologic reactions. Rabbit platelets store large quantities of histamine and serotonin, and most of the histamine in the blood is found in these cells. Other platelet constituents that are potentially injurious include lysosomal enzymes, permeability factors unrelated to the vasoactive amines, epinephrine, and clotting factors.

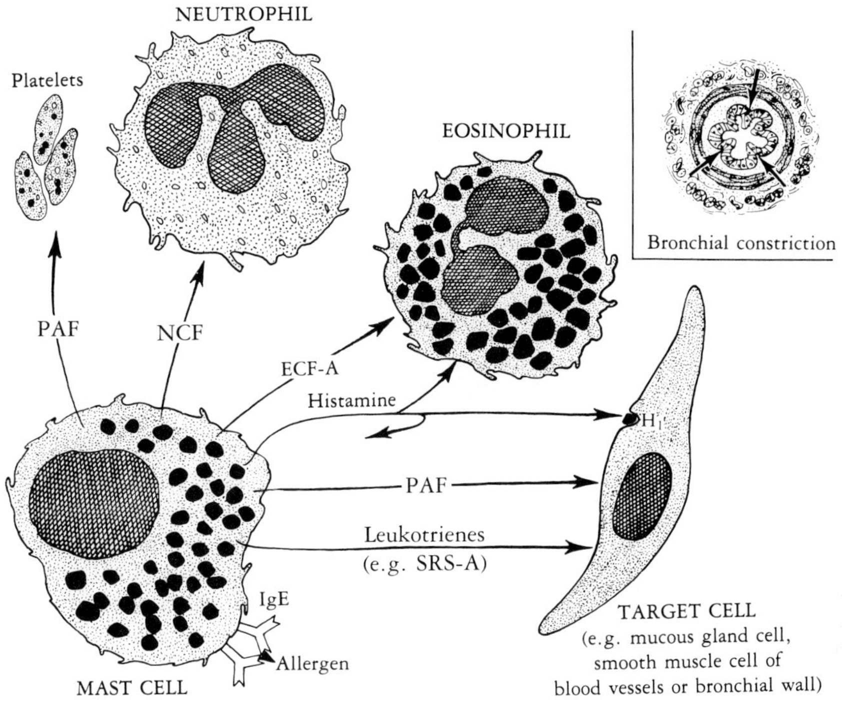

Figure 13–19. Schematic representation of the release of mediators from the mast cells and their effects on other cells involved in the inflammatory response.

Platelets may be involved in the deposition of circulating immune complexes in the rabbit by releasing vasoactive amines and thus increasing vascular permeability. Other permeability reactions may also result from the reactions of these cells. Aggregates of platelets and leukocytes are common findings in the blood vessels of patients with acute inflammatory reactions (e.g., Arthus reaction) and may also be seen in kidney homografts that are being rejected (Chapter 20B).

RELEASE OF CONSTITUENTS FROM PLATELETS BY IMMUNE COMPLEXES

A number of immunologic mechanisms for release of histamine from rabbit platelets are shown in Figure 13–20. Rabbit platelets have

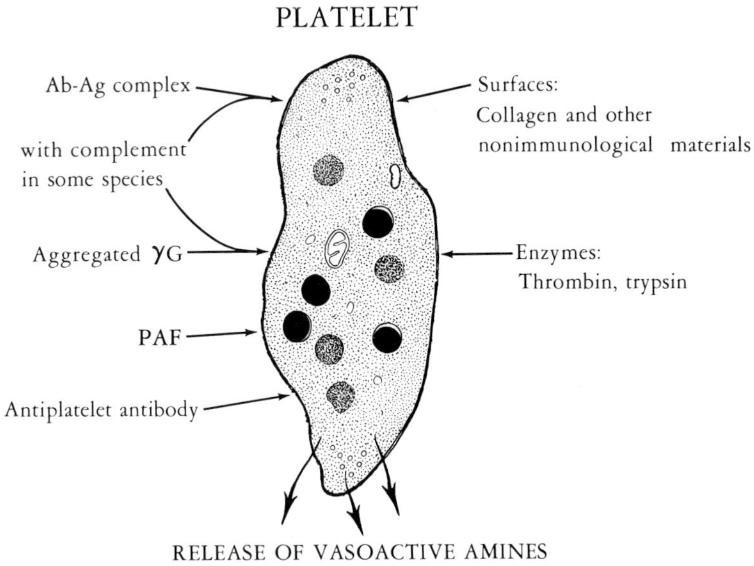

Figure 13–20. Some stimuli that can induce release of vasoactive amines from platelets.

the property of adhering to immune complexes that have fixed complement through C3. This is prominently seen with particulate antigens. The ability to undergo C3 immune adherence is shared by neutrophils, eosinophils, and macrophages. Following adherence, the platelet may be stimulated to release histamine, serotonin, and nucleotides (ATP, ADP, and AMP). Since ADP is a potent platelet-aggregating agent, its release causes additional platelet clumping. Most of these reactions of platelets may thus be divided into two phases—an initial adherence and then aggregation that leads to an amplification of the effect by bringing more platelets into the reaction, i.e.:

Immune complexes→ Adherence of platelets → Release of ADP→ Aggregation of more platelets

This effect is also true of reactions of platelets with nonimmune materials, such as collagen, or inert surfaces. The release of histamine from rabbit platelets following immune adherence may be augmented by the presence of neutrophils that can also react with immune complexes. It may be significant that *in vivo,* both cell types are often found together.

The vasoactive amines within the platelet are contained within specialized granules, distinct from the lysosomes. Their release requires platelet energy metabolism, platelet esterases, and environmental calcium. Since platelet lysis is minimal, an active release process is involved. It is of interest that the active release of substances from many different cell types appears to involve similar mechanisms, although the initiating events for release may be different (see below).

Another reaction of rabbit platelets is with soluble immune complexes in antibody excess, with activation of the total complement sequence. This results in the complete lysis of platelets, the liberation of lysosomal and cytoplasmic enzymes, and the release of vasoactive amines and nucleotides. Immune adherence brings together platelets and complexes that have fixed complement up to the C3 stage. Then, the fixation of complement to complexes closely adherent to the platelet surface leads to lysis of the platelet. The platelet in this type of reaction has been termed an innocent bystander.

In man, platelets cannot be shown to undergo C3 immune adherence. By contrast, in the human, erythrocytes can adhere to fixed C3b (Chapter 6). Platelets from other species, e.g., ruminants and pigs, also fail to react with C3; however, such platelets, including those from the human, will react with immune complexes, in this case adhering to the Fc region of the gamma globulin. Since the adherence results in the release of vasoactive amines (serotonin) and ADP, the end result is similar to that in the rabbit, although the mechanism is different. Allergy in man to certain drugs also involves platelets. Thus, drug reactions to quinidine and apronalide (Sedormid) sometimes result in thrombocytopenia. It has been suggested that antibody-drug complexes adhere to the platelets, which in the presence of complement results in platelet lysis by the innocent bystander mechanism. However, since only certain antigens (drugs) do this, another more likely possibility is that the Sedormid combines with the platelet surface, providing a new antigen with which specific antibody can react and cause cytolysis (Chapter 20A).

Neutrophils

Polymorphonuclear neutrophilic leukocytes have a number of properties that are important in the mediation of tissue damage. As described earlier, these typical inflammatory cells are essential for the pathogenesis of acute necrotic reactions, such as the Arthus reaction, vasculitis of immune-complex disease, severe glomerulonephritis of nephrotoxic nephritis, and many others. Neutrophils are also involved in inflammatory reactions of nonimmunologic origin and are instrumental in the defense of the body against bacterial infection (Chapter 15). The reactions of neutrophils that will be briefly described here are chemotaxis, adherence, phagocytosis, and the release of constituents (Fig. 13–21).

CHEMOTAXIS

For years it has been known that neutrophils migrate actively toward certain stimuli by a process referred to as chemotaxis (Fig. 13–21). This, of course, is a property of many phagocytic cells, including unicellular organisms such as amebae. The phenomenon in regard to neutrophils has been studied by a technique in which neutrophils migrate through a micropore filter with pores of a specified size toward a chemotactic stimulus (Chapters 2 and 26). Neutrophils are placed in an upper chamber, separated from the

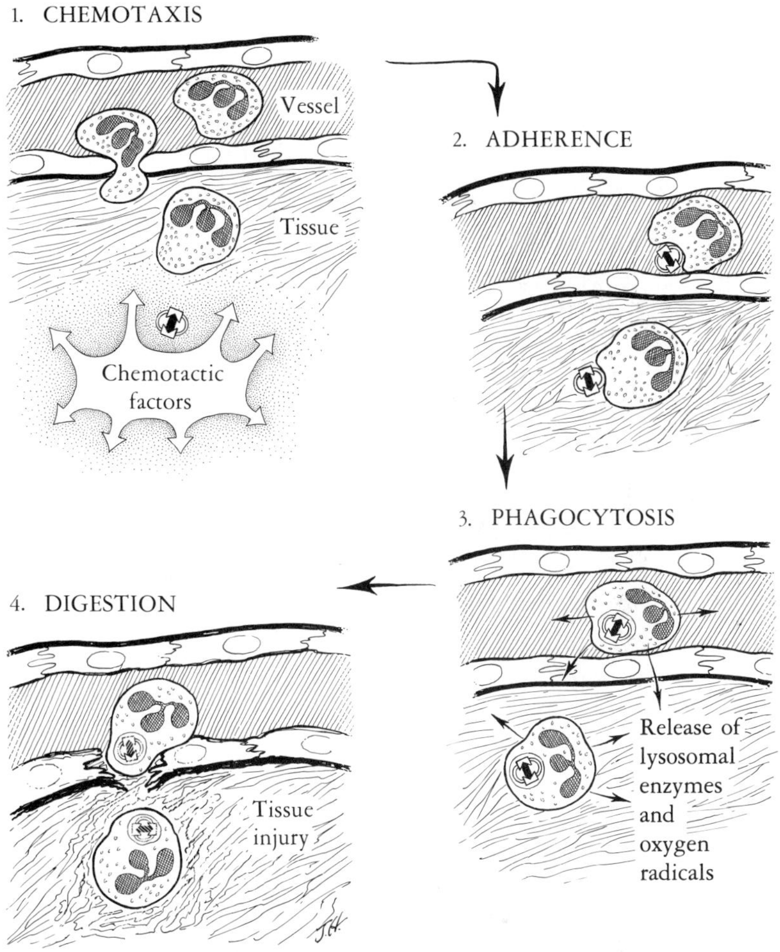

Figure 13–21. Sequence of reactions leading to tissue injury associated with PMN influx. Note that in addition to chemotaxis, adherence, phagocytosis, and digestion processes that normally result in particle inactivation, there may also be the release of neutrophilic constituents (lysosomal enzymes) that result in tissue injury.

source of chemotactic factors by the micropore filter. The number of neutrophils that negotiate the narrow pores of the filter and emerge on the lower surface is an indication of the strength of the chemotactic stimulus.

Activation of the complement sequence by antigen-antibody complexes leads to the liberation of factors that are chemotactic to neutrophils (Chapter 6). The small fragments of C5 (C5a and C5a des arg) can cause neutrophils to migrate through the filter, when placed in the lower chamber. The cells move up the concentration gradient of the chemotactic factor, and the migration may be prevented if the factor is mixed with the neutrophils in the upper chamber.

When antibody combines with antigen in the tissues and the complex fixes complement, the chemotactic factors generated will diffuse away from the complex and set up concentration gradients. Neutrophils contacting the factors and stimulated by them can migrate toward their source until they reach the immune complexes. In the Arthus reaction, this accumulation takes but a few hours. A wide variety of bacteria also liberate a peptide during growth that is chemotactic for neutrophils and may account for the early accumulation of neutrophils at sites of local infection in the absence of an immunologic reaction. It is also of interest that tissue damage (e.g., infarction) can liberate proteolytic enzymes capable of splitting chemotactic fragments from complement components. Other chemotactic materials include a number of denatured proteins, small peptides containing formylated methionine, a factor derived from neutrophils themselves, and the important enzyme of the coagulation and kinin-forming systems, kallikrein.

NEUTROPHIL ADHERENCE

Neutrophils have the ability to adhere to antigen-antibody-complement complexes (Figs. 13–21 and 13–22). The reactions may be easily demonstrated by reacting antibody with particulate antigens, such as erythro-

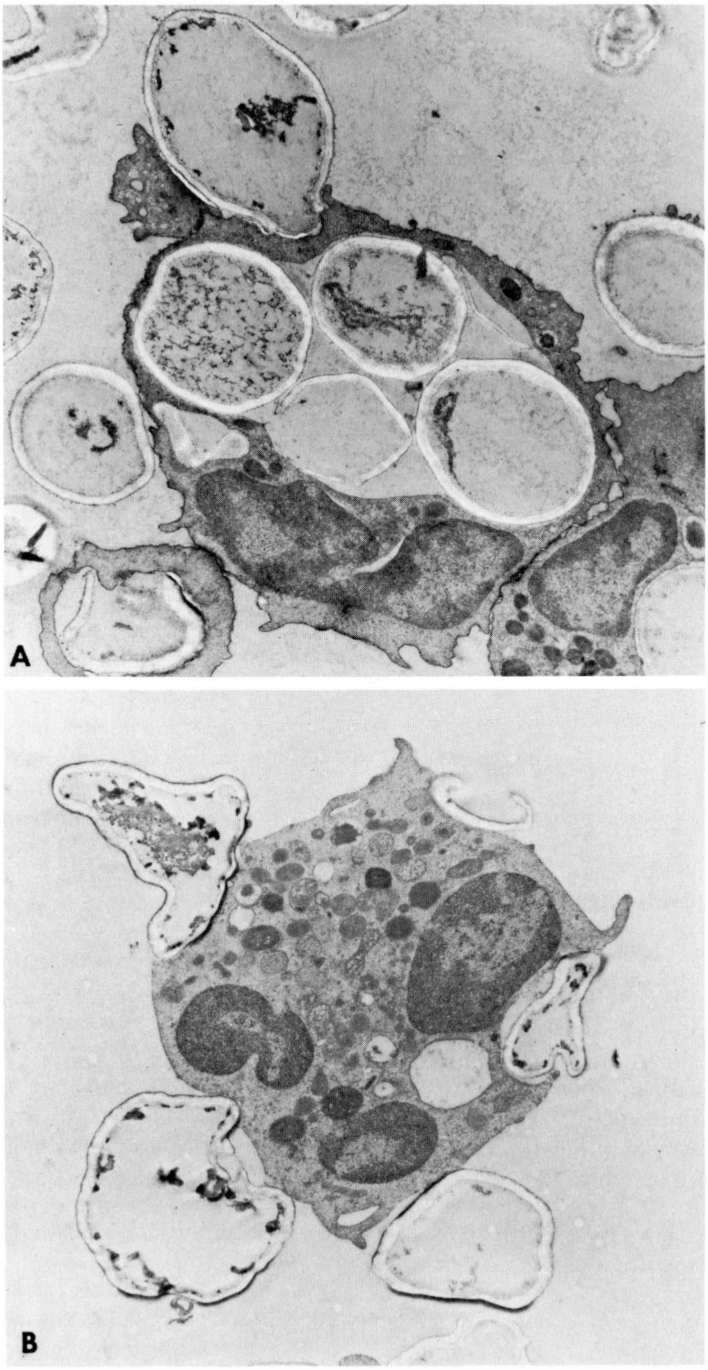

Figure 13–22. Adherence and phagocytosis by rabbit neutrophils. *A,* Electron photomicrograph of a neutrophil that has phagocytosed zymosan particles (yeast cell walls) that have fixed complement. Four particles are seen within a large vacuole, and the cell is adherent to a fifth. Note the paucity of granules in the cytoplasm. ×7500. *B,* A similar cell adherent to zymosan particles with fixed complement. The cell's metabolic pathways have been inhibited to prevent ingestion of the particles and to demonstrate the adherence process. If the zymosan has no fixed complement, neither adherence nor phagocytosis occurs. ×9300.

cytes, and then observing the ability of the antibody-coated particle to bind to neutrophils. In this way it has been shown that neutrophils adhere to immunoglobulin either as specific antibody bound to antigen or to previously aggregated gamma globulin. This reactivity is dependent upon the presence of the Fc fragment of the immunoglobulin. Since this process results in phagocytosis of the complexes under suitable conditions, it represents one form of what was originally called opsonization.

Neutrophil adherence can also be induced by C3 fixation (Fig. 13–22*B*). This can be shown by using IgM antibody to erythrocytes in relatively low quantity and by fixing complement as far as the C3 step. Since a large number of C3b or iC3b molecules are fixed for every antibody molecule, the C3 acts as an amplification of the adherence reactivity of the immune complex. The receptors on the neutrophil for the C3 adherence are different from those for gamma globulin but are antigenically similar to these on macrophages, monocytes and primate erythrocytes.

PHAGOCYTOSIS

Following adherence of the neutrophil surface to the immune complex, the cell is stimulated to phagocytose the complex (Fig. 13–21). An esterase in the cell is involved, energy metabolism is stimulated, and by an invagination process the complex is taken into the cell within a phagocytic vacuole (Chapter 2). The increase in the surface area of membrane produced by the presence of membrane-bounded vacuoles or phagosomes is provided by increased lipid synthesis and by recycling of membrane back to the plasmalemma.

Once inside the cell, the complex, bacteria, or other foreign material has to be degraded. The neutrophil contains at least two, and possibly three, types of granules, each bounded by a membrane and containing degradative enzymes separated from the cell cytoplasm. Following phagocytosis, the granule membranes fuse with those of the phagocytic vacuole and thus liberate the granule contents into the vacuole, where they can digest the phagocytosed materials. The pH within the vacuole falls, probably because of the lactic acid production, and, since many of the granule enzymes work best in an acid medium, conditions are ideal for the digestive process. By employing radiolabeled antibody in the phagocytosed immune complex, the degradation of proteins to small peptides in the neutrophil can easily be demonstrated.

Release of Oxygen Radicals. Following phagocytosis, neutrophils (and monocytes and macrophages) are stimulated to undergo a burst of oxygen consumption, followed by the generation of extremely toxic oxygen radicals (Chapter 2). By sequential reduction steps, molecular oxygen is converted to superoxide anion (O_2^-, hydrogen peroxide [H_2O_2], hydroxyl radical [OH^-]) and then to water. These molecules are so reactive that they have short half-lives in biologic fluids. They are responsible for a major portion of the bactericidal activity of inflammatory cells. Moreover, it is becoming increasingly apparent that many of the toxic effects of neutrophils in immune complex–mediated and inflammatory reactions are due to release of these radicals, which can also damage mammalian cells. Of particular importance are the reactions of H_2O_2 with neutrophil myeloperoxidase in the presence of chloride, and the direct effect of hydroxyl radical. It should be noted that tissue cells are not without protection against these injurious agents. Superoxide dismutase and catalase rapidly convert the O_2 to water, and are found in the cell cytoplasm. It appears, therefore, that only when massive amounts of oxygen radicals are generated does cell injury ensue.

RELEASE OF NEUTROPHIL CONSTITUENTS

If all the neutrophil constituents were carefully contained within the phagocytic vacuoles it would be difficult to see how these cells could be responsible for the tissue damage attributed to them. There is a release, however, of constituents to the extracellular environment during the phagocytic process (Fig. 13–21). This can be shown *in vitro* by feeding immune complexes or particles coated with antibody or complement, or both, to neutrophils and measuring materials in the supernatant afterwards. There are many potentially harmful neutrophil constituents (Table 13–4). In recent studies, many of these have been shown to be released. Proteolytic enzymes (cathepsins, collagenase, elastase, and so forth) are of particular importance, since they could be instrumental in the damage to basement membranes and connective tissue.

Another group of materials released include basic protein materials of low molecular weight that have bactericidal activity and also induce increased vascular permeability. The production of leukotrienes and PAF has been attributed to neutrophils and could contribute to the wealth of the pharmacologically active mediators mentioned. Likewise, kinins can be generated by neutrophil kininogenase. Neutrophil proteases can cleave C5 to generate C5a, which itself can stimulate neutrophil secretion, as well as functioning as a potent chemotactic agent. In addition, neutrophils contain substances that interact with the coagulation system and may initiate the fibrin deposition, which is a common consequence of neutrophil accumulation.

The mechanisms involved in the release processes are yet to be pieced together. These same processes are probably also involved in

Table 13–4. **Injurious Constituents of Neutrophils**

Constituent	Activity
Collagenase Elastase Cathepsin A	Hydrolysis of basement membranes, internal elastic laminae, cartilage and other connective tissue, generation of C5 fragments, angiotensin II
Basic proteins (3)	Increased vascular permeability
Basic protein (1)	Activation of mast cells, release of vasoactive amines
Leukotrienes C_4 and D_4	Increased vascular permeability, contraction of smooth muscle
Kininogenase	Hydrolysis of kininogen with release of vasoactive kinin
Procoagulant activity	(?) Generation of fibrin, activation of platelets
Platelet activation factor (PAF)	Activation of platelets Increased vascular permeability Contraction of smooth muscle Activation of neutrophils
Leukotriene B_4	Attraction of leukocytes
Lysosomal enzymes	Digestion of tissue constituents
Oxygen radicals	Damage to cells

secretion from the other inflammatory cells considered in this section. Neutrophils adherent to immune reactants along a surface too large to be phagocytosed, such as is found along the glomerular basement membrane in nephrotoxic nephritis, will also release some of their lysosomal enzymes. Other contributions to severe tissue damage arise from neutrophil death and disintegration, possibly resulting from such factors as anoxia, lowered pH, and the large amounts of degradative enzymes present at a site of such severe inflammation.

Monocytes and Macrophages

Monocytes and macrophages (monocytes that have undergone a maturation process in the tissues and have also undergone phagocytosis with the development of secondary lysosomes) are cells characteristic of delayed hypersensitivity. They are also found in many inflammatory reactions, particularly later in the course of the inflammation, i.e., after the neutrophil-dependent reaction. Study of the biologic activities of mononuclear phagocytes (the generic term for monocytes and various types of macrophages) represents a major effort for a large number of laboratories. A great deal is known of these cells, but their functions are so many and so varied that it is not possible to describe them all herein. Some of these properties, including their involvement in the immune response, are discussed in other chapters (Chapters 2 and 7). A few of the activities of these cells will be mentioned below. It is important to recognize the great adaptability of the mononuclear phagocyte line. They are truly pluripotential cells, whose final expressed phenotype will reflect the environment in which they are found (or placed).

Like neutrophils, these cells also respond to chemotactic stimuli *in vitro*. Monocytes are phagocytic cells, and they will adhere to immune complexes, both to the fixed immunoglobulins and to the C3b. Following the adherence, phagocytosis, granule discharge into the phagocytic vacuole, and digestion of the complexes occur. Like neutrophils, mononuclear phagocytes also discharge preformed lysosomal enzymes to the outside of the cell during phagocytosis. It may be presumed that the biochemical processes involved are very similar. A difference from neutrophils is that macrophages are more versatile. They can actively synthesize and secrete new enzymes, make more granules, and can also undergo mitosis and divide under special conditions. The role played by macrophages in removal of tissue damage and in repair has already been mentioned.

The secretion of macrophage factors plays an important role in the tissue damage of delayed hypersensitivity, since in the reaction these are the cells that invade the tissues and are considered to be the chief mediators of delayed hypersensitivity reactions. Various *in vitro* models of delayed hypersensitivity involve the macrophage and use its migration, aggregation, or disappearance as end points. Factors released from lymphocytes (e.g., MIF) have been implicated in the retention of macrophages at a site of delayed hypersensitivity once they have arrived there. Other lymphocyte factors can be involved in attraction of monocytes in the first place and in activation of these cells to a state in which they are able to kill tumor cells and resist infections by certain facultative intracellular pathogens (e.g., tuberculosis). This last factor has been termed macrophage activating factor (MAF) and has recently been suggested to be identical with γ-interferon. "Activated" macrophages make more oxygen radicals; secrete more proteases, other enzymes, and growth factors; and are often more actively phagocytic.

Among the secreted products of these cells that are of particular interest to immunologically induced tissue injury may be included the following. (1) Collagenase and elastase result in tissue degradation. (2) Leukocyte pyrogen raises body temperature and may account for the fever seen, for example, in serum sickness. This molecule may also be identical or similar to interleukin 1 (Chapter 9) and fibroblast growth factor (which is presumably involved in repair). (3) Most of the complement components (Chapter 6) *can* be made by macrophages. How important this source is for local sites of immune-complex formation, by comparison with the major source in the liver, has yet to be determined.

The role of the macrophage in antigen uptake and processing has been described in Chapters 2 and 7.

Lymphocytes

The lymphocyte is now regarded as the keystone of immunology. Upon reaction with specific antigen, B-cells can differentiate into plasma cells and produce antibody. This simplified statement, however, covers a multitude of steps, a number of which, at the moment, are purely hypothetical. These processes are described more fully in Chapters 2 and 7. The T-lymphocytes are also instrumental in the production of cell-mediated immunity or delayed hypersensitivity (Chapter 9). It is thought that this type of cell reacts with antigen by means of a receptor on its surface. The nature of the receptor is known, but its great specificity argues for an antibody-like molecule incorporated into or on the cell membrane (Chapter 7). Knowledge of the importance of the specifically sensitized lymphocyte in the mediation of delayed hypersensitivity comes from cell transfer studies. The consequences of its reaction with antigen in the tissue include macrophage emigration, further lymphocyte accumulation, and tissue injury. A number of *in vitro* studies of lymphocytes have revealed properties that may be involved in these processes.

RELEASE OF LYMPHOCYTE FACTORS

It is apparent that lymphocytes can also release a battery of materials, the lymphokines, when they react with antigen *in vitro* (Chapter 9). Although not fully characterized, these effector molecules are thought to represent the *in vitro* correlates of delayed hypersensitivity (cell-mediated) reactions *in vivo.* A list of some of these factors is shown in Table 13–5. Their known physical and biologic properties are given in Chapter 9 (Table 9–3).

DIRECT CYTOTOXIC ACTIVITY OF LYMPHOCYTES

The reaction of cellular elements with target cells has been described in Chapter 9 and is composed of a heterogeneous set of reactions involving many subclasses of lymphocytes, e.g., killer (K) and natural killer (NK) cells, and reactions mediated by macrophages. The reaction of sensitized T-lymphocytes with target cells bearing foreign antigens may lead to direct cytotoxic effects of the lymphocytes. The first step in this reaction involves the clustering of lymphocytes around target cells, after which killing occurs by mechanisms that involve close contact between these cells. It is not yet clear whether locally produced cytotoxic factors might be

Table 13–5. Some Factors (Lymphokines) Released from T-Lymphocytes

Macrophages activating factor (MAF) (probably = γ interferon)
Macrophage migration inhibition factor (MIF)
Specific chemoattractants for monocytes, T-lymphocytes, neutrophils, eosinophils, and basophils
Lymphotoxin
Factors that stimulate lymphocytes (e.g., interleukin II)

causing the cell death. Nonsensitized lymphocytes may be induced to kill target cells by nonspecific mitogens, e.g., phytohemagglutinin, that bring the lymphocyte and target cells together and may also activate the lymphocytes to release lymphokines. Consequently, contact appears to play an important role in lymphocyte cytotoxicity.

This phenomenon of T-cell cytotoxicity may be distinguished from two other forms of lymphocyte-mediated cytotoxicity (Chapter 9): (1) T-lymphocytes that produce soluble cytotoxic factors, e.g., lymphotoxin, and (2) a subpopulation of lymphocytes—the killer or K lymphocytes that react with antibody on a target cell and kill the cell in the so-called antibody-dependent cellular cytotoxic (ADCC) reactions. As mentioned previously, macrophages can also exhibit cytotoxic properties, as can neutrophils, under certain circumstances, particularly when the target cells are coated with antibody.

SUMMARY

Immunologic tissue injury may result from three main types of reaction. (1) Reaction of antigen with certain types of homocytotropic antibody fixed to mast cells and basophils results in the release of some of the pharmacologic mediators of immediate hypersensitivity reactions (Type I reaction). (2) Humoral antibody can initiate damage either by reacting with tissue antigens directly (Type II reaction) or as a result of the inflammatory properties of antigen-antibody complexes (Type III reaction). The damage is generally a consequence of complement and/or cellular interaction with the complexes, and the neutrophil is the cell most clearly implicated. (3) In delayed hypersensitivity, the recognition of antigen occurs at the cellular level, and the T-lymphocyte is responsible (Type IV reaction). Tissue damage results from an accumulation of lymphocytes and macrophages (and basophils) at the site of antigen localization.

Suggestions for Further Reading

Becker, E. L., Simon, A. S., and Austen, K. F. (eds.): Biochemistry of the Acute Allergic Reactions. New York, Alan R. Liss, 1981.

Henson, P. M.: Secretion of lysosomal enzymes induced by immune complexes and complement. *In* Dingle, J. T., and Dean, R. T. (eds.): Lysosomes in Biology and Pathology. Vol. 5. Amsterdam, North-Holland Publishing Company, 1976.

Lachman, P. J., and Peters, D. K. (eds.): Clinical Aspects of Immunology. 4th ed. Vols. I and II. Oxford, Blackwell Scientific Publications, 1982.

van Furth, R. (ed.): The Mononuclear Phagocyte. Part I and II. London, Martinus Nijhoff Publishers, 1980.

Waksman, B. H.: Cellular hypersensitivity and immunity: Inflammation and cytotoxicity. *In* Parker, C. W. (ed.): Clinical Immunology. Vol. I. Philadelphia, W. B. Saunders Company, 1980.

Weissman, G.: Handbook of Inflammation. Vols. 1, 2, and 3. New York, Raven Press, 1979.

Part II

Protective Mechanisms Involved in the Immune Response to Infectious Agents

Chapter 14

Host-Parasite Relationships

Joseph A. Bellanti, M.D.

Two factors are implicit in the term "host-parasite relationship": (1) the properties of the infecting microorganisms, and (2) the host's total response to the infecting agents. The eventual outcome of the host-parasite struggle will be the net result of the interaction of both.

Immunity is a condition that exists in the host, not in the parasite. The immunity with which the host responds may be influenced by an alteration of the microorganism or by deleterious changes in the environment that predispose the host to parasitic invasion. Changes in age, nutrition, environmental pollution, and underlying disease processes, for example, may have profound effects on the host-parasite relationship. Thus, the host-parasite relationship must be viewed from the standpoint of the host, the parasite, and the environment in which the interaction occurs.

BASIC CONCEPTS

INFECTIONS VERSUS INFECTIOUS DISEASE

The process of *colonization* of organisms in or on the host is termed *infection.* An infection may or may not result in an illness; e.g., the colonization of the intestinal flora of the newborn is an infection. The term *infectious disease* refers to the signs and symptoms of frank illness caused by the infection of tissues normally free of significant numbers of organisms.

The mechanisms by which parasites colonize epithelial surfaces are complex but can be separated into two general categories: (1) those concerned with properties of the epithelial surface, e.g., ciliated versus nonciliated, mucoprotein content, presence of secreting IgA; and (2) those associated with characteristics of the pathogen, e.g., viral neuraminidase, bacterial pili, elaboration of extracellular products interfering with host immunity (Chapters 15 to 18). These will be described more fully further on.

PATHOGENICITY VERSUS VIRULENCE; OPPORTUNISTIC INFECTIONS

Microbes that are usually incapable of penetrating natural defenses and therefore normally fail to produce disease are referred to as *nonpathogenic* organisms. Conversely, those that are capable of overwhelming these defenses and producing disease are termed *pathogenic.* Some microbes are so highly pathogenic that whenever they infect they are capable of producing disease; these are referred to as *virulent* organisms. From a prac-

Table 14–1. Opportunistic Infections in Patients with Compromised Defense Mechanisms

Agents	Predisposing Factor	Mechanism
Staphylococcus epidermidis, Escherichia coli	Indwelling catheter or prosthesis	Foreign body
Staphylococcus aureus, Pseudomonas aeruginosa	Extensive burns	Breach in body perimeter, diminished cell-mediated immunity (?)
Cytomegalovirus, *Pneumocystis carinii*	Allograft recipients, patients with malignant disease receiving chemotherapy	Diminished cell-mediated immunity
Candida albicans	Newborn	Diminished cell-mediated immunity, (?) diminished macrophage function
Streptococcus (Diplococcus) pneumoniae, Salmonella paratyphi	Absence or malfunction of the spleen (splenectomy, sickle cell anemia)	Diminished IgM (opsonic) antibody synthesis, diminished clearance

tical point of view, the terms *pathogenic* and *virulent* are often used synonymously. It is becoming increasingly apparent, however, that many microorganisms that are not ordinarily considered pathogenic or virulent may, under certain circumstances, become so when the immunologic capacity of the host is impaired. These infections are referred to as *opportunistic infections* (e.g., candidiasis) and are assuming increasing clinical importance as the number of patients with compromised defense mechanisms continues to increase (Table 14–1). Perhaps one of the most striking examples of opportunistic infections has been in association with the recent epidemic, acquired immunity deficiency syndrome (AIDS) (Chapter 22). In this condition there is profound inhibition of cell-mediated immunity with lymphopenia and reversal of the helper cell (T4):suppressor cell (T8) ratio, which makes the patient susceptible to opportunistic infections caused by a wide variety of microorganisms. Shown in Table 14–2 are some of the opportunistic infections seen in AIDS. Virulence thus represents the interaction between the properties of the host and the pathogen that permits expression of the pathogenic properties of a parasite to the detriment of the host.

ORGANOTROPISM

Organotropism refers to the high degree of selectivity of infection for certain tissues that organisms display. For example, certain viruses are neurotropic and infect primarily the central nervous system, e.g., rabies. Other viruses have a predilection for the respiratory tract, e.g., influenza. The mechanism for tropism is poorly understood but may be explained by metabolic requirements of certain organisms, the protective characteristics that certain tissues afford, or the availability of essential receptor sites on host cells. The mechanisms by which organisms attach to and penetrate epithelial surfaces represent an important step in the initiation of infection and are described below.

PATTERNS OF DISEASE: CLINICAL, SUBCLINICAL, OR LATENT INFECTIONS

Infectious disease may be considered a state in which an infection has become sufficiently active to involve normally uninfected tissues, thus giving rise to signs and symptoms of the illness. These are conditions, however, in which infection is present but not sufficiently active to give rise to recognizable signs and symptoms. These types of infection are referred to as *inapparent* or *subclinical infections.* Inapparent or subclinical infections are exemplified by viral illnesses such as Type A hepatitis, rubella, and mumps. In such cases, infection may be so mild that it does not give rise to recognizable signs or symptoms of disease. An alternative explanation for infection being only subclinical is a pre-existent immunity in the host. For example, the passive administration of gamma globulin to individuals exposed to Type A hepatitis will prevent the overt clinical disease, as manifested by an absence of jaundice, but may not prevent a subclinical infection, shown by a characteristic rise in serum liver enzymes. Subclinical infections are of great medical importance, since they may induce immunity without the overt mor-

Table 14–2. Opportunistic Infections Seen in Acquired Immunodeficiency Syndrome (AIDS)

Viral	
Cytomegalovirus	
	Disseminated
	Pneumonia
	Retinitis
	Encephalitis
Herpes simplex	
	Progressive
Herpes zoster	
	Limited cutaneous
Progressive multifocal leukoencephalopathy	
Fungal	
Candida albicans	
	Oral thrush
	Esophagitis
	Disseminated
Cryptococcus neoformans	
	Meningitis
	Disseminated
Histoplasma capsulatum	
	Disseminated
Petriellidium boydii	
	Pneumonia
Aspergillus	
	Pulmonary
Protozoal	
Pneumocystis carinii	
	Pneumonia
	Retinal infection
Toxoplasma gondii	
	Encephalitis
Cryptosporidium	
	Enteritis
Isospora belli	
	Enteritis
Mycobacterial	
Mycobacterium avium-intracellulare	
	Disseminated
Mycobacterium tuberculosis	
	Disseminated
Others	
Nocardia	
Legionella	

Reproduced with permission of publishers (Gottlieb, M. S., et al., The acquired immunodeficiency syndrome. Ann. Int. Med. 99:208, 1983).

bidity of the disease. Furthermore, they may pose a problem for the physician by obfuscating the problems associated with the disease. For example, administration of gamma globulin to a pregnant female exposed to rubella may convert a clinical case of rubella to a subclinical case. In this instance, a viremia may still occur, with spread to the fetus and resultant production of the congenital rubella syndrome in the absence of overt clinical disease in the mother.

A special case of subclinical infection is the *carrier state.* This refers to the excretion of an organism, ordinarily considered to be a pathogen, following recovery from a clinical disease. For example, a patient recovering from streptococcal pharyngotonsillitis may excrete the organism for several weeks after recovery. In the case of typhoid fever, most individuals stop excreting the organism in the stool by two months, but some continue to excrete the organism for many years and are therefore contagious. Collectively, these individuals are referred to as carriers and are important reservoirs of infection.

Latent infections are persistent inapparent infections in which the presence of the microbe cannot readily be detected by any of the methods currently available. This type of infection is known to flare up from time to time under various conditions. Herpes labialis (cold sores) caused by herpes hominis (simplex) viruses is a good example of a latent-type infection that may be exacerbated by such factors as excessive sunlight, menstruation, stress, or infection. During the interim, the virus cannot be readily detected. Recent evidence suggests that a diminution of specific cell-mediated immunity may be associated with exacerbations of these latent infections. Recent application of molecular hybridization techniques has permitted the identification of viral genome integrated in host cell DNA for several latent viral infections, e.g., hepatitis B, cytomegalovirus (CMV) (Chapter 16).

COMMUNICABILITY

Communicability refers to the ease with which an infection is transmitted from one individual to another. Although communicability may be exhibited by nonpathogenic organisms, it is a prerequisite for the important pathogenic organisms of man.

The efficiency of transmission depends upon four factors: (1) an adequate source, (2) a large enough inoculum, (3) a means of survival for the organism in transit, and (4) a susceptible host (Fig. 14–1).

The communicability of a disease is an important consideration for the physician. It provides both a basis for the containment of disease and a rationale for vaccine prophylaxis. In the case of rubella, for example, the concern is largely with the individual's immunity; in the case of poliomyelitis, the production of population immunity (herd immunity) is of greater importance.

It should be emphasized that the hands of medical care personnel remain an important vehicle for the transmission of infectious dis-

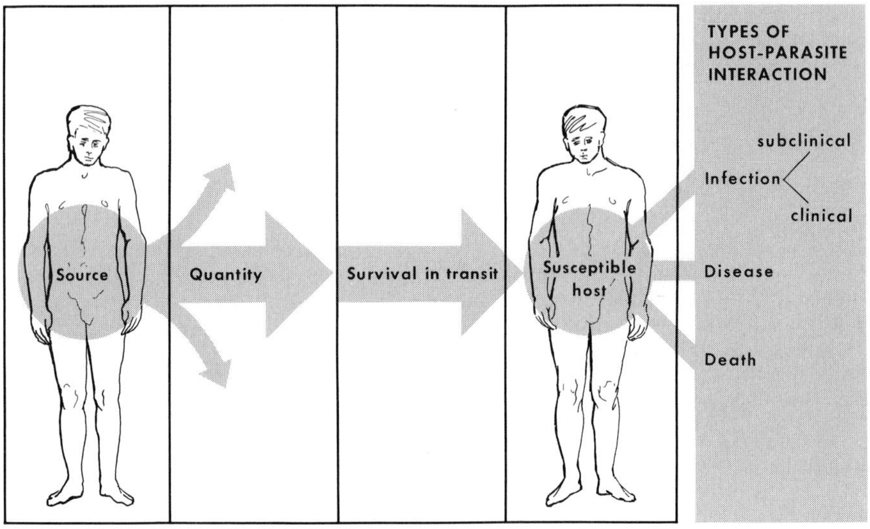

Figure 14–1. Requirements for parasitism.

ease. Ironically, hand washing represents the best and most often neglected preventive measure in the control of infectious diseases, particularly those acquired in hospitals, the so-called nosocomial infections. Recently, intimate forms of contact, such as kissing and sexual intercourse, have been recognized as important vehicles for the transmission of a wide variety of infectious agents, e.g., EB virus and herpes hominis viruses (Chapter 16). Other forms of contact or sexual habits may be important in the recently described AIDS.

PROPERTIES OF THE PARASITE

Modes of Infection

Generally speaking, the pathogenic microorganisms that give rise to disease may be divided into two groups: (1) the *extracellular parasites* and (2) the *intracellular parasites* (Table 14–3). This arbitrary classification is based upon the site of replication of the organism relative to certain cellular elements of the immune system, e.g., phagocytes.

The *extracellular parasites* are those that establish infection by replicating outside of phagocytic cells and that generally produce an acute, fulminating type of infection of relatively short duration. These organisms are, for the most part, bacteria, such as the staphylococcus and the streptococcus. For destruction of these organisms, phagocytosis, particularly by the polymorphonuclear leukocytes, followed by intracellular killing is a critical event. The subsequent production of opsonizing antibody together with complement may enhance these processes.

The second group of parasites are those that establish an *intracellular* domicile within phagocytes (Table 14–3). These can be subdivided further into (1) the *facultative intracellular parasites,* and (2) the *obligate intracel-*

Table 14–3. Classification of Pathogenic Microorganisms

Type	Characteristics	Example of Causative Organism
Extracellular parasites	Acute, fulminating, of short duration	*Staphylococcus aureus*
Intracellular parasites		
Facultative intracellular	Chronic, taken up by phagocytes but not killed	*Mycobacterium tuberculosis* *Histoplasma capsulatum* *Toxoplasma gondii*
Obligative intracellular	Chronic, require intracellular parasitism for their replication	*Mycobacterium leprae* *Rickettsia rickettsiae* viruses

lular parasites. The facultative intracellular parasites are those organisms that, although readily taken up by phagocytic cells, particularly the macrophages, are relatively resistant to subsequent intracellular digestion. These organisms include many bacteria (e.g., *Mycobacterium tuberculosis*), fungi *(Histoplasma capsulatum),* and protozoa (e.g., *Toxoplasma gondii*) that establish chronic infections. Once these organisms have been phagocytosed, the macrophage shows a heightened metabolic state with increased reactivity, not only toward the infecting organism but also toward nonrelated organisms and tumor cells. Knowledge of this heightened state of macrophage activity, "cellular immunity" toward tumor cells has been utilized in cancer immunotherapy, e.g., use of BCG (Chapter 19).

The obligate intracellular organisms are those that show an absolute requirement for intracellular parasitism for their replication. These include some bacteria (e.g., *Mycobacterium leprae*), rickettsiae, (e.g., *Rickettsia rickettsii*), chlamydia (e.g., *Chlamydia psittaci*), and all viruses. Many of these organisms show a tropism for cells of the reticuloendothelial system, and cellular immunity and cell-mediated immunity (delayed hypersensitivity) are prominent features of these interactions.

A third type of interaction representative of certain viruses, including the oncogenic viruses, leads to the incorporation of part of the viral genome with host nucleic acid. These segments encode for the production of proteins or fully infectious viral particles. The oncogenic viruses are believed to play a role in the malignant transformation (Chapter 19). Cell-mediated immunity is also a prominent feature of these complex interactions.

Virulence

The basic mechanisms through which pathogens cause disease are the following: (1) attachment to epithelial surfaces, (2) penetration and invasiveness of tissues, (3) production of toxic materials (toxins), and (4) capacity for genetic alteration.

ATTACHMENT TO EPITHELIAL CELLS

In order for a microorganism to establish infection it must first breach the primary line of defense provided by the intact skin and mucous membranes and become attached to an epithelial surface, such as the skin, the respiratory tract, the gastrointestinal tract, the genitourinary tract, or the eye. These sites have primary importance as attachment sites for most pathogenic organisms. There are a number of mechanisms by which organisms have been shown to attach to these epithelial cells.

The attachment of microorganisms to epithelial surfaces is remarkably cell-specific. The selectivity of attachment of many viruses and bacteria appears to be related to cell surface properties of both the microorganism and the host cells. In the case of certain viruses, for example (Chapter 16), the presence of neuraminidase, an enzyme that cleaves the terminal sialic acid residues from glycoprotein, appears to be related to the preferential attachment and subsequent infection of the epithelial cells within the respiratory system. Similarly, bacterial adherence appears to be mediated by the attraction of species-specific microbial adhesins (also called lectins) to complementary host cell-specific receptors. These adhesins are microbial products that frequently exist in many bacteria as filamentous projections called pili or fimbriae. These adhesins bind to specific receptors on the surface of epithelial cell membranes. A surface glycoprotein referred to as fibronectin is likewise involved in surface attachment and, when released in the circulation together with complement and specific antibodies, amplifies the opsonic function. Recently, a decrease of this protein has been described following splenectomy, in severe burns, and in the newborn. Other microbial structures important to attachment include certain surface proteins of a bacterium, e.g., M protein of *Streptococcus pyogenes,* or certain structures, e.g., pili (fibriae) of *Neisseria gonorrhoeae* and *Shigella.* Other organisms such as the *Streptococcus mutans* elaborate certain products, e.g., glucans and fructans, that can attach to the enamel surface of teeth and have been implicated in the causation of dental caries. Following attachment, the organisms can either replicate locally and produce localized infection or penetrate the epithelial cell with systemic spread and produce more generalized disease. At times the local attachment and colonization by organisms leads to disease, as in the case of *Pseudomonas* infection of the respiratory tract in cystic fibrosis patients, in whom the presence of mucoid strains of the organism adds to the burden of the obstructive characteristics of the disease.

There are a number of host factors that are directed against this phase of microbial virulence. The integrity of the body perimeter, e.g., skin and mucous membranes, can protect against attachment. The normal microbial flora and the acidity of the gastrointestinal tract may also prevent attachment of these organisms. The defense provided by local IgA immunoglobulins in restricting the spread of organisms in the respiratory tract, the gastrointestinal tract, and possibly the genitourinary tract may provide a highly efficient localized type of defense (Chapter 5). The mechanisms by which secretory IgA functions are not entirely clear, but several possibilities exist: (1) direct neutralization, (2) direct lysis of organisms, (3) their opsonic effect, or (4) the direct coating of mucosal cells, preventing surface attachment. However, the microbial virulence is capable of overcoming many of these host defense mechanisms. There is evidence, for example, that certain bacteria elaborate enzymes capable of cleaving the IgA molecule.

PENETRATION AND INVASIVENESS

Following the encounter of a pathogen with a susceptible host, invasiveness is a requirement for the production of disease. The factors that contribute to virulence vary with different organisms. In the case of acute bacterial infections, these factors consist of the elaboration of *capsules* and the production of *enzymes* that facilitate invasion.

Encapsulated microorganisms, such as *Streptococcus (Diplococcus) pneumoniae* and *Haemophilus influenzae,* and also certain fungi are protected from the effects of phagocytosis. In contrast, unencapsulated organisms are readily phagocytosed. The mechanism for this phenomenon is not well understood but may be due to the inability of binding at the capsule-phagocytic interface owing to characteristics related to hydrophobicity and surface tension properties of the capsule. Of interest is the finding that when the capsule is removed or when the organism is treated with specific antibody (opsonins), the organisms are rendered susceptible to phagocytosis and subsequent intracellular digestion.

A number of bacteria elaborate enzymes that may enhance their invasive properties. For example, certain of the gram-positive bacteria produce hyaluronidase, which is capable of hydrolyzing the hyaluronic acid material of the ground substance of cells, and this may be important as a "spreading factor." Coagulases, which clot plasma, are produced by staphylococci; streptokinases, which catalyze the lysis of fibrin, are produced by certain strains of streptococci. Clostridia and anaerobic gas-producing organisms elaborate collagenases, which destroy the collagen matrix of muscle and are believed to be important in the spread of these organisms. Illustrative enzymes, their actions, and their bacterial sources are listed in Table 14–4. Other enzymes elaborated by pathogens play a detrimental role for the host, such as the hemolysins, which can cause transient hemolytic anemias in patients with infectious disease. Paradoxically, certain enzymes produced by microorganisms may facilitate their own destruction. For example, the respiratory burst with production of peroxide and activated forms of oxygen is a well-known metabolic pathway in neutrophils important for the killing of bacteria (Chapter 2). Children with the inborn deficiency of neutro-

Table 14–4. Examples of Enzymes Elaborated by Microorganisms Contributing to Virulence

Enzyme	Bacteria	Action	Potential Effect
Hyaluronidase	Gram-positive (e.g., *Streptococcus pyogenes)*	Depolymerizes hyaluronic acid	"Spreading factor"
Coagulases	Gram-positive (e.g., *Staphylococcus aureus)*	Clots plasma	Builds up a fibrin network
Streptokinase	Gram-positive (e.g., *Streptococcus pyogenes)*	Lyses fibrin	Allows the streptococci to spread
Collagenases	Gram-positive (e.g., *Clostridium perfringens)*	Destroys collagen	Allows proliferation of the clostridia, with production of gas gangrene
Hemolysins	Gram-positive (e.g., *Streptococcus pyogenes)*	Lyses red blood cells	Anemia

phils, chronic granulomatous disease, are predisposed to infections with peroxide-negative organisms (Chapter 22). Bacteria deficient in catalase (peroxide-positive) appear to provide bacterial sources of peroxide, replacing the defect found in these leukocytes.

TOXIN PRODUCTION

Once the organism has successfully invaded the host, toxic materials may be elaborated by the organism. There are two types: (1) exotoxins and (2) endotoxins.

Exotoxins are proteins elaborated by bacteria as extracellular products that have the capacity of acting as cell poisons. Examples of exotoxins are the diphtheria and the tetanus toxins. *Endotoxins* are composed of a lipid-polysaccharide complex.

The biologic effects of exotoxins are of clinical importance. Exotoxin activities are revealed by such diverse effects as cytotoxic effects, inhibition of protein synthesis (diphtheria toxin), interference with neuronal transmission (botulinus toxin), and transport of ions and water across cell membranes (possible mechanism of cholera toxin). Exotoxins do not induce an inflammatory response, although the organisms that produce them are phlogistic (inflammation-producing). Exotoxins are soluble proteins that bind to tissue and, once bound, cannot be neutralized readily by circulating antibody. These proteins are capable of producing an antibody response (antitoxin). Moreover, they can be altered (denatured) to form substances that retain their immunogenicity but lose their toxicity. These denatured forms of toxins are referred to as *toxoids* and are important sources for bacterial vaccines (Chapter 23). Antitoxin may be assayed by *in vivo* techniques, e.g., toxin neutralization, or by *in vivo* techniques, e.g., Schick and Dick tests (Chapter 8).

The biologic effects of endotoxins are equally important. It is now recognized that most biologic activity of endotoxins resides in the lipid protein (lipid A) of the molecule. When injected into the experimental animal, endotoxin produces the biologic effects of shock, fever, leukopenia, hyperglycemia, and intravascular coagulation. Endotoxins are also capable of eliciting the Sanarelli-Shwartzman reaction.

If two small subcutaneous doses of endotoxin are given 24 hours apart, the second injection results in a localized vasculitis and a hemorrhagic necrosis (localized Shwartzman reaction); however, if the injections are given intravenously, the animal dies within 24 hours and bilateral cortical necrosis of the kidneys is seen (generalized Shwartzman reaction).

The clinical counterpart of this phenomenon is seen in septicemias due to gram-negative organisms such as the meningococcus and in the hemolytic-uremic syndrome. Autopsy findings show similar bilateral cortical necrosis of the adrenals or kidneys, respectively. Disseminated intravascular coagulation, seen in many overwhelming septicemias, is also believed to be related to effects of endotoxin. Recently, this knowledge of the structural and biologic functions of endotoxin has had clinical application in the treatment of acute shock due to bacteremia by gram-negative bacteria by the use of human antisera to the lipid moiety of endotoxin (Chapter 24).

CAPACITY FOR GENETIC CHANGE

A factor that contributes to the maintenance of the virulence of an organism in a population is the ability of certain pathogens to undergo mutation periodically. The influenza virus represents the pathogen *par excellence* that manifests this phenomenon and has caused the most frequent epidemics. Influenza can be maintained in nature only within a susceptible population. Following an epidemic, a population that has developed immunity to any given serotype is no longer susceptible. Many variants of influenza, e.g., A2 Victoria, are known to occur owing to antigen shifts or drifts in the composition of the viral genome (Chapter 16). These viral mutations are responsible for new waves of epidemics, since the population is again susceptible. Similar mutations among other pathogens permit maintenance of virulent strains in nature.

The exploitation of microbial genetics has potential for future vaccine development. Recently, genetically attenuated (e.g., temperature-sensitive or biochemically defective) mutants of bacteria and viruses have been developed and show promise as new vaccines (Chapter 23).

PROPERTIES OF THE HOST

To counter the vast array of virulence factors of the microbes, the protective mechanisms of the host show an equal array of complex immunologic responses to maintain homeostasis. This homeostasis or immunologic balance must be as variable as the mechanisms expressed by the organisms that establish the infections. The homeostasis of man's immunologic system is different from that seen in other metabolic processes of the body, however, in the sense that it is much more heterogeneous. For example, the maintenance of normal concentration of blood sugar is achieved through complex metabolic processes that regulate the quantity of one product, sugar. In the case of the immune response, one type of microbial invasion affects many immune mechanisms that involve the interplay between a variety of cell types and a multitude of structurally unrelated products differing in quantity and function (heterogeneity). The pathogens against which the immunologic surveillance is directed are constantly undergoing changes in virulence. These changes therefore must be countered swiftly and efficiently by the recognition system of the host so as to reinstate immunologic homeostasis, or balance (Chapter 2).

The physician must evaluate the many factors that affect the responses of the host to infectious agents. These include age, genetic predisposition to infection, nutrition, the psychologic state of the host, and the environment (Chapter 1).

Age

The maturation of man, from fetal life to senescence, is accompanied by a corresponding development of the immunologic responses. With regard to the protective mechanisms against infecting agents, the fetus is a unique host. It is now recognized that the fetus is not immunologically incompetent; it is immunologically pristine. If the fetus is exposed to an infectious agent *in utero,* it is capable of a limited but specific immunologic response. Specific antibody synthesis to agents such as those that produce toxoplasmosis, rubella, cytomegalovirus, herpes, and syphilis (TORCHS syndrome) has been demonstrated early in gestation. All immunoglobulins can be synthesized as early as the twelfth week of fetal life; however, the mature lymphoid tissues are not fully developed and, as a result, the full expression of cell-mediated immunity is not optimal in the fetus and neonate. Consequently, convalescence from infections, recovery from which is dependent upon this mechanism, e.g., infections of cytomegalovirus or rubella virus, may be delayed and lead to devastating effects in the infant. These infants are known to excrete virus for prolonged periods of time after birth and become silent reservoirs of virus, capable of infecting susceptible individuals.

The polymorphonuclear responses are likewise less efficient in the newborn and young infant. Passive transfer of IgG-associated antibodies to many viruses and bacteria occurs, so that the infant is protected from many of the common pathogenic organisms; however, there is no transfer of IgM-associated antibodies, such as those to the gram-negative bacteria. These findings may explain in part the well-known susceptibility of the newborn infant to infection with gram-negative organisms. In older infancy and childhood the spectrum of disease changes. With a changing maturation, additional immunologic responses are available to the older child. The susceptibility to gram-negative enteric organisms disappears after the first month of life. This is associated with the increased synthesis of IgM immunoglobulin. Concomitant with the disappearance of maternal IgG immunoglobulin during the first six months of life, there is a susceptibility to infection with organisms such as the *Haemophilus influenzae, Streptococcus (Diplococcus) pneumoniae,* and beta-hemolytic streptococci and other common respiratory viruses.

It has been suggested by several workers that the presence of this passively acquired IgG-associated antibody may at times be harmful to the host. It has been considered that bronchiolitis in the young infant may be due in part to the viral antigen-antibody complexes formed during the course of viral infection. The complexes, formed between the maternally derived antibody and viral antigen within the respiratory tract, may contribute to immunologic injury of the lungs during bronchiolitis. Alternatively, the cell-mediated immunity and IgE antibody have been suggested to participate in the pathogenesis of the bronchiolitis syndrome. The changing spectrum of infection with age is seen with other organisms, such as the Group A beta-hemolytic streptococci (streptococcosis). In the newborn infant, Group A streptococcal infection may be restricted to the skin; in children two to three years old, it may be restricted to the nasopharynx; and in the five- to six-year-old child, the classic pharyngotonsillitis is seen. Another possible factor contributing to localized infection seen in the developing child is the delayed development of the IgA immunoglobulins, which do not assume adult capability until adolescence (Chapter 3).

Within a wide range of normality, the mature adult expresses full immunologic competence that is due to previous immunizing exposure to an immense variety of infections and noninfectious stimuli. As a consequence, re-exposure to a previously encountered pathogen usually results in an anamnestic stimulation of the immunologic response with minimal or no sequelae.

Finally, in later adult life, reinfection occurs in spite of prior infection. For example, herpes zoster is known to occur in patients who have recovered from varicella infection. In fact it has been stated that "whooping cough is a disease of infants and grandmothers." It has been reported that there is a measurable diminution in serum gamma globulins in persons over the age of 50. Finally, the increase in autoimmunity and malignancy known to occur in the elderly may reflect a waning immunity or an increase in errors of the immunologic mechanisms.

Genetic Predisposition to Infection

Several genetic factors affect host susceptibility to infection in man and other species. The defects may or may not involve the immunologic system. Recently, a relationship has been demonstrated between histocompatibility types and susceptibility to certain infectious diseases (Chapter 3).

Within the immunologic defects, there are two compartments of resistance: those concerned with nonspecific immune responses and those concerned with specific immune responses (Fig. 14–2). The genetic predisposition to infection in a normal population is expressed by the wide variations in both types of resistance mechanisms. The extreme aberrations of this variation are best exemplified in the immune deficiency diseases (Chapter 22).

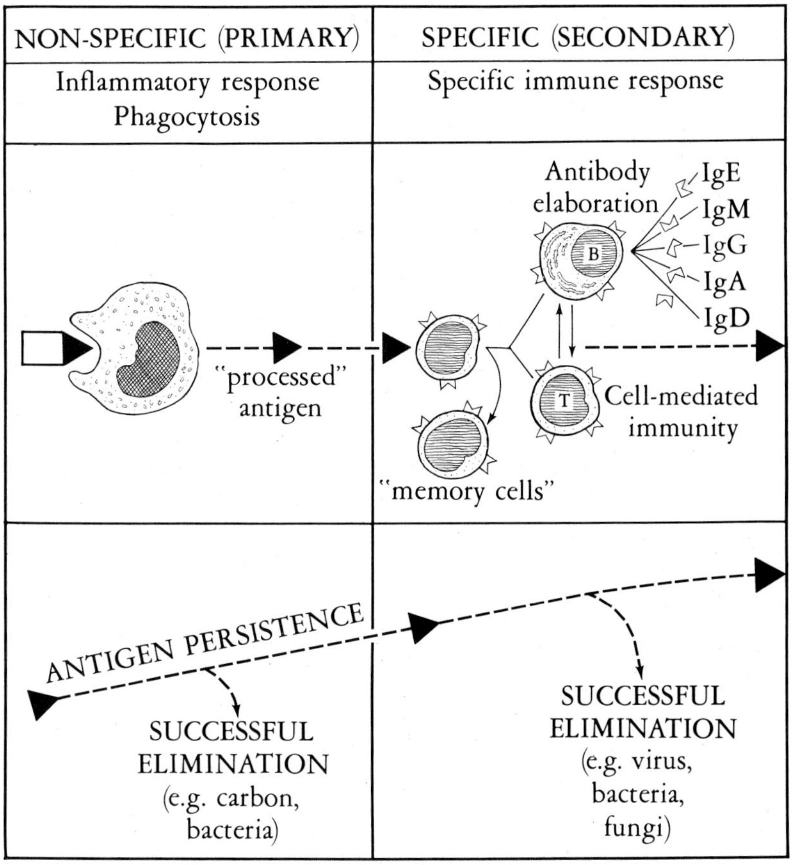

Figure 14–2. Compartments of the resistance mechanisms.

The genetic defects unrelated to the immune response that affect the susceptibility or resistance to infection include such entities as sickle cell anemia, glucose-6-phosphate dehydrogenase deficiency, and many hemoglobinopathies. In areas of the world where malaria is endemic, individuals who possess these defects have less severe malaria than individuals without these defects. In the case of sickle cell disease, the homozygote is at a disadvantage from the primary disease. Individuals with the sickle cell trait, however, appear to have a survival advantage when living in malaria-infested areas; the trait confers a disadvantage in nonmalarious areas and in adverse environments, e.g., high altitudes. Thus, environmental differences can affect the expression of a single hereditary factor in infectious disease susceptibility. Another aspect is that of the deficiency of pneumococcal opsonins, which have been demonstrated in individuals with sickle cell disease.

Genetic susceptibility, correlated with racial factors and sex factors, is seen in the increased incidence of tuberculosis in nonwhites. Furthermore, a greater proportion of male infants than female infants are known to be victims of serious bacterial infections.

Thus, genetic susceptibility to infectious disease appears to be under the control of many genes (polygenic). The effect of defects in specific immunologic and nonimmunologic systems and the role of the environment must be evaluated in the total expression of genetic predisposition to infection.

Nutrition

The nutritional status of the host plays an important role in the prevalence and severity of infectious diseases, particularly among those suffering from nutritional deficiency. Although malnutrition does not depress antibody formation or phagocytosis in the adult, such a nutritional deficit can lead to a profound deficiency in cell-mediated reactivity in the developing infant and child. For example, in patients with marasmus and kwashiorkor there is a high susceptibility to viral, bacterial, and parasitic diseases as a consequence of protein malnutrition.

Malnutrition may also interfere with recovery from infectious diseases. For example, the walling-off processes initiated by an infecting agent require the synthesis of fibrin, polysaccharides, and collagen. During malnutrition, these responses are retarded because of an inadequate intake of essential precursors, including protein. The rate of healing of wounds, for example, is markedly retarded by dietary deficiencies.

Psychologic Status of the Host

The psychologic status of the patient with infectious disease can markedly affect the course of the disease. In those diseases that are not readily treated by antibiotic therapy, the psychologic state of the host becomes a major factor in the recovery of the individual. In addition, the effect of stress in such disease states can be associated with a more prolonged convalescent course through physiologic alterations. For example, in recruits in basic training who are known to be susceptible to adult respiratory distress syndrome (ARDS), hormonal levels of 17-hydroxy-corticosteroid increase markedly during the early weeks of basic training. The timing of this event coincides with the period of increased susceptibility to many of the ARDS agents.

Pregnancy

Pregnancy represents a special category of an altered metabolic state. Pregnant women are more prone to certain infections than are nonpregnant women for a variety of causes, including anatomic and metabolic ones. For example, the compression of ureters with obstruction due to fetal positioning predisposes the patient to urinary tract infections. The reasons for the susceptibility to other infectious diseases, e.g., influenza and poliomyelitis, are not apparent. Recently, a diminution in cell-mediated immunity during pregnancy has been demonstrated, which provides yet another basis for susceptibility to certain infectious diseases, e.g., viral diseases, during this period. The precise basis for this transient diminution is unknown, but several hormones, e.g., alpha-fetoprotein, human gonadotropin, and progesterone, have been shown to exert an immunosuppressive effect on lymphocytes.

MANIFESTATIONS OF HYPERSENSITIVITY AS A COMPLICATION OF INFECTIOUS DISEASES

During the course of the host parasite interaction in infectious diseases, the immune response to the microorganisms may not be beneficial but at times may be responsible for tissue injury through hypersensitivity reactions (Chapters 13 and 20C). Although many of the Gell-Coombs reactions may be operative, foremost among these are the reactions caused by immune complex injury (Type III reactions). The production of antigen-antibody complexes, in which complement is activated, leads to the development of inflammation through the release of soluble mediators, including many of the phlogistic components of complement (Chapter 5). These manifestations are particularly prominent when pathogens persist and there is failure of elimination of the antigen. Immune complex complications of infectious diseases have been documented in such entities as viral hepatitis (in which persistent antigenemia due to HBsAg is involved), in infectious endocarditis with the persistence of bacteria (e.g., *Streptococcus viridans*), in acute glomerulonephritis following infection caused by Group A hemolytic streptococci or by *Plasmodium malariae.*

ENVIRONMENT OF THE HOST AND PARASITE

The host-parasite relationship is influenced directly by the external environment. In the case of the parasite, the environment affects the type of parasite, its rate of mutation, its geographic distribution, and its transmissibility. Man-made alterations in the external environment result in a disturbed ecologic balance in the natural flora and fauna; for example, the widespread use of fertilizers and insecticides produces changes in parasitic forms and the clustering of disease-causing parasites. In addition to this, the artificial and rather complete dissemination of parasites occurs in our modern world through modern transportation. Thus, one can easily see the potential for widespread epidemics of disease, e.g., smallpox and influenza. Moreover, the recent emergence of opportunistic infection from the use of immunosuppressive drugs or that seen in the epidemic of AIDS represents another example of the effects of environment and lifestyle on the host-parasite relationship. The indiscriminate use of antibiotics has added to the problems, because of the development of antibiotic-resistant strains of bacteria that present a very real therapeutic difficulty for the physician. Thus, the physician should be aware of these and other variables that can affect the host-parasite relationship in his patients.

The external environment of the host affects the host-parasite relationship to disadvantage, either by self-administered toxic substances such as drugs, alcohol, tobacco impurities, or a deficient diet (e.g., malnutrition) or from substances imposed upon him such as pollutants, insecticides, food additives, and toxic substances used in certain manufacturing industries.

Alterations of the external environment as well as life systems clearly affect both the host and the parasite. Thus, the physician is faced with expressions of disease that may take unexpected form or emerge as a new disease entity because of altered form and condition of the parasite, e.g., AIDS.

SUMMARY

The host-parasite relationship represents the overall interplay between the factors controlling the changing virulence of an organism and the immense variability of the host's surveillance system, which must swiftly and efficiently counteract in order to maintain immunologic balance (homeostasis). The many factors that influence the host-parasite relationship include the age, genetic predisposition, nutrition, metabolic state, and psychologic state of the host as well as the environment in which the host-parasite relationship occurs.

Suggestions for Further Reading

Bellanti, J. A. (ed.): Acute Diarrhea: Its Nutritional Consequences in Children. New York, Raven Press, 1983.

Chandra, R. K.: Nutrition, immunity and infection: present knowledge and future directions. Lancet, *1*:688, 1983.

Drutz, D. J., and Mills, J.: Immunity and infection. *In* Stites, D. P., Stobo, J. D., Fudenberg, H. H., et al. (eds.): Basic and Clinical Immunology. Los Altos, Lange Medical Publications, 1982.

Gottlieb, M. S., et al.: The acquired immunodeficiency syndrome. Ann. Intern. Med., *99*:208, 1983.

Mackowiak, P. A.: The normal microbial flora. N. Engl. J. Med., *307*:83, 1982.

Quinn, T. C., Stamm, W. E., Goodell, S. E., et al.: The polymicrobial origin of intestinal infections in homosexual men. N. Engl. J. Med., *309*:576, 1983.

Ziegler, E. J., McCutchan, J. A., Fierer, J., et al.: Treatment of gram negative bacteremia and shock with human antiserum to a mutant *Escherichia coli.* N. Engl. J. Med., *307*:1225, 1982.

Chapter 15

Mechanisms of Immunity to Bacterial Diseases

Joseph A. Bellanti, M.D.

Bacterial infections in man best illustrate the mechanisms involved in the host-parasite relationship, the outcome of which is determined by the genetic endowment of the host and the genetic capability of the bacteria. It is now generally accepted that bacteria possess an extreme degree of variability and have great potential for adaptation through such mechanisms as mutation, metabolic alterations induced by a changing environment, lysogenization with bacteriophage, production of toxins, and capability for prolonged survival (sporulation). Such complex responses from the bacterial pathogen are met with equally complex and diverse immune responses in man.

The field of immunology is a direct outgrowth of the study of host responses to bacterial infection, and, in fact, the early successes of bacteriology are the foundations upon which modern immunology rests. *Immunoprophylaxis*, the prevention of disease by vaccines, and *immunotherapy*, the prevention and treatment of disease through the use of immune sera or gamma globulin, are the tools of the physician in assisting the patient (i.e., the host) to enhance the natural immune responses to bacteria and other pathogens (Chapters 23 and 24).

In the early days of bacteriology, research emphasis was on humoral factors. This restriction of interest was due to a primary concern with the protective role of serum antibody, particularly as related to antitoxic immunity. It is now known, however, that cellular responses are also involved in the immune responses to bacteria and these play perhaps the most critical and decisive role in certain host-parasite interactions. Thus, immunity to bacterial diseases must include a very broad biologic view, encompassing the vast interplay of humoral and cellular factors that compose the total immunologic responses of the host.

CLASSIFICATION OF BACTERIAL INFECTIONS

Three broad categories of bacterial infections are recognized: (1) the *acute* or highly productive type of infection; (2) the *chronic* type, exhibiting the capacity of certain bacteria, e.g, intracellular parasites, to establish intracellular parasitism (Chapter 14); and (3) the *toxigenic* or *toxin-producing* type of infection, usually seen in acute infections (Table 15–1).

Acute

The first type of infection is exemplified by bacteria, e.g., *Staphylococcus* or *Streptococcus*, that may gain access to the body through any of the natural portals of entry, including the respiratory tract, the gastrointestinal tract, or the genitourinary tract or through breaks in the continuity of the skin or mucous membranes. The bacteria may undergo a limited replication and cause a localized lesion, which may be accompanied by abscess formation (a collection of polymorphonuclear leukocytes). Some bacteria are effectively killed by polymorphonuclear leukocytes; others require the presence of antibody and complement (opsonins) (Chapters 5 and 6). If host defense mechanisms are sufficient to contain this pyogenic (pus-forming) response locally, resolution and healing will occur. If, on the other hand, host defense mechanisms are insufficient to restrain these

Table 15–1. Classification of Bacterial Infections

			Immunity Mechanisms				
			Nonspecific		Specific		
			Phagocytosis	Inflammatory Response	Antibody		Cell-mediated
Type	**Examples**	**Histopathology**			Serum	Local	
Acute							
Localized	Staphylococcal abscess, streptococcal pharyngitis	Polymorphonuclear leukocytes ("abscess")	+	+	+	?	?
Generalized	Meningococcemia	Varied	+	+	+	0	?
Chronic	Tuberculosis, leprosy, brucellosis	Macrophage ("granuloma")	+	+	0	0	+
Toxigenic	Diphtheria, tetanus, cholera	Exotoxin—none	0	0	+	+	0
		Endotoxin—varied	?	0 to +	?	?	0

bacteria locally, the infection could spread regionally or gain access into the systemic circulation, causing a fulminating sepsis. Other organs may be "seeded" as a result of the latter process. Strains of various bacteria, e.g., *Staphylococcus*, vary in their ability to produce a number of toxins and digestive enzymes, which may contribute to their virulence and invasive potential. Organisms causing acute infection may be completely disposed of or may enter into chronic infection.

Chronic

The second type of bacteria-host interaction is that characterized by a protracted or chronic course of infection, in which bacteria enter into a mutualism with the host (Table 15–1). These types of infection are caused by such organisms as *Mycobacterium tuberculosis, Mycobacterium leprae*, and the Brucellae and may be protracted over long periods of time. Such infections establish a delicate balance with the host and evoke an inflammatory response characterized by macrophage and lymphoid accumulation with granuloma formation (Chapter 12). The infections are characterized by the intracellular residence of organisms within phagocytes (macrophages) for extended periods of time. An example of chronic infection of significance to the physician is the carrier state, which represents a specialized example of inapparent infection (Chapter 14). In this state, an infection exists (e.g., staphylococcus nasal carrier) in the absence of overt disease; hence, the pathogen is not deleterious to the host but can be transmitted to susceptible individuals. A carrier state can be seen as a further manifestation of acute infections such as typhoid fever and streptococcal and meningococcal infections. The mechanism for this phenomenon is unknown.

Toxigenic

A third type of bacteria-host interaction involves production of toxin, after a limited replication of the bacterium. The toxin may be one of two types: endotoxin or exotoxin (Chapter 14). The effects of exotoxin account not only for many of the consequences resulting from classic infectious diseases such as the myocarditis of diphtheria and the paralysis of tetanus but also for many of the less obvious disease expressions more recently identified, e.g., toxic shock syndrome. Exotoxins may be elaborated after only limited bacterial replication but may have wide distribution through the circulation and may exert highly specific effects. In general, the tissue response to exotoxins is minimal, while the response to endotoxin may be more prominent and include a variety of vascular changes and effects on the hematopoietic system (Chapter 14).

Certain strains of bacteria produce many exotoxins that, in turn, are associated with specific clinical entities. For example, the staphylococcus produces a variety of enterotoxins (A, B, C, D, E, F) that are responsible for staphylococcal food poisoning, staphylococcal enterocolitis, exfoliative skin disorders, and, most recently, the toxic shock syndrome. Similarly, enteropathogenic strains of *Escherichia coli* are known to elaborate different classes of enterotoxins. These so-called enterotoxigenic *E. coli* (ETEC) produce heat-stable enterotoxin (ST) and heat-labile enterotoxin (LT), which are responsible for such diverse clinical entities as infantile enteritis and sepsis as well as travelers' diarrhea.

Thus, the antibacterial mechanisms of host defense vary according to the nature of the bacterial infection (Table 15–1). The relative roles of nonspecific factors (e.g., phagocytosis and the inflammatory response) and specific factors (e.g., antibody and cell-mediated events) will vary according to the nature of the infection.

ANTIBACTERIAL IMMUNITY MECHANISMS OF THE HOST

Antibacterial immunity mechanisms operative in man are directly influenced by the environment in which he lives and the lifestyle he chooses. There are certain predisposing physical and emotional conditions that may alter the expression of the immune response. Noteworthy are the occupational hazards (e.g., pneumoconiosis, pollutants, drugs, chemical additives, and insecticides) that may overtax the immune response. Alcohol, for example, directly depresses the functional and metabolic activities of phagocytes, e.g., chemotaxis and microbicidal activities. In addition, malnutrition is known to adversely affect the immune response to bacterial agents. Recent examples of this include the opportunistic infections seen in AIDS (Chapter 22), the toxic shock syndrome caused by toxemic staphylococcal infections resulting from use of tampons, and legionnaires' disease caused by *Legionella pneumophila* in contaminated water from air conditioners.

Many bacteria found on the body surfaces are in a state of balance with the host and are restricted to superficial sites of the body. If these bacteria gain access to deeper tissues, symptoms and signs of disease will result. Thus, the defense function of the lymphoreticular tissues must be active in order to restrict these bacteria and maintain a state of health.

The mechanisms involved in a primary or immediate encounter of the host with a bacterial pathogen are termed *nonspecific immunologic mechanisms;* those involved in encounters subsequent to the primary encounter are the *specific immunologic responses*. It should be noted that both processes are stimulated in all infections and the expressions will vary.

Nonspecific Factors

The intact skin and mucous membranes offer a mechanical barrier against invasion by bacteria. When the integrity of the skin is broken, e.g., because of burns or eczema, bacterial skin infections (pyoderma) may result. These infections are most often associated with organisms that normally colonize the skin, e.g., *Staphylococcus aureus*. Similarly, the well-known secondary staphylococcal pneumonia that occurs following influenza may be explained, in part, by loss of respiratory epithelium, which is a sequela of the viral infection and offers entry to the *Staphylococcus aureus*. There may also be direct effects of viral infection on the activity of phagocytes, which may be incriminated in staphylococcal pneumonia.

There are several other nonspecific factors important in antibacterial defense. The gastric juice, because of its acidity, may destroy many types of bacteria, whereas certain pathogenic bacteria, such as *Salmonella typhosa*, may survive this acid medium and produce gastrointestinal or systemic infections. Humoral factors important in antibacterial defense include the unsaturated fatty acids of the skin, which kill many surface bacteria. Also, lysozyme, an enzyme found in tears, saliva, and nasal secretions, is capable of degrading the mucopeptide layer of cell walls of many bacteria. This appears to be an important nonspecific defense mechanism of the host, which cleanses the normal mucous membranes of the upper respiratory passages.

Microbial antagonism is a factor important in maintaining an ecologic balance of microorganisms on the body surface. The balance may be upset by disease or by treatment. For example, the overgrowth of pathogenic *Staphylococcus aureus* following the use of the broad-spectrum antibiotics is one type of interaction in which homeostasis is altered.

PHAGOCYTOSIS AND THE INFLAMMATORY RESPONSE

If bacteria overcome the initial barriers, primitive responses of the host are stimulated, i.e., phagocytosis and the inflammatory response (Chapters 2 and 12). After invading deeper tissues, bacteria may be engulfed by wandering tissue macrophages (histiocytes), a random encounter that is not an efficient process (Fig. 15–1). More commonly, the organisms undergo limited replication and then trigger the inflammatory response with mobilization and emigration of neutrophils toward the infection site (Fig. 15–1). These cellular elements confront the microorganisms and, in the case of many acute pyogenic infections, the microorganisms are engulfed and digested efficiently. The capsules of some bacteria, e.g., pneumococcus, resist phagocytosis and contribute to increased pathogenicity; however, with the subsequent development of antibody (opsonin), the bacteria are coated and phagocytosis is facilitated (see Fig. 15–4). The familiar abscess or furuncle, which is a collection of polymorphonuclear leukocytes, is an example of this type of phagocytic mechanism important in antibacterial defense. In addition, a number of other factors are triggered by the inflammatory response, such as activation of the complement sequence and the coagulation system, with deposition of fibrin. These factors may also facilitate phagocytosis and the repair processes.

If bacteria are not successfully killed at the local sites, they may continue to replicate locally or further invade the host by way of the lymphatics to the regional lymph nodes (Fig. 15–2). The well-known "red streaks" that extend up the arm (lymphangitis) with enlarged epitrochlear or axillary lymph nodes are examples of this response. Within

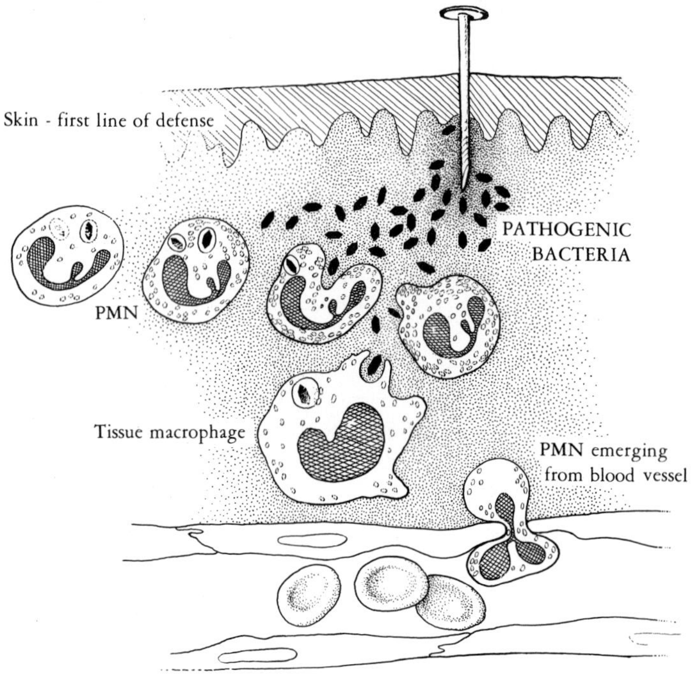

Figure 15–1. Schematic representation of phagocytosis by polymorphonuclear leukocytes (PMN) and tissue macrophages following penetration of the skin and introduction of pathogenic bacteria into deeper tissues. The PMN's are more efficient in phagocytosis than are the macrophages. Note that the PMN's are mobilized into tissues from blood vessels during the inflammatory response.

lymph nodes, the bacteria encounter elements of the phagocytic system (macrophages) that may be prerequisite to the initiation of specific immune responses (Fig. 15–3). Those organisms escaping phagocytosis may initiate an acute inflammatory response within the lymph node (lymphadenitis).

Bacteria may overcome the lymphatic-associated barriers and gain access directly into the blood stream. Here they come into contact with circulating phagocytes (polymorphonuclear leukocytes and monocytes), or they may reach organs such as the liver and the spleen, where they can interact with fixed phagocytic elements. Enlargement of the spleen (splenomegaly) is an important clinical finding in sepsis and reflects this increased phagocytic function. Although a powerful defense system of the host, the final reticuloendothelial barrier may also be overcome with seeding of such organs as the bone (osteomyelitis), the brain (brain abscess), or

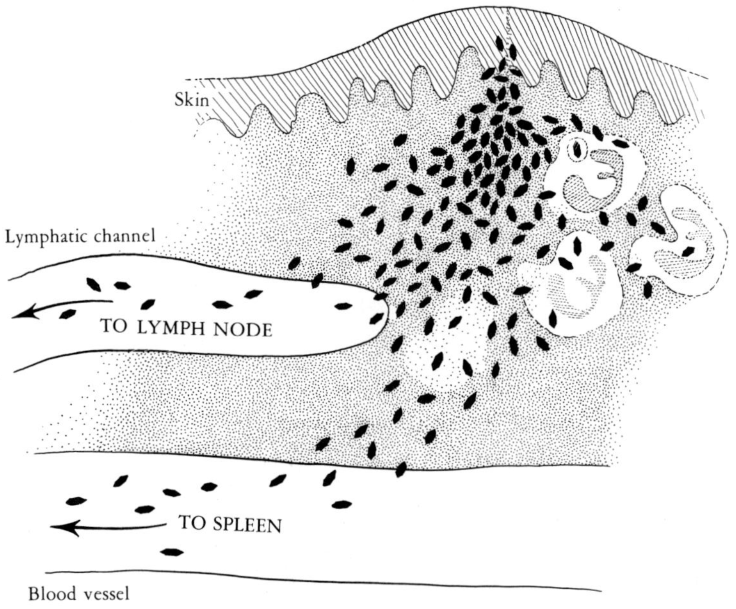

Figure 15–2. Schematic representation of the cellular events occurring if the PMN leukocytes are unsuccessful in killing the bacteria. The organisms are shown replicating in the tissues and entering a lymphatic channel and a blood vessel.

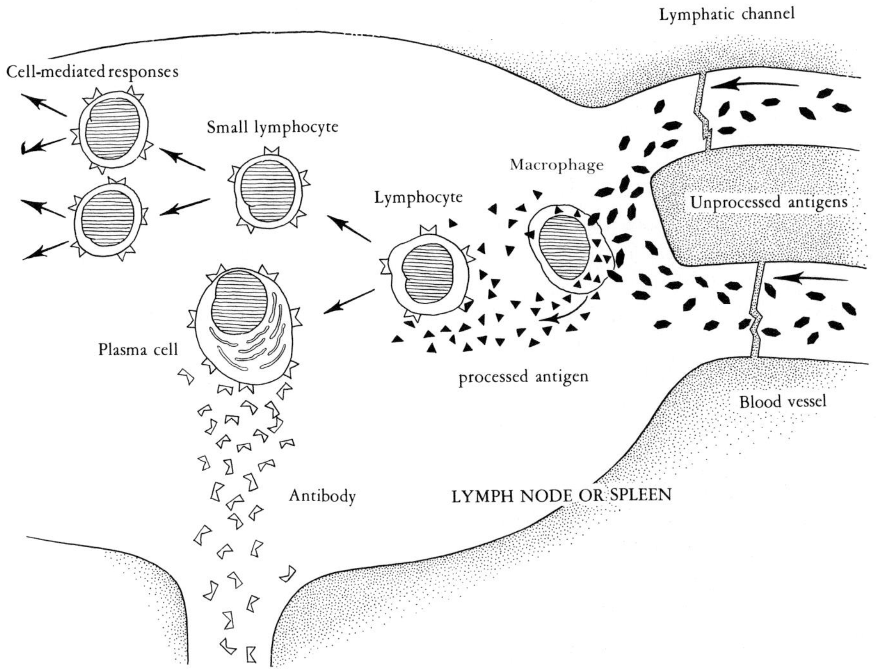

Figure 15–3. Schematic representation of the induction of a specific immune response in a lymph node or the spleen with elaboration of cell-mediated (delayed hypersensitivity) responses and antibody.

the kidney (renal abscess), terminating in fatal septicemia. Thus, the first encounter of the host with a bacterial pathogen of the acute pyogenic type summons elements of the nonspecific defense system, with participation by the products of the specific immune system that may interact in bodily defense.

Specific Antibacterial Mechanisms

During the course of bacterial infection or immunization, elements of the specific immune response are activated via cells of the lymphoid tissues. Involvement of the following may occur: regional lymph nodes, in the case of localized infection (skin); specialized lymphoid nodules lining the respiratory, gastrointestinal, and genitourinary tracts, in the case of organisms that infect at these sites; or the spleen, in the case of organisms invading the blood stream. Although all elements of the specific immune response may be activated in every type of infection, the relative roles vary with the type of invading organism. In the case of highly productive acute types of infection, antibody, primarily of the IgG variety, is stimulated. Certain bacteria, however, such as the gram-negative enteric bacteria, stimulate antibody that is primarily of the IgM class. Furthermore, in certain types of localized infections, particularly those of the respiratory and gastrointestinal tracts, there is evidence that local IgA antibody synthesis occurs. For example, in the case of cholera, local IgA antibody is produced within the gastrointestinal tract (coproantibody) that appears to be an important antibacterial mechanism at mucosal surfaces, as described in the following section.

ANTIBODY

The host response to infection by bacteria or to immunization leads to a sequential appearance of specific antibodies. The antibody appearing initially is usually of the high molecular weight IgM variety and is followed by IgG antibody. These differences, in order of appearance, however, may be laboratory artifacts and may reflect sensitivity of the antibody-detecting system. There is now evidence that on a molar basis, IgM antibodies have greater relative opsonizing, bactericidal, and agglutinating abilities than IgG; the IgG antibodies, on the other hand, possess greater relative precipitating abilities (Chapter 8).

From an operational standpoint, each of these antibodies seems to be well suited to perform specific functions. For example, IgM antibody, which is formed early in the immune response, appears to function best as an opsonin, facilitating and cooperating with the phagocytic events described earlier. Additionally, this class of antibody can immobilize bacteria by agglutination or, in the case of gram-negative bacteria, can lyse cell walls in the presence of complement (Chapters 5 and 6). Further, since IgM antibody is confined largely to the vascular compartment, it seems to be uniquely well suited to perform its function within the blood vascular system. IgG antibody, on the other hand, appears to diffuse quite readily between vascular and extravascular compartments. These IgG antibodies, which show good precipitating capacity, are effective in neutralizing toxins that might be found both in blood and in the tissues. The IgA antibody in secretions appears to have a number of novel features that make it well suited to function at body surfaces. The secretory IgA antibody, with its additional secretory component, is endowed with a unique stability, allowing it to function within the milieu in which other immunoglobulins would be degraded, e.g., the gastrointestinal tract (Chapter 5). Recently, some bacterial strains have been identified that are capable of elaborating proteases capable of degradation of IgA. These IgA mucosal antibodies, therefore, appear to be an important "first line of defense" in body secretions.

Upon subsequent encounter between a host and a bacterial pathogen, there occurs a secondary or anamnestic response that results in elaboration of antibody in an enhanced fashion, i.e., markedly increased quantity. This rapid "recall" of immunity terminates the infection quite rapidly. There are infections, however, the nature of which makes them insusceptible to these host defenses. These include infections such as abscesses or other chronic infections that by their nature prevent the ready access of antibody into areas of infection.

CELL-MEDIATED IMMUNITY (DELAYED HYPERSENSITIVITY)

Those bacterial infections that overcome the nonspecific factors of the host induce a tissue response that is characterized by the production of cell-mediated events (delayed hypersensitivity). The reactivity is induced during a primary encounter with a bacterial pathogen and is seen in all subsequent encounters with the same pathogen. Although this response occurs in all bacterial infections, it is most prominent in infections of the chronic type, e.g., intracellular infection. The presence of reactivity is also useful in the diagnosis of certain chronic infections, e.g., tuberculosis.

In certain chronic infections, e.g., leprosy, a state of anergy is seen in which there is a loss of delayed hypersensitivity skin testing. The diminished reactivity is proportional to the progression of disease. A loss of primary bacterial delayed hypersensitivity is also seen when there are concurrent infections such as measles. These findings indicate a possible explanation for the aggravation effect of concurrent viral infection on the course of a preexisting bacterial infection. For example, influenza is known to exacerbate an old quiescent tuberculosis into an active form.

INTERRELATIONSHIPS BETWEEN THE COMPARTMENTS OF THE IMMUNE RESPONSE DURING THE PATHOGENESIS OF BACTERIAL INFECTIONS

The compartments of the immunologic system work in concert so that, when the primitive defense mechanisms of the host have been surmounted and the specific immunologic responses are stimulated, the products of the latter will enhance the former (Fig. 15–4). In stimulating the specific immune response, the resultant production of opsonins and simultaneous stimulation of cell-mediated events (delayed hypersensitivity) result in products that can enhance phagocytosis by macrophages or polymorphonuclear (PMN) leukocytes (Chapters 8 and 9). Both responses are stimulated in all infections. It must be emphasized that although there is a predominant expression of one or the other mechanism, depending upon the type of infection, there is a quantitative relationship between the mechanism expressed and the infective characteristics of the pathogen. The three types of bacterial infection in man exemplify these relationships: (1) the acute bacterial infection, (2) the chronic infection, and (3) the toxigenic infection.

Acute Infection

In Figure 15–5 it can be seen that in an acute infection a nonencapsulated organism

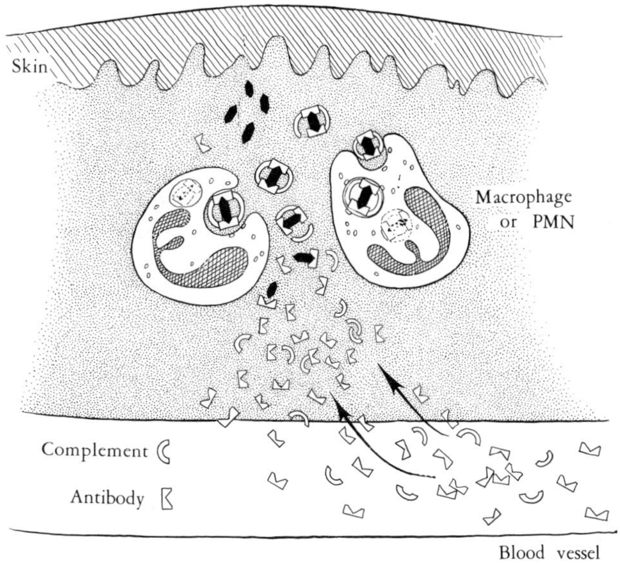

Figure 15–4. Schematic representation of the enhancement of phagocytosis, occurring with the development of specific antibody together with the participation of complement.

will be readily phagocytosed. In contrast, in the case of the encapsulated organism following the subsequent production of antibody and the initiation of the complement cascade (opsonins), phagocytosis by PMN leukocytes will be greatly enhanced. Simultaneously, there is stimulation of cell-mediated immunity, which enhances phagocytosis by macrophages. Since such organisms are not regularly phagocytosed by macrophages, this scheme normally appears to be of relatively lesser importance (Fig. 15–5).

However, in clinical situations in which the PMN leukocytes are deficient, as in the newborn or in CGD (chronic granulomatous disease), a prominent but low-efficiency macro-

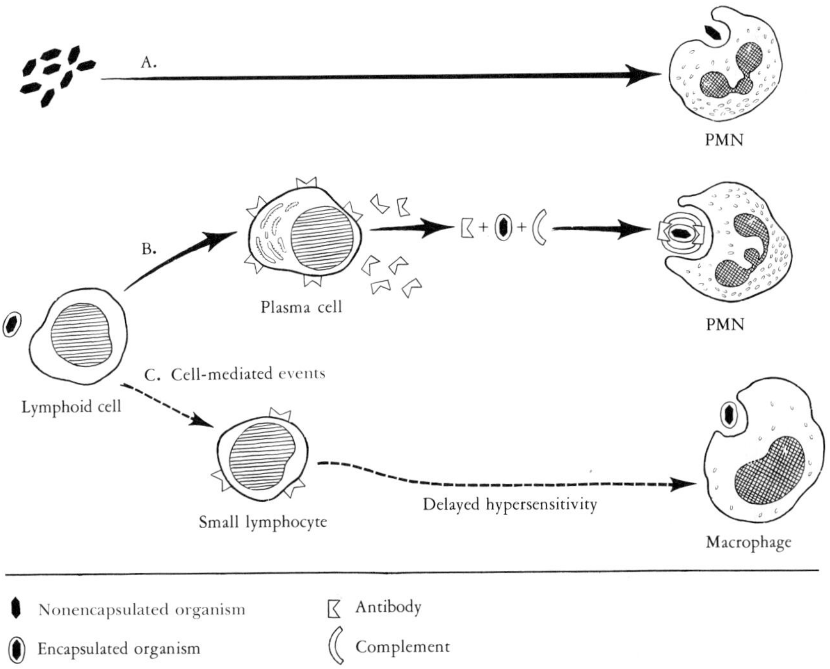

Figure 15–5. Schematic representation of relative roles of antibody and cell-mediated events in enhancement of phagocytosis in *acute* bacterial infections. *A*, Phagocytosis of an unencapsulated organism through an unenhanced process; *B*, the enhanced process of phagocytosis through antibody and complement; and *C*, the relatively lesser importance of cell-mediated events during acute infection. Note the interrelationship of antibody and phagocytosis by PMN leukocytes and its relatively greater importance than cell-mediated events during acute infections.

phage interaction is seen, indicating that this mechanism can be utilized (Chapter 22).

Chronic Infection

The chronic type of infection is best exemplified by tuberculosis in man (Fig. 15–6). In the initial encounter between tubercle bacillus and polymorphonuclear leukocytes, a paradoxical situation arises. This cell can ingest the organism but cannot degrade the lipid capsule. Thus the invading microorganism has an advantage, since transport is provided to deeper tissues along with nutriment for necessary life processes and protection from the extracellular effects of antibody. The short-lived cells (PMN) provide only a limited period of intracellular parasitism, however. The major cellular response in the infection is subsequent phagocytosis by macrophages, in which the organisms survive for an even longer period of time. In addition, upon ingestion, there is a simultaneous stimulation of cell-mediated events (delayed hypersensitivity), with the elaboration of products such as the macrophage inhibitory factor (MIF) and chemotactic factors (Chapters 9 and 13) (Fig. 15–6) that can further enhance the activity of macrophages. If these pathogens remain viable, further response of the host is manifested through granuloma formation, which serves to wall-off or localize the infected area. Any breakdown in bodily defense, such as concurrent viral infection, is known to permit dissemination of the tubercle bacillus with exacerbation of the disease. Some individuals can terminate infection successfully during macrophage phagocytosis and show no granuloma formation. Evidence indicates that termination of intracellular parasitism is coincident with the development of increased macrophage efficiency ("activated macrophages"), which seems to be under the control of the effector molecules released from sensitized lymphocytes, e.g., MIF. Such increased efficiency also confers an increased ability of the macrophage to kill nonrelated organisms.

Of importance in the host-parasite relationship is the recognition that the expressions of certain bacterial diseases may reflect the relative status of cell-mediated immunity. For example, in lepromatous leprosy, a diminution of cell-mediated immunity is known to exist, whereas in the tuberculid form a heightened cell-mediated immunity is found.

Toxigenic Infection

A third type of bacterial infection involves toxin production (Fig. 15–7). Exotoxins are proteins elaborated as extracellular products of microorganisms. The extracellular metabolites may be produced in toxic quantities after even minimal infection of the host or may be produced outside the host and enter via ingestion, e.g., botulism. The prime defense of the host against toxins is through neutralization by production of specific antibody (antitoxin). This detoxification process leads to the production of toxin-antitoxin complexes that are usually removed by phag-

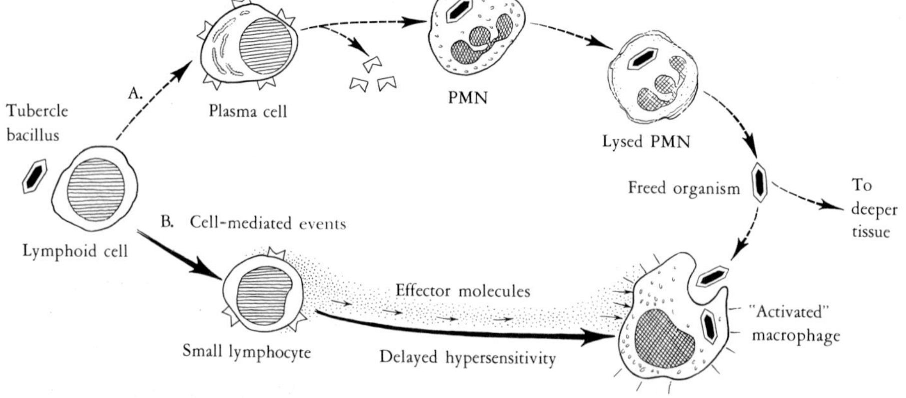

Figure 15–6. Schematic representation of relative roles of antibody and cell-mediated events in enhancement of phagocytosis during *chronic* bacterial infections. *A* shows limited activity of the polymorphonuclear leukocytes, and *B*, the major cellular response in chronic infection, carried out through macrophages with simultaneous stimulation of cell-mediated events, further enhancing immunity. Note the interrelationship between the cell-mediated immunity effector molecules with phagocytosis by macrophages and its relatively greater importance than antibody-enhanced phagocytosis by PMN leukocytes in chronic infection.

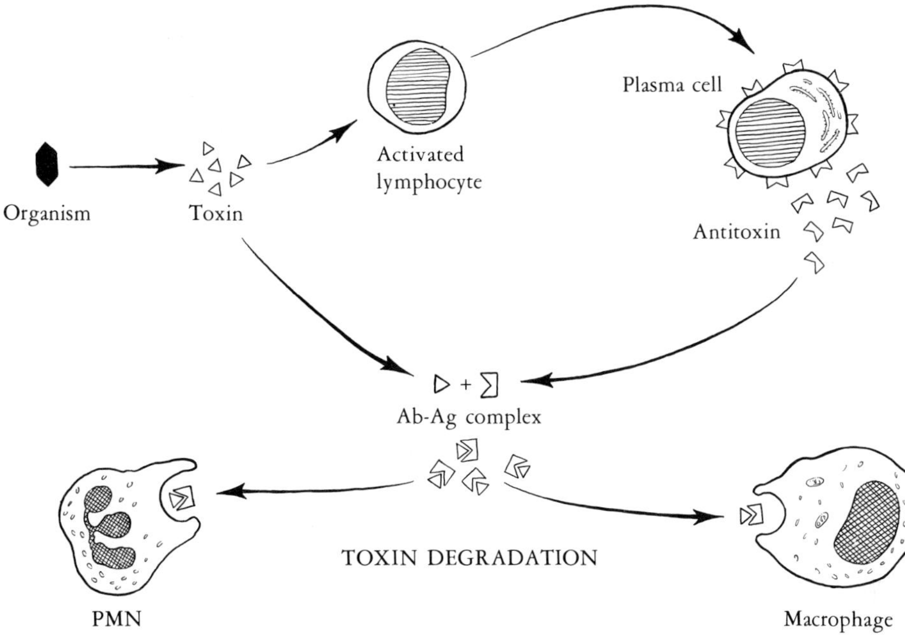

Figure 15–7. Schematic representation of the immunologic mechanism of toxin neutralization by antibody. The neutralized toxin-antitoxin complexes are shown being taken up and degraded within both types of phagocytic cells.

ocytic degradation (Fig. 15–7). However, under conditions of antigen excess, these complexes can be injurious to the host (Chapter 13) and lead to immunologically mediated disease (Chapter 20). The endotoxins exhibit a more generalized effect on the host, including pyrogen release by polymorphonuclear leukocytes resulting in fever, leukopenia by destruction of PMN leukocytes, and the initiation of the coagulation sequence resulting in intravascular coagulation and sometimes shock (Chapter 14). Obviously, the host is placed at great risk, since many of these effects, e.g., leukopenia, lead to impaired phagocytic defense. In addition, although they are formed against endotoxins, antibodies do not appear to be as protective as those against exotoxins. Furthermore, the mechanisms of response to endotoxins appear to be as varied as the generalized effect of the endotoxins themselves. Recent studies using antiserum to endotoxin of *E. coli* suggest a beneficial effect in the treatment of gram-negative bacteremia and shock (Chapter 24).

IMMUNOLOGIC INJURY SECONDARY TO BACTERIAL INFECTION

If the response of the host to any of the types of microorganisms is inappropriate, inadequate, or aberrant, the pathogen is placed at distinct advantage with respect to the host. Factors altering host responsiveness, such as age, pre-existing disease, nutrition, and concurrent infections, obviously will have a significant effect on the outcome of the host-bacteria interaction.

When the host response is aberrant, products of the immune response may result in immunologically mediated tissue injury (Chapters 13 and 20). For example, following Group A beta-hemolytic streptococcal infection, rheumatic heart disease can result, presumably through cross reactions of cardiac tissue with the organism (Chapter 20). Similarly, acute glomerulonephritis may occur following infection with these organisms owing to injury mediated by antigen-antibody complexes. The physician must be aware of these potential tertiary manifestations of the immune response when assessing the course of a bacterial infection.

SUMMARY

The immune mechanisms displayed by the host in bacterial defense are best viewed according to the type of host-parasite interaction—*acute, chronic,* or *toxigenic* types of infection. Bacterial pathogens as a group evoke in the host all the known types of immune effector mechanisms. Some of the processes are poorly understood, and others are completely unknown. In general, the participation of both nonspecific and specific immune mechanisms occurs in all bacterial infections in man. The relative roles of each, however, vary with the type of infection. At times, the products of the immune response can be harmful and are manifested as immunologically mediated diseases of man.

Suggestions for Further Reading

Bass, J. W.: The spectrum of staphylococcal disease. From Job's boils to toxic shock. Postgrad. Med., *72*:58, 69, 75, 1982.

Dondero, T. J., Jr., Rendtorff, R. C., Mallison E. G., et al.: An outbreak of Legionnaires' disease associated with a contaminated air-conditioning cooling tower. N. Engl. J. Med., *302*:365, 1980.

Editorial: Mechanisms in enteropathogenic *Escherichia coli* diarrhea. Lancet, *1*:1254, 1983.

Gorbach, S. L.: Travelers' diarrhea. N. Engl. J. Med., *307*:881, 1982.

Harvey, M., Horwitz, R. I., and Feinstein, A. R.: Toxic shock and tampons: evaluation of the epidemiologic evidence. JAMA, *248*:840, 1982.

Mackaness, G. B., and Blanden, R. V.: Cellular immunity. Progr. Allergy, *11*:89, 1967.

Mudd, S.: Infectious Agents and Host Reactions. Philadelphia, W. B. Saunders Company, 1970.

Ziegler, E. J., McCutchan, J. A., Fieres, J., et al.: Treatment of gram negative bacteremia and shock with human antiserum to a mutant *Escherichia coli*. N. Engl. J. Med., *307*:1225, 1982.

Chapter 16

Mechanisms of Immunity to Viral Diseases

Joseph A. Bellanti, M.D.

Viruses are a unique class of infectious agents that are obligate intracellular parasites. They differ from all other types of microorganisms in their organization, composition, and mechanism of replication. A complete viral particle, or virion, may be regarded as a basic block of genetic material, consisting of either DNA or RNA and surrounded by a protective coat of protein, i.e., capsid, that may also serve as a vehicle for its transmission from one host cell to another. In addition, some viruses are surrounded by a viral envelope, which consists of a lipid bilayer membrane containing viral glycoproteins that protrude as spikes (Fig. 16–1). The increased awareness during the past 50 years of the prevalence of viruses and their frequency as etiologic agents of human infectious diseases has stimulated widespread interest in their pathogenicity and immunogenicity. The spectrum of diseases produced ranges from acute viral infections (in which the interaction of virus and host immune response leads to virus clearing and immunity or to dissemination, infection, and death) to more chronic forms of viral infection (in which a prolonged viral replication, in concert with the immune response, may lead to tissue injury and result in disease). Moreover, the discovery of an association between viruses and tumors has initiated areas of intensive research (Chapter 19).

The eradication of many viral infections has been made possible through the use of effective vaccines that stimulate specific immunologic responses (Chapter 23). Rapid advances in immunology are providing new tools with which the immunologic system may be modulated ("up" or "down" regulation) and which are being actively evaluated for the prevention, diagnosis, and treatment of viral infections as well as tumors and the autoimmune diseases. These include interferon(s), interleukins, thymic hormones, and monoclonal antibodies (Chapters 7, 9, 10, 19, and 20C). Thus, it is important for the student of medicine to have a fundamental grasp of immunologic mechanisms. Not only do they play a major role in the normal processes of antiviral immunity but also they provide a clearer understanding of atypical responses seen during viral infection and of adverse effects seen following immunization.

CLASSIFICATION OF VIRAL INFECTIONS

The outcome of an encounter between a virus and an appropriate host cell will depend upon the properties of the *virus,* the *cell,* and the *environment* in which the virus–host cell interaction occurs. In general, the properties of the virus that are of prime importance are (1) the ability of virus produced in one cell to invade another, causing a spreading infection; and (2) the ability of the virus to produce functional alterations within infected cells.

For ease of discussion, the responses seen following viral infection may be divided into the following: (1) *cytolytic,* (2) *steady-state,* and (3) *integrated* (Table 16–1; Fig. 16–2). Rapid viral replication leads to early cell death (cytolytic effect), with release of virus into the extracellular fluid. (No maturation occurs at cell surfaces.) In this response, viral progeny spread extracellularly to nearby or distant uninfected cells. Steady-state infections are characterized by slow intracellular replication, during which the cell may or may not die. In this interaction, most of the virus is

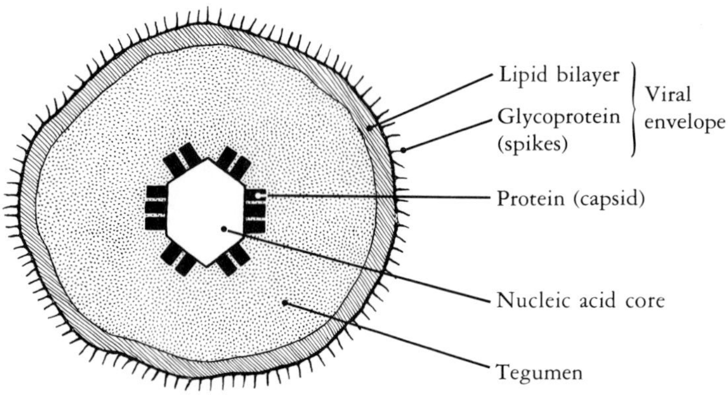

Figure 16–1. Schematic representation of a viral particle.

intracellular, and release occurs as a "budding" process at the cell surface (steady-state effect). In this response, viral progeny not only may spread to uninfected cells through the extracellular release of virus but also may infect neighboring cells through intercellular bridges without passage through extracellular fluids. The integrated effect is differentiated in that part of the viral nucleic acid that becomes incorporated into the DNA of the host cell and passes to daughter cells by meiosis. In the latter case, there is an initial brief interaction of virus with a cell, after which accelerated cell growth commences and persists indefinitely in the absence of fully infectious virus. The presence of the integrated viral genome may or may not express antigens on the surface of the virus-bearing cell. Given these three modes of viral transmission, it will become apparent that the corresponding immunologic responses of the host, i.e., humoral versus cell-mediated immune responses, will be determined by the nature of these viral–host cell interactions.

Cytolytic Effect

Perhaps the most common and best studied virus–host cell interaction is the type in which a virus first infects a susceptible cell and then, after a brief intracellular phase of replication, destroys the cell (Fig. 16–2). This type of interaction leads to a highly productive type of acute infection with high release of fully infectious virus into the extracellular fluid following cell death. There are two important points in this type of interaction: (1)Infection leads to cell death and release of infectious virus, and (2) the assembly and maturation of viral particles occur intracellularly with extracellular release of virus occurring only following cell death (cytolysis).

Table 16–1. Virus–Host Cell Interactions

Host-Cell Response	Target Organ	Examples
Cytolytic		
Localized	Skin Respiratory tract Gastrointestinal tract Genitourinary tract	Warts Rhinoviruses Enteroviruses Enteroviruses
Generalized	Multisystemic	Poliomyelitis Smallpox
Steady-State Effect		
Localized	Skin Mucous membranes	Herpes simplex Varicella-zoster
Generalized	Multisystemic	Rubella, rubeola Varicella
Integrated Effect		
	Seen in experimental animals; humans	DNA viruses, Papova (adenovirus, SV 40) Herpes viruses

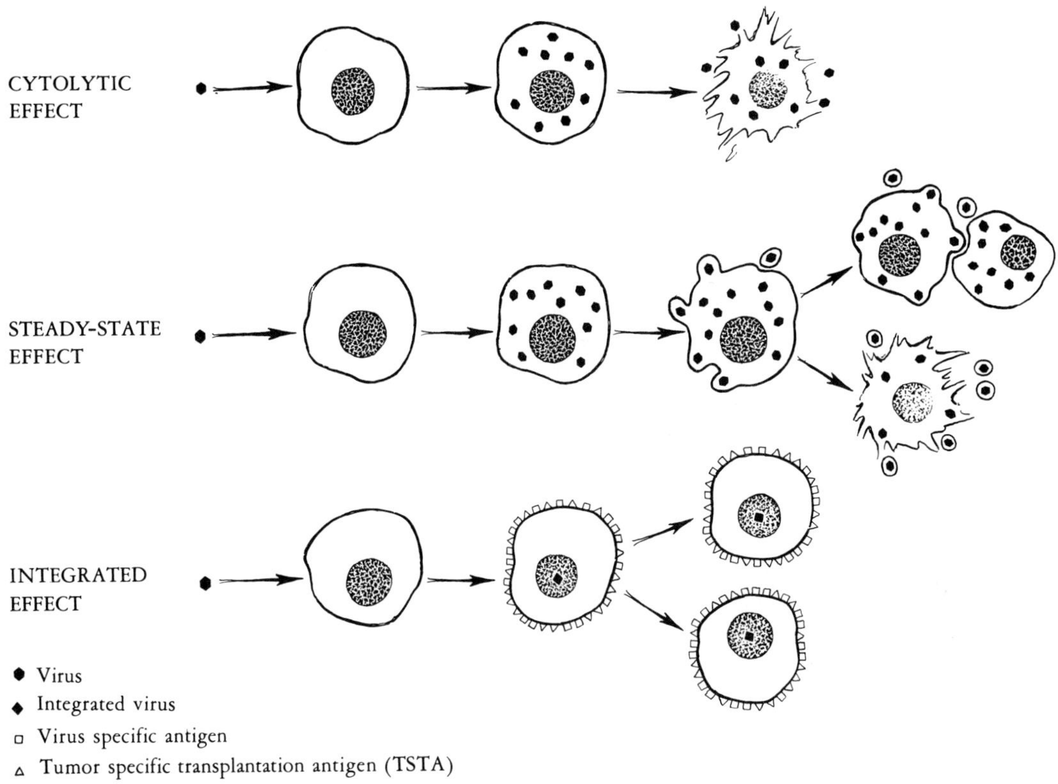

Figure 16–2. Schematic representation of three types of virus–host cell interactions.

If cell death occurs on a sufficient scale, the results of tissue damage become obvious and symptoms of disease result. If damage is restricted to the portal of entry, localized symptoms are seen, such as with common respiratory tract infection (Table 16–1). On the other hand, if virus is disseminated and damage is more widespread, the symptoms of disease are of a more generalized nature, e.g., smallpox or poliomyelitis.

Steady-State Infections

A second type of virus-host cell interaction is the type in which there may or may not be cell death. In either case, however, extracellular release of virus occurs as a membrane-associated event, and virus is released into the extracellular fluids through a "budding" process at cell surfaces (Fig. 16–2). Many viruses enter into this type of interaction, including the RNA viruses, e.g., influenza, and certain DNA viruses, e.g., herpes (simplex) hominis. Both of these virus types are rich in lipid in their outer envelope. They lead to cell death in some cases; in others, they persist in a steady-state interaction in which infected cells synthesize and release new virus while the host cell continues to survive. Moreover, under certain conditions, the cells may divide, with transmission of virus to daughter cells (Fig. 16–2). In that case, the cells go on multiplying or carrying out their normal functions without apparent disturbance, although fairly large quantities of virus are produced. In steady-state infections, cell death does not appear to be prerequisite to the release of fully infectious virus. Dissemination of certain of these viruses is by contiguous spread from cell to cell through intercellular bridges (desmosomes). This may explain how such viruses, e.g., herpes (simplex) hominis, can persist in the presence of circulating antibody.

Other types of viruses that display these characteristics are those that produce congenital infections, e.g., lymphocytic choriomeningitis (LCM) in mice and avian leukemia in chickens. Mice infected *in utero* with LCM virus sustain a high level of viremia throughout life and excrete virus in all their secretions. Most of their tissues contain large amounts of infectious virus, since every cell type appears to be infected from the time of conception. The mouse infected congenitally is able to maintain viral antigen in all somatic cells without detectable antiviral antibody, i.e., they are "immunologically tolerant" (Chapter 10). More recent evidence, however, suggests that antibody is formed but is not detectable because it is complexed. Infection of adult mice, on the other hand, produces a rapidly fatal disease. A similar situation obtains in chickens infected congenitally with leukemia virus. However, unlike mice infected with LCM, these congenitally infected chickens suffer other consequences from their infection. Although infection is not cytocidal, certain infected cells become transformed and the bird may develop leukemia or other types of solid tumors. Certain congenital infections of mice with murine leukemia virus also appear to follow a similar course (Chapter 19).

Infection of the human fetus with rubella virus exemplifies the generalized steady-state, noncytocidal type of infection. Cells are not destroyed but instead are infected and pass on large quantities of virus to daughter cells in the presence of circulating antibody. Since this type of infection occurs *in utero* at a time when the immunologic system is incompletely developed, it may explain the anomalous relationship between virus and host cells in a steady-state infection. Moreover, it may explain the rare cases of agammaglobulinemia seen in early infancy that appear to result from an intrauterine viral infection, e.g., rubella, that occurred when the immunologic system was developing (Chapter 22).

Infections of the human with any of the members of the herpes virus family, e.g., herpes (simplex) hominis 1 or 2 (HSV-1 or HSV-2), varicella-zoster (V-Z), Epstein-Barr (EBV), or cytomegalovirus (CMV), may be considered examples of latent steady-state infections of a localized nature that are reactivated by certain stimuli. HSV or V-Z may remain latent in nerve cells of sensory ganglia for months or years. Although the mechanism by which reactivation occurs is poorly understood, it seems that the virus travels down Schwann cells by contiguous growth from cell to cell until it reaches the skin, where vesicular eruptions appear (Fig. 16–3). Herpes zoster infections are believed to represent a reactivation of varicella virus infections that have occurred previously and remained latent in sensory ganglia. The pathogenesis of recurrent herpes simplex follows a course similar to that of the varicella-zoster group. In both activated zoster and herpes (simplex) hominis infections, virus replicates successfully and produces disease despite the presence of high levels of serum antibody. Protection of virus owing to its intracellular location may explain this phenomenon. Of particular importance in immunity to this type of infection are the cell-mediated responses.

Integrated Infections

The third type of virus-host interaction is referred to as an integrated virus infection

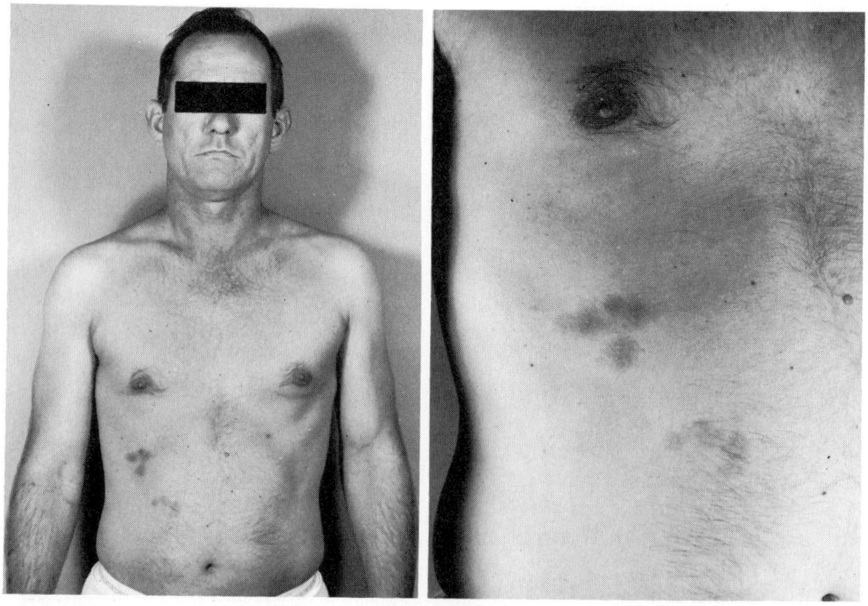

Figure 16–3. Lesions of herpes zoster in a patient with lymphoma. (Courtesy of Dr. S. Gerald Sandler.)

(Table 16–1; Fig. 16–2). The viral DNA, or part of it, appears to become integrated into the host cell DNA in a fashion analogous to lysogenic bacteriophage interactions with bacterial cells. This type of interaction differs from the previous two in that fully infectious virus is neither assembled nor released from the host cell. As described above, some steady-state viruses may enter into an integrated state, e.g., herpes viruses, which explains the inability to culture infectious virus from individuals with recurrent herpetic infections during periods of remission. Thus far, most integrated infections have been observed only in experimental animals and under specialized circumstances, e.g., inoculation of virus into a host at birth or shortly thereafter. In most integrated infections, the transformed cells do not release fully infectious virus; however, other stigmata of the presence of viral DNA can be detected, for example, the appearance of new antigens, including viral-specific and tumor-specific transplantation antigens (TSTA) as described in Chapter 19.

PATTERNS OF DISEASE

Based upon this biologic classification, we may arbitrarily divide the types of infection due to viruses according to their clinical appearance into the following classes: *localized, generalized, inapparent,* and *"slow" virus* infections.

Localized Infections

Localized infections are those in which viral multiplication and cell damage remain at the portal of entry. The virus may first infect and then spread from cell to cell either directly, in the case of cytolytic viruses, or by contiguity, as with some steady-state viruses. The virus may then exert its effect by forming a single lesion or a group of lesions at the portal of entry. For example, warts represent a type of localized infection of the skin, and the common cold is a type of localized infection of the respiratory tract (Table 16–1).

Generalized Infections

Other viruses undergo a progression through a number of steps, including the following: (1) primary multiplication at the portal of entry and spread to regional lymph nodes; (2) spread of progeny virus through blood to internal organs (viremia); (3) replication at an internal site; and (4) secondary viremia with spread to target organs, causing cell damage, pathologic lesions, and clinical disease (Fig. 16–4).

Generalized infection may be seen either with the cytolytic infections (poliovirus) or with the steady-state viruses (measles). In the case of the cytolytic viruses, the effects of disease appear to be caused by the direct spread of virus and cell death. In the case of the membrane-associated steady-state viruses, the disease pattern appears not only to be related to the spread of virus and to cell death, but additionally, some of the manifestations may be due to hypersensitivity, e.g., rash of measles. Still other manifestations of disease may be mediated by the effects of humoral antibody, e.g., renal injury mediated by viral-antiviral complexes in the mouse, or by the effects of cell-mediated immunity or meningeal infiltration in lymphocytic choriomeningitis. These will be described more fully later.

Inapparent Infections

Many infections of both cytolytic and steady-state varieties may occur without symptoms of disease. These appear to be of great importance in medicine because they confer immunity without overt clinical disease. This may be due to the nature of the virus or the status of host immunity.

For example, passive administration of gamma globulin can convert a clinical disease such as rubella or hepatitis Type A into a subclinical disease. In the case of rubella, for example, administration of gamma globulin to a pregnant female may prevent the overt signs of disease but not the subclinical infection. The congenital rubella syndrome can occur in the fetus without overt disease in the mother (Chapter 24).

Failure of the virus to reach the target organ may be another cause of inapparent infection. In some cases of poliomyelitis in which limited replication of virus occurs in the gastrointestinal tract, the infection may not spread to the central nervous system. Instead, a localized infection may occur within the gastrointestinal tract that may be abortive or productive of few signs and symptoms within the infected host and yet capable of transmission to another susceptible indi-

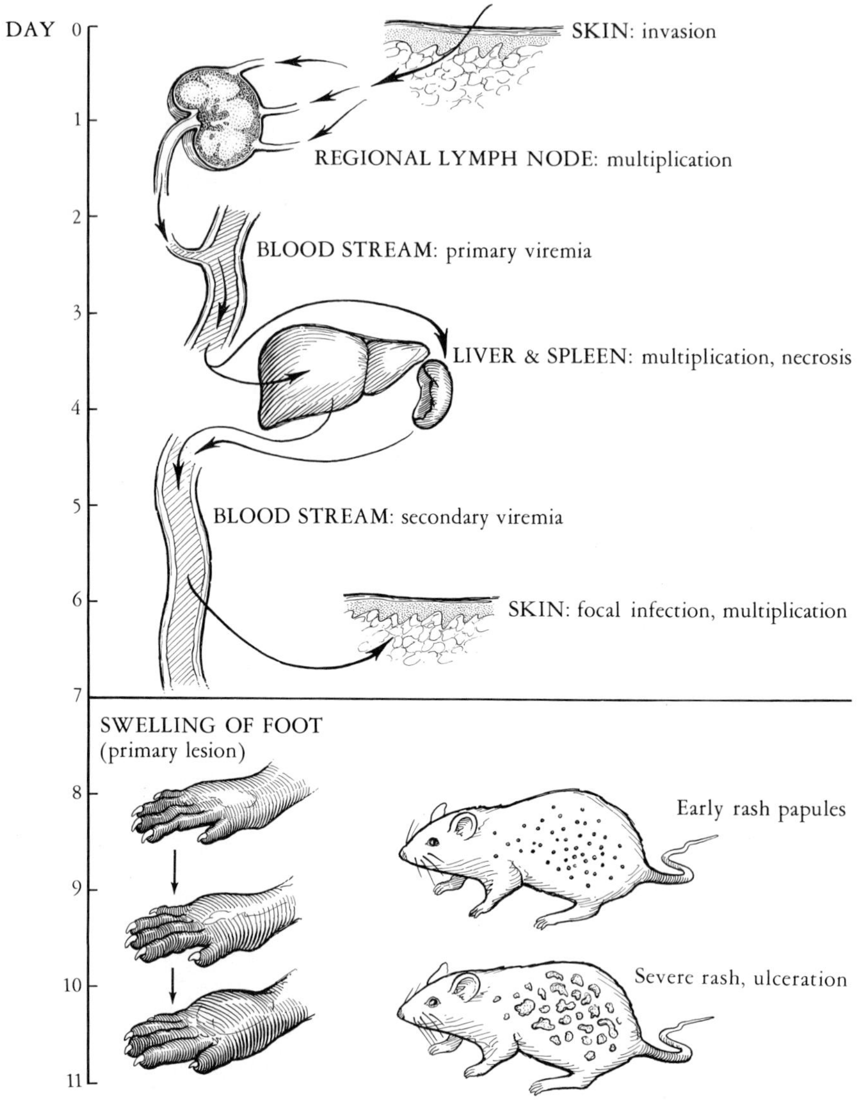

Figure 16–4. Sequential events in pathogenesis of viral infection. (After Fenner, F.: Pathogenesis of acute exanthems. Lancet, *2*:915, 1948.)

vidual with the production of overt paralytic disease. The use of live attenuated viral vaccines may be considered as a special case of inapparent infection, in which a purposeful attempt is made to produce a subclinical infection with resultant protective immunity without disease (Chapter 23).

Slow Virus Infection

Slow virus infections may be defined as a group of entities, putatively caused by viruses, in which the incubation periods are very long and the clinical expressions of disease are relatively slow in progression. The hallmark of these infections is the persistence of a viral agent or genome in a host that ultimately sustains cellular and tissue injury from the effects of the virus. Thus, the immunologic responses in the host that are normally efficient in eliminating conventional viruses are either not stimulated or rendered inoperable. Moreover, in some cases, cellular and tissue damage may actually develop as a result of the immune response itself. Thus, the term "slow virus infection" may refer at times to the speculated slowness of replication of the putative viral agent and at other times to the delayed onset and protracted course of the disease in the host. Such slow virus infections have been found both in man and in animals (Table 16–2).

Agents associated with slow virus infections

Table 16–2. **Slow Virus Infections**

	Target Organ	Cardinal Features
Man		
Kuru	CNS	Neurologic
Creutzfeldt-Jakob	CNS	Neurologic
Subacute sclerosing panencephalitis (SSPE)	CNS	Neurologic
Progressive rubella panencephalitis	CNS	Neurologic
Progressive multifocal leukoencephalopathy (PML)	CNS	Neurologic
Multiple sclerosis	CNS	Neurologic
Animals		
Scrapie	CNS	
Visna	CNS	Neurologic
Transmissible mink encephalopathy	CNS	
Aleutian mink disease	Generalized connective tissue	Generalized
Lactic acid dehydrogenase (LDH)	Liver	Liver failure
Lymphocytic choriomeningitis (LCM)	Generalized	Renal, CNS

have been conveniently classified by Hanson into two major categories: (1) those that are fairly *conventional* in their behavior, and (2) those that are distinctly *unconventional* (Table 16–3).

The conventional viruses include such agents as those associated with subacute sclerosing panencephalitis (SSPE), progressive multifocal leukoencephalopathy, rabies, lymphocytic choriomeningitis (LCM), and visna. The herpes group of viruses, including herpes (simplex) hominis Types 1 and 2, cytomegalovirus (CMV), the varicella-zoster (V-Z) virus, and the Epstein-Barr (E-B) virus, and the hepatitis viruses, particularly Type B, should also be added to this list, since they, too, can produce a lingering persistent infection with a slow progression of disease. These agents all have in common morphologic evidence of either complete viral structure or substructure that can be inhibited by metabolic antagonists. In some cases, a complete virus can actually be rescued from its incomplete precursor form, e.g., rubeola or rubella viruses. The conventional viruses all elicit immune responses in the infected host. In some cases, the viruses may actually diminish the immune response; in others, the expression of disease may be modified by the state of the immunity of the host. These viruses induce either degenerative or inflammatory changes in a wide variety of tissues. Because of their capacity to exist in more than one set of conditions, these viruses are sometimes referred to as facultatively slow viruses.

In contrast, the "unconventional viruses,"

Table 16–3. **Classification of Agents Associated with Slow Virus Infections***

	Conventional Agents	Unconventional Agents
Examples	Subacute sclerosing panencephalitis (SSPE), progressive multifocal leukoencephalopathy, rabies, lymphocytic choriomeningitis, visna, herpes, hepatitis Type B	Scrapie, kuru, Creutzfeldt-Jakob disease, transmissible mink encephalopathy
Morphologic properties	Definite evidence of viral structure	No evidence of viral structure
Biochemical properties	Have nucleic acid genomes, can be inhibited by inhibitors, some can be "rescued" (SSPE); usual liability	No evidence of nucleic acid; unusual stability
Immunologic properties	Immunogenic manner of other viruses; some may modify the immune response; the immune response may modify expression of disease	Nonimmunogenic
Tissue tropism	Many organs and tissues	Only CNS disease; viral agents may be detected also in other tissues
Tissue pathology	Degenerative and/or inflammatory changes	Only degenerative changes

*After R. P. Hanson as modified by D. L. Walker: Behavior and properties of viruses associated with slow virus infections. *In* Slow Virus Infections, Sixty-Fourth Ross Conference on Pediatric Research. Columbus, Ohio, Ross Laboratories, 1972, p. 3.

which include the agents of scrapie, kuru, Creutzfeldt-Jakob disease, and transmissible mink encephalopathy, present striking differences from the conventional viruses. Thus far, all attempts at demonstrating virion or viral nucleic acids in these diseases have been uniformly unsuccessful. The unconventional viruses appear to be nonimmunogenic, and no immune response has been detected thus far in the infected host. Moreover, these agents are usually stable to a wide variety of physical and chemical agents, and they produce only degenerative changes that are confined primarily to the central nervous system. Thus, the evidence for consideration of these agents as true viruses is indirect at best and is based primarily on their transmissibility to other hosts.

The importance of these slow virus infections is in their possible application to other human diseases of unknown etiology that affect large segments of the population. Such neurologic diseases as multiple sclerosis, the leukodystrophies, and Parkinson's disease are being assessed for a possible slow virus pathogenesis. There are also implications for other diseases of unknown etiology such as malignant and autoimmune diseases (Chapters 19 and 20). The recently described AIDS also may fulfill certain of the criteria of a slow virus infection, e.g., long incubation period, protracted course. Until the causative agent(s) is identified, this remains a hypothesis.

CLASSIFICATION OF IMMUNITY MECHANISMS

Immunity is defined as encompassing all those mechanisms that are concerned with the recognition of foreignness, and includes both the primary encounter of a host who is susceptible and nonimmune and the subsequent encounters of a host who is immune. Those mechanisms the host may employ upon initial encounter with a virus are the *recovery mechanisms,* or nonspecific immunity; those employed upon all subsequent encounters with the same virus are the *resistance mechanisms,* or the specific immunologic responses (Table 16–4).

Mechanisms of Recovery: Nonspecific Immunity

There are a number of nonspecific elements that the host has at its disposal for initial encounter with virus. The first line of defense against viral invasion is usually provided by the intact skin or mucous membranes. In addition to the passive barrier of the skin, other factors such as sweat (containing lactic acids), sebaceous secretions (fatty acids), lysozyme, ciliated epithelium, and mucous secretions play a significant role. The protective effect of these factors appears to be nonspecific except for the specific virus-inactivating properties of mucous secretions that are associated with the secretory IgA globulins (s-IgA).

Blood contains a number of substances that act in a nonspecific manner. One such factor is properdin, a serum protein that in the presence of the third component of complement (C3 or β_1C) and magnesium ions has been shown to have bactericidal and viricidal properties (Chapter 6). Although originally properdin was thought to be different from antibody and related to a natural mechanism of host resistance, it is now felt that the presence of minute amounts of antibody may account for the properdin effect.

Many tissues of the body, including brain, lung. and intestine, have receptors to which viruses attach during the first stage of infection. When cells have been treated with a receptor-destroying enzyme (RDE) from *Vibrio comma* prior to exposure to influenza virus, infection is prevented, since cellular receptors essential for virus attachment have been removed. The influenza virus itself contains neuraminidase, an enzyme that hydrolyzes the neuraminic acid linkages of many mucoproteins in the body, including those

Table 16–4. Mechanisms of Viral Immunity

Type of Encounter	Immunity Mechanisms	Effector Mechanisms
Primary	Nonspecific (recovery)	Skin, mucous membranes, fever, nonspecific inhibitors, interferon
Subsequent	Specific immunity (resistance)	Cell-mediated responses, antibody-mediated responses

on cell surfaces. This enzyme, with the hemagglutinin, plays an important role in the genetic variability leading to new serotypes.

The influence of the inflammatory response on viral infection has been investigated. It would appear that such factors as acid metabolites, elevated temperature (fever), and lowered oxygen tension may adversely affect the multiplication of some viruses and thus be beneficial to the host in overcoming the infection. Phagocytosis, widely known to be an important defense mechanism in bacterial infections, may also be important in resistance to viral infections. Macrophages remove antibody-neutralized virus from the circulation and degrade the complexes to low molecular weight substances. In some cases, virus may enter a macrophage and be unable to replicate; in others, the macrophages may serve as potential vehicles for infection. In the case of herpes (simplex) hominis virus, it has been suggested that the macrophages from newborns are more susceptible to infection with this virus than those of the adult. It has been suggested that age-dependent resistance to certain viruses may be related to maturation processes.

INTERFERONS

It is now well established that certain phases of resistance to viral infection are mediated by nonantibody substances. Of prime importance in this regard is the factor called interferon, first discovered by Isaacs and Lindenmann in 1957. They showed that chick allantoic tissue exposed to inactivated influenza virus produced a soluble substance that rendered fresh chick membranes resistant to challenge by fully infectious virus. Since then, interferon production has been demonstrated with many viruses. However, interferon induction is not restricted to viruses but also includes a markedly diverse collection of bacterial, rickettsial, and synthetic polymers (Table 16–5).

Table 16–5. **List of Substances That Can Induce the Production of Interferon***

I. Microorganisms
Viruses
Rickettsiae
Bacteria
Protozoa
Chlamydia
II. Microbial Extracts
Bacterial extracts (endotoxins)
Viral extracts (double-stranded RNA)
Rickettsial extracts
Fungal extracts
Plant extracts (phytohemagglutinin, pokeweed)
III. Synthetic Polymers
Polyphosphates (polyinosinic acid/polycytidylic acid)
Polysulfates
Polycarboxylates
Polythiophosphates

*After DeClercq, E., and Merigan, T. C.: Current concepts of interferon and interferon induction. Annu. Rev. Med., *21*:17, 1970.

Recently, three distinct types of interferon have been identified according to their cells of origin and functional characteristics. These are referred to as alpha, beta, and gamma (immune) interferons (Table 16–6). In addition to their direct antiviral properties, the interferons have been shown to have an immunoregulatory function, e.g., enhancement of natural killer production and activation as well as a cell regulatory function, e.g., inhibition of cellular growth. The alpha and beta interferons are primarily antiviral; the gamma has mainly an immunoregulatory function. The term "interferon system" has been suggested to describe the antiviral mechanism, since it is now thought that the interferon effect is divisible into at least two components (Fig. 16–5). It is generally accepted that interferon is a protein produced or released by cells following viral infection or after exposure to certain inducers, shown in Table 16–5. Interferon is not directly antiviral but produces an antiviral effect in cells by reacting with them and inducing the

Table 16–6. **Various Types of Interferon and Their Properties**

Type	Cell of Origin	Inducing Agents	Activity
Alpha (leukocyte)	Lymphocytes	Viruses, foreign cells	Antiviral activation of NK cells
Beta (fibroepithelial)	Fibroblasts, epithelial cells, macrophages	Viruses, nucleic acids	Antiviral
Gamma (immune)	T-lymphocytes	Mutagens and antigen	Immunoregulatory

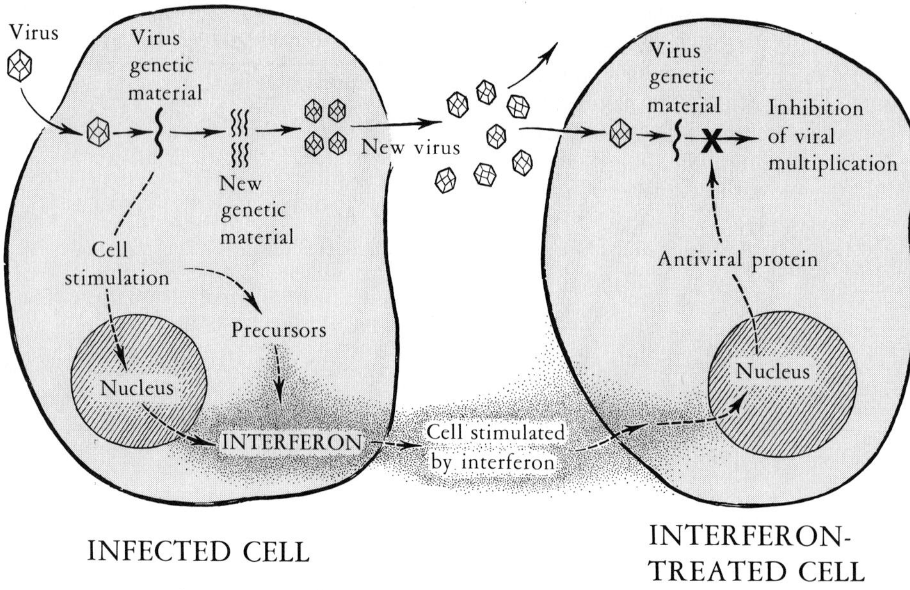

Figure 16–5. Schematic representation of interferon activity.

formation of a second protein. The latter may be a polypeptide or a protein and is referred to as the antiviral protein (Fig. 16–5). Following infection of a cell, interferon production is thought to occur by derepression of the interferon cistron, leading to the formation of interferon mRNA, which then results in the production of interferon protein. Completed interferon is then rapidly released from the cells and reacts with surrounding cells that are uninfected. The interferon reacts with the uninfected cells and produces the proposed antiviral protein by a derepression of another cistron and the formation of mRNA for this polypeptide. This second antiviral protein is thought to mediate the antiviral action of interferon by altering the cell's protein synthesis. In this way, the viral infection of the cell that is protected by interferon still leads to the release of viral genetic material, but new viruses remain unassembled.

It is believed that interferon, as in the case of hormones, may also be distributed throughout the body via the blood stream and may exert its effects at sites distal to the site of production.

Early studies by a number of investigators documented the facts that interferon is a nonglobulin protein, relatively resistant to heat and acid, and only weakly antigenic. Recently, an acid-labile form of alpha interferon has been found in autoimmune diseases and in AIDS. The important properties of interferon are given in Table 16–7.

Interferon appears to be species-specific to a great extent; that is, interferon produced by rabbit tissue culture is more effective when applied to other rabbit cells than to chick cells. Interferon produced in response to one virus, however, is just as effective against other viruses. For example, interferon produced by influenza virus Type A is active against eastern equine encephalitis virus and vaccinia virus, as well as influenza Type A.

Certain cells appear to be better producers of interferon than others. Embryonic tissues do not appear to produce interferon as well as adult tissues do. There is also some evidence that the attenuated viruses, such as vaccine strains, may induce infected cells to produce interferon in higher concentration than fully virulent strains. One explanation for the increased virulence of certain viruses is their relative resistance to the effects of interferon. Interferon differs from serum antibody in a number of respects, as indicated in Table 16–8.

Recently, technologic advances have made possible one large-scale production of interferon, e.g., recombinant DNA in bacteria and use of human-cell cultures. This has resulted

Table 16–7. Properties of Interferon

Nonglobulin protein
Molecular weight = 25,000–100,000
Destroyed by proteolytic enzymes (i.e., trypsin)
Not affected by amylase, lipase, deoxyribonuclease, or ribonuclease
Relatively insensitive to heat
Stable between pH 2 and pH 11
Only weakly antigenic
Nondialyzable

Table 16–8. Comparison of Antibody and Interferon

Antibody	Interferon
Globulin	Nonglobulin
Produced by B-lymphocytes	Produced by infected host cells
Specific—for one antigen	Nonspecific—for many viruses
Inactivates virus extracellularly	Acts on host cells to inhibit virus replication

in the production of different species of all three types of interferon. A number of these interferon preparations, e.g., alpha interferon, are being tested in the human in a variety of clinical situations, including patients with neoplasms, with chronic viral infections (e.g., hepatitis), in renal transplant recipients to minimize CMV infection, and, most recently, in patients with AIDS who present with Kaposi's sarcoma.

Mechanisms of Resistance: Specific Immunity

In contrast to the stereotyped responses that the host has at its disposal for a primary encounter with virus, all subsequent encounters with a viral agent call forth the specific immunologic responses, both antibody-mediated and cell-mediated. They are characterized by their exquisite specificity, heterogeneity, and memory (Chapter 1).

CELL-MEDIATED IMMUNE RESPONSES

The cell-mediated immune (CMI) responses are important in viral resistance and include cellular responses that may directly destroy virally infected cells or result in the elaboration of specific cell products that can enhance viral clearance (Chapter 9). Upon interaction with immunogen, specifically sensitized T-cells of the lymphoid series are capable of responding to the virally infected cell either directly or through the release of a number of effector molecules, including interferon, macrophage inhibitory factor (MIF), lymphotoxin, and interleukins 1, 2, 3 (Chapters 9 and 13). Moreover, activated macrophages, in addition to their role in phagocytic and viricidal activity, can participate directly in the destruction of virus-infected cells. Of importance in the cytotoxic effects of lymphocytes are the requirements for certain histocompatibility restrictions that appear to exist in cytotoxic activity (Chapter 9). In the mouse, these have been identified at the H-2 D or H-2 K locus and they require identity for both the effector lymphocyte and the target cell. Alternatively, the release of cytotoxin from sensitized T-lymphocytes may also facilitate the destruction of virus-infected cells. Recently, the recognition of antibody-dependent cytotoxicity (ADCC) mechanisms has been made in connection with cell-mediated immune responses. This presumably occurs through K cells that have receptors for Fc fragments of immunoglobulins, which are attached to virus-specific antigens on infected target cells (Chapter 9). Alternatively, the coating of virus particles with antibody or the coating of macrophages with virus-specific cytophilic antibody (armed macrophages) could enhance the phagocytic processes. Recently, the use of interleukin 2 as well as interferon has been shown to enhance the activity of natural killer cells, which are active in killing of virus-infected cells.

The role of cell-mediated immunity is believed to be an important component of the specific immunologic response, particularly in the type of infection caused by noncytolytic agents, including both steady-state and integrated-type infections. Intracellular replication and cell-to-cell transfer of virus occur in spite of circulating antibody. The recurrence of herpes labialis (cold sores) in patients with circulating antibody illustrates this point. The overwhelming and devastating effects of vaccinia in infants with thymic-dependent immunologic deficiencies are also examples of the importance of this parameter in host resistance (Chapter 22).

The precise mechanism by which cell-mediated events are involved in viral immunity is not clear. It would appear that cell-mediated events are particularly well suited for infections in which viral antigens are produced at cell surfaces. This would allow greater cell-to-cell interaction with an increasingly efficient elimination of intracellular virus by the effector substances released by the interaction of lymphocyte and cell-bound antigen. In the case of cytolytic infections, cell-mediated events appear to be of lesser importance than antibody, although this remains to be shown.

ANTIBODY-MEDIATED IMMUNITY

As shown in Table 16–9, there exist in the human at least five major classes of immunoglobulin— IgG, IgM, IgA, IgD, and IgE globulins (Chapter 5). All of these except IgD and IgE have known functions in virus-host

Table 16–9. **Human Serum Immunoglobulins**

Class	Serum Concentration* (mg/100 ml)	MW/S Rate	Examples
IgG	1240	150,000 (7S)	Most "late" viral antibodies
IgM	120	1,000,000 (19S)	Early "viral" antibodies, heterophil, cold agglutinin
IgA	280	170,000 (7S–14S)	Some serum antibody; local secretory antibody
IgD	3	150,000 (7S)	Unknown
IgE	0.03	196,000 (8S)	Reaginic-type antibody

*Normal adult values

interactions. The most thoroughly studied of the serum immunoglobulins are the IgG globulins, which contain most of the antiviral activity in serum. This class of immunoglobulin has many interesting properties, such as the ability to fix complement, which is believed to be necessary for certain steps in viral neutralizaton. Perhaps one of the most important biologic functions in the human is the ability of IgG to be transported across the placenta, a property not shared by the other immunoglobulins. In this manner, the newborn infant is endowed with a vast variety of preformed antibody at birth, including practically all the maternal antiviral antibodies. In addition, it is this type of passive transfer that may inhibit active immunization of the infant with live-virus vaccines. A knowledge of this must be taken into account when planning immunization schedules in the young infant (Chapter 23). The IgG class of immunoglobulins is also the type that is administered in immunotherapy against many of the viral infectious diseases (Chapter 24).

The serum IgA globulins have been studied somewhat less, mainly because of technical difficulties encountered in their characterization. Recently, however, it has been possible to demonstrate IgA viral antibody in the serum. One of the most important recent discoveries in immunology is that a unique form of IgA is found in the external secretions of the body, i.e., in the external secretory system (Chapters 2 and 5). These secretory antibodies have been shown to be an important part of the protection of the host against viruses, particularly those that produce localized infections.

The secretory IgA globulins are found in relatively large quantities in the external secretions of the body that bathe organs and tissues in continuity with the external environment. These globulins have structural and functional properties significantly different from those of the serum IgA globulins (Chapter 5). The relevant properties of the secretory IgA globulins compared with those of serum are summarized in Table 16–10.

Many types of antiviral activity have been described in various external secretions, including those from the respiratory, gastrointestinal, and genitourinary tracts. These immunoglobulins are believed to be synthesized locally. As a prerequisite to immunoglobulin production, an immunogen must gain access to local cells in continuity with the external environment. The production of secretory IgA globulins is favored after natural infection and immunization with live attenuated vaccines. In the normal respiratory tract, the IgA globulins have been shown to be the prime mediators of antiviral activity. Under experimental conditions, IgA antibody in secretions appears to correlate better with immunity than circulating antibody, particularly in infections whose pathogenesis is localized. This class of immunoglobulin has also been produced after administration of attenuated vaccines, such as measles vaccine and live oral poliovirus vaccine. Although inactivated vaccines appear to be effective in producing serum antibody, they are less effective in producing local IgA antibody when administered parenterally. This compartmentalization of serum and local antibody may lead to tertiary manifestations of hypersensitivity that are responsible for adverse immunologic reactions, as described later.

Table 16–10. **Properties of Serum and Secretory IgA Globulins**

Property	Serum IgA	Secretory IgA
Sedimentation rate	7S	11.4S
Molecular weight	170,000	390,000
Presence of secretory component	None	Present
Effect of proteolytic enzymes	Destroyed	Resistance
Sites of production	Systemic, local	Local

Various new approaches have been suggested for the production of this IgA antibody for immunoprophylaxis in the human, such as the local application of viral antigen directly into the respiratory tract. This enhanced antibody production has been demonstrated in the case of influenza vaccines (Chapter 23).

The IgM globulins are the largest of the immunoglobulins and include antiviral antibodies produced early in the immune response. These globulins have also been shown to be phylogenetically and ontogenetically primitive forms of antibody that are characteristic of the fetal or newborn antibody response in man (Chapter 2). Other viral antibodies of this type include the cold agglutinins found in viral pneumonia and the heterophile antibody seen in infectious mononucleosis (Table 16–9).

Following immunization or infection with viruses, there appears to be a sequential appearance of the molecular varieties of antibody. Initial antibody is usually associated with the IgM class and is followed later by IgG antibody. The precise timing of the IgA antibody is unknown, but it appears within a few days or several weeks after the appearance of IgM and IgG antibody. Macroglobulin is more pronounced in the fetal or newborn response than in that of the adult. Elevated levels of IgM globulins as seen in intrauterine infections, such as rubella, and cytomegalovirus (CMV) syndromes have been suggested as an aid in diagnosing intrauterine infection (Chapter 26).

WORKING HYPOTHESIS OF THE ROLES OF VARIOUS ELEMENTS OF THE IMMUNE RESPONSE DURING THE PATHOGENESIS OF VIRAL INFECTIONS

It may now be possible to construct a hypothesis of the interactions of the factors of immunity that may be involved in the host-parasite defense against viral agents. For a nonimmune and susceptible host, primary encounter with a virus of any type may be countered by the nonspecific defense mechanisms. If these are successful, infection will be prevented; if not, the virus may establish a *localized* infection, or it may become disseminated as a consequence of viremia and seed a number of target organs, producing a *generalized* infection. Prevention of local dissemination or viremia may be accomplished by the interferon system, which is activated by any of the cells invaded by virus, especially the phagocytes. The effect of interferon in the blood stream and of interferon-producing leukocytes may be amplified, since these cellular elements are continuously circulating; i.e., the interferon effect may be transmitted to noninfected cells in advance of actual virus spread.

Within 24 to 48 hours after infection, the stage is set for the development of specific immunologic events that consist of antibody- and cell-mediated immunity. In cytolytic and noncytolytic interactions, it appears that both humoral and cell-mediated events are stimulated upon release of sufficient virus from infected cells. The induction of the specific immune response occurs with the subsequent appearance of *antibody.* In serum, the predominant antibody is associated with IgG, and in secretions it is associated with the secretory IgA immunoglobulins. Thus, it would appear that following natural infection, both compartments of the antibody response—circulating and local—are stimulated. The same dual response is seen following immunization with live vaccine. The duration of IgA antibodies in secretions is much shorter than the duration of IgG antibody in serum. The role of the IgE immunoglobulins in secretions is unknown, but it may be to amplify the immune response during infection. Another role of antibody is in ADCC reactions, as described above.

The development of cell-mediated immunity may precede antibody production. It is associated with many of the signs and symptoms of the disease itself. For example, the rash of many childhood exanthems (e.g., measles) is thought to represent a cell-mediated attack on virus localized within cells of the skin. Here again, it should be pointed out that the term "cell-mediated immunity" is more appropriate than the term "delayed hypersensitivity," which implies that the event is something undesirable. It would appear that infections that lead to noncytolytic relationships with host cells, i.e., steady-state or integrated infections, stimulate cell-mediated events to a much greater degree than cytolytic types of infection, since all steady-state viruses mature at cell surfaces and, therefore, have sites with which the effector mechanism of cell-mediated immunity can interact (Fig. 16–6).

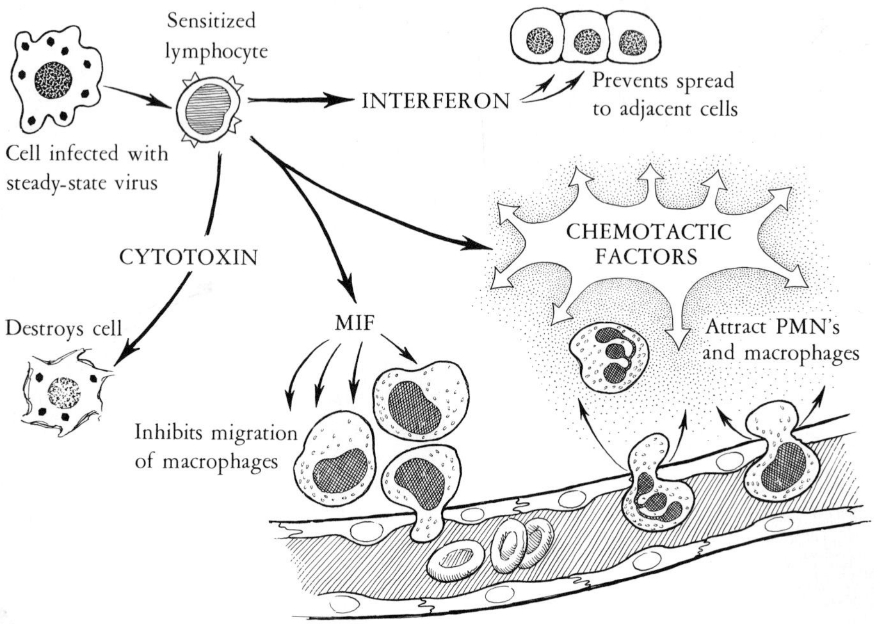

Figure 16–6. Schematic representation of cell-mediated events in viral infections. MIF: migration inhibitory factor.

The interaction between the cellular elements of the immune system and the virus-infected target cell includes any or all of the mechanisms described in Chapters 9 and11, including: (1) direct lymphocytotoxicity by T-cells; (2) elaboration of lymphotoxin; (3) participation of K cells in antibody-dependent cellular cytotoxic (ADCC) reactions; (4) action of macrophages; and (5) natural killer (NK) cells. In addition the production of lymphokines, e.g., chemotactic factors, and interleukins involved in several biologic processes is important in antiviral defense. These include the recruitment and containment of phagocytic cells by chemotactic factors, the enhancement of natural killer (NK) cells by interferon and the interleukins, and the activation of macrophages by macrophage activating factor (MAF).

Since it is known, for example, that there is an increased risk of malignant disease and autoimmune events in individuals with depressed cell-mediated immunity (Chapter 22), the importance of cell-mediated immunity in man is becoming more prominent. Thus, there appears to be an interaction of the various components of immunity, conferring an advantage to the host. (The relative roles of specific immunologic mechanisms are summarized in Table 16–11.) It seems clear that serum antibody confers protection in the generalized types of cytolytic or steady-state infections such as measles, poliomyelitis, and hepatitis Type A; when relatively small quantities of antibody contained in gamma globulin are inoculated into susceptible individuals, temporary resistance is provided against these three viral diseases. It should be pointed out that although clinical disease is prevented, subclinical disease may occur. These events indicate that serum antibody provides resistance to infection or, if infection occurs, resistance to overt illness. The explanation for this protection is that virus must pass once or twice through the blood. Antibody in serum is therefore extremely effective in neutralizing or in inactivating viruses that have a blood-borne phase.

Table 16–11. Relative Roles of Specific Immunologic Mechanisms in Viral Infection

	Cytolytic Type		Steady-State Type	
	Localized	Generalized	Localized	Generalized
Virus-released	+	+	0 or +	0 or +
Cell death	+	+	0 or +	0 or +
Humoral	+	+ + + +	+	+ + +
Local IgA	+ + + +	+	+ + +	+
Cell-mediated	+	+	+ + + +	+ + + +

In localized infections, however, protection from infection does not correlate with serum antibody, but it does correlate with the presence of local IgA antibody. For example, studies of experimental infection in volunteers, using parainfluenza Type I, clearly demonstrated that protection against challenge with this virus correlated much better with the presence of local IgA in secretions than with the presence of circulating IgG antibody. This has been shown in a number of other localized types of infections that are restricted to the respiratory tract (e.g., respiratory syncytial virus and influenza) or to the gastrointestinal tract (e.g., poliomyelitis). At times, the presence of serum antibody, in the absence of local IgA, may lead to an aberration of the immune response, resulting in hypersensitivity rather than in protective immunity.

In steady-state types of infection, too, such as varicella-zoster and recurrent herpes (simplex) hominis, it is clear that serum antibody may fail to provide protection. In these instances, however, the virus may be protected by virtue of its intracellular residence. As mentioned before, cell-mediated events may be of greater importance in immunity to these kinds of viral disease.

There is evidence that in certain types of steady-state infections, antibody itself may lead to undesirable effects. For example, in some of the slow virus infections, such as LCM in mice and leukemia virus in birds, minute amounts of antibody that are too small to be detected may be produced in serum. However, these serum antibodies form a complex with virus, and the resulting antigen-antibody complexes may localize in the kidney, leading to immune-complex disease (Chapter 8). There is accumulating evidence that a similar pathogenesis for nonstreptococcal nephritis may occur in the human during the course of certain viral infections.

In summary, serum antibody seems to be effective in preventing infections of a generalized nature in both cytolytic and steady-state types of interaction; however, in localized infection of both varieties, the presence of local IgA antibody appears to correlate much better with protection than does circulating IgG antibody. In steady-state infections, serum antibody may restrict virus replication but does not abolish the steady state. Indeed, serum antibody may be responsible for certain of the long-term adverse sequelae of these infections.

ABERRATIONS OF THE IMMUNE RESPONSE SEEN IN VIRAL IMMUNITY: IMMUNOLOGIC IMBALANCE

The definition of immunologic imbalance presented in Chapter 1 included aberrations of the immune response that may occur when the nature of either the immunogenic stimulus (virus) or the immunologic response is inappropriate to the other.

Aberrations Due to Immaturity of the Immune Response: Congenital Infections

The first to be considered concerns cases in which the immunologic stimulus is greater than the response of the host, on the basis of developmental immaturity. It is now clear that certain intrauterine infections due to viruses such as rubella and cytomegalic inclusion disease virus (cytomegalovirus) lead to a progressive chronic infection of the host in which large amounts of virus are disseminated in many tissues. These infections occur early in embryogenesis when the immunologic system is incompletely developed. In the case of congenital rubella, maternal disease during the first trimester leads to a clinical state in which multiple congenital defects occur involving virtually every system of the body, including the lymphoreticular system. Infection can occur unimpeded by any of the specific immunologic components. Later, a steady state is established in which large amounts of virus are produced and excreted by the infant in the presence of circulating antibody. The humoral component appears adequate, and large amounts of antibody are produced, particularly of the IgM variety. An impaired proliferative response of cell-mediated immunity, as measured by lack of responsiveness to phytohemagglutinin, has been demonstrated in these congenital viral infections. Recently, impairment in specific cell-mediated immunity has been demonstrated in the congenital rubella syndrome.

Slow Virus Infections

Another kind of immunologic imbalance is the type that occurs in certain slow viral infections, as described previously. Two types of slow virus infections illustrate certain of the mechanisms of immunity and immune injury involved in these interactions: lymphocytic choriomeningitis of mice and subacute sclerosing panencephalitis (SSPE) of man.

LYMPHOCYTIC CHORIOMENINGITIS

LCM virus infection of mice serves as a prototype of a slow viral infection in which the host sustains immunologic injury. Mice infected with LCM *in utero* or in the newborn period go on to a carrier state in which they sustain a high level of viremia throughout their lives and excrete large quantities of infective virus in all their secretions. In this steady-state infection, the mouse maintains viral antigens in many tissues. Since conventional serologic methods in the past have failed to detect circulating antibody in these neonatal mice, they were thought to represent the classic example of immunologic tolerance produced by a viral agent. For many years it was thought that these animals were "tolerant", i.e., no antibody was seen in the presence of large amounts of virus. Recent studies have shown that infant mice infected early do produce small amounts of antibody that, when complexed with a massive amount of antigen, form circulating complexes that are deposited in tissue such as the renal glomeruli and induce renal disease later in the animal's life through a Type 3 immune-complex injury. Histologic examination of the brains of neonatally infected carriers has shown little or no evidence of choroidal, meningeal, or parenchymal damage; however, such animals develop a mild and transient choroiditis during the second week of life. Immunofluorescence staining of tissue from the carrier mouse has revealed minimal antigen within cells in the choroid plexus, ependyma, and meninges but widespread infection in several regions of the brain. Other types of viruses that display these characteristics include lactic dehydrogenase virus, Aleutian mink disease virus, and equine infectious anemia virus. This, then, is an example of the effect of an incompletely developed immunologic system on the progress of an immunologically mediated disease in which the host sustains injury not as a result of the virus *per se* but as a result of the effects of the immune response.

Infection of adult animals with LCM, on the other hand, leads to a rapidly fatal disease in which the virus regularly produces a lethal disease within six to eight days. Histologic examination of the brain reveals marked mononuclear cell infiltration in all membranes (meninges, ependyma, and choroid plexus) but little pathologic change in neurons. In contrast to the neonatally infected mouse, fluorescent antibody staining in tissues of the adult infected with LCM demonstrates a heavy antigen concentration that is localized primarily in the choroid plexus and meninges with little involvement of the brain parenchyma.

Studies have shown that treatment of adult mice with cyclophosphamide converts potentially lethal choriomeningitis in the adult mouse into a nonfatal carrier infection similar to that seen in the neonatally infected mouse, with persistence of viral antigen in the carrier. These studies have indicated that the adoptive transfer of immune, but not normal, lymphoid cell into the drug-induced carriers results in acutely fatal choriomeningitis, histologically similar to classic LCM. These results are summarized in Table 16–12.

The results suggest that in the adult mouse the manifestations of acute choriomeningitis may be the result of cell-mediated immune injury by sensitized lymphocytes and not the effects of antibody as in the neonatal model. Thus, in LCM the status of the immune response has been shown to affect the manifestations of the disease.

SUBACUTE SCLEROSING PANENCEPHALITIS

SSPE is a chronic, fatal, inclusion body encephalitis of children and adolescents that usually develops several years after an initial exposure to natural measles virus or possibly live measles vaccine. Recently, the disease has been shown to follow the congenital rubella syndrome. The relationship of these viruses to SSPE is now well established. Fibroblast cultures of brain tissues of SSPE patients have shown the presence of suppressed intracellular measles or rubella virus and viral antigen on the surface of cells. Completely enveloped virus has not been detected in the fluid from these cultures. SSPE therefore represents an abortive type of measles infection occurring in partially permissive cells. (The immune response that is directed to this virus stands in marked contrast to that described for LCM. These differences are illustrated in Table 16–13).

Table 16–12. **Comparison of Effects of Age or Immunosuppression on Manifestations of LCM in the Mouse**

Mouse	Site of Virus Replication Membranes	Site of Virus Replication Parenchyma	Pathology	Chorio-meningitis	Disease Entity
Adult	+ + + +	±	−	+	Acute choriomeningitis
Newborn	±	+ + + +	−	−	Carrier state
Adult and cyclo-phosphamide	±	+ + + +	−	−	Carrier state
Adult and cyclophospha-mide and adoptive transfer of immune lymphocytes	+ + + +	±	−	+	Acute choriomeningitis

In newborn hamsters inoculated intracerebrally with human measles virus, neurologic signs of encephalitis developed. When the virus was inoculated into hamsters containing maternally derived measles-neutralizing antibody, the onset of acute encephalitis was blocked, but a chronic silent infection was established. When these chronically infected animals were treated with cyclophosphamide, however, several developed tremors, and infectious virus was isolated from the brain at autopsy. Thus, the effects of cyclophosphamide in this animal model were exactly opposite those seen in LCM. More recent studies have indicated that a chronic infection can be established *in vitro.*

There are a number of conflicting reports in the literature regarding the role of immune factors in the pathogenesis of SSPE. Originally, an immunologic imbalance between humoral and cell-mediated immunity was suggested as a pathogenetic mechanism for the progressive disease SSPE. Burnet suggested that an altered state of immunity (tolerance) might exist in which selective inhibition of cell-mediated immunity to measles virus resulted, while measles antibody-forming capacity remained intact. More recently, cell-mediated immunity has been shown to be normal and alterations of immunity may stem from the presence of "blocking factors" that interfere with the expressions of immunity. These blocking factors may be similar to those described in cancer and appear to consist of free antigen or complexes of viral antigen and antibody (Chapter 19).

Aberrations Involving the Specific Immunity Mechanisms

Another type of immunologic imbalance leading to severe clinical sequelae results when one compartment of the specific immunologic apparatus, either humoral or cell-mediated, is selectively stimulated or, alternatively, when one compartment is congenitally absent or deficient.

ABERRATIONS OF THE ANTIBODY COMPONENT

In addition to their protective role in viral immunity, it is now well established that antibodies are important in the pathogenesis of viral disease. If serum IgG antibody is stimulated in the absence of local secretory IgA, severe reactions can occur. For example, respiratory syncytial virus (RSV) disease occurs most frequently during the first six months of life, at a time when circulating maternal IgG antibody is present in the infant's serum. Since IgA antibody does not cross the pla-

Table 16–13. **Comparison of Two Experimental Slow Virus Infections**

	LCM	Measles
Virus	LCM	Measles virus or SSPE variant
Animal	Mouse	Hamster, man
Age	Fetal or newborn; *chronic infection* Adult: *acute infection*	Newborn or weanling: *fatal infection* Adult: *silent infection*
Effect of maternal antibodies	Form antigen-antibody complexes with resultant disease	Prevent acute encephalitis; lead to latent infection
Effect of cyclophosphamide	Convert acute infection in adult into asymptomatic infection	Convert latent infection into acute infection

centa, the infant is susceptible to such localized infections as RSV. When infection occurs, maternal IgG antibody permits the formation of antigen-antibody complexes that damage the lungs. Thus, even the maternal gift of IgG can be deleterious in certain types of viral infection.

Another type of immunologic imbalance is known to occur following the use of inactivated (killed) vaccines and results in the selective stimulation of serum IgG without a concomitant stimulation of secretory IgA antibody. This effect has been seen in children immunized with either killed RSV or measles virus vaccines. Following natural infection with RSV or measles virus, these children develop a severe disease that is more intensified than that seen in unimmunized children. It has been suggested that this type of immunologic imbalance occurs because of an anomalous situation in which the killed vaccine stimulates predominantly serum IgG antibody but not secretory antibody. Because of the secretory antibody deficiency, upon subsequent exposure to natural virus, a viral replication can occur within the respiratory tract. Since only limited IgG antibody is available and the viral antigen is in relative excess, antigen-antibody complexes occur that lead to immunologic injury. This damage may be restricted to the lungs, in the case of RSV infection, or may be generalized, as in the case of measles, with skin and pulmonary manifestations (atypical measles) (Chapters 20A and 23).

ABERRATIONS INVOLVING THE CELL-MEDIATED COMPONENT

A deficiency in the host's cell-mediated immunity may render him susceptible to repeated or protracted infections. For example, infants born with defects of the thymic-dependent immune system are prone to viral infections, including vaccinia necrosum following the use of smallpox vaccine and Hecht cell pneumonia following natural measles. The well-known exacerbation of herpes zoster in older individuals with malignant disease may represent a failure of the surveillance mechanism of the host; in any patient with herpes zoster, a very careful search for malignant conditions should be made. These examples illustrate the effect of impaired cell-mediated function on viral susceptibility of the host whose resistance is dependent upon this mechanism of immunity.

ABERRATIONS DUE TO VIRUSES THAT PERSIST: IMMUNE-COMPLEX DISEASE AND VIRUS-INDUCED CELL-MEDIATED IMMUNOPATHOLOGY

In certain chronic virus infections of man and animals the interplay of ongoing viral replication and a continuing host immune response have been shown to lead to an immune-complex (Type 3) or cell-mediated immune (Type 4) form of immunopathology. These mechanisms, described in greater detail in Chapters 13 and 20, seem to contribute to tissue injury because of the persistence of viral antigen. In addition, virus antibody complement (V-Ab-C) complexes have been shown to act as blocking factors, inhibiting cell-mediated immunity in a fashion analogous to that seen in malignant disease (Chapter 19). Listed in Table 16–14 are some viral infections in which these various mechanisms of injury have been shown to occur.

Aberrations Due to Herpes and Hepatitis Viruses

The herpes and the hepatitis viruses are two groups assuming increasing importance in medicine today because of their frequency and their ability to become latent or persistent in the host, with clinically apparent sequelae. The following discussions will briefly highlight some of the recent observations concerning these viruses, together with their immunologic implication and disease processes.

THE HERPES VIRUSES

There are four currently known types of viruses in the herpes group. These are listed in Table 16–15 with their common clinical characteristics.

Herpes (Simplex) Hominis Viruses—Types 1 and 2. There are two known types of herpes (simplex) hominis viruses: Type 1 usually produces an oral infection, and Type 2 produces a genital infection. In addition, these viruses can sometimes infect a wide variety of other tissues, such as the skin, the cornea, and the central nervous system, and lead to a generalized form of disease in the newborn or the immunosuppressed patient. Maternal genital infection presents a partic-

Table 16–14. **Pathogenetic Mechanisms of Tissue Injury in some Viral Infections***

Species	Infection	Evidence for Immune Complexes In Injury	Blocking Factors	CMI
Man	Hepatitis B	+	−	?
	Epstein-Barr (E-B)	+	−	±
	Dengue hemorrhagic fever	+	−	?
	Subacute sclerosing panencephalitis (measles rubella)	+	+	+
	Multiple sclerosis	−	+	?
Animal	Lactic dehydrogenase	+	−	
	LCM—infant mouse	+	−	
	—adult mouse	−	−	+
	Oncornaviruses	+	+	+
	Aleutian disease	+	−	
	Equine infectious anemia	+	−	
	Hog cholera	+	−	

*After Oldstone, M. B. A., and Dixon, F. J.: Immune complex disease associated with viral infections. In Notkins, A. L. (ed.): Viral Immunology and Immunopathology. New York, Academic Press, 1975.

ular risk to the neonate because of immature immunologic responses. The most significant features of these herpetic viral infections are their ability to become latent in the nervous system (e.g., dorsal root ganglia) and their capacity to cause recrudescent infections at other sites (e.g., skin, eyes, and central nervous system). As stated previously, the mechanisms of immunity involved in these herpetic infections appear to involve mainly the cell-mediated immune responses and the interplay of both macrophages and lymphocytes. Antibody appears to play a relatively minor role, although it may facilitate antibody-dependent cytotoxicity reactions or may directly affect antibody-mediated lysis (Chapters 6 and 9). In addition, the herpes hominis viruses have been implicated in certain forms of malignant disease in the human (Chapter 19). Women with recurrent herpes genitalis show a threefold increase in cervical carcinoma. Conversely, women with cervical carcinoma have significantly elevated titers of antibody to herpes (simplex) hominis virus.

The immunologic implications of herpetic infections stem largely from the fact that these infections are more frequent in the immunologically compromised host, which includes pregnant women, the newborn, and patients receiving tumor chemotherapy or immunosuppressive agents. In each of these clinical situations, a diminution in specific cell-mediated immunity appears to contribute to the enhanced infection rate.

Cytomegalovirus. Another ubiquitous member of the group of herpes viruses of man is cytomegalovirus. The major interest in this virus was initially stimulated because of its teratogenic role. The virus is now considered to be the major cause of congenital birth defects. An estimated 1 of 1000 infants sustains some form of functional disability as a result of intrauterine or perinatal infection. In the older child and adult, the virus may produce a wide spectrum of clinical diseases ranging from a mild form of heterophil-negative infectious mononucleosis with atypical lymphocytes to more severe forms of

Table 16–15. **The Herpes Viruses of Man**

Type	Usual Age of Onset (Years)	Usual Clinical Manifestations
H. hominis Type 1	0–20	Cold sores (herpes labialis)
Type 2		Genital herpes (herpes genitalis)
		Neonatal herpes
Cytomegalovirus	0–20	Congenital CNS
		Infectious mononucleosis (heterophil-negative)
Varicella-zoster (V-Z)	0–10	Chickenpox
		Shingles (herpes zoster)
Epstein-Barr (E-B)	0–10	Infectious mononucleosis (heterophil-positive)

hepatitis and hematologic disorders. Primary or recurrent infection occurs in the vast majority of patients with renal or bone marrow transplantation, as well as in patients with malignant disease, particularly those receiving cancer chemotherapy. As with the herpes (simplex) hominis infections, all of these appear to be related to depressed cell-mediated immunity. Although not proven, the role of CMV in oncogenesis has been suggested by the recent findings of the capacity of the virus to induce *in vitro* transformation and by the elevated titers of antibody to CMV seen in patients with cancer of the cervix.

Varicella-Zoster Virus. The varicella-zoster (V-Z) virus is the causative agent for both varicella (chickenpox) and herpes zoster. Like the other herpes infections, primary infection is usually seen in childhood, after which the virus becomes latent in dorsal ganglia. In this location the virus may be activated and lead to a recrudescent type of infection consisting of localized vesicular lesions restricted to the dermatomes. The V-Z viruses pose a twofold significance with regard to malignant disease. The significance of the V-Z virus is seen in either primary or secondary immune deficiency states in which the virus is a major cause of opportunistic infection.

Epstein-Barr Virus. The Epstein-Barr (E-B) virus is now recognized as the causative agent of primary E-B infection in man. The manifestations of this infection appear to be age-related. In the infant, the disease is associated with an upper respiratory infection; in the older child and adult, it causes the syndrome of infectious mononucleosis. Originally identified in the lymphocytes of patients with Burkitt's lymphoma, its precise relationship to this malignant disorder is still unknown. The virus appears to have a selective affinity for infection of the B-lymphocyte, which contains specific receptors for this virus. The subsequent reaction of the T-cell to E-B virus–specific antigens on the B-cell appears to be responsible for the atypical lymphocytes seen in this disease.

A wide variety of antibodies of both virus-specific and heterogeneic antibody responses can be detected in individuals with infectious mononucleosis. The virus-specific antibodies include VCA, EA, MA, and EBNA. In addition to the classic heterophil antibodies, cold agglutinins may be generated during the course of the disease, particularly the anti-I antibodies that occasionally may be associated with hemolytic anemia.

THE HEPATITIS VIRUSES

Another major group of viruses that produce latent or chronic infections with immunologic sequelae are the hepatitis viruses. At present, there is evidence for several classes of hepatitis viruses. These are shown in Table 16–16 with some of their characteristics.

Type A. The agent responsible for what was originally known as "infectious" or "short-incubation hepatitis" is now known as hepatitis virus A. The disease is usually transmitted by the fecal-oral route and produces a self-limited illness that is often subclinical in the young and more severe in the elderly. Unlike other forms of hepatitis, chronic hepatitis is rarely seen, if it occurs at all. Several

Table 16–16. Viral Hepatitis: Characteristics

Characteristic	Type A	Type B	Type Non-A, Non-B
Disease			
Incubation period (days)	30 (15–50)*	90 (21–180)	50 (15–160)
Severity (acute)	Mild to moderate	Moderate to severe	Mild to moderate
Chronicity	Probably no	Yes	Yes
Epidemiology			
Mode of spread			
Blood, blood products	Rare	Yes	Yes
Fecal contamination	Yes	Probably no	Probably no
Close personal contact	Yes	Yes	Probably yes
Etiologic agent			
Size (nm)	27	42	?
Nucleic acid	? Probably RNA	DNA	?
Classification	? Picornavirus	No existing classification	?

*Average and range
(After Dr. Robert H. Purcell)

antibody tests are now available for the detection of hepatitis Type A, including complement fixation, immune electron microscopy, immune adherence, and radioimmunoassay. The control of hepatitis A depends on interrupting the transmission of virus, e.g., improved personal and public hygienic measures. The administration of immune serum globulin (ISG) to exposed individuals before or shortly after exposure is also recommended (Chapter 24).

Type B. The second type of virus, responsible for what was known originally as "serum hepatitis," is hepatitis Type B. As with Type A, infection is more commonly seen in the lower socioeconomic groups and occurs primarily at an early age. Unlike infection with hepatitis A, the acute illness is more severe and has a greater predilection for producing chronic infection. Up to 10 per cent of clinical cases are associated with a chronic carrier state that is sometimes manifested in apparent chronic carriage of the virus, or more frequently as chronic active or chronic passive hepatitis (Chapter 20).

Although Type B hepatitis was originally thought to occur only following the parenteral administration of blood or blood products, e.g., transfusion, recent studies have demonstrated that the virus can be passed perinatally from mother to newborn by venereal transmission and by any of a variety of external secretions such as saliva, breast milk, or genital secretions.

The virus consists of two basic components: (1) a core, which contains the hepatitis B core antigen (HB_cAg), and (2) the coat, which contains the hepatitis B surface antigens (HB_sAg). There is a group-specific antigen common to all hepatitis B surface antigens that is classified "*a*." In addition, there are subtype antigenic specificities referred to as *d, y, w,* and *r.* These occur as allelic pairs—*adw, ayw, adr,* and *ayr.* All of the evidence indicates that antibody to the *a* antigen appears to afford protection against all subtypes. Other minor antigenic variations, consisting of four subspecificities of *w* (*w*1, *w*2, *w*3, *w*4), have also been detected. These major and minor specificities have epidemiologic importance since they suggest that several types of hepatitis virus B may exist in a worldwide distribution, in comparison with Type A, in which only a single type has been described.

An additional antigen, E (HB_eAg), appears during many hepatitis virus infections. Although not part of the surface of the hepatitis virus B, it is now thought to be part of the core antigen (HB_cAg). The detection of HB_eAg and virus-specific DNA polymerase in the serum correlates well and is an important marker of infectivity.

A large number of immunologic tests have been developed for the detection of hepatitis B antigens and antibodies. The most widely used include radioimmunoassays and enzyme-linked immunoassays (ELISA), usually based on the identification of HB_sAg in acute-phase sera. Although several reports have appeared concerning cell-mediated immune responses to hepatitis virus B, they have not been substantiated and their specificity and significance await further clarification.

Once HBV infection has been diagnosed and confirmed by clinical and immunologic testing, it is essential to establish the stage of infection by use of the various specific hepatitis B antigen or antibody profiles. This is important in determining the stage of infectivity for infection control measures among contacts as well as to determine long-term prognosis. Shown in Table 16–17 are the several patterns of various hepatitis B antigen and antibody responses and their clinical interpretations.

The control of Type B transfusion-associated hepatitis has been effectively acheived by screening for the presence of HB_sAg by very sensitive immunologic techniques. The screening of donor blood for HB_sAg by blood banks has resulted in a decrease in the incidence of transfusion-associated hepatitis from as high as 50 per cent to less than 10 per cent in some studies.

The significance of persistent excretion of hepatitis B antigens is seen in certain forms of chronic hepatitis. This will be described in greater detail in Chapter 20.

Although hepatitis virus B has not been cultured *in vitro,* "subunit" vaccines have been prepared from HB_sAg that has been purified from the plasma of individuals chronically infected with the virus. Such vaccines have proved to be safe, immunogenic, and effective in preventing hepatitis in chimpanzee experiments and in studies in the human. Such vaccines are now licensed for human use. Second-generation vaccines developed by recombinant DNA technology have now appeared and are undergoing preliminary clinical evaluation (Chapter 23).

Type Non-A, Non-B Hepatitis. A third type of hepatitis appears to be caused by an

Table 16–17. Serologic Interpretation of HBsAg, HBeAg, Anti-HBc, Anti-HBe, and Anti-HBs in Type B Hepatitis

HBsAg	HBeAg	Anti-HBc	Anti-HBe	Anti-HBs	Interpretation
+	−	−	−	−	Very early acute phase of hepatitis, indicative of onset of viremic state.
+	+	−	−	−	Very early acute phase of hepatitis, very infectious, within 3–5 days after onset of viremic state.
+	+	+	−	−	Acute phase of hepatitis, very infectious, usually 7–14 days after onset of viremic state. The same profile is found in serum of patient who is a chronic carrier.
+	+	+	+	−	Infrequently found (<3%). Patient is underging HBeAg/Anti-HBe seroconversions. Prognostic for resolution of viral disease. This profile also can be found in chronic hepatitis, in which case the interpretation is different.
+	−	+	+	−	Acute phase of hepatitis; patient still potentially infectious. Good prognostic sign of pending resolution of viremic state. This profile can also be found in serum of patient who is a chronic carrier, in which case clinical interpretation is different.
−	−	+	+	−	Patient is in convalescence state of disease; may still be infectious owing to shedding of virus not detected by current HBsAg assays.
−	−	+	+	+	Patient is in recovery state of disease; is no longer considered infectious.
−	−	+	−	+	Patient is in recovery state of disease. Anti-HBe levels are no longer detectable; usually occurs several years after original acute viremic state.
−	−	+	−	−	Patient is usually in recovery state of disease; anti-HBe, anti-HBs levels are no longer detectable. This state is usually present years after original acute viremic state. Another example is seen when anti-HBe levels are not immediately detectable after loss of HBeAg. This is infrequently seen (3–5%). Also depicts "low-level" carrier state.

agent that is unlike that of Type A and Type B viruses. This agent has been arbitrarily designated "non-A, non-B" virus or viruses. Serologic tests for this virus are nonexistent, but several epidemiologic studies indicate that the agent more closely resembles the agent for hepatitis Type B than Type A.

Delta (δ) agent. Recently, another type of hepatitis virus has been identified, referred to as the δ (delta) *agent.* This virus appears to be a defective agent and requires coinfection with hepatitis B. Recent studies have indicated that 25 to 50 per cent of fulminant hepatitis thought to be caused by hepatitis B virus are associated with the δ agent.

Neoplasia and Autoimmunity

It appears that neoplasia and autoimmunity occur as frequent sequelae in individuals with deficiencies of cell-mediated immunity. Many have speculated that this increase in incidence of both neoplasia and autoimmunity may reflect an increased susceptibility to infections—more frequently with viral agents—due to defects in immunologic surveillance. The continued persistence of antigen may in turn lead to an "autoimmune" state or the transformation to a malignant state. The recent application of molecular hybridization techniques employing restriction endonucleases has permitted the identification of parts of viral genomes integrated in host DNA for several of the latent viral infections, e.g., herpes simplex, CMV, EBV, and hepatitis virus. Recently, the human retroviruses (e.g., human T-cell leukemia viruses [HTLV]) have been linked to human malignancies and, most recently, they have been suggested as a strong candidate for the cause of AIDS (e.g., HTLV-III).

PROJECTIONS FOR THE FUTURE

The immunologic mechanisms described make it apparent that the major emphasis for the management of viral infection is on prevention. This has been made possible through the use of vaccines (Chapter 23), the most effective of which are those viral vaccines that most closely mimic natural disease. Experience has shown that some inactivated viral vaccines may have harmful effects, since they selectively lead to an immunologic imbalance that leads to a state of hypersensitivity rather than to protective immunity.

The therapeutic use of interferon has become available for the treatment of viral infections and neoplasms. In our lifetime, the increased knowledge of virus-host relationships may eventually lead to the elucidation of the underlying causes and prevention of malignant disease and autoimmune diseases in man.

Suggestions for Further Reading

Adams, D. H., and Bell, T. M.: Slow viruses. Advanced Blood Program. Reading, Mass., Addison-Wesley, 1976.

Bellanti, J. A.: Immune defenses. *In* Baron, S. (ed.): Medical Microbiology. Menlo Park, Calif., Addison-Wesley, 1982.

Bellanti, J. A.: Biologic significance of the secretory IgA globulins. Pediatrics, *48*:715, 1971.

Bellanti, J. A., and Artenstein, M. S.: Mechanisms of immunity to virus infection. Pediatr. Clin. North Am., *11*:558, 1964.

Davis, B. D., Dulbecco, R., Eisen, H. A., et al.: Microbiology. 2nd ed., New York, Harper & Row, 1973.

DeClercq, E., and Merigan, T. C.: Current concepts of interferon and interferon induction. Annu. Rev. Med. *21*:17, 1970.

Evans, A. S.: Viral Infections of Humans. Epidemiology and Control. New York, Plenum Medical Book Company, 1976.

Feinstone, S. M., Kapikian, A. Z., Purcell, R. H.: Transfusion-associated hepatitis not due to viral hepatitis type A or B. N. Engl. J. Med., *292*:767, 1975.

Fenner, F.: The Biology of Animal Viruses. Vol. 1. Molecular and Cellular Biology. Vol. 2. The Pathogenesis and Ecology of Viral Infections. New York, Academic Press, Inc., 1968.

Finter, N. B.: Interferons. Philadelphia, W. B. Saunders Company, 1966.

Gajdusek, D. C., Gibbs, C. J., Jr., and Alpers, M.: Slow, Latent and Temperate Virus, Infections. United States Department of Health, Education and Welfare, Public Health Service, 1965.

Gallo, R. C., et al.: Frequent detection and isolation of cytopathic retroviruses (HTLV-III) from patients with AIDS and at risk for AIDS. Science, *224*:500, 1984.

Gillis, S.: Interleukin biochemistry and biology: summary and introduction. Fed. Proc., *42*:2635, 1983.

Hilleman, M. R.: Prospects for the use of double stranded ribonucleic acid (Poly I:C) inducers in man. J. Infect. Dis., *121*:196, 1970.

Johnson, R. T.: Subacute sclerosing panencephalitis. J. Infect. Dis., *121*:227, 1970.

Krugman, S., and Gershon, A. A.: Progress in Clinical and Biological Research. Vol. 3. Infections of the Fetus and the Newborn Infant. New York, Alan R. Liss, Inc., 1975.

McCollum, R. W.: Infectious mononucleosis and the Epstein-Barr virus. J. Infect. Dis., *121*:347, 1970.

Merigan, T. C.: Human interferon as a therapeutic agent—current status. N. Engl. J. Med. *308*:1530, 1983.

Nahmias, A. J., and O'Reilly, R. J. (eds.): Immunology of Human Infection. Part II. Viruses and Parasites; Immunodiagnosis and Prevention of Infectious Diseases. New York, Plenum Medical Book Company, 1900.

Notkins, A. L.: Viral Immunology and Immunopathology. New York, Academic Press. 1975.

Peterson, J. M., Dienstag, J. L., and Purcell, R. H.: Immune response to hepatitis viruses. *In* Notkins, A. L. (ed.): Viral Immunology and Immunopathology. New York, Academic Press, 1975.

Remington, J. S., and Klein, J. O.: Infectious Disease of the Fetus and Newborn Infant. Philadelphia, W. B. Saunders Company, 1976.

Rizzetto, M.: The delta agent. Hepatology, *3*:729, 1983.

Stagno, S., Pass, R. F., Dworsky, M. E., et al.: Congenital cytomegalovirus infection: the relative importance of primary and recurrent maternal infection. N. Engl. J. Med., *306*:945, 1982.

Stewart, W. E., II: The Interferon System. New York, Springer Verlag, 1979.

Tomasi, T. B., Jr., and Bienenstock, J.: Secretory immunoglobulins. Adv. Immunol., *9*:2, 1968.

Vilcek, J., Gresser, I., and Merigan, T. C. (eds.): Regulatory functions of interferons. Ann. N.Y. Acad. Sci., *350*:1, 1980.

Youmans, G. P., Paterson, P. Y., and Sommers, H. M.: The Biologic and Clinical Basis of Infectious Diseases. Philadelphia, W. B. Saunders Company, 1975.

Chapter 17

Mechanisms of Immunity to Parasitic Diseases

Raymond H. Cypess, D.V.M., Ph.D.

Parasitic diseases continue to result in large-scale morbidity, mortality, and economic loss to humans and their domestic animals in both industrialized and developing countries. Essentially, the immunologic responses of the host to parasitic infection are governed by the same principles that govern responses to other infectious agents, but they involve more complex host-parasite interactions.

Although parasitic organisms were among the first disease agents to be studied, a great deal of the early interest in this field centered upon morphologic descriptions, elucidation of life cycles, studies of mechanisms of transmission, and development of new chemotherapeutic agents. In recent years, increased attention has been focused on the biochemical aspects of these organisms, their virulence factors, and the response of the host to infection with these agents as well as methods by which these parasites circumvent, modulate, or turn off the host's immune responses. Despite the progress in the prevention and control of some parasitic diseases, these advances have not matched those made with other infectious agents. The slow development of the field of immunoparasitology can be attributed largely to several factors. First, the difficulty in culturing these agents *in vitro* not only limits the availability of antigenic materials for analysis but also, coupled with their complex life cycles and strict host-specificity, limits the availability of these agents for experimental models of infection and immunity. Second, the complexity of their developmental cycles results in multiphasic antigenic stimulation of the host and a diversified immune response both functional (e.g., protective) and nonfunctional in type. Moreover, there has been to date little success in developing attenuated strains suitable for immunization employing methods normally used in other fields of microbiology (such as bacteriology and virology), in producing temperature-sensitive mutants, or in growing organisms by *in vitro* cultivation. Finally, the lack of understanding of the genetic structure and function of these complex eukaryotes and their respective hosts coupled with a lack of communication between parasitologists and immunologists has impeded progress in immunoparasitology. Nevertheless, the current renaissance in the fields of immunology and immunopathology has begun to stimulate greater interest in the role of immunologic factors in these host-parasite systems and the use of these agents as models for immunologic responses.

MAJOR GROUPS OF ANIMAL PARASITES

The parasites affecting man are a heterogeneous group and based on cell number and morphology can be separated into four groups: the Protozoa (eukaryotic protists, i.e., unicellular organisms with a true membrane-bound nucleus); the Nematodes (multicellular organisms with rounded shapes); the Platyhelminths (multicellular organisms with flattened shapes); and the Arthropoda (multicellular organisms with jointed appendages). Besides morphologic and physiologic differences, the location of the agent in the host (i.e., intestinal, oral, and genital versus blood and tissue sites) and its ability to survive in extracellular versus intracellular host environments, determine the degree and type of pathologic and immunologic responses (Tables 17–1 and 17–2).

Table 17–1. Protozoan Infections

Location in Host	Group
Oral, Intestinal, Genital	Rhizopoda (amoebae)
Oral	*Entamoeba gingivalis**
Intestinal	*Entamoeba histolytica* *Entamoeba coli** *Endolimax nana** *Iodamoeba bütschlii** *Dientamoeba fragilis**
	Ciliata (ciliated protozoa)
	Balantidium coli
	Mastigophora (flagellated protozoa)
	*Chilomastix mesnili** *Trichomonas hominis** *Giardia lamblia*
Genital	*Trichomonas vaginalis*
Blood and Tissue	
Intracellular	Sporozoa
	Plasmodium spp. *Toxoplasma gondii*
	Mastigophora
	Leishmania donovani *Leishmania tropica* *Leishmania braziliensis*
	Unknown Classification
	Pneumocystis carinii
Blood and intracellular	*Trypanosoma cruzi* (Mastigophora)
Blood	*Trypanosoma gambiense* (Mastigophora) *Trypanosoma rhodesiense*

*Nonpathogenic commensals

Infections produced by a number of the medically important protozoans are often intracellular in several or all of the tissue-invading stages of the life cycle of the organism. This location in an intracellular site not only provides the parasite with a host environment for survival or replication but also shields it from the immune response. Many of these agents undergo multiplication within the host, and the disease spectrum may proceed from a localized tissue involvement to a rapidly fulminating syndrome. In contrast, the metazoa are primarily extracellular, do not usually multiply in the definitive host, and often produce a more chronic localized disease accompanied by nonspecific symptoms. Because the sexual stages of metazoan agents do not generally replicate within the definitive host, the host's parasite load becomes a function of the number of stages that survive following each infection as well as the frequency of infection. Parasitic load, in turn, influences the patient's clinical response, antigen burden, and treatment selection.

IMMUNE RESPONSE TO PARASITIC INFECTIONS

The events that result from the interaction between these agents and mammalian hosts

Table 17–2. Metazoan Infections

Location in Host	Group
	Nematoda (roundworms)
Intestinal	*Enterobius vermicularis* *Trichuris trichiura*
Intestinal and Tissue	*Ancylostoma duodenale* *Necator americanus* *Strongyloides stercoralis* *Trichinella spiralis** *Ascaris lumbricoides*
Tissue	*Wuchereria bancrofti* *Brugia malayi* *Onchocerca volvulus* *Loa loa* *Dipetalonema* spp. *Mansonella ozzardi* *Dracunculus medinensis*
	Platyhelminths (flatworms)
	Cestoda (tapeworms)
Intestinal (adult stages)	
	Diphyllobothrium latum *Taenia saginata* *Taenia solium* *Hymenolepis nana*
Tissue (larval stages)	
	Taenia solium *Hymenolepis nana* *Echinococcus granulosus* *Echinococcus multilocularis*
	Trematoda (flukes)
Tissue	
	Schistosoma haematobium *Schistosoma mansoni* *Schistosoma japonicum* *Paragonimus westermani* *Fasciola hepatica*
Intestinal	
	Fasciola buski *Clonorchis sinensis*

*Intracellular stages in life cycle

vary greatly, ranging from the extreme of noninvasion of the host by the agent to the other end of the spectrum, the vulnerability of the host to the presence of the agent. The two major forces that determine the eventual outcome of the host-parasite encounter are the recognition of nonself (parasite) by the host and the capacity of the parasite to evade the host's resistance factors (both immune and nonimmune). With the exception of a few of the protozoan and several of the atypical metazoan infections that can result in high mortality, most of the host-animal parasite systems that the clinician encounters today have evolved to the point that neither the host nor the parasite is eliminated and both species survive and replicate. For those agents that remain in tissue for long periods, resulting in chronic infections and persistent antigenic stimulation, serologic and other laboratory assays are important diagnostic aids. The clinician should be aware of the availability and validity of these tests for parasitic diseases.

Much of the information on immunoparasitology has come from studies of both laboratory and domestic animal populations. These studies have shown that just as with other host-parasite relationships, i.e., bacteria (Chapter 15), viruses (Chapter 16), and fungi (Chapter 18), resistance to multicellular and unicellular parasites is conditioned by both innate and naturally acquired factors. These experimental studies also indicate that manifestations of immunity operate in two ways: (1) those that affect the parasite directly, i.e., inhibition of penetration and infection, retardation of development, decrease of the duration of patency, inhibition of multiplication resulting in a slower increase in parasitemia, reduction of fecundity, elimination of residual parasitic populations, and alterations of structural and physiologic components; and (2) those that operate indirectly to modify the effects of the parasite within the host and that result in reduction of morbidity and mortality of the host. The extent to which these same phenomena occur in humans has not been fully established.

There is ample evidence that man exhibits innate resistance to many of the animal parasites. This resistance may vary depending on the host characteristics of race, age, and physiologic and nutritional status. It has been difficult to document whether individuals develop acquired immunity to many of the metazoa, and much of the information concerning this question has been derived indirectly from epidemiologic studies. If acquired immunity does develop, its expression probably would not result in complete removal of the parasitic (i.e., sterile immunity) agent. It is only in rare instances that one sees sterile immunity against these agents in any host system, and in many parasitic infections the immune state is defined as one in which parasite numbers are controlled at a low pathogenic level and hyperinfection of the host does not occur. One could hypothesize that sterile immunity does not occur with *any* group of agents, but since animal parasites are large, their presence in low numbers is more readily apparent.

Parasites contain a variety of somatic and metabolic antigens, some of which are stage-specific and transitory in nature, and others that persist throughout the life cycle of the parasite and may continually stimulate a diversity of immunologic responses. Host responses to these agents are further complicated by the fact that many parasites share antigenic moieties not only with other infectious agents but also with antigens of the host. Extracts of *Trichinella spiralis,* for example, have been reported to cross react with A_2 human isoantigen, *Ancylostoma, Ascaris, Filaria, Onchocerca, Trichuris, Echinococcus, Fasciola, Schistosoma, Salmonella typhi, Treponema, Giardia,* and human serum albumin. It is therefore not surprising that these agents stimulate a multitude of both humoral and cell-mediated immune (CMI) responses, which can be detected by a variety of *in vitro* and *in vivo* assays. To date, the role of these responses in the pathogenesis of parasitic diseases is not clear, nor is the relationship between these responses and immunity to these agents well defined. In spite of an often rapid and exaggerated humoral and CMI response to infection with these agents, many of these parasites remain viable within the host for extended periods (Fig. 17–1). The failure of a host to develop acquired immunity under natural conditions may be the result of the following factors:

1. Limited tissue invasion or tissue contact by the agent, which results in little or no stimulation of the immune system by the surviving stage (intestinal helminths): *Enterobius vermicularis, Taenia* spp., adult *Ascaris;* protozoa: *Entamoeba histolytica, Giardia lamblia.*
2. The inaccessibility of the agent to the immune system: (a) among intracellular pro-

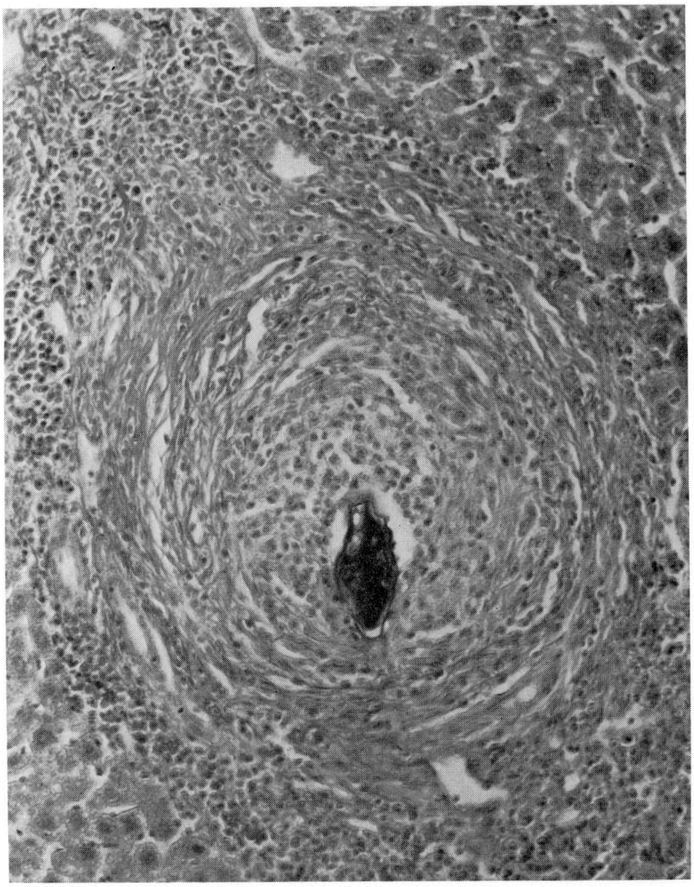

Figure 17–1. Section of liver from a patient with schistosomiasis. Egg of *Schistosoma mansoni* is seen within the center of a granuloma, containing a heavy infiltration of eosinophilic leukocytes. Hematoxylin and eosin stain, ×100.

tozoa, *Toxoplasma gondii* in macrophages and neurologic tissue, *Trypanosoma cruzi* in macrophages and myocardium, *Leishmania donovani* in macrophages, *Plasmodium vivax* in exoerythrocytic and erythrocytic stages; (b) tissue helminths: *Trichinella spiralis* in striated muscle, *Echinococcus granulosus* in hepatic tissue, *Toxocara canis* in somatic and neurologic tissue. In several of the examples cited, encapsulation of the parasite stage may protect the parasite from host defenses, although leakage of antigen and stimulation of the host take place.

3. Infection of the host in subthreshold doses. Since metazoa do not normally multiply within the host, the amount of antigen available for stimulation of the immune system may be limited by the size of the infecting dose.

4. The ability of the agent to alter its antigenic composition (antigenic variation): in protozoa, African trypanosomes, *Plasmodium* spp., *Babesia* spp. Sequential changes in the surface glycoproteins of trypanosomes have been observed, and these phenotypic variations may contribute to the ability of trypanosomes to survive in the face of high titers of circulating antibody.

5. The incorporation of host (self) antigens on the parasite surface, resulting in a coating of the agent, e.g., *Schistosoma* spp. Host components that may be incorporated on this trematode surface have been reported to include blood group antigens, histocompatibility complex antigens and immunoglobulin fragments.

6. The shedding of antigens from the surface of parasite stages: *Leishmania enriettii, Schistosoma mansoni.*

7. The release of large amounts of soluble and particulate antigens, resulting in the synthesis of ever increasing quantities of nonfunctional antibody and the possible development of tolerance: blood and tissue protozoa: *Plasmodium* spp., *Leishmania donovani;* blood and tissue metazoa: filariae, *Schistosoma* spp., *Toxocara canis.*

8. The ability of the agent to tolerate the arsenal of primary and secondary immune responses: many of the metazoa: *Toxocara* and other atypical migrating larval stages, schistosomes, and so forth. It may be impos-

sible for activated macrophages, phagocytic cells, antibodies, lymphokines, and a complement-mediated reactions to engulf, aggregate, or lyse metazoa or cysts, which are also protected by external barriers. One of the enigmas puzzling parasitologists relates to the effector mechanisms by which humoral or cellular immune factors operate to either expel or destroy parasite stages.

Depending on the specific host-parasite relationship, one or several of these factors may account for the failure of the host to develop acquired immunity.

Immunity to Metazoa (Helminths)

HYPERSENSITIVITY REACTIONS TO HELMINTHS

Immediate and delayed hypersensitivity are commonly associated with helminth parasites in both man and animals (Table 17–3). Why this group of agents so frequently stimulates these reactions is unknown. Possible explanations for this association may be related to the nature of their antigens, the chronicity of their infections (which permits persistence of antigens), the route of infection, or the presence of developmental or adult stages at mucosal membranes, thereby allowing the interaction of the proper immune receptors with parasite antigens. For example, there are different portals of entry for different organisms. The skin is an important and common portal of entry for some of the helminthic infections, e.g., hookworm. For others, the gastrointestinal tract is paramount, e.g., ascariasis. The significance of this is that different routes of presentation of antigen may selectively favor the stimulation of one or another type of immune response, e.g., humoral *versus* cellular immunity, and may also influence the sequence of involvement of immunologic responses, e.g., local *versus* systemic antibody.

Intradermal tests of the immediate, delayed, and mixed types have been described for ancylostomiasis (human and animal origin), ascariasis, dracontiasis, enterobiasis, filariasis, strongyloidiasis, trichinosis, paragonimiasis, clonorchiasis, schistosomiasis, diphyllobothriasis, echinococcosis, and taeniasis. Much of the data on hypersensitivity reactions to helminths in human needs to be re-examined and verified, since many of the antigens used for skin testing used in the past were often inadequate with regard to their method of preparation, purity, and standardization.

Since many helminths are potent inducers of homocytotropic antibodies, e.g., IgE and immediate hypersensitivity reactions (Chapter 20A), it is not surprising that localized or systemic eosinophilia is often observed in parasitized hosts (Table 17–3). The development of eosinophilia is most marked in helminthic infections in which developmental stages invade and migrate in tissues, e.g., ascariasis, dracontiasis, filariasis, strongyloidiasis, trichinosis (Fig. 17–2). Eosinophils often persist at high levels in infections of humans involving nonhuman helminths *(Angiostrongylus, Toxocara, Brugia, Strongyloides, Ancylostoma, Gnathostoma).* The precise role that these hypersensitivity reactions play in the pathogenesis and the development of acquired immunity in these diseases is not known, but parasitized hosts often exhibit a variety of symptoms that may be manifes-

Table 17–3. Hypersensitivity Reactions Associated with Helminthic Infections in Man

	Immune Reactions		
Type	Antibody Circulating	Reagin (IgE)	Delayed Hypersensitivity
Intestinal			
Taenia spp.	0	0	0
Enterobius vermicularis	0	?	?
Intestinal and tissue			
Ascaris lumbricoides	+	+	?
Toxocara canis	+	+	?
Ancylostoma duodenale	+	+	?
Necator americanus	+	+	?
Trichinella spiralis	+	+	+
Tissue			
Schistosoma spp.	+	+	+

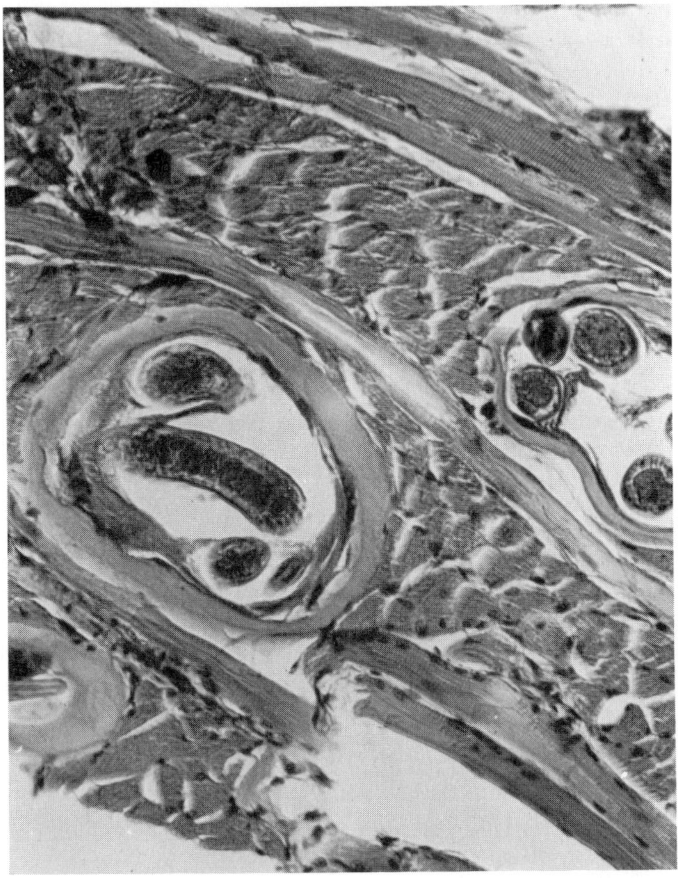

Figure 17–2. *Trichinella spiralis,* rat. Larvae encapsulated in the skeletal muscle of a rat. The intense inflammatory reaction that characterized the early stages of the infection is no longer present and has been replaced by a protective fibrous capsule, within which the larvae may remain quiescent but infective. Hematoxylin and eosin, ×100.

tations of both immediate and delayed hypersensitivities. In the case of immediate hypersensitivity, these include the urticaria, pruritus, asthma-like signs, abdominal pain, and acute diarrhea observed in ascariasis; the muscle pain, fever, rashes, and edema in trichinosis; and the urticaria, asthma-like signs, subcutaneous edema, and generalized lymphadenopathy in schistosomiasis. In the case of delayed hypersensitivity, the symptoms include the formation of associated granulomas with the egg stage in schistosomiasis and capillariasis; the granulomas associated with the larval stages of *Toxocara, Trichinella,* and *Filaria;* and a component of the intestinal inflammation observed in trichinosis, trichostrongyloidosis, and other gastrointestinal helminthiases.

Of interest has been the observation that under certain experimental conditions several helminths, i.e., *Nippostrongylus, Fasciola,* and *Trichinella,* potentiate immediate hypersensitivity responses to nonrelated antigens. This potentiating effect by helminths may be of clinical significance in the etiology of urticaria, asthma, and other related phenomena, but further investigations need to be undertaken in human populations before these associations can be substantiated.

Schistosomiasis. Granuloma formation and fibrosis are serious sequelae of chronic infection with *S. mansoni, S. haematobium* and *S. japonicum,* and it has been hypothesized that the extensive tissue granulomata associated with these infections are caused by cell-mediated immunologic reactions to specific egg antigens in the case of *S. mansoni* and *S. haematobium,* and by antibody-mediated mechanisms in *S. japonicum.* In this parasite infection, therefore, the occurrence and severity of disease would appear to be influenced by the number of schistosome eggs in the tissues and the immune response of the host.

Trichinosis. Unlike most intestinal nematodes, *T. spiralis* appears to be an intracellular parasite in all stages of development, is relatively non–host specific, and completes all stages of its life cycle in a single host. From studies in rodents it has been determined that the murine host responds independently and specifically to different developmental stages in the parasite's life history. These experimental infections clearly illustrate the complex sequence of events that accompany infection of mammalian hosts with antigenically diverse metazoan parasites. Although there has been extensive experimental work dealing with laboratory infections, there is no evidence to indicate whether or not humans develop resistance to infection with this agent. Following infection in humans, specific IgM, IgG, and IgA antibodies can be detected. In addition, immediate and delayed hypersensitivity reactions to a variety of *Trichinella* antigens can be elicited in most hosts. Serologic testing is an important diagnostic tool in this infection since parasitic stages are not routinely detected in stools. Because of its excellent specificity, the most reliable of the available diagnostic tests has been the bentonite flocculation assay. Perhaps the most exciting advance to date in experimental studies has been the observation that in laboratory rodents, resistance and susceptibility to infection have an immunogenetic basis. Major histocompatibility (MHC)–linked genes, along with genes mapping outside of the MHC, act collectively to control the relative degree of susceptibility or resistance expressed by given strains of mice (Chapter 3). The role of genetic factors in controlling levels of susceptibility and in mediating the immunopathologic sequelae observed in a variety of parasitic diseases is an area that has received only limited attention.

Ascariasis. *Ascaris lumbricoides,* the giant roundworm of humans, contains antigens that are potent inducers of hypersensitivity reactions in a variety of hosts. The life cycle of this nematode involves an obligatory tissue migration phase, in which developing larval stages undergo two molts in the lung accompanied by the release of highly allergenic metabolic products. Thus, acute hypersensitivity reactions involving pulmonary tissue are characteristic of infections with this nematode, and asthma-like symptoms with high tissue and circulating eosinophilia are not infrequent findings in *Ascaris* infections. The nature of the parasite antigens responsible for induction of hypersensitivity is not clear, but it is believed that *Ascaris* contains substances that can degranulate mast cells either directly or through the mediation of IgE-*Ascaris* allergens at the surface of mast cells.

Immunity to Protozoa

The type and level of immune responses induced by protozoan infections are influenced by their site of colonization and the extent of tissue involvement, e.g., intracellular versus extracellular, and intestinal versus blood or tissue location. In general, humoral responses are elicited in response to stages that circulate in the blood, and cell-mediated reactions are seen with those agents with intracellular development. In contrast to the metazoa, these parasites generally do not induce immediate-type hypersensitivity skin responses and eosinophilia is not a common feature of these infections.

INTESTINAL PROTOZOA

In the human alimentary tract, the lumen is the most frequent site of colonization. Tissue invasion occurs only with the ciliate *Balantidium coli* and the amoeba *Entamoeba histolytica.* The third intestinal protozoan of clinical importance to humans, the flagellate *Giardia lamblia,* occurs either free in the lumen, intracellularly, or attached to the mucosal surface of the villi of the small intestine.

The most frequently studied intestinal amoeba is *E. histolytica,* the cause of both acute and chronic amebiasis in humans. The amoeba, ingested with contaminated food or water, encysts and colonizes in the intestinal tract. Occasionally, it may become invasive and penetrate tissues locally (intestinal amebiasis) or systemically (extraintestinal amebiasis). The infection may be asymptomatic or symptomatic. Of the latter, the most frequent manifestation is intestinal amebiasis. Hepatic amebiasis is the most common form of extraintestinal amebiasis (Fig. 17–3). The prevalence of this disease has been difficult to assess because of the lack of a simple, direct diagnostic test. Very little is known about acquired immunity, and the lack of an adequate animal model has limited experimental studies. There is no evidence for the development of resistance to reinfection, which may be related to the inaccessibility of the parasite to the immune mechanisms of the host. The principal success of immunologic studies to date has been in the development of serodiagnostic tests (indirect hemagglutination, precipitin, particle agglutination, fluorescent antibody). Because antibody response follows the invasion of the intestinal mucosa or colonization within the liver, serologic tests are most useful in establishing tissue exposure to the parasite. Negative results with the indirect hemagglutination and precipitin tests are of clinical importance in excluding cases of extraintes-

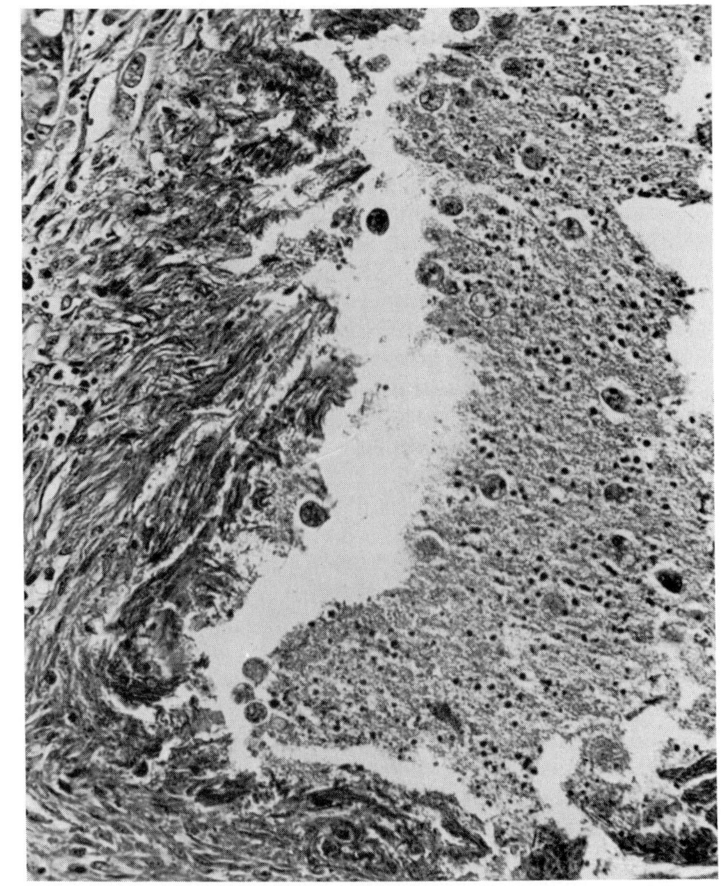

Figure 17–3. Section of liver from a patient with an amoebic liver abscess. Note the massive destruction of liver parenchyma with minimal surrounding cellular reaction. Hematoxylin and eosin stain, × 125.

tinal amebiasis. Nonetheless, the occurrence of cases in which no antibody titers can be detected sometimes limits the diagnostic value of these tests. Both immediate and delayed hypersensitivity skin reactions to *Entamoeba* antigens have been reported in patients, but the specificity and sensitivity of these antigens need careful evaluation. Of interest is the recent report that a depression in specific cell-mediated immunity to parasite antigens occurs in patients with amoebic liver abscess. After successful treatment, delayed skin reactivity apparently returns, suggesting that the skin test may have value as a therapeutic index.

The protective effect of local antibody in a number of systems, including those involving bacterial, fungal, and viral agents, has been demonstrated. However, a protective role for secretory IgA or local cellular immunity against intestinal protozoa has not been established. A few patients with selective IgA deficiency have been reported to develop giardiasis, but this observation requires confirmation. The functions of IgA in localized immunity to microbial agents have been described previously (Chapter 14); they include its neutralizing or coating effect on epithelial surfaces, which prevents attachment or penetration of the organism.

BLOOD AND TISSUE PROTOZOA

Trypanosoma. There are two major groups of trypanosomes that contain species that parasitize man. The first group, *Stercoraria,* is characterized by transmission from host to host of infective forms that occur in the feces of insect vectors and multiply intracellularly in muscle and in macrophages and other cells. An example is *T. cruzi,* the agent of American trypanosomiasis, or Chagas' disease. The second group, *Salivaria,* is characterized by transmission from host to host of infective forms that occur in the saliva or mouth parts of the insect vector and do not multiply intracellularly but in the lumen of blood vessels and in tissue spaces (*T. gambiense* and *T. rhodesiense,* the agents of African trypanosomiasis). Protective antibodies can be demonstrated in the sera of animals following experimental and natural infections with *Sal-*

ivaria, but to date there is no immunizing procedure that will protect man against natural infection. Patients with African trypanosomiasis may exhibit a rapid marked increase in IgM globulins in serum and cerebrospinal fluid (CSF), but most of this immunoglobulin response is nonspecific. The elevation of IgM globulin in CSF is of diagnostic importance. In several animal models, infection with *Salivaria* produces selective IgG immunosuppression to nonrelated antigen. Whether infection of man with trypanosomes causes immunosuppression is not clear, but recent studies have shown that patients with sleeping sickness have impaired humoral and cell-mediated immune responses to some antigens.

Leishmania. The leishmaniases are important protozoan diseases that affect large numbers of humans in a variety of countries. The diseases evolve in several clinical forms that appear to depend on the host's immunologic response to the parasite. The two major forms of disease are a cutaneous and a visceral type. Cutaneous leishmaniasis is caused by a variety of *Leishmania* species and is expressed clinically as a spectrum of disease. The three major forms are (1) diffuse cutaneous leishmaniasis (DCL), characterized by an absence of specific delayed hypersensitivity to leishmania, disseminated nodules, and poor response to treatment; (2) lupoid leishmaniasis, characterized by a well-developed specific delayed hypersensitivity, local scar formation with peripheral spread of lesions but no metastases, and a variable response to treatment; and (3) cutaneous leishmaniasis (Oriental sore), the moist form in which delayed hypersensitivity develops after a variable period of time and single lesions may take one to two years to heal. In DCL, the patients handle intercurrent infections normally, respond positively to skin tests with nonrelated antigens, and exhibit no apparent alterations in serum immunoglobulin levels.

Visceral leishmaniasis (kala-azar) is caused by infection with *L. donovani.* This form of the disease is characterized by heavy parasitization of systemic macrophages, a lack of specific delayed hypersensitivity, and a massive hyperglobulinemia. After successful treatment of kala-azar, the delayed hypersensitivity response returns and the host exhibits an immunity to reinfection. The intradermal test for delayed hypersensitivity reactions in leishmaniasis is termed the leishmanian skin (Montenegro) test and a positive reaction correlates with *in vitro* lymphocyte transformation to leishmanian antigens.

Plasmodium. The infectious cycle of malaria is illustrated schematically in Figure 17–4. Following the bite of an infected *Anopheles* mosquito, sporozoites are introduced into the blood stream and migrate directly to the liver, where they multiply within parenchymal cells. In experimental studies in rodents and primates, the administration of inactivated sporozoites has been shown to induce species- and strain-specific immunity to subsequent challenge against sporozoite-initiated infections. The application of this procedure to humans is currently under investigation and holds great promise for the development of an effective vaccine. The exoerythrocytic stages apparently do not stimulate an immune response, and, following exoerythrocytic development, the liver cells burst, releasing merozoites into the peripheral circulation. Rapidly multiplying erythrocytic stages release an abundance of antigens, resulting in the induction of specific and nonspecific host responses. This situation is expressed as a rise in specific and nonspecific immunoglobulins, a marked proliferation and hyperactivation of the reticuloendothelial system, and alterations in various lymphoid organs. What function these various responses play in the cessation or promotion of the parasite cycle is not clear. However, vaccination of monkeys with either killed or inactivated merozoites induces a strain- and species-specific protection, which appears to function through the mediation of antibody directed against infected erythrocytes. Since in endemic populations the newborn is protected from infection by maternally transferred antibody, and the passive transfer of high doses of antiserum will protect humans, humoral antibody clearly plays some role in the development of acquired immunity.

In addition to acquired immunity, there is strong evidence that innate host factors contribute resistance against malarial infection in some populations. Thus, African or American blacks lacking Duffy blood group antigen are resistant to infection by *P. vivax;* individuals with sickle cell hemoglobin exhibit less severe clinical manifestations to *P. falciparum;* and persons with persistent fetal hemoglobulin, e.g., thalassemia minor, or with glucose-6-phosphate dehydrogenase deficiency do not support the growth of *P. falciparum* in their red cells. In many parasitic infections, the immune state is defined as one

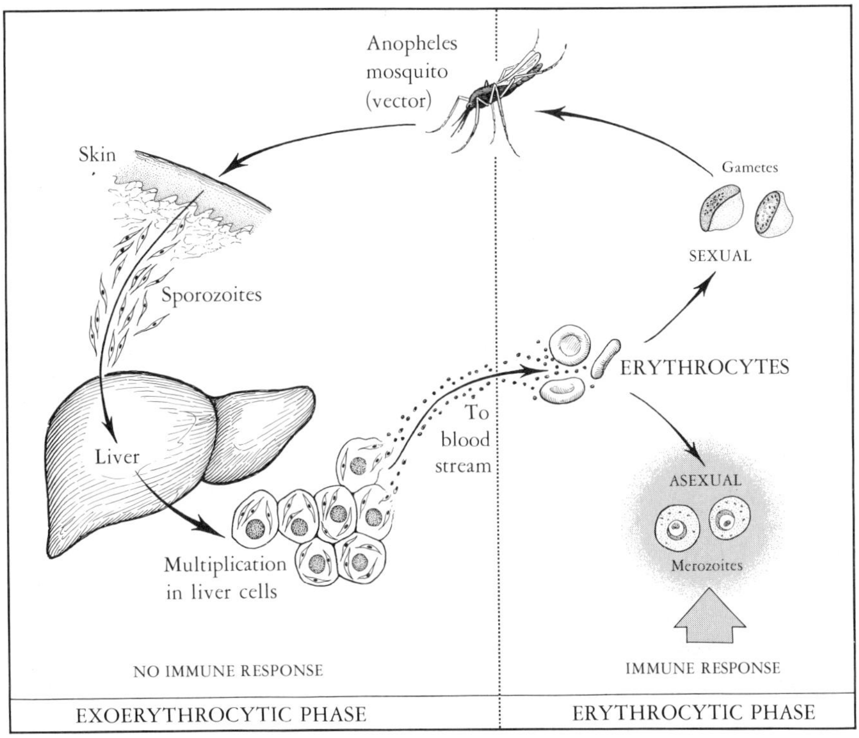

Figure 17–4. Schematic life cycle of malaria. Note that detectable immune responses are directed against erythrocytic phase.

in which the parasite numbers, despite their persistence, are controlled at a low pathogenic level and hyperinfection of the host does not occur. This state, referred to as premunition, appears to be a common finding in human populations residing in hyperendemic malarial areas, and the host-parasite relationship permits survival of the host in the face of continuous exposure to infected mosquitoes.

Field reports in areas where malaria is endemic indicate that children produce low tetanus antibody titers in response to vaccination with tetanus toxoid. This association of immunosuppression has also been observed in experimentally induced malaria in rodents. A depression of various components of the complement system is also observed in humans and animals, and it is clear that infection with this parasite results in multiple alterations of the immune system.

Toxoplasma. One of the most important of the intracellular parasitic infections in the United States is toxoplasmosis. *T. gondii* is an obligate intracellular infection primarily of cats (i.e., the definitive host), and human infection is usually acquired by the ingestion of oocysts from cat's excreta or cysts present in inadequately cooked meat. The type and degree of the immune response to infection of the human with this parasite are complex and influence the course of infection, its clinical manifestations, and its diagnosis. The disease may take several forms ranging from the most common asymptomatic form to an acute syndrome resembling infectious mononucleosis to a more acute disseminated infection or congenital infection. Congenital infection, the most serious form, occurs as a result of maternal infection with parasitemia and transmission of the organisms to the fetus (Fig. 17–5).

Humoral Response. Infection results in the production of several classes of specific antibodies whose detection serves as the basis for serologic diagnosis. The serodiagnostic assays most commonly utilized are (1) the Sabin-Feldman dye test (DT), (2) the complement-fixation (CF) test, (3) the indirect hemagglutination (IHA) test, and (4) the indirect fluorescent antibody (IFA) test. The IHA test has often been found to be negative in cases of congenital toxoplasmosis and is best utilized for serologic surveys and for diagnosis of acute acquired infections. The IFA and IgM–fluorescent antibody tests appear to be

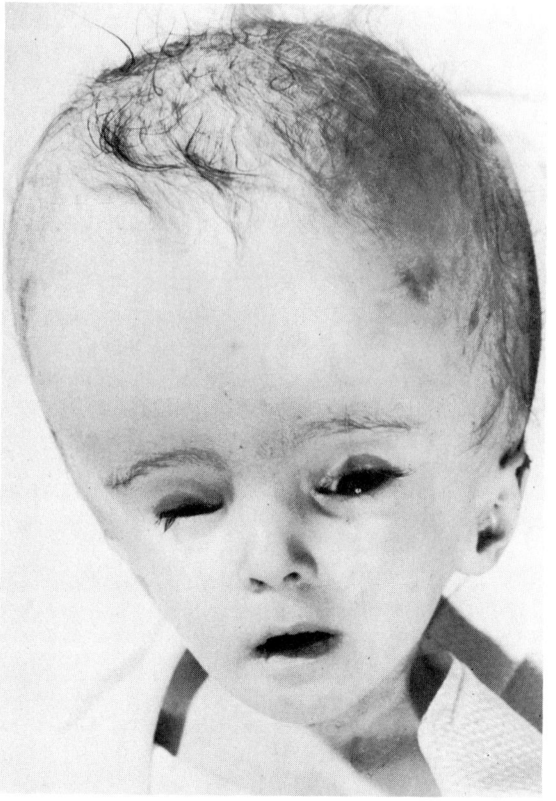

Figure 17–5. Photograph of an infant with congenital toxoplasmosis. Note extreme hydrocephalus. (Courtesy of Dr. Leon Jacobs.)

comparable in specificity to the DT, but false positive reactions in the IFA can occur in sera that contain antinuclear antibodies and in the IgM-IFA system with sera that contain rheumatoid factor. The IgM-IFA has particular value in the diagnosis of congenital and active acute acquired toxoplasmosis, but the diagnostic value of the IgM-IFA is dependent on the availability of specific antiserum for IgM. As in all serologic tests, the interpretation of results depends on a number of factors. Also, because of the varied clinical expressions observed in toxoplasmosis and the high prevalence of toxoplasma antibodies in the population, several serologic tests may have to be employed to establish a diagnosis of active or congenital infection, clinical disease, or previous infection. In acute or subclinical congenital toxoplasmosis, neonates may exhibit variations in their serologic response to diagnostic antigens as well as alterations in immunoglobulin development. Thus, although some neonates with congenital toxoplasmosis have an elevation in IgM and IgM *Toxoplasma* antibody, a majority of these neonates exhibit no detectable specific IgM antibody in their sera. In some cases, development of serum IgA is retarded and excessive production of IgM and IgG occurs, the degree of increased IgM and IgG possibly being associated with the severity of infection. A similar elevation in levels of IgM and IgG is seen in congenital rubella, cytomegalovirus disease, syphilis, and some chronic parasitic infections (Chapter 26).

Cell-Mediated Immune Response. A delayed hypersensitivity skin response and lymphocyte transformation (LT) to *toxoplasma* antigens have been induced in toxoplasmosis. The toxoplasmin skin test response appears to correlate closely with the detection of humoral antibody, but both delayed hypersensitivity and lymphoproliferation responses seem to develop after antibody production during the chronic stage of infection and remain detectable for many years. The long duration of detectable cell-mediated responses to *Toxoplasma* antigens following *Toxoplasma* infections has been hypothesized to be the result of antigenic stimulation of the immune system by the persistence of obligate or facultative intracellular stages of organisms in the host's tissue.

There is substantial evidence that immunocompetent hosts develop immunity to toxoplasmosis and that the basis for this immunity involves both humoral and cellular components. It appears that humans and other animals respond to *Toxoplasma* infection by producing antibodies that, together with complement, are directed against extracellular organisms free in the blood or in extracellular fluid; these antibody-mediated responses appear to be unable to penetrate cysts or cells containing intracellular parasites. Since the organism is killed by macrophages and since several defects in cellular immunity—e.g., Hodgkin's or other lymphomatous diseases, acquired immunodeficiency syndrome (AIDS), or following corticosteroid therapy or other intense immunosuppressive treatment—predispose to a recrudescence of active generalized toxoplasmosis, a role for CMI is strongly suggested in immunity to this organism.

THE ROLE OF ANIMAL PARASITES IN THE IMMUNOLOGICALLY COMPROMISED HOST

As is the case with certain fungi, bacteria, and viruses, the compromised host can develop a fatal disseminated disease following initial infection or relapse of latent infection with certain parasitic agents. Of particular significance in this regard are *Pneumocystis carinii, Strongyloides stercoralis,* and *Toxoplasma gondii.*

Pneumocystis Carinii

The classification of *P. carinii* is uncertain, since morphologic, histologic, and serologic studies have not clarified whether this organism is a protozoan or a fungus. Because of the lack of a reliable serologic or *in vitro* method for identification of the organism, its prevalence in human populations is unknown. The organism is an example of a parasite of low-grade virulence, believed to occur as a latent infection in both animals and humans, and in the United States the disease is most frequently observed in populations with impaired host immunity. These include hosts with inherited or acquired immune deficiency as well as both children and adults who have certain malignancies or who are receiving immunosuppressive therapy. In Europe, the agent causes epidemic pneumonia in newborn nurseries, suggesting possible differences between the European and American strains. In Europe, a complement-fixation test has been developed that is reportedly positive in 75 to 85 per cent of the cases by the second week of the disease. In contrast, sera from known American patients give a much lower rate of positivity. Whether this is because the European strain differs antigenically from the American or because the European disease affects debilitated but immunologically intact children whereas the American disease is primarily one of immunosuppressed or immunologically deficient patients is not known. Although intrauterine and person-to-person transmissions of the agent have been reported, these observations require confirmation and the exact modes of transmission are unknown. The organism does not appear to invade tissue or to have an intracellular mode of existence. It produces little necrosis, and, although commonly found in association with mononuclear cells, it is not associated with the formation of granulomas. It is often observed embedded in a heavy matrix of PAS-positive cellular debris, the source and nature of which is unknown. Whether these substances play a role in protecting the organism from host destruction is unclear. Although the organism is found in hosts with a variety of impaired immune functions, the relationship between the impaired humoral or cellular components and the biology of the agent is not clear.

Pneumocystis carinii pneumonitis has a characteristic clinical course. In infants and in individuals with primary immunologic deficiency diseases, the onset is insidious, with an increasing state of dyspnea and progressive cyanosis and a dry, nonproductive cough. In individuals with secondary immunologic deficiencies, such as those treated with immunosuppressive agents, the onset may be sudden and the pulmonary symptoms progressive within several days. Physical examination usually reveals rales and rhonchi and decreased breath sounds. Most remarkable is the lack of systemic reaction to this infection; many patients are usually dyspneic and cyanotic even in the absence of fever, malaise, or anorexia. The laboratory findings include the demonstration of a ventilation-perfusion deficit with a relatively normal pH and pCO_2 in the face of severe cyanosis. Pulmonary compliance is markedly decreased; low arterial oxygen saturation can be brought to near-normal levels or normal levels by high concentrations of oxygen.

The disease is mainly confined to the lungs. Although infiltration of the spleen and liver with cysts has been reported, little or no dysfunction of these tissues occurs. A severe interstitial fibrosis and a characteristic intra-alveolar exudate are the pathologic lesions induced by *Pneumocystis carinii.* The parasites are difficult to demonstrate in tissue with conventional staining, but may be readily visualized with silver impregnation techniques such as the Gomori methenamine silver stain (Fig. 17–6). The cyst is approximately one fifth the size of an erythrocyte. The double outer membrane of the cyst distinguishes it from other cells within the lung parenchyma (Fig. 17–6). The cyst can sometimes be seen in sputum specimens or tracheal washings. Since there is diffuse involvement of both lungs, an open lung biopsy and frozen section may be necessary to confirm the diagnosis. The x-ray findings parallel the pathologic process. The lung parenchyma reveals a diffuse interstitial infiltration involving the lower lung fields of the hilum (Fig. 17–7). Rupture of the lung parenchyma with spontaneous pneumothorax has also been reported.

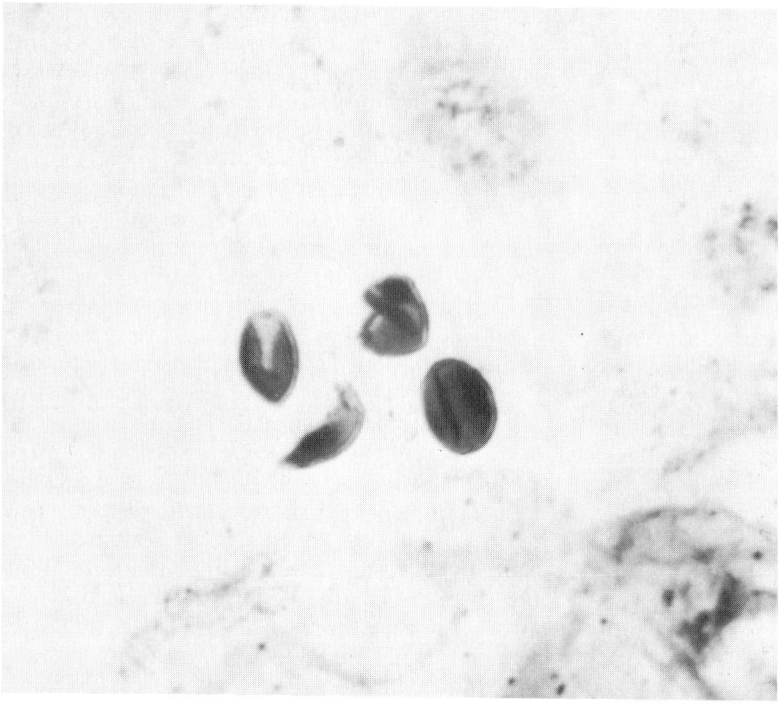

Figure 17–6. Cyst of *Pneumocystis carinii* from a frozen section of an open lung biopsy stained with Gomori's methenamine silver. The double outer membrane of the cyst helps to distinguish this structure from other cell types. Original magnification, ×930. (From Bradshaw, M., Myerowitz, R. L., Schneerson, R., et al.: *Pneumocystis carinii* pneumonitis. Ann. Intern. Med., *73*:775, 1970.)

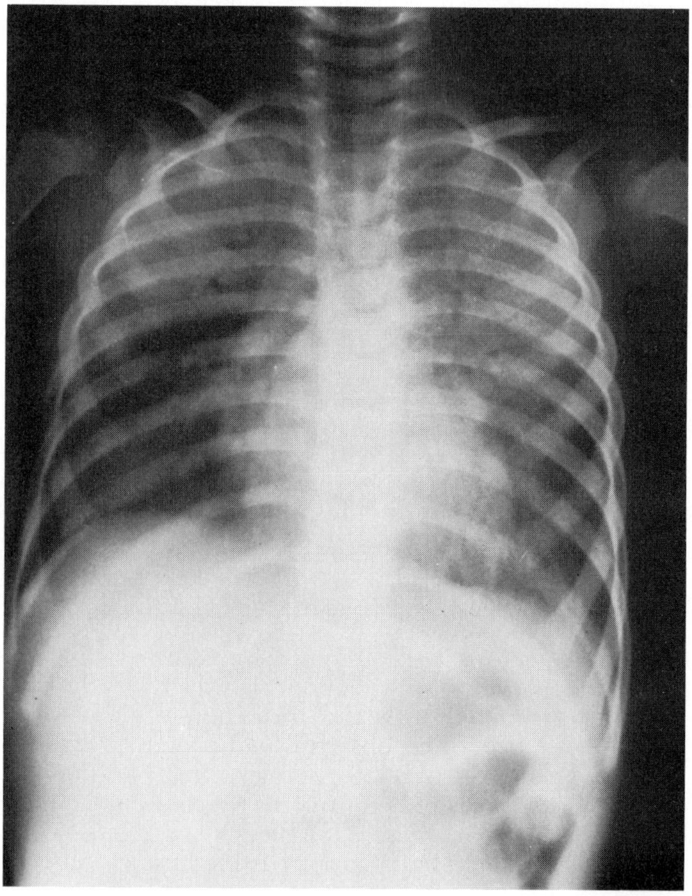

Figure 17–7. Chest roentgenogram of a five-year-old child with *Pneumocystis carinii* pneumonitis. (From Bradshaw, M., Myerowitz, R. L., Schneerson, R., et al.: *Pneumocystis carinii* pneumonitis. Ann. Intern. Med., *73*:775, 1970.)

Successful treatment of affected individuals with pentamidine isethionate has been reported. This drug may produce some toxic effects, particularly a bleeding diathesis secondary to a thrombocytopenia. More recently, the use of trimethoprim-sulfadiazine has been introduced; its toxicity is considerably less.

The nature of the infecting parasite is unknown. Information concerning the pathogenesis of human infection has been hampered by the inability to grow the organism *in vitro*. Recently, an *in vitro* method has been introduced, but additional studies have not been completed. The disease may be induced in laboratory animals by treating them with immunosuppressive drugs or cytotoxic agents, e.g., cyclophosphamide. Serologic techniques for the diagnosis of the disease are hindered in humans, since most affected individuals have immunologic deficiency states and are therefore incapable of an antibody response. Since the detection of the organism in the environment is not possible, the mode of spread of this parasite in nature unknown.

Recently, an increase in the rate of several opportunistic infections, including those by *Pneumocystis, Toxoplasma,* herpes simplex, *Candida,* and *Cryptococcus,* has been observed in individuals with acquired immune deficiency syndrome (AIDS) (Chapter 14). These individuals had not been recognized previously to have an immunosuppressive illness. Although both male and female patients have been involved, the infection rate has been predominantly observed in four groups of males (homosexuals, Haitians, drug abusers, and hemophiliacs). These same population groups also demonstrated an increased rate of an aggressive form of Kaposi's sarcoma (Chapter 19), and immunologic evaluation of these individuals has demonstrated profound defects in their cellular immune functions. The underlying immunologic syndrome in AIDS is characterized by diminished numbers of circulating lymphocytes, diminished percentage of T-lymphocytes, and reversal of the ratio of helper T-cells to suppressor T-cells, but levels of immunoglobulin and complement remain normal. Although the cases of these immunologic defects are unclear, the occurrence of *Toxoplasma* and *Pneumocystis* infections in these individuals supports the hypothesis that cell-mediated immunity plays a pivotal role in acquired immunity to toxoplasmosis and pneumocystis infection in human populations.

ATYPICAL PARASITISM IN HUMANS

It is becoming increasingly evident that even in the industrialized urban environment, humans are exposed to a number of zoonotic animal parasites. The isolation of a nematode larva from the liver of a two-year-old girl with chronic eosinophilia in 1952 led to the discovery that nematodes of domestic animals have the ability to penetrate and invade the human host. This syndrome has been termed larva migrans, the migration of larvae through the tissues of unsuitable hosts. In most instances the migrating larva is a nematode, and the infection results in a nonpatent nematodiasis. Depending on the location of the migrating stages, larva migrans may be separated into three groups: cutaneous, visceral, and subcutaneous-visceral. A number of helminths have since been shown to induce this syndrome (Table 17–4). Within this group, visceral infections by dog and cat ascarids of the genus *Toxocara* have received the most attention.

Transmission of *Toxocara* to humans occurs either directly by contact with infective puppies or indirectly by ingestion of contaminated food, water, fomites, or soil. Children are particularly at risk of infection because of their frequent and close contact with puppies and their habits of pica. This may explain the observation that the average age of the patient with acute visceral larva migrans (VLM) is one to four years. Ocular involvement in VLM was reported in 1950, when it was observed that 24 of 46 enucleated eyes with a histologic diagnosis of pseudoglioma, first diagnosed clinically as retinoblastoma, actually contained either nematode larvae or

Table 17–4. **Agents Reported to Cause Larva Migrans**

Visceral Larva Migrans	Cutaneous-Subcutaneous Larva Migrans
*Toxocara cati** *Toxocara canis**	*Ancylostoma caninum** *Ancylostoma braziliense**
Angiostrongylus cantonensis *Angiostrongylus costaricensis*	*Dirofilaria conjunctivae* *Dirofilaria repens*
Anisakis spp.	*Anatrichosoma cutaneum*
Phocanema spp.	*Rhabditis niellyi*
Terranova spp.	*Lagochilascaris minor*
Oesophagostomum stephanostomum *Oesophagostomum bifurcum*	*Gnathostoma spinigerum*
Gnathostoma spinigerum	*Thelazia callipaeda*
Dirofilaria immitis	

*Majority of cases.

their remnants (Fig. 17–8*A*). The diagnosis of VLM is based on the presence of a constellation of clinical symptoms and laboratory findings. However, the five most common findings associated with VLM patients with positive serology have been eosinophilia, leukocytosis, hypergammaglobulinemia, elevated isohemagglutinin titers, and a history of pica. Definitive diagnosis is currently based upon the positive identification of larvae from biopsied tissues, enucleated eyes, or autopsied material (Fig. 17–8*B*). The difficulty in recovering and identifying *T. canis* larvae in biopsied tissues, the risk associated with open biopsy in patients with clinical VLM, and the lack of an effective therapeutic regimen stimulated research efforts to develop a reliable serologic test. Although a variety of serologic tests have been offered for the detection of *T. canis* antibodies, most have been found to lack sensitivity and specificity. In particular, they fail to distinguish between individuals infected with *Toxocara* spp., *Ascaris lumbricoides, Trichinella spiralis,* and *Filaria* spp. In addition, false positive reactions are not uncommon owing to cross reactivity of the ascarid antigens with the heterophile antibodies, isohemagglutinins, and C-reactive protein. The recent development of an enzyme-linked immunosorbent assay (ELISA) and a double diffusion in agar method for the serodiagnosis of VLM using an antigen prepared from the embryonated eggs of *T. canis* has provided clinicians with a reliable serologic assay; a positive ELISA titer of >1:32 is accepted as confirmation of infection with *Toxocara canis.*

Another atypical parasitism accompanied by significant mortality for humans and other accidental hosts in many parts of the world is infection caused by the canine cestode *Echinococcus granulosus.* Transmission occurs when eggs passed by dogs are ingested by humans, resulting in the release of larval stages into the intestinal lumen and their subsequent penetration of the mucosa and migration to the liver and lungs. In these tissues the larvae become encapsulated fluid-filled cysts (hydatid), and the host responds by the production of antibodies, including high levels of IgE. Rupture of these cysts can release cyst fluid containing allergens into

A

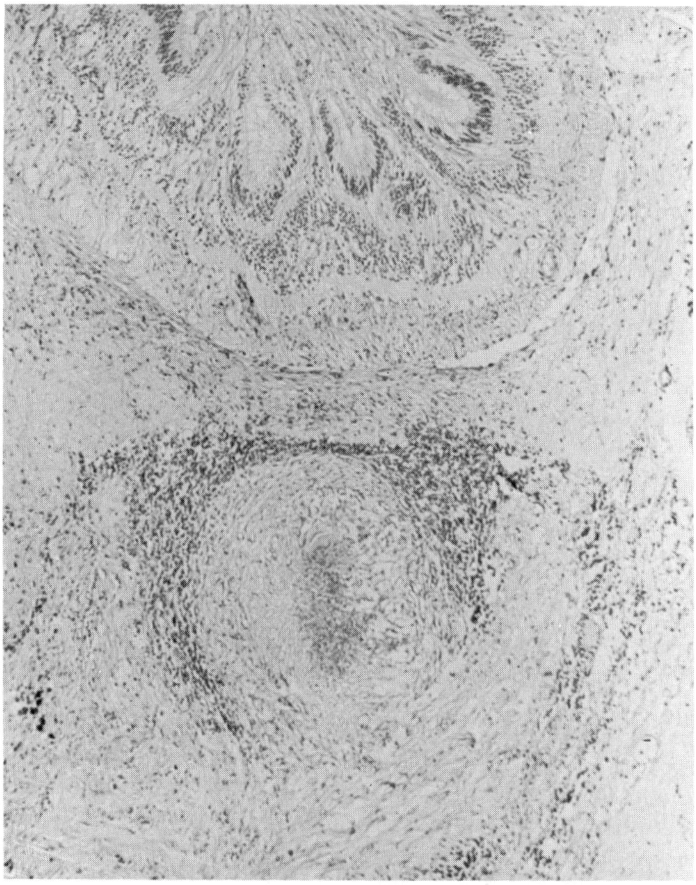

Figure 17–8. *Toxocara canis,* human. *A,* Section of retina from a child diagnosed as having retinoblastoma. Larvae of *Toxocara canis* are seen within a granuloma surrounded by lymphocytic infiltrations. Hematoxylin and eosin stain, ×44.

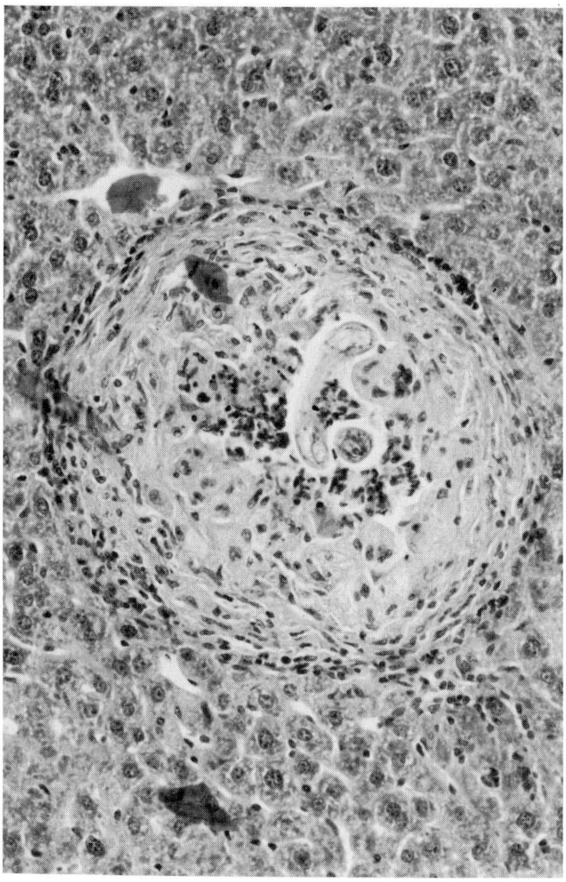

B

Figure 17–8. *Continued. B,* Section of liver from a 23-month-old child whose only clinical finding was a marked eosinophilia. Larvae of *T. canis* are seen within a granuloma surrounded by a fibrous capsule. Minimal cellular reaction surrounds the capsule. Hematoxylin and eosin stain, ×250.

the tissues, resulting in anaphylactic shock to the host. When hydatid cyst fluid is injected into the skin of infected hosts (Casoni skin test), an immediate and delayed hypersensitivity reaction is observed, suggesting infection with *Echinococcus* or related helminth species.

IMMUNOPATHOLOGIC ELEMENTS IN PARASITIC INFECTIONS

The parasitic infections represent the example *par excellence* for conditions of tissue damage by any of the four mechanisms of immunologic injury (Chapters 13 and 20). This stems, in large part, from the persistence or release of parasites or host-cell antigens during the course of infection and the relative inefficiency of the host in eliminating these antigens or cross-reacting antibodies to the host, e.g., Chagas' disease.

Certain immunologic factors observed in conjunction with parasitic infections have also been associated with the development of immunopathologic phenomena in other infectious diseases. These include (1) the release of large amounts of antigen during the course of infection, (2) the persistence of antigen in many tissues and in the circulation, (3) the alteration and destruction of host tissue, (4) the presence of shared antigenic components between the host and the parasite, and (5) the chronicity of the infections. Nevertheless, direct evidence for immunopathologic complications in many of these infections is limited and as yet not fully understood. Most of the investigations in autoimmunity in parasitic infections have been directed to malaria and trypanosomiasis, in which the presence of cold agglutinins, rheumatoid factor, antinuclear factors, and heterophil antibodies has been observed. In addition, the presence of soluble malaria antigen, the renal deposition of specific immunocomplexes, and the formation of autoantibody have been observed in malaria patients. In the case of *Schistosoma mansoni* and *S. japonica,* both experimental studies in animals and observations on natural infections in humans support the concept of immune complexes in the pathogenesis of schistosomal renal disease. Other parasitic diseases in which autoimmune factors are suspected are filariasis and ascariasis.

Suggestions for Further Reading

Bloom, B. R.: Games parasites play: How parasites evade immune surveillance. Nature, *279*:21, 1979.

Cohen, S.: Mechanisms of malarial immunity. Trans. R. Soc. Trop. Med. Hyg., *71(4)*:283, 1977.

Cypess, R. H., Karol, M. H., Zidian, J. L., et al.: Larva-specific antibodies in patients with visceral larva migrans. J. Infect. Dis., *135*:633, 1977.

Mansfield, J. M.: Immunobiology of African trypanosomiasis. Cell. Immunol., *39*:204, 1978.

Masur, H., Michelis, M. A., Greene, J. B., et al.: An outbreak of community-acquired Pneumocystis pneumonia. Initial manifestations of cellular immune dysfunction. N. Engl. J. Med., *305(3)*:1431, 1981.

Mitchell, G. F.: Responses to infection with metazoan and protozoan parasites in mice. Adv. Immunol., *28*:451, 1979.

Phillips, S. M., and Colley, D. G.: Immunologic aspects of host responses to schistosomiasis: Resistance, immunopathology and eosinophil involvement. Prog. Allergy, *24*:49, 1978.

Playfair, J. H. L.: Effective and infective immune responses to parasites: Evidence from experimental models. Curr. Top. Microbiol. Immunol., *80*:37, 1978.

Remington, J. S., and Krahenbuhl, J. L.: Immunology of *Toxoplasma gondii*. *In* Nahmias, A. J., and O'Reilly, R. J. (eds.): Immunology of Human Infection, Part II. New York, Plenum Press, 1982, pp. 327–371.

Turk, J. L., and Bryceson, A. D. M.: Immunological phenomena in leprosy and related diseases. Adv. Immunol., *13*:209, 1971.

Wassom, D. L., David, C. S., and Gleich, G. J.: MHC-linked genetic control of the immune response to parasites: *Trichinella spiralis* in the mouse. *In* Skamene, P. A., Kongshaun, L., and Landy, M. (eds.): Genetic Control of Natural Resistance to Infection and Malignancy. New York, Academic Press, 1980, pp. 75–82.

Wyler, D. J.: Malaria—resurgence, resistance and research. N. Engl. J. Med., *308*:875, 934, 1983.

Chapter 18

Mechanisms of Immunity to Fungal Diseases

Joseph A. Bellanti, M.D., and John P. Utz, M.D.

Fungi are a class of infectious agents that have classically been regarded as "plantlike" in their organization and structure. One of their outstanding properties, which is not shared by any of the other microorganisms, is the ability to exist in nature as a branching, twiglike structure (vegetative or a mold form) and in the tissues of the host as a unicellular, oval, or spheric form (the yeast phase). This property, termed dimorphism, is one of several properties of fungi that differentiate them from bacteria.

The effects of fungi on man have been both beneficial and harmful. As a class of microorganisms, they have a diverse number of properties that are beneficial to man, including their role in fermentation reactions and their biosynthetic capability in the production of antibiotics and in maintaining the geochemical structure of the earth's soil. Their pathogenic relationship to man, however, often poses serious problems for the physician. In this chapter we shall focus on the host defense mechanisms involved in the immunity to fungus infections.

In contrast to his success with bacteria, parasites, and some viruses, which have been controlled by chemotherapy, immunization, and public health measures, man has shown a notable lack of success in removing fungal pathogens from his environment. In fact, with the advent of chemotherapy for bacterial diseases there has been a change in the flora within the host, resulting in some cases in fungal overgrowth. The fungi present a second problem to the physician because of the limited number of therapeutic measures available for the treatment of fungal diseases. Thus, in spite of the widespread prevalence and occurrence of fungi, the mechanisms of immunity to them have been only recently elucidated, and considerably less is known of fungal immunology than of viral or bacterial immunology.

PATHOGENESIS OF FUNGAL DISEASES

In order to understand the mechanisms of immunity involved in fungal diseases, it is necessary first to describe the various types of interaction that a fungus can have with a host. The eventual outcome of such an interaction will depend upon (1) the properties of the fungus and (2) the status of the host in which the interaction occurs.

Localized Versus Generalized Infection

The properties of fungi that are important in pathogenicity include their ability to establish localized infection at the portal of entry and their ability to become invasive and establish generalized infection. Examples of localized infection include those fungal infections restricted to body surfaces, such as those caused by the *Candida* or the dermatophytes. Fungal infections of a more generalized nature include histoplasmosis, coccidioidomycosis, and blastomycosis. Certain fungi have a polysaccharide capsule that may be of importance in resisting phagocytosis in a manner similar to that described for the encapsulated bacteria (Chapter 15).

Acute Versus Chronic Infection

A second important consideration in the pathogenesis of fungal infections is whether a disease is *acute* or *chronic*. The chronicity reflects adaptation of the fungus to its host. Those fungal infections that are characterized by the initiation of an acute inflammatory process have been most responsive to disposal by the host's immune mechanisms and also to treatment; those that establish quiet residence with minimal tissue damage are most apt to continue as parasites in man. In general, if the defense mechanisms of the host are adequate to resist the initial attack by fungus, the disease will be acute and self-limiting. If, on the other hand, the nature of the virulence factors of the organism or the size of the initial inoculum can overwhelm the host defense factors, or if the defense mechanisms are incompletely developed or suppressed, then the eventual outcome will be unfavorable for the host and will lead to chronic systemic, and sometimes fatal, infection. With the development of chronic infection, there is development of a prominent delayed cutaneous hypersensitivity with granuloma formation.

Effect of Environmental Factors

Environmental conditions affect the host-fungus relationship. For example, the aridness of the western United States is associated with high incidence of fungal diseases such as coccidioidomycosis (San Joaquin Valley fever). It seems that the immune system of otherwise normal individuals is ineffective under these environmental conditions. It may be related to either a high concentration of pathogen in these areas or diminished efficiency of the nonspecific immune responses in the host. A pathogen in high enough concentration can overwhelm the defense mechanisms of the normal host. Other types of fungal infections are more commonly seen with different environmental conditions, such as occupations in which the skin is subjected to immersion in water, predisposing the host to superficial fungal infections of the skin. These two examples illustrate the effect of the external environment on the host-parasite relationship involved in fungal infections.

CLASSIFICATION OF FUNGAL DISEASES

The various types of fungal diseases, the mycoses, may be classified according to the following types: (1) opportunistic, (2) cutaneous, (3) subcutaneous, and (4) systemic (Table 18–1).

Opportunistic Fungi

Perhaps the most common of the fungi infecting man are the so-called opportunistic fungi (Table 18–1). These fungi are normally nonpathogenic in healthy humans but may behave as virulent organisms in individuals with depressed immune function: the newborn, patients with lymphoreticular malignancy, patients receiving immunosuppressive therapy, or patients in other clinical situations, e.g., diabetes mellitus or the use of broad-spectrum antibiotics. The fungi included in this group are the *Candida, Aspergillus*, and *Phycomycetes*. Under circumstances in which either nonspecific or specific factors are depressed, these fungi may establish a variety of localized or generalized, acute or chronic types of infection (Fig. 18–1). Of

Table 18–1. **Types of Mycotic Diseases of Man Caused by the Pathogenic Fungi**

Type of Infection	Fungus	Portal of Entry	Type of Disease
Opportunistic	*Candida albicans, Aspergillus* spp., *Phycomycetes (Mucor, Rhizopus)*	Mucous membranes, skin and respiratory tract	Thrush, vulvovaginitis, pneumonitis
Cutaneous	*Microsporum, Trichophyton, Epidermophyton*	Skin, hair, and nails	Tinea corporis, tinea capitis, onychomycosis
Subcutaneous	*Sporothrix schenckii*	Break in skin and lymphatics	Ulcerating nodular abscess with lymphangitic spread
Systemic	*Cryptococcus neoformans* *Coccidioides immitis* *Histoplasma capsulatum* *Blastomyces dermatitidis*	Respiratory tract, skin	Pneumonia, skin, CNS, or other systemic involvement

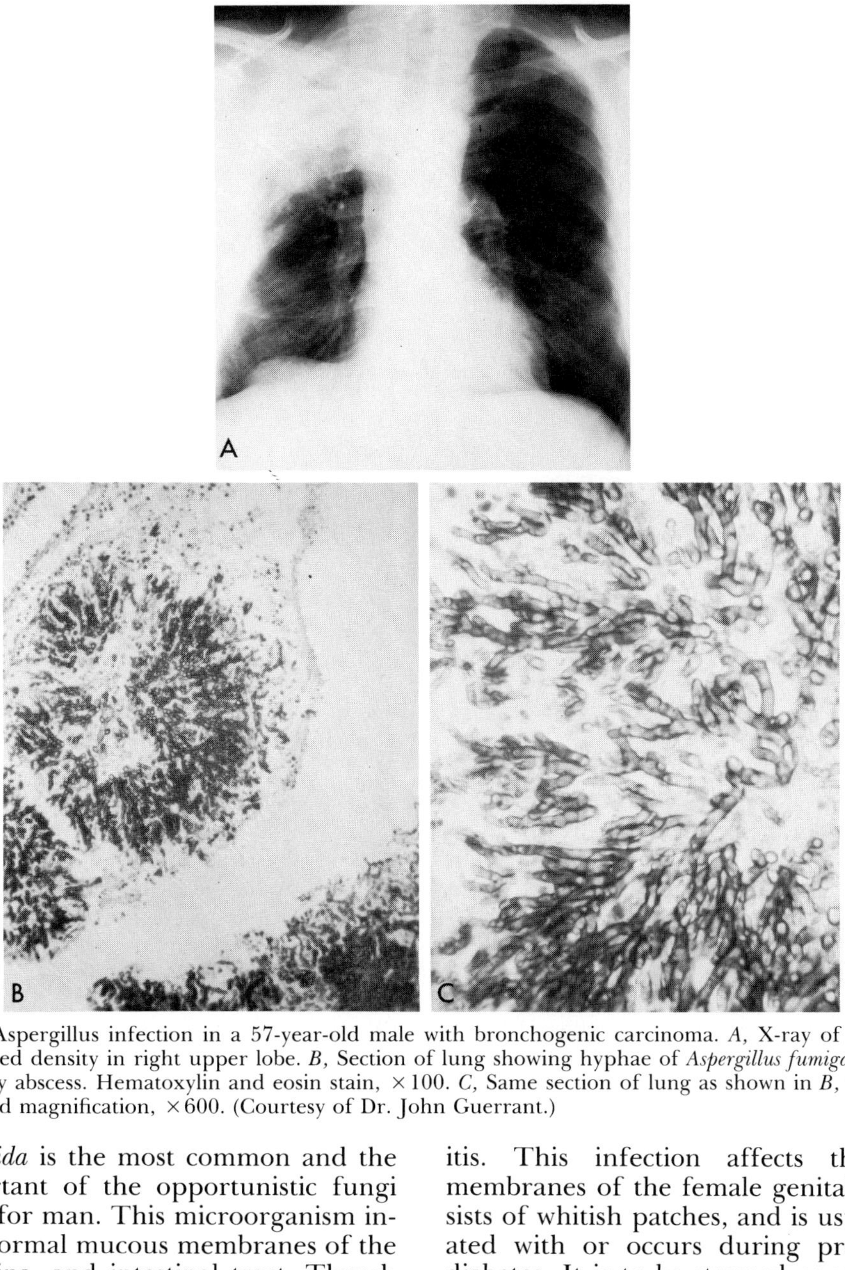

Figure 18–1. Aspergillus infection in a 57-year-old male with bronchogenic carcinoma. *A*, X-ray of chest showing area of increased density in right upper lobe. *B*, Section of lung showing hyphae of *Aspergillus fumigatus* in the wall of a pulmonary abscess. Hematoxylin and eosin stain, ×100. *C*, Same section of lung as shown in *B*, photographed under increased magnification, ×600. (Courtesy of Dr. John Guerrant.)

these, *Candida* is the most common and the most important of the opportunistic fungi pathogenic for man. This microorganism inhabits the normal mucous membranes of the mouth, vagina, and intestinal tract. Thrush and vaginitis are examples of infections of the mucous membranes caused by *Candida*. Thrush, a localized infection of the mucous membranes of the mouth and pharynx, consists of discrete whitish patches, is seen during the early newborn period and in young infants, and is presumably acquired by passage through the birth canal. It is also seen in individuals receiving broad-spectrum antibiotics or with depressed specific immunity, such as in patients receiving immunosuppressive therapy. A second type of involvement of the mucous membrane is vulvovaginitis. This infection affects the mucous membranes of the female genital tract, consists of whitish patches, and is usually associated with or occurs during pregnancy or diabetes. It is to be stressed once again that the pattern of disease cannot be described merely as a function of the pathogen but rather must be viewed in total perspective with the host response.

These opportunistic fungal infections may be acute and self-limited or chronic and occasionally disseminated, particularly in very immature infants or individuals with severely depressed immune functions. These opportunistic fungi may become invasive and involve virtually every tissue of the body. A particular form of candidiasis is seen in children with immune deficiency diseases involving the thymic-dependent tissues (Chapter 22). This is associated with a chronic form of mucocutaneous candidiasis, involving the mucous membranes of the mouth, the respiratory and gastrointestinal tracts, and the skin and the nails, that is often serious and life-threatening. This presenting clinical picture is so common that if candidiasis is seen beyond the newborn period in individuals not receiving antibiotics a diligent search should be made for diseases of the lymphoproliferative system or for an immunologic deficiency, particularly of the thymic-dependent limb of immunity.

Another type of involvement with these opportunistic fungi is seen in clinical situations in which prosthetic valves or devices are used in the human, e.g., the use of cardiac valves or ventricular valves in the treatment of hydrocephalus. These prostheses act as foci of infection and, since they are avascular, are not accessible to the normal clearing mechanisms available to the host, i.e., phagocytosis.

Cutaneous Fungi

A second type of infection produced by fungi involves the epidermis and its appendages (hair and nails). These infections are referred to as the *dermatophytoses;* the fungi responsible for these infections are referred to as dermatophytes (Table 18–1). Included within this group are members of the following genera: *Microsporum, Tricophyton,* and *Epidermophyton.* These fungi have a predilection for keratin-rich tissues such as the skin, hair, and nails. They appear to have the capacity to degrade keratin and use its breakdown products as a nutritional source.

These fungi can produce infections of the scalp (tinea capitis), of the skin (tinea corporis), or of the nails (onychomycosis) (Table 18–1). Infection of the scalp due to *Microsporum canis* or *Microsporum audouini* occurs most frequently in childhood. Conversely, infection of the skin (e.g., athlete's foot) very rarely occurs in children and is more commonly seen in adults. The immune mechanisms controlling these types of infection are poorly understood but appear to involve both nonspecific and specific immunologic events. For example, the resistance of adults to tinea capitis, i.e., ringworm of the scalp, has been attributed mainly to the increase in secretion of saturated fatty acids with antifungal activity at puberty. The increased susceptibility of adults to infection of the skin may be related to factors that promote fungal growth, e.g., excessive sweating (hyperhidrosis).

Immunity cannot always be explained in terms of classic specific immunologic reactions. Although fungistatic factors have been noted in the sera of individuals with and without infection, they are not associated with the immunoglobulins. Cell-mediated immunity appears to be an important immune mechanism during the course of most fungal infections. Since antibody occurs in individuals with and without an infection, antibody determinations offer little diagnostic or prognostic value. Certain localized manifestations of the skin occur during the course of fungal infections and are referred to as "id" reactions. The mechanism of these reactions is one of delayed hypersensitivity. The role of these reactions in immunity is unclear.

Subcutaneous Fungi

A third type of infection caused by fungi is the *subcutaneous* type of infection. An example of these fungi is *Sporothrix.* They are distributed in soil and on plants and are introduced into the body by penetration of the skin with contaminated splinters, thorns, and soil. Once established, infections tend to be localized in subcutaneous tissues and become associated with chronic draining ulcerated lesions. There may be involvement of the lymphatics and, occasionally, systemic spread. Immune mechanisms appear to include nonspecific and specific antibody and cell-mediated factors.

Systemic Fungi

The systemic mycoses, the fourth type of infection caused by fungi, are the most serious. Fungal infections of this type include cryptococcosis, coccidioidomycosis, histoplasmosis, and blastomycosis (Table 18–1). Specific immune responses are stimulated in these diseases and appear to be important mechanisms of resistance. Thus, the development of serum antibody, including precipitins, agglutinins, and complement-fixing antibodies, offers both diagnostic and prognostic value.

The pathogenesis of these infections usually invokes entry of the pathogen by inhalation into the respiratory tract or by introduction through a break in the skin (Fig. 18–2). Following a limited replication at a local site, the organism may be removed by nonspecific factors (macrophages) in which it may persist for long periods of time. Following infection, an inflammatory response characterized by granuloma formation is seen (Chapter 12). In many of the infections, such as histoplasmosis, caseous necrosis may develop, and recovery may be associated with roentgenographic evidence of calcification.

In addition, cell-mediated immunity (delayed hypersensitivity) may develop. Thus, the injection of purified blastomycin, coccidioidin, or histoplasmin is associated with the development of a cutaneous delayed-hypersensitivity reaction. The effector mechanisms by which these cell-mediated events effect recovery have been described (Chapter 9).

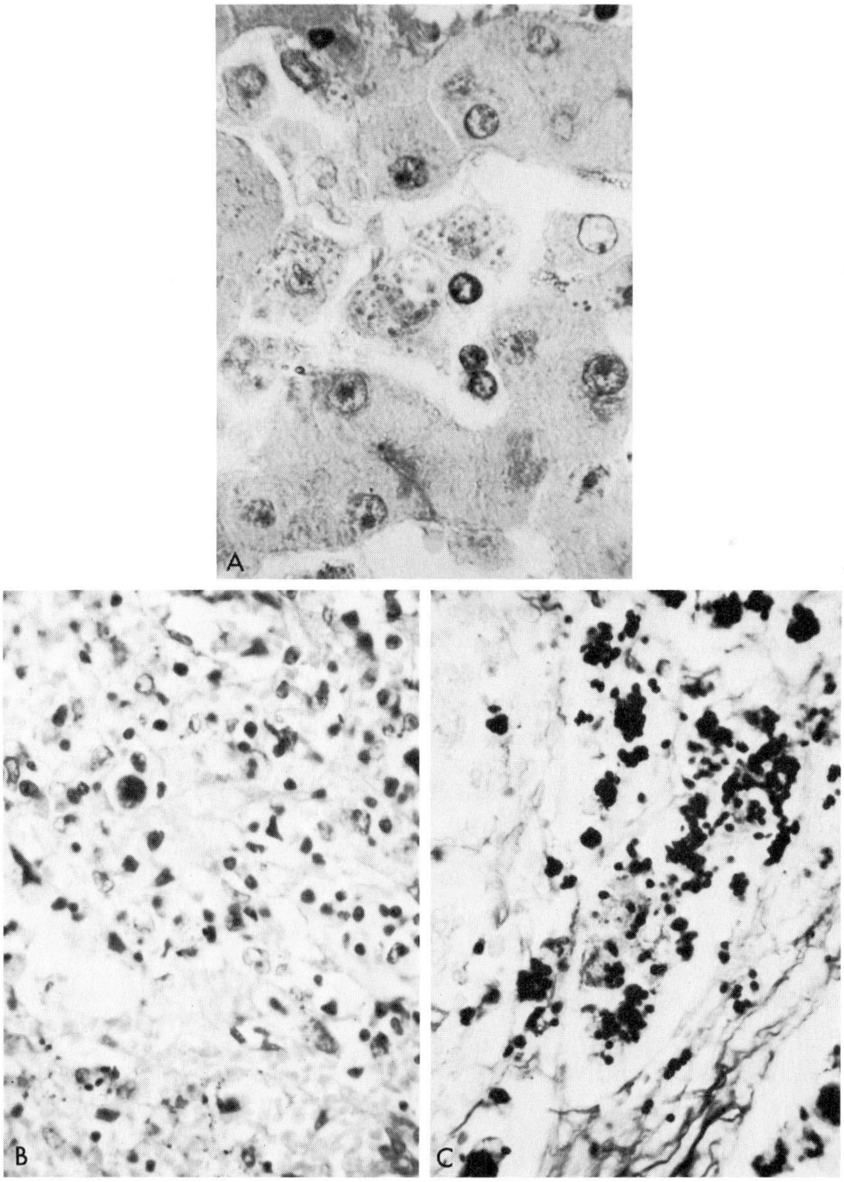

Figure 18–2. Disseminated histoplasmosis in a 60-year-old male who died of myeloid metaplasia. *A,* Section of liver showing the *Histoplasma capsulatum* within Kupffer cells. Hematoxylin and eosin stain, ×600. *B,* Section of spleen showing *Histoplasma capsulatum* within macrophages. Hematoxylin and eosin stain, ×100. *C,* Section of lymph node showing *Histoplasma capsulatum* in tissue. Silver methenamine stain, ×100. (Courtesy of Dr. Daniel Mohler.)

These cell-mediated responses also offer important diagnostic aid.

WORKING HYPOTHESIS OF THE ROLES OF THE VARIOUS ELEMENTS OF THE IMMUNE RESPONSE DURING FUNGAL INFECTIONS

Starting with a nonimmune susceptible host, a primary encounter with fungus would be countered by the nonspecific barrier presented by the intact skin and mucous membranes. If these are surmounted, the next barriers encountered are the nonspecific humoral factors, such as antifungal properties of sebum. If these are overcome, an infection may be initiated. This might take the form of a *localized* infection, e.g., thrush; or it may be more extensive, as in the case of cutaneous and subcutaneous infections; or it may be even more extensive, with systemic involvement. The pulmonary lesions of systemic infections may be localized within macrophages, e.g., granuloma formation. If these barriers are not effective, however, there may be widespread generalized dissemination of the fungus to deep-seated organs, such as the brain. In all these host-fungus interactions, but particularly in the case of the more extensive infections, there are stimulated specific immunologic factors consisting of antibody and delayed hypersensitivity. The precise role of these specific factors in the recovery of these infections is unclear. Cell-mediated immunity, however, appears to be an important effector mechanism in these deep-seated chronic infections and probably exerts its effect by the same interactions with macrophages as described for bacterial diseases (Chapter 15).

CLINICAL STATES IN WHICH ABERRATIONS OF THE IMMUNE RESPONSE LEAD TO PREDISPOSITION TO FUNGAL INFECTIONS

Trauma

Trauma appears to be a predisposing condition in the successful establishment of many fungal infections, especially those of the chronic granulomatous type. Trauma to either the mucous membranes or the skin provides a portal of entry for fungi.

Age

The very young and the very old are predisposed to fungal infections, particularly the opportunistic fungi, presumably owing to either immaturity or senescence of the immune system. In the case of infants, infections are usually self-limited and disappear as the child grows. Whereas most adults possess agglutinins and delayed-hypersensitivity reactions to *Candida*, the neonate usually manifests neither. The development of both antibody and delayed hypersensitivity occurs with maturation because of an exposure to these pathogens.

Metabolic States

Many types of metabolic derangements, including diabetes and pregnancy, are associated with overgrowth of fungi. The precise role of the metabolic derangement is incompletely understood but might be related to enhanced growth as a result of increased glucose in extracellular fluids.

Acquired Immune Deficiency Syndrome (AIDS)

The occurrence of opportunistic infections caused by a variety of microorganisms, including fungi, has been seen in patients with defective cell-mediated immunity in the recent epidemic of AIDS (Chapter 22). The fungal agents that are found in greatest frequency include *Candida albicans, Aspergillus* species, and *Cryptococcus neoformans*.

Treatment with Antibiotics or Immunosuppressive Agents

The overgrowth of fungi is widely known to occur during the course of treatment with broad-spectrum antibiotics, wherein the ecologic balance of microbial growth is disturbed. The opportunistic fungi are usually involved in these interactions. As described earlier, the specific defects of the immunologic system, particularly those involving the thymic-dependent system, may present with overwhelming fungal infections, e.g., mucocutaneous candidiasis. Patients receiving immunosuppressive therapy, e.g., metabolites or steroids, or with lymphoproliferative diseases, e.g., leukemia or lymphomas, may also present with these fungal infections. Therefore, with any patient who develops fungal infection, these factors should be taken into consideration and diligent search made for underlying diseases.

CLINICAL CONDITIONS THAT RESULT FROM HYPERSENSITIVITY TO FUNGI

There are three probable outcomes that result from the interaction between the host immune response and fungus. The degree to which fungal antigen persists or is reintroduced will determine the expression of the host's reaction. If fungal antigen is successfully eliminated by the inflammatory response and phagocytosis, or if a specific immune response is stimulated with the development of delayed hypersensitivity and antibody, then no further host interaction is seen. If the fungus is not successfully eliminated or is reintroduced in either a live or a killed form, the persistence of fungal antigen causes further host interaction. For example, if the IgE reagins are stimulated, the patient could express symptoms of asthma (Type I reaction). If precipitating antibody is stimulated and fungal antigen is reintroduced via the respiratory tract, antigen-antibody complexes might result and could be associated with such diseases as farmer's lung (Type III reaction); the persistence of fungal antigen could also result in granuloma formation, with the development of delayed hypersensitivity locally or at distal sites in the skin, e.g., "id" reactions (Type IV reaction).

SUMMARY

The immune mechanisms displayed by the host in antifungal defense are best viewed according to the type of fungal infection that occurs: (1) opportunistic, (2) cutaneous, (3) subcutaneous, and (4) systemic. The fungal pathogens as a group evoke both nonspecific and specific factors of immunity, and the participation of these various factors is directly correlated with the degree of penetration of the fungus into the host. Cell-mediated immunity (delayed hypersensitivity) appears to be a most important defense mechanism in most types of fungal infections. Congenital or iatrogenic depression of the immune function predisposes the host to fungal infections.

Suggestions for Further Reading

Catanzaro, A.: Immunology of fungal diseases. *In* Handbook on Fungal Diseases. Park Ridge, Ill., American College of Chest Physicians, 1981, pp. 12–16.

Cohen, M. S., Isturiz, R. E., Malech, H. L., et al.: Fungal infection in chronic granulomatous disease. The importance of the phagocyte in defense against fungi. Am. J. Med., *71*:59, 1981.

Drutz, D. J., and Huppert, M.: Coccidioidomycoses: Factors affecting the host-parasite interaction. J. Infect. Dis., *147*:372, 1983.

Penn, R. L., Lambert, R. S., and George, R. B.: Invasive fungal infections: The use of serologic tests in diagnosis and management. Arch. Intern. Med., *143*:215, 1983.

Richardson, M. D., and Warnock, D. W.: Mechanisms of resistance to fungal infection in the non-compromised host. *In* Warnock, D. W., and Richardson, M. D. (eds.): Fungal Infection in the Compromised Patient. New York, John Wiley & Sons, 1982, pp. 1–28.

Rippon, J. W.: Medical Mycology. Philadelphia, W. B. Saunders Company, 1982.

Wientzen, R. L., and Utz, J. P.: The mycoses other than histoplasmosis. *In* Kendig, E. L., and Chernick, V.: Disorders of the Respiratory Tract in Children. Philadelphia, W. B. Saunders Company, 1983, pp. 732–762.

Chapter 19

Immune Defense Mechanisms in Tumor Immunity

Ronald B. Herberman, M.D., and Joseph A. Bellanti, M.D.

An aberration or imbalance in the surveillance mechanisms of the host immune system is now believed to be involved in the development of neoplasms. Such an association has been investigated in animals for decades and may be applicable to man. One of the lines of evidence in support of this comes from observations that the widespread use of immunosuppressive agents in graft recipients is associated with an increased incidence of malignant disorders after organ tranplantation. In addition, accumulated data have shown that children with immunologic deficiency diseases have a greater risk of neoplasia (Chapter 22). This increased incidence is shown in Table 19–1. A further example of the likely role of the immune system in resistance to development of tumors is the high incidence of Kaposi's sarcoma in male homosexuals or other individuals with the acquired immunodeficiency syndrome (AIDS) (Chapter 22).

There are several possible explanations for an association between immune depression and increased tumor growth. Initially, almost all attention was focused on the role of specific T-cell–mediated immunity in reacting against new or altered antigens on the surface of tumor cells. More recently, however, it has become clear that there is also a natural immune system that may play an important role in resistance against the development and progressive growth of tumors.

THE CONCEPT OF TUMOR ANTIGENICITY

A tumor cell, either transplanted or induced, represents a foreign configuration to the host in which it arises. The immune mechanisms operable against tumor cells are basically the same as those marshaled in response to any other foreign configuration.

Most of the responses in tumor antigenicity and in specific tumor immunity closely resemble those that apply to allograft rejection phenomena involving relatively weak transplantation antigen systems. Antigens arise in many tumors as a consequence of the neoplastic change and are specific for each tumor or group of tumors. These antigens are referred to as tumor-associated transplantation antigens (TATA) or tumor-associated antigens (TAA). They are cell-surface antigens and evoke a specific immune response when injected into an appropriate host. The implication of these findings is that the origins of these newly acquired antigens are influenced by the oncogenic agent. The antigens are

Table 19–1. Evidence of Malignancy in Primary Immunodeficiency Syndromes

Disease	Incidence	Estimated Risk (Per Cent)
Congenital X-linked immunodeficiency	6/approx. 100	6
Severe combined system immunodeficiency	9/approx. 400	2
IgM deficiency	6/approx. 70	8
Wiskott-Aldrich syndrome	24/approx. 300	8
Ataxia-telangiectasia	52/approx. 500	10
Common variable immunodeficiency	41/approx. 500	8
Total	138/approx. 1870	7

From Kersey, J. H., Spector, B. D., and Good, R. A.: Primary immunodeficiency diseases and cancer: the immunodeficiency-cancer registry. Int. J. Cancer, *12*:333, 1973.

under genetic control and are transmitted to the descendants of these altered tumor cells. A knowledge of them may allow for their ultimate utilization in the diagnosis and treatment of certain human neoplasms.

During the early part of this century, many attempts were made to develop a "cancer vaccine." These efforts, using outbred strains of animals, met with almost uniform failure because of the histocompatibility differences, which were unknown at that time. Immunity induced against the histoincompatible tumors was directed largely against the foreign histocompatibility antigens and only to a lesser and ill-defined extent to the TAA. By using a genetic approach with inbred animal strains that are histocompatible, the activity of TAA could be studied. Such techniques have made it possible to identify the host reaction to determinants on the tumor that may distinguish it from normal cells.

Responses to Allogeneic Tumor Transplantation

In two dissimilar individuals, the transplantation of tumor tissue can have one of three outcomes: (1) *rejection* due to incompatibility, (2) *acceptance* and growth (*enhancement*) of the tumor transplant, or (3) inhibition due to a nonspecific tumor cytolytic effect (*allogeneic inhibition*). These are shown schematically in Figure 19–1.

With the first outcome, if a normal tissue, such as skin, were transplanted between two genetically dissimilar animals, A and B, the graft would be rejected as a result of the dissimilarity of the normal transplantation antigens (Chapter 3). If tumor cells were transplanted from A to B, the graft would be rejected owing to two types of incompatibility: (1) that due to the dissimilarity of normal histocompatibility antigens and (2) that due to the tumor graft itself, which contains TAA foreign to the recipient host. As a result of either response, the graft would be promptly rejected because of tissue incompatibility.

A paradoxical effect is seen in the second outcome, in which animal B is *preimmunized* to the tumor antigens either actively or, more typically, by passive transfer of immune serum (Fig. 19–1). Although preimmunization of the recipient usually leads to accelerated rejection of the tumor graft, in some circumstances the net effect is one of increased tumor growth, or enhancement. Two mechanisms have been proposed to explain this anomalous effect: (1) The antibody may combine with the tumor antigens before reaching a lymph node, thereby preventing an immune response (afferent blockade), or (2) the antigen-combining sites on the tumor may be masked by being coated with antibody (efferent blockade) (Chapter 24). It must again be stressed, however, that preimmunization does not usually cause tumor enhance-

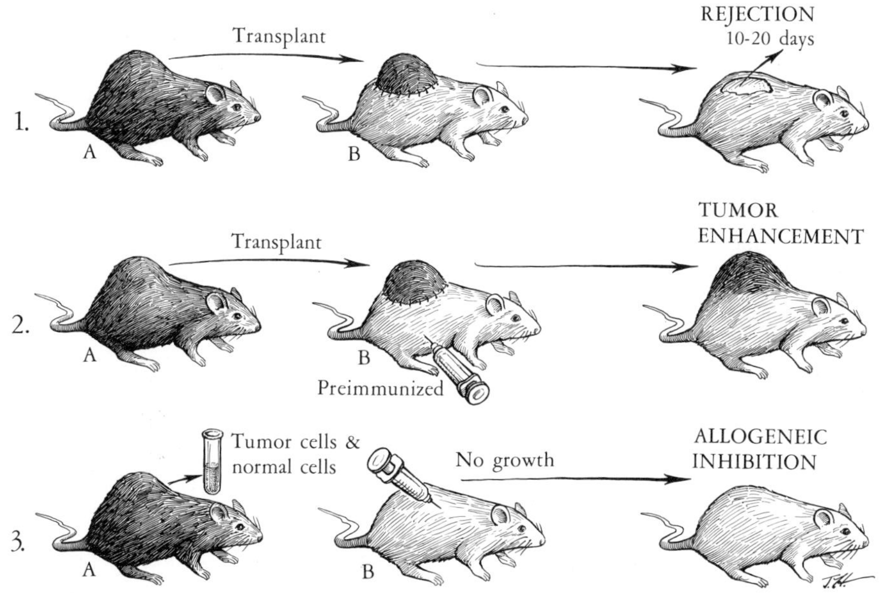

Figure 19–1. Types of responses seen after allogeneic tumor transplantation in the mouse.

ment; more often, tumor growth is delayed and animals are protected. Apparently, the quality of immunity in the sensitized animals and the relative dose of transplanted tumor cells determine the outcome.

Yet another consequence of tumor transplantation between two dissimilar hosts is seen in the third outcome (Fig. 19–1). Mixing of tumor cells with normal cells prior to tumor implantation may result in tumor cell destruction or inhibition. This phenomenon, referred to as allogeneic inhibition, was originally believed to represent a reaction between dissimilar cell surfaces but now may be explained by the action of cells of the natural immune system (see below).

Responses to Syngeneic Tumor Transplantation

In contrast to the responses seen between allogeneic hosts, syngeneic hosts provide genetic similarity so that the effects of the TAA's are their major difference. Thus, these experimental animal systems provide an opportunity to gain insight into immune responses to tumors in a situation that is similar to that of the individual in which the tumor arose and which, in the human, could be duplicated only by experiments with identical twins.

Although spontaneous tumors with no known etiology may arise in man and in animals, it has been convenient to utilize experimentally induced tumors, which arise more rapidly and consistently, that may serve as models for malignant tumors in man (Table 19–2).

Methylcholanthrene (MCA) produces tumors that are representative of those induced by chemical and physical agents. These agents induce unique TAA's. Regardless of morphologic similarity, each new tumor induced by the same agent possesses a TAA specificity unique to that tumor (Fig. 19–2). Thus, resistance to one chemically induced tumor does not prevent growth of a second tumor induced by a different chemical, even though the two tumors may be morphologically identical. The strength of the tumor-associated antigens on the cell surface is thought to be directly related to the length of the latent period between the application of the oncogen and the development of the tumor—the shorter the latent period, the greater, in general, the strength of the antigen. The mechanism for emergence of the unique TAA is unknown, but, based on recent evidence, it seems more likely to be related to induction of expression of a so-called oncogene.

In contrast, these characteristics differ from those seen in tumors induced by virus (Fig. 19–3). The virus-induced tumors have antigens that cross-react with other tumors induced by the same or similar viruses, even though morphologic appearance differs. Such cross-reactivity, seen with both DNA and RNA viruses, is presumably due to the ability of viral nucleic acid to be incorporated into the genetic material of the host. In spite of the cross-reactivity, there are fundamental differences in the ability of viruses to induce tumors (Fig. 19–4). The DNA viruses produce an *integrated infection* through which the host cell's properties are transformed; however, cell growth persists in the absence of fully infectious virus (Chapter 16). From within the cell, the virus specifies the production of unique transplantation antigens on the cell surface as well as the production of other virus-specific antigens (Fig. 19–4).

The integrated type of infection is not seen in hosts normally infected with the virus; it is seen only in an unnatural host (e.g., newborn) to which it is artificially transmitted. For example, the SV-40 virus normally infects monkeys and results in an inapparent or respiratory infection. When this virus is transferred to the newborn hamster, however, sarcoma develops in the absence of its usual disease expression. Since the virus seems to be restricted to the nucleus, there is no shedding of infectious virus and consequently no development of a state of tolerance (Chapter 10). As the newborn develops, there is an increased incidence of tumor with little demonstrable evidence of antibody formation. In adult animals, however, the DNA-virus infections lead to a state of immunity, with elimination of virus and no evidence of tumor formation. Adults previously thymectomized during the neonatal period show an increased tumor incidence when infected during adult life. The implication of this model for the physician is that many human tumors may be related to expression of oncogenes that are integrated pieces of DNA of the host himself but that resemble the integrated virus DNA. Such expression of oncogenes in human cells may come from translocations of these pieces of DNA to other chromosomes where they are more likely to be translated and expressed.

Table 19–2. **Types and Antigenic Characteristics of Tumor Formation**

Group	Example of Agent	Type of Tumor Induced	Antigenic Specificity (TATA)	Result of Primary Infection or Exposure: In Newborn	In Adult	In Adult Thymectomized as Newborn
Chemical or physical agents	Methylcholanthrene (MCA)	Sarcoma Leukemia Carcinoma	Individual for each tumor	Tumors after maturity; no tolerance	Solid immunity	Increased tumor incidence
Viruses						
DNA viruses	Polyoma SV-40 Adenoviruses	Heterogeneous Sarcoma Undifferentiated sarcomas	Cross react within group	Tumors after maturity; no tolerance	Solid immunity	Increased tumor incidence
RNA viruses	Rous sarcoma virus (RSV) and avian leukosis viruses	Avian leukemia and sarcoma	Cross react within group, generally	Tumors after maturity; no primary response; animals can be immunized	Not susceptible to infection	
	Murine-leukemia-sarcoma complex (Friend, Maloney, Rauscher [FMR], and Gross*)	Murine leukemia, sarcoma	Cross react within group	Tumors after maturity;* tolerance	Solid immunity	Leukemia prevented when infected in newborn
	Mammary tumor virus	Mammary carcinoma	Cross react within group, but also some individual TAA	Tumors after maturity; tolerance	Solid immunity	Decreased tumor incidence
Spontaneous	Unknown	Many types	Undetectable, or individual for each tumor	Unknown	Unknown	Unknown

*Gross virus capable of inducing tumors in newborn; virus contains type-specific antigens.

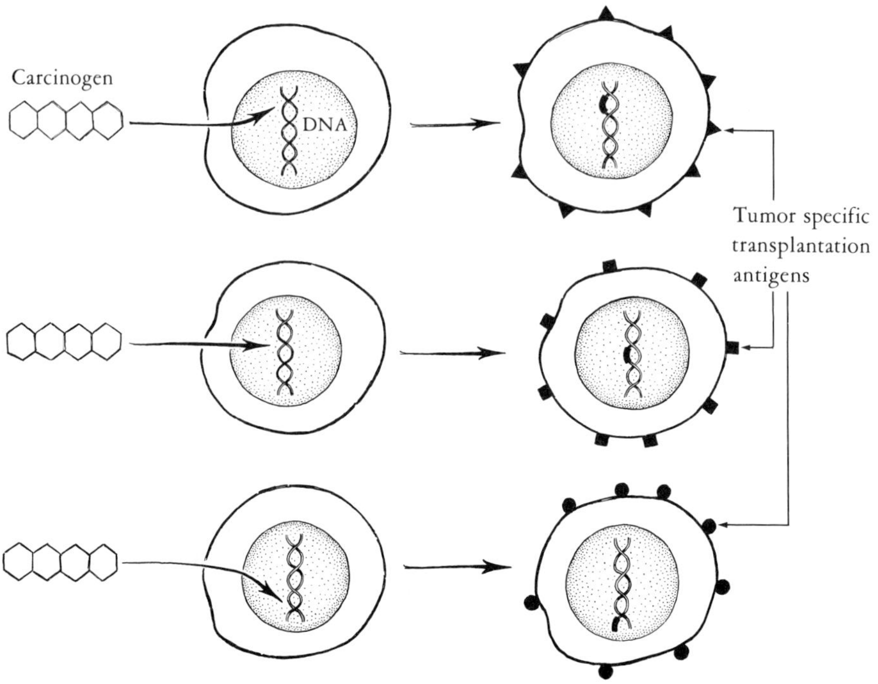

Figure 19–2. Schematic representation of development of tumor antigens by a chemical carcinogen. Note that when cells of identical genetic identity are transformed by the same chemical carcinogen, each new tumor has its own unique antigenic specificity regardless of morphologic appearance.

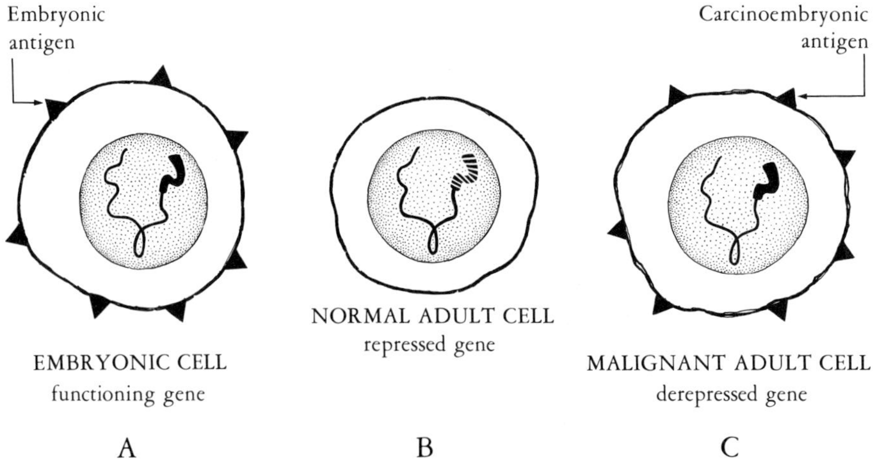

Figure 19–3. Postulated mechanism of emergence of carcinoembryonic antigens. *A*, A normal embryonic antigen produced by a functioning gene within an embryonic cell. *B*, Repression of the gene *(dotted line)* with no further elaboration of the embryonic antigen in the adult cell. *C*, Derepression of the gene in the malignant cell with reappearance of the embryonic antigen (carcinoembryonic antigen) on the surface of the cell.

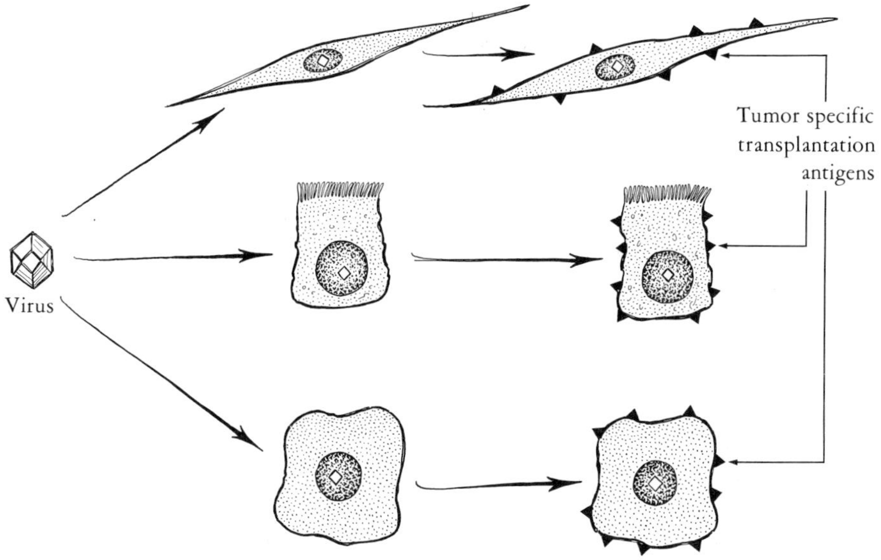

Figure 19–4. Schematic representation of the development of tumor-specific antigens (TSA) by a tumor virus. Note that although the morphologic appearance may vary, each tumor induced by a single virus contains the same TSA on the cell surface.

The pathogenesis of malignant disorders in the case of the RNA viruses is somewhat different. With the notable exception of RSV, RNA viruses produce steady-state infections (Chapter 16). The maturation of these lipid-rich viruses occurs at cell surfaces, where they are extruded by "budding" (Fig. 19–5). These viruses are fully infectious and are acquired congenitally by "vertical transmission"; they freely circulate and produce a state of tolerance (Chapter 10). In contrast to the DNA viruses, they produce in their natural hosts a high level of viremia that is sustained. Thus, the steady-state viruses show

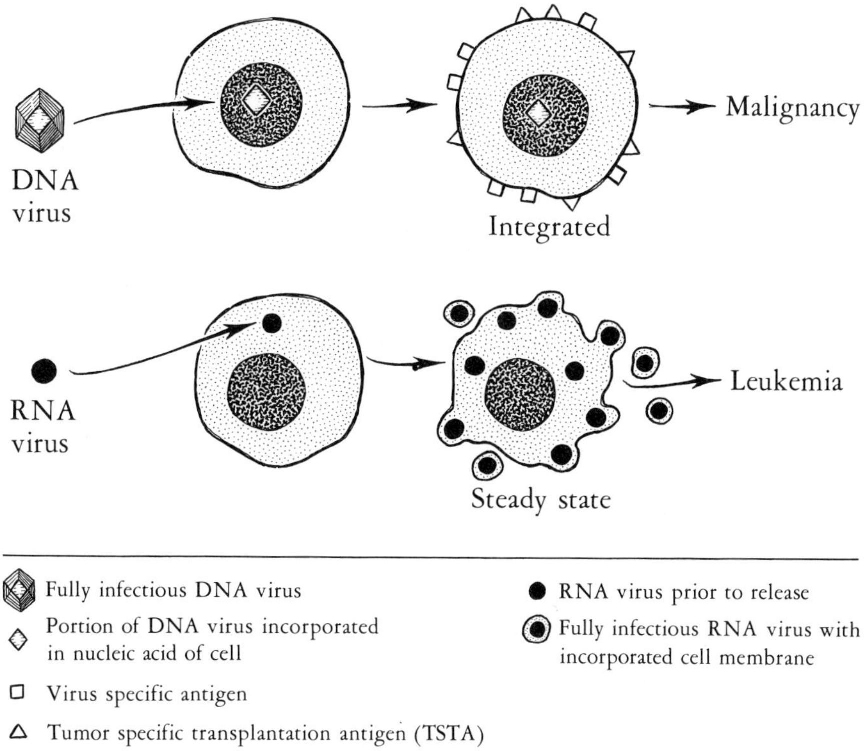

Figure 19–5. Schematic representation of the types of tumors seen in response to oncogenic viruses.

the criteria for the induction of tolerance as follows: (1) a high-dose inoculum of viral antigen, (2) the persistence of virus-specific antigen, and (3) the development and persistence of tumor-specific antigens. Infection of adults who have a fully developed immunologic system results in active immunity, elimination of virus, and a reduced incidence of tumor formation. In contrast to the response to DNA viruses, adults previously thymectomized in neonatal life show a decreased tumor incidence when infected with RNA viruses during adult life.

It appears that RNA viruses themselves can carry oncogenes, which closely resemble those detected in host cells. Animal RNA tumor viruses are able to reverse the normal flow of transmission of genetic information from DNA to RNA to protein by using an enzyme to produce DNA from RNA messenger molecules. The enzyme is an RNA-dependent DNA polymerase and is also called reverse transcriptase. The fact that high levels of reverse transcriptase activity have been found in human leukemia cells and other neoplastic cells suggests associated RNA viruses. This finding is not unique to neoplasia; elevated enzyme activity can also be found in embryonic tissues, normal cells, and cells infected with nononcogenic tumor viruses.

EVIDENCE FOR VIRUS INVOLVEMENT IN HUMAN ONCOGENESIS

No virus has as yet been proved to be the etiologic agent causing any human cancer, although several viruses from human and animal sources have oncogenic abilities in laboratory animals. Recent demonstration of C-type particles in human and nonhuman primate placentas suggests the presence of vertically transmitted potentially oncogenic RNA viruses. There has also been some suggestion for a role of DNA herpesvirus in causing human cancer. This has been supported by findings that herpesvirus hominis Type 2 can induce tumors in hamsters. However, although elevated levels of antibody to herpesvirus hominis Type 2 in women with cervical cancer are consistent with an etiologic association, the evidence remains circumstantial.

Burkitt's Lymphoma

Burkitt's lymphoma provides the most suggestive evidence for a human malignancy of viral etiology. The disease was first described by Burkitt in 1958 as a multiple visceral and jaw tumor in children who lived in restricted areas of Africa (Fig. 19–6). Since then, Burkitt's lymphoma has been reported in other parts of the world, including North America.

Evidence has been obtained for a viral etiology of the tumor by the demonstration of membrane-bound virus particles (Epstein-Barr or EB particles) in tissue culture cells derived from tumor biopsy material (Fig. 19–7). The evidence suggests that it is a DNA virus of the herpes group (Chapter 16). In many ways, this virus–host cell interaction resembles an integrated infection.

Serologic studies have revealed a high incidence of EB antibody in the sera of normal American children (35 per cent) and adults (85 per cent), as demonstrated by immunofluorescence. These data suggest that either the same virus or a similar one is occurring with a high frequency in the United States. Of African patients with Burkitt's lymphoma, close to 100 per cent have high serum titers of antibody to the EB virus. In Far East Asia, a similar frequency of EB antibody has been detected among patients with nasopharyngeal carcinoma.

Study of individual EB virus–induced antigens on Burkitt lymphoma cells differentiates immune responses in patients. Antibodies to membrane antigens correlate with the clinical course and are highest in tumor regression and lowest in tumor progression. Antibodies to (cytoplasmic) *capsid* antigens have no clinical relevance and are found in humans with a wide variety of disorders. Antibodies to *early* antigens (EA) and *precipitating* antigens are found during active phases of Burkitt's lymphoma only (Chapter 16).

On the basis of serologic findings, EB virus has subsequently been shown to be related to infectious mononucleosis. Lymphocytes from patients with infectious mononucleosis behave in many respects like the lymphoma cells from patients with Burkitt's disease. Both appear as transformed cells and acquire the propensity for increased growth potential *in vitro*. Recently, a receptor for the EB virus was demonstrated on the surface of the B-cell, which appears to be closely related to

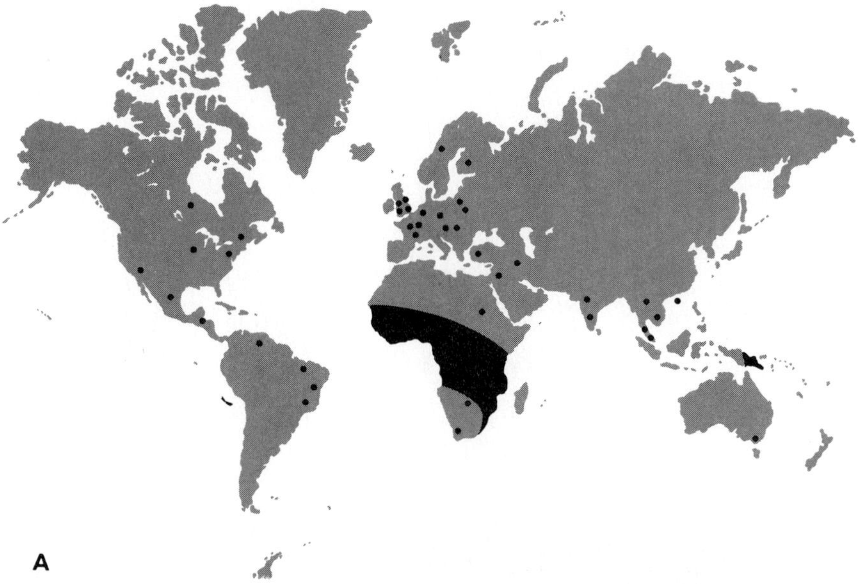

A

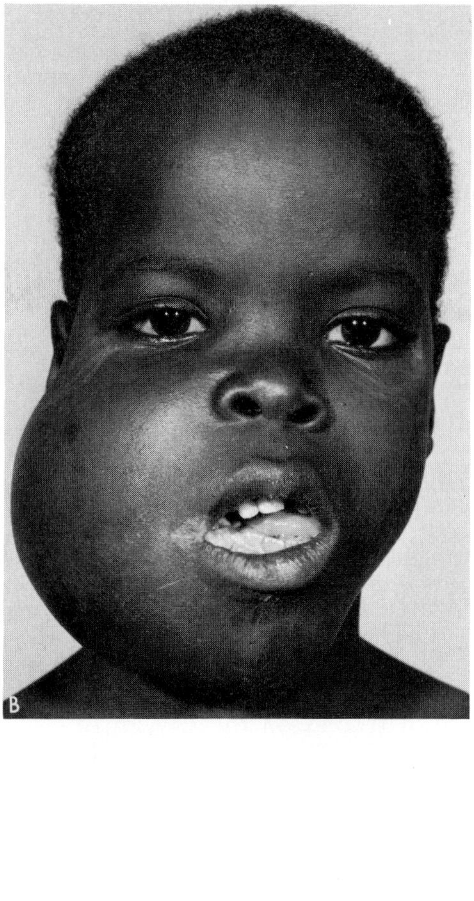

Figure 19–6. *A,* Map of world showing worldwide distribution of Burkitt's lymphoma. *B,* Photograph of a seven-year-old boy with Burkitt's lymphoma of the mandible. (Courtesy of National Institutes of Health.)

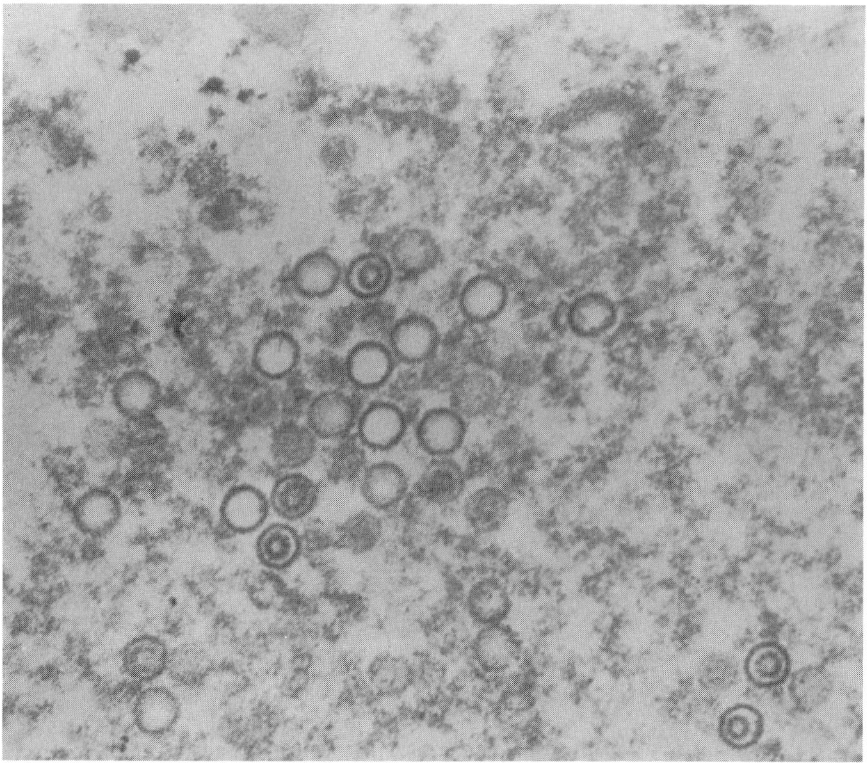

Figure 19–7. Electron micrograph of EB virus from a patient with Burkitt's lymphoma. ×32,000. (Courtesy of Dr. Paul H. Levine.)

the complement receptor. The atypical lymphocytes of infectious mononucleosis resemble very closely the morphology of normal large granular lymphocytes, which mediate natural killer cell activity (see below), and these cells may represent a component of the effective host control of the infection. Overall, the evidence suggests an etiologic role for EB virus in Burkitt's lymphoma, nasopharyngeal carcinoma, and infectious mononucleosis.

T-Cell Leukemias and Lymphomas

Recently, a similar association has been noted by Gallo and others between some T-cell leukemias and lymphomas and a Type C RNA virus, termed human T-cell leukemia virus (HTLV). This virus was discovered during the course of studies on the growth of normal and malignant T-cells in culture, in the presence of T-cell growth factor or interleukin 2 (IL-2). It was noted that the cultured cells from some patients with Sézary's syndrome had abundant Type C virus particles. This virus, which has been isolated and characterized, appears to selectively infect T-cells.

Serologic studies have revealed a high incidence of anti-HTLV antibodies in the sera of most patients in Japan with adult T-cell leukemia or lymphoma, and a lower frequency in relatives of these patients and in American patients with these diseases. Overall, although no etiologic link has been demonstrated and it has not been possible to demonstrate oncogenicity by HTLV in nonhuman primates or other animal models, the available circumstantial evidence strongly indicates a close association between HTLV and some forms of T-cell leukemia and lymphoma.

CHARACTERISTICS OF THE IMMUNE RESPONSE IN HOST RESISTANCE TO TUMORS

The host possesses both nonspecific and specific mechanisms of response to tumor formation. In tumor rejection, as in protection from infecting agents, the host immune response is directed toward the maintenance of homeostasis (Chapter 2). The homeostasis can be altered toward establishment of the tumor or in favor of the host.

Nonimmunologic Factors

There is evidence that nonspecific, nonimmunologic factors may be of paramount importance in determining the fate of neoplastic cells in a host. Presumably, mutations induced by viruses, chemicals, physical factors, and radiation occur frequently. Why, then, are occasional clones able to evade recognition long enough to establish themselves as cancerous disease? The cancer cell appears to have a metabolic edge: It has lost contact inhibition and no longer responds normally to controlling influences that regulate the activity of other cells. It manufactures a variety of unique products: Some are transplantation-type antigens (TATA); some reflect an expressed virus; and some are fetal, indicative of a derepressed state. Other products of the tumor cell may be of crucial importance to the survival of the cancer cell. For example, many tumor cells have been shown to produce an enzyme, Type IV collagenase, which can selectively degrade the collagen at the basement membrane of endothelial cells and thereby facilitate the extravasation of tumor cells and subsequent metastatic growth. In addition, the tumor cells may have novel properties or may produce factors that help to evade many facets of host defense, such as chemotaxis; phagocytosis; and killing by macrophages, killing by lymphocytes, and lymphocyte transformation with release of mediators necessary for expression of cell-mediated immunity (Chapter 9). Several suppressive products of cancer cells have been found (e.g., inhibitor of chemotaxis); some are dialyzable and thermolabile, and others are heat-stable proteins. Their significance in the establishment and maintenance of the cancer state *in vivo* remains speculative.

Immunologic Factors

THE CASE FOR IMMUNOLOGIC SURVEILLANCE

The concept of "immunologic surveillance" states that malignant disorders occur when there is failure of the immune system to recognize and destroy neoplastic cells before they become established in the body. This concept is supported by the observed higher incidence of malignancy in patients with immunologic deficiency syndromes or immune suppression secondary to drugs.

IMMUNOLOGIC DEFICIENCY STATES

The immunologic deficiency states comprise a heterogeneous group of inborn and acquired defects of the lymphoreticular tissues that may involve defects of the humoral (B) and/or the thymic (T) system (Chapter 22) or of the natural immune system. These diseases are characterized by an increased susceptibility to infection as a common clinical sign that reflects a defective defense function. The same defects that lead to this aberration in defense from infectious disease also give rise to defects in surveillance and result in an increased risk of neoplastic change. Children with immunologic defects have a high incidence of tumors, which constitute one of the major causes of death. These tumors usually involve malignant disorders of the lymphoreticular tissues, especially the thymus. Although the group as a whole is at risk, the apparent increase in malignancy appears to affect primarily those subjects with defects of the thymic-dependent tissues. These tumors have been described in patients with ataxia-telangiectasia, Wiskott-Aldrich syndrome, and acquired hypogammaglobulinemia (see Table 19–1). Similarly, patients with the Chédiak-Higashi syndrome, who have a selective deficit in granulocyte function and in the activity of their natural killer cells, have a high incidence of lymphoproliferative disorders. This increased susceptibility to neoplastic change provides clinical support for a relationship between resistance mechanisms and tumor formation.

IMMUNOSUPPRESSION

Patients whose immune systems have been suppressed are vulnerable to viral and bacterial infections and are also susceptible to neoplasia. In the several thousand organ transplants that have been performed throughout the world, an increased incidence of subsequent neoplasia has been reported. The possibilities exist that unsuspected neoplastic tissue may have been transplanted or that immunosuppression led to the genesis of a primary tumor.

It has been suggested that, in humans, Burkitt's lymphoma might represent an inadequate immunologic defense against EB virus infection, with most normal infected individuals limiting the viral expression to the benign disease, infectious mononucleosis. The EB virus appears to infect B-lymphocytes; normally, the T-lymphocytes and natural killer cells make an appropriate immunologic response, perhaps including antimitotic suppressor cells. Plasma from convalescent infectious mononucleosis patients contains factors that inhibit incorporation of tritiated thymidine in normal resting lymphocytes *in vitro*; such activity is not present in plasma from normal patients or from those in the acute phase of infectious mononucleosis. It may be that the lymphoma occurs only in those patients who are relatively immunologically deficient, either innately or as a result of malarial infection, malnutrition, or other factors. In support of this, Purtilo has described an X-linked form of childhood leukemia in which children with the syndrome, before developing tumors, have a deficient ability to adequately control infections by EB virus.

THE CASE AGAINST IMMUNOLOGIC SURVEILLANCE

Because many cancer patients appear to be immunologically intact and do make an appropriate, vigorous immune response to their cancer, many workers have begun to question the validity of the concept of immunologic surveillance. They note that bona fide immune deficiency is chiefly associated with lymphoreticular malignancy and not with solid tumors of other organ systems. A further and more direct challenge to the immune surveillance hypothesis has come from evidence in mice and rats that congenital absence, or neonatal removal, of the thymus is not associated with increased susceptibility to the development of spontaneous or chemical carcinogen-induced tumors. It is not yet understood how a clone of transformed cells is able to "sneak through" the host's multiple recognition mechanisms to become established. In individuals with essentially normal immune function, it may be that the neoplastic cells possess protective advantages. In some instances, tumor-specific antigens may be weak and of low density on the cell membrane (Table 19–3); in such cases, the host's immune response could not be vigorous.

Immunoselection. A possible immunologic effect that may be applicable to man is *immunoselection.* Antigenic specificity does not appear to be altered during serial passage. It has been postulated that immunologic factors suppress those cells with the most surface antigenicity and "select" those cells with the least surface antigenicity. For example, if a tumor is passed repeatedly through animals immune to TATA, a tumor is obtained that has lessened antigenicity and lessened susceptibility to the effects of cell-mediated and/or antibody-mediated cytotoxicity. In a manner consistent with the phenomenon of immunoselection, tumors with the highest concentration of surface antigen, such as the RNA-induced tumors, are most likely to lose antigenicity, as contrasted with DNA tumors with weak antigens, which lose little or no antigenicity through passage. This phenomenon has been used in the laboratory in selecting clones of tumor cells with varying concentrations of surface antigen. The importance of immunoselection in the growth of human tumors has yet to be demonstrated, but it may represent a mechanism by which a neoplastic cell with low antigenicity may "sneak through" the specific immune surveillance mechanisms of the host.

In other cases, the tumor may induce an inappropriate immune response. In multiple myeloma, macrophages are induced to make a material that suppresses antibody formation by normal B-lymphocytes (a feedback inhibition?) (Chapter 21). In other cases, the tumor appears to stimulate suppressor T-lymphocytes or macrophages more than it

Table 19–3. The Relationship Between Relative Concentration of Tumor-Specific Antigens and Biologic Effects

Relative Surface Concentration	Types of Tumors	Susceptibility to Complement-Mediated Cytotoxicity *in vivo*	Enhancement
High	RNA viruses	+ + + +	+
Low	DNA viruses, chemical, spontaneous	±	+ + + +

does killer lymphocytes and helper T-lymphocytes. It is obvious that most human patients with cancer of any sort possess specific cell-mediated immunity and specific antibodies against tumor-associated antigens (TAA) of their autochthonous tumors. It is not clear why, in those individuals with progressing or disseminating cancer, such demonstrable immune responses are not adequate to control the tumor; some of the probable explanations are described in later sections.

SPECIFIC CELL-MEDIATED IMMUNITY IN CANCER

In many animal tumor systems and in some cancer patients, specific lymphocyte killing of autochthonous or syngeneic tumor cells (Chapter 9) can be demonstrated. Newer radioisotope cytotoxic assay procedures have replaced the more cumbersome colony-inhibition method in many laboratories. As with cytotoxic T-lymphocytes reactive against other cell surface antigens, specifically tumor-immune T-cells recognize the TAA in association with antigens of the major histocompatibility complex (MHC), and their reactivity is usually restricted to tumor cells with compatible MHC determinants. Tumor immunity has also been demonstrated against membrane-bound or solubilized antigens by lymphocyte transformation or by release of mediators such as MIF and LIF from sensitized lymphocytes. Moreover, it is likely that other mediators, such as blastogenic factor, transfer factor, immune RNA, and interferon, participate in the *in vivo* cell-mediated response against tumor antigens (Chapter 9). It should be emphasized that since these cell-mediated immune responses to tumor antigens can be demonstrated in appropriate tests *in vitro,* and *in vivo* by delayed cutaneous hypersensitivity reactions, during all stages of disease, central or afferent tolerance to TAA does not exist (Chapter 10).

ANTIBODY-MEDIATED IMMUNITY IN CANCER

In many tumor-bearing individuals, specific antibodies can be demonstrated. Antibodies specific for tumor antigens have been shown to kill tumor target cells in two ways, and some evidence exists for both mechanisms operating *in vivo.* The first way is complement-dependent; IgG and IgM antibodies fix to antigenic sites on target cells and activate the complement cascade. Terminal C8 and C9 components bring about lysis by the classic pathway. The second cytocidal pathway is independent of complement and is known as antibody-dependent, cellular cytotoxic (ADCC) reaction (Chapter 9). Once tumor-specific IgG antibody fixes to target cell membrane, there is an alteration of the Fc portion of the heavy chain. Various effector cells with receptors for the Fc portion of IgG can then bind to the antibody-coated tumor cells and cause their lysis. The main effector cells with such potential are macrophages and K-cells, which have been shown recently to be large granular lymphocytes and which in most cases can also mediate natural killer cell activity.

Some evidence suggests that such antibodies can be detrimental to the host. In experimental situations, antibodies administered before transplantation of tumor or infection by oncogenic virus lead to tumor enhancement (afferent limb—suppression of response). Other studies suggest that antibodies attach to the surface of tumor cells, thereby blocking or masking attachment sites for cytotoxic lymphocytes and cytolytic antibodies (efferent limb).

Natural Immune Responses in Cancer

In addition to the above-described classic components of the immune response to cancer, it has recently become clear that there is a family of natural immune effector mechanisms that may also play an important role in resistance to tumor growth. In contrast to specific T- and B-cell–mediated immunity, which is not present in normal individuals and develops after a latent period of one to two weeks after sensitization by TAA, natural immunity is present spontaneously in normal individuals and does not depend upon exposure to tumor cells.

The natural immune system is a multifaceted compartment, including macrophages, natural killer (NK) cells and related cytotoxic effector cells, granulocytes, and natural antibodies. Since natural immunity exists prior to the development of tumor cells, and since its activity usually can be augmented very rapidly (within hours to days after certain stimuli), it has been suggested that these components of the immune system may form the first line of defense against tumor cells and other foreign materials such as microbial agents.

Monocytes and macrophages from normal individuals may have spontaneous cytotoxic reactivity against a wide variety of tumor cells. Upon activation by various signals, particularly the T-cell–mediated lymphokine, macrophage activating factor, and interferon, these cells can become highly cytotoxic. Their reactivity against tumor cells does not appear to depend on recognition of TAA's but rather on recognition of some cell surface structures that are expressed on a large proportion of tumor cells and that are usually undetectable on normal cells of the same individual. This allows activated monocytes and macrophages to exert strong, selective killing activity against tumor cells and to leave surrounding or adjacent normal cells unharmed.

NK cells were discovered about ten years ago as lymphoid cells with spontaneous cytotoxic activity against many tumor cells. For quite some time, their characterization was elusive, and it could be stated only that they lacked the characteristic features of macrophages, T-cells, or B-cells. Recently, however, it has been found that a small subpopulation of cells, termed large granular lymphocytes (LGL) and representing about 5 per cent of the mononuclear cells in human or rodent blood or spleen, account for virtually all of the NK activity. These LGL are morphologically distinguishable from typical lymphocytes, having a kidney-shaped nucleus and more abundant cytoplasm and numerous azurophilic granules, and, by virtue of their lower density, can be highly purified. NK cells, in contrast to cytotoxic T-lymphocytes, react with tumor cells independently of MHC antigens but rather appear to recognize a few broadly distributed target cell structures. Although NK cells primarily react only with tumor cells, they have been found to also lyse small subpopulations of normal cells, especially undifferentiated cells in the thymus or bone marrow or embryonic cells. The activity of NK cells can be rapidly increased by treatment with interferon or interferon-inducers and, on the other hand, can be inhibited by prostaglandins of the E series and by certain macrophages or T-suppressor cells.

Natural and antitumor antibodies are also widely expressed in the sera of normal individuals. These provide yet another possible mechanism for interaction with tumor cells. As described earlier for immune antibodies, they might have direct complement-dependent cytotoxic effects or they might be involved in ADCC reactions against tumor cells.

IMMUNOLOGIC PHENOMENA ASSOCIATED WITH STATE OF DISEASE

At any stage of cancer, including early localized disease, factors that inhibit phagocyte chemotaxis, phagocytosis, and target cell killing can be found in the plasma of a significant number of patients. These factors are produced either by tumor cells or by immune regulatory cells.

During active progression or dissemination of some tumors, certain other phenomena have been noted that probably occur generally (Table 19–4). There is seeding of interstitial fluid and blood with cancer cells, cell fragments, and membrane-associated soluble antigens. These neutralize lymphocytes and combine with specific antibody, blocking an effective immune response at the site of tumor cells. Plasma levels of antibody to TAA are low or not measurable. With advanced or disseminated cancer, specific or general immune suppression may occur, possibly manifested by diminished numbers of circulating T-lymphocytes, disappearance of delayed hypersensitivity in the skin (anergy), and decrease in lymphocyte transformation and release of mediators after mitogen or antigen stimulation *in vitro*. These phenomena persist as long as the tumor progresses; their presence at the time of diagnosis portends a poor prognosis.

During remission of tumor, findings are the opposite. In the plasma, there are no TAA or immune complexes; the levels of specific antibodies for tumor-associated membrane antigens are found to be high. Levels of antibodies to membrane antigens appear to be more relevant than do those nuclear or cytoplasmic antigens measured by other techniques such as complement fixation. Tumor-specific immunity and general immune function are intact; there usually is no anergy *in vivo* or *in vitro*. Subsequent appearance of TAA or immune complexes in the plasma and decline in cell-mediated immune reactivity or in titer of tumor-specific antibody may be indicative of tumor exacerbation. These changes in immunologic parameters may precede clinical manifestations of tumor recurrence by weeks or months.

Table 19–4. The Relationship Between Various Immunologic Parameters and the Clinical State in Cancer Patients

Immunologic Parameter	Material Tested	Tumor Progression or Dissemination	Tumor Remission
Delayed hypersensitivity to multiple agents	*In vivo* (skin)	Often decreased	Normal
Number of T-lymphocytes	Blood	May be decreased	Normal
Tumor-associated antigens (TAA)*	Plasma or serum	Present	Absent
Cytotoxic antibodies to TAA	Plasma or serum	Absent or low titer	Present
Immune complexes	Plasma or serum	Usually present	Absent
Suppressor cells (T-cells and/or monocytes)	Blood	Often present	Usually absent
Lymphocyte transformation by antigens and mitogens		May inhibit	No effect
Release of lymphokines		May inhibit	No effect
Phagocyte function: chemotaxis, phagocytosis, target cell killing		May inhibit (even in early, localized cancer)	No effect

*TAA = Tumor-associated antigens, dispersed on cell membrane or solubilized from cell membranes.

IMPLICATIONS FOR THERAPY

For a variety of cancers, cure rates and incidence of remission have been steadily improving. This is due in part to the cooperation of surgeons, radiologists, oncologists, and immunologists who jointly manage cancer patients, applying multiple modalities at appropriate times. Surgical removal and radiation therapy probably serve to reduce the bulk of tumor mass; chemotherapy eliminates the majority of persisting tumor cells (Table 19–5). The expectation is that the host's natural and acquired defenses will be able to control surviving cancer cells or eliminate them entirely.

The aim of immunotherapy or biologic response modification is to augment such antitumor defenses (Chapter 10). Many approaches are under study, and thus far there have been varying degrees of questionable or limited success (Table 19–5). One approach is the augmentation of nonspecific phagocytosis and of killing of tumor cells by macrophages and/or NK cells. Application of infectious BCG mycobacteria has been the most widely used approach; administration of nonliving *Corynebacterium parvum* is increasingly being employed. Glucan, a glucose polymer derived from microorganisms, is also being evaluated. Levamisole is an anthelmintic drug that appears to be efficacious in stimulating CMI and macrophage function. In leukemia and some solid tumors, beneficial results have been demonstrated with such prolonged adjuvant treatments. Recently,

Table 19–5. Therapeutic Goals in Treatment of Cancer

A. Primary: Reduction of tumor mass (antigen load)
   1. Surgical extirpation
   2. Radiation
   3. Chemotherapy
B. Secondary: Augment body defenses (immunotherapy or biologic response modification)
   1. Nonspecific
      a. Adjuvants of CMI and of macrophage and NK cell function
         —BCG
         —*C. parvum*
         —glucan
         —levamisole
      b. Topical delayed hypersensitivity to unrelated antigen (DNCB)
   2. Specific
      a. Passive—transfer of antibodies to TAA
      b. Active—immunization with autologous or homologous processed tumor cell antigens, with or without adjuvant
      c. Adoptive
         —thymus-soluble products
         —transfer factor or immune RNA
         —immune cells, NK cells, macrophages
         —transplantation of fetal thymus or immunocompetent cells, e.g., bone marrow

there have been major efforts to evaluate the therapeutic efficacy of interferon, which might be expected to act by augmenting the cytotoxic reactivity of NK cells and monocytes and macrophages.

A related approach has been carried out successfully in such localized tumors of the skin as keratoses, basal cell carcinoma, squamous carcinoma, and melanoma. Dinitrochlorobenzene (DNCB) is a contactant that induces cell-mediated immunity readily. When applied topically to skin tumor sites, the ensuing DNCB-specific delayed hypersensitivity reaction brings about the "nonspecific" regression of tumor by local accumulations of killer lymphocytes and activated macrophages.

Augmentation of tumor-specific immunity can be passive, active, or adoptive. Passively administered serum containing a high titer of antibodies to TAA has been attempted with limited success. Recently, much renewed interest has been focused on this approach, because of the growing availability of monoclonal antibodies to human TAA's. Such antibodies might be expected to have some antitumor effects, especially when attached to highly toxic proteins or radioisotopes. It is hoped that the specific antibodies will selectively deliver the toxins to the tumor site and thereby avoid systemic toxicity.

Much effort has been extended toward increasing active immunity to tumor antigens. At surgery, tumor sites have been cauterized, frozen, chemically burned, and enzymatically treated to alter endogenous TAA *in situ. In vitro,* tumor cells have been irradiated, freeze-thawed, and treated with neuraminidase to expose more antigen sites or to denature tumor antigens. Upon injection of treated cells or solubilized TAA into the same or a homologous host, with or without adjuvant, the expectation is that the host can make a more vigorous and varied immune response to the tumor.

Adoptive measures remain the most alluring, with the hope of transferring to the host missing ingredients of defense from a healthy immune donor. Thymosin, a hormone extracted from bovine or human thymus (Chapter 2), has been shown to enhance T-lymphocyte immunity in individuals with primary or secondary immune deficiency and has recently been reported to have antitumor effects in some clinical trials with cancer patients. Transfer factor, a dialyzable, nonimmunogenic message material from T-lymphocytes, seems to transfer specific reactivity to new antigens *de novo* as well as to boost pre-existing immunity in the manner of an adjuvant (Chapters 9 and 22); it is under study in patients with cancer. Immune RNA in animals protects against otherwise fatal infectious disease in susceptible hosts; its applicability to the human is currently under study. The ability to grow T-cells and NK cells *in vitro* in the presence of IL-2 and to clone and select for specifically immune cells or active NK cells offers a new approach to adoptive immunotherapy, and clinical trials are just being started. Similarly, transfer of immunocompetent lymphoid tissue in the form of bone marrow transplants has been used in the treatment of leukemia. This approach has some serious problems: The tumor-bearing recipients will reject a bone marrow graft unless the recipient is immunosuppressed. There is always the risk of serious overwhelming infection, and if the bone marrow "takes," a graft-versus-host reaction is possible. Recently, some promising results have been obtained by treatment of the bone marrow with anti–T-cell antibodies, to eliminate cells with the potential of mediating graft-versus-host disease. Although bone marrow transplantation remains an experimental approach, the results of several research groups with patients with leukemia, especially during the first drug-induced remission, are highly encouraging and appear better than other available approaches.

At this time, it is fair to say that the efficacy of biologic response modification in the treatment of tumors is not yet proved. Indeed, the vital role of specific immunity in control of most tumors in most individuals is not defined. It is possible that nonimmunologic, nonspecific defense mechanisms or even tumor cell characteristics per se will prove to be more critical in determining the success of host defense against neoplasms.

Suggestions for Further Reading

Alexander, P.: The nature of the immunological interaction between the host and the tumor. Can. J. Otolaryngol., *4*(1):36, 1975.

Alexander, P., Eccles, S. A., and Gauci, C. L. L.: The significance of macrophages in human and experimental tumors. *In* Friedman, H., and Southam, C. (eds.): International Conference on Immunobiology of Cancer. Vol. 276. New York, New York Academy of Sciences, 1976, pp. 124–133.

Anderson, V., Kuer, M., and Bendixen, G.: In vitro

demonstration of cellular hypersensitivity to tumour antigens in man. Ser. Haematol., *5*:3, 1972.

Baldwin, R. W., Embleton, M. J., Jones, J. S. P., et al.: Cell-mediated and humoral reactions to human tumors. Int. J. Cancer, *12*:73, 1973.

Chang, R. S., and Spiva, C. A.: Suppression of spontaneous in vitro transformation of autologous leukocytes by plasma from convalescent and post-convalescent injection mononucleosis patients. J. Natl. Cancer Inst., *55*:803, 1975.

Currie, G.: Immunological aspects of host resistance to the development and growth of cancer. Biochim. Biophys. Acta, *458*:135, 1976.

Harris, J., and Copeland, D.: Impaired immunoresponsiveness in tumor patients. Ann. N. Y. Acad. Sci., *230*:56, 1974.

Hellström, I., Hellström, K. E., Sjögren, H. O., et al.: Serum factors in tumor-free patients. Cancelling the blocking of cell-mediated tumor immunity. Int. J. Cancer, *8*:185, 1971a.

Hellström, I., Sjögren, H. O., Warner, G. A., et al.: Blocking of cell-mediated tumor immunity by sera from patients with growing neoplasms. Int. J. Cancer, *7*:226, 1971b.

Herberman, R. B. (ed.): NK Cells and Other Natural Effector Cells. New York, Academic Press, 1982.

Herberman, R. B., and Ortaldo, J. R.: Natural killer cells: Their role in defenses against disease. Science, *214*:24, 1981.

Irie, K., Irie, R. F., and Morton, D. L.: Evidence for in vivo reaction of antibody and complement to surface antigens of human cancer cells. Science, *186*:454, 1974.

Kerbel, R. S.: Mechanisms of tumor-induced immunological deficiencies and their possible significance in relation to the use of immunopotentiators in tumor-bearing hosts. Biomedicine, *20*:253, 1974.

Khoo, S. K., Warner, M. L., Lie, J. T., et al.: Carcinoembryonic antigenic activity of tissue extracts: A quantitative study of malignant and benign neoplasms, cirrhotic liver, normal adult and fetal organs. Int. J. Cancer, *11*:681, 1973.

Kniker, W. T., Ganaway, R. L., and Smith, K. O.: Suppression of lymphocyte transformation by fetal and tumor factors. Fed. Proc., *33*:749, 1974.

Lewis, M. G., Hartman, D., and Jerry, L. M.: Antibodies and anti-antibodies in human malignancy: an expression of deranged immune regulation. *In* Friedman, H., and Southam, C. (eds.): International Conference on Immunobiology of Cancer. Vol. 276. New York, New York Academy of Sciences, 1976, pp. 316–327.

Morton, D. L., Holmes, E. C., Eilber, F. R., et al.: Immunological aspects of neoplasia: a rational basis for immunotherapy. Ann. Intern. Med., *74*:587, 1971.

Nelson, D. S.: Immunity to infection, allograft immunity and tumor immunity: Parallels and contrasts. Transplant. Rev., *19*:226, 1974.

Perlmann, P., Perlmann, H., and Wigzell, H.: Lymphocyte-mediated cytotoxicity in vitro. Induction and inhibition by humoral antibody and nature of effector cells. Transplant. Rev., *13*:91, 1972.

Perlmann, P., O'Toole, C., and Unsgaard, B.: Cell-mediated immune mechanisms of tumor cell destruction. Fed. Proc., *32*:153, 1973.

Pilch, Y. H., and Golub, S. H.: Lymphocyte-mediated immune responses in neoplasia. Am. J. Clin. Pathol., *62*:184, 1974.

Smith, R. T.: Tumor specific immune mechanisms. N. Engl. J. Med., *287*:439, 1972.

Snyderman, R., and Pike, M. C.: Defective macrophage migration produced by neoplasms. *In* Fink, M. A. (ed.): The Macrophage in Neoplasia. New York, Academic Press, 1976.

Ting, C. C., and Herberman, R. B.: Humoral host defense mechanisms against tumors. Int. Rev. Exp. Pathol., *15*:93, 1976.

Vanky, F., Stjensward, J., Klein, G., et al.: Tumor-associated specificity of serum-mediated inhibition of lymphocyte stimulation by autochthonous human tumors. J. Natl. Cancer Inst., *51*:25, 1973.

Waldmann, T. A., Strober, W., and Blaese, R. M.: Immunodeficiency disease and malignancy. Various immunologic deficiencies of man and the role of imune processes in the control of malignant disease. Ann. Intern. Med., *77*:606, 1972.

Wilson, R. E., Alexander, P., Rosenberg, S. A., et al.: Horizons in tumor immunology. A seminar. Arch. Surg., *109*:17, 1974.

Winters, W. D.: Immunovirology. *In* Shottenfield, D. (ed.): Cancer Epidemiology and Prevention. Springfield, Ill., Charles C Thomas, 1975, pp. 207–230.

Wybran, J., Hellström, L., Hellström, K. E., et al.: Cytotoxicity of human rosette-forming blood lymphocytes on cultivated human tumor cells. Int. J. Cancer, *13*:515, 1974.

Section Three

CLINICAL APPLICATIONS OF IMMUNOLOGY

Chapter 20

Immunologically Mediated Diseases

Joseph A. Bellanti, M.D.

Introduction: The Concept of Immunologically Mediated Disease

The basic function of the immunologic system is to detect and eliminate from the body any substance recognized as *foreign*. In performing this function, the host employs a wide variety of cells and cell products, each interacting with one another in the removal of this material (Chapter 11). Usually, such interactions are efficient and successful without detriment to the host. Occasionally, however, when the type of antigen presented to the system or the reactivity of the host is inappropriate, perturbations occur that lead to harmful sequelae—the *immunologically mediated diseases*.

The summation of the total immunologic capability of the host to all foreign matter is shown schematically in Figure 20–1.

There are three types of responses through which all foreign substances can proceed, the progression of which depends upon two factors: (1) the nature of the substance (Chapter 4), and (2) the genetic constitution of the host (Chapter 3) (Fig. 20–1).

The *nonspecific (primary)* response, the most primitive type, consists of those ancient responses to the first encounter with a foreign configuration—*phagocytosis* and *inflammation*. If the substance (e.g., carbon particles) is completely eliminated at this stage, the host's response terminates. Some substances, however, are not completely eliminated at this stage and reflect antigen persistence.

If the primary encounter leads to a processed product (antigen), the *specific (secondary)* or more sophisticated responses are stimulated (Fig. 20–1). These consist of two possible effector mechanisms: (1) B-lymphocyte-mediated humoral immunity with the elaboration of antibody (IgE, IgM, IgG, IgA, and IgD), and (2) T-lymphocyte–mediated antigen elimination. A sophisticated addition to these mechanisms is the capacity to enhance the immunologic responses through the actions of complement, the coagulation sequence, and a bank of "memory cells" if antigen is re-encountered. If antigen is successfully eliminated, the immunologic response terminates. Normally, most antigens are successfully eliminated at this stage without detriment to the host.

If antigen still persists, the *tissue-damaging (tertiary)* responses are called into play. Antigen persistence may result from the nature of the antigen itself or from some genetic defect in antigen processing. If antigen persists, four types of immunologic interactions can be elicited: Types I, II, III, and IV (Chapter 13). These responses are no longer beneficial to the host and are manifested

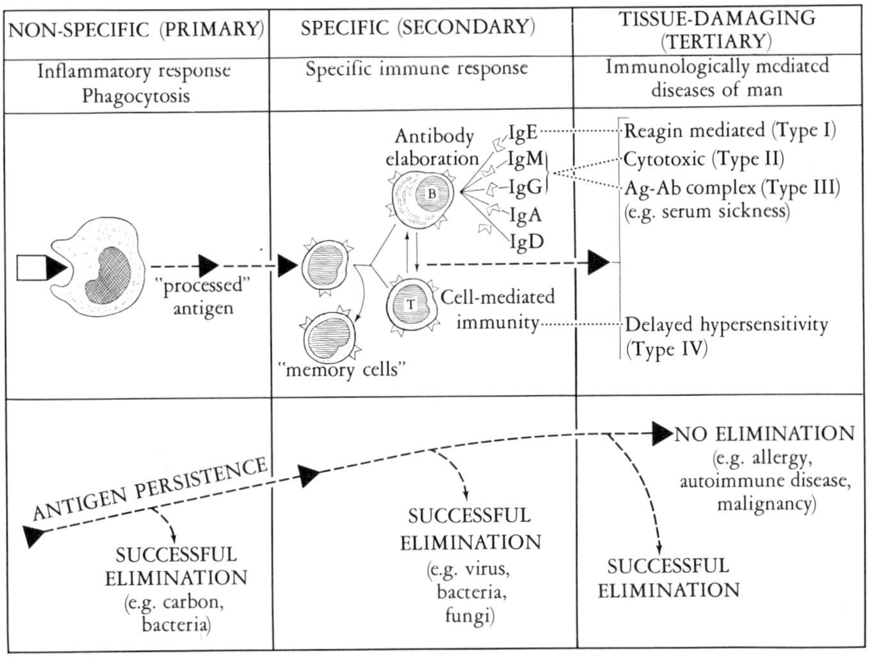

Figure 20–1. Schematic representation of the total immunologic capability of the host based upon efficiency of elimination of foreign matter.

as disease phenomena, the *immunologically mediated diseases* (IMD). These may be either temporary or permanent, depending upon the efficiency of antigen elimination (Fig. 20–1). If antigen can be removed or eliminated, the tertiary response is terminated with minimal discomfort to the patient (e.g., penicillin hypersensitivity). However, if the tertiary response is ineffective and antigen still persists, the more harmful sequelae of the immune response emerge, e.g., "autoimmune disease." This represents a maximal deleterious, self-perpetuating attack of an aberrant immune response in which the host sustains injury. It has been postulated that a failure in surveillance with persistence of antigen could also be involved in malignant disorders (Chapter 19).

TYPES OF IMMUNOLOGICALLY MEDIATED DISEASES

It should be recalled that the immune response does not occur as an isolated event *(in vacuo)*; every foreign configuration may stimulate several immunologic systems. Certain compartments of the immunologic system, however, may be selectively stimulated, depending upon the nature of the antigen, its configuration, the degree of macrophage processing, and the route by which antigen is introduced into the host (Chapter 7).

Immunologically mediated diseases may be viewed as three general types, depending upon the nature of the antigen—those involving *exogenous, allogeneic,* or *autologous* antigens. Examples of each are listed in Table 20–1.

Thus, antigens that make contact topically may favor the stimulation of the secretory immunoglobulin system (IgA or IgE). These responses serve useful functions normally. In some individuals, the local production of IgE may lead to undesirable allergic symptoms characteristic of atopic diseases, e.g., hayfever reaction to pollen. Also, the genetic controls of the immunologic system are expressed as variations in immunologic responsiveness between individuals (Chapter 3). These variations depend not only on the nature of the antigen but also on a number of modifying

Table 20–1. The Immunologically Mediated Diseases of Man

Type of Antigen	Example of Disease Response
Exogenous	Atopic diseases and reactions to environmental allergens, e.g., tree and grass pollens
Allogeneic	Alloantigens (including transplantation, blood transfusions, and erythroblastosis fetalis)
Autologous	Autoimmune diseases, e.g., systemic lupus erythematosus (SLE)

factors, including age and the emotional and nutritional status of the host. The association of the HLA system and immune responsiveness, as well as the recent knowledge of the cellular interactions of T-helper and T-suppressor cells, has been implicated in the expression of allergic disease (Chapters 3 and 7). Regardless of the precipitating factors, whether involving host or antigen, if aberrations are established, *immunologic imbalance* is created, with resultant IMD (Chapter 2).

EFFECTOR MECHANISMS OF IMMUNOLOGIC INJURY

Basically, the mechanisms responsible for immunologically mediated diseases comprise four categories that were presented in Chapter 13 and are summarized in Table 20–2.

The first of these, the anaphylactic (cytotropic), or Type I, reaction, is mediated primarily by the IgE reaginic antibodies. These immunoglobulins are cytotropic and have a characteristic property of binding to mediator cells, e.g., mast cells or their circulating counterpart, the basophils. Following reaction with antigen, subsequent release of pharmacologically vasoactive amines accounts for the clinical symptoms of these diseases (Chapter 13). The target organs most commonly involved are the *gastrointestinal tract,* the *skin,* and the *respiratory tract.* This reaginic response is seen in the normal individual but, when aberrant, is responsible for most of the atopic allergic diseases of man (atopy).

The cytolytic (cytotoxic), or Type II, reaction is usually mediated through complement-fixing properties of antibody. Also included in this type are the antibody-mediated reactions that require the participation of cellular elements. This may occur by any of three mechanisms, each of which involves the cytotoxic effect of antibody with antigen on a cell surface. In one type, the reaction of antibody with antigens on the surface of a particle enhances the phagocytosis of the particle (opsonization) with its subsequent intracellular destruction. A second cytotoxic effect of antibody is its direct reaction with surface antigens that together with complement lead to the destruction of the cell through antibody-mediated cytolysis (Chapter 6). The third type of cytotoxic reaction is that in which antibody, through its participation with killer cells, can function in antibody-dependent cellular cytotoxicity (ADCC) reactions (Chapter 9). The best studied of these cytotoxic reactions are the antibody-

Table 20–2. Mechanisms of Immunologically Mediated Diseases According to Gell and Coombs

Type	Target Organs	Clinical Manifestations	Mechanisms
I. Anaphylactic (cytotropic)	Gastrointestinal tract Skin Lungs	Gastrointestinal allergy, urticaria, atopic dermatitis, rhinitis, and asthma	IgE and other immunoglobulins, e.g., IgG_4
II. Cytolytic (cytotoxic)	Circulating blood elements (red cells, white cells, and platelets)	Hemolytic anemia, leukopenia, thrombocytopenia, hemolytic disease of newborn, and Goodpasture's disease	IgG, IgM, and phagocytes (opsonization) and mononuclear cells (ADCC) reactions, or antibody-mediated complement cytolysis
III. Arthus: immune complex (serum sickness)	Blood vessels of: Skin, joints, kidneys, and lungs	Serum sickness, systemic lupus erythematosus, nephrosis of quartan malaria, and chronic glomerulonephritis	Antigen-antibody complexes (IgG)
IV. Cell-mediated (delayed hypersensitivity)	Skin Lungs CNS Thyroid Other organs	Contact dermatitis Tuberculosis Allergic encephalitis Thyroiditis Primary homograft rejection	Sensitized T-lymphocytes, K cells, NK cells, macrophages
V. Mixed types: I and III		Allergic bronchopulmonary aspergillosis	IgE and precipitating IgG antibodies
III and IV		Extrinsic allergic alveolitis	Antigen-antibody complexes and cell-mediated immunity

mediated, complement-directed cytotoxic reactions. The effector mechanisms in these cases are mediated primarily by IgG or IgM antibody directed toward target cells, e.g., circulating blood cells (Table 20–2). The clinical manifestations of these diseases may present as hemolytic anemia, leukopenia, or thrombocytopenia.

A third category of immunologically mediated diseases is the immune complex, or Type III (Arthus), type. These reactions have assumed increased clinical significance and have been implicated in several immunopathologic states, including a variety of vasculitides, systemic lupus erythematosus, and glomerulonephritis. The mechanism of injury is mediated by antigen-antibody complexes that form in moderate antigen excess (Chapter 8). In this form, the soluble aggregates fix complement, circulate in the vascular system, and then may deposit in vascular endothelium, where they initiate a sequence of destructive inflammatory reactions in tissues, e.g., blood vessels, skin, joints, kidneys, and lungs, or may participate in the destruction of circulating cellular elements. The resultant clinical entities are exemplified by acute glomerulonephritis, serum sickness, and certain drug reactions.

The fourth mechanism of immunologic injury is the cell-mediated (delayed hypersensitivity), or Type IV, reaction. Unlike the previous three mechanisms, this response does not involve humoral antibody but is mediated by the action of sensitized T-lymphocytes. As described in Chapters 9 and 11, the action of T-cells may involve direct cytotoxic effects; the participation of other cells, e.g., killer (K) or natural killer (NK) cells; the elaboration of lymphokines; and the recruitment of other cells, e.g., macrophages.

In addition to these four types of mechanisms of immunologic injury, which may be considered "pure," there is a fifth type, which consists of mixed types, e.g., I and II, III and IV. These mixed types are assuming clinical significance in such entities as allergic bronchopulmonary aspergillosis and extrinsic allergic alveolitis (Table 20–2), which will be described in greater detail below.

A. Immunologically Mediated Disease Involving Exogenous Antigens (Allergy)

Robert T. Scanlon, M.D., and Joseph A. Bellanti, M.D.

Classically, the term "allergy," coined by von Pirquet, referred to a state of altered reactivity (Chapter 13). Subsequent modifications of the term's meaning have equated allergy with hypersensitivity. Since the concept of immunity presented throughout this book has been one of a reaction to foreignness, allergy is best viewed as a specialized case of immunity in which the reaction to foreign material terminates in a deleterious outcome. Allergy may be considered as one of several types of immunologically mediated disease of man directed at exogenous antigens.

There are four general types of allergic diseases seen in man. These include the *atopic reactions,* the *drug sensitivities, serum sickness,* and *contact dermatitis.*

Allergic diseases manifest imbalance primarily through three target organs—the *gastrointestinal tract,* the *skin,* and the *respiratory tract.* A common feature to all three is their exposure to the external environment, which provides a common route of entry for exogenous agents.

The most common routes and types of antigens that give rise to allergic manifestations are shown in Table 20–3, together with their suspected immunologic mechanisms and disease manifestations.

CLINICAL MANIFESTATIONS OF GASTROINTESTINAL ALLERGY

Gastrointestinal (GI) allergy may be defined as hypersensitivity to certain exogenous substances, usually foods, that gain access to the body via the gastrointestinal tract. This hypersensitivity is manifested primarily through vomiting, diarrhea, or abdominal pain, and at times may be of such severity as to result in malabsorption or protein-losing enteropathy. These may also be accompanied by skin manifestations (e.g., atopic eczema and urticaria) and respiratory tract manifes-

Table 20–3. **Routes and Types of Antigens That Give Rise to Allergic Manifestations**

Route	Example of Antigen	Immunologic Mechanism	Disease Manifestation
1. Ingestants	Foods	Type I	Gastrointestinal allergy
	Drugs	Types I, II, III	Urticaria, atopic manifestations Immediate drug reaction Hemolytic anemia Serum sickness
2. Inhalants	Pollens Dusts Molds	Type I	Allergic rhinitis Bronchial asthma
	Aspergillus fumigatus	Types I, III	Allergic bronchopulmonary aspergillosis
	Thermophilic actinomycetes	Types III, IV	Extrinsic allergic alveolitis
3. Injectants	Drugs	Types I, II, III	Immediate drug reaction Hemolytic anemia Serum sickness
	Bee stings	Type I	Anaphylaxis
	Vaccines	Type III	Localized Arthus reaction
	Serum	Type I	Anaphylaxis
4. Contactants	Poison ivy	Type IV	Contact dermatitis

tations (e.g., rhinitis and asthma) (Fig. 20–2). This symptom complex of diarrhea and vomiting after the ingestion of certain foods encompasses a syndrome of varying etiology of which GI allergy may be a component. Conditions other than allergy to food that can produce this same clinical picture include the following entities: disaccharidase deficiency, gluten-sensitive enteropathy (celiac disease), cystic fibrosis, and galactosemia. Foods most frequently implicated in gastrointestinal allergy are milk, chocolate, citrus fruits, eggs, wheat, nuts, peanut butter, and fish.

Gastrointestinal allergy is manifested clinically by the rejection of the foreign antigen through vomiting and diarrhea. The small infant may present with restlessness, spasmodic pain, and crying characteristic of colic. Although some of these symptoms are thought to be mediated through the IgE reaginic response via the liberation of vasoactive substances (Chapter 13), other non–IgE-mediated mechanisms may also be operative in some cases. In addition, the clinical syndrome of growth retardation, gastrointestinal symptoms (e.g., bleeding), iron deficiency anemia, and recurrent pulmonary disease with hemosiderosis has been reported in association with the finding of milk precipitins in sera of small infants (Heiner's syndrome). Although a Type III antigen-antibody complex response has been suggested as a possible mechanism of injury in this syndrome, the evidence is indirect and inconclusive.

Several difficulties exist in attributing this symptom complex to gastrointestinal allergy. When food is the offending agent, the active immunogen may be the degradative product of the food, whose identity may escape detection. Further, antigens may be added to foods in the form of drugs, additives, or preservatives. For example, cows with mastitis are treated with penicillin and yield milk containing trace amounts of this antibiotic. Thus, a penicillin hypersensitivity unrelated to milk protein may occur by the ingestion of trace amounts of the drug. Also, current nutritional practices including food additives such as preservatives, sweeteners, and coloring agents, e.g., tartrazine (yellow dye 2), may further complicate the identification of the etiologic agent. A second difficulty in establishing the diagnosis of gastrointestinal allergy is a lack of incontrovertible immunologic evidence. Although precipitating antibody has been found in the sera and stools of infants suspected of being sensitive to milk, similar antibodies are also present in otherwise normal infants and in individuals recovering from gastroenteritis. Nonetheless, there is suggestive evidence that hypersensitivity to food substances may play a role in the pathogenesis of gastrointestinal allergy. For example, isolated segments of guinea pig ileum sensitized by exposure to serum antibody manifest smooth muscle contracture after exposure to antigen (Shultz-Dale reaction) (Chapter 13). More recently, although RAST has been employed to measure IgE-

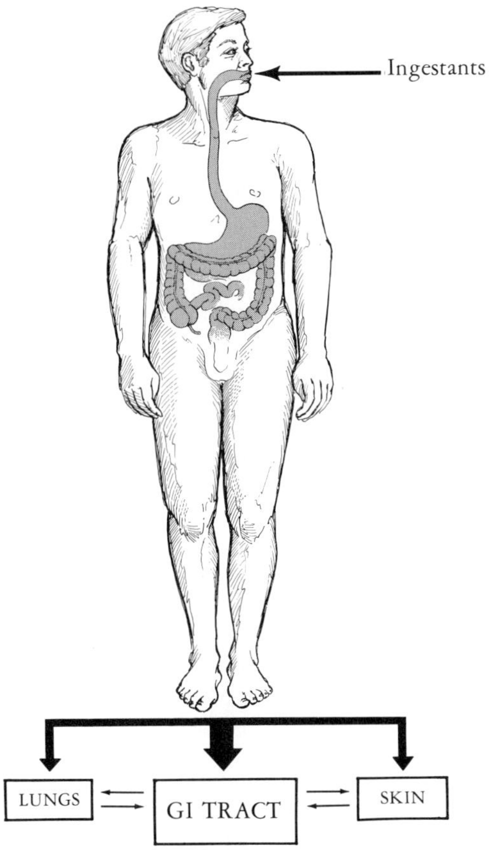

Figure 20–2. Schematic representation of the clinical manifestations of gastrointestinal allergy.

associated antibodies to a variety of allergens, including foods, and has been found to correlate significantly with clinical presentation, RAST testing has not been generally found to be more contributory to diagnosis than skin testing. The significance of these observations awaits further elucidation.

As described in Chapter 5, the secretory IgA immunoglobulins (s-IgA) are found in abundance at mucosal surfaces such as the gastrointestinal tract, where they appear to function primarily in local immunity to infectious agents. The attachment of these immunoglobulins to mucosal cells may also protect the intestinal cell from penetration by other antigens, e.g., allergens. For example, a decrease in s-IgA content in the infant may occur in severe diarrheal diseases and in marasmus, as well as in isolated IgA deficiency, conditions that may favor the development of allergic sensitization. The precise relationship of the secretory IgA system and the IgE system is unknown, but it has been suggested that the deficiency of IgA could allow the absorption of potentially allergenic substances that could result in IgE production with subsequent local or systemic reactions. Conversely, the presence of s-IgA in breast milk may be important in preventing the absorption of antigen and may explain its beneficial effect in the prevention of food allergy in the breast-fed infant.

Although gastrointestinal allergy is primarily a reaction to dietary antigen, it should be emphasized that dietary antigen need not manifest itself solely by gastrointestinal symptoms but can also lead to involvement of other shock organs, such as the *skin* and *lungs.*

CLINICAL MANIFESTATIONS OF ALLERGIC DISEASE OF THE SKIN

The skin is another frequently involved shock tissue. The manifestations of allergic reactions in skin may be classified under two broad categories: (1) the *immediate,* e.g., urticaria, and (2) the *delayed,* e.g., contact dermatitis. These disorders may be induced by ingested food, drugs, or contactants. Although the main shock organ is the skin, secondary involvement may also include the respiratory tract and the gastrointestinal tract (Fig. 20–3).

The mechanisms underlying the immediate reaction involve the release of vasoactive amines primarily through the IgE reagin Type I response; the "delayed" reactions may involve other types, including Type IV (delayed hypersensitivity), independent of circulating antibody. The immediate reactions are triggered primarily by ingestants and injectants and, at times, inhalants; the delayed reactions are caused primarily by contactants (Table 20–3).

Atopic Eczema and Contact Dermatitis

The clinical appearance and the histologic features of the lesions of atopic and contact dermatitis are similar; the two differ in their mechanisms of production and their distribution. Atopic dermatitis is commonly grouped with the immediate-type hypersensitivities, and elevated serum levels of IgE are commonly seen. The basic defects of atopic dermatitis are unknown but may be due to sebum deficiency allowing free skin water to absorb edema fluid, transepidermal

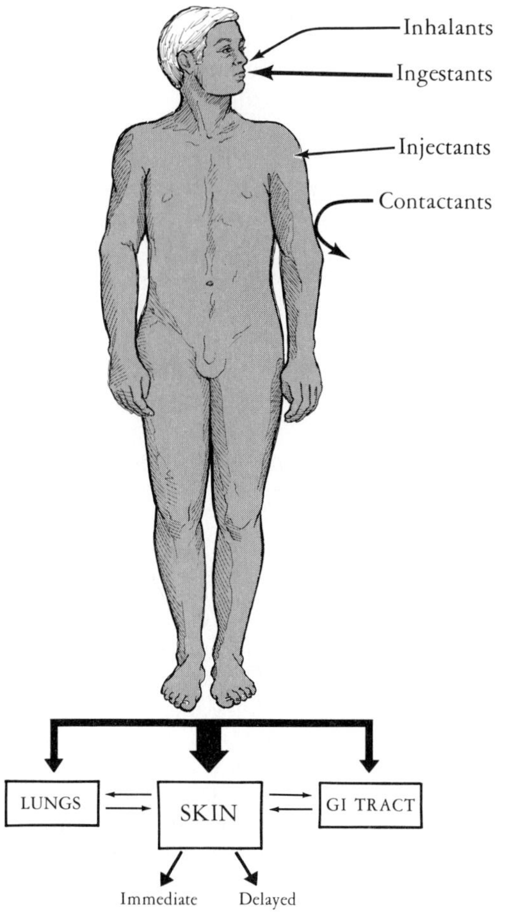

Figure 20–3. Schematic representation of the clinical manifestations of allergy affecting the skin.

water loss by evaporation due to deficiency of water-binding agents (e.g., urea), and a very low pruritic threshold perhaps resulting from a genetic difference in pain fiber associated with pruritus (cyclic nucleotide imbalance). The immunologic basis for atopic dermatitis, however, is even less well understood. Although elevated levels of IgE are commonly seen, the histopathologic features in no way represent those of a Type I reaction. The lesions of atopic dermatitis may be generalized and are characterized by erythematous, papular, vesicular lesions that may weep and ooze, particularly in the small infant. In this age group, the lesions are usually distributed on the cheeks, forehead, wrists, extensor surfaces of the forearms, and lower extremities (Fig. 20–4). After the age of two years, the skin tends to be thickened, scaly, and lichenified, and the distribution becomes confined predominantly to the flexor surfaces of the antecubital and popliteal areas (Fig. 20–5).

The lesions of contact dermatitis may also show erythema, papules, vesicles, and bullae in the acute stage and, when chronic, become thickened, scaly, and lichenified. Histopathologically, both atopic and contact dermatitis demonstrate vasodilatation of blood vessels of the corium, resulting in intracellular edema in the malpighian layer of the epidermis. This is followed by an inflammatory reaction in the underlying dermis and subsequent parakeratosis, scaling, and acanthosis (Fig. 20–6). An important differentiating point is the distribution of the two lesions; the multiple-area involvement of atopic dermatitis stands in marked contrast to the localization of lesions generally found in contact dermatitis. This restriction and localization is the key differentiating point between the two entities (Fig. 20–7).

The immunologic mechanisms for the two conditions are known to differ. Contact dermatitis expresses itself through the Type IV mechanism of delayed hypersensitivity mediated by sensitized T-lymphocytes. The etiologic agent is a simple chemical or other compound of low molecular weight, e.g., hapten, including the many substances that characterize our complex environment. These include plants (poison ivy), cosmetics, industrial products, detergents, topical medications, clothing, food, and metals. These agents act as haptens and combine firmly and irreversibly with tissue protein to form a complete antigen (immunogen).

The immunologic mechanism underlying atopic eczema is thought to be associated with the immediate Type I hypersensitivity (Chapter 13). It appears that the reaction of the offending antigen with cell-bound IgE antibody might lead to the release of vasoactive substances with a resultant increased vascular permeability. However, there are a number of other abnormal skin findings seen in patients with atopic eczema whose relationship with the primary disorder is unclear. These include blanching of the skin on stroking (white dermatographism), delayed blanching after injection of acetylcholine, in contrast to the normal erythema, and an exaggerated response in the cold pressor test. Although cellular cyclic AMP has been found to be reduced in the skin of atopic individuals, levels of adenyl cyclase are normal.

Urticaria

Urticaria, or hives, is a skin manifestation that has an immediate onset and is character-

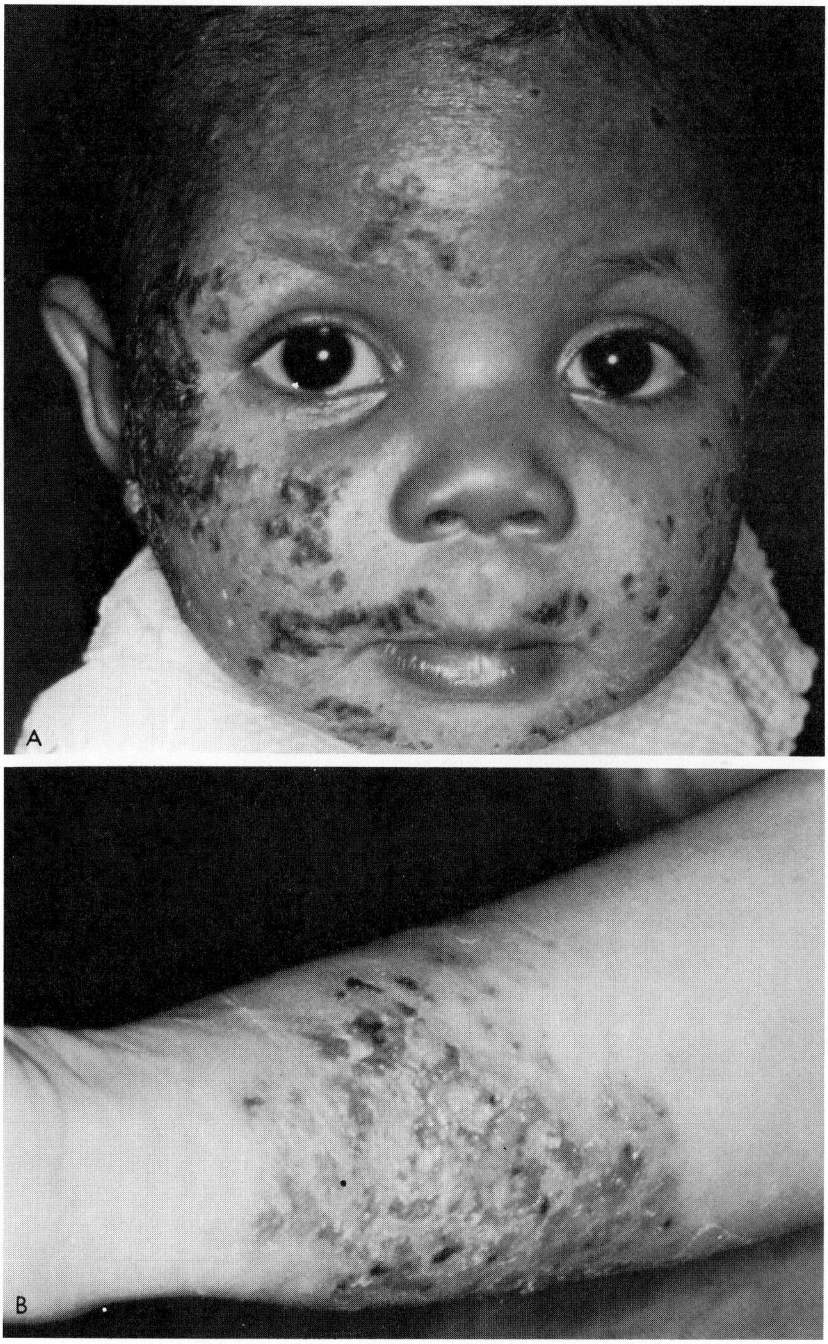

Figure 20–4. Photographs of the lesions of atopic eczema in the infant. Note the distribution on the face *(A)*, on the surfaces of the lower forearms *(B,)* and on the back *(C)*, (Courtesy of Dr. James P. Rotchford.)

Illustration continued on following page.

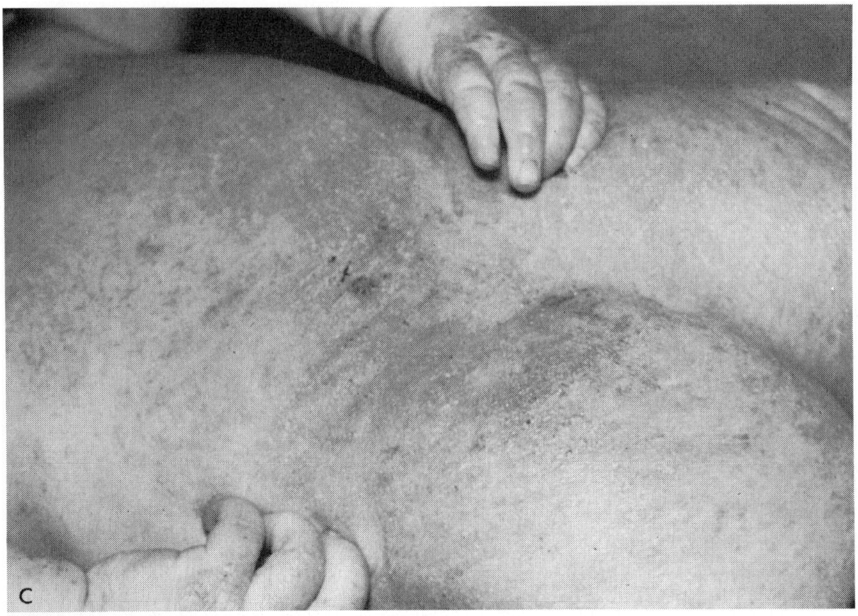

Figure 20–4 *Continued.*

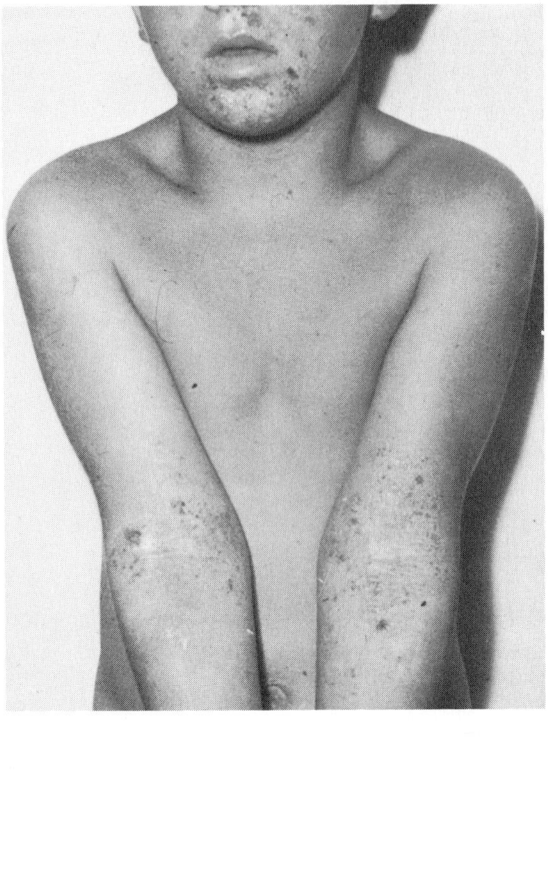

Figure 20–5. Photograph of the lesions of atopic eczema in an older child showing the distribution on the face and flexor surfaces of the antecubital areas. (Courtesy of Dr. James P. Rotchford.)

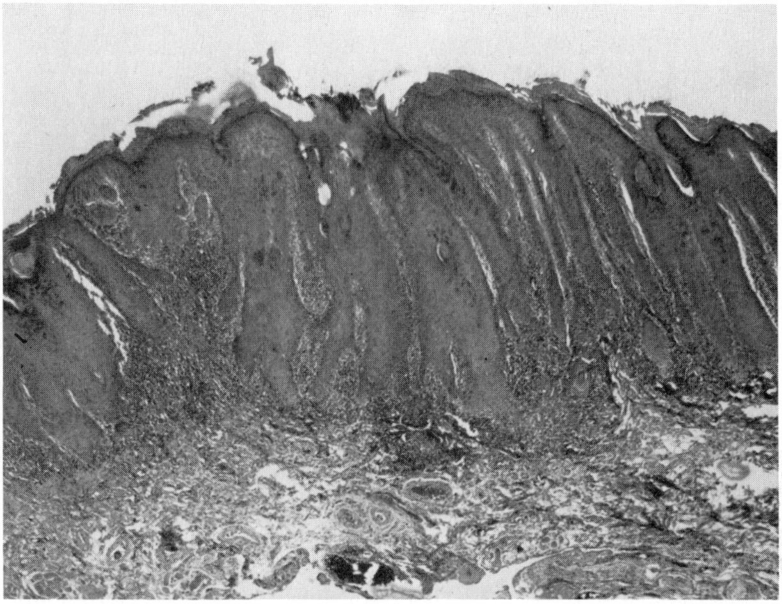

Figure 20–6. Photomicrograph of the skin lesion of atopic dermatitis showing the characteristic inflammatory reaction in the dermis with parakeratosis and acanthosis. Hematoxylin and eosin stain, ×120. (Courtesy of Dr. George H. Green.)

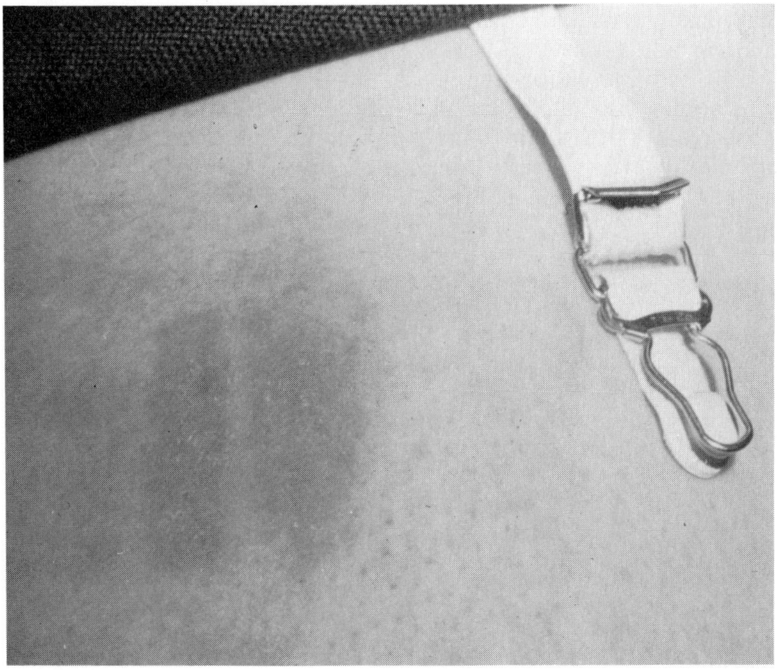

Figure 20–7. Photograph of the thigh of a patient with contact dermatitis due to nickel sensitivity (garter). Note the localization of the lesion to the area in contact with the metallic surface. (Courtesy of Dr. James P. Rotchford).

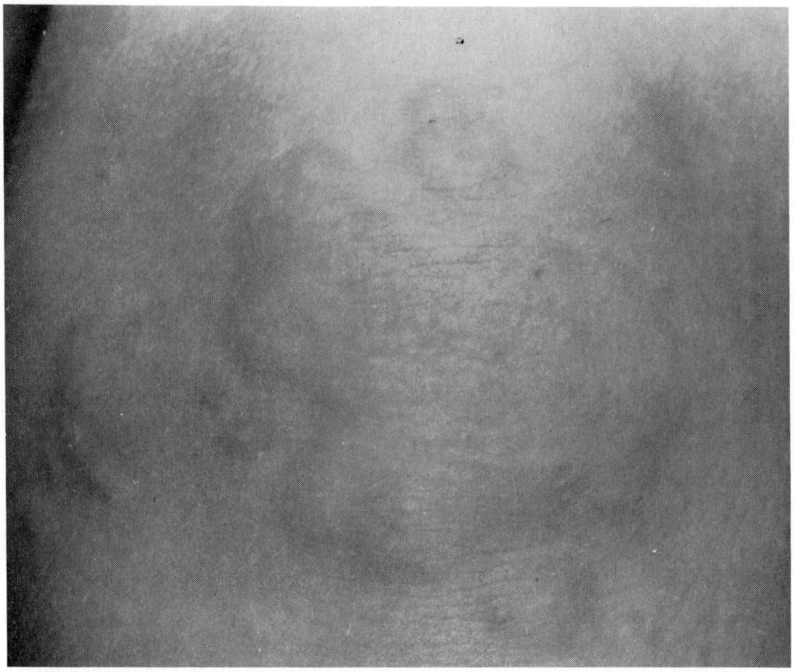

Figure 20–8. Photograph of the knee of a patient with urticarial lesions of the skin. (Courtesy of Dr. James P. Rotchford.)

ized by erythema and wheal formation (Fig. 20–8). The lesions are characteristically evanescent, vary in size and shape, and are pruritic.

From a clinical standpoint, the urticarias are classified as (1) immunologic and (2) nonimmunologic, e.g., physical (cold urticaria), cholinergic, emotional, or produced by histamine-releasing drugs, e.g., codeine, or systemic diseases, such as lymphomas, hyperthyroidism, and malignant disorders. The basic mechanism underlying all of the urticarias involves the localized increase in vascular permeability that occurs through the release of vasoactive amines, e.g., histamine, via any of a number of mechanisms.

The urticarial lesion is explained by the triple response of Lewis: (1) localized vasodilatation (erythema), (2) transudation of fluid (wheal), and (3) flaring due to local axon reflex.

In the immunologic type of urticaria, the release of vasoactive substances from mast cells occurs by any of a number of immunologic reactions, e.g., IgE response, antigen-antibody complexes, or cytophilic mechanisms (Chapter 13). Thus, urticaria can be seen after a penicillin reaction (IgE), during a serum sickness–like reaction (IgE or antigen-antibody complex), or during an incompatible blood transfusion (cytotoxic antibodies). However, the most common causes of urticaria are immunologically related and appear to be associated with infection (acute, e.g., streptococcal and parasitic, or chronic, e.g., dental and genitourinary), foods, and drugs (Table 20–4).

There are two other entities that enter into the differential diagnosis of chronic urticaria: urticaria pigmentosa and hereditary angioedema. Urticaria pigmentosa is characterized by discrete pink papules that are infiltrated by mast cells. When the lesions are stroked, the presence of these cells causes visible wheal and flare formation. This rare and self-limited disease is mediated by mediator release (Fig. 20–9).

Hereditary angioedema (HAE) is a familial disease transmitted as an autosomal dominant trait (Chapter 22). The basic defect is a deficiency of the inhibitor or a nonfunctional inhibitor of C1 esterase that expresses itself

Table 20–4. Common Causes of Urticaria

Type	Examples
Infection	Bacteria Viruses Parasites Fungi
Foods	Berries Shellfish Chocolate Nuts
Drugs	Penicillin Laxatives Tranquilizers Aspirin

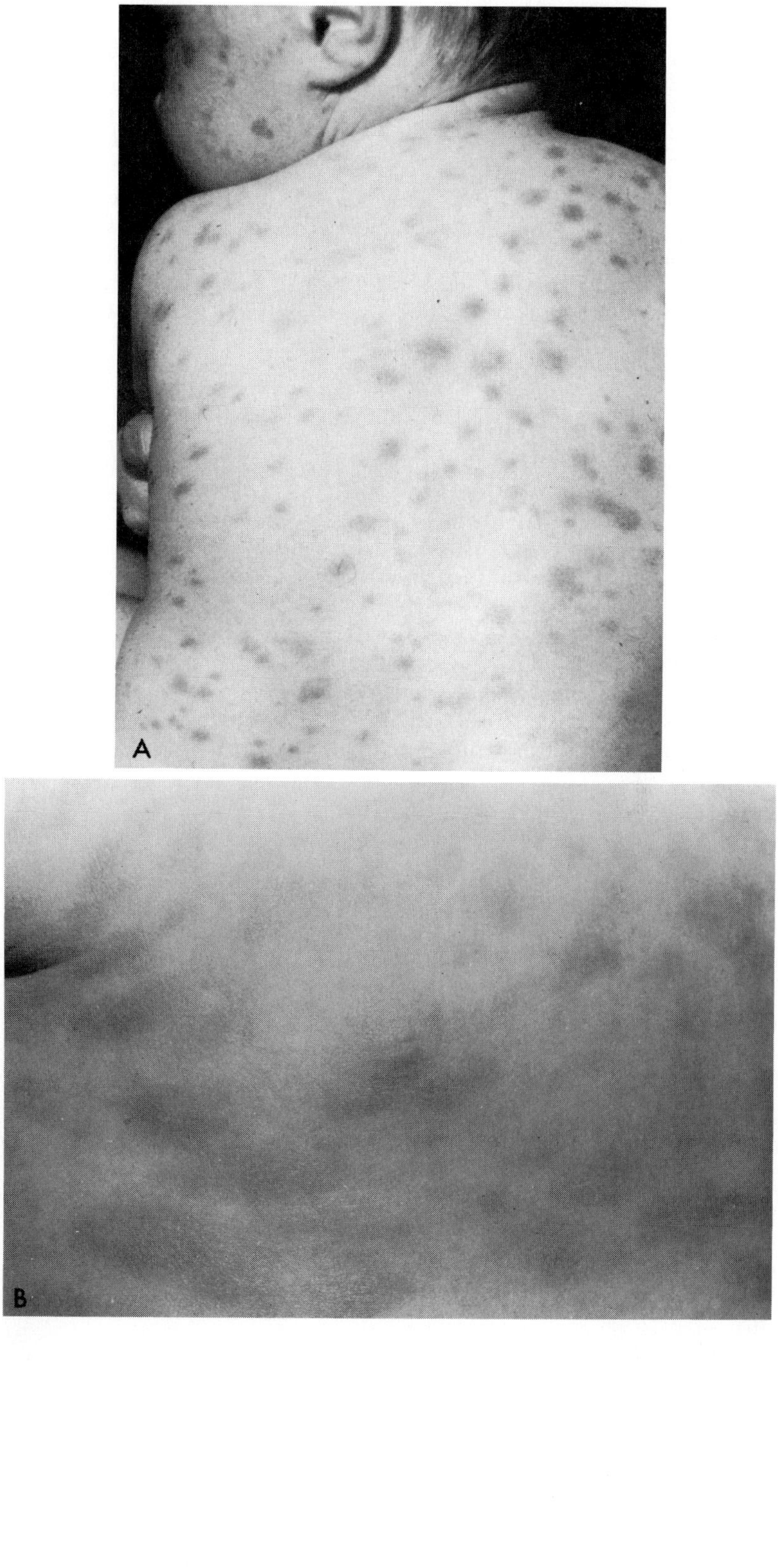

Figure 20–9. Photograph of a patient with urticaria pigmentosa. Note the wide distribution of the lesions *(A)* and the development of visible wheal and flare formation after stroking the affected areas *(B)*. (Courtesy of Dr. James P. Rotchford.)

as a marked increase in vascular permeability. It presents as a sudden onset of painless urticarial edema, which at times can be life-threatening. It should be pointed out that patients with this disease do not have the classic circumscribed lesions of urticaria (Fig. 20–10) but rather have massive collections of fluid in the subcutaneous tissues (angioedema) (see Fig. 22–8). The diagnosis can be suspected by demonstration of C1q inhibition or decrease in C4 with normal C3 activities. The definitive diagnosis can be made only by measurements of C1 esterase activity, and these procedures are available only in research laboratories. Treatment of this disorder has traditionally rested with the use of epsilon-aminocaproic acid. The use of danazol has shown quite promising results and is considered the treatment of choice.

ALLERGIC DISEASE OF THE RESPIRATORY TRACT

Further hostility of the environment is manifested through exposure of the host to a variety of noxious agents that assault the respiratory tract. The majority of these insults occur by inhalation of organic and inorganic substances, including dust, pollen, molds, animal dander, silica, organic dusts, and living organisms (Fig. 20–11). These allergic diseases of the lung may also be triggered by *ingestants* (foods and drugs) or by *injectants* (drugs and vaccines). Examples of allergic diseases of the respiratory tract and their mechanisms of injury are given in Table 20–5.

Allergic diseases of the respiratory tract include several of the mechanisms of immunologic injury. The majority of clinical entities are produced by Type I reactions. Delayed hypersensitivity is a prominent feature of many infectious diseases of the respiratory tract, e.g., tuberculosis. Although such reactivity is not the primary cause of the disease, it contributes to the excessive tissue destruction commonly seen in these infections. In other forms of allergic disease of the lung, mixed forms of immunologic injury are operative.

Type I Response

The major localized anaphylactic categories of disease that affect the respiratory tract include conjunctivitis, rhinitis, and asthma. These respiratory insults are resented by the host, who expresses symptoms of the disease through the harmful action of cytotropic antibodies found at local sites. Although these reactions are primarily IgE-mediated, there is some recent evidence to

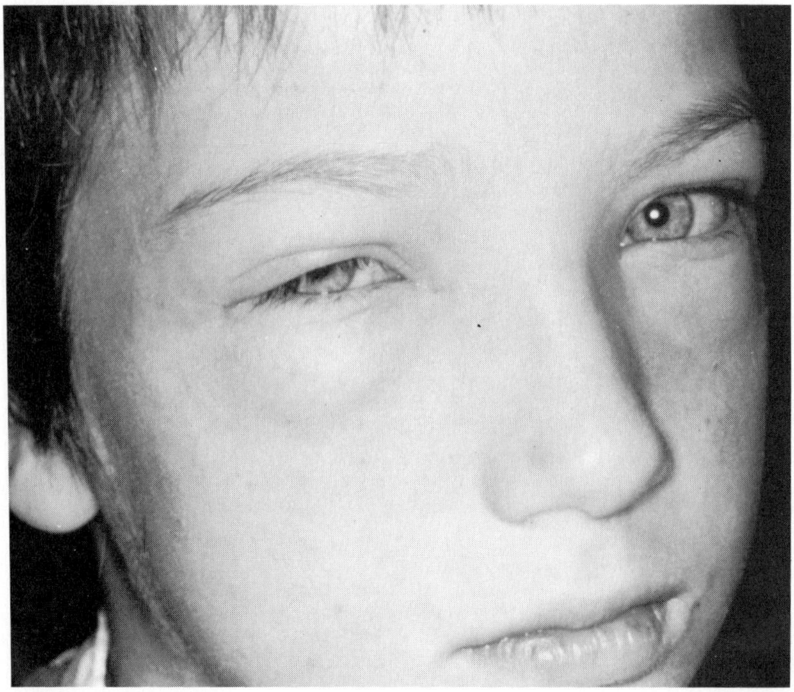

Figure 20–10. Photograph of a patient with angioedema showing the affected eyelids. (Courtesy of Dr. James P. Rotchford.)

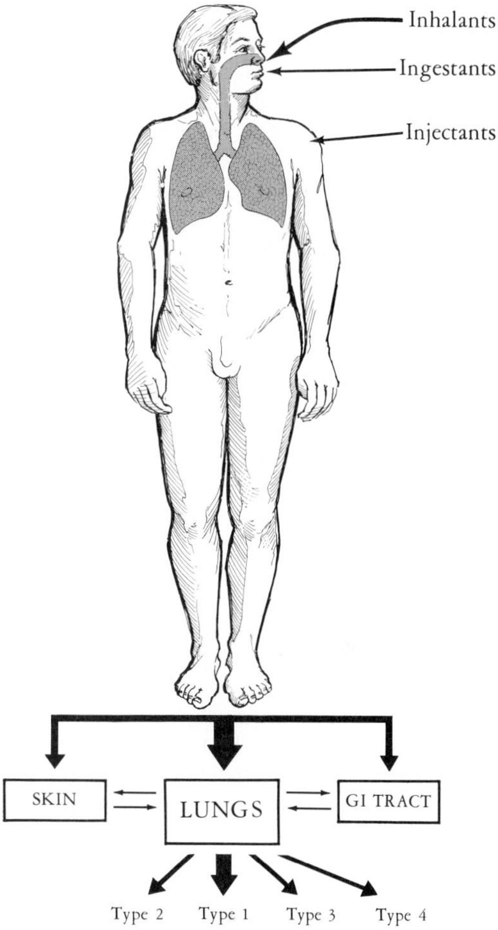

Figure 20–11. Schematic representation of the clinical manifestations of allergic diseases of the respiratory tract.

suggest a pathogenetic role of IgG reagins, e.g., IgG4. After the interaction of antigen with cell-bound reagin, there is the release of vasoactive amines, e.g., histamine, SRS-A, ECF-A, PAF, prostaglandins and other arachidonic acid metabolites, and other mediators (Chapter 13), which cause vasodilatation, hypersecretion, edema, and swelling of the (respiratory) mucosa or contribute to the inflammatory reaction. Since there is a continuity of the mucous lining membranes of all components of the respiratory tract (accessory sinuses, nasopharynx, and upper and lower respiratory tract), all components are adversely affected in this allergic attack. The degree to which each is affected will determine the clinical manifestation of the disease. Thus, in the young child, obstruction with nasal blockage and eustachian tube impedance frequently is accompanied by otitis media, e.g., secretory otitis media.

ASTHMA

Asthma may be defined as acute, intermittent, reversible obstructive airway disease.

Table 20–5. Allergic Diseases of the Respiratory Tract

Type	Example of Disease	Example of Antigen	Mechanism
Type I	Allergic rhinitis Bronchial asthma	Pollen	IgE antibody
Type II	Goodpasture's syndrome	Glomerular basement membrane (GBM) antigen	Anti-GBM
Type III	Farmer's lung	Dust of molding hay	Antigen-antibody complexes (together with Type IV)
Type IV	Tuberculosis	Tuberculoprotein	Sensitized lymphocytes

The entity has been classically divided into *extrinsic* asthma, in which an exogenous allergen can be identified, and *intrinsic* asthma, in which no identifiable causative agent can be demonstrated. It should be pointed out, however, that this classification is inadequate, since intrinsic defects may be demonstrated in extrinsic asthma, and extrinsic factors, e.g., microorganisms, have been suggested in intrinsic asthma. Indeed, both show a β-adrenergic blockade, as will be described below. Moreover, certain forms of chronic obstructive pulmonary disease (COPD) may have a bronchospasmic component.

The central defect in allergic diseases of the lung of atopic individuals is caused by obstruction of the lumen of the large and small airways of the lower respiratory tract by bronchospasm, edema, thick secretions, and hyperplasia of smooth muscle and mucus-secreting glands. This leads to ventilatory insufficiency due to obstruction, with wheezing and dyspnea (Fig. 20–12). This insufficiency presents with hyperinflation, expiratory wheezes, and musical rales characteristic of lower tract involvement. Radiographic changes may show hyperinflation (Fig. 20–13). There is a striking similarity between these responses of the host and the bronchiolitis seen after infection with respiratory viruses, e.g., respiratory syncytial virus. Indeed, in clinical onset they may be so similar as to create diagnostic confusion until a subsequent course of the disease clarifies the issue. These viral agents have been associated with exacerbation of pulmonary symptoms in the atopic host, e.g., wheezing in asthmatic children.

Type II Response

The classic example of a Type II hypersensitivity reaction involving the lung is Goodpasture's syndrome. The disorder is characterized by diffuse proliferative glomerulonephritis, pulmonary hemorrhage, anemia, and a rapidly progressive course that usually ends in death within a few weeks to months. The pulmonary manifestations are clinically indistinguishable from those seen in idiopathic pulmonary hemosiderosis, and both are associated with pulmonary hemorrhages, hemoptysis, iron deficiency anemia, and hemosiderin-laden macrophages, which are usually demonstrable in smears of the sputum or gastric washings. The character-

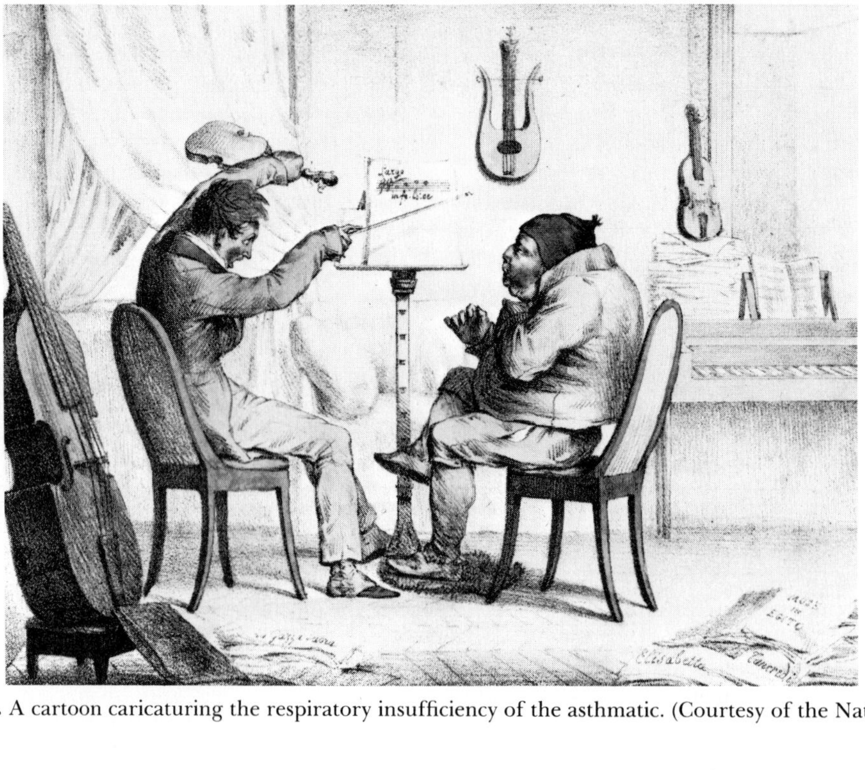

Figure 20–12. A cartoon caricaturing the respiratory insufficiency of the asthmatic. (Courtesy of the National Library of Medicine.)

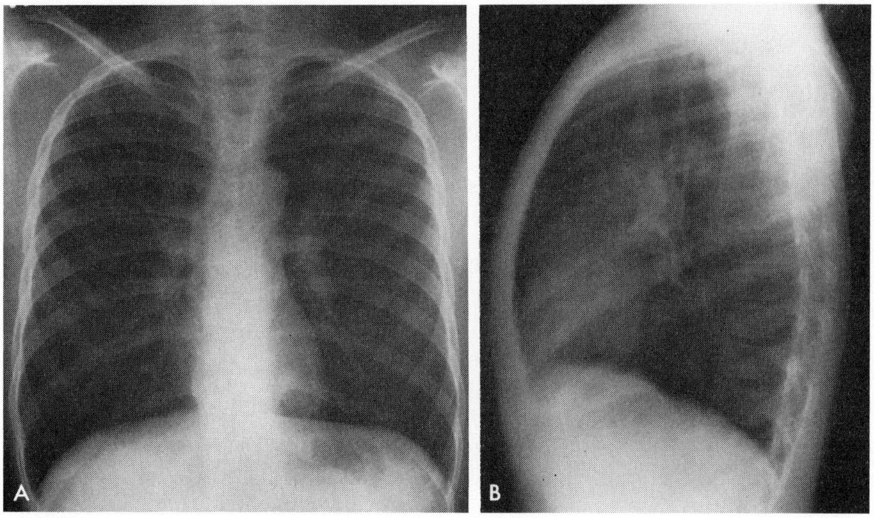

Figure 20–13. An x-ray of the chest of a patient with bronchial asthma showing the hyperinflation *(A)* and depressed diaphragm *(B)* characteristic of the disease.

istic immunologic feature of Goodpasture's syndrome is the finding of antibodies in the serum that are reactive with glomerular basement membrane of the lung and the kidney. These anti-GBM antibodies have been shown to deposit in the kidneys and in the lungs with a characteristic linear pattern of deposition (Chapter 20C).

The course of Goodpasture's syndrome is nearly always fatal. Treatment with corticosteroids may induce temporary remission, but it does not alter the ultimate outcome. A variety of other approaches, including immunosuppressive cytotoxic agents, e.g., azathioprine, exchange transfusion, and plasmapheresis have been used but with limited success. Bilateral nephrectomy with subsequent renal transplantation has been used in some patients.

Type III Response

Several hypersensitivity reactions of the lung involve a Type III immune complex–type injury (Table 20–5). They occur in concert with other types of immunologic mechanisms and are described below with allergic diseases of the lung involving injury caused by mixed immunologic responses.

Type IV Response

The classic example of the Type IV hypersensitivity reaction in the lung is that seen after infection with tuberculosis. The basic histopathologic feature of this condition is the formation of granulomata containing collections of epithelioid cells, fibrous tissue, and lymphocytes. In this reaction, the sensitized lymphocytes play the major role, independent of circulating antibody. There are other exogenous agents that elicit similar responses. These include silica, coal dust, and beryllium, as well as drugs, e.g., nitrofurantoin (Furadantin). The response to these materials may represent a simple inflammatory episode, although evidence for participation of special immunologic events is suggested by the similarity in histopathologic appearance of the lesion.

There are a number of other poorly defined pulmonary diseases seen in other clinical conditions, such as rheumatoid arthritis. The association with exogenous agents in these diseases has not been clearly established. The physician should be constantly alert to the possibility of new pollutants and industrial by-products that may produce new immunologically mediated diseases.

Mixed Immunologic Responses: Extrinsic Allergic Alveolitis, Types III and IV, and Allergic Bronchopulmonary Aspergillosis, Types I and III

Another set of responses of the host to exogenous antigens is that caused by the extensive inhalation of proteinaceous material, as seen in extrinsic allergic alveolitis, or that resulting from the effects of aspergillus, as seen in allergic bronchopulmonary aspergillosis. These diseases appear to involve mixed immunologic responses that allow a basis for classification of their clinical presentations (Tables 20–2 and 20–6).

EXTRINSIC ALLERGIC ALVEOLITIS (PULMONARY HYPERSENSITIVITY DISEASE)

This form of hypersensitivity disease results from special circumstances of occupational or environmental exposure. A wide variety of thermophylic actinomycetes, molds, and proteinaceous materials have been implicated in this disorder. Examples of the antigens that give rise to these clinical entities are shown in Table 20–7. Unlike the Type I responses, which affect only about 15 to 20 per cent of genetically predisposed individuals under conditions of everyday exposure, these reactions are seen predominantly in the nonatopic individual under conditions of intensive exposure. Moreover, there appears to be a direct relationship between the intensity of the clinical symptoms and the circumstances of exposure. For example, a more acute form of the disease is seen after intensive exposure, whereas a low-grade exposure leads to a more chronic presentation. The effect of such agents in extrinsic allergic alveolitis is to stimulate IgG precipitating antibody in the serum, which then forms complexes with antigen and complement in the interstitial tissues of the lung, mediating injury in a Type III reaction (Table 20–6). Recent evidence suggests that a Type IV–mediated reaction may also be involved. The primary effect of these immunologic reactions is to induce an inflammatory reaction in the lungs with primary involvement of bronchioles and alveoli leading to an interstitial pneumonitis. In contrast to the Type I reaction, this type of allergic disease of the lung is characterized by a restrictive ventilatory defect rather than an obstructive defect. These abnormalities consist of decreased carbon monoxide diffusion, decreased lung compliance, and increased residual volume. Clinically, the condition is characterized by cough, dyspnea, and cyanosis. Wheezing is usually absent, but systemic findings of fever and chills, malaise, and loss of weight are common. Radiographic changes include micronodular infiltrations followed by diffuse fibrosis and "honeycomb" changes affecting particularly the upper lobes (Fig. 20–14). The diagnosis should be

Table 20–6. Comparison of the Clinical and Laboratory Findings in Extrinsic Allergic Alveolitis and Allergic Bronchopulmonary Aspergillosis*

	Extrinsic Allergic Alveolitis	Allergic Bronchopulmonary Aspergillosis
Basic nature	Nonatopic	Atopic
Immunologic basis	Immune complexes and hypersensitivity (Types III and IV)	Immediate hypersensitivity and immune complexes (Types I and III)
Physical examination	±	Wheezing
Skin test	±	Dual positivity (immediate Type I and Type III Arthus in 4–6 hours)
X-ray	Pulmonary infiltrates—interstitial	Pulmonary infiltrates—lobar
Complications	Pulmonary fibrosis	Atelectasis, bronchiectasis
Blood	Normal	Eosinophilia
Sputum	Normal	Eosinophilia, mycelia
IgE	Normal	Elevated
Pulmonary function	Restrictive	Obstructive
Bronchial provocation	Delayed (5–6 hours)	Immediate and late
Antibody	Precipitating (IgG)	Precipitating (IgG), nonprecipitating (IgE)

*Adapted from Slavin, R. G.: Allergic bronchopulmonary aspergillosis. *In* Middleton, E., Reed, C. E., and Ellis, E. F. (eds.): Allergy: Principles and Practice. St. Louis, C. V. Mosby Company, 1983.

Table 20–7. **Causes of Hypersensitivity Pneumonitis***

Disease	Source of Antigen	Probable Antigens
Vegetable Products		
Farmer's lung	moldy hay	thermophilic actinomycetes *Micropolyspora faeni* *Thermoactinomyces vulgaris*
Bagassosis	moldy pressed sugarcane (bagasse)	thermophilic actinomycetes *Thermoactinomyces sacchari*
Mushroom worker's disease	moldy compost	thermophilic actinomycetes *Micropolyspora faeni* *Thermoactinomyces vulgaris*
Suberosis	moldy cork	unknown
Malt worker's lung	contaminated barley	fungi *Aspergillus clavatus*
Maple bark disease	contaminated maple logs	fungi *Cryptostroma corticale*
Sequoiosis	contaminated wood dust	fungi *Graphium* sp. *Pullularia* sp. other fungi
Wood pulp worker's disease	contaminated wood pulp	fungi *Alternaria* sp.
Humidifier lung	contaminated home humidifier and air conditioning ducts	thermophilic actinomycetes *Thermoactinomyces vulgaris* *Thermoactinomyces candidus*
Paprika slicer's lung	moldy paprika pods	fungi *Mucor stolonifer*
Grain measurer's lung	cereal grains	unknown
Thatched roof disease	dried grass and leaves	unknown
Tobacco grower's disease	tobacco plants	unknown
Tea grower's disease	tea plants	unknown
Coffee worker's lung	green coffee beans	unknown
Hypersensitivity pneumonitis	sawdust	unknown
Coptic disease	cloth wrappings of mummies	unknown
Animal Products		
Pigeon breeder's disease	pigeon droppings	pigeon serum protein (albumin, gamma globulin, and others)
Duck fever	bird feathers	chicken proteins
Turkey handler's disease	turkey products	turkey proteins
Insect Products		
Miller's lung	wheat weavils	*Sitophilus granarius*
Bacterial or Viral Products		
Hypersensitivity pneumonitis	*B. subtilis* enzymes[a]	*Bacillus subtilis*
Smallpox handler's lung	smallpox scabs	unknown

[a]Probably induces IgE mediated obstructive airways disease in the great majority of cases.

*From Lopez, M., and Salvaggio, J.: Hypersensitivity pneumonitis: Current concepts of etiology and pathogenesis. Annu. Rev. Med., *27*:453, 1976.

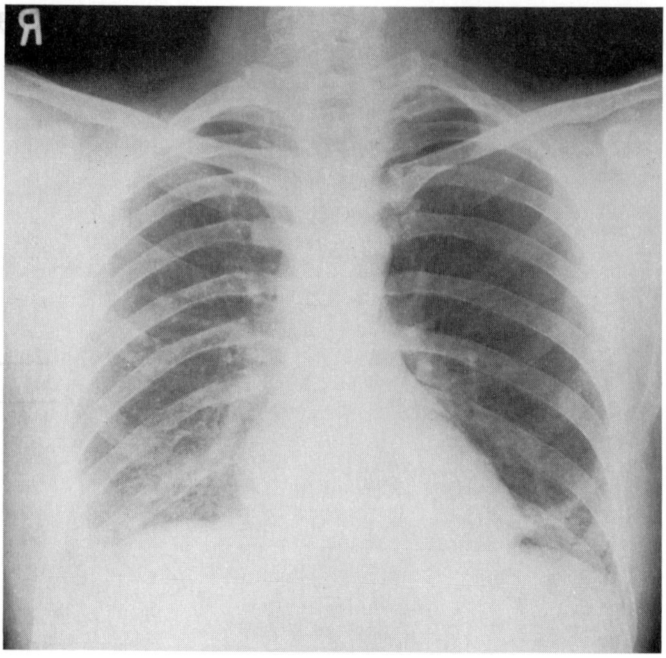

Figure 20–14. An x-ray of the chest of a patient with farmer's lung, showing the "honeycomb" changes in the lungs. (Courtesy of Dr. Sol Katz.)

suspected on the basis of history, pulmonary function tests, and the finding of precipitins in the serum. Skin tests are of limited value since most antigens, e.g., thermophylic actinomycetes, lead to nonspecific dermal responses. A delayed response to bronchial challenge is usually obtained after five to six hours. This procedure should be used with great caution, however, because of the dangers of systemic and pulmonary reactions. Although these responses are mediated primarily by antigen-antibody complexes, as described above, more recent evidence suggests that the late-acting effects of IgE may also be involved.

ALLERGIC BRONCHOPULMONARY ASPERGILLOSIS (ABA)

A second type of allergic lung disease whose pathogenesis involves a mixed immunologic response is allergic bronchopulmonary aspergillosis (ABA) (Table 20–6). This is one of several conditions that compose the so-called Loeffler syndrome or pulmonary infiltration with eosinophilia (PIE) syndrome. Shown in Table 20–8 are the three manifestations of infestation of the host with aspergillus. Aspergilloma, or fungus ball, is an accumulation of the organisms in a pulmonary cavity that can result from a variety of causes, e.g., congenital or bronchiectatic cysts. The disseminated form of aspergillosis occurs as a complication seen primarily in immunosuppressed hosts or in chronic debilitating conditions. Allergic bronchopulmonary aspergillosis is a form of hypersensitivity reaction involving primarily the lung. In contrast to extrinsic allergic alveolitis, ABA occurs primarily in the atopic individual who usually has a long-standing history of bronchial asthma (Table 20–6). The disease occurs as a result of normal exposure to various species of *Aspergillus,* e.g., *A. niger* or *A. fu-*

Table 20–8. Manifestations of the Host After Infestation or Exposure to Aspergillus

Manifestation	Predisposing Condition
Aspergilloma	Cysts, e.g., congenital or bronchiectatic
Disseminated aspergillosis	Immunosuppressed host, e.g., patients receiving azathioprine or with chronic debilitating condition (e.g., malignant disorder)
Allergic bronchopulmonary aspergillosis (ABA)	Exposure of the atopic host to aspergillus

migatus. The net effect of such exposure is the production of both IgE nonprecipitating and IgG precipitating antibodies that then participate in immunologic reactions contributing to the tissue injury characteristic of the clinical entity. The most characteristic symptoms of the disease are mediated by Type I IgE-mediated responses, which give rise to the obstructive pulmonary component of the disease. IgG precipitating antibody may also participate in a Type III reaction. A dual skin response is commonly seen, including an immediate Type I (IgE) response and a Type III (Arthus) response seen in four to six hours. The clinical presentation is characterized by low-grade fever, episodic wheezing and dyspnea, and a typical expectoration of golden brown plugs that consist primarily of eosinophils and mycelia. Hyperimmunoglobulinemia E and blood eosinophilia, as well as the finding of positive precipitating antibody to aspergillus by Ouchterlony double diffusion in agar, are helpful diagnostic aids. The chest roentgenogram classically reveals transient lobar pulmonary infiltrates that affect different lung areas at different times. Bronchial provocation, when performed, reveals a dual response (immediate and late), as will be described below.

The management of both extrinsic allergic alveolitis and allergic bronchopulmonary aspergillosis rests with the identification of the offending antigen, its removal from the environment where possible or its avoidance, and the use of anti-inflammatory agents, e.g., steroids.

A specialized form of allergic disease of the lung involving mixed immunologic responses is believed to be the basis for the atypical reaction seen after the injection of killed viral vaccines in children (Chapter 23). The two major offenders observed are measles virus and respiratory syncytial virus. After immunization with killed viral vaccines, natural infection resulted in a typical and more devastating disease than occurs in previously nonimmunized children. One hypothesis for these reactions is that selective stimulation of serum IgG antibody had occurred in the absence of local secretory IgA antibody in the respiratory tract. This immunologic imbalance leads to an atypical disease that may have a basis similar to that described for extrinsic allergic alveolitis. Following subsequent exposure to natural measles, an anomalous situation is believed to occur in which viral antigen within the respiratory tract could complex with serum IgG antibody. Such complexes would initiate a Type III reaction in the lung (Fig. 20–15). Children previously immunized with killed measles vaccine who subsequently received live measles vaccine show a localized Arthus reaction at the site of injection (Chapter 23). Immunopathologic staining of biopsy material from these children has revealed the

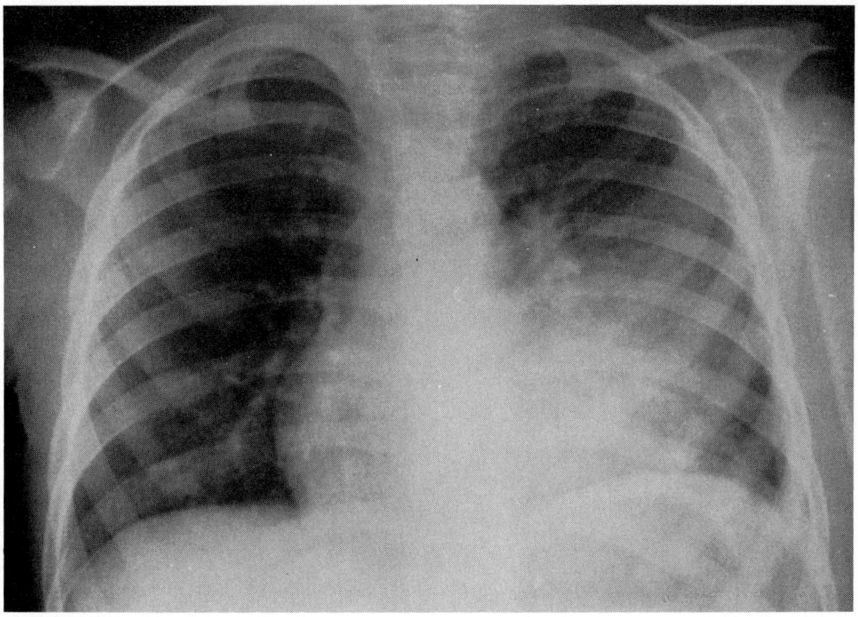

Figure 20–15. An x-ray of the chest showing a pulmonary infiltrate attributed to a Type III reaction occurring in a child with atypical measles who had been previously immunized with killed measles vaccine.

presence of C3, measles, and IgG globulin, all present simultaneously within blood vessel walls. Although these histopathologic findings provide direct evidence for the participation of these immune complexes in the pathogenesis of this type of disease, other mechanisms of immunologic injury, e.g., Type I or Type IV, may also be operative in the pathogenesis.

IMMUNOLOGICALLY MEDIATED DISEASES OF UNKNOWN ETIOLOGY ASSOCIATED WITH INFECTION

In many infections caused by various organisms (bacteria, viruses, fungi, and parasites), there are a number of hypersensitivity reactions that occur (Chapters 15 to 18). Some of these are transitory and occur during the course of the disease; others are more protracted and lead to more severe sequelae, e.g., rheumatic fever or acute glomerulonephritis after group A beta-hemolytic streptococcal infection. Some acute expressions of acute viral infection might also result in hypersensitivity reactions, e.g., RSV infections that mimic attacks of acute asthma. Indeed, it is still uncertain whether the virus may be infecting selective populations, e.g., atopic individuals, in the expressions of bronchiolitis. These immunologically mediated diseases that are triggered by exogenous agents but affect autologous tissues will be described under the section on autologous antigens.

In summary, the gastrointestinal tract, the skin, and the respiratory tract constitute the primary target organs of the common allergies of man. Although the composition of the initiating agent varies, they are all exogenous in nature. It should be noted that they are all mediated by any of the four mechanisms of immunologic injury. There frequently occurs a transition from one target organ to another. In the most severe case of this nature, i.e., the dermal respiratory syndrome, severe eczema progresses to intractable asthma. Indeed, the more elevated levels of IgE immunoglobulins, for example, are seen in those patients with eczema who also have respiratory tract disease. Factors that foster the progression from one target organ to another may be an expression of the genetic constitution of the host, may be related to the quantitative load of antigen, or may represent an insult that overwhelms the immunologic capacity of the individual. It is clear that exogenous antigens evoking these responses should be identified and eliminated from the environment if immunologic balance is to be maintained.

NONIMMUNOLOGIC MECHANISMS INVOLVED IN ALLERGY

Although the immunologic basis of allergic disease has been highlighted in this section, it should be emphasized that another type of imbalance may exist in the allergic individual, i.e., an imbalance of the autonomic nervous system upon which the immunologic imbalance may be superimposed.

The autonomic nervous system is composed of the parasympathetic (cholinergic) and the sympathetic (adrenergic) systems. These two systems generally exert opposing effects on various organs. Between these two systems there appears to exist a balance that maintains a homeostatic control over *mediator cells* and *target cells.* In mediator cells such as the mast cell, for example, the release of vasoactive amines (mediators) can be modulated by both adrenergic and cholinergic agonists; similarly, smooth muscle tone in target cells such as in the bronchial tree can be determined by the balance between sympathetic and parasympathetic activity.

According to current concepts, sympathetic and parasympathetic responses exert their effects through the second messenger system, the cyclic nucleotide system (Fig. 20–16). Stimulation of the parasympathetic system, e.g., vagus, leads to the production of acetylcholine, which converts an inactive form of guanylate cyclase to its active form. This enzyme, in turn, converts guanosine triphosphate (GTP) into cyclic guanine monophosphate (cGMP). This effect of parasympathetic stimulation can be blocked by the muscarinic antagonist atropine.

In a manner similar to that in which the parasympathetic system affects the levels of cGMP, sympathetic stimulation affects the quantities of cyclic AMP (cAMP). Stimulation of the sympathetic nervous system leads to two types of effects: (1) stimulation of the α receptors leads to decreased intracellular levels of cAMP, and (2) stimulation of the β receptors leads to an elevation of cAMP that occurs through the conversion of the inactive form of adenyl cyclase to its active form,

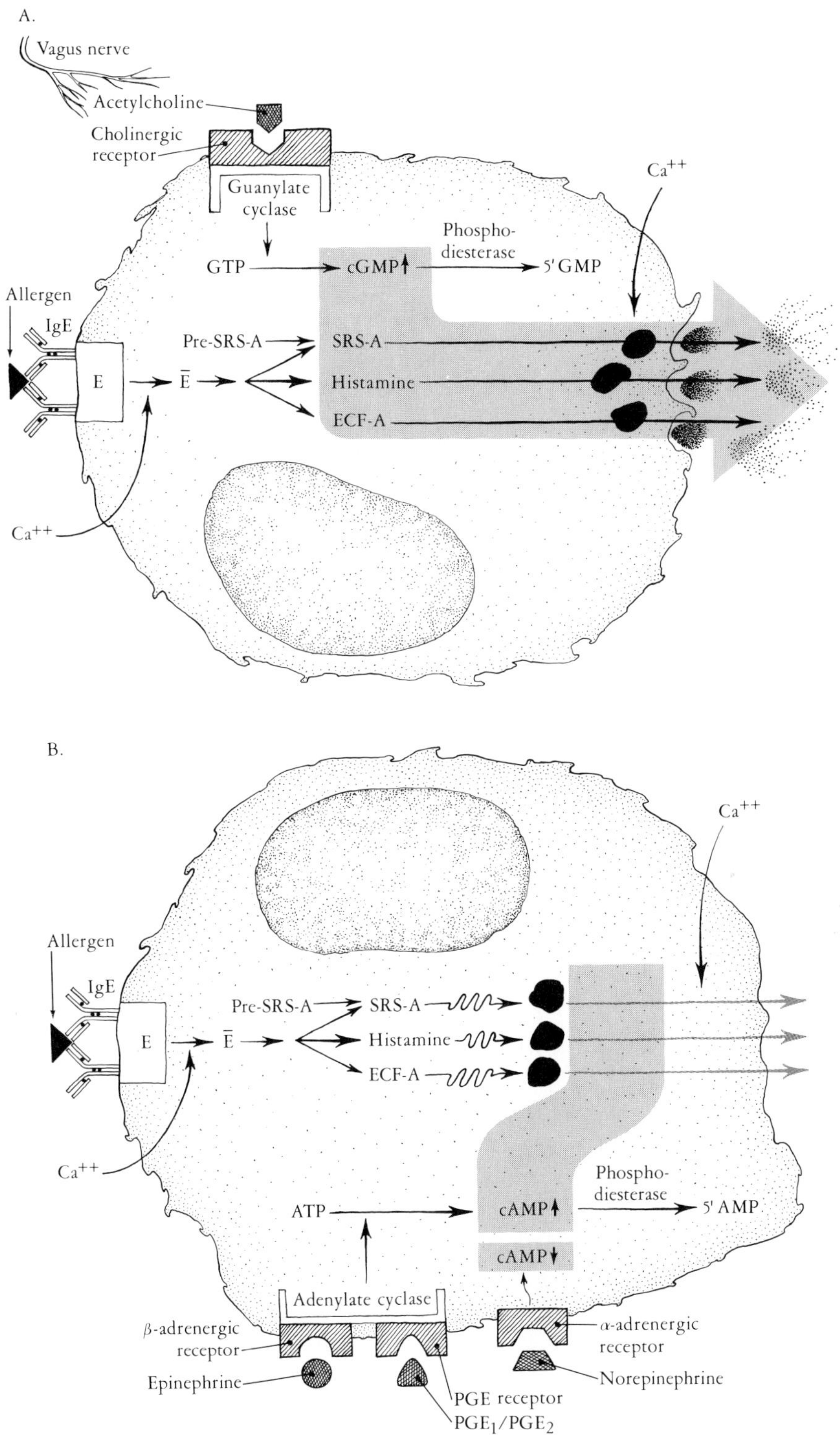

Figure 20–16. Schematic representation of the effects of the sympathetic and parasympathetic responses in allergic mediator release that are mediated through the cyclic nucleotide system. *A*, Effects of elevated cGMP on increased mediator release. *B*, Effects of elevated cAMP on decreased mediator release. *C*, Effects of pharmacologic agonists and antagonists on mediator release. *D*, Role of microtubules in mediator release and inhibiton. (*A*, *B*, and *C* adapted from Dr. T. Hubscher.)

Illustration continued on following page.

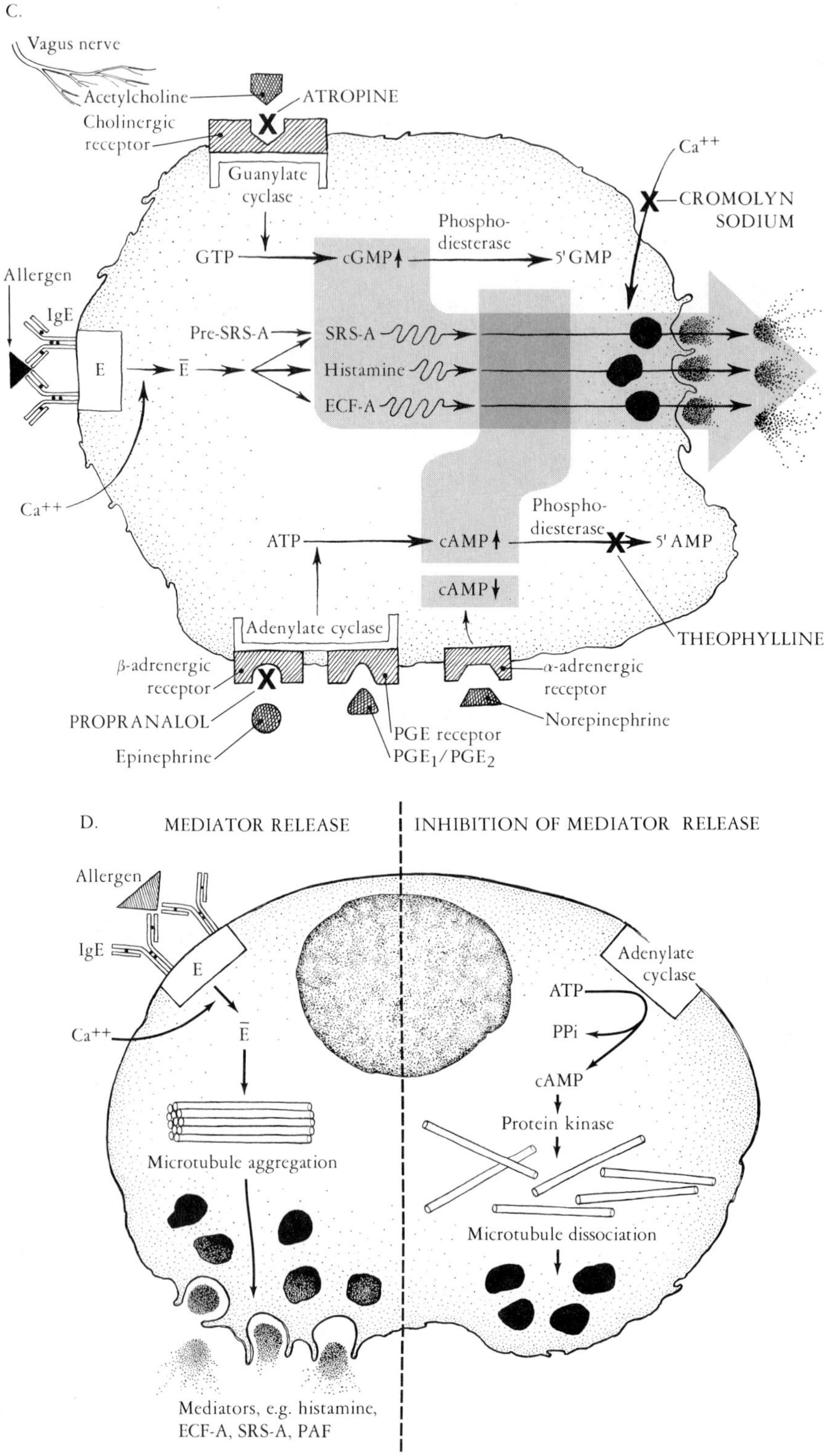

Figure 20–16C and D *Continued.*

which in turn catalyzes the conversion of ATP to cyclic AMP. The breakdown of both cGMP and cAMP occurs through the actions of the enzyme phosphodiesterase.

The α and β receptors of the sympathetic nervous system are stimulated differentially by various endogenous effector molecules (agonists). Norepinephrine, for example, secreted at the noradrenergic nerve terminals, acts at both α and β receptors, with the α effect predominating. Epinephrine, released by the adrenal medulla, likewise acts on both α and β receptors, but the β effects predominate. There are, in addition, exogenous adrenergic agonists that are specific for the β receptor, e.g., isoproterenol. More recently, it has been demonstrated that there are two types of β receptors, β_1 and β_2, whose distribution in tissues varies. For example, the β_2 receptor is found predominantly in lung tissue, and the development of specific β_2 agonists, e.g., albuterol, has had particular therapeutic significance in the treatment of bronchial asthma.

PROPOSED MECHANISMS OF RELEASE OF MEDIATORS AND THEIR EFFECTS ON TARGET CELLS

Normally, a balance appears to exist between intracellular levels of cAMP and those of cGMP, the effects of cAMP predominating (Fig. 20–17). As just described, this balance is influenced by both parasympathetic and sympathetic activity, as well as by a variety of other reactants, including inflammatory mediators, e.g., histamine, prostaglandins, and the actual levels of cAMP and cGMP (Fig. 20–17). The relative amounts of these reactants appear to maintain a homeostatic control over both *mediator cells,* e.g., basophils and mast cells, and *target cells,* e.g., smooth muscle cells and mucosal cells. The arbitrary use of these latter terms throughout this book has been defined in Chapters 2, 11, and 13.

Following the interaction of at least two membrane-associated IgE molecules with antigen, a sequence of biochemical events occurs that ultimately leads to the secretion of mediators (Fig. 20–16). This occurs in several steps that include the activation of a proesterase (E) to an active esterase ($\bar{E}$), microtubular aggregation, and finally, the movement of granule-containing mediators to the surface of these cells with the subsequent release of mediators (Fig. 20–16*D*). Concomitant with these events is a decrease in cellular levels of cAMP. The release of mediators is an energy-requiring step for which ions, e.g., Ca^{++}, must be present. Some mediators (e.g., histamine and ECF-A) are found preformed in the cell; others (e.g., leukotrienes C_4, D_4, E_4, formerly known collectively as SRS-A) are synthesized from precursors (Fig. 20–16) (Chapter 13). It is now established that agents capable of stimulating adenyl cyclase, e.g., the β-adrenergic agonists, increase the intracellular levels of cAMP and inhibit mediator generation or release, or both (Fig. 20–18). Phosphodiesterase inhibitors such as aminophylline also block mediator release; this occurs because of the elevated levels of cAMP that result from the failure of cAMP catabolism by the inhibition of phosphodiesterase

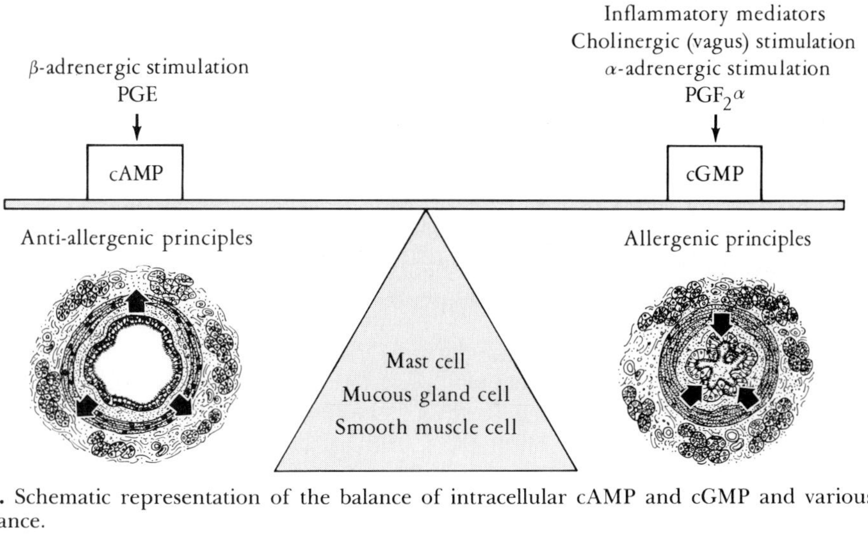

Figure 20–17. Schematic representation of the balance of intracellular cAMP and cGMP and various factors that affect this balance.

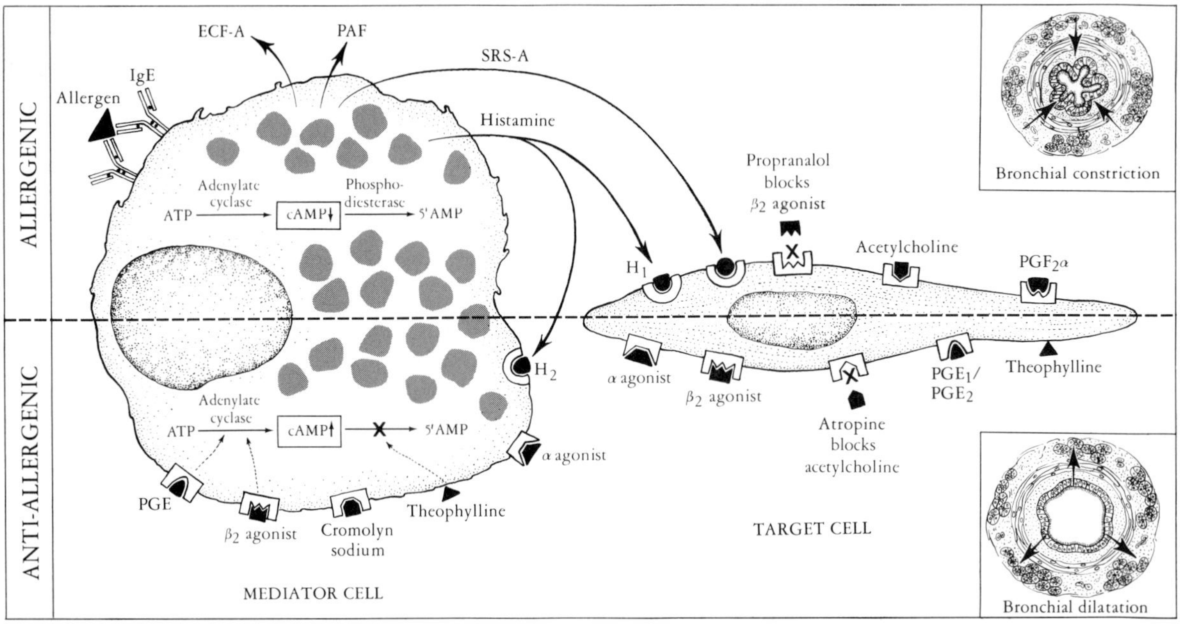

Figure 20–18. Schematic representation of the pharmacologic control of allergic responses by various agents that affect mediator release from mediator cells or the effects of mediators on target cells. (Adapted from Dr. T. Hubscher.)

(Fig. 20–16). The net effect of this intracellular buildup of cAMP is microtubular dissociation and an inhibition of mediator release (Fig. 20–16). It should be pointed out that the release of histamine itself can have a negative feedback on this process, since histamine, through its action on the H_2 receptors (Chapter 13), leads to a decreased secretion of mediators (Fig. 20–18).

The relative balance of the cyclic nucleotides also exerts its effect on target cells by modulating the physiologic state of the cell, e.g., bronchial smooth muscle tone (Fig. 20–18). The effects of raised levels of cAMP lead to a relaxation of smooth muscle, vasoconstriction of blood vessels, or decreased secretion of mucus from target cells; decreased levels of cAMP have the opposite effect. In addition, the release of mediators also has an effect on the target cell, acting presumably through receptors on the surface of the target cell (Fig. 20–19). The mediators can also exert their effects secondarily by affecting subepithelial irritant receptors that can exert a cholinergic effect, e.g., through the vagus, on the target cell (Fig. 20–19).

Thus, the effects of the autonomic balance are twofold: (1) They effect the release of mediators, e.g., histamine, and (2) they lead to effects on target cells, e.g., relaxation of smooth muscle, vasoconstriction of blood vessels, or decreased secretion of mucus. Although less well studied, the effects of cGMP appear to be opposite to those of cAMP.

THE NATURE OF THE AUTONOMIC IMBALANCE IN THE ALLERGIC (ATOPIC) INDIVIDUAL

It has been proposed that owing either to a partial β-adrenergic blockade, as originally suggested by Szentivany, or to an inefficiency of the β receptor, an imbalance between intracellular levels of cAMP and cGMP exists in the atopic individual. Such an imbalance would lead to an aberration in the homeostatic regulation of both mediator and target cells in the atopic individual having a tendency toward hyperactive release of mediators and a hyperresponsiveness of target cells. It is known, for example, that the airways and the skin of the atopic individual are more responsive to a wide variety of both specific and nonspecific stimuli than the airways and skin of the normal individual. In the patient with bronchial asthma, one can see the results of this dual effect. The exaggerated response of the airways of the allergic individual that is known to occur after the inhalation of such nonspecific exogenous irritants as smoke, sulfur dioxide, and drugs (e.g., methacholine), as well as endogenous products, e.g., $PGF_{2\alpha}$, could be accounted for by the hypothesized autonomic imbalance. This response, which appears to be mediated by the irritant receptors (Fig. 20–19), traces its origin from the afferent vagus to the medulla, with completion of the cycle through the efferent vagal nerve endings.

The autonomic imbalance of the allergic individual would also explain the responses of mediator cells. The release of mediators from the mast cells of the allergic individual, for example, would be enhanced by the β blockade owing to decreased intracellular levels of cAMP. This would lead to a further assault on the target cell by the augmentation of target cell responsiveness through these released mediators.

MODIFYING FACTORS

Genetic Predisposition. It is well established that there is a genetic predisposition for the development of the atopic diseases of man. These diseases are grouped together, since they are all mediated by a prominent IgE reaginic antibody response. It should be noted, however, that what appears to be heritable is not the specific allergic disease but the capacity to become sensitized to an allergen with which the patient has repeated contact. For example, a mother with asthma whose attacks are precipitated by ragweed may give birth to a child who subsequently suffers from allergic rhinitis, with house dust being the prime offending agent. Furthermore, there is no correlation of an allergen with a specific shock organ. For example, ragweed may trigger allergic rhinitis in one individual and bronchial asthma in another. Recently, there have been associations of allergic disease made with certain histocompatibility types (Chapter 3). Although not definitively proved, a relationship has been suggested between HLA 7 and ragweed hypersensitivity. More recent studies suggest subtle defects in T-lymphocytes (e.g., suppressor cells) that may account for heightened IgE production.

Age. In achieving immunologic balance, the age of the individual is of critical importance. This is particularly true of the small child in whom the allergic insult may occur prior to complete maturation of the immunologic system. With maturation, the child will develop increasing resistance to many of the infectious agents that at a younger age may be important in initiating his allergic disease. The importance of maturation is also illustrated by the manner in which various diseases present. Tuberculosis in the young infant very often presents in a disseminated miliary form with extrapulmonic involvement; in the older child it is largely restricted to the lungs. These differences are thought to reflect expressions of immunologic maturity. Of particular importance to allergy is the age-related maturation of the IgE system. Age differences have implications in diagnosis, therapy, and predictive value of future disease (Chapter 26).

Role of Infection. The role of infection in complicating and triggering allergic disease (asthma) is clear and must be considered in management. Severe bronchospasm and wheezing may initially be triggered by a va-

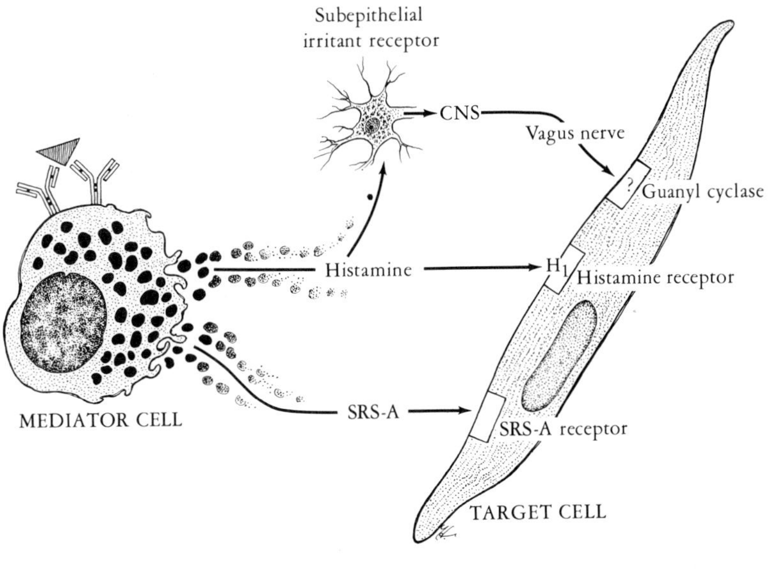

Figure 20–19. Schematic representation of the effects of released mediators on target cells and the indirect mediators in irritant receptors.

riety of microorganisms, particularly the respiratory viruses, e.g., respiratory syncytical virus (RSV). In other situations, after stimulation by the primary exogenous antigen, these infectious agents may be superimposed upon a primary allergic reaction. Although the mechanism of the precipitation of asthma by infection is not completely understood, it may reflect the stimulation of the irritant receptors of the vagus nerve, as described above.

Emotional Factors. An important concept in the management of the allergic individual is the appropriate consideration of the role of the emotional factors as both triggering and exacerbating events. It is well known that an attack of asthma may be evoked by an emotional upset. Similarly, the allergic disease may have profound effects on the psychologic development of the individual. As described above, these emotional factors too may exert their effects by way of the autonomic nervous system.

Physical Factors. In addition to the aforementioned factors, a variety of physical factors, including heat, cold, exercise, and changes in barometric pressure, may trigger allergic attacks. Although the precise mechanism of these factors is not completely understood, they are believed to be mediated primarily through the parasympathetic nervous system and initiated by irritation of the afferent receptors in various shock organs.

MANAGEMENT

More than in any other immunologically mediated disease, the causal relationship to persistent antigen is best demonstrated in allergic disease. Symptoms persist precisely as long as the antigen persists. Upon removal of the antigen or blockage of its effect there is a disappearance of the harmful expressions of the immune response. When undertaking the management of the allergic diseases, therefore, there are four points to consider: (1) prevention of the immunologic imbalance, (2) recognition of the immunologic manifestation, (3) identification and removal of the offending agent, and (4) therapy.

Prevention of Immunologic Imbalance

Elimination of potential antigens, e.g., foods, animals, and other offending substances, even before the clinical evidence of disease occurs is an important preventive measure. Prior experience, either within a family or derived from prior therapeutic practices, can indicate the preferential avoidance of potential substances known to be allergenic. For example, in other family members in which atopic disease occurs, the use of breast feeding or milk substitutes may prevent the subsequent development of allergy to milk protein. Moreover, since immunologic maturity of the gastrointestinal tract occurs at approximately five months of age, it would seem reasonable to delay, when possible, the introduction of solid foods, or at least the most frequently allergenic foods, until this time. Furthermore, it has been postulated that the absorption of food proteins or other macromolecules from the gastrointestinal tract may lead to sensitization and subsequent immunization of the older patient manifesting a variety of hypersensitivity diseases, particularly in the IgA-deficient individual. The use of active immunization or the use of human hyperimmune sera rather than foreign sera, e.g., horse serum, in immunotherapy will prevent the development of a serum sickness reaction. Finally, the avoidance of undue exposure to environmental allergens in some of the environmentally induced allergies, e.g., dermatitis and extrinsic allergic alveolitis, may be an important preventive measure in the management of these diseases.

Recognition of the Immunologic Manifestation

In order to recognize the immunologic manifestations of immunologically mediated disease, a thorough *history* and *physical examination* must be performed and appropriate *laboratory tests* must be made.

A family history is helpful in identifying patterns of allergic disease in parents or grandparents. Thus, in about 40 per cent of children with severe atopic allergy, a history can be elicited of one parent's having manifest allergy; if both parents have atopic disease, the incidence is raised to approximately 80 per cent in the offspring. In addition to genetic expression, a history of environmental exposure should be obtained. Agents to be looked for include a panorama of foods, inhalants, contactants, or infecting organisms that may be responsible for immunologic imbalance. The history of repeated respiratory–middle ear infections may provide the first clue to the diagnosis of allergic disease, particularly in small children.

Physical examination will reveal signs that vary with the age of the individual and with the length of exposure to the offending exogenous agent. In general, the type and degree of tissue involvement will determine the variety of physical signs. Similarly, appropriate labotatory tests, including nasal smears for eosinophilia, eosinophil counts, sedimentation rates, and appropriate radiographs, may help substantiate the diagnosis of allergic disease (Chapter 26).

Identification of the Offending Antigen

TESTS OF IMMEDIATE HYPERSENSITIVITY

***In Vivo* Tests.** The most commonly applied technique for the determination of sensitivity to a number of offending agents employs the demonstration of a reaginic effect when small amounts of antigen are introduced either into *(intradermal)* or onto (epicutaneous or prick test) the skin (Chapters 13 and 26). The principle underlying the procedure is based on the immediate-type hypersensitivity reaction that is mediated primarily by cell-bound IgE reaginic antibody. Following the encounter with specific antigen, there is a release of vasoactive substances from the tissue mast cells that results in erythema, induration, and wheal and flare reaction at the site of injection. This response is immediate (within minutes) and its timing assumes diagnostic importance. Occasionally, one encounters late cutaneous allergic reactions (LCAR) that occur four to six hours after the application of the test antigen and appear to be associated with the immediate IgE cutaneous responses. This LCAR may also contribute to the late bronchial provocation reaction as described below.

The P-K, or Prausnitz-Küstner, test represents the passive counterpart of this test and is performed by injecting serum from a positive individual into the skin of a normal recipient. After a latent period of 24 hours, the skin site is injected with specific antigen. If the serum contains reagin, an immediate hypersensitivity reaction is seen. The test is not as commonly used because of the risk of transmitting hepatitis B virus and the development of newer techniques of *in vitro* testing, e.g., RAST. The importance of an immediate skin test reaction is that it is diagnostic in ascertaining the atopic hypersensitivity. This has been particularly useful in the inhalatory antigens but is of limited value in the immunologic imbalance caused by food substances and drugs. The commonly used skin test allergens in allergy include extracts of dusts, molds, pollens, and animal dander.

Immediate-type skin reactivity is not to be confused with other skin tests, such as the Dick and Schick tests, that measure circulating antitoxin (toxin-neutralization) to erythrogenic toxin and diphtheria toxin, respectively, and not mediator release (Chapter 8). These are not mediated by IgE antibody but by classic IgG antibody.

Provocation Tests. Provocation challenge is another method of *in vivo* diagnosis that is sometimes used to further document immediate hypersensitivity states. These procedures include conjunctival, nasal, and bronchial challenge, as well as oral challenge in the case of ingestants. In addition to the use of specific antigens, pharmacologic agents, e.g., methacholine, have also been employed to demonstrate the autonomic imbalance.

There are basically three types of reactions commonly seen after bronchial challenge (Table 20–9, Fig. 20–20). These include the immediate, late, and dual responses. The immediate responses

Table 20–9. **Types of Responses Seen After Bronchial Provocation in Various Allergic Diseases of the Lung**

Type	Functional Response	Mechanism	Example of Disease
Immediate	Fall in FEV_1 within minutes	IgE (Type I)	Bronchial asthma
Late	Fall in FEV_1 within 4–6 hours	Type III or late IgE	Pulmonary hypersensitivity
Dual	Both immediate and late	Type I Type III or IgE	Allergic bronchopulmonary aspergillosis

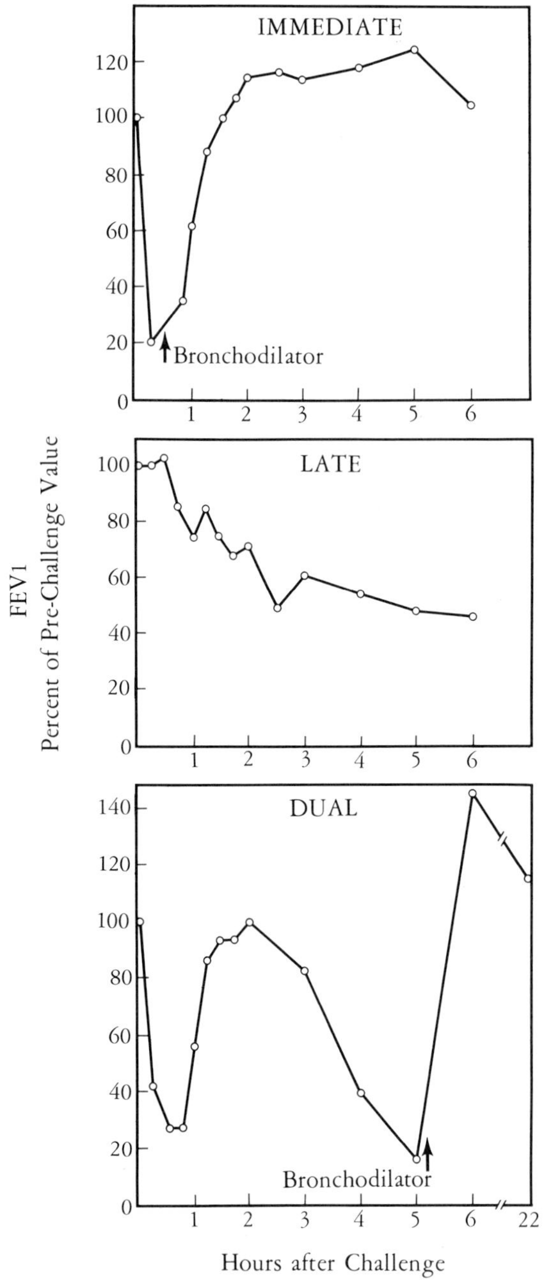

Figure 20–20. Schematic representation of various bronchial provocation responses (immediate, late, and dual) seen in allergic diseases of lung.

are characterized by a fall in FEV_1 within minutes of challenge, are triggered by the IgE Type I mechanism, and are classically seen in bronchial asthma. Late responses are characterized by a fall in FEV_1 within four to six hours after challenge, are mediated classically by antigen-antibody complexes (Type III) or the late effects of IgE antibody, and are classically seen in extrinsic allergic alveolitis. The dual responses involve both immediate and late reactions, are triggered by the immediate Type I responses of IgE, the late responses of IgE, or the responses of antigen-antibody complexes (Type III), and are classically seen in acute allergic bronchopulmonary aspergillosis.

***In Vitro* Tests.** There are a variety of *in vitro* tests for the detection of IgE globulin and IgE-associated antibody (Chapter 26). The most commonly employed test for the determination of serum IgE concentrations is the PRIST test. This assay is based on a radioimmunoassay and has the additional advantages of increased sensitivity and specificity. The principles underlying these procedures have been described in Chapter 8 and are shown schematically in Figure 20–21. Elevated concentrations of IgE are seen in atopic individuals, particularly in older children and adults. In addition, a wide variety of other nonatopic conditions have been associated with elevated IgE concentrations (Table 20–10). The most widely employed test for the detection of IgE-associated antibody is the radioallergosorbent test (RAST), which is represented schematically in Figure 20–21.

TESTS OF ARTHUS HYPERSENSITIVITY (TYPE III)

At times, it may be diagnostically helpful to examine for the presence of Type III (Arthus) reactions after the introduction of antigen into the skin. These responses are seen particularly in the mixed forms of hypersensitivity diseases of the lung, e.g., extrinsic allergic alveolitis or allergic bronchopulmonary aspergillosis. The principle underlying this response is based on the formation and subsequent deposition of antigen-antibody-complement complexes that initiate an inflammatory dermal reaction within four to eight hours.

TESTS OF DELAYED HYPERSENSITIVITY (TYPE IV)

***In Vivo* Tests.** Other skin tests of the delayed type are used for the assessment of accompanying infectious disease (Chapter 26). These include delayed-hypersensitivity reactions to histoplasmosis, blastomycosis, coccidioidomycosis, cat scratch disease, tuberculosis, and atypical mycobacteria.

Patch Tests. Patch test techniques evoke a skin response in sensitized individuals to surface contactants and represent a form of delayed-type hypersensitivity (Type IV).

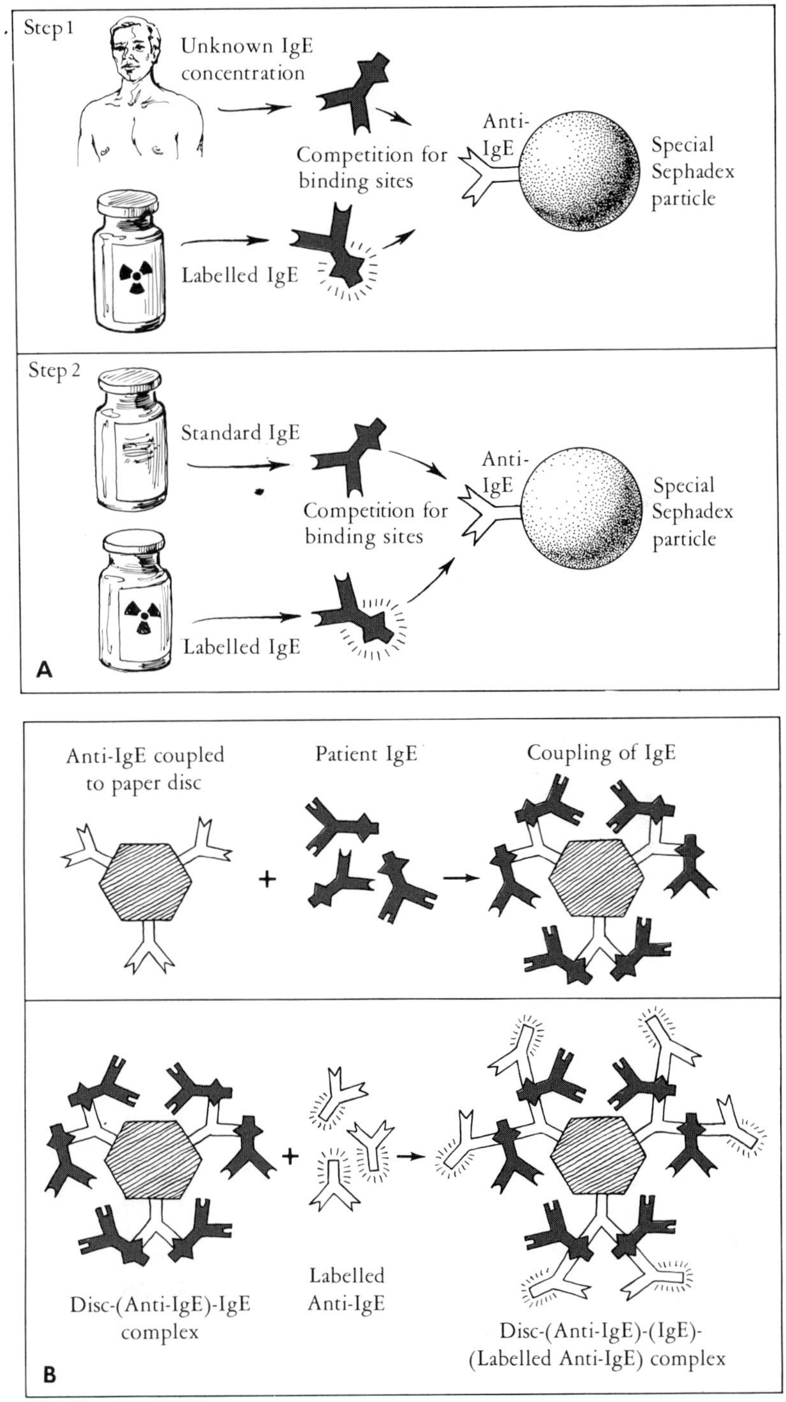

Figure 20–21. Schematic representation of the RIST *(A)*, the PRIST *(B)*, and the RAST *(C)*.

Illustration continued on following page.

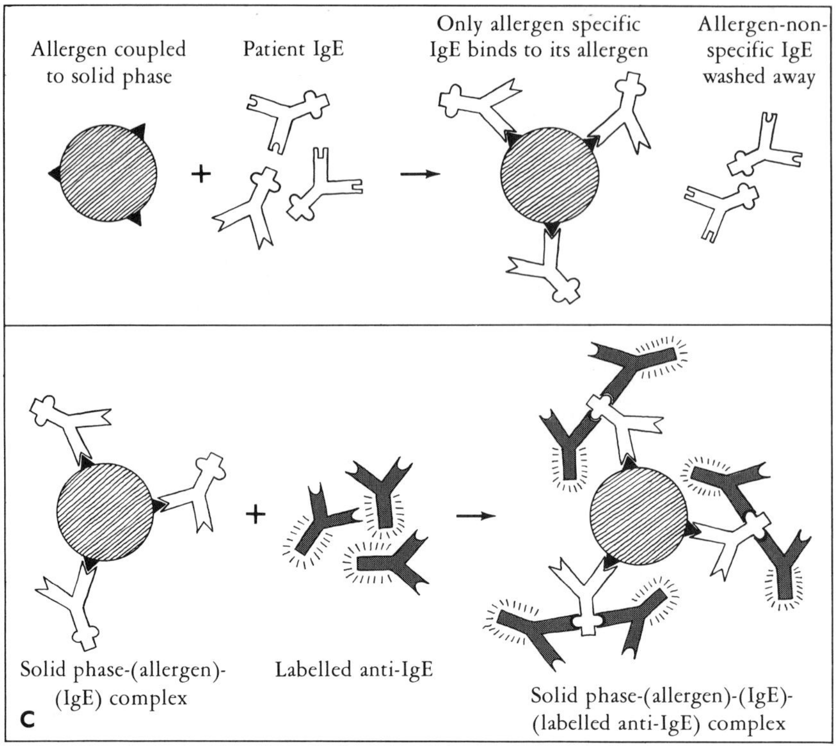

Figure 20–21C *Continued.*

After application of 24 to 48 hours, an erythematous reaction can be elicited at the site of contact with the offending material. This test is of value in determining contact hypersensitivity. In this situation, the offending agent acts as a hapten conjugated to tissue protein. The offending agents include a variety of dyes, metals, plastics, and organic materials.

***In Vitro* Tests.** *In vitro* tests of delayed hypersensitivity may also be performed.

Table 20–10. Clinical Conditions Associated with Elevations of IgE

Atopic
Eczema
Allergic rhinitis
Bronchial asthma
Food allergy (?)
Nonatopic
Parasitic infections
IgE myeloma
Immune deficiency:
Hypergammaglobulinemia E with recurrent infections
Wiskott-Aldrich
Thymic dysplasia
Pulmonary infiltrates with eosinophilia (PIE)
Loeffler's syndrome
Bronchopulmonary aspergillosis

These tests are described in greater detail in Chapter 26 and rely upon the detection of surface markers or morphologic and biochemical responses of T- and B-lymphocytes.

Therapy

Management of immunologically mediated disease in response to exogenous antigens rests on efforts to adequately identify the causative agent by history, physical examination, and laboratory procedures. If this is to be accomplished, the first role of the physician is to remove the offending agent from the patient. In some cases this is possible, e.g., the removal of household pets, an offending food, or the offending contactant. In other cases, such as with household dust or pollen, total elimination is a physical impossibility. In these cases, a regimen of allergic hyposensitization is often recommended. When the agent is identified as a susceptible bacterium, the offending agent can be eliminated by appropriate antibiotic or chemotherapeutic agents. The use of gamma globulin as a nonspecific adjunct in the treatment of allergic diseases rests on tenuous ground and must be condemned.

HYPOSENSITIZATION (IMMUNOTHERAPY)

After identification of the offending exogenous antigen, immunotherapy is frequently employed. This procedure has been shown to be of greater benefit in allergic rhinitis than in bronchial asthma. The procedure involves the injection into the host of gradually increasing doses of antigen, usually to maximal tolerated doses, at varying intervals in an attempt to develop blocking (IgG) antibody protection against these agents. The mechanism of this therapy is thought to be primarily due to the blocking effects of this antibody against reaginic IgE antibody. The demonstration of IgA blocking antibody in the nasal secretions of individuals undergoing immunotherapy has suggested another possible mechanism for immunotherapy. During the course of immunotherapy, elevated levels of IgE are seen initially; with continued therapy, however, there is a gradual decrease in IgE antibody that generally accompanies the elevation of IgG blocking antibody in the serum. In addition, evidence suggests that the development of IgA and IgG blocking antibody in nasal secretions occurs during immunotherapy, and its presence may correlate with improvement. These events are represented schematically in Figures 20–22 and 20–23. The recent observation of the development of antigen-specific suppressor cells following immunotherapy with ragweed antigen suggests a possible mechanism for the decrease in IgE known to occur with this form of therapy. It is obvious that such therapy may be ineffective unless accompanied by elimination of other agents to which the patient is sensitive.

PHARMACOLOGIC THERAPY

With the increased knowledge of the pathophysiologic mechanisms underlying allergic disease, it is possible to provide a more rational approach to the pharmacologic treatment of these diseases.

Antihistamines are frequently used to prevent the symptoms of IgE-mediated atopic allergies. They appear to modify the response and to interrupt the chemical mediation of a number of symptoms of allergic disorders, such as coryza, edema, and itching, characteristic of these entities. They act by antagonizing the effects of histamine. Their use in asthma may further enhance the degree of viscosity of mucus owing to their atropine-like effect and may further complicate the obstructive phenomenon characteristic of the asthmatic state. Their use alone in the treatment of this entity has not been recommended. Recently, however, this cholinergic effect of antihistaminics has been questioned; therefore, if required in therapy, they may be used in conjunction with other antiasthmatic medications. In addition, other drugs, such as the hydroxyzines, are of benefit in the treatment of urticaria and serum sickness. These drugs have a diverse action that includes an antihistaminic, anticholinergic, and antiserotonin activity.

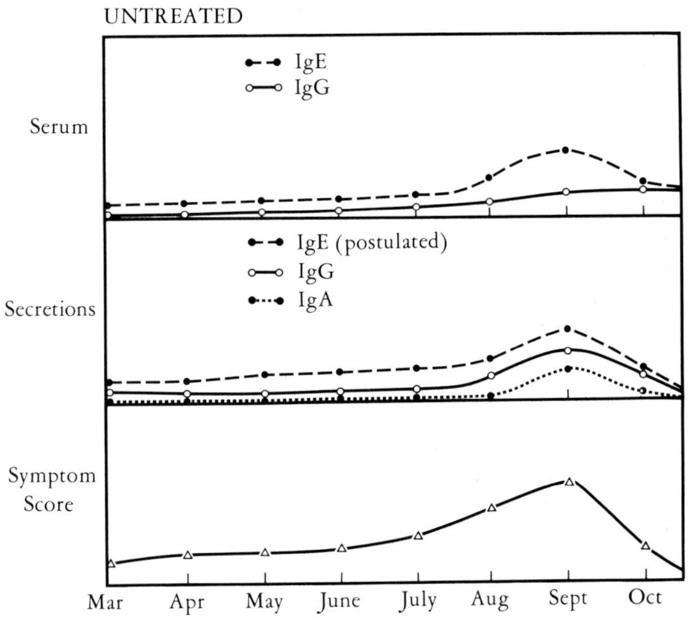

Figure 20–22. Schematic representation of the changes in serum and secretory immunoglobulins and symptom score in untreated allergic individuals.

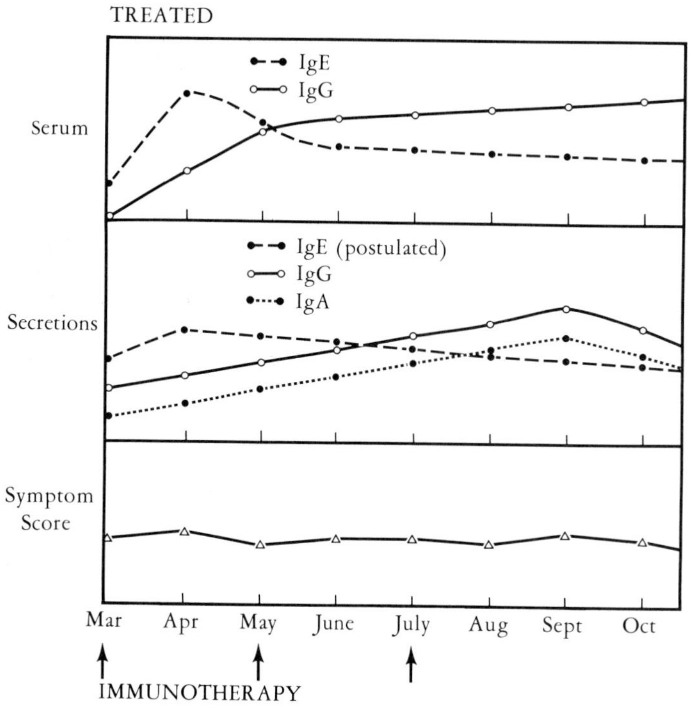

Figure 20–23. Schematic representation of the changes in serum and secretory immunoglobulins and symptom score in treated allergic individuals.

Another group of drugs is the β agonists that act by stimulating the β receptors (Fig. 20–16). The most efficacious drug for the treatment of immediate hypersensitivity reactions, particularly the anaphylactic, is epinephrine. This drug acts on both β_1 and β_2 adrenergic receptors: (1) β_1 stimulation affects such organs as the heart and skeletal muscle, and (2) β_2 stimulation affects the smooth musculature, blood vessels, and mucus-secreting glands of the lung, for example. The β_1 stimulatory effects of epinephrine are a disadvantage, and various sympathomimetic drugs have been developed by alterations in the basic structure of the epinephrine moiety. These drugs have resulted in agents that contain more β_2 and less β_1 activity and are available both for aerosolization and for systemic use, e.g., isoetharine, metaproterenol, terbutaline, and salbutamol (albuterol).

Another group of drugs that act on the cyclic nucleotide system are the xanthine drugs. Theophylline is one of the most useful drugs in the treatment of asthma. It acts primarily by inhibiting the effects of phosphodiesterase, leading to enhanced levels of cAMP. The drug is best utilized orally or parenterally (5 to 7 mg per kilogram per six hours in children or half the dose in adults); however, owing to pharmacokinetic differences in drug metabolism, particularly in children, it is important that blood levels be obtained in order to prevent toxicity; optimal blood levels are usually achieved within the range of 10 to 20 μg per milliliter.

Disodium cromoglycate (cromolyn) is used in the prevention of bronchial asthma (Fig. 20–16). It is particularly effective in extrinsic asthma and exercise-induced asthma. Its mode of action is to prevent the release of mediators from mediator cells, presumably by preventing calcium influx after the allergen-IgE reaction. Reports have suggested toxic reactions to the drug consisting of hypersensitivity pneumonitis, which is reversible upon cessation of the drug.

The corticosteroids have also been useful in preventing or modifying many of the hypersensitivity manifestations of several allergic states, primarily through their anti-inflammatory effect (Chapter 25). They may be applied locally in atopic and contact dermatitis but also have been used systemically in all allergic diseases. Because of side-effects, however, the systemic use of the medication has been reserved for cases refractory to other modes of therapy. The recent development of corticosteroid drugs that can be administered by aerosolization, e.g., beclomethosone and triamcinolone, has provided new approaches to the use of these agents, which have the advantage of producing few or no systemic side effects when used by the aerosol route. Although local candidiasis and mucosal cell atrophy have been reported after use of these local steroidal preparations, these do not appear to be serious side effects.

Although systemic use of atropine-like drugs for the treatment of asthma has been avoided in the past because of their drying effects, recent studies have indicated that atropine administered via the aerosol route may be a valuable adjunct in the treatment of bronchial asthma. This approach provides relief of the cholinergic stimulation through its parasympatholytic effect.

INSECT ALLERGY

A specialized group of allergic reactions are those caused by insects. These include those that result from stinging insects (e.g., bees, wasps, yellow jackets, and hornets), from biting insects (e.g., deerfly, blackfly, and the fire ant), or from insect emanations (e.g., caddis fly and cockroach). The mechanisms of these reactions vary with each and may result from the venom (stinging insects), from the salivary secretions (the biting insects), or from inhalation of the allergen (insect emanations). These reactions are for the most part IgE-mediated and may be localized or systemic. The stinging insects produce most serious reactions, which may be life-threatening anaphylactic reactions. The management of these reactions requires a careful history or direct examination of the site (some produce a distinctive lesion, e.g., the fire ant). Preventive measures include avoidance, when possible; however, for those in certain occupations, e.g., agricultural workers and bee keepers, this may not be possible. Purified specific venom is more effective than whole-body extracts for testing and appears to be the treatment of choice. Several enzymes have been found in the venom that appear to be potent allergens, e.g., phospholipase A. The continuing development of RAST and ELISA procedures that can measure the specific antibodies to these allergens may be useful in the future in diagnosis and evaluation of treatment regimen.

ALLERGIC DRUG REACTIONS

Adverse drug reactions have become increasingly common as the number and variety of therapeutic agents have multiplied. It is estimated that between 5 and 10 per cent of hospital inpatients have drug reactions during their stay and that in the general population there is an incidence of approximately 0.1 to 1 per cent of allergic reactions to any given drug. Moreover, as many as 15 per cent of individuals in the general population believe themselves to be allergic to one or more drugs and therefore may be unnecessarily deprived of an effective drug in a subsequent therapeutic situation. Clearly, it is important to recognize such adverse reactions and to understand their immunologic basis in order to prevent their occurrence or to ameliorate their disease expressions.

Classification of Drug Reactions

A drug may be defined as any agent used in the diagnosis, treatment, or prevention of disease. In addition to the wide range of drugs currently available to the physician for the treatment of disease, e.g., antibiotics (penicillin), anti-inflammatory drugs (aspirin), anticonvulsant drugs (phenytoin), and local anesthetics (lidocaine), all of which may be associated with adverse reactions, other agents used in the diagnosis of disease, e.g., contrast media (diatrizoate), can also give rise to adverse reactions. The subject of adverse reactions to biologicals used in the prevention of disease, e.g., sera and vaccines, will be discussed in Chapters 23 and 24. Thus, adverse drug reactions can arise during the course of normal therapeutic or diagnostic procedures and can be superimposed upon already existing clinical conditions to create two clinical problems instead of one.

For ease of discussion, the adverse drug reactions are commonly divided into the following groups: (1) *overdosage,* (2) *intolerance,* (3) *idiosyncrasy,* (4) *side effects,* (5) *secondary effects,* (6) *drug interactions,* and (7) *allergy (hypersensitivity).* Overdosage refers to the symptoms that occur after excessive intake or failure of normal metabolism or excretion of a drug. When the symptoms of overdosage occur at normal pharmacologic doses of the drug, the adverse reaction is referred to as *intolerance. Idiosyncrasy* refers to a qualitatively abnormal response after drug administration that differs from its pharmacologic effect but is not immunologically determined. Idiosyncratic effects generally result from a biochemical variation in drug metabolism. For example, in individuals with G-6-PD deficiency, the ingestion of primaquine results in enhanced red cell hemolysis. A *side effect* is defined as a therapeutically undesirable but often unavoidable action of a drug, e.g., drowsiness associated with antihistamine therapy. In addition to the primary action of a drug, *secondary effects* occasionally are seen, e.g., candidiasis in patients receiving tetracycline. Another category of adverse drug reactions that is assuming increased clinical importance is that of *drug interaction.* This is defined as the action of one drug upon the effectiveness or toxicity of another. Drug interactions may occur *in vitro* owing to incompatibility of drugs when mixed, or *in vivo* when one drug affects the absorption, protein binding, metabolism, excretion, or interactions at the binding site of another drug. Finally, *allergic (hypersensitivity)* reactions are similar to the idiosyncratic reactions in that both are qualitatively abnormal reactions occurring in small numbers of patients. However, unlike idiosyncrasy, the allergic reactions are immunologically mediated. This section will focus primarily on these allergic drug reactions.

Factors Influencing the Development of Drug Allergies

Basically, two groups of factors appear to influence the development of drug hypersensitivity: (1) *drug factors* and (2) *host factors.*

DRUG FACTORS

The immunogenicity of the drug will be affected by its basic nature. For example, some inert drugs, such as the antacids that are composed of simple inorganic chemicals, rarely produce adverse reactions. The capacity to induce an immune response depends upon the capacity of the drug or one of its reactive metabolites to bind to tissue proteins and to then function as a complete immunogen.

Drugs initiating allergic manifestations are usually chemicals of low molecular weight (< 1000 MW) and therefore are not immunogenic in themselves. They act as haptens and must form a firm covalent bond with a tissue protein before an immunologic response can be generated. In some cases, the drug administered is not directly immunogenic, but its degradation products are. The prime example of this is penicillin (Fig. 20–24).

The most frequently used penicillin, benzylpenicillin, produces several distinct breakdown products (Fig. 20–24). When benzylpenicillin is allowed to interact with protein, the major proportion (approximately 95 per cent) forms the benzylpenicilloyl (BPO) haptenic group, the "major" haptenic group. A small proportion of the benzylpenicillin degrades further to produce a number of metabolites, including benzylpenicilloic acid, benzylpenaldic acid, and penicillamine. These may all act as haptens, combining with protein to form antigenic determinants collectively known as the "minor" determinants. These "minor" haptenic groups have major clinical importance, however. Although IgE antibodies are directed against both major and minor antigenic determinants, most of the IgE reaginic antibodies responsible for severe immediate hypersensitivity drug reactions are directed against the minor determinants.

Other clinical reactions related to these metabolic degradation products of drugs are seen. Drugs may cross react because their basic structures are similar or the degradation products are antigenically related. For example, multiple semisynthetic penicillins have been produced by the modification of the side chain attached to the beta-lactam ring of the penicillin nucleus. Since most of the immunologic reactivity of the penicillin nucleus is directed to the 6-aminopenicillanic acid nucleus common to all, variations of the side chain have little effect in decreasing cross allergenicity between penicillin and other homologs. Thus, oxacillin, nafcillin, ampicillin, and carbenicillin produce the same types of allergic reactions in penicillin-allergic individuals as does benzylpenicillin.

Although a wide variety of drugs have been implicated in hypersensitivity drug reactions, the more common drug allergens include: *antibiotics* (e.g., penicillin), *anti-inflammatory agents* (e.g., aspirin), and *chemotherapeutic agents* (e.g., sulfonamides). Collectively, these drugs account for 80 to 90 per cent of allergic drug reactions encountered in the human.

Another factor influencing drug allergy is the route by which the drug is administered. Topical application of a drug has the greatest capacity for inducing sensitivity, e.g., contact sensitivity; oral administration has the least.

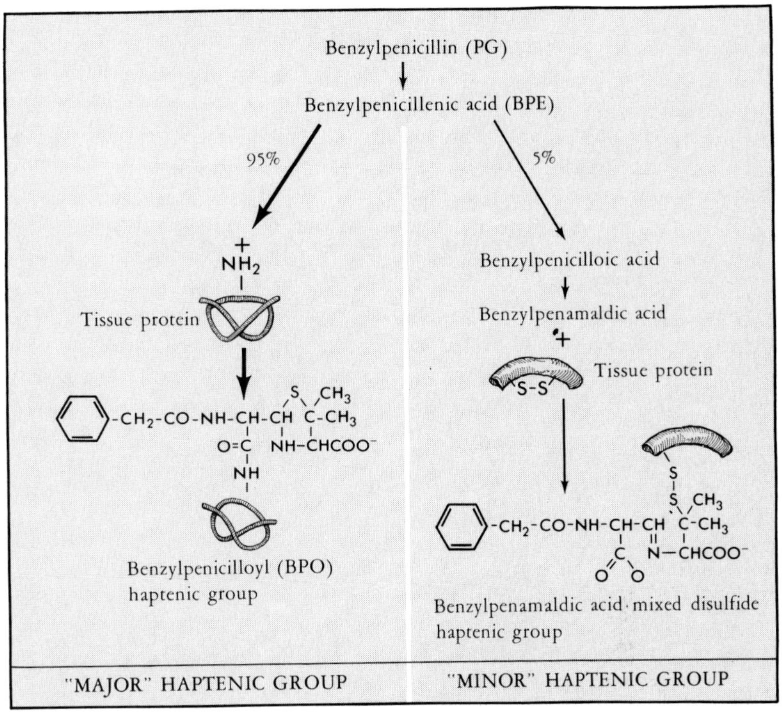

Figure 20–24. Schematic representation of the breakdown products of penicillin thought to be important in penicillin hypersensitivity. (After Levine B.: Genetic factors in hypersensitivity reactions to drugs. Ann. N.Y. Acad. Sci., *151*:988, 1968.)

The likelihood of reactions following parenteral administration is considered intermediate. Thus, commonly used effective antibiotics that have a potential systemic use should not be used topically, and, except in serious life-threatening infections, the oral route is preferred.

The degree of exposure to a drug may also affect the likelihood of sensitization. The induction period, the time between drug administration and onset of symptoms, varies from one individual to another. In general, the immediacy of onset of the allergic drug reaction is proportional to the degree of prior exposure. Reactions of later onset may reflect the results of an ongoing sensitization. Although prolonged administration of drugs at higher doses would suggest a greater likelihood of sensitization, clinically this does not appear to be the case. The more a drug is used, however, the more likely that a drug reaction will develop in any susceptible individual. Furthermore, it should be noted that a drug reaction can be seen in individuals without known prior administration of the drug. For example, penicillin reactions have been observed in individuals who have received the drug for the first time. This presumably represents sensitization by trace amounts of penicillin in food, milk, or nature.

HOST FACTORS

Age. Drug allergy, although appearing in all ages, is seen less frequently in the young. This may reflect the developmental immunologic deficiency of the younger patient or simply the lower degree of exposure to drugs required for sensitization at this age.

Genetic Makeup of the Individual. The fact that only a small proportion of the population is affected indicates a genetic predisposition to drug hypersensitivity rather than a drug effect *per se.* Information concerning genetic controls operative in drug hypersensitivity is limited. However, many clinical and experimental observations have been made recently that suggest the relationship between drug hypersensitivity and genetic regulation. Although allergic drug hypersensitivity, particularly to penicillin, has been thought to occur with greater frequency in atopic individuals, more recent evidence has not confirmed this impression. Furthermore, the atopic state does not predispose to the development of contact sensitivity or the immune-complex type of drug allergy.

Conceptually, genetic controls may be operative in any of the following types of mechanisms (Fig. 20–25): (1) the metabolic degradation of a drug, (2) the capacity to

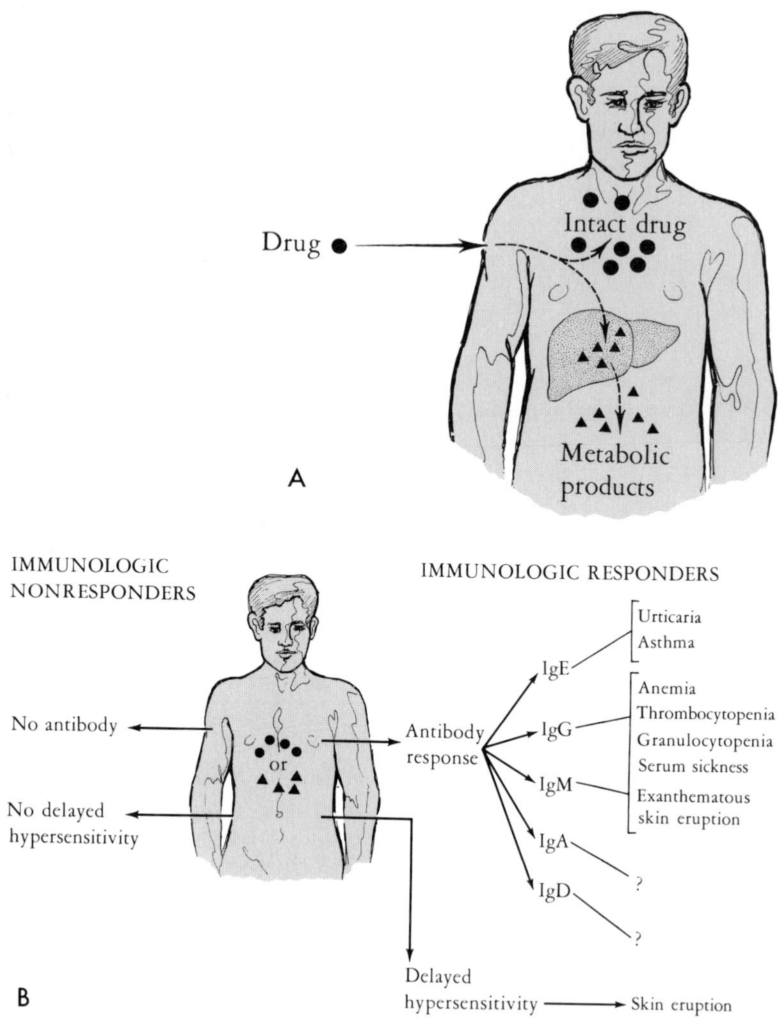

Figure 20–25. Schematic representation of the points at which genetic mechanisms may be operative in drug hypersensitivity: (1) metabolic degradation of a drug *(A),* (2) the capacity to respond with the elaboration of components of the imunologic array *(B),* (3) the structural integrity of the receptor sites on tissue cells *(C),* and (4) the elaboration of pharmacologically active mediators *(C)* as shown in the four types of mechanisms of immunologic injury.

elaborate components of the immunologic array, (3) the structural integrity of the receptor site on tissue cells, and (4) the elaboration of pharmacologically active mediators.

Metabolic Degradation of a Drug. As described above, the allergic drug reaction is often directed against metabolic degradation products of the drug. Thus, it is apparent that in the allergic individual, the development of drug hypersensitivity may be a function of genetically determined differences in drug metabolism.

Elaboration of the Immunologic Array. The varieties of reactions to a drug are as different as the genetic constitutions of the individuals who receive it. Again, penicillin serves to illustrate this variation of immunologic response (Fig. 20–25*B*). Some individuals produce IgE antibodies that result in various urticarial reactions. Others produce IgM antibodies complexed with penicillin that have been associated with exanthematous skin reactions. In still others, destruction of hematopoietic cells is produced, resulting in hemolytic anemia, granulocytopenia, or thrombocytopenia. The nature of the control of these mechanisms is still unclear.

The mechanisms by which a drug produces blood dyscrasias are unknown. Five mechanisms have been proposed (Fig. 20–25*C*). The first mechanism is that of IgE-mediated injury. Anaphylactic reactions are those reactions that involve the release of vasoactive amines from mediator cells and can involve Type I (homocytotropic), Type II (cytotoxic), or Type III (anaphylotoxic) responses, as described in Chapter 13. The most frequent and most serious are the IgE responses. Mimicking the anaphylactic reactions are those in which the release of vasoactive substances from mediator cells occurs by nonimmunologic mechanisms, e.g., bee venom, anesthesia, or drugs. These reactions are sometimes termed *anaphylactoid.*

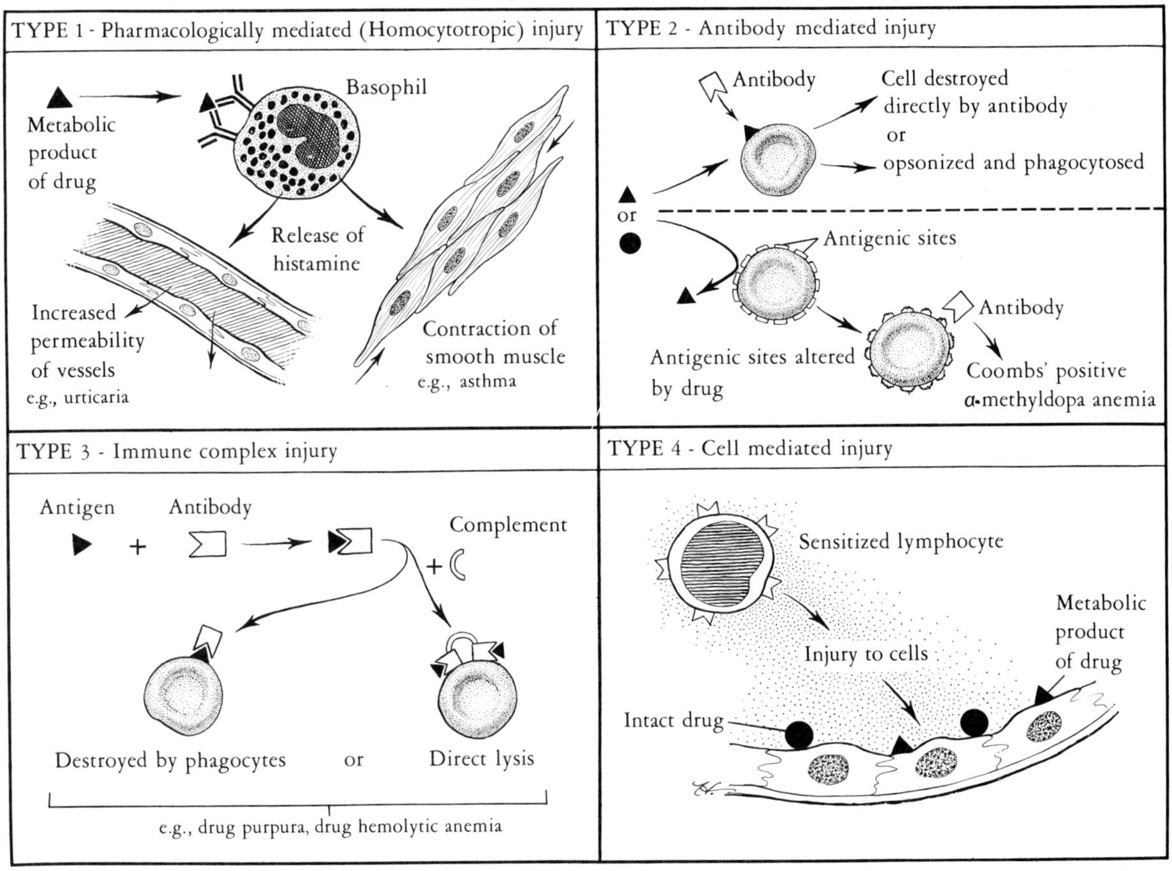

C

Figure 20–25 *Continued*

Another mechanism was postulated by Ackroyd, who demonstrated the presence of platelet-lysing antibodies in the sera of patients who had received the drug apronalide (Sedormid). When platelets, drug, and complement were added *in vitro,* the platelets were lysed. The platelet cell was assumed to contain the carrier protein that complexed with the drug (hapten), and then antibodies were developed against the platelets (Fig. 20–25*C*, Type II); antibodies to the drug were not demonstrated, however. The nature of this reaction is unexplained on the basis of classic hapten immunology, in which antibodies are usually formed to the hapten, and, therefore, the nature of this reaction is still unclear.

Another mechanism is Type II of hemolytic anemia seen in penicillin hypersensitivity, in which the major haptenic antigen (BPO) attaches firmly to the red cell surface and antibodies are directed to the hapten. This antibody then coats cells, which produce a positive Coombs test, after which the red cells are removed. This phenomenon has been referred to as "passive" hemagglutination or "passive" hemolysis (Fig. 20–25*C*, Type II).

The fourth mechanism is one of antigen-antibody complexes in which antibodies to the drug and the hapten form soluble complexes (Fig. 20–25*C*, Type III). Subsequent injury of the target cell occurs through the direct cytotoxic effect of these complexes. This phenomenon is reminiscent of the leukopenia and thrombocytopenia seen in serum sickness, in which it has been shown that immune complexes with complement lead to the rapid elimination of these cells from the circulation.

Another mechanism involves alteration of cell surface antigens by drugs such as alpha-methyldopa (Fig. 20–25*C*, Type II). This mechanism leads to autoantibody formation, and this will be described later.

The complexes of drug with antibody can also result in a more generalized serum sickness reaction with involvement of skin, joints, and kidneys. Finally, contact hypersensitivity to penicillin has resulted from the repeated handling of the drug by medical personnel. While the capacity to become allergically sensitive to all drugs probably is under complex genetic control, it has been postulated that a genetic polymorphism exists to respond to certain immunogens with the production of reaginic antibody, the atopic condition. Atopic individuals appear to be more susceptible to reactions mediated by reaginic antibody than nonatopic individuals. Recent studies in humans and animals suggest the existence of genes that control the capacity to respond to specific allergens and others that regulate the amounts of IgE synthesized under the influence of suppressor T-cells (Chapter 3). Moreover, in the case of contact hypersensitivity, recent work suggests that the expression of these hypersensitivity states can be regulated by suppressor T-cells (Chapter 10). This knowledge concerning the genetic controls of immunologic reactivity should provide new approaches to the prevention and therapy of allergic drug reactions in the future.

Receptor Sites. Several explanations have been proposed to explain drug allergies on the basis of variability of tissue receptor sites or differences in binding of the drug with products of the immune response (Fig. 20–25*C*). For example, alpha-methyldopa administration has been associated with the appearance of a positive Coombs test in certain individuals. The autoantibody has been shown to be of the IgG warm active type and has shown specificity for the Rh locus. Presumably, tissue receptors at the Rh locus are modified by the drug or its products. These observations suggest that a genetic control may exist at the tissue receptor sites, accounting for drug hypersensitivity in some individuals.

Elaboration of Pharmacologically Active Mediators. The elaboration of pharmacologically active mediators may also be a controlling factor in the development of drug allergy. Inbred strains of animals show striking variations in histamine release. Variations in response to a single drug also occur within a strain. These observations have not been substantiated in man, but the great variability in urticarial lesions, for example, from individual to individual suggests that the elaboration of these mediators may be under genetic control and may account for the variability of drug reactions in man (Fig. 20–25*C*). As described above, the anaphylactic reaction may be an example of this phenomenon.

Clinical Varieties of Drug Reactions

The clinical manifestations of drug reactions are varied and can affect virtually every tissue of the body. For ease of discussion, the clinical varieties of drug reactions can be divided into: (1) *systemic* and (2) *cutaneous.* The common manifestations of both are shown in Table 20–11 and Table 20–12, together with examples of drugs known to cause these various manifestations.

SYSTEMIC VARIETIES OF DRUG REACTIONS

Drug Fever. One aspect of drug reactions is drug fever. This condition is characterized by a temperature elevation seen during the course of drug administration. The diagnosis of this condition may be at times perplexing, since the drug is usually an antibiotic, e.g., penicillin, that is being used in the treatment of an ongoing infection in which fever may also be seen. Drug fever should always be suspected if a prolonged febrile response occurs in the patient after adequate antibiotic therapy. Drug fever may be associated with a vasculitis characterized by multiple small vessel inflammation. If allowed to continue, the drug can lead to severe organ damage. Early recognition of the condition is therefore mandatory.

Anaphylactic, Accelerated, and Late Reactions. Classification of allergic drug reactions can be based on the time of onset of symptoms after administration of the drug (Table 20–13). The most serious drug reactions occur within minutes of drug administration and are characterized by urticaria, hypotension, and shock. When the reaction is life-threatening, it is termed *anaphylactic* or *anaphylactoid.* These reactions are *immediate* and are mediated primarily by the IgE reaginic antibodies, which in the case of penicillin hypersensitivity are directed toward the minor haptenic groups of the molecule. *Accelerated* reactions begin from 1 to 72 hours after drug administration and are almost always manifested by urticaria. They occasionally take the form of morbilliform eruptions and laryngeal edema, which are associated with antibodies directed toward the major antigen. The *late* reactions begin three days after therapy and are seen as various forms of skin eruptions, serum sickness, and drug fever (Fig. 20–26). More rarely, the unusually late reactions, which are listed in Table 20–13, are seen. Although it is not known with certainty, the accelerated drug allergies are thought to be mediated by IgE, and the late allergic reactions are thought to be mediated by soluble antigen-antibody complexes in which the antibodies are pri-

Table 20–11. **Clinical Patterns of Adverse Drug Reactions: Systemic**

Manifestation	Example of Drug
Drug fever	Para-aminosalicylic acid
Anaphylaxis	Penicillin
Serum sickness syndrome	Penicillin, serum
Pulmonary manifestations	
Bronchial asthma	Aspirin
	Nitrofurantoin
Hypersensitivity lung disease	Cromolyn
Loeffler's type syndrome (pulmonary infiltrate with eosinophilia [PIE])	Para-aminosalicylic acid
Interstitial fibrosis	
Vasculitis	Sulfonamides
Hematologic-lymphoreticular manifestations	
Eosinophilia	Phenytoin (Dilantin)
Thrombocytopenia	Chlorothiazides
Hemolytic anemia	Alpha-methyldopa (Aldomet)
Lymphadenopathy	Phenytoin (Dilantin)
Hepatic manifestations	
Cholestasis	Phenothiazines
Hepatocellular damage	Iproniazid
Collagen-vascular manifestations	
Vasculitis	Penicillin
Polyarteritis	Sulfonamides
SLE–like	Hydralazine

marily of the IgG and IgM varieties. The unusually late reactions are triggered by a variety of immunologic mechanisms and are less readily classified. For example, some are associated with IgG cytolytic (Type II) reactions, e.g., hemolytic anemia; others with antigen-antibody complexes (Type III), e.g., thrombocytopenia; and still others with unknown mechanisms, e.g., the Stevens-Johnson syndrome.

Serum Sickness Syndrome. The syndrome of serum sickness was originally described after the use of foreign serum in passive immunization. The reaction resulted from the vehicle of the heterologous serum (Chapter 24). This response is no longer commonly seen after the use of heterologous serum, since, whenever possible, human sources of antibody are now used in immunotherapy. It has since been observed that some drugs may

Table 20–12. **Clinical Patterns of Adverse Drug Reactions: Cutaneous**

Manifestation	Example of Drug
Contact dermatitis	Penicillin, paraben esters
Urticaria and angioedema	Salicylates
Exanthematous eruptions	Barbiturates
Erythema multiforme–like eruptions (Stevens-Johnson syndrome)	Phenytoin (Dilantin)
Erythema nodosum	Iodides and bromides
Purpuric eruptions	Sulfonamides
Exfoliative dermatitis	Barbiturates
Fixed drug eruptions	Phenolphthalein
Photosensitivity	
Phototoxicity	Chlorpromazine
Photoallergy	Sulfonamides

Table 20–13. Clinical Types of Allergic Drug Reactions*

Immediate	Accelerated	Late	Usually Late
Urticaria	Urticaria	Urticaria	Hemolytic anemia
Hypotension	Morbilliform eruptions	Exanthematic skin reactions	Thrombocytopenia
Asthma	Laryngeal edema	Serum sickness–like reactions	Granulocytopenia
Laryngeal edema		Drug fever	Stevens-Johnson syndrome
			Acute renal insufficiency
			Lupus-like syndrome
			Cholestatic jaundice

*After Levine, B. B.: Genetic factors in hypersensitivity reactions to drugs. Ann. N.Y. Acad. Sci., *151*:988, 1968.

also induce a serum sickness–like syndrome. Clinically, the syndrome is characterized by low-grade fever, urticaria, facial edema, pain and swelling of the joints, and lymphadenopathy. Occasionally, other complications occur, such as periarteritis nodosa, Guillain-Barré syndrome, brachial plexus neuritis, optic neuritis, and nephritis.

Pulmonary Manifestations. The lung is occasionally the primary target organ of injury during the course of many adverse drug reactions (Table 20–11). Bronchial asthma, which is the most common pulmonary manifestation of a drug reaction, can occur following the systemic use of drugs such as aspirin. Other forms of hypersensitivity lung disease have been seen following the administration of drugs used in therapy, e.g., nitrofurantoin. Some pulmonary drug reactions are accompanied by the pulmonary infiltration with eosinophilia (PIE) syndrome, e.g., para-aminosalicylic acid. Other drugs can lead to chronic forms of pulmonary injury with fibrosis, e.g., busulfan. Although the precise mechanisms of immunologic injury involved in lung injury are unknown, it has been suggested that with some drugs, e.g., nitrofurantoin, Types II and III injury may be involved in the acute form of the disease and Type IV mechanisms may be operative in the chronic forms. The lung may also be involved in allergic vasculitis, which is usually one of the systemic manifestations of the collagen-vascular diseases.

Hematologic-Lymphoreticular Manifestations. Each of the circulating blood elements can be adversely affected in allergic drug reactions by any of the mechanisms described previously (Table 20–11). Eosinophilia may accompany other adverse drug reactions or may be the sole manifestation of drug hypersensitivity. Its presence, therefore, should alert the clinician to the possibility of an adverse drug reaction. Thrombocytopenia is also a well-known complication; it presents clinically with petechiae or, rarely, with hemorrhage. A wide variety of drugs can produce this clinical syndrome, e.g., chlorothiazides.

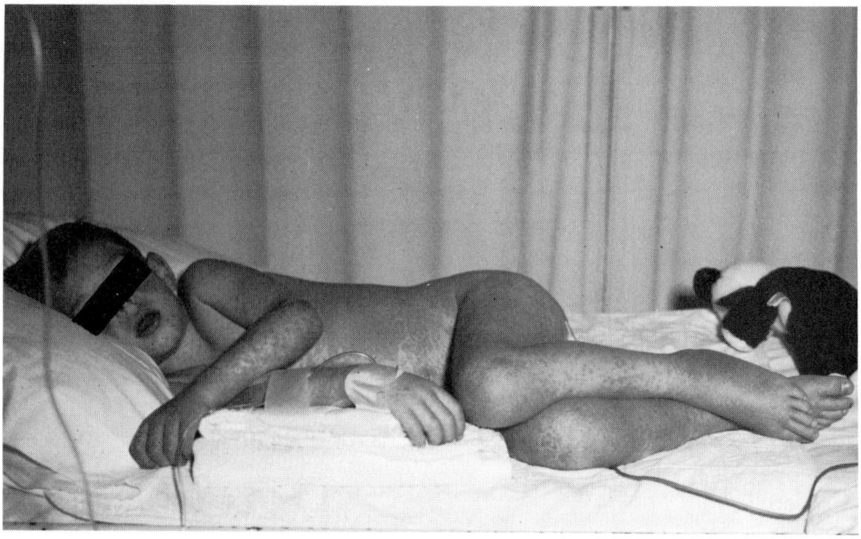

Figure 20–26. Photograph of a child with a late drug reaction due to ampicillin. Note the generalized exanthem, edema of the extremities, and involvement of the joints characteristic of a serum sickness–like reaction.

Hemolytic anemia due to immunologically mediated injury of red cells, e.g., alpha-methyldopa (Aldomet), must be differentiated from the idiosyncratic form that stems from a deficiency of the enzyme glucose-6-phosphate dehydrogenase, e.g., primaquine. Lymphadenopathy is also a common feature of many allergic drug reactions, particularly as part of the serum sickness syndrome. However, it may be present as an isolated event ("pseudolymphoma"), particularly with the anticonvulsant drugs, e.g., phenytoin.

Hepatic Manifestations. The liver can be involved in two types of adverse drug reactions: (1) *cholestasis* and (2) *hepatocellular damage*. Intrahepatic cholestasis is associated primarily with the phenothiazines, which give rise to a clinical picture of biliary obstruction that is usually reversible upon cessation of the drug. The second type of hepatic reaction is that of hepatocellular damage resembling the clinical picture of viral hepatitis. This is a more serious sequela and may not be reversible; it is seen with drugs such as the monoamine oxidase inhibitors, e.g., iproniazid.

Collagen-Vascular Manifestations. Drug allergy should be suspected in the differential diagnosis of all collagen-vascular diseases, since the two diseases can mimic each other. A clinical picture of vasculitis including polyarteritis nodosa with involvement of the skin, musculoskeletal system, kidneys, lungs, and peripheral nerves has been seen after the use of penicillin and the sulfonamides, as well as with a wide variety of other drugs. Other vascular involvements, e.g., Wegener's granulomatosis, allergic granulomatosis, and temporal arteritis, also occur and are less commonly associated with drug administration.

The drug-induced systemic lupus erythematosus–like picture is a well-recognized syndrome following the administration of several drugs, e.g., hydralazine and procainamide (Chapter 20C). This presents with manifestations indistinguishable from those of systemic lupus erythematosus (SLE), e.g., fever, rash, arthritis, and the presence of antinuclear antibodies. It is uncertain whether the mechanism of this reaction is a drug effect *per se* or whether the drug is selecting the individual genetically predisposed to the natural disease.

Nephropathy. The kidney may be affected in adverse drug reactions either as a glomerulonephritis or as an interstitial nephritis. Several of the anticonvulsants, e.g., trimethadione (Tridione), have been associated with the development of the clinical picture of the nephrotic syndrome indistinguishable from that of the minimal disease type. An interstitial nephritis with tubular damage has been observed after the administration of the penicillins, particularly methicillin. Although a Type III mechanism of injury has been implicated, antitubular membrane antibodies (ATM) have also been demonstrated in this entity.

Neurologic Manifestations. The nervous system has also been involved as the adventitious target of injury in adverse drug reactions. Several drugs have been known to produce a postvaccinal encephalomyelitis–like picture, as well as a peripheral neuritis, either alone or as part of the serum sickness–like syndrome (Table 20–11).

CUTANEOUS VARIETIES OF DRUG REACTIONS

Contact Dermatitis. An allergic eczematous contact dermatitis may be produced by drugs that are applied topically to the skin or mucous membranes and can be exacerbated after the systemic administration of drugs (Table 20–12). Physicians, nurses, and pharmacists are particularly likely to develop such reactions during the course of handling such drugs, e.g., penicillin; dentists are susceptible to similar problems from handling local anesthetics. A particular problem of increasing importance associated with contact sensitization is that of the paraben esters, which are used as preservatives in creams and lotions.

Urticaria and Angioedema. Urticaria and angioedema can occur as isolated events but may be part of the serum sickness–like reaction. In either case, a diligent search for a drug etiology should be made in every patient. A long list of drugs is associated with this clinical picture; the most common are penicillin and the salicylates.

Exanthematous Eruptions. A wide variety of exanthems may accompany adverse drug reactions. These range from erythematous macular, papular lesions to petechial purpuric lesions and very often may be confused with the common viral exanthems (Fig. 20–26). A wide variety of drugs may produce these lesions; the most common offenders are the barbiturates, penicillin (particularly ampicillin), and the anticonvulsants, e.g., phenytoin.

Of special interest are the two major types of drug eruptions due to ampicillin: (1) a toxic reaction, and (2) an immunologic reaction. After the administration of ampicillin, a florid erythematous eruption may be seen within the first week of therapy. This may be exaggerated in patients with infectious mononucleosis or other viral infections. These toxic reactions associated with ampicillin are not immunologically mediated, and the eruptions subside promptly after the drug is stopped. These reactions may be triggered by toxic impurities in the preparations. With recent improvements in the preparation of ampicillin, however, more purified preparations of the drug are available that have fewer of these toxic reactions. In addition to these toxic reactions, the truly immunologically mediated reactions to ampicillin may occur because of the cross-reacting 6-aminopenicillenic acid nucleus. These reactions may present clinically with urticaria or with more life-threatening sequelae characteristic of true penicillin hypersensitivity.

A particularly important variant of cutaneous drug eruptions is that of the erythema multiforme eruption due to drug allergy and its malignant variant that affects the mucous membranes, the Stevens-Johnson syndrome. Erythema multiforme should be suspected whenever the classic features of erythema with typical bull's eye, sharply circumscribed lesions with central clearing (iris lesions) are present. The Stevens-Johnson syndrome should be suspected whenever the mucous membranes are involved, e.g., mouth, anus, vulva, and conjunctivae. A wide variety of drugs have been implicated in the pathogenesis of these diseases, e.g., phenytoin.

Exfoliative Dermatitis. Extensive erythema and scaling with shedding of the superficial skin characterize the severe adverse drug reaction exfoliative dermatitis. Death is frequent, particularly in the debilitated or the elderly. Commonly involved drugs include the heavy metals, the barbiturates, and the sulfonamides.

Fixed Drug Eruptions. Fixed drug eruptions consist of isolated lesions recurring in the same site each time the specific drug is given. This finding is virtually pathognomonic of this type of drug hypersensitivity. Common causes include phenolphthalein, barbiturates, and sulfonamides.

Photosensitivity Reactions. After being exposed to sunlight, patients receiving drugs may exhibit adverse reactions. These reactions presumably involve the interaction of a drug and light energy at a restricted wave length (2800–4300 Å). This may occur with direct sunlight or with filtered or artificial light. There are two types of photosensitivity reactions: (1) phototoxic and (2) photoallergic. The phototoxic reactions are nonimmunologic and occur in a significant number of individuals after the first exposure to a drug when adequate light and drug concentrations are present. Clinically, the reaction resembles an exaggerated sunburn, occasionally with vesiculation. Demethylchlortetracycline (Declomycin) and chlorpromazine (Thorazine) have been associated with these reactions. The photoallergic reactions, on the other hand, generally present with an eczematous phase and can also mimic allergic contact dermatitis. These reactions appear to have an immunologic basis and can be differentiated from phototoxic reactions by the fact that only a small fraction of patients exposed to the drug and light will exhibit them. They usually do not occur immediately but may require incubation periods of days or months. Further, the concentration of drug required to elicit these reactions is usually lower than with phototoxic reactions, and there appears to be a significant cross reactivity with other drugs of similar structure.

LOCAL ANESTHETICS

Another important aspect of drug reactions is that of adverse reactions to local anesthetics. The three major types of adverse reactions to these agents, in the order of decreasing frequency, are: (1) toxic, (2) vasovagal, and (3) allergic. The toxic reactions arise primarily from overdosage, e.g., rapid absorption after accidental intravascular injection. The manifestations of toxic reactions include central nervous system stimulation, excitement, nausea, vomiting, and, occasionally, convulsions with coma and respiratory and cardiac failure. Other undesirable side effects are the manifestations arising from the sympathomimetic effects of epinephrine, which is often mixed with the local anesthesia to delay absorption. The symptoms consist of anxiety, tremor, tachycardia, and occasionally hypertension; syncope may accompany a vasovagal reaction following dental anesthesia. The allergic reactions, which are relatively infrequent, are immunologically mediated and range from the immediate Type I reaction, e.g., urticaria, to contact hypersensitivity (Type IV).

The local anesthetics are commonly divided into two groups, based upon the presence or absence of the para-aminophenyl nucleus. Group I, the "procaine group," contains the para-aminophenyl nucleus and includes such drugs as procaine (Novocain), benzocaine, and tetracaine (Pontocaine); Group II drugs lack the para-aminophenyl nucleus and include lidocaine (Xylocaine), mepivacaine (Carbocaine), and dibucaine (Nupercaine). The clinical importance of this division is that patients allergic to drugs in one group can safely receive drugs in the other.

CONTRAST MEDIA

Reactions to contrast media, although mimicking allergic reactions, do not appear to have an immunologic basis. They occur within the first few hours after administration of the contrast medium and range from vasomotor reactions, e.g., lightheadedness, syncope, pruritus, and urticaria, to the serious sequelae of coma and death. Although the precise mechanism is unknown, these agents are believed to initiate their effects through mediator release in susceptible individuals. Although these reactions occur three to five times more frequently in atopic individuals, this does not prove that they have an allergic origin. It appears that there are fewer reactions occurring after intra-arterial injection than after intravenous administration. The reactions are not more commonly seen in allergic individuals, and the use of intradermal, ocular, and oral tests is not reliable. Preadministration of antihistamines and steroids to individuals with previous reactions may lessen the severity of these adverse reactions.

RESPONSE TO PROTEIN HORMONES

A variety of reactions to protein hormones have been described. Of particular importance are the reactions to insulin. These may take two forms: (1) insulin allergy and (2) insulin resistance. Although both may involve antibody to insulin, insulin allergy involves an IgE-mediated reaction, and insulin resistance involves circulating IgG, IgA, and IgM antibodies.

Insulin allergy may be characterized by immediate hypersensitivity, e.g., urticaria or anaphylaxis. The management of insulin allergy includes the change of insulin from one species to another or the use of recrystallized insulin. If these procedures are ineffective, the judicious use of desensitization has been suggested. The use of highly purified forms of insulin, e.g., monocomponent or single-peak insulin, has been shown to be associated with a significantly lower incidence of insulin allergy; this suggests that these reactions may be more related to contaminating proteins than to the insulin itself.

The presenting features of insulin resistance are the appearance of excessive requirements for insulin, i.e., greater than 200 units daily, in the absence of other complications, e.g., diabetic acidosis. The management of insulin resistance usually involves the use of steroids.

It has been shown that protein hormones, e.g., insulin, ACTH, and growth hormone, require binding to a membrane receptor for their action. Conditions of hormone resistance have been shown to be related to impairment in hormone-receptor interaction. In the case of insulin resistance, a cause of this interference relates to two effects of antibody: (1) antibody directed to the insulin molecule, preventing the interaction of insulin with its receptor; and (2) antibody directed to the receptor itself, which blocks the hormone receptor from interacting with the insulin. In myasthenia gravis, antibody to the acetylcholine receptor has been demonstrated to be associated with interference of neurotransmission characteristic of this disease. Paradoxically, in certain patients with thyrotoxicosis, antibody to TSH receptors may actually be responsible for the disease state. For example, in certain patients with Graves' disease, thyroid-stimulating immunoglobulins (TSI), which may represent autoantibodies to the thyroid thyrotropin receptors, are present and lead to a stimulation of thyroxine production (Chapter 20C).

Diagnosis and Treatment

The diagnosis of drug hypersensitivity rests primarily on a high index of suspicion and on disappearance of symptoms upon discontinuance of the drug. Except in the case of penicillin hypersensitivity and hypersensitivity of protein hormones, skin tests are usually unreliable. This lack of reliability is related to the lack of knowledge of the precise nature of the haptenic determinants responsible for these reactions.

In the case of penicillin hypersensitivity, skin tests employing both major and minor antigenic haptenic groups may be used in a predictive way. Only the major haptenic groups are available commercially. Recently, it has been suggested that as an alternative to the use of the minor haptenic determinants, which are not available commercially, skin testing may be performed with freshly prepared solutions of benzylpenicillin, which conjugates with skin proteins to form the appropriate minor antigenic determinants. Skin tests are limited to IgE reactions. There are no assays that can predict risk with the other immunopathologic states associated with drug hypersensitivity. On the basis of retrospective analysis of the results of skin testing with these preparations, it has been estimated that approximately 95 per cent or more of the potential anaphylactic reactors can be identified. Scratch tests are usually performed prior to intradermal testing. Negative skin tests, however, do not rule out the possibility of late drug reactions, e.g., morbilliform or exanthematic skin reactions, or serum sickness–like reactions, since these are mediated by non-IgE mechanisms, e.g., IgG or IgM.

Other tests of drug hypersensitivity include *in vitro* tests of histamine release and lymphoproliferative responses to the drug. These tests also suffer from a general lack of availability and a lack of reliability. The radioallergosorbent test (RAST) for penicillin and the major BPO antigen allows the detection of some IgE antibodies. Although this provides some additional information, it cannot be used solely for the exclusion of IgE responses.

TREATMENT

The treatment of drug hypersensitivity, as in other cases of immunologically mediated disease, rests upon removal of the offending agent (drugs). In life-threatening situations, epinephrine is the drug of choice, along with other supportive measures. In the other types of drug hypersensitivity, symptomatic treatment using antihistaminics and corticosteroids may be employed.

B. Immunologically Mediated Disease Involving Allogeneic Antigens

Chester M. Zmijewski, Ph.D.

Alloantigens are genetically controlled characteristics that differentiate one member of a given species from another (Chapter 3). When alloantigens are involved in immunologically mediated disease, the process is referred to as alloimmunization and the predominant effector mechanisms may be an antibody-mediated (cytolytic) reaction (Type II), a cell-mediated reaction (Type IV), or a combination of the two.

Alloantigens are important in clinical medicine. Immunologically mediated diseases related to these antigens form three broad categories: (1) disorders due to blood donor incompatibility encountered in transfusion or pregnancy, (2) disorders due to organ or tissue transplantation, and (3) disorders due to postulated tumor-specific transplantation antigens (TSTA) that may develop during the course of malignant transformation (Chapter 19). The immunologically mediated diseases associated with alloantigens are listed in Table 20–14 with examples.

In describing alloimmunization, a clear distinction should be made between the response of the host to alloantigens from another member of the same species and the response to alloantigens that have been altered within the host by exogenous agents. For example, multitransfused patients may develop antibodies to red cell, white cell, and platelet alloantigens that can lead to systemic reactions; viral infections, such as measles, may alter the host platelet alloantigens so as to induce an immunologically mediated attack on the host's platelets (thrombocytopenic purpura). The development of antibody to platelet alloantigens from other individuals is clearly different from the development of antibody to altered platelet alloantigens within the same individual.

The most frequent and most clinically important alloimmunizations result from allosensitization to red blood cell antigens of the ABO and Rh_o systems not present in the host. They present as hemolytic disease of the newborn (erythroblastosis fetalis) or as transfusion reactions. The genetic principles that underlie such potential incompatibilities were presented in Chapter 3.

Table 20–14. **Immunologically Mediated Diseases Associated with Alloantigens**

Category	Example of Antigen	Example of Diseases
Transfusion or pregnancy	Red blood cell (ABO, Rh_0 incompatibility)	Hemolytic transfusion reactions, hemolytic disease of newborn
	White blood cell	Nonhemolytic transfusion reactions, neonatal granulocytopenia
	Platelets	Thrombocytopenic purpura, neonatal thrombocytopenia
	Gamma globulin	Hypersensitivity reactions to gamma globulin, prolonged physiologic hypogammaglobulinemia, nonhemolytic anaphylactoid transfusion reactions
Organ transplantation	Histocompatibility antigens (HLA)	Graft rejection; graft-versus-host reaction (GVH)
Tumor antigens	Tumor-specific transplantation antigens (TSTA)	Malignant disorders

In the case of Rh_0 and ABO alloimmunization, IgG and IgM antibodies seem to be of primary clinical importance. The naturally occurring anti-A and anti-B antibodies are IgM and are the result of exposure to antigens of similar structure that are ubiquitous in nature. Blood group antibodies acquired as a consequence of alloimmunization are "immune," or IgG in type. On a molecular basis, the IgM antibodies have twice the hemolytic activity of IgG antibodies. Only the IgG antibodies, however, can cross the placenta and give rise to hemolytic disease of the newborn. In contrast, both IgM and IgG antibodies have been associated with transfusion reactions.

TRANSFUSION REACTIONS

The generic term *transfusion reaction* refers to a variety of immune and nonimmune complications occurring during or after the transfusion of whole blood or blood products (Fig. 20–27). Examples of nonimmune complications include infections secondary to transfusion of contaminated blood (hepatitis) and cardiac failure due to the rapid transfusion of blood. The immune complications result from the interaction of antibodies present in the plasma of the recipient with foreign alloantigens expressed on transfused red cells, white cells, platelets, or gamma globulin. Less commonly, immune complications may result from the passive transfusion of allergic antibodies that can initiate hypersensitivity phenomena in the recipient (e.g., reagin-mediated urticaria).

Immunologic Aspects

From a practical standpoint, the most commonly occurring and clinically important types of transfusion reactions are those that result in the destruction of red blood cells—the hemolytic transfusion reactions (Table 20–15). The signs and symptoms of these reactions are due to the massive hemolysis of red blood cells along with release of vasoactive substances triggered by the antigen-antibody reaction and consist of chills, fever, pain in the lower back, and hemoglobinuria. The hemolytic reactions may be either *immediate* or *delayed* in onset (Table 20–15).

The immediate reactions are due to the presence of preformed antibody and may occur as the result of two situations: *major* and *minor* incompatibilities. The distinguishing feature between these two types of reactions is the origin of the antibody. The more severe transfusion reactions are seen when antibody is present in the recipient's plasma (major incompatibility). If the antibody is in the donor's plasma, it is diluted upon entering the recipient's circulation and is less likely to produce a severe reaction (minor incompatibility). In contrast, in the delayed type, the transfusion reaction is late in onset and occurs only after antibody is induced, usually through an active secondary response.

The prevention of a hemolytic transfusion reaction begins with proper compatibility testing (cross matching). These tests reveal the presence of antibodies directed against either donor or recipient red blood cell antigens. Blood group antibodies have a wide

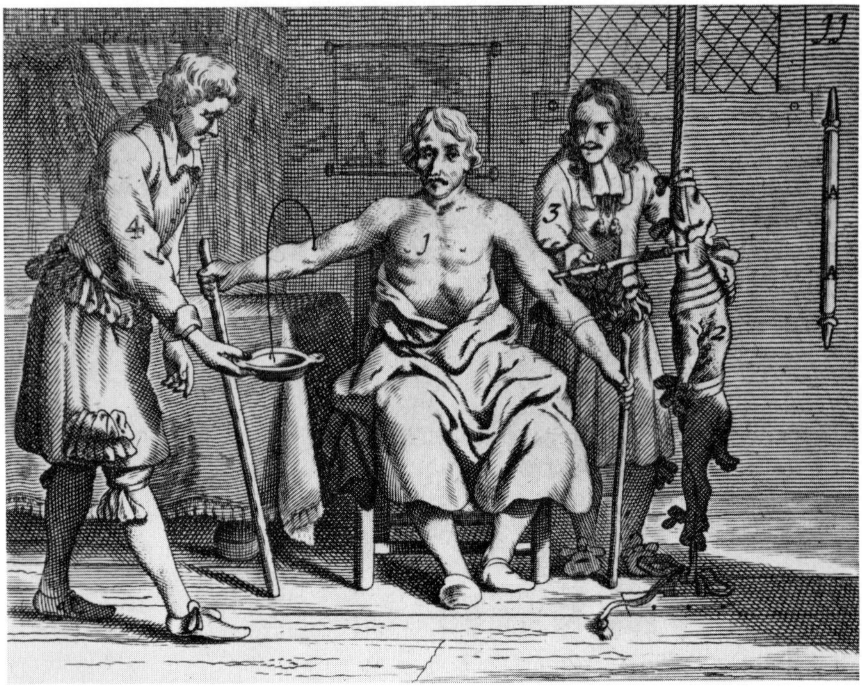

Figure 20–27. Engraving of a blood transfusion from an animal donor to man by Johann Scultetus, Leyden, 1693. (Courtesy of National Library of Medicine.)

spectrum of serologic activity dependent upon their immunochemical properties. Therefore, these tests are carried out under a variety of conditions, usually consisting of tests at room temperature in saline to detect primarily IgM antibodies, tests at 37°C in albumin or low ionic strength solution (LISS) to detect certain IgG antibodies, and the antiglobulin (Coombs) technique to detect other IgG antibodies directed against deeply situated receptors in the erythrocytes.

Clinical Management

The immediate management of a transfusion reaction requires the prompt cessation of the transfusion at the earliest signs suggesting a reaction while maintaining a continuous intravenous infusion for the direct administration of medications, if necessary (Table 20–16). After the blood has been stopped, plasma hemoglobin, which is potentially toxic to the kidney, is removed by osmotic diuretics (10 per cent mannitol) and liberal fluids. This is continued until hemoglobinuria has ceased. If a diuresis does not occur, the possibility of acute renal failure secondary to renal tubular necrosis should be entertained and a program of appropriate fluid restriction instituted. Vasopressor drugs, which may reduce renal perfusion and clearance of hemoglobin, should be avoided.

If it is anticipated that a patient will receive multiple transfusions, e.g., for aplastic anemia, the use of buffy coat–poor red cells without platelets and white cells will reduce the probability of alloimmunization to non–

Table 20–15. **Types of Hemolytic Transfusion Reactions**

	Type	Symptoms
Immediate		
Major incompatibility	Antibody in recipient's plasma; antigen on donor's cells	Chills, fever, pain, and shock
Minor incompatibility	Antibody in donor's plasma; antigen on recipient's cells	Mild transient hemolytic anemia, self-limiting
Delayed	Delayed onset of antibody production	Late onset of hemolytic anemia

Table 20–16. Immediate Treatment of Hemolytic Transfusion Reactions

1. Stop transfusion of blood.
2. Give 1000 ml of 10 per cent mannitol solution, or
3. Give 1000 ml of normal saline.
4. If diuresis continues, repeat Steps 2 and 3 until hemoglobinuria occurs.
5. If diuresis does not occur, suspect renal tubular necrosis and anticipate hemodialysis with concurrent exchange transfusion.
6. Do not use vasopressor drugs.

red cell antigens. This will, in turn, reduce the incidence of nonhemolytic transfusion reactions caused by this type of alloimmunization, which will be described later.

HEMOLYTIC DISEASE OF THE NEWBORN

Hemolytic disease of the newborn (HDN) is a condition characterized by enhanced fetal red cell destruction due to the hemolytic action of maternal antibody transferred across the placenta (see Fig. 4–1). The clinical signs of HDN are explicable on the basis of the hemolytic process (anemia and jaundice) or the sequelae of increased red cell regeneration (erythroblastosis and hepatosplenomegaly). The consequences of anemia are the major causes of intrauterine death and include heart failure and, in severe cases, generalized edema (hydrops fetalis).

Mechanisms of Sensitization

Although the most frequent fetomaternal incompatibility is that of the ABO system (fetal A and maternal O), the symptoms of the disease are usually relatively mild. Severe hemolytic disease of the newborn is more commonly caused by Rh incompatibility. The antibody most frequently responsible for the disease is the anti-Rh_0(D); as previously described, only the IgG antibody can cross the placenta and express this disorder.

Antibody formation in the mother can occur through prior transfusion of incompatible cells or, more commonly, as a consequence of previous pregnancies (Fig. 20–28). It has been shown that fetal red cells can be detected in the blood of randomly selected

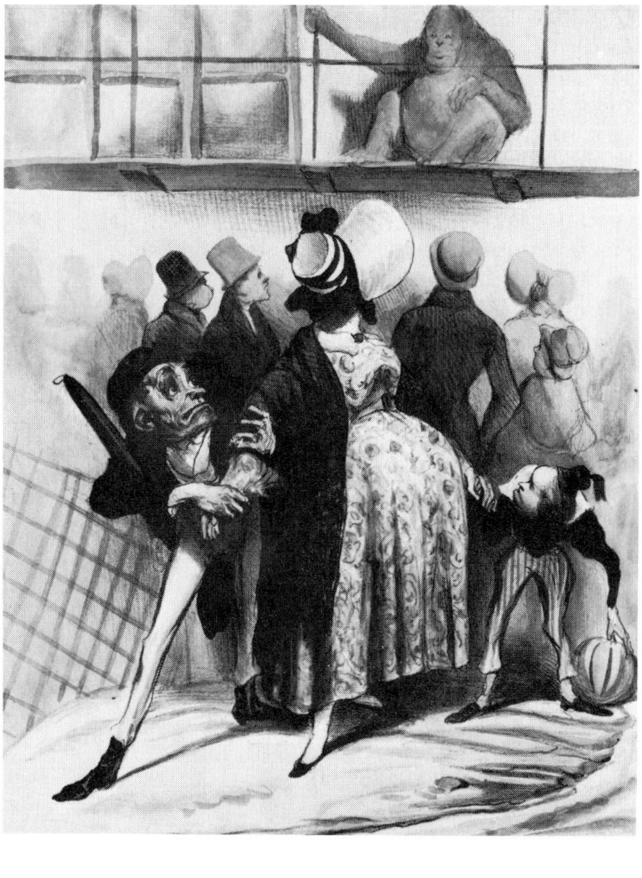

Figure 20–28. Caricature illustrating superstitious fears of prenatal influences on the fetus. A hunchbacked husband and son urge the pregnant mother not to look at an orangutan to avoid malformation in the unborn infant. (Courtesy of National Library of Medicine.)

postpartum women in approximately 71 per cent of cases. Currently, it is felt that the large doses of fetal cells introduced into the maternal circulation as a result of the trauma of parturition is the primary source of immunogen. There is a variability in maternal production of antibody to these cells that appears to be dependent upon genetic constitution, the number of immunizing cells, and the type of red cell antigen transferred. In general, in the case of Rh_o incompatibility, the severity of the disease is directly proportional to the number of affected pregnancies. The risk of Rh_o immunization is diminished if a concurrent ABO incompatibility exists between the mother and the fetus. Any Rh_o-positive cells that enter the Rh_o-negative mother's circulation are destroyed immediately, preventing maternal anti-Rh_o antibody formation. This observation has formed the basis for the most effective method of prevention of Rh_o sensitization by immunosuppression through the use of specific anti-Rh_o antibody. This will be described more fully later.

Regardless of the blood group incompatibility responsible for HDN, an anemia develops that is characterized by a fall in hemoglobin concentration and an increase in the number of nucleated red cells (erythroblasts) in the peripheral circulation; this latter finding gives rise to the term "erythroblastosis fetalis." The anemia is more severe in the case of Rh_o incompatibility.

In addition to anemia, the hemolysis of erythrocytes causes increased amounts of bilirubin pigments to appear in the infant's circulation. In intrauterine life, potentially toxic quantities of indirect bilirubin are excreted through the placenta and are conjugated to direct water-soluble bilirubin in the maternal liver. Postnatally, however, the excess indirect bilirubin cannot be conjugated by the immature neonatal liver, and toxic quantities of indirect bilirubin may accumulate. If they attain sufficiently high concentrations in plasma, the lipid-soluble indirect bilirubin pigment may deposit in brain tissue, resulting in kernicterus with permanent cerebral damage.

Diagnosis

IMMUNOLOGIC TESTS

Routinely, the red blood cells of expectant mothers are typed for ABO and Rh_o blood types. Their sera are screened for the presence of "irregular" antibodies (other than the normally expected anti-A or anti-B) that may have been induced by a previous pregnancy or transfusion. If the mother is Rh_o-negative, the father should be tested to determine his Rh_o status. If he is found to be Rh_o-negative, no possible incompatibility exists as far as Rh_o (D) is concerned; if he is Rh_o-positive, the possibility exists that the child may also be Rh_o-positive. Although the probability of HDN in the first newborn child is quite low, it is possible that this pregnancy could induce alloimmunization of the mother. In subsequent pregnancies the possibility of the child's being Rh_o-positive remains the same, but the disease probability increases. The risk depends upon whether the father is homozygous or heterozygous for Rh_o(D) antigen. After delivery and after every subsequent delivery of an Rh_o-positive baby, the mother should be given anti-Rh_o globulin within 72 hours of delivery in order to prevent sensitization (Chapter 24).

In addition, during the pregnancy of an Rh_o-negative woman who has a chance of carrying an Rh_o-positive fetus, Rh_o serum titers should be measured to determine whether active immunization is taking place. Once stimulation has occurred, significant antibody titers persist for many years. Therefore, in such a situation, a single specimen would be uninformative. However, a rise in anti-Rh_o antibody titer during the course of an individual pregnancy would indicate that an active alloimmunization is in progress. Thus, the possibility of HDN can be assessed from antenatal antibody titers, although the definitive diagnosis can be made only by other techniques.

In patients with a high probability of HDN, prenatal diagnosis can also be established by amniocentesis and spectrophotometric examination of the amniotic fluid for the presence of hemoglobin breakdown pigments. If the diagnosis is established, the risk of fatal HDN can be reduced by the use of intrauterine transfusion of compatible red blood cells. Care should be taken to use blood that has been treated to remove lymphocytes, e.g., irradiated blood. Transfusion of lymphocyte-contaminated blood has given rise to graft-versus-host reactions subsequent to the course of intrauterine transfusions.

After birth, the diagnosis of HDN is established on the basis of clinical and laboratory findings. Jaundice within the first 24 hours of life accompanied by an anemia almost invariably indicates HDN. Evidence to substantiate the diagnosis rests on immunohematologic and chemical laboratory tests. The immunohematologic techniques are employed for the detection of antibody sensitization of red blood cells. Fetal erythrocytes may be tested directly for antibody coating using the direct Coombs test. Indirect evidence for antibody sensitization may be obtained by screening the maternal serum against a panel of red blood cells with known antigenic specificity to identify antibodies that would be potentially harmful to the fetus.

In addition, through the combined use of the direct antiglobulin test and the adult serum-albumin slide sensitization test (Witebsky test), it may be possible to further differentiate ABO sensitization from Rh_0 sensitization. Both tests can be performed on cord blood in every suspected case. Both tests are usually positive in the case of HDN due to Rh_0 sensitization; usually only the Witebsky test, however, is strongly positive in ABO sensitization (Table 20–17). A positive direct antiglobulin test in the absence of obvious Rh_0 incompatibility may be indicative of sensitization with one of the other less common blood group systems, e.g., Duffy or Kell. Since the mother is the source of antibody, a specimen of her blood should be obtained in every case for cross matching with prospective donors for exchange transfusions and also for further characterization of the injurious alloantibodies.

CHEMICAL TESTS

Since the intensity of a positive antiglobulin test does not indicate the severity of the disease, hemoglobin and bilirubin determinations are often performed as indicators of red cell destruction. These tests should always be performed in conjunction with the preceding serologic tests. Cord hemoglobin values below 14 gm per 100 ml are considered abnormal. Bilirubin levels require an accelerated rate of rise as an index for exchange transfusion. Although a level in excess of 20 mg per 100 ml has been used as a guide for exchange transfusion, the decision is more complex, since several other critical factors will influence the therapy, e.g., anoxia, prematurity, low birth weight, and serum albumin concentration.

Table 20–17. Immunologic Tests for Detection of Red Cell Sensitization in Hemolytic Disease of Newborn

Type of HDN	Coombs	Witebsky
Rh_0	+	+
ABO	0 or weakly positive	+

Treatment

Exchange transfusion has literally saved the lives of thousands of children and prevented untold numbers of infirmities, such as mental retardation, deafness, and cerebral palsy. The purpose of exchange transfusion is to (1) correct the anemia and restore cardiac function, (2) remove sensitized red cells and therefore the source of additional bilirubin, and (3) remove the accumulated bilirubin.

Prevention

The use of specific antibody in suppressing the immune response is a well-established technique. It has been used successfully in the prevention of Rh_0 alloimmunization in the human. The clinical use of the material is described in Chapter 24.

Rh_0 immune globulin is indicated in Rh_0-negative mothers whose newborns are shown to be Rh_0-positive. The preparation is administered within 72 hours of delivery, since this is the time that the greatest number of fetal cells are in the maternal circulation. The material can also be used to prevent immunization due to the transfusion of Rh_0-positive blood to Rh_0-negative women of childbearing age. This has been done successfully in many cases with Rh_0-negative women. Once sensitization has occurred, however, this form of therapy is ineffective.

IMMUNOLOGICALLY MEDIATED DISEASE INVOLVING WHITE CELL AND PLATELET ALLOANTIGENS

Alloimmunizations to white cell and to platelet antigens are analogous in their clinical expressions. Both are seen in multitransfused patients and may occur in multiparous women. They account for nonhemolytic transfusion reactions after blood transfusions. These reactions consist of chills, fever, dyspnea, cardiac abnormalities, and pulmonary edema. These antibodies, when present in the sera of pregnant women, have been shown on occasion to cause neonatal granulocytopenia and neonatal thrombocytopenia.

IMMUNOLOGICALLY MEDIATED DISEASE INVOLVING GAMMA GLOBULIN

Alloimmunization to gamma globulin has been observed in individuals receiving gamma globulin injections and also in multiparous females. These antibodies have been associated with hypersensitivity reactions, such as localized reactions consisting of swelling and tenderness, and with generalized anaphylactic reactions. In addition, they have been implicated in the prolonged physiologic hypogammaglobulinemia of infancy, owing presumably to the passive transfer of antibody directed to paternal gamma globulin types (Chapter 22). These data indicate that gamma globulin therapy should not be used indiscriminately, since it may have undesirable effects. Furthermore, the development of antibodies to IgA globulins has been reported to account for approximately 80 per cent of nonhemolytic transfusion reactions. These antibodies can be of two types: (1) one type that reacts with all forms of IgA (panreactive) and usually occurs in individuals lacking IgA, and (2) another type that is directed against a single genetic form of IgA and can arise in anyone who has been sensitized by transfusion or by some other means (Chapter 5).

ORGAN TRANSPLANTATION

Michael C. Gelfand, M.D.

The science of organ transplantation originated more than a thousand years ago with the grafting of skin to repair congenital defects. Today, organ transplantation from one individual to another or within the same individual from one location to another is an accepted therapeutic measure of modern medicine. Virtually every organ except the central nervous system has been transplanted (Table 20–18). In the treatment of end-stage kidney disease alone, over 60,000 renal transplants have been performed, and each year more than 10,000 new kidney transplants will be done throughout the world. Productive years have been added to the lives of patients seriously debilitated with severe heart disease, liver failure, or chronic obstructive pulmonary disease through transplantation. Essentially normal lives have been restored to patients with end-stage kidney disease or a variety of forms of bone marrow failure by transplantation of kidneys or bone marrow cells. Sight may be re-established by the grafting of cornea, one of the most exciting organ transplants of all, since the cornea may be preserved for extended periods of time in organ banks, may be freely transplanted between individuals, and is not readily rejected. Moreover, the privileged condition of the corneal transplant not only has provided evidence for the importance of lymphatic drainage in inducing sensitization of the host but

Table 20–18. **Organ Transplants**

Type of Transplant	Example of a Clinical Indication	Complications
Skin	Burns	Rejection, infection
Bone marrow, thymus	Severe combined immune deficiency (SCID), DiGeorge syndrome	Rejection, graft-versus-host reaction
Kidney	End-stage kidney disease	Destruction of graft due to underlying disease process, rejection, infection due to overzealous immunosuppression
Heart	Arteriosclerotic heart disease, congenital heart disease	Rejection
Liver	Congenital biliary atresia	Rejection
Lungs	Chronic obstructive pulmonary disease	Rejection
Pancreas	Pancreatic insufficiency, diabetes, chronic pancreatitis	Rejection
Cornea	Cornea destruction	Opacification

also, more importantly, represents the desired ideal situation for future transplantation in which organs might someday be preservable and used interchangeably among patients.

In spite of increasingly expanding experience, organ transplantation remains, at best, an imprecise science. This is partly because our knowledge of the various technical, biochemical, and immunologic aspects of transplantation remains incomplete and partly because the clinical aspects of every transplant are different. In experimental organ transplantation in animals, many of these variables are controlled by the use of highly inbred animals as recipients or donors, or both. Factors such as age, sex, environmental exposure, tissue antigens, diet, and so forth may be standardized. Since this is not readily accomplished in human organ transplantation, each transplant situation must be approached with considerable individualization.

Nevertheless, the careful analysis of data from experimental and clinical organ transplantation has provided a number of useful general principles of organ transplantation. This section will present the guiding principles that are largely applicable to all organ transplants, highlighting problems of special clinical interest concerning the transplantation of specific organs.

Terminology

LIVING AND CADAVERIC DONOR GRAFTS

The term by which a graft is known depends on the origin of the graft and its relationship to the recipient. Thus, in human organ transplantation, a graft may be obtained from a living donor (in the case of duplicated organs such as the kidney) or from a recently deceased individual (as is necessary in the case of an essential organ such as the heart or liver). Grafts from the former category are called living donor grafts and those from the latter are called cadaveric donor grafts.

AUTO-, ISO-, ALLO-, AND XENOGRAFTS

Four types of grafts may be identified, depending on the relationship of the donor to the recipient (Chapter 3). An autograft is a graft taken from and transplanted to the same individual, for example, skin transplanted from the thigh to the chest in a patient with a severe burn. Autografts are not rejected since they are derived from the recipient himself. A graft from an identical twin is called an isograft. This type of graft is also not rejected, since it is antigenically identical to the recipient and is similar to transplantation between inbred littermate animals.

The vast majority of grafts are allografts, exchanged between individuals of the same species but having different tissue antigens. With the exception of the identical twin transplant, all human-to-human organ grafts are allogeneic grafts.

The xenograft is not often used in clinical organ transplantation. In this situation, the graft is transplanted between individuals of different species, for example, a baboon liver transplanted into a human with liver failure. Xenografts are generally rapidly rejected since we are not yet successful in transplanting across species lines.

HISTOCOMPATIBILITY ANTIGENS

The cell surface proteins that give an organ its recognizable antigenicity and evoke the rejection phenomenon are referred to as histocompatibility antigens (Chapter 3). In most animal species studied sufficiently, similar antigens have been identified on the surface of the nucleated cells of the transplanted tissue. These glycoprotein molecules are responsible for the induction of rejection and appear to be inherited in a systematic fashion, in all cases bearing a relationship to parental antigens.

HISTOCOMPATIBILITY COMPLEX

The chromosome region that codes for the histocompatibility antigens of man is known as the major histocompatibility or HLA complex (Chapter 3). Mice and rats have analogous systems known as H-2 and AGB, respectively, that have been carefully studied and have provided much of our understanding of the HLA complex of man. In these systems, there are genes capable of coding for the production of cell surface antigens, which can be recognized by the recipient as self or foreign. On each of two chromosomes there are at least four known loci, each containing a series of codominant allelic forms. At present, in man, 51 antigens have been recognized in the HLA system: 20 on locus A, 20 on locus B, 5 on locus C, and 6 on locus D (see Table 3–3). Each individual inherits one chromosome from each parent and thus one allele from each of these four loci from each parent. A parent will share exactly half of the antigens with an offspring, and siblings may share all, some, or none of these antigens.

Histocompatibility antigens have been designated as Class I and Class II antigens (Chapter 3). The Class I antigens are the antigens of the HLA-A and HLA-B series. Class II antigens are the antigens of the D/Dr series. This latter series is considered to provide the "first" antigenic signal and stimulation of antigen-reactive T-helper cells to recognize the foreignness of the graft. The helper T-cells then stimulate B-cells to produce antibody against the Class I antigens. Class II antigens are capable as well of stimulating the mixed lymphocyte response, an *in vitro* test of immune recognition.

Donor-Recipient Matching

The closer the match between the donor and the recipient, the more likely it is that the transplant will be successful. This is clearly apparent when graft survival in identical twin donor-recipient pairs is compared with that in unrelated pairs. Indeed, bone marrow transplantation almost invariably met with dismal failure until the development of methods of typing and matching donor bone marrow. Histocompatibility matching is not as critical in liver and heart transplantation.

The general principles of donor-recipient matching are illustrated in Table 20–19. The first two principles are inviolable, whereas the remainder are relative requisites. Transplantation will not be successful in the presence of ABO incompatibility. It can, however, be performed in the presence of incompatibilities of minor blood group, including Rh. A positive T-cell cross match, i.e., when the recipient has demonstrable circulating antibodies against the T-cell antigens of the donor, is also a contraindication to transplantation. Such circulating cytotoxic antibodies are routinely tested for by incubating donor lymphoid cells in recipient serum in the presence of a source of complement. After a period of incubation, a marker of cell death (such as trypan blue) is added to the cell suspension and the proportion of dead cells is counted. The presence of significant numbers of dead cells indicates a positive cross match. Recently, it has been suggested that certain antibodies may not prevent successful transplantations. These include anti–B cell antibodies, in particular those reacting at 4°C ("cold" B-cell antibodies).

The lack of histocompatibility between recipient and donor is not a contraindication to transplantation; however, in most cases, especially in renal transplantation, every effort is made to obtain the closest possible antigenic match for the recipient. This is done by tissue typing, i.e., identifying the antigens of loci A, B, C, and DR on the cells of the recipient by means of monospecific antisera obtained from sensitized individuals and by performing a series of individual cross-match tests with the recipient's lymphoid cells. The same is done with the cells of all potential donors, and in the absence of other critical factors, the closest match is selected to be the donor. Critical factors that might eliminate a potential donor include ABO incompatibility, antibodies in the recipient against the donor's cells, medical disability of the donor, and unwillingness to donate an organ.

Living related donors may be further

Table 20–19. Principles of Donor-Recipient Matching

Principle	Method Used for Testing
1. No transplantation across ABO incompatibility	Hemagglutination
2. No transplantation in presence of positive T-cell crossmatch, i.e., anti–T-cell antibodies; avoid transplantation in presence of warm anti–B-cell antibodies	Lymphocytotoxicity, leukagglutination
3. Attempt to obtain best HLA match from ABO-compatible potential donors (not critical in liver or heart transplantation)	Lymphocytotoxicity
4. Attempt to obtain transplant from donor inducing least mixed lymphocyte response from ABO-compatible, satisfactorily matched, potential donors	Mixed lymphocyte culture reactivity

matched to recipients by evaluating D locus compatibility. Compatibility for this locus is evaluated by mixed lymphocyte culture reactivity (MLC), i.e., the degree to which recipient lymphocytes undergo blast transformation on exposure to donor lymphocytes (Chapter 7 and 9). To date, the mixed lymphocyte response of the recipient is only evaluated prospectively in living donor transplantation situations. In cadaver transplantations, Class II antigens are evaluated by identifying DR antigens. The MLC test requires a number of days to perform and therefore requires too much time to evaluate the recipient's response to cells of a cadaveric donor. In studies done retrospectively, low response of recipient lymphocytes to cadaveric donor cells is associated with better allograft survival.

Immunobiology of Rejection

Rejection may be defined as the process by which the immune system of the host recognizes, becomes sensitized against, and attempts to eliminate the antigenic differences of the donor organ. With the exception of autografts and isografts, some degree of rejection occurs with every transplant. For the present, until clinically applicable methods of inducing unresponsiveness are developed (Chapter 10), the function of immunosuppression is to control the host's natural response and to prevent rejection of the graft.

The prototype of the immunobiology of rejection is primary (first-set) rejection (Chapter 10). In this form of rejection, the host encounters the histocompatibility antigens on the surface of the cells of the transplant for the first time. In some as yet poorly described manner locally or within regional lymph nodes, macrophages process antigenic material and present it to B- and T-lymphocytes for sensitization (Fig. 20–29). Recent evidence suggests that the process of sensitizing lymphocytes is facilitated by the antigen-stimulated release of soluble factors called interleukins (Chapters 7 and 9). Sensitized lymphocytes may then enter the peripheral circulation directly or may proceed via lymphatics to the thoracic duct and then enter the peripheral circulation. Upon arriving in the grafted organ and encountering the specific antigens of the graft, sensitized lymphoid cells initiate immune injury. The immune injury may be mediated by either the humoral or the cellular limb of the immune response in a variety of ways: (1) directly, by cytotoxic T-cells (or NK cells); (2) indirectly, by soluble T-cell mediators of immune injury (lymphokines); (3) by B-cell–mediated (humoral) antibody; or (4) by antibody-dependent cellular cytotoxicity (ADCC) attack on the target organ (K cells). This process of primary rejection is the classic model and can become clinically evident after the first week post transplantation.

In contrast to primary rejection is hyperacute rejection. In this type of rejection, the recipient has been sensitized to the histocompatibility antigens of the graft by previous transfusions, pregnancy, or transplantation. Circulating cytotoxic antibodies to the HLA antigens of the graft may be found in the serum of recipients hyperacutely rejecting their grafts. Upon completion of the vascular anastomosis, there is prompt deposition of antibody along the vascular endothelium with activation of the complement and the coagulation systems, resulting in fibrin deposition, polymorphonuclear leukocyte infiltration, platelet thrombosis, and prompt coagulative necrosis with invariable loss of the graft (Fig. 20–30).

Acute rejection describes the clinical situation associated with the abrupt onset of signs and symptoms of rejection. The graft is tender and it is heavily infiltrated with mononuclear and inflammatory cells. Nevertheless, this type of rejection may respond to immunosuppressive therapy with resolution. In acute rejection, both cellular and humoral immunity are involved.

Chronic rejection occurs after an extended period of time and is characterized by gradual loss of function of the graft. On histopathologic examination, the chronically rejected organ appears infiltrated with large numbers of mononuclear cells predominantly of the T-cell line, although B-cells may also be involved. This type of rejection is indolent and is often unresponsive to immunosuppressive therapy (Fig. 20–31).

Diagnosis and Treatment of Rejection

The clinical diagnosis and treatment of allograft rejection are extremely challenging for the transplantation immunologist, since there is neither a precise method to make

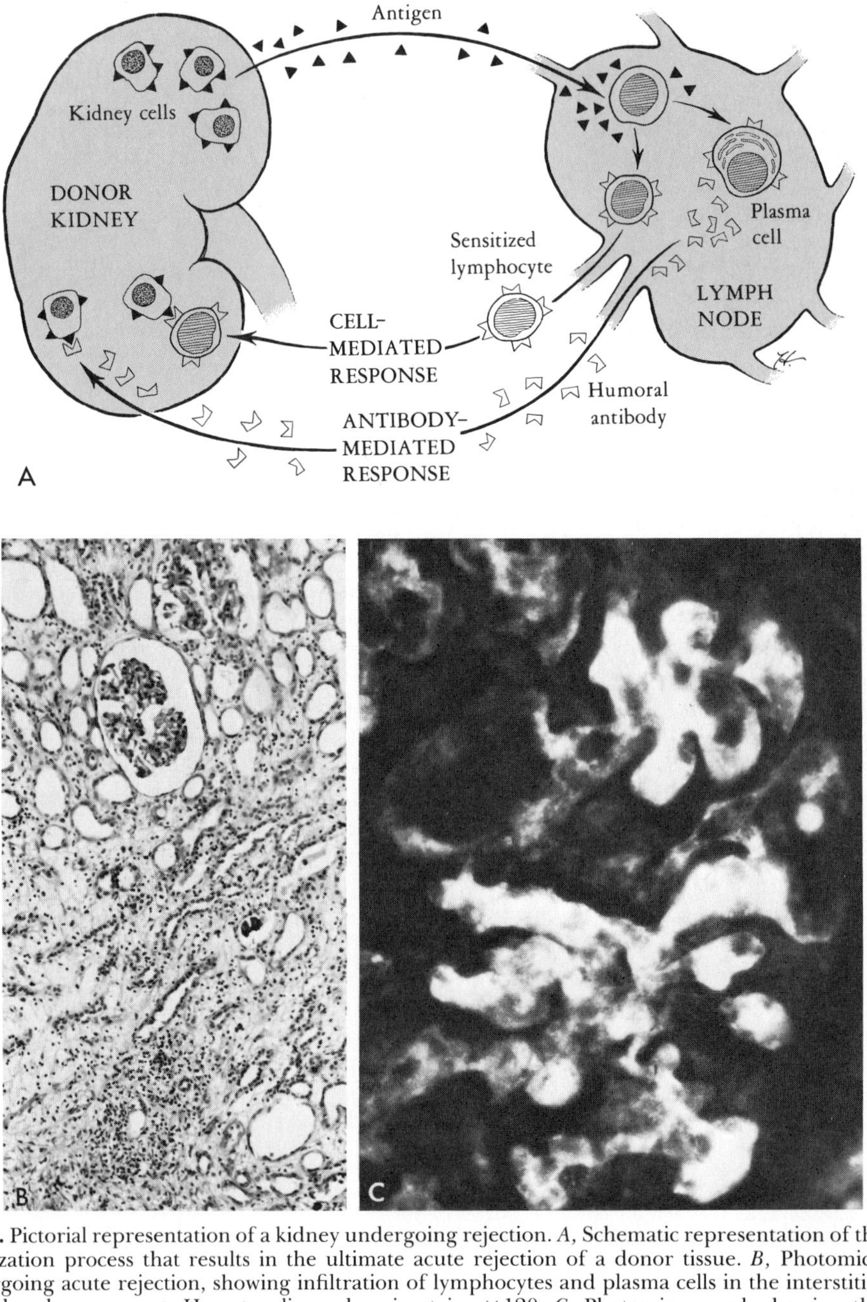

Figure 20–29. Pictorial representation of a kidney undergoing rejection. *A*, Schematic representation of the mechanism of the sensitization process that results in the ultimate acute rejection of a donor tissue. *B*, Photomicrograph of a kidney undergoing acute rejection, showing infiltration of lymphocytes and plasma cells in the interstitial tissues with tubular atrophy also apparent. Hematoxylin and eosin stain, ×120. *C*, Photomicrograph showing the fluorescent antibody staining of a kidney undergoing acute rejection. Note the localization seen along glomerular basement membranes. Original magnification × 800. (*B*, Courtesy of Dr. Abner Golden; *C*, courtesy of Dr. Heinz Bauer.)

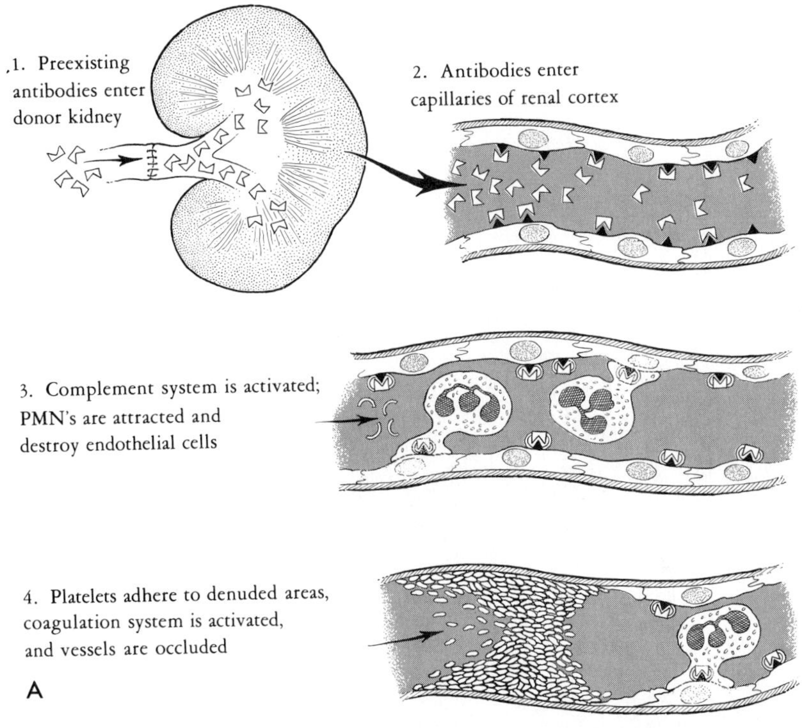

1. Preexisting antibodies enter donor kidney
2. Antibodies enter capillaries of renal cortex
3. Complement system is activated; PMN's are attracted and destroy endothelial cells
4. Platelets adhere to denuded areas, coagulation system is activated, and vessels are occluded

A

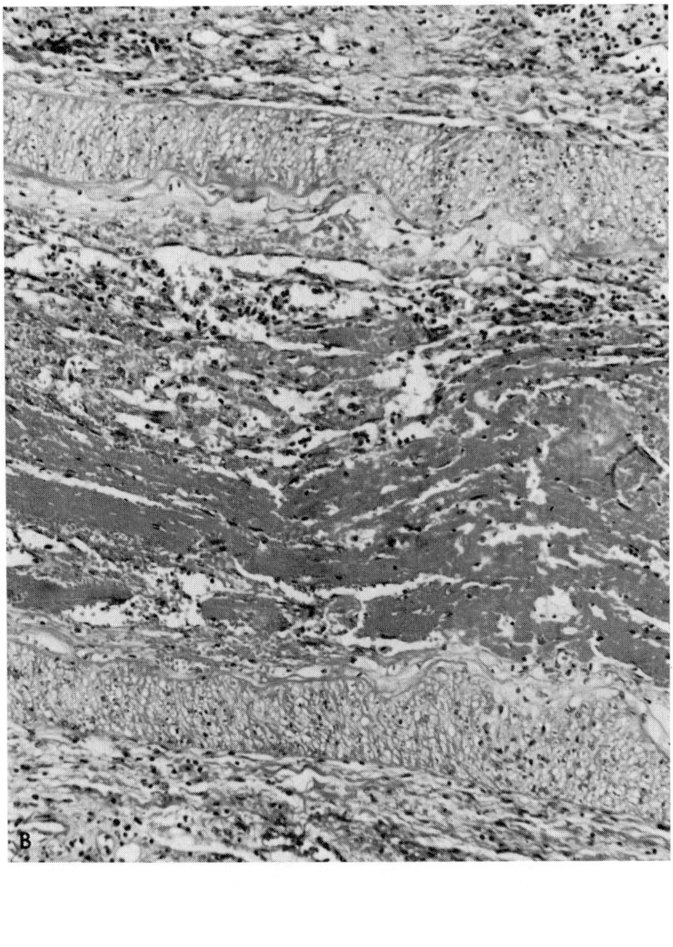

B

Figure 20–30. Pictorial representation of a kidney undergoing *hyperacute* rejection within minutes of transplantation. *A*, Schematic representation of the mechanism of blood vessel occlusion. *B*, Photomicrograph of a kidney undergoing hyperacute rejection and showing thrombosis of a major interlobar renal artery. Hematoxylin and eosin stain, × 120. (Courtesy of Dr. Abner Golden.)

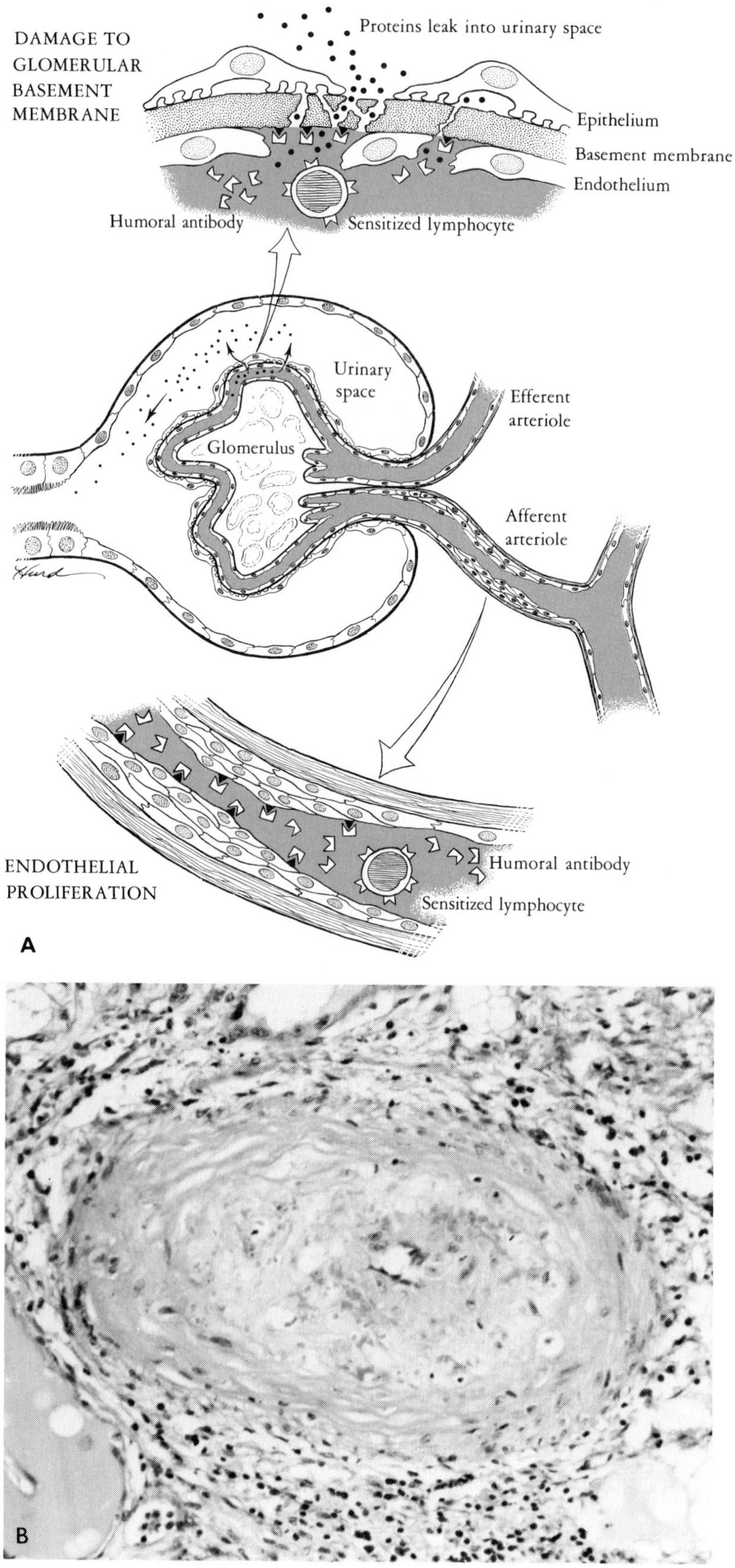

Figure 20–31. Pictorial representation of a kidney undergoing *chronic* rejection. *A,* Schematic representation of the tissue destruction seen in the chronic rejection of a kidney. *B,* Photomicrograph of a kidney undergoing chronic rejection and showing marked intimal thickening with constriction of the lumen of a renal artery. Note the mucinous appearance of the intima. Hematoxylin and eosin stain, ×360. (Courtesy of Dr. Abner Golden.)

the diagnosis nor any universally accepted or "correct" treatment. This is, in part, related to the fact that no two recipients, donors, or recipient-donor pairs are identical. For example, the underlying state of health of one recipient will differ from that of another, or the type of organ being transplanted might differ. Some of these variables are listed in Table 20–20. Nevertheless, a number of clinically helpful symptoms and signs of rejection have been identified and are listed in Table 20–21. Fever, myalgias, and localized graft tenderness are frequently observed symptoms; hypertension, leukocytosis, and hypocomplementemia are useful biochemical signs in the diagnosis of graft rejection. In addition, depending on the type of organ being transplanted, there are more specific signs and symptoms to be observed. In renal transplantation, for example, oliguria, lymphocyturia, hematuria, proteinuria, and rising serum urea nitrogen and creatinine may be seen. In heart transplantation, the development of cardiac arrhythmias may signal incipient rejection.

The treatment of rejection varies considerably depending on the type of transplant and the institution; however, there are a number of generally applicable principles of immunosuppression, which are described in Chapter 25 and shown in Table 20–22. The goal of immunosuppression is to prevent or minimize sensitization, because once sensitization has occurred, the suppression of the immune response becomes considerably more difficult. For this purpose, the recipient receives the largest dose of immunosuppression just prior to or during the first week after transplantation, the period during which primary sensitization occurs. In the unfortunate instance in which the recipient has been presensitized, prompt graft rejection (hyperacute or accelerated) will ensue, defying in most cases the most strenuous attempts at immunosuppression. If no early rejection occurs, the drugs used for immunosuppression are tapered over succeeding days to weeks until a stable maintenance dose is achieved.

In the event of the development of an acute rejection episode, the dose of immunosuppressive agents being used may be in-

Table 20–20. Some Factors Affecting Organ Transplantation Between Individual Donor-Recipient Pairs

Recipients

1. Immunologic integrity
2. Previous sensitization
3. Presence of other diseases affecting immune response (e.g., uremia)
4. Presence of disease that might affect metabolism of immunosuppressive drug (e.g., liver disease)
5. Presence of systemic condition that might be exacerbated (e.g., diabetes or hypertension)
6. Need for other medication (e.g., allopurinol)
7. Nutritional status
8. Patient compliance

Donors

1. Type of organ being transplanted
2. Relationship to recipient
3. Degree of match with recipient
4. If cadaver donor, cause of death

Table 20–21. Symptoms and Signs of Organ Transplant Rejection

Symptoms
- Fever
- Malaise
- Graft tenderness

Signs

General
- Hypertension
- Eosinophilia
- Leukocytosis
- Hypocomplementemia
- Elevated sedimentation rate
- ↑ T4/T8 ratios
- ↑ Spontaneous blastogenesis
- β-2 microglobulinemia
- ↑ C-reactive protein

Organ-Specific Signs

Renal:	Rising BUN
	Rising β-2 microglobulins
	Rising creatinine
	Lymphocyturia
	Hematuria
	Proteinuria
	Oliguria
	Thromboxanuria
Heart:	Arrhythmias
	Rising cardiac enzymes
Liver:	Rising alkaline phosphatase
	Rising bilirubin
	Rising liver enzymes

Table 20–22. Principles of Immunosuppression

1. Use highest dose of treatment during early post-transplantation period to prevent sensitization.
2. Combination drug regimens are often more effective than a single-drug regimen.
3. Taper immunosuppression when possible.
4. If effective, low-dose or alternate-day regimens are associated with reduced side effects.
5. Treat rejection promptly and aggressively.
6. In severe infection or leukopenia, immunosuppression may have to be greatly reduced or stopped to prevent patient death.
7. Do not overtreat.

creased or different drugs may be added to the regimen until the rejection is brought under control or the graft is lost.

IMMUNOSUPPRESSIVE AGENTS

The drugs used for immunosuppression fall into three general categories: anti-inflammatory agents, antimetabolites, and cytotoxic agents (Chapter 25). Table 20–23 lists the commonly used immunosuppressive agents and their mechanisms of action.

Anti-Inflammatory Agents. The major anti-inflammatory and perhaps the major agents used for immunosuppression are the adrenocortical steroids, e.g., prednisone, prednisolone, and methylprednisolone. These agents provide broad, nonspecific, anti-inflammatory action by stabilizing lysosome membranes. In addition, steroids have a variety of other functions in suppressing the immune response, including prevention of antigen recognition and the effector limb of lymphocyte function (Chapter 25).

Antimetabolites. A number of agents with antimetabolic properties have been used in immunosuppression. The purine antagonist azathioprine and its active metabolite 6-mercaptopurine competitively inhibit effective purine nucleotide synthesis, thereby resulting in faulty RNA synthesis. The alkylating agents cyclophosphamide and chlorambucil also have antimetabolic effects, since these agents induce breaks in the cross linkage of the DNA helix with faulty relinkage and subsequent cell death.

Cytotoxic Agents. This large category includes a variety of agents. X-irradiation, whether total-body, local to the graft, or delivered extracorporeally to cells of the blood stream, has cytolytic properties, especially on rapidly reproducing cellular elements such as lymphoid cells undergoing sensitization. In addition, antilymphocyte serum or globulin, an antibody produced in animals (usually the horse) against human lymphocytes, is of help in suppressing the immune response by destroying or inactivating circulating lymphocytes (Chapter 24). Monoclonal antibody to human T-cell surface antigens produced by hybridoma technology (Chapter 5) is now being evaluated as an immunosuppressive agent (Chapter 24). Steroids, azathioprine, the alkylating agents, and certain antibiotics such as actinomycin D also have cytotoxic capabilities. The steroids are predominantly effective in ablating recirculating lymphocytes, the alkylating agent cyclophosphamide is effective against both T- and B-lymphocytes, azathioprine predominantly affects T-lymphocytes, and actinomycin D is cytotoxic for a variety of dividing cells.

Cyclosporine. This agent has only very recently been approved by the United States Food and Drug Administration for use in clinical transplantation. However, clinical trials in the United States and Europe have suggested that this agent represents perhaps the most powerful single immunosuppressive agent discovered to date. A product of a fungus, cyclosporine is capable of profound prolongation of a variety of organ grafts. Its mechanism of action, while not clear, may be through increasing the activity of suppressor T-lymphocytes. Others maintain that cyclosporine inhibits helper T-cell functions.

IMMUNOSUPPRESSIVE TREATMENT REGIMENS

Most treatment regimens are designed to combine the effects of various immunosuppressive agents so as to provide a multifocal

Table 20–23. Immunosuppressive Agents Used in Organ Transplantation

Type of Agent	Mechanism
I. Anti-inflammatory	
Adrenocortical steroids: Prednisone, prednisolone, methylprednisolone	Stabilizes lysozomes, impairs antigen recognition and processing Lymphocytolysis, impairs antibody synthesis
II. Antimetabolites	
Azathioprine, 6-mercaptopurine	Impairs nucleic acid synthesis and pyrimidine ribonucleotide
III. Cytotoxic	
Alkylating agents: Cyclophosphamide, chlorambucil	Causes inter- and intrastrand DNA crosslinkage with alteration of DNA helix
X-irradiation	Karyorrexis, destruction of DNA helix
Antilymphocyte globulin	Immune cytolysis
IV. Cyclosporine A	Activates suppressor T-cells or inhibits helper T-cells

attack on the immune response. For example, many regimens include a corticosteroid to prevent sensitization, ablate lymphocytes, impair antibody synthesis, and suppress inflammation plus an antimetabolite to inhibit the transmission of the message of antigen sensitization and to provide additional lymphocytolysis. An alkylating agent such as cyclophosphamide may be included for its additional cytotoxic properties, especially against B-lymphocytes. X-irradiation or antilymphocyte serum may be added to enhance cytotoxicity. In the treatment of rejection episodes, boluses of intravenous corticosteroids are frequently added to the standard regimen, with tapering upon successful reversal of rejection. With the approval of cyclosporine for transplantation, most immunosuppressive regimens will soon probably add this agent in some way.

Table 20–24. Consequences of Immunosuppression

1. Infections
Common organisms
Pneumococcus
Escherichia coli
Uncommon organisms (i.e., opportunistic)
Pneumocystis carinii
Cytomegalovirus
Candida albicans
2. Neoplasms
Lymphomas
Reticulum cell sarcoma
Skin and lip carcinomas
3. Graft-versus-host disease
Dermatitis
Diarrhea
Fever
Failure to thrive
Death (if severe)

CONSEQUENCES OF SUPPRESSION OF IMMUNE RESPONSE

Immunosuppressive therapy provides one of the rare opportunities in clinical medicine to be *too* successful. Since most immunosuppressive regimens are nonspecific assaults on immune responsiveness, successful efforts to prevent normal graft rejection must invariably be accompanied by depression of host immune reponses. Fortunately, in most instances, alterations in immunocompetence do not result in major complications. For example, delayed hypersensitivity to an intradermal antigen such as PPD may disappear during immunosuppressive therapy. This is a rather trivial consequence; however, the reactivation or new acquisition of tuberculosis during therapy is an example of a more significant complication.

There are three major complications of immunosuppression: (1) increased susceptibility to infection; (2) development of neoplasms; and (3) graft-versus-host disease (Table 20–24). Infection represents the most important category and includes common and uncommon infectious agents. When approaching the diagnosis of infection in the immunosuppressed host, it is appropriate to consider first the more common organisms. Pneumonia is still more likely to be caused by pneumococcus, and urinary tract infection is more likely to be caused by *Escherichia coli.* Nevertheless, the immunosuppressed individual has a considerably increased risk of having pneumonia caused by *Pneumocystis carinii* or cytomegalovirus and having urinary tract infection caused by *Candida.*

In most instances, infections in the transplant recipient can be successfully treated with routine antimicrobial therapy. In the event of overwhelming infection or infection caused by an uncommon organism for which treatment may be ineffective (such as disseminated herpes), it may be of utmost importance to restrict or even stop immunosuppressive treatment to allow recruitment of host immune defenses or to employ antiviral chemotherapy, e.g., ARA-a. In some cases, such infections result in loss of the graft; however, the ultimate survival of the host must be the primary objective. Frequently, the goals of host survival and graft survival are not easily separated. In renal transplantation, the host may be kept alive by returning to hemodialysis in the event of graft failure; however, in cardiac transplantation, it is virtually impossible to save the patient who loses his graft.

The second category of undesired consequences of immunosuppression is neoplastic transformation. Since the normal immune response provides surveillance against the development of neoplasms, it is not unexpected that the immunosuppressed host is at higher risk to develop neoplasms (Chapter 19). The risk of lymphoma developing in the immunosuppressed transplant recipient appears to be increased 35-fold, with reticulum cell sarcoma occurring at 300 times the expected frequency. Of less serious clinical consequence, but also occurring with considerably increased frequency in the transplant recipient, are cancers of the skin and lip.

Perhaps the clearest example of excessive immunosuppression of the host is the development of graft-versus-host (GVH) disease. This entity lies at the far end of the spectrum of host-graft symbiosis and results when the host is so totally immunosuppressed that the donor lymphoid cells transplanted along with the graft are able to become sensitized and mount an unchallenged immune response against the host. The GVH phenomenon is well described in experimental transplantation where immunoincompetent neonatal F_1 hybrid mice are injected with parental immunocompetent spleen cells. The parental cells recognize and mount an immune response against the F_1 host cells, but the neonatal host cells fail to recognize the parental cells as foreign. In the ensuing reaction, recipient mice develop a clinical syndrome characterized by failure to thrive, runting, diarrhea, dermatitis, and eventually death. In effect, in GVH disease, the host is "rejected" by the uninhibited immune assault of donor lymphoid cells. GVH occurs infrequently (or only subclinically) in most instances; however, in bone marrow transplantation, because the recipient is often spontaneously or intentionally severely depleted of immunocompetent cells, GVH disease is not an uncommon complication. More recently, treatment of the bone marrow inoculum with monoclonal antibody to remove a subpopulation of T-lymphocytes (e.g., T8) has diminished the likelihood of GVH reactions and has enhanced the likelihood of successful engraftment.

SPECIFIC ORGAN TRANSPLANTATION

In this section, the problems relating to specific organ grafts will be presented. In most cases, general principles of organ transplantation are appropriate; however, each organ transplanted provides specialized challenges to the transplantation surgeon and immunologist.

Renal Transplantation. The successful renal transplant provides the most effective rehabilitative therapy for patients with end-stage renal disease. This is because the kidney provides not only excretory function but also a number of metabolic functions such as vitamin D metabolism and erythropoietin production. Hemodialysis or peritoneal dialysis may provide satisfactory substitution for excretory function, but metabolic functions are not adequately replaced. A dramatic example of this is transplantation of a normal kidney into a patient with Fabry's disease, in which renal failure results from the deposition of glycolipid in the kidney due to absence of α-galactosidase. After renal transplantation, levels of the enzyme as high as 10 per cent or more have been observed, suggesting that renal transplantation has resulted not only in restoration of renal function but also in partial reversal of the underlying enzyme deficiency.

Over 100,000 renal transplants have now been performed, providing the majority of current clinical experience in organ transplantation. This experience has emphasized the importance of careful management of the transplant recipient with avoidance of excessive immunosuppressive therapy. With good matching, the current success rate at two years approaches 85 per cent for living related donor transplants and 60 per cent for the cadaveric donor transplants (Fig. 20–32). Moreover, living related donor transplantation is generally associated with fewer and more easily reversible complications, allowing for a smoother post-transplantation course. For these reasons, many transplant centers prefer to do living related donor transplantation whenever possible. Graft survival statistics in renal transplantation actually have not changed significantly in a number of years; however, patient survival rates have increased, suggesting progress in medical management of the transplant recipient. It is expected, however, that the availability of cyclosporine in clinical renal transplantation will result in a significant improvement in the outcome of this form of transplantation.

The general principles of organ transplantation described above are applicable in renal post-transplantation follow-up; however, two types of complications are of special importance in renal transplantation. In a small number of patients, technical or surgical problems such as leakage of urine from the newly implanted ureter, stenosis of the newly anastomosed renal artery, or the collection of lymph around the kidney may occur. These technical problems may result in graft loss; however, prompt corrective surgical intervention is usually successful.

A second complication specific for renal transplantation is graft loss secondary to return of the original disease. This was first noted in identical twins in whom no rejection

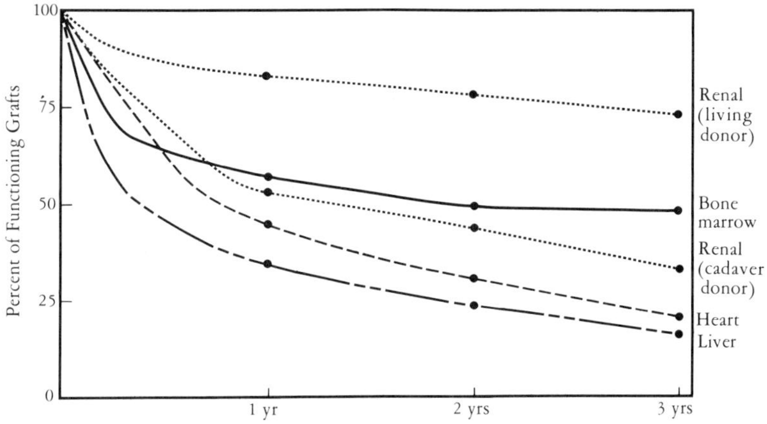

Figure 20–32. Survival of various cadaver and living related donor transplants.

should occur, yet a large proportion of recipients of twin renal grafts had loss of function. Analysis revealed that the loss of function in the transplant resulted from return of glomerulonephritis, the original disease. More recently, the list of diseases that recur after renal transplantation has been expanded to include such diseases as anti-glomerular basement membrane disease, diabetes, and oxalosis (Table 20–25).

Bone Marrow Transplantation. Over 1000 bone marrow transplants have been performed throughout the world for a variety of conditions of bone marrow failure but primarily for severe combined immunodeficiency disease (SCID) and aplastic anemia.

SCID is a rare congenital disorder in which the functional capacities of both T- and B-cell lines are absent or severely depressed (Chapter 22). Prior to 1968, the disease was incurable and invariably fatal, usually within the first year of life. Over the last decade, more than 70 children with this disorder have been treated by bone marrow transplantation. Of those treated in this way, nearly 30 per cent remain alive as long as eight years after transplantation. Almost two thirds of children who receive HLA-A and B identical and mixed lymphocyte culture unreactive bone marrow cells survive for at least six months. Children receiving HLA-A or B nonidentical but MLC unreactive marrow have a 38 per cent chance of six months' survival; however, of those receiving MLC-incompatible marrow, only 5 per cent survive six months. These results emphasize the critical importance of MLR matching and the less critical but additional importance of HLA matching.

Of those children who did not survive, nearly all died of infection within the first four months after transplantation. A second major problem in bone marrow transplantation for SCID is GVH disease. GVH is more severe in males, in males receiving bone marrow from females, and in older children (over six months of age) than it is in females and younger children.

Bone marrow transplantation in the treatment of aplastic anemia is associated with approximately a 50 per cent one-year survival. In those patients surviving a year there is virtually no increased mortality at two or three years, showing that a full "take" has occurred by one year. Younger patients (under 21 years) have better survival rates than older patients. Again, sepsis and GVH disease are the most common causes of death.

Cardiac Transplantation. The era of cardiac transplantation was ushered in with fantastic excitement, perhaps because of the mystique attributed to that organ; however, the overall results of cardiac transplantation have been somewhat disappointing. Approximately 500 heart transplants have been performed, and although there are many long-term survivors, sudden death from myocardial infarction or complete atrioventricular conduction block in patients apparently doing well has prevented the proliferation of centers performing this procedure. Nevertheless, groups actively pursuing cardiac transplantation report 50 per cent one-year

Table 20–25. Diseases Found to Recur After Renal Transplantation

Glomerulonephritis
1. Focal sclerosing glomerulonephritis
2. Membranoproliferative glomerulonephritis
3. Rapidly progressive glomerulonephritis (Anti-GBM type)
Henoch-Schönlein purpura
Polyarteritis
Oxalosis
Diabetes
Hypertension

survival and 30 to 40 per cent two-year survival.

The same general principles hold true with heart transplants as with other organ transplants; however, there are some special problems. The recipient cannot lose his graft and still survive, as he can in kidney transplantation. Except in rare circumstances, there can be no living donor heart transplantation. In cardiac transplantation, the recipient is, in most instances, otherwise uncompromised. This is different from the recipient in kidney or bone marrow transplantation, in which the recipient is immunosuppressed by uremia in the former instance or by the absence of immunocompetent cells in SCID or aplastic anemia in the latter.

It is probably too early to draw any significant conclusions regarding the future of cardiac transplantation. Certainly, heart disease is a major public health problem, and when successful, cardiac transplantation has provided from months to many years of added functional life. The vital nature of the heart, and thus the lack of available time in which to reverse the effects of rejection, make successful cardiac transplantation exceedingly difficult.

Transplantation of Other Organs. More than 500 liver transplants have now been performed with increasing success, perhaps as a result of the use of cyclosporine for liver transplantation. It has been suggested that the difficulty with liver transplantation is in part related to the surgical difficulty encountered in the procedure. Nevertheless, survivals as long as five years have been reported, and hepatic transplantation has been lifesaving in the presence of irreversible hepatic failure without major secondary systemic decompensation.

Other organs that have been transplanted include the lung and the pancreas. Experience with transplantation of these organs is still too small to provide significant conclusions as to their success rates.

Future Prospects

A major breakthrough in the field of organ transplantation has now been eagerly awaited for a number of years. Some feel that the new drug cyclosporine will represent this breakthrough. Others feel that the careful use of blood transfusions will be of benefit to transplantation survival. Still others point to the use of monoclonal antibodies to control the immune response.

From the present viewpoint, any future advances in organ graft survival will out of necessity be derived from some form of specific or selective alteration of immune responsiveness of the recipient-graft pair. One way this might occur is through immunologic tolerance—the induction of a state of immunologic unresponsiveness to a specific antigen but not to others (Chapter 10). Such states have been achieved experimentally by the induction of blocking antibodies, by a noncytotoxic form of specific antibody, and by the establishment of tolerance in the recipient through high- or low-dose antigen administration or the creation of chimerism in the recipient. All these methods are very exciting experimentally and applicable in theory but have not been successfully applied to clinical organ transplantation.

Another area that may be ultimately more difficult is the alteration or removal of the antigens of the donor organ with replacement of these antigens by those of the recipient. This would in effect result in an autograft or isograft situation and, if maintained, indefinite graft survival.

Whatever method is achieved, it is clear that the future of organ transplantation requires some form of more specific control of the immune response. If more specific immunoregulation is not forthcoming in the near future, allograft organ transplantation might well be replaced by functional artificial organ implantation, if or when technologic advances provide safe, reliable artificial hearts, kidneys, livers, or lungs.

SUMMARY

Immunologically mediated diseases involving homologous antigens include disorders resulting from immunization to those antigens that differentiate one member of the species from another, the alloantigens. The process by which this occurs is called alloimmunization. These disorders may arise as a consequence of a maternal-fetal relationship surrounding pregnancy, transfusions, or transplantation.

Since all these entities are expressions of the host's response to genetically controlled antigenic specificities, a knowledge of these genetic factors is essential for the prevention and management of these disorders.

C. Immunologically Mediated Disease Involving Autologous Antigens

Joseph A. Bellanti, M.D., John J. Calabro, M.D., and Michael C. Gelfand, M.D.

In a minority of the population there occur disorders known as autoimmune diseases. In these, the cardinal feature is tissue injury caused by an apparent immunologic reaction of the host with its own tissues. In most individuals, there exist within the host "self-recognition" and tolerance of all body components; however, in autoimmune disease, there exists the anomalous condition that Ehrlich referred to as "horror autotoxicus," in which a self-destructive process occurs directed by one's own immune system.

A clear distinction must be made between *autoimmune response* and *autoimmune disease.* The term "autoimmune response" refers to the demonstration of an autoantibody directed to a "self" antigen or reactivity of lymphocytes sensitized to a "self" antigen. The autoimmune response may or may not be associated with autoimmune disease. Although it is thought that autoimmune diseases result from tissue damage by autoimmune responses, it is not known whether the autoimmune phenomena are a cause, a result, or a concomitant finding in autoimmune disease. In spite of extensive animal experimentation, the autoimmune responses as a cause of human disease remain a hypothesis.

It is common to see autoimmune phenomena in association with infectious diseases. Cold hemagglutinins are commonly seen after infection with *Mycoplasma pneumoniae* and are sometimes associated with hemolysis. Yet there exists no evidence that this autoimmune response results in a self-perpetuating protracted autoimmune disease.

The unfortunate use of the term "autoimmune disease," implying a primary attack of the host against itself, arose prior to current knowledge of immunologic mechanisms of tissue injury (Chapter 13). The terms "collagen," "collagen-vascular," and "connective tissue" diseases have likewise imposed additional semantic problems. These terms focus undue attention on the connective tissue, which is only one of several tissues involved. The immunopathology of autoimmune disease may manifest itself by any of the mechanisms of tissue injury described in Chapter 13. Autoimmunity may be considered a tertiary manifestation of the immune response directed at antigen whose inappropriate processing leads to destruction of host tissues. This view differs from the classic concept of a primary attack of the host against its own tissues.

THEORIES OF PATHOGENESIS OF THE AUTOIMMUNE DISEASES

Three hypotheses have been proposed to explain the mechanism and manifestations of autoimmune disease (Fig. 20–33).

The first hypothesis, the *forbidden-clone theory,* postulates a clone of mutant lymphocytes arising through somatic mutation (Fig. 20–33*A*). Mutant cells that carry a surface antigen recognized as foreign (antigenically positive mutant) would be normally destroyed. However, according to this theory, mutant cells that lack surface antigen (antigenically negative mutants) would not be destroyed. With the proliferation of these antigen-deficient mutants (forbidden clones), these cells would be capable of reacting with target tissues because of genetic dissimilarity. The phenomenon is analogous to a genetically incompatible lymphocyte graft-versus-host reaction (Chapter 3).

The second hypothesis, the *sequestered-antigen theory,* is based on the phenomenon of tolerance induction in the fetus (Chapter 3) (Fig. 20–33*B*). According to this theory, during embryonic development, tissues that are exposed to the lymphoreticular system are recognized as "self." Those that are anatomically separated or sequestered from the lymphoreticular system are not identified as "self." These antigens occur in tissues such as the lens of the eye, the central nervous system, the thyroid, and the testes. In later life, exposure, through trauma or infection, of the sequestered tissue antigens to the lymphoreticular system results in autoimmune disease.

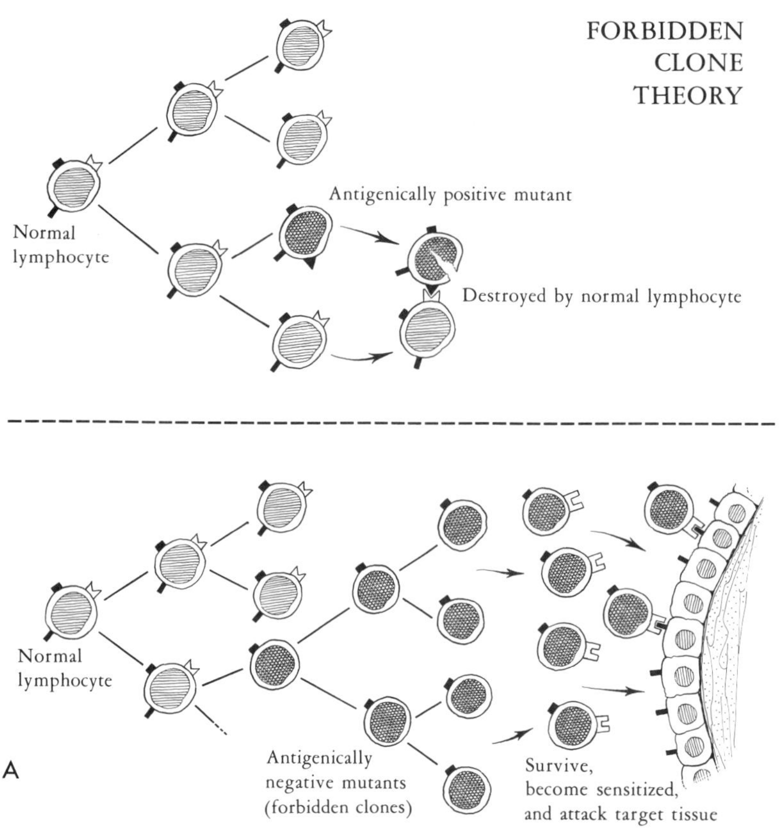

Figure 20–33. Schematic representation of possible mechanisms of development of autoimmunity. *A,* Forbidden-clone theory. *B,* Sequestered-antigen theory. *C,* Immunologic deficiency theory. Note that immunologic deficiency can lead to emergence of deleterious clones or to immunologic injury secondary to persistence of microbes.

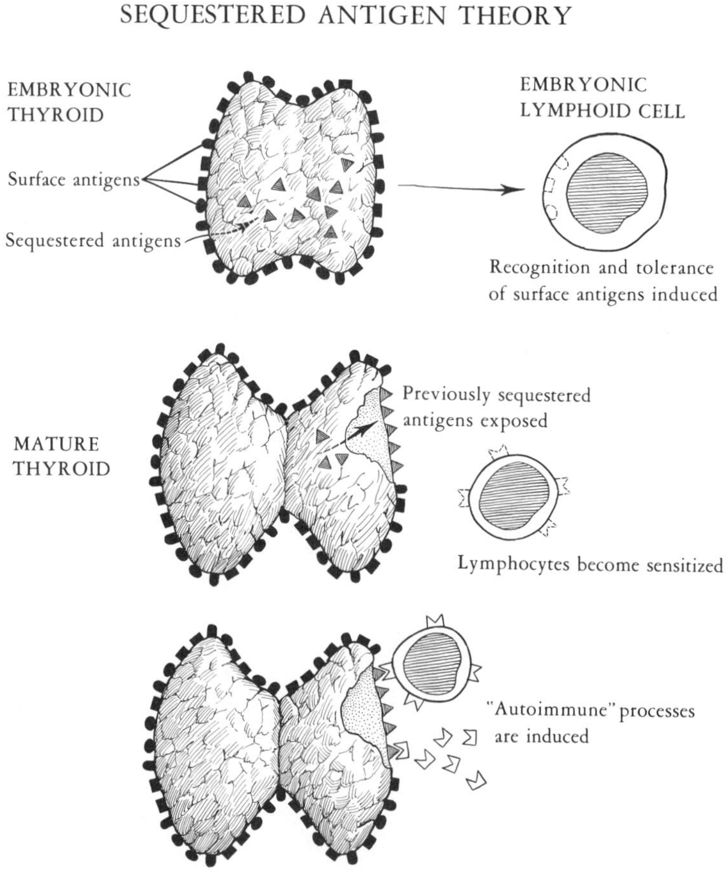

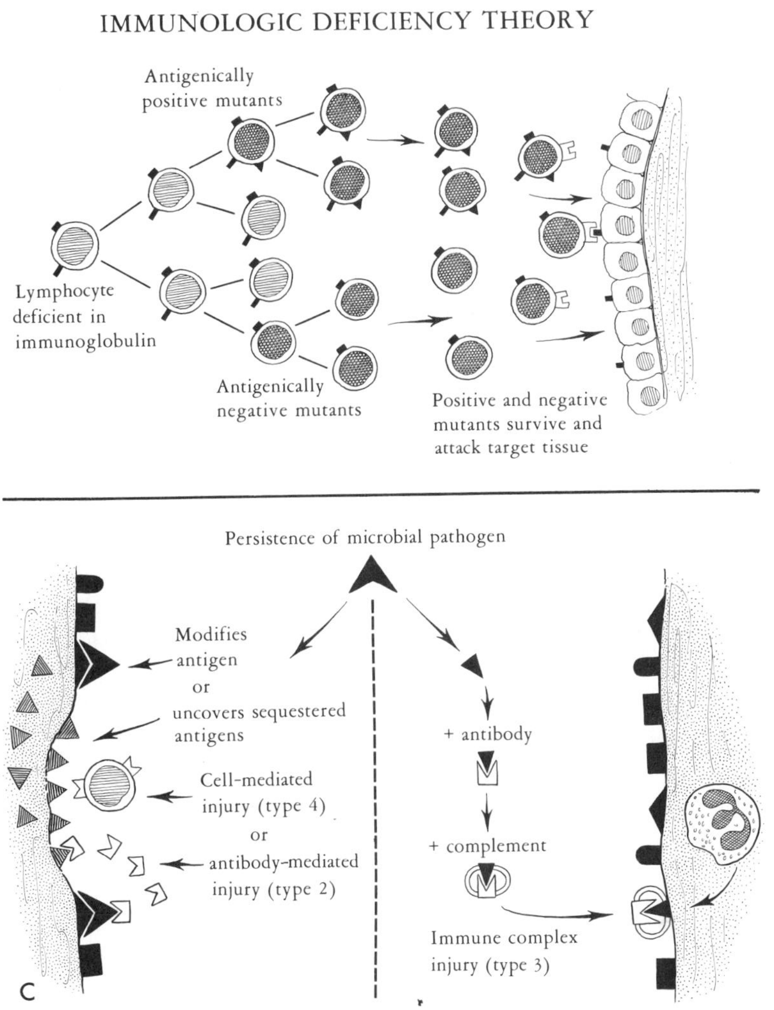

Figure 20–33 *Continued.*

Both these concepts are based on the premise of *hyperactivity* of the immune response, which through autoantibody formation or sensitized lymphocytes (delayed hypersensitivity) would lead to the production of an autoimmune disease.

A third hypothesis, the concept of *immunologic deficiency,* is based on a hypoactive or a deficient immunologic system (Fig. 20–33*C*). It derives its support from the clinically observed relationships between immunologic deficiency syndromes and the increased incidence of autoimmune abnormalities (Chapter 22). These relationships have been extrapolated largely from data obtained in experimental animals. Injury would occur through the emergence of mutant lymphocytes or as a consequence of persistence of microbial antigen (Fig. 20–25*C*). From these observations, it has been postulated that otherwise normal individuals who develop autoimmune disease may, in fact, have a more subtle form of underlying immune deficiency predisposing them to the autoimmune states.

Finally, any concept that seeks to explain the development of the autoimmune state must take into account the genetic control of the immune system (Chapter 3). Familial patterns and sex distributions (for example, showing a female predominance) characterize most of the autoimmune disorders. The discovery of the association of certain histocompatibility antigens with a variety of diseases suggests that the immune response (Ir) gene in humans may be closely linked to the HLA loci on the sixth chromosome (Chapter 3). The most notable association is the relatively high risk of the development of ankylosing spondylitis or Reiter's syndrome in HLA-B27–positive individuals, who have an inherited susceptibility to develop spondylitis or Reiter's syndrome from a variety of antigenic stimuli. Other associations between human diseases and HLA antigens are shown in Table 20–26.

Recent evidence in both the experimental animal and the human suggests a disordered immune regulation based upon genetically determined imbalances of the T-cell subpopulations (i.e., T_4 helper/inducer and T_8 cytotoxic/suppressor cells) as an important determinant in the development of autoimmune diseases as well as the allergic diseases (Chapter 20A).

CLASSIFICATION

The autoimmune diseases are grouped into the *systemic* and *organ-specific* diseases (Table 20–27). Systemic disorders are those in which major involvement is seen in more than one organ, and the organ-specific diseases are those in which the major effect involves a single organ.

SYSTEMIC AUTOIMMUNE DISEASES

Systemic Lupus Erythematosus (SLE)

Seen mainly in females, SLE is a generalized disorder that expresses itself as a vasculitis involving many organ systems. The primary target cells are the hematopoietic system, skin, joints, and kidney (Fig. 20–34). These are involved in a variety of ways by a vast array of antibodies (Table 20–28). Antibodies to red cells, white cells, and platelets account for the hemolytic anemia, leukopenia, and thrombocytopenia, respectively. A prolonged prothrombin time and partial thromboplastin time are occasionally seen because of a "lupus anticoagulant"; in some cases, antibodies to coagulation factors may be observed. Antibody to nuclear material or other unknown antigens may complex with antigen and lead to injury of vascular tissues, glomerular membrane of the kidney, or synovial lining of the joints (Fig. 20–35). The extensive antibody formation is reflected by the hypergammaglobulinemia, i.e., polyclonal gammopathy, characteristic of many of the autoimmune diseases. Except for damage to blood cells, the autoantibody alone does not seem to initiate tissue damage directly. Damage is thought to occur primarily through the deposition of these antigen-antibody complexes (Type III reaction). As in many of the complex-induced vascular disorders, certain tissues are more vulnerable to injury than others. These tissues include the small blood vessels, glomeruli, joints, spleen, and heart valves.

Pathogenesis. A genetic predisposition, termed "lupus diathesis," has been implicated on the basis of increased incidence in twins

Table 20–26. **HLA Antigens and Human Disease**

Disease	Antigen	Disease	Antigen
Ankylosing spondylitis	B27	Psoriasis	B13, B17, B27, B37, Cw6, D11, DR7
Reiter's syndrome	B27	Pemphigus	B13
Reactive arthritis (*Yersinia, Salmonella,* and *Shigella* infections)	B27	Multiple sclerosis	A3, B7, B18, D2
Rheumatoid arthritis	Dw4, DRw4	Myasthenia gravis	B8
Systemic lupus erythematosus	A1, B8, DR3	Acute anterior uveitis	B27
Diabetes mellitus (insulin-dependent)	B8, B15, Dw3	Chronic glomerulonephritis	A2
Graves' disease	B8	Hodgkin's disease	B5
Addison's disease	B8, Dw3	Chronic myelogenous leukemia	A3
Celiac disease	Dw3, B8	Acute lymphocytic leukemia	A2, B12
Chronic active hepatitis	B8	Lymphosarcoma	B12
Pernicious anemia	B7	Primary Sjögren's syndrome	Dw3

Table 20–27. **Autoimmune Diseases**

I. Systemic

Systemic lupus erythematosus (SLE)
Rheumatoid arthritis, ankylosing spondylitis
Sjögren's syndrome
Polyarteritis nodosa
Polymyositis and dermatomyositis
Progressive systemic sclerosis (scleroderma)
Mixed connective tissue disease

II. Organ-Specific

Organ	Disease Manifestation
Blood	Anemia, leukopenia, thrombocytopenia
Central nervous system (CNS)	Allergic encephalitis, demyelinating diseases
Endocrine	Thyroiditis, Addison's disease, hypoparathyroidism
Gastrointestinal	Pernicious anemia, ulcerative colitis, regional ileitis, gluten-sensitive enteropathy
Liver	Chronic liver disease
Kidney	Goodpasture's syndrome, acute poststreptococcal nephritis
Muscle	Myasthenia gravis
Heart	Rheumatic fever
Eye	Uveitis, sympathetic ophthalmia
Skin	Dermatitis herpetiformis, lupus erythematosus, bullous pemphigoid, pemphigus vulgaris

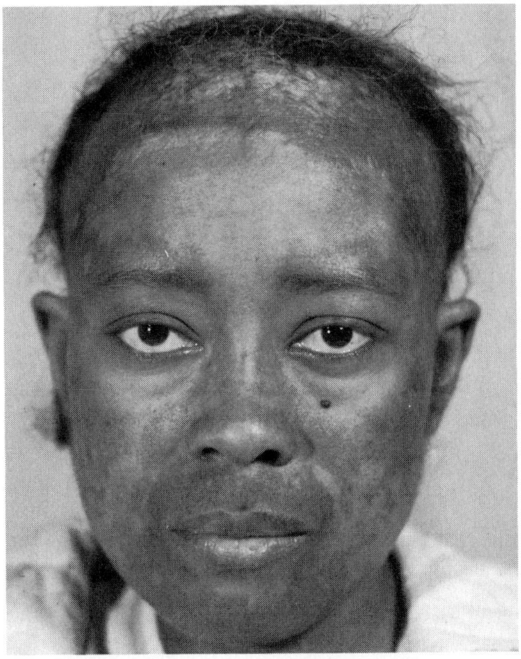

Figure 20–34. Photograph of a patient with systemic lupus erythematosus (SLE) showing the skin lesions and alopecia. (Courtesy of Dr. F. Paul Alepa.)

Table 20–28. **Common Manifestations of SLE**

Mechanism	Manifestation
Antibody to RBC	Coombs + hemolytic anemia
Antibody to WBC	Leukopenia
Antibody to platelets	Thrombocytopenia
Antibody to clotting factors	Prolonged clotting time
Extensive antibody formation	Hypergammaglobulinemia
Antigen-antibody complex: blood vessels	Vasculitis
Antigen-antibody complex: glomeruli	Nephritis
Antigen-antibody complex: synovial membrane	Arthritis

and the existence of autoimmune disease in the families of patients with lupus erythematosus. Additionally, there appears to be an increased incidence in patients who are HLA-DR2 or DR3 positive. Transient lupus-like syndromes have occurred after prolonged use of drugs such as hydralazine and procainamide (Chapter 20A). In the genetically susceptible individual, certain exogenous factors such as ultraviolet light, certain drugs, and a variety of infectious agents may serve as antigens or produce antigens that trigger self-destructive immunologic responses.

Evidence obtained from the experimental animal also suggests a genetic etiology. In inbred New Zealand black (NZB) strains of mice, a lupus-like syndrome occurs consisting of LE cells and glomerular lesions. In addition to a genetic predisposition, the finding of virus-like particles in these mice raises the possibility of an infectious etiology leading to the autoimmune state. There is recent evidence that suppressor T-cells or a soluble immune response suppressor (SIRS) substance may be deficient in NZB mice (Chapter 10). Although the precise function of suppressor T-cells in the human is unknown, they seem to play an important role in immunologic regulation and in the prevention of autoantibody production. It might follow, then, that a deficiency of suppressor cell function might allow B-cells to escape from this normal regulatory mechanism and proceed to produce autoantibodies. The descriptions of myxovirus subparticles in renal biopsy material from human cases of systemic lupus erythematosus accentuate this possibility in man (Fig. 20–36). The significance of these findings is as yet unknown.

Immunologic Tests. The lupus erythematosus (LE) cell is a polymorphonuclear leukocyte that has ingested nuclear material complexed with antinuclear antibody (Fig. 20–37). Tests for the presence of these cells may be used to verify the diagnosis of SLE. Peripheral blood or bone marrow is incubated at 37° C, and LE cells are then sought. Because of their nonspecificity, these tests are rarely performed today. More frequently, antibodies directed against protein or other nuclear materials are sought in the diagnosis of SLE. Some antibodies are detected by

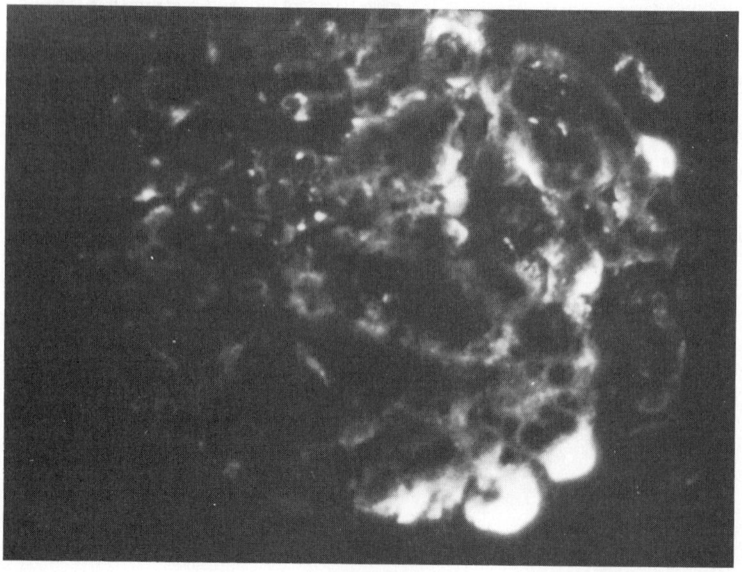

Figure 20–35. Photomicrograph of a kidney of a patient with SLE showing the characteristic irregular immunofluorescent deposition of IgG globulins along the glomerular basement membrane. Original magnification ×100. (Courtesy of Dr. Heinz Bauer.)

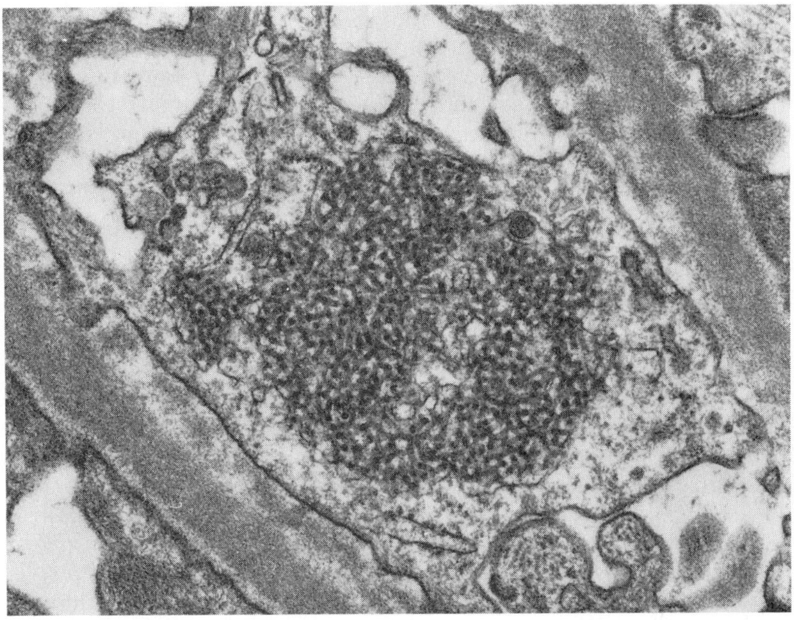

Figure 20–36. Microtubular structures seen in a kidney biopsy of a patient with SLE. ×32,000. (Courtesy of Dr. Theodore Pincus; from Pincus, T., Blacklow, N. R., Grimley, P. M., et al.: Glomerular microtubules of systemic lupus erythematosus. Lancet, *2*:1058, 1970.)

fluorescence (fluorescent antinuclear antibody); others are detected by ammonium sulfate precipitation techniques (Chapter 8).

Antinuclear antibodies (ANA) have the capacity of complexing with antigen and fixing complement. When the disease is most active, particularly with renal involvement, there is diminished circulating complement (e.g., C3) in the sera of these individuals, which assumes both diagnostic and therapeutic significance since levels become normal with successful therapy.

Tests for ANA are currently being used to screen for SLE. Since ANA and LE cells also occur in patients receiving drugs, a careful history of drug ingestion should be obtained. Complement levels may provide a useful guide in both the diagnosis and the management of the disease, particularly with renal involvement. Rare SLE patients with defi-

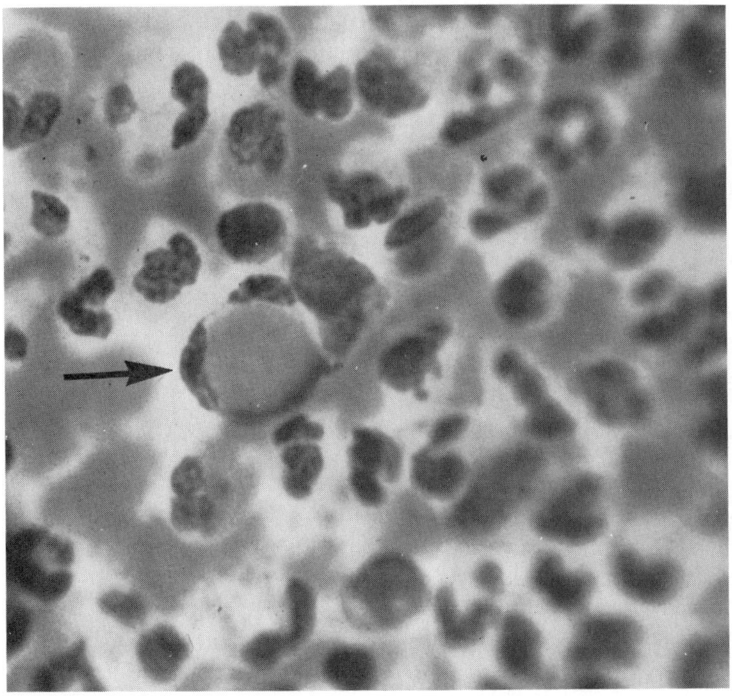

Figure 20–37. Photomicrograph of a lupus erythematosus (LE) cell. Note the amorphous intracytoplasmic inclusion within the polymorphonuclear leukocyte. ×1200. (Courtesy of Dr. S. Gerald Sandler.)

ciency of the early components of complement should also be identified (Chapters 6 and 22). Anti-DNA antibody and DNA binding are additional tests that have a high specificity for SLE and are used serially to assess disease activity. Among these are the antibodies to extractable nuclear antigens (ENA), such as ribonucleoprotein (RNP), Sm, Ro, and La antigens. It is of interest that immunofluorescent microscopy of skin reveals immunoglobulin deposition at the dermoepidermal junction in over 90 per cent of specimens from involved skin and in over 50 per cent from uninvolved skin in patients with SLE. In contrast, in discoid lupus, the deposits are noted only in involved skin.

The treatment of SLE is variable. In some patients, nonsteroidal anti-inflammatory drugs may provide adequate control of disease activity. In others, particularly those with major organ system involvement, corticosteroids and, in some cases, cytotoxic drugs are necessary (Chapter 25).

Rheumatoid Arthritis (RA)

Rheumatoid arthritis is another disease that may involve many organ systems by producing vasculitis (Fig. 20–38). The most frequent site of injury is the synovial lining of joints (Fig. 20–39). More widespread lesions may occur, particularly in systemic RA.

Pathogenesis and Etiology. The etiology of RA is unknown. Several etiologies have been postulated, including metabolic derangements and infectious agents (bacteria and mycoplasma). Indirect evidence has been presented for viruses in synovial membranes of patients with RA. However, there is no direct proof that these play a role in the pathogenesis of RA. A mild arthritis is known to accompany some viral infections. For example, following natural rubella or rubella immunization, approximately one third of adults develop transient rheumatoid arthritis–like effects.

Genetics. Families of probands affected with RA show an increased incidence of connective tissue disorders (e.g., SLE). Furthermore, children with immune deficiency (e.g., agammaglobulinemia) have an increased incidence of connective tissue diseases (e.g., rheumatoid arthritis). Additionally, there is an increased incidence of HLA-DR4 in RA patients. Hence, there may exist underlying genetic factors determining the susceptibility of patients to RA, but they are complex and, at present, ill understood.

Immunologic Findings. Rheumatoid factors (RF) is an IgM globulin that has the capacity to react with IgG globulins *in vitro.* There are other antiglobulins of the IgG, IgE, and IgA variety. The stimulus for the production of RF is not known. This factor is found in the sera and synovial fluid of most adult patients with established rheumatoid arthritis but is seldom seen in juvenile RA. Although RF is diagnostically useful, it is not specific for the disease and is found in a host of other diseases, including the connective tissue disorders. The test for RF is carried out using various carrier substances as a vehicle for the gamma globulin (latex, bentonite, and erythrocytes).

Because of the rheumatoid factor–gamma globulin–complement complex has been found in synovial fluids, RF has been implicated as a causative factor of the chronic inflammatory joint disease of RA. Unlike the case of SLE, a lowered serum complement level is rarely seen in the sera of patients with RA. Since the complexes are localized primarily within the joints, lowered complement levels have been found in the joint fluids of patients with RA. Synthesis of RF has also been demonstrated within the synovia of affected joints.

Immunologic Tests. In adults, the major differentiating test for RA is the serum RF test. In the systemic or acute febrile form of juvenile RA, the onset of illness often resembles that of an acute infectious process with high fever, rash, leukocytosis, and a rapid sedimentation rate. In children, the definitive diagnosis of RA may have to await the development of joint manifestations.

Treatment of RA is directed primarily at relieving joint pain and inflammation. Commonly used drugs include the salicylates and other nonsteroidal agents. Most patients are benefited by these agents and physiotherapy. Patients with progressive RA may require gold, antimalarials, D-penicillamine, steroids, or even the cytotoxic drugs. These agents may have "remittive" effects in that they may halt the progression of RA.

Ankylosing Spondylitis (AS)

Ankylosing spondylitis (AS) is a systemic rheumatic disorder characterized by inflammation of the sacroiliac and spinal apophys-

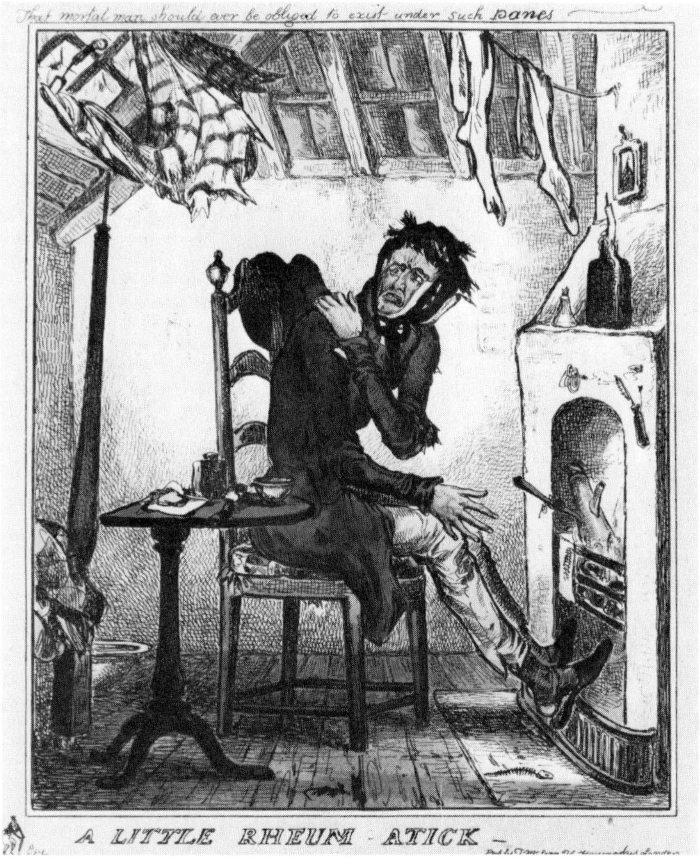

Figure 20–38. Caricature of a patient with "rheum-atick"; "that mortal man should ever be obliged to exist under such panes." (Courtesy of National Library of Medicine.)

eal (synovial) joints. Consequently, back pain is a frequent presenting complaint, although the disease can begin in peripheral joints and, rarely, even with acute iridocyclitis. AS affects ten times more men than women and begins most often between the ages of 20 and 40.

Although the precise etiology of AS remains uncertain, evidence for the influence of genetic factors appears to be mounting. AS has long been suspected of having a genetic background, first because of the striking familial clustering observed among patients, and second because of a high concordance rate found in monozygotic twins. More recently, the disclosure of an unusually high frequency of the inherited antigen HLA-B27

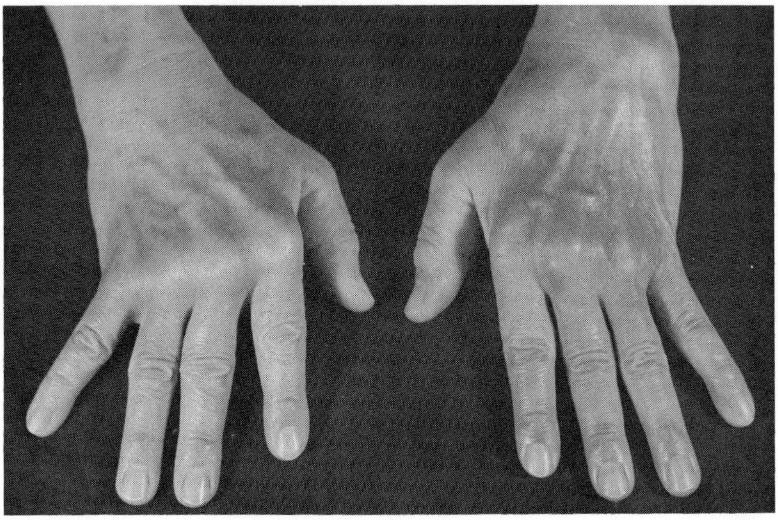

Figure 20–39. Photograph of the hands of a patient with moderately advanced rheumatoid arthritis. Note the deformities of the metacarpal-phalangeal joints with atrophy of the hypothenar muscles and ulnar deviation. (Courtesy of Dr. F. Paul Alepa.)

in up to 96 per cent of patients and 50 per cent of first-degree relatives as compared with 9 per cent of controls provides overwhelming evidence of a genetic linkage in this disorder.

The frequent associations between AS and such seemingly unrelated disorders as ulcerative colitis, regional enteritis, Reiter's syndrome, and psoriasis have, until recently, been unexplained. It now appears that among these underlying disorders, patients with the B27 antigen are those who are primarily destined to develop AS. In fact, it has been estimated that the risk of developing AS is 40 times greater in patients with ulcerative colitis carrying the B27 antigen than in those without the antigen.

Precisely how this genetic relationship links the susceptible individual to the eventual development of AS is unknown. However, recent reports provide evidence of antibody formation and immune complex deposition in AS. Consequently, the pathogenesis of AS may evolve in the following manner. Variable inciting factors, such as ulcerative colitis, might precipitate the evolution of spondylitis in a genetically predisposed individual having the B27 marker. The disease may then be perpetuated by a self-destructive attack of the immune response against "altered self."

Key drugs in management include indomethacin and phenylbutazone, each of which promptly suppresses joint inflammation and discomfort, thereby allowing patients to undertake lifelong supportive measures such as postural training and therapeutic exercise. These drugs, however, do not prevent progression of AS. For rare patients with advanced kyphoscoliosis, vertebral wedge osteotomy may prove beneficial.

SJÖGREN'S SYNDROME (SS)

Sjögren's syndrome (SS), in its primary form, consists of keratoconjunctivitis sicca (dry eyes) and xerostomia (dry mouth). However, SS more often occurs secondary to RA or one of the connective tissue disorders such as SLE, scleroderma, or polymyositis. One of the most characteristic features of SS is the remarkable immunologic reactivity detected in serum. LE cells, ANA, RF, and hypergammaglobulinemia are frequently present; antibodies against RNA, salivary duct, lacrimal gland, smooth muscle, mitochondria, and thyroid gland may also be found. Additionally, antibodies against antigens termed SS-A and SS-B are found in a high percentage of SS patients. There is an increased frequency of renal tubular acidosis in SS. Lymphoma may also develop in these patients, particularly in those with the primary form of SS.

Anti–salivary duct antibodies, demonstrated by indirect immunofluorescence of human salivary and lacrimal glands, occur more frequently in patients with SS and RA than in those with primary SS. These antibodies appear to block (react with and cover) determinants on ductal lining cells that might otherwise be attacked by sensitized lymphocytes. Recently, an association of HLA-DW3 has been made with the primary Sjögren's syndrome.

Diagnosis is confirmed by salivary technetium pertechnetate scintiscanning, which is more sensitive than sialography, and labial biopsy. Treatment includes supportive measures such as the use of artificial tears and steroids or immunosuppressive drugs for serious systemic manifestations such as vasculitis.

Necrotizing Angiitis

Necrotizing angiitis encompasses a group of entities characterized by segmental inflammation of arteries. Polyarteritis nodosa (PN) has a predilection for males and involves both median and small arteries whereas hypersensitivity angiitis involves only small vessels. Clinically, it is often difficult to distinguish PN from hypersensitivity angiitis except that marked cutaneous involvement suggests hypersensitivity angiitis, which is often caused by drugs, notably sulfonamides and penicillin. The toxic appearance of patients with either disorder reflects the variable and widespread organ involvement that results from diffuse vascular occlusion. Treatment includes high doses of steroids and occasionally the addition of other immunosuppressive drugs. The prognosis is better for hypersensitivity angiitis; surviving patients should avoid implicated drugs.

Henoch-Schönlein's purpura affects small vessels of the skin, joints, and gastrointestinal tract (Fig. 20–40). Purpura, gastrointestinal bleeding, and focal glomerulonephritis frequently accompany the angiitis. Recently, biopsies of purpuric lesions have revealed bright granular deposits of IgA, C3, and fibrin-fibrinogen in capillaries and connective tissue of the dermis, findings that may be

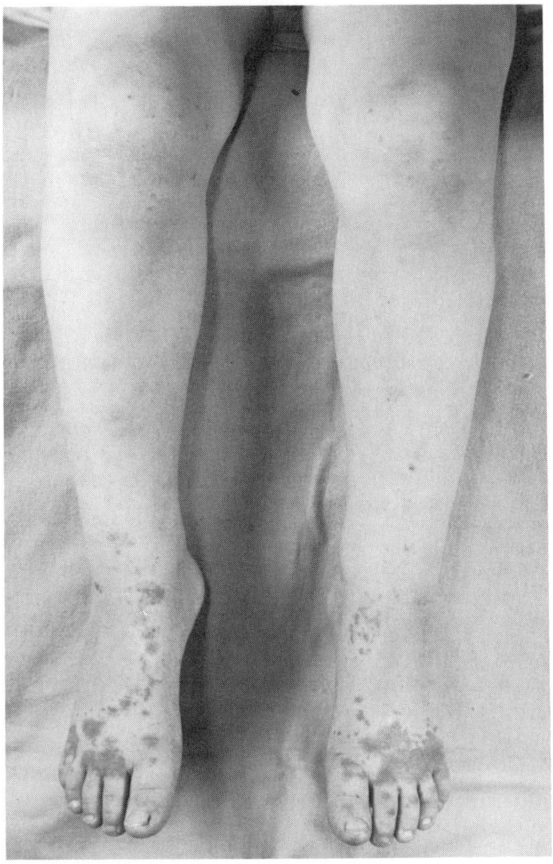

Figure 20–40. Photograph of the lower extremities and feet of a child with Henoch-Schönlein purpura. Note the purpuric lesions characteristically localized to the skin of the lower extremities.

useful diagnostically, particularly in atypical cases. In Wegener's granulomatosis, vasculitis occurs in the upper respiratory tract, lung, and kidney; in Kawasaki disease, it occurs chiefly in the coronary arteries; in Takayasu's (pulseless) disease, it occurs in the aorta and its major branches; and in giant cell arteritis, it occurs in the temporal and other cranial arteries.

Pathogenesis and Etiology. The presence of immune complexes of the hepatitis B antigen (HB_sAg) in affected tissues, including the kidney, has recently been demonstrated in 30 to 40 per cent of patients with PN. Otherwise, the etiology of these conditions remains unknown. The immunopathologic hallmark of these entities, however, is a vasculitis similar to an immune complex–type injury. Laboratory findings include a leukocytosis and occasionally eosinophilia. With kidney involvement, there may be a heterogeneity of cellular elements found within the urinary sediment ("telescoped urine"). Biopsy is the sole means of confirming a diagnosis and should be obtained from an affected area.

Polymyositis (Dermatomyositis)

Polymyositis is another systemic autoimmune disorder characterized pathologically by degeneration and inflammation of skeletal muscle. Clinically, the disease is manifested by weakness of the shoulder and pelvic girdle muscles. Dermatomyositis is a form of polymyositis in which there is also involvement of the skin (Fig. 20–41).

Pathogenesis and Etiology. The etiology of these conditions is obscure, although evidence for a cell-mediated mode of immune injury of muscle continues to mount. Of interest is an overall incidence of a malignant disorder seen in up to 20 per cent of cases,

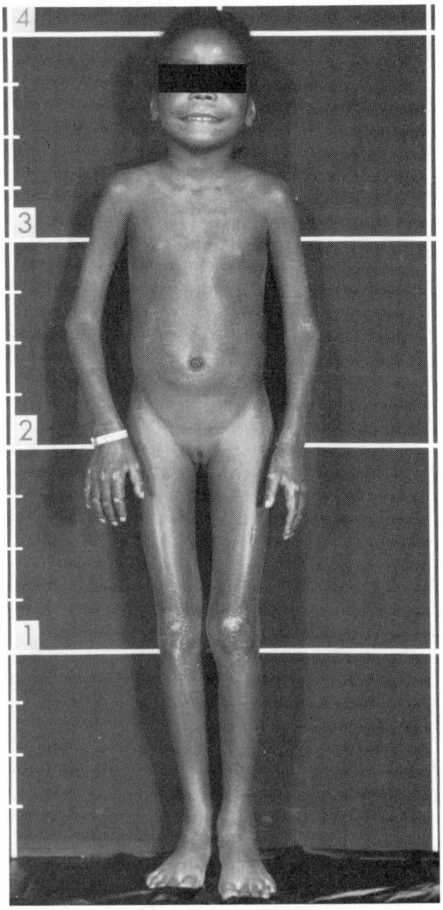

Figure 20–41. Photograph of a patient with dermatomyositis. Note the atrophy of the skin and the wasting of the proximal musculature. (Courtesy of Dr. F. Paul Alepa.)

usually in patients with dermatomyositis. This incidence is related to the age of the host, being highest in the aged. Therefore, in any older adult with these diseases, a diligent search for neoplasm should be undertaken, particularly when the onset is acute. Laboratory findings include elevated serum muscle enzymes (transaminase, aldolase, and creatine phosphokinase) and abnormal electromyographic tracings. The diagnosis can be substantiated by muscle biopsy. Treatment includes the use of immunosuppressants, e.g., steroids.

Progressive Systemic Sclerosis (PSS; Scleroderma)

PSS is a chronic illness of unknown etiology characterized by a fibrous thickening of the skin (scleroderma) and several internal organs (gastrointestinal tract, heart, kidney, and lungs). Two thirds of the patients are female.

Increased levels of immunoglobulins, ANA (particularly of the speckled and nucleolar patterns), and DNA binding in children with PSS and localized scleroderma (morphea and hemiatrophy) are evidence for an antigen-mediated pathogenesis. *In vitro* examination of scleroderma skin fibroblasts demonstrates an increase in collagen synthesis, suggesting that the basic defect in PSS is one of disordered regulation or activation of the fibroblast. Currently, there is no effective therapy, although D-penicillamine holds some promise, particularly for the skin disease of PSS.

Mixed Connective Tissue Disease (MCTD)

This designation is reserved for patients with combined clinical features of RA, SLE, PSS, and polymyositis. Patients exhibit polyarthritis, diffusely swollen hands, Raynaud's phenomenon, disturbed esophageal motility, myositis, lymphadenopathy, and hypergammaglobulinemia. Typically, patients have positive ANA of the speckled pattern. Diagnosis is confirmed by the demonstration of high titers of antibody to extractable nuclear antigen (ENA), particularly the RNP antigen. MCTD serum antibody does not react with the antigen when it is pretreated with ribonuclease, unlike the case in SLE. In MCTD, serum complement levels are normal. Many patients respond readily to corticosteroids. Prognosis seems favorable, but long-term follow-up indicates that many patients evolve into a classic connective tissue disease, such as PSS.

Summary

In these systemic diseases, it is apparent that the etiology has remained obscure. With the exception of polyarteritis nodosa, they are often manifested as a group of diseases in which a preponderance of females is seen. In cases in which immunopathologic data are available, there also exists a vasculitis that seems to be the hallmark of these diseases. This is reminiscent of damage seen in the experimental form of immune complex–type injury (Chapter 13). The diagnosis is established by the clinical pattern and, in some cases, by appropriate laboratory tests. Treatment in most of these pateints is accomplished by the use of immunosuppressive agents. An autoimmune etiology is suggested by the multiplicity of immune phenomena that often accompany these disorders and account for their protean manifestations.

SPECIFIC ORGAN DISEASES

Autoimmune Hemolytic Anemias (AHA)

The AHA are a heterogeneous group of anemias characterized by a hemolytic process associated with red cell–specific antibodies in the serum. Some of the antibodies agglutinate red cells (agglutinins); others lyse them (hemolysins) in the presence of complement. Since these antibodies are directed against the patient's own red cells, they are called autoantibodies. The AHA are classified according to physical characteristics of the antibodies (Table 20–29).

The most common of the AHA are the warm agglutinin group, consisting of idiopathic and secondary types. In these patients, the antibodies are of the IgG class and show limited complement-fixing ability. In the *idiopathic* type, which accounts for more than half of all cases of AHA, the etiology remains obscure. On long-term follow-up, however, some of these patients develop lymphoma. In the secondary type, anemia occurs in association with one of many diseases or after the use of drugs.

Table 20–29. **Characteristics of Red Cell Autoantibody**

Type	Antibody Type	Ability to Fix C′	Type of Disease
Warm agglutinins (37° C)	IgG	Rare	Idiopathic: > 50 per cent; secondary: lymphoproliferative diseases, tumors, viral diseases, sarcoidosis and drugs, SLE
Cold agglutinins (4° C)	IgM	Frequent	Infectious mononucleosis (anti-i), *M. pneumoniae* (anti-I), cold agglutinin disease (kappa chain)
Cold hemolysins (4° C)	IgG	Usually	Donath-Landsteiner antibody (variable infections)

In the cold agglutinin group, antibodies of the IgM class have the ability to fix complement and react in the cold (4° C), primarily against the I blood group. These anti-I autoantibodies are found in such diseases as atypical pneumonia *(Mycoplasma pneumoniae),* infectious mononucleosis, and cold agglutinin disease (Chapter 21).

The cold autohemolysins (Donath-Landsteiner type) are found in a third group of AHA associated with paroxysmal cold hemoglobinuria and variable infections, including viral. This disease was first described in patients with tertiary syphilis. The antibodies are IgG and uniformly fix complement. Owing to avid complement fixation, most red cells are lysed before they reach phagocytic cells, producing rapid intravascular hemolysis with the hemoglobinemia and hemoglobinuria characteristic of the disease.

Etiology. The etiology of AHA is unknown. It has been postulated that exogenous agents (drugs and viruses) may alter antigenic structure of the red cell membrane, resulting in susceptibility of the erythrocyte to hemolysis. In patients who develop AHA there may be a genetically determined susceptibility to develop autoantibodies that in some cases may be associated with immunologic abnormalities, e.g., an inherited or acquired partial failure to form immunoglobulins.

Diagnosis. The major diagnostic criteria used in differentiating the AHA from other forms of anemia are the presence of spherocytes in the peripheral smear and a positive antiglobulin reaction (Coombs' test) for autoantibody. Temperature-dependent agglutination reactions will help identify the specific type of autoantibody (Table 20–29).

Therapy. In the warm agglutinin types, steroids are useful drugs, but other immunosuppressive agents, such as azathioprine, may be employed if the patient fails to respond. Splenectomy may also benefit some patients who are unresponsive to steroids. In the cold agglutinin group, no specific treatment is required for the postinfectious type; cytotoxic agents are useful in the idiopathic variety. In paroxysmal cold hemoglobinuria, drug therapy has been unsuccessful, although transfusions with blood previously warmed to 37° C are often beneficial.

Endocrine

Autoimmune antibodies have been found in disorders of the thyroid, adrenal, pancreas, and parathyroid glands. The most extensively studied and most frequently occurring are diseases involving the thyroid gland.

THYROID GLAND

The diseases of the thyroid gland in which autoimmune factors have been found are *thyroiditis* and *Graves' disease.*

Thyroiditis is a condition in which varying degrees of destruction of the gland with inflammatory infiltration occur. The patient may present with *acute, subacute,* or *chronic* manifestations of the disease, which are defined by the degree of inflammation and its duration. The immunologic nature of thyroiditis was clarified by studies in which the disease was produced in rabbits by injecting thyroid tissue emulsified in complete Freund's adjuvant. Although originally thought to be mediated by antibody, it is now felt that the primary mechanism of immunologic injury may involve other mechanisms, e.g., cell-mediated injury.

Acute thyroiditis may be either suppurative or nonsuppurative. There is evidence that the nonsuppurative form may have an immunologic basis. It presents with fever, sore throat, and an enlarged, tender thyroid gland. Symptoms of hyperthyroidism may be present, and the serum thyroxine concentration may be elevated. Symptoms may resemble those of infection, and there may be an elevated white count and a rapid sedimentation rate. The possibility of thyroiditis should be seriously considered in any patient who presents with hyperthyroidism. The female to male ratio is 6:1.

A less fulminating clinical picture occurs in *subacute thyroiditis.* This may or may not be preceded by acute thyroiditis. In this condition, there occurs a tender nodular thyroid gland or a localized goiter that may be confused with carcinoma. Although at one time considered a rare entity, subacute thyroiditis is now being recognized more commonly. Characteristically, patients are euthyroid and no abnormalities in thyroid function are detected.

In chronic lymphocytic thyroiditis (Hashimoto's thyroiditis), the patient has progressed through acute and subacute phases (Fig. 20–42). He may remain euthyroid or may develop varying degrees of hypothyroidism. Depletion of the gland may be total, resulting in myxedema. In the classic form, a diffusely enlarged, nontender gland is found. In cases with myxedema, physical examination may reveal either a goiter or a small, firm thyroid gland with the findings of depressed thyroid function.

As a result of newer immunologic discoveries, Graves' disease is now considered to be a multisystem disorder in which three clinically distinct entities exist: (1) hyperthyroidism due to a diffuse goiter, (2) infiltrative ophthalmopathy (exophthalmos), and (3) infiltrative dermopathy ("localized pretibial myxedema"). These three components may present individually or in combination with each other. The manifestations of infiltrative ophthalmopathy and infiltrative dermopathy are more commonly seen in the adult patient in whom a higher incidence of antibodies is encountered.

The association between Graves' disease and Hashimoto's disease is becoming more frequently recognized. The two entities frequently coexist and indeed may represent different manifestations of a common spectrum. Circulating antibodies as well as *in vitro* lymphoproliferative responses to various constituents of thyroid are commonly found in both. Moreover, pathologic changes of Hashimoto's disease are frequently seen in the thyroid gland of patients with Graves' disease. In addition to circulating antibodies, which may represent autoimmune phenomena, antibodies have been described in these two diseases that appear to regulate cellular activity and may actually contribute to the hyperthyroidism. These include a long-acting thyroid stimulator (LATS), a LATS protector activity (LPA), and thyroid-stimulating immunoglobulins (TSI). It is unclear at present whether these activities represent three distinct antibodies or whether they may all be different manifestations of the same antibody specificity, differing only in the methods employed for their detection. These antibodies are detected by means of bioassay–LATS by

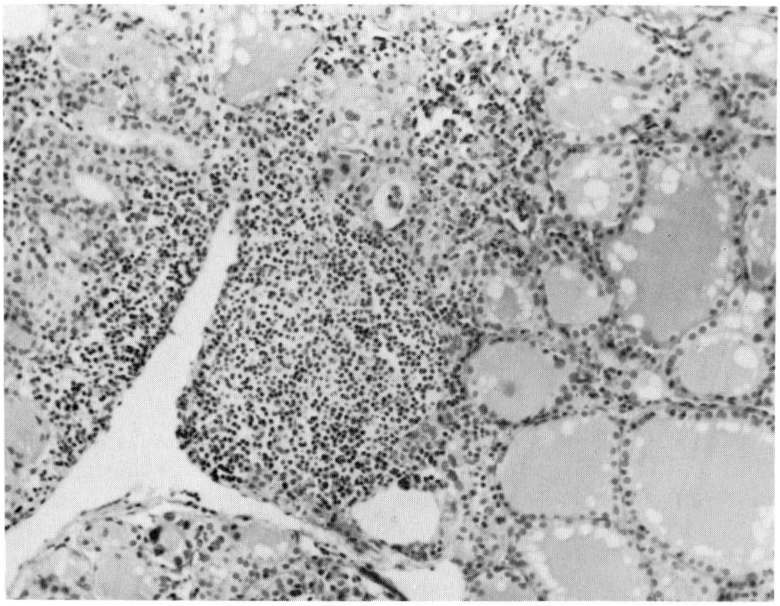

Figure 20–42. Photomicrograph of the thyroid gland showing the characteristic changes of chronic thyroiditis (Hashimoto's thyroiditis). Note the destruction of the normal architecture of the gland with heavy infiltration of mononuclear cells. Hematoxylin and eosin stain, ×100. (Courtesy of Dr. Byungkyu Chun.)

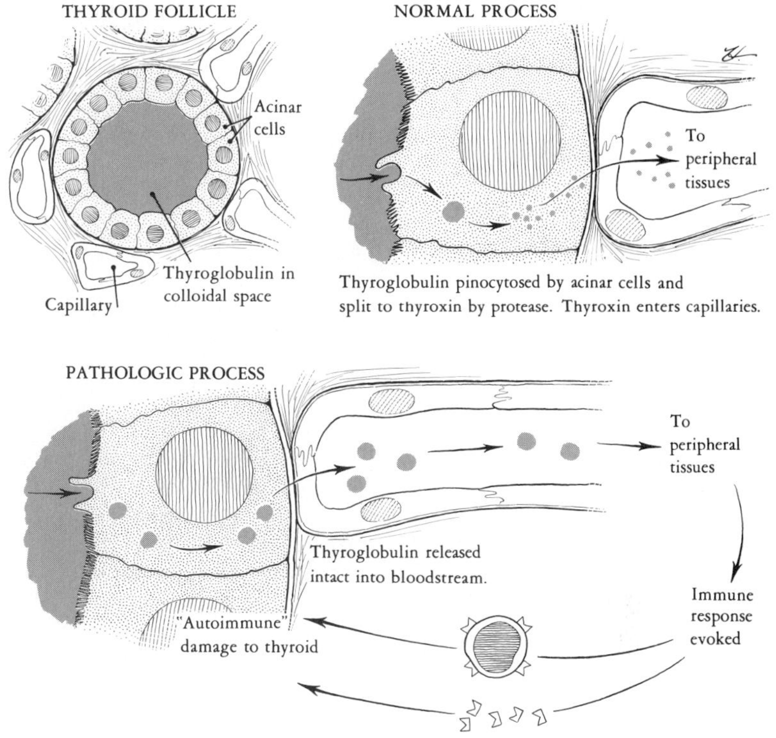

Figure 20–43. Schematic representation of points at which aberrations might occur in immunologic disease of the thyroid gland.

its *in vivo* ability to enhance the release of thyroid hormone and LPA by its ability to prevent the neutralization of LATS by an inactivator normally present in human thyroid extract. TSI appear to represent autoantibodies directed to thyrotropin receptors, capable of binding to the receptor and stimulating the production of cyclic AMP and the excessive production of thyroid hormone. Patients may also have antibodies directed against thyroglobulins and microsomal antigens.

Pathogenesis. The points at which aberrations might occur in immunologic disease of the thyroid are depicted schematically in Figure 20–43. Thyroglobulin is normally transported from the colloidal space into acinar cells by means of a process of pinocytosis. Within the acinar cells, a protease releases thyroxine from a macromolecular protein complex. Normally, thyroglobulin does not enter the circulation in significant amounts. The released thyroxine enters capillary structures surrounding the acinar cells and is transported to peripheral tissues. If the macromolecular complex is not cleared by the protease or is released intact, it may pass into the circulation and induce an immune response with resultant "autoimmune" damage to the thyroid (Fig. 20–43). This may be seen after trauma or infection. More recently, genetic factors have been implicated in the pathogenesis of chronic thyroiditis both in the human and in the experimental animal. With the recent descriptions of LATS, LPA, and TSI, it is thought that these additional antibodies may play a role in the pathogenesis of both Graves' disease and chronic lymphocytic thyroiditis.

Immunologic Tests. There are several immunologic tests useful for the detection of antibodies to thyroid tissues. Antithyroglobulin antibodies can be detected by precipitation techniques, latex agglutination, the tanned red cell (TRC) test, and radioimmunoassay. Microsomal antibodies are detected by complement fixation, cytotoxicity tests, immunofluorescence of unfixed thyroid epithelial cells, radioimmunoassay, and hemagglutination tests. The microsomal antigen is intimately associated with lipoproteins of thyroid extracts and is attached to the membranous portion of smooth endoplasmic reticulum. The second antigen of acinar colloid, a protein distinct from thyroglobulin, is also detected by immunofluorescence (Fig. 20–44). The staining for this antibody is brightest in Hashimoto's thyroiditis, although it is not specific for this disorder and can be seen frequently in the sera of patients with thyrotoxicosis and cancer of the thyroid. Thyroid-specific cell surface antibodies have been

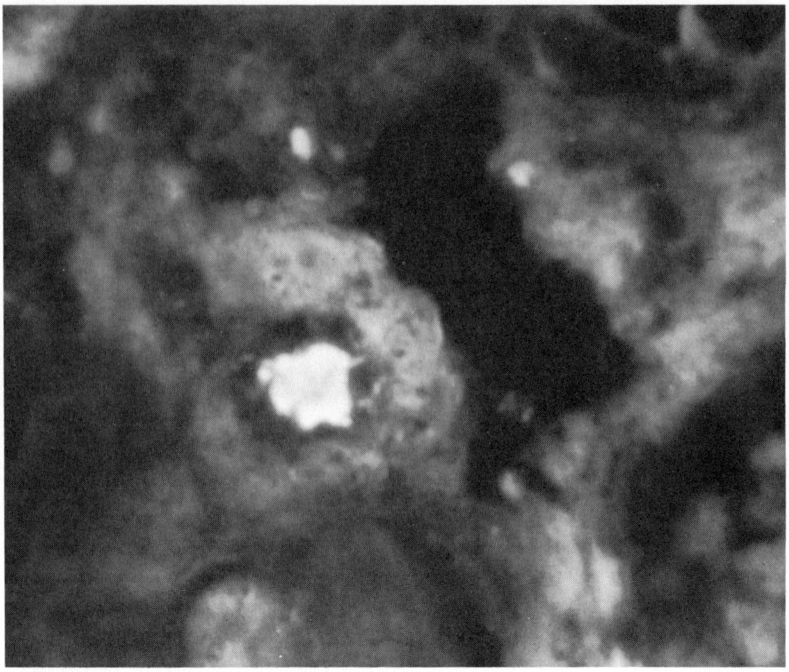

Figure 20–44. Presence of antibody to thyroid colloid in the serum of a patient with chronic thyroiditis as revealed by indirect immunofluorescence. (Courtesy of Dr. Heinz Bauer.)

detected by immunofluorescence on living suspensions of human thyroid cells. The significance of these antibodies is unknown.

Long-acting thyroid stimulator (LATS) has been detected in approximately 50 per cent of patients with Graves' disease. Circulating thyroid-stimulating immunoglobulins (TSI) have been detected in 90 per cent of patients with Graves' disease and in 15 per cent of patients with Hashimoto's thyroiditis. Although hyperthyroidism may characterize certain phases of thyroiditis, the overall thrust of the self-destructive process of Hashimoto's disease appears to be directed toward the relentless production of chronic inflammation with lymphocytic infiltration and glandular destruction and the eventual attrition of thyroid function and hypothyroidism. The cause of the exophthalmos of Graves' disease is unknown. However, recent studies demonstrating the presence of thyroglobulin in the orbital muscle of patients with this disease may substantiate a basis for cell-mediated immune injury in the pathogenesis of this entity.

The various forms of thyroiditis can be distinguished by means of a variety of thyroid function and antibody studies (Table 20–30). In the acute form, the most common pattern is that of an increased total T_4 along with a diminished iodine-131 uptake. Antithyroid antibodies are usually not detected in acute thyroiditis. In subacute thyroiditis, thyroxine levels are frequently normal, but an increase in circulating nonthyroxine iodinated compounds may be detected. Iodine-131 uptake is frequently normal. Antithyroid antibodies are not usually present in subacute thyroiditis. In the chronic form, thyroid function may be normal or decreased, depending upon the degree of thyroid involvement. Antithyroid antibodies are usually detected. In Graves' disease, the total T_4 is elevated, the radioactive uptake of ^{131}I is increased, and antithyroid antibodies, particularly LATS and TSI, are present.

PANCREAS

Circulating antibodies to insulin have been found in the sera of diabetic patients, which may contribute to insulin allergy (IgE) or insulin resistance (IgG, IgA, or IgM) (Chap-

Table 20–30. Thyroid Function and Antibody Studies in Various Thyroid Diseases

	T4*	RAI†	Thyroid Antibodies
Thyroiditis			
Acute	N or ↑	N or ↓	0
Subacute	N	N	0
Chronic	N or ↓	N or ↓	+
Graves' disease	↑	↑	±

*T_4—serum thyroxine determination.
†RAI—radioactive ^{131}I uptake.

ter 20A). However, antibodies have not been regularly encountered in untreated patients. More recently, insulin resistance has been described in untreated patients and appears to be related to two types of antibody: (1) antibody directed to the insulin molecule, and (2) antibodies directed to the insulin receptor. In both situations, the interaction of insulin with its receptor appears to be blocked. Insulin antibodies produced in animals have also provided the basis for a useful test for the radioimmunoassay of insulin concentrations.

Recently, thyroid and gastric autoantibodies have been found in the sera of diabetic patients without clinical thyroid disease or pernicious anemia. These autoantibodies were more commonly detected in the insulin-dependent (juvenile-onset) type and more frequently detected in females. These findings may be one aspect of the heterogeneity of this endocrine disorder.

ADRENALS

The finding of antibody to adrenal tissues in patients with Addison's disease has been reported. These antibodies have been detected by immunofluorescence or complement fixation. The significance of these findings is at present obscure.

PARATHYROIDS

Idiopathic hypoparathyroidism occurs with greater frequency in children than in adults and is more common in females than in males. Associated disorders may accompany hypoparathyroidism, including idiopathic Addison's disease, alopecia totalis, pernicious anemia, and moniliasis. Antibodies to thyroid, adrenal, and gastric tissues have been detected. Reasonably conclusive evidence has been obtained for an autosomal recessive mode of transmission of a defect underlying these variably associated disorders when clusters of two or more are present. It should be noted that there is also an association of hypoparathyroidism with developmental failure of the thymus-dependent immune system in the DiGeorge syndrome (Chapter 22).

Central Nervous System

Autoimmune diseases of the central nervous system may occur spontaneously or may follow immunization or infectious diseases. Autoimmune encephalitis in the human was first described after the use of Pasteur rabies vaccine grown in rabbit spinal cord. These early observations led to experimental studies in rabbits showing that experimental autoimmune encephalitis (EAE) could be produced by the injection of neurologic tissue homogenates incorporated in Freund's complete adjuvant. It was subsequently demonstrated that this experimental disease could be transferred by the adoptive transfer of lymphocytes but not by serum, suggesting that EAE is a disease of delayed-type hypersensitivity. While the role of circulating antibrain antibodies is not understood, it is possible that antibodies may also be operative in immunologic injury.

The demyelinating diseases of man are of three major types, including (1) acute hemorrhagic encephalopathy, (2) acute disseminated encephalomyelitis, and (3) a chronic form, e.g., multiple sclerosis. These disease entities are shown in Table 20–31, together with their histopathologic features.

Acute hemorrhagic encephalopathy is the most fulminating form and closely resembles EAE. It is primarily a disease of adults and is seen usually in association with an upper respiratory tract infection. There is an explosive onset followed by a relatively short course of illness that is almost uniformly fatal. Histopathologic features include perivascular infiltrates of polymorphonuclear leukocytes in brain tissues.

The second clinical form is the acute disseminated encephalomyelitis seen after inoculation of rabies vaccine; it is also a sequela of a variety of infectious diseases (postinfectious type). One distinguishing feature is the relatively long latent period between infection or immunization and appearance of the disease. This period of time may range from a few days to two weeks. Unlike the case in the acute hemorrhagic variety, the onset of encephalitis is not explosive, and the clinical course is characterized mainly by signs of increasing intracranial pressure. Histopathologic features include a perivascular infiltration of mononuclear cells in brain tissues with fewer polymorphonuclear leukocytes than in the acute hemorrhagic form. Mortality rates vary from 20 per cent in the case of measles to as high as 50 per cent in the case of postvaccinal encephalitis. Survival is the rule, although most patients are left with residual changes or have relapses over a number of months.

Table 20–31. **Demyelinating Diseases of Man***

	Acute Acute Hemorrhagic Encephalopathy	**Subacute** Acute Disseminated Encephalomyelitis, Rabies, Postinfectious	**Chronic** Multiple Sclerosis
Type of illness:	Explosive	Acute	Chronic
Duration:	Hours or days	Days or weeks	Weeks or years
Histopathologic features:	Focal disseminated perivascular	Focal disseminated perivascular	Focal disseminated perivascular
Cell type:	RBC; PMN	Mononuclear, histiocytes	Very few monocytes and histiocytes
Myelin destruction:	± to +	+ to + +	+ + to + + +
Axon and nerve cell damage:	±	±	±
Astrocyte proliferation:	±	+	+ + to + + +
Outcome:	Death	Recovery	Chronic relapsing progressive disease

*From Paterson, P. Y.: The Demyelinating Diseases. *In* Samter, M. (ed.): Immunological Diseases. Boston, Little, Brown & Company, 1978.

Multiple sclerosis is characterized by a chronic course with many relapses. A number of infectious disease pathogens have been implicated but none have been confirmed. The finding of an elevated spinal fluid gamma globulin in 80 per cent of patients is a distinguishing feature. Histopathologic features include degeneration of myelin with considerably less perivascular infiltration than that seen in the other forms. The Guillain-Barré syndrome is another form of neurologic disease with immunologic features. It is a polyneuritis of unknown etiology characterized by peripheral nerve involvement. This entity may follow a variety of infectious diseases or may occur as a sequela of immunization, e.g., swine influenza immunization (Chapter 23).

Working Hypothesis. Immunologically mediated diseases affecting the central nervous system include a consideration of "slow virus" infections (Chapter 16). In virus infections of the central nervous system, the physician is confronted with a spectrum of diseases that may be either a manifestation of the viral infection itself or an expression of the immunity mechanisms directed against it. These events are shown schematically in Figure 20–45. At one end of the spectrum, the pathologic events of encephalitis resulting from herpes simplex infection represent a direct invasion of the central nervous system by virus. Mumps virus also invades the central nervous system before or after parotitis appears. Varicella and measles encephalitis usually follow a viremia, and clinical findings are referred to as postinfectious types. In the postinfectious encephalitides, it has been difficult to culture virus directly from central nervous system tissue, although inclusion bodies have been observed in brain tissue of children with encephalitis (Fig. 20–46). At the other end of the spectrum, the encephalitis that follows administration of rabies vac-

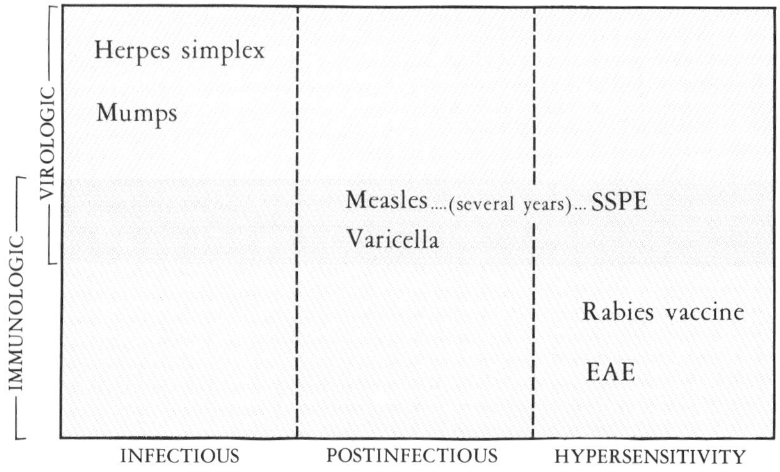

Figure 20–45. Schematic representation of etiologic factors in viral encephalitis.

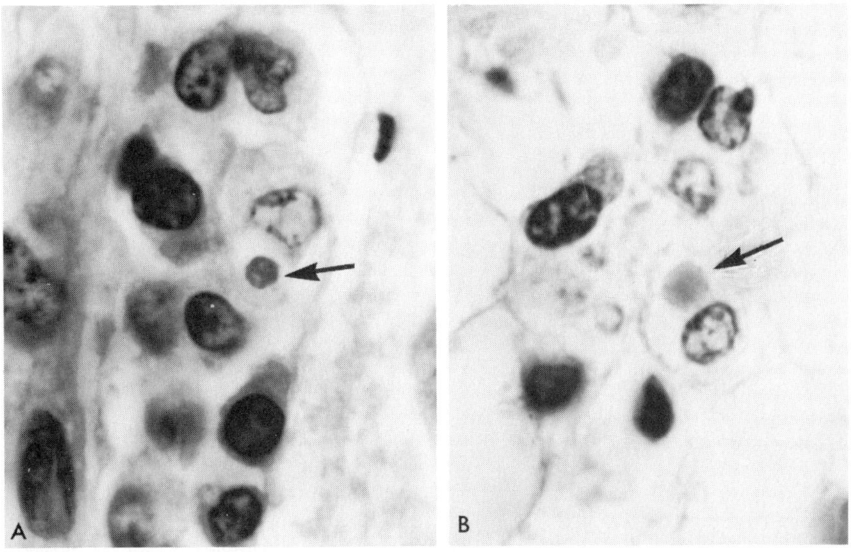

Figure 20–46. Photomicrograph of brain of child who died of measles encephalitis, showing measles inclusion bodies after natural measles *(A)* and after immunization with live measles vaccine *(B)*. Hematoxylin and eosin stain, ×2100. (Courtesy of Dr. John Adams.)

cine represents an example of a pathologic process resulting from hypersensitivity. The isolation of measles virus from brain biopsy specimens of children with subacute sclerosing panencephalitis (SSPE) suggests that measles virus may be present in an incomplete or masked form (Fig. 20–47). These recent observations concerning incomplete (slow) viral infections offer interesting explanations for what were previously considered autoimmune diseases of the nervous system.

Gastrointestinal

Many lines of evidence suggest that both the stomach and the intestines may be involved in autoimmune processes. Diseases that are triggered by immunologic processes are listed in Table 20–32 and include pernicious anemia, regional ileitis, ulcerative colitis, and gluten-sensitive enteropathy.

PERNICIOUS ANEMIA (PA)

Pernicious anemia is a disorder characterized by inflammation and subsequent atrophy of the gastric mucosa with inability to secrete hydrochloric acid, intrinsic factor, and pepsin. This is followed by the development of a megaloblastic anemia. Up to 95 per cent of patients with this disorder have serum antibody directed against parietal cells or intrinsic factor. Recently, antibody has been found in the gastric juice, and lymphoid cells have been found to infiltrate gastric mucosa. The sera of patients with pernicious anemia contain antibody that, when mixed with intrinsic factor, interferes with the absorption of vitamin B_{12}. It is not known whether these antibodies are the result or the cause of the disease. The fact that some patients improve after treatment with steroids reinforces the possibility of an autoimmune basis for PA. This effect, however, may merely be a consequence of anti-inflammatory action of steroids.

Family studies in first-degree relatives of patients with PA indicate a threefold increase in the incidence of gastric parietal antibody, gastritis, and achlorhydria. In addition, there are thyroid antibodies in about 50 per cent of patients with PA and their relatives. About one third of patients with Hashimoto's disease have antibodies to gastric parietal cytoplasm with no clinical manifestations of PA.

Immunologic Tests. Antibodies in the sera of individuals with PA are of two types: (1) those directed against the microsomal fraction of gastric mucosal cells (these are detected by complement-fixation test or by immunofluorescence), and (2) those directed against intrinsic factor. These antibodies bind with preformed intrinsic factor B_{12} complex (binding antibody) or those that block the combination of intrinsic factor with antibody (blocking antibody) (Table 20–33). The application of these tests in clinical medicine is

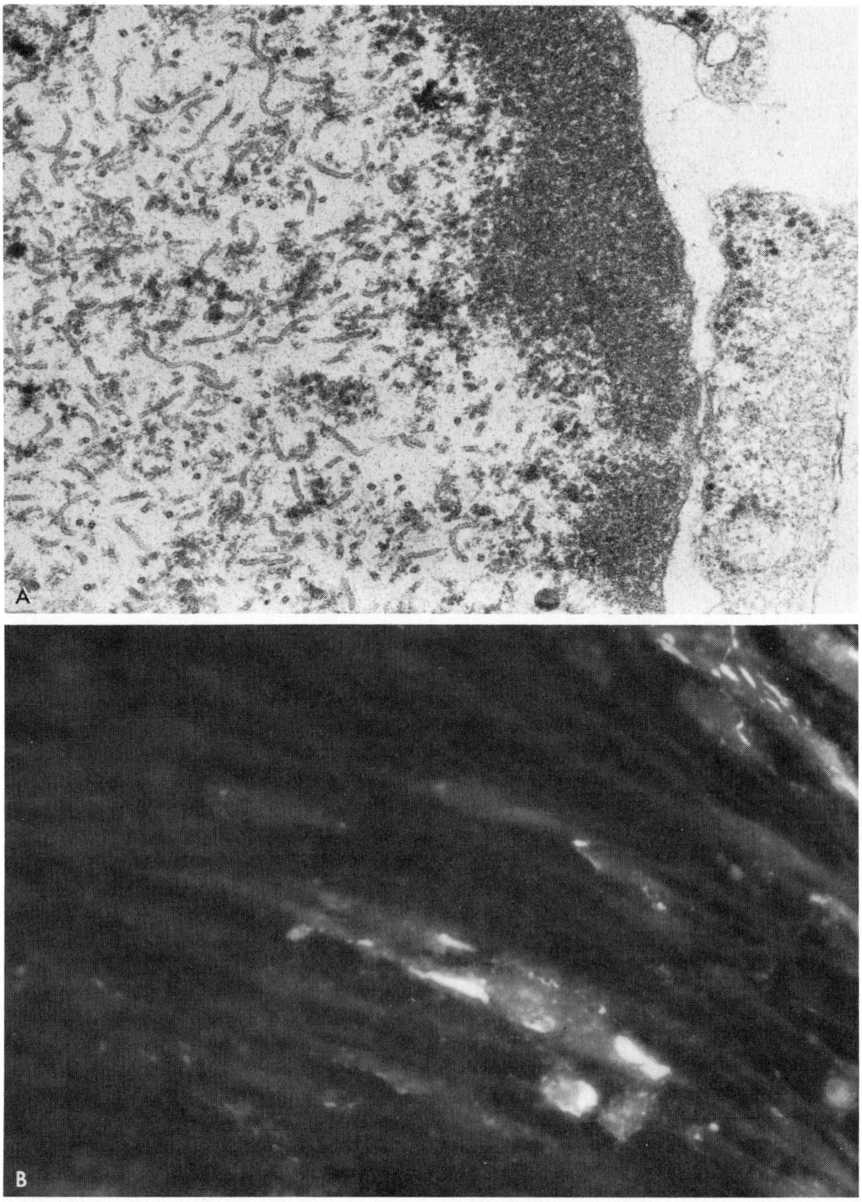

Figure 20–47. Demonstration of measles antigen in brain biopsy of patient with subacute sclerosing panencephalitis (SSPE). *A,* Demonstration of measles virus nucleocapsids (microtubules) in the cytoplasm of glial cells by electron microscopy ×74,250. *B,* Demonstration of measles antigen within glial cells by direct immunofluorescence. (Courtesy of Dr. Luiz Horta-Barbosa.)

important in differentiating PA from other causes of megaloblastic anemia.

ULCERATIVE COLITIS

Ulcerative colitis is a chronic disease affecting primarily the large bowel and is characterized by bloody diarrhea, abdominal pain, weight loss, and anemia. The pathogenesis is unknown but thought to be autoimmune on the basis of circulating antibody to colonic tissue. Enteric infection may be the triggering event. There is evidence for a genetic predisposition to this disorder with a slightly increased female to male ratio among those affected.

Immunologic Tests. Three types of antibodies have been demonstrated against colonic tissue: (1) an IgM hemagglutinin, (2) a precipitating antibody, and (3) an immunofluorescent antibody. Their importance in the pathogenesis of ulcerative colitis is uncer-

Table 20–32. **Autoimmune Diseases Affecting the Gastrointestinal Tract**

Region	Disease
Stomach	Pernicious anemia
Intestine	Regional ileitis Ulcerative colitis Gluten-sensitive enteropathy (celiac disease)

tain. Antibody-containing serum does not cause cytotoxicity to cells in culture, whereas lymphocytes from affected patients do. This suggests that cell-mediated immune mechanisms may be more important than humoral antibody in the pathogenesis of ulcerative colitis.

REGIONAL ILEITIS (CROHN'S DISEASE)

Regional ileitis is a chronic disease of unknown etiology characterized by granulomatous inflammatory changes of the ileum that sometimes involve other parts of the gastrointestinal tract as well. Antibodies to heterologous colon have been demonstrated in regional ileitis. Although suspected, an autoimmune basis has never been substantiated.

GLUTEN-SENSITIVE ENTEROPATHY (GSE; CELIAC DISEASE)

This syndrome is characterized by malabsorption of fats and carbohydrates. Diarrhea appears to be triggered by ingestion of the gliadin fraction of gluten, a protein found in grains. It is not known precisely how this effect is mediated. There may also occur a hpersensitivity reaction to the gliadin fraction itself. Recently, HLA-Dw3 and B8 have been associated with GSE. High antibody titers to gliadin have also been detected in affected patients. The antibodies that mediate these reactions are of the IgA and IgM type, which are also the principal immunoglobulins at mucosal sites. Moreover, IgA deficiency occurs more frequently in celiac patients than in the general population. This is probably related to common factors underlying both IgA deficiency and GSE.

IMMUNOLOGIC MECHANISMS OF THE GASTROINTESTINAL TRACT

The gastrointestinal tract is endowed with specific defense mechanisms in addition to nonspecific defense mechanisms provided by the intact mucosa: pH unfavorable for the growth of most pathogens, proteolytic enzymes, and competitive inhibition of commensal bacteria. These specific defense mechanisms include humoral IgG antibodies and secretory IgA antibodies (coproantibody), which are synthesized locally (Chapter 5). Recent evidence indicates that lymphocytes that can mediate immunologic reactions alone (T-cell–mediated immunity) or in conjunction with antibody (ADCC reactions) are known to exist in the lamina propria of the gastrointestinal tract.

Autoimmune Disease of the Liver

Immunologic disorders have been implicated as a cause of a number of different acute and chronic diseases of the liver (Table 20–34).

INFECTIOUS HEPATITIS (TYPE A) AND SERUM HEPATITIS (TYPE B)

At least four viruses have been found to cause hepatitis: hepatitis virus A (infectious hepatitis) and hepatitis virus B (serum hepatitis). Other cases of hepatitis, although not well characterized, appear to be caused by at least two non-A, non-B viruses (Chapter 16). Type A virus is commonly associated with fecal-oral spread and a disease of short duration; Type B virus is transmitted via the parenteral route and is associated with a disease of considerably longer incubation.

Table 20–33. **Types of Serum Antibody Found in Patients with Pernicious Anemia**

Autoantigen	Antibody Test
Gastric parietal cell antigen	Complement-fixation (CF) Immunofluorescence (FA)
Intrinsic factor	Blocking antibody Binding antibody

Table 20–34. **Liver Diseases with Immunologic Features**

1. Hepatitis
   a. acute
   b. chronic
2. Drug-induced liver disease
3. Biliary cirrhosis
4. Portal cirrhosis

Immunologic phenomena have long been thought to play a role in the pathogenesis of diseases caused by these viruses. Antibody to extracts of liver have been detected in the sera of patients with both forms of hepatitis. In more chronic forms of hepatitis, elevated levels of serum gamma globulin are found, and there is a lymphocytic infiltration of the liver, suggesting an immunologic component.

An antigen originally termed the Australia antigen, Au/SH, and now known as hepatitis B surface antigen (HB_sAg) (Chapter 16), has also been detected in the sera of patients with hepatitis. Recent findings have suggested that the HB_sAg represents a subunit of the surface protein of hepatitis B virion, and a variety of techniques are available for its detection, including precipitation, counterimmune electrophoresis, and radioimmunoassay. There is evidence to suggest a genetic predisposition controlling the prevalence and persistence of this antigen in certain individuals, e.g., those with Down's syndrome. The original description of Australia antigen among inbred Australian aborigines itself suggested a genetic expression.

It has been reported that the severity of hepatitis may vary according to the amount and persistence of HB_sAg antigen in the host. In one study in which the presence of virus alone was detected, it was not associated with active disease. When smaller amounts of antibody were produced, viral antibody complexes and free excess antigen were found, indicating antigen excess. In this case, chronic active disease resulted, resembling in many respects a serum sickness–type of immunologic injury (Chapter 13). In a fatal case, viral antibody complexes were detected in the serum, indicating relative antibody excess. These data offer interesting possibilities for a basis of immunologic injury of the liver mediated by antigen-antibody complexes. Several recent reports also suggest, but do not prove, the participation of cell-mediated injury. HB_sAg has also been detected in affected tissues of patients with polyarteritis nodosa.

CHRONIC LIVER DISEASE

Hepatitis virus B infection can serve as a model of an infection in which immunologic factors may play a role in the pathogenesis of chronic liver disease. Liver involvement after hepatitis B infection can be divided into the following categories: (1) acute fulminating hepatitis (acute liver necrosis and acute yellow atrophy), (2) acute hepatitis (classic hepatitis B, serum hepatitis, and acute subclinical hepatitis), (3) chronic active hepatitis, (4) chronic persistent subclinical hepatitis with exacerbations, (5) asymptomatic chronic carrier state of HB_sAg, and (6) neonatal hepatitis. At one end of the spectrum is acute fulminant infection with massive hepatocellular destruction and rapid death. The vast majority of cases of hepatitis B follow a second pattern characterized by a variable incubation period, a short episode of clinical symptoms,. HB_sAg antigenemia, and fairly rapid clinical and biochemical recovery within four to six weeks, followed by a rapid reversion to an HB_sAg-negative state. In some cases, particularly in children, the acute infection may be entirely subclinical. A third category is chronic active hepatitis, characterized by a variable symptomatology with a protracted debilitating course with biochemical evidence of disease, HB_sAg antigenemia, and progressive liver destruction and cirrhosis. Chronic persistent hepatitis is associated with intermittent symptomatology with exacerbations, abnormal biochemical findings, but chronic liver disease that is usually not progressive. In young women, a variant of chronic hepatitis has been described in which clinical and laboratory manifestations were suggestive of SLE (lupoid hepatitis or plasma cell hepatitis) (Fig. 20–48). Originally thought to be a variant of SLE, the entity is now considered to be a form of chronic active hepatitis. Another category is the asymptomatic chronic carrier state in which the patient is free of symptoms and normal biochemical findings in the face of persistent HB_sAg in the blood and secretions. The chronic carrier state constitutes a risk for transmission via blood, saliva, and genital secretions and poses a significant risk in certain professions, e.g., dentistry. The last category is neonatal hepatitis (which can take two forms depending on the time of maternal infection). This can present as an acute fulminant infection or as a more protracted disease with a subclinical course and persistent antigenemia. The expression of the disease appears to be dependent upon the timing of maternal infection. Neonatal infection can be acquired in one of three ways: (1) transplacental infection from a chronic carrier mother during the last trimester, (2) perinatal transmission of the virus from a mother with acute hepatitis, or (3) perinatal infection from a mother through breast milk or genital secretions.

DRUG-INDUCED LIVER DISEASE

A number of drugs induce liver disease on the basis of hypersensitivity. There are basically two forms of drug-induced liver damage: a toxic and a true hypersensitivity reaction (Chapter 20A). No circulating antibodies have been detected in the hypersensitivity type. Treatment is limited to discontinuing the drug.

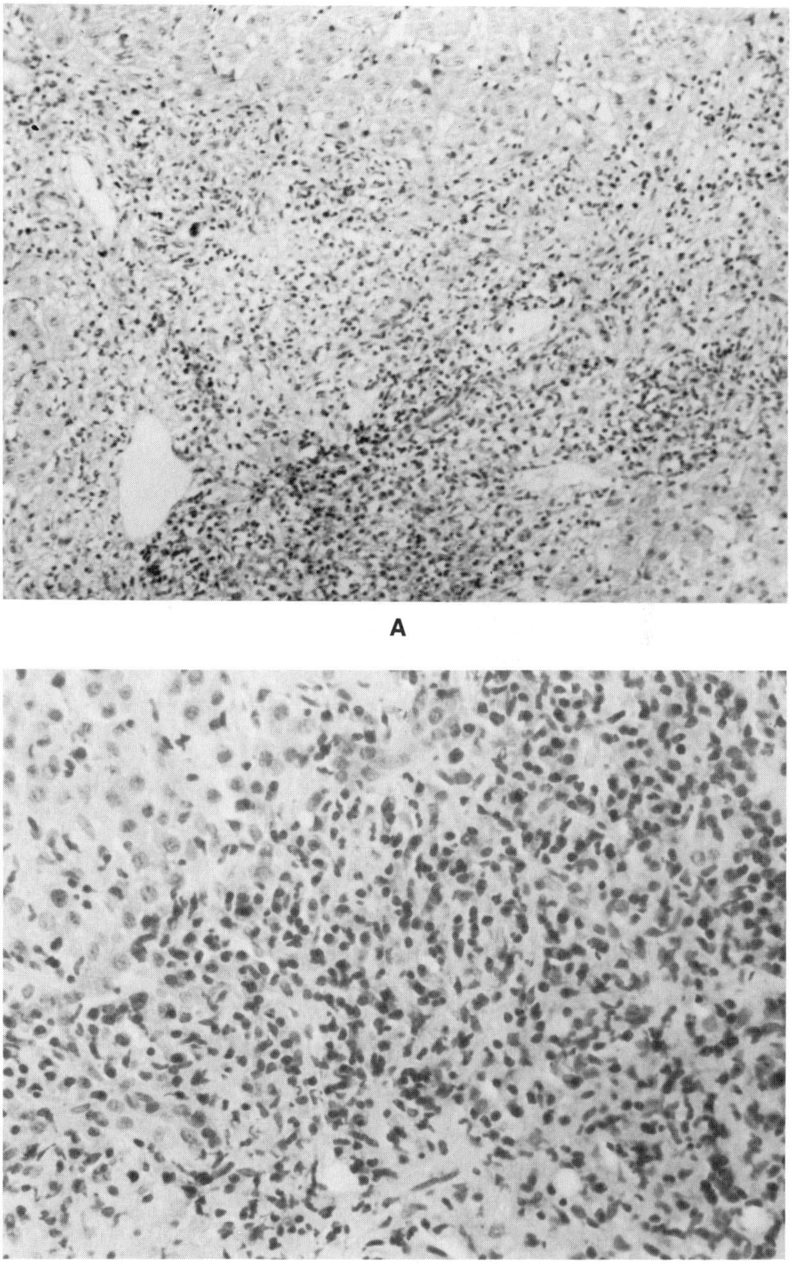

A

B

Figure 20–48. *A*, Photomicrograph of a liver biopsy from a patient with chronic active hepatitis showing liver cell destruction, beginning fibrosis, and prominent infiltration with round cells. Hematoxylin and eosin, ×100. (Courtesy of Dr. Byungkyu Chun.) *B*, Higher magnification of a periportal area of a liver biopsy from a patient with chronic active hepatitis showing infiltration of lymphocytes and plasma cells. Hematoxylin and eosin, ×400. (Courtesy of Dr. Kornel L. Terplan.)

Kidney

Immunologically mediated renal diseases result from the triggering of an inflammatory reaction within the kidney. Inflammation, in most instances, proceeds via immune activation of the complement, coagulation, and kinin systems. Since renal parenchymal tissue is capable of responding to immune inflammatory injury in only a limited number of ways, such as hyperplasia, reduplication, necrosis, and fibrosis (Table 20–35), the nature of the resultant immune injury depends basically upon two factors: (1) the type of immune response and (2) its location within the kidney.

Hypersensitivity reactions occurring within the kidney of Types II (cytotoxic), III (immune-complex), and IV (cell-mediated) are associated with development of a variety of recognizable renal diseases. These types of hypersensitivity reactions may occur in glo-

Table 20–35. **Renal Parenchymal Tissues and Their Responses to Immune Injury**

Renal Parenchymal Tissue	Response
Glomerulus	PMN, mononuclear cell infiltration; sclerosis
Glomerular capillary endothelial cell	Hyperplasia
Glomerular basement membrane	Thickening
Mesangial cell	Hyperplasia
Glomerular visceral epithelial cell	Hyperplasia
Epithelial cell of Bowman's capsule	Hyperplasia (crescent formation)
Interstitium	Cellular infiltration; fibrosis
Tubular epithelial cells	Swelling, necrosis
Interstitial macrophages	Hyperplasia

merular or tubulointerstitial locations, or both, thus defining the pattern of the disease. Type I (anaphylactic) hypersensitivity has not, as yet, been definitively demonstrated to be associated with specific renal injury (Table 20–36).

TYPE I (ANAPHYLACTIC) IMMUNE RENAL DISEASE

Although no specific renal disease has been definitively ascribed to Type I hypersensitivity, IgE-mediated release of vasoactive amines from mast cells may be of importance in the propagation of a variety of immune inflammatory reactions in the kidney. This concept has been supported by the therapeutic effectiveness of antihistamines in suppressing experimental immune renal injury in animals (Chapter 13).

It is likely, however, that Type I hypersensitivity plays at least a contributing role in the interstitial nephritis of methicillin-induced nephritis as well as in some forms of reversible renal transplant rejection.

TYPE II (CYTOTOXIC) IMMUNE RENAL DISEASE

In this form of hypersensitivity, injury to the kidney results from the attack of antikidney antibodies against kidney antigens, with subsequent local activation of the complement and other systems of inflammation. If, for example, antibody is produced with specificity for glomerular basement membrane (GBM), the result is anti-GBM disease. This form of immune renal injury is characterized by the deposition of antibody and complement in a linear fashion along the GBM, as can be shown by direct immunofluorescence (Fig. 20–49 and Chapter 13). Occasionally, the anti-GBM antibody also reacts with other basement membranes, such

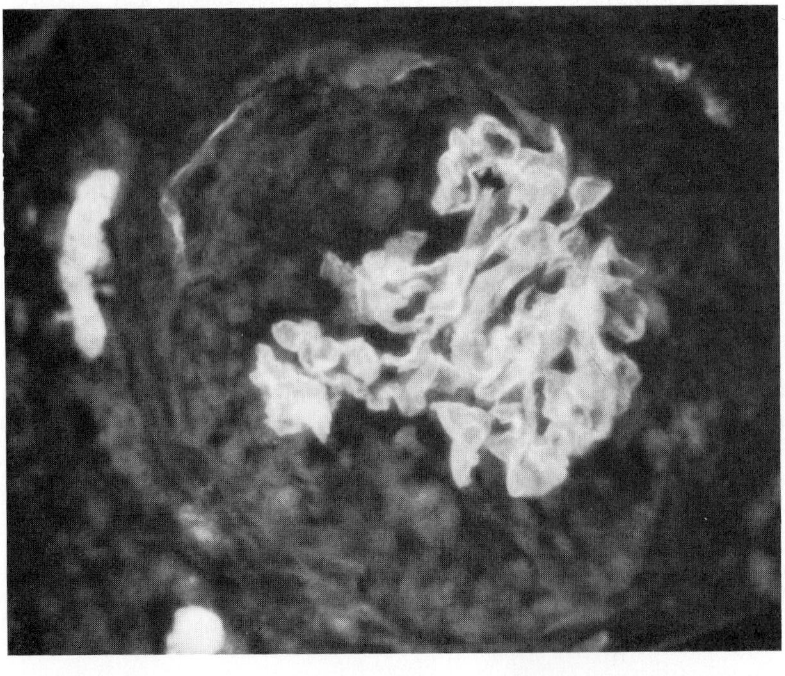

Figure 20–49. Photomicrograph of a kidney of a patient with Goodpasture's syndrome, demonstrated by direct fluorescence microscopy. Note the linear distribution of IgG globulin along the basement membrane and the absence of immunoglobulin in a surrounding crescent. (Courtesy of Dr. Heinz Bauer.)

Table 20–36. Patterns of Immunologically Mediated Renal Diseases

Type of Immune Response	Associated Renal Disease	Antigen	Pattern of Deposition of Immune Components: Ig	Complement	Fibrin	Cells
Type I (Anaphylactic)	1. Methicillin-nephritis	Pencillin-hapten	Focal mesangial IgE (?)	—	—	Eosinophils
Type II (Cytotoxic)	1. Anti-GBM disease	GBM	Linear along GBM	Linear along GBM (sometimes absent)	Extracapillary	—
	2. Anti-TBM disease	TBM	Linear along TBM	Linear along TBM	—	—
	3. Hyperacute rejection	HLA	Diffuse vascular	—	Diffuse cortical vascular	PMN's
Type III (Immune-complex)	1. Immune-complex GN, e.g., poststreptococcal, serum sickness, hepatitis B, SLE, etc.	Variety of exogenous and endogenous	Lumpy-bumpy in capillary wall	Lumpy-bumpy in capillary wall	Minimal	Endothelial and epithelial hypercellularity
Type IV (Cell-mediated)	1. Chronic renal allograft rejection	HLA	Diffuse granular	Diffuse granular	Vascular	Lymphocytes
	2. Chronic GN	Renal	Variable	Variable	Vascular	—
Miscellaneous	1. Membranoproliferative GN	None	Often none, occasional IgG in mesangium	C3, subendothelial or intramembranous	Rare	Endothelial, epithelial, and mesangial hypercellularity
	2. IgG-IgA nephropathy	(?)	IgG and IgA in mesangium	Mesangial, scattered	—	Mesangial hypercellularity

as lung, producing injury to the pulmonary capillary bed. The syndrome of anti-GBM antibody–mediated immune renal failure and pulmonary hemorrhage is known as Goodpasture's syndrome.

If the anti–basement membrane antibody is directed against tubular basement membrane, the resulting renal disease is predominantly tubulointerstitial. As in anti-GBM disease, the antibody is deposited in a linear fashion along the antigenic tissue for which it is specific (in this case, tubular basement membrane). Anti-TBM antibodies are associated with diseases such as systemic lupus erythematosus (SLE) and renal transplant rejection.

In some instances, Type II immune renal injury may result from the deposition of cytotoxic antibody specific for nonrenal, "planted" antigens. This may, for example, represent an alternative explanation for the pathogenesis of methicillin-induced nephritis. According to this theory, the antigenic penicillin-hapten is concentrated by the renal tubular cells and becomes "planted" along the tubules. Cytotoxic IgM or IgG antibody against the penicillin-hapten then localizes in the tubules in association with the antigen, triggering an inflammatory response by complement activation and recruitment of components of inflammation.

A form of Type II–mediated renal disease that affects the entire kidney is hyperacute renal allograft rejection (Chapter 20B). This form of immune renal injury is associated with high levels of pre-existing antibodies to the histocompatibility antigens (HLA) of the transplant. Upon completion of the vascular anastomosis, there is prompt thrombotic occlusion to the vessels throughout the kidney. It is likely that this diffuse injury results from Type II attack by anti-HLA antibodies against the widely distributed HLA antigens of the renal transplant.

TYPE III (IMMUNE-COMPLEX) IMMUNE RENAL DISEASE

Immune renal diseases associated with Type III hypersensitivity reactions constitute by far the majority of immunologically mediated renal diseases. In this form of hypersensitivity, inflammation and complement activation result from activation by antigen-antibody complexes. In Type III immune renal disease, these antigen-antibody complexes deposit in the glomerular capillary wall (immune-complex glomerular disease) or in the tubulointerstitium (immune-complex tubulointerstitial renal disease). The antigens that induce the immune-complex glomerulonephritis may be any of a variety of exogenous or endogenous antigens (Table 20–37). In the prototypic disease, poststreptococcal acute glomerulonephritis, the antigen resides in the wall of the streptococcus. Infection with a nephritogenic strain of streptococcus induces production of antibody that combines with the streptococcal antigens to form an immune complex. When these complexes deposit in the glomerular capillary wall, an acute glomerular inflammatory response results with activation of complement, generation of chemotactic components of complement, e.g., C567, release of lysozymes from polymorphonuclear cells, and subsequent tissue injury. Since the immune complexes probably deposit in a more sporadic fashion in Type III injury than in Type II antibody–mediated anti-GBM disease, it is reasonable that, on immunofluorescence, antibody and complement components appear as lumpy-bumpy structures in the capillary wall (Fig. 20–50).

Table 20–37. Antigens Associated with Type III Immune Renal Injury

Antigen	Examples
Exogenous	
Bacterial	Poststreptococcal GN
	Staphylococcal
Viral	Chickenpox
	Hepatitis B
Parasitic	Malaria
	Toxoplasmosis
Foreign serum	Serum sickness
Drugs	Heroin nephropathy (?)
Endogenous	
Nuclear antigens	SLE
Tumor antigens	CEA

Endogenous antigens may also cause immune complex–type renal disease, as in the prototypic immune-complex nephritis of SLE. Except for the more diffuse distribution of immune-complex deposition in some forms of lupus nephritis, poststreptococcal and lupus glomerulonephritis look very much alike. In lupus and other immune-complex diseases, the complexes may deposit additionally or preferentially in interstitial structures, resulting in immune injury in tubulointerstitial areas of the kidney.

In contrast to anti-GBM–mediated or anti-TBM–mediated renal diseases, in which an-

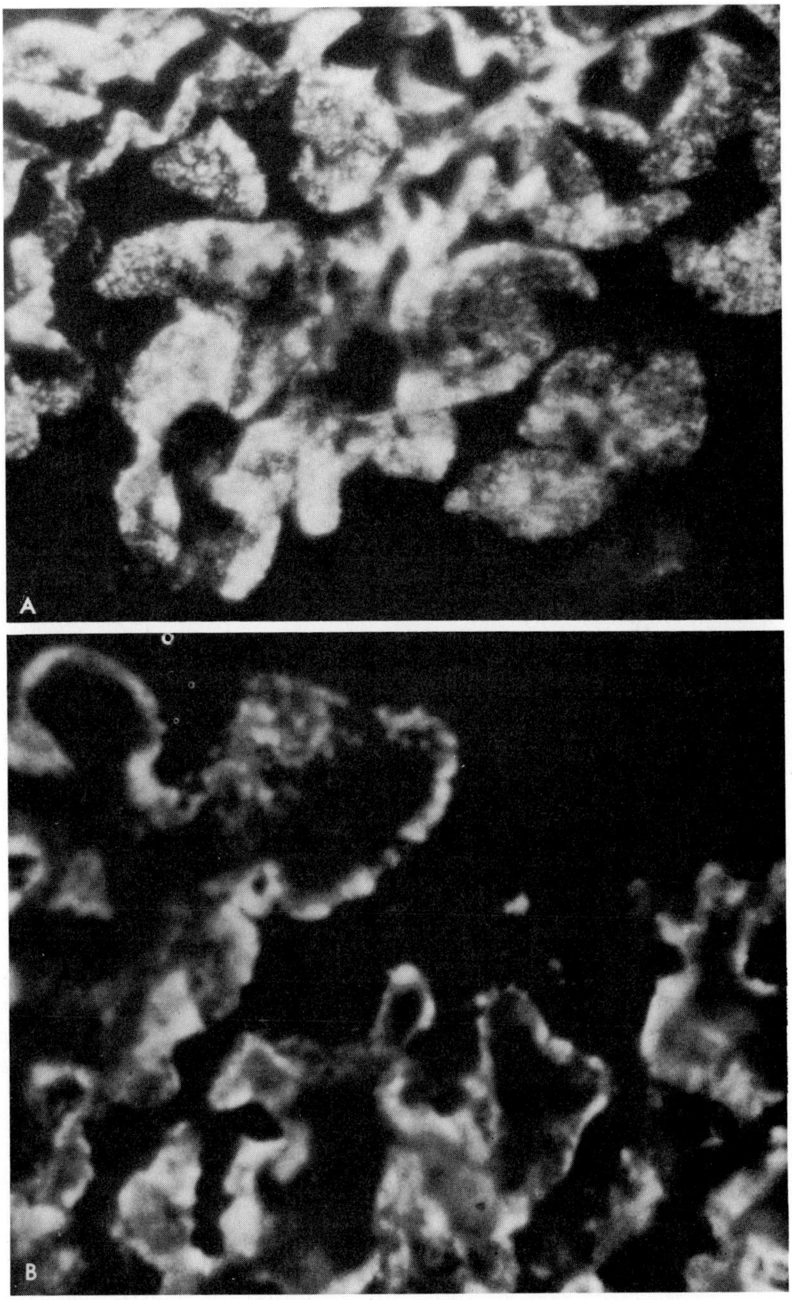

Figure 20–50. Photomicrograph of a kidney of a patient with membranous glomerulonephritis demonstrated by direct fluorescence microscopy. *A,* When capillaries are viewed from above, note the diffuse deposition of the complexes. Original magnification, ×400. *B,* Note the subepithelial localization and lumpy character of the immune-complex deposition. Original magnification, ×400. (Courtesy of Dr. Heinz Bauer.)

tibody fixes directly to antigenic sites, the cause of immune-complex deposition in the glomerular capillary wall is less easily understood. Renal blood flow may explain the delivery of immune complexes to sites of deposition, and the influence of factors such as vasoactive amines to increase permeability of the capillary wall for the movement of antigen-antibody complexes out of the vascular space may help explain how immune complexes arrive at subepithelial sites, where deposition characteristically occurs (Fig. 20–51). Recently, receptors for activated complement have been demonstrated on the visceral epithelial cells of the renal glomerular capillary. These glomerular complement receptors (GCR) may provide the pathogenetic mechanism to explain the fixation of antigen-antibody-complement complexes in these subepithelial sites. The demonstration of specific glomerular receptors for C3 suggests that immune complexes are transported to

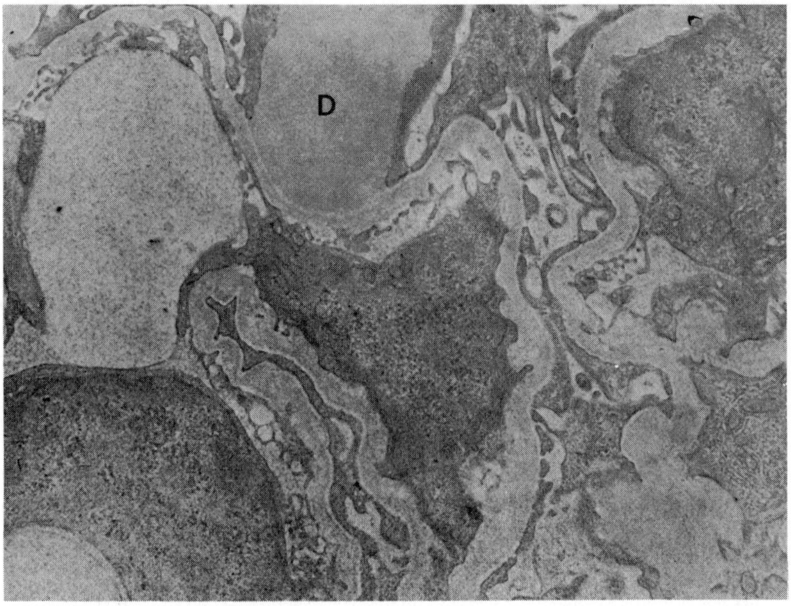

Figure 20–51. Electronmicrograph of a kidney biopsy from a patient with poststreptococcal glomerulonephritis. Note the subepithelial deposit *(D)* "hump" along the border of the basement membrane. ×6000. (Courtesy of Dr. Leticia U. Tiña.)

the glomerulus via the blood stream, traverse the capillary wall because of the effect of vasoactive amines, and become fixed to subepithelial sites by means of the attraction of C3 within the complex to GCR (Fig. 20–52). This hypothesis is supported by studies of renal biopsies from patients with immune renal diseases. In those biopsies in which *in vivo* deposition of immune complexes in subepithelial sites is demonstrated, the GCR are blocked, suggesting occupation of available binding sites by the complexes.

TYPE IV (CELL-MEDIATED) IMMUNE RENAL DISEASE

Type IV immune reactions are characterized by cell-mediated attacks on the target organ. This type of immune renal injury is best exemplified in renal allograft rejection, in which sensitized lymphoid cells attack the graft and result in immune renal injury (Chapter 20B). This type of immune reaction is diffusely distributed throughout the kidney and proceeds via the release of soluble substances by sensitized lymphoid cells (Chapter 9). These soluble lymphoid cell products, called lymphokines, are capable of propagating an inflammatory immune response and inducing immune injury (Chapter 9).

Another form of renal disease that may fall within the category of Type IV hypersensitivity is chronic glomerulonephritis. One hypothesis to explain this progressive destruction of renal tissue is that cell-mediated hypersensitivity to renal antigens occurs when injured renal tissue antigens are released after acute glomerulonephritis (e.g., poststreptococcal). Renal injury is then propagated by cell-mediated attack on renal tissue. Support of this pathogenesis of chronic glomerulonephritis has been provided by studies showing the release of migration inhibitory factor (MIF) on exposure to renal tissue antigens by lymphoid cells from patients with chronic glomerulonephritis.

MISCELLANEOUS FORMS OF IMMUNE RENAL DISEASE

A number of renal diseases appear to have immunologic bases that do not fit precisely into one of the foregoing categories. Two such diseases are IgG-IgA nephropathy (Berger's disease) and membranoproliferative (or mesangiocapillary) glomerulonephritis.

In IgG-IgA nephropathy, the patient may present with proteinuria and hematuria. The renal biopsy shows deposition of IgG and IgA immunoglobulin in mesangial areas of the glomerulus, with subsequent reactive mesangial cell hyperplasia. The precise cause of the immunoglobulin deposition in this disease is not known; however, in rabbits given repeated injections of bovine serum albumin (BSA) in amounts to balance antibody production, antibody deposition is prodominantly localized to the mesangial region during the first few weeks of antigen administration. It is only subsequently that im-

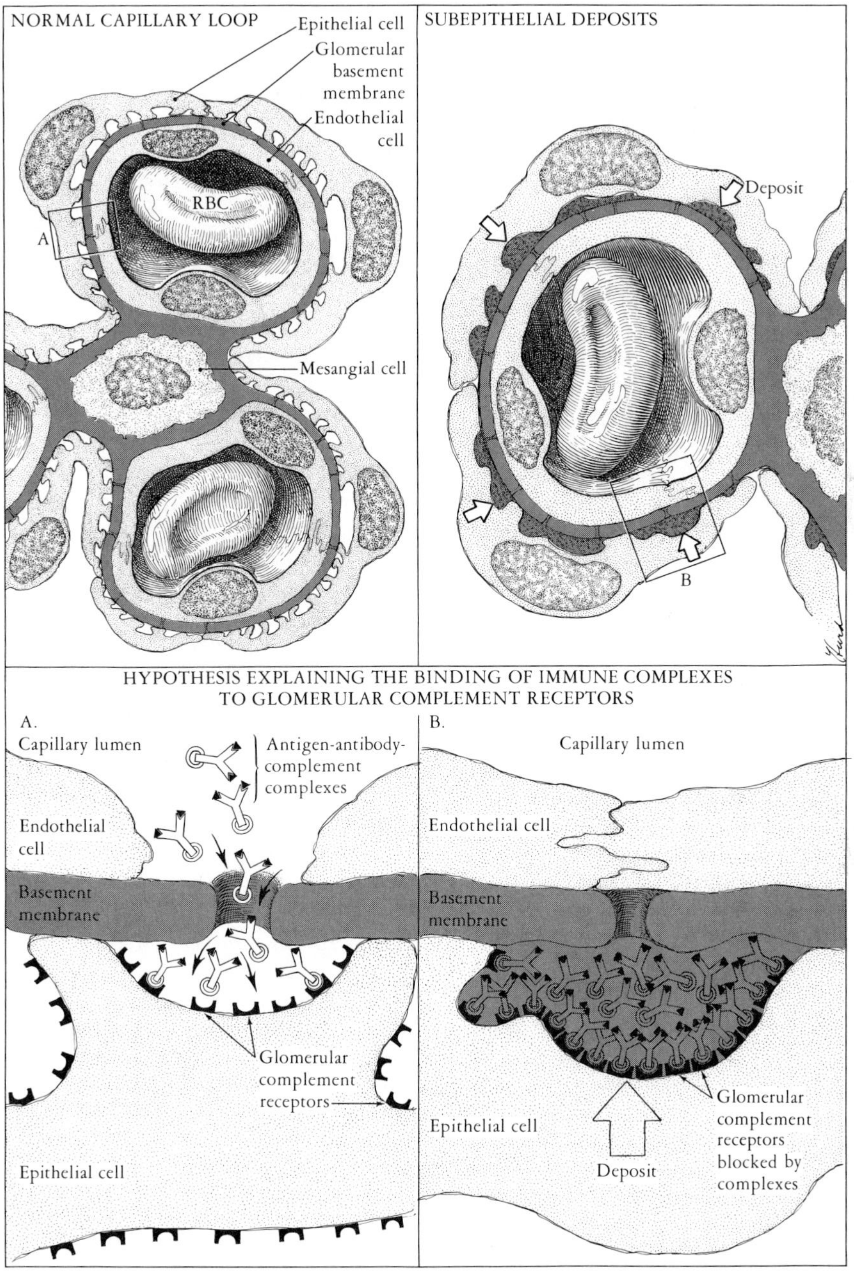

Figure 20–52. Hypothesis to explain development of subepithelial immune deposits as a result of binding of immune complexes to complement receptors on the visceral epithelial cell. Inset *A* shows the complexes, composed of antigen, antibody, and complement (C3), migrating through the basement membrane to come in contact with complement receptors on the surface of the visceral epithelial cell. Inset *B* depicts the accumulation of immune complexes to form a subepithelial deposit with the blocking of all available complement receptor sites that have migrated to the site of the deposit.

mune-complex deposition may be observed in the capillary wall or extraglomerular (tubulointerstitial) locations. These results suggest that the mesangium may function to clear small amounts of immune complexes early during antigen-antibody production or when the level of complexes is relatively small. Later perhaps, after saturation of other mononuclear phagocytic systems such as in the liver and spleen, complexes may begin to accumulate in capillary wall and extraglomerular sites.

Membranoproliferative glomerulonephritis is a very interesting form of renal disease that appears to result from deposition of activated complement components within the kidney. It is probable that in this form of renal disease, activation of the complement system proceeds predominantly via the alternative pathway (Chapter 6), i.e., as a result of direct activation of C3 to C3b. The direct activation of C3 is likely to be related to a factor in the serum known as nephritic factor, a 7S gamma globulin (MW 150,000) that is heat-stable. Nephritic factor is capable of cleaving C3 to C3b directly. In this form of renal disease (although two variants have been described), C3 is deposited densely within the capillary wall of the glomerulus, possibly by fixation to GCR. It is of note that the membranoproliferative form of glomerulonephritis has been found clinically associated with other complement system abnormalities and susceptibility to infections in patients with partial lipodystrophy. Although membranoproliferative glomerulonephritis does not proceed to renal failure in all instances, patients who develop renal failure and receive a renal transplant are at very significant risk of experiencing the recurrence of the disease in the transplant.

Muscle

Myasthenia gravis is a disorder of voluntary muscles characterized by muscle weakness and fatigability. A transitory neonatal form has been described occurring in infants born of myasthenic mothers (Chapter 26). Rarely, it is congenital and persists. Juvenile and adult cases are chronic, although signs and symptoms may be variable. There are thymic abnormalities consisting of hyperplasia and plasma cell infiltration in at least 80 per cent of patients. Evidence suggests that there is a thymic polypeptide factor that acts to inhibit neuromuscular transmission at the myoneural junction. More recently, antibodies to neuromuscular receptors have been described.

Immunologic Factors. Serum antibodies directed against muscle may be detected by a variety of tests, including direct and indirect immunofluorescence (Fig. 20–53), complement fixation, precipitation, and tanned-cell hemagglutination. Delayed hypersensitivity does not appear to be impaired in these patients.

The presence of these antibodies may be useful in diagnosis, prognosis, and therapy. If found, they may provide a differential point in distinguishing myasthenia gravis from other disorders characterized by muscle weakness. If they are detected, the physician is well advised to persist in a careful search for thymic abnormalities (e.g., thymoma), even if there is an absence of x-ray evidence of an enlarged gland. Antibodies may also serve in a prognostic way, aiding in the follow-up of the patient after surgery, since it is sometimes difficult to detect and remove aberrant thymic tissue.

Treatment of the disorder includes the use of anticholinergic drugs, thymectomy, and, in certain cases, the use of steroids, x-irradiation of the thymus, and plasmapheresis.

Heart

Antibodies directed against heart tissues are found in two clinical situations: (1) antibody produced to cardiac antigen released into the serum after damage or trauma and (2) antibody produced to a cross-reacting antigen, such as following Group A beta-hemolytic streptococcal infections.

In the first situation, antigen may be released into the circulation after trauma, myocardial infection, myocardial infarction, or surgery. This is a normal reaction to the release of cardiac antigen. These antibodies have been implicated in the postcardiotomy syndrome and postmyocardial infarction syndrome, in which the patient may have retrosternal pain, pleuritis, and pericarditis. In the second type, the antibody is directed primarily against antigens of the infecting microorganisms and secondarily against cardiac tissue because of its structural similarity to the microorganism. Rheumatic fever has been classified as an autoimmune disease and is thought to result as a consequence of these

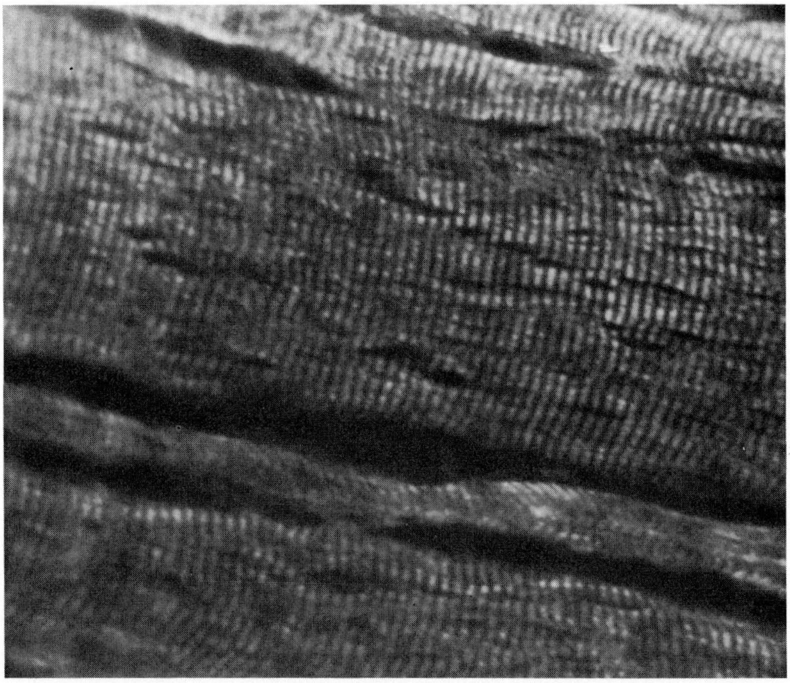

Figure 20–53. The presence of serum antibody to cross-striations of skeletal muscle in a patient with myasthenia gravis demonstrated by indirect immunofluorescence. (Courtesy of Dr. Heinz Bauer.)

cross-reacting antibodies. Only a small percentage of patients with Group A beta-hemolytic streptococcal infections develop rheumatic fever (from 2 to 3 per cent). However, once it has been initiated, the incidence of recurrence after a subsequent streptococcal infection increases to 50 to 60 per cent. Since there is no way of identifying individuals at risk for rheumatic fever and acute glomerulonephritis, the physician should promptly diagnose and adequately treat Group A beta-hemolytic streptococcal infections in order to lower the risk of these sequelae.

Skin

The diseases in which an autoimmunologic basis has been described include dermatitis herpetiformis, lupus erythematosus, bullous pemphigoid, and pemphigus vulgaris. Shown in Table 20–38 are typical immunologic fluorescent staining patterns seen in these various diseases.

Dermatitis herpetiformis is a disease characterized by grouped vesicles surmounted on an erythematous base involving predominantly the extensor surfaces of the back and arms (Fig. 20–54). The disease is characterized by an incapacitating burning pruritus, and patients have also been shown to have a patchy duodenal-jejunal atrophy indistinguishable from that of adult celiac disease. However, this gastrointestinal lesion is generally asymptomatic and has not been associated with an increased incidence of steatorrhea or malabsorption. HLA-B8 antigen has been found in approximately 75 to 80 per

Table 20–38. Immunofluorescence Staining Pattern in Autoimmune Diseases of the Skin, Illustrating Demonstration of Immunoglobulins (Ig) and Complement (C)

	Direct						Indirect	
	Intercellular		Basement Membrane					Basement
Disease	IgG	C	IgG	IgA	IgM	C	Intercellular	Membrane
Dermatitis herpetiformis	—	—	+	+ + + +	0	+	0	0
Lupus erythematosus								
Systemic lupus (SLE)*	—	—	+ + + +	+	+	+	0	0
Discoid lupus†	—	—	+ + + +	+	+	+	0	0
Bullous pemphigoid	—	—	+ + + +	+	+	+	0	+
Pemphigus vulgaris	+ + + +	+	—	—	—	—	+	0

*Involved and uninvolved skin
†Uninvolved skin only

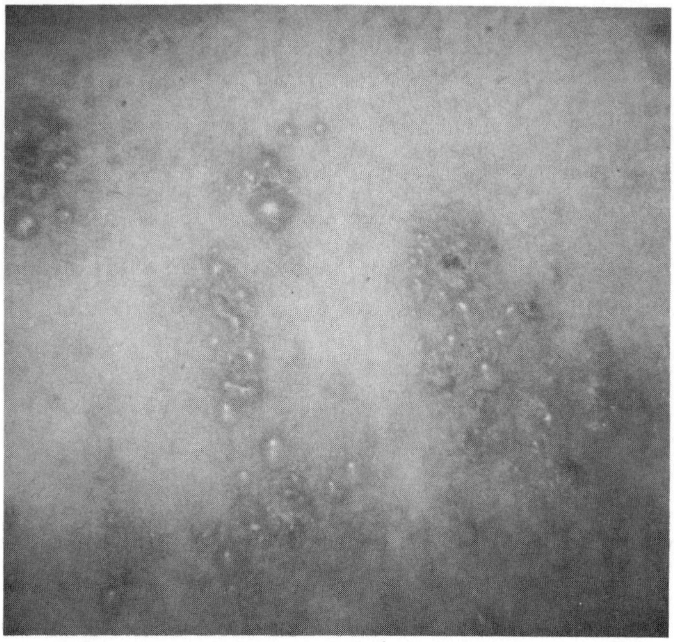

Figure 20–54. Characteristic lesions from a patient with dermatitis herpetiformis. Note the characteristic grouped vesicles surmounted on an erythematous base. (Courtesy of Dr. Thomas T. Provost.)

cent of patients with dermatitis herpetiformis. The examination of the perilesional skin of patients with dermatitis herpetiformis has revealed a granular deposition of IgA in 95 per cent of patients thus far examined (Fig. 20–55). The IgA deposition is virtually pathognomonic for dermatitis herpetiformis (Table 20–38). In addition, C3, C5, properdin, and properdin factor B have been frequently noted in a granular deposition along the dermal-epidermal junction; IgG and early components of the complement system, i.e., C1q and C4, are infrequently noted (Table 20–38). These direct immunofluorescent findings suggest that the major activation of the complement system in dermatitis herpetiformis may be via the alternative complement pathway (Chapter 6). The disease is responsive to sulfapyridine and diaminodiphenylsulfone (dapsone). Within a short time after either of these two drugs is instituted, the patient's burning pruritus and lesions

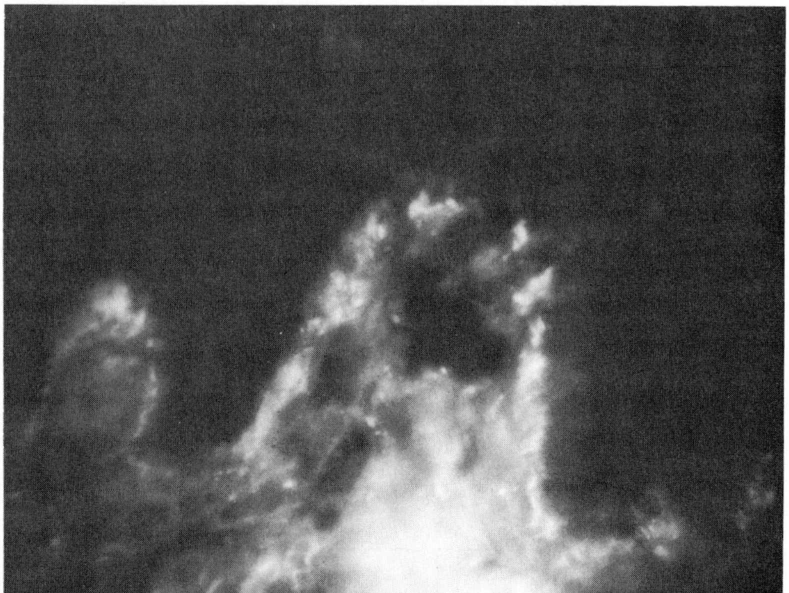

Figure 20–55. Photomicrograph of a biopsy of skin from a patient with dermatitis herpetiformis, illustrating the granular deposition of IgA that appears to be virtually pathognomonic for the disease. (Courtesy of Dr. Thomas T. Provost.)

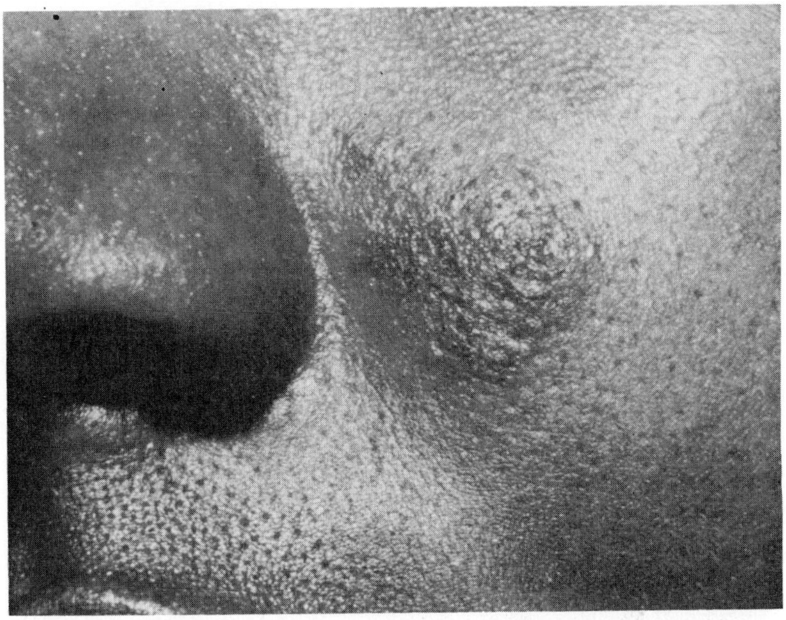

Figure 20–56. Photograph of a patient with chronic discoid lupus erythematosus, illustrating a sharply circumscribed scaly erythematous dermatitis. (Courtesy of Dr. Thomas T. Provost.)

often disappear. Surprisingly, the examination of asymptomatic patients receiving these two drugs has consistently revealed the continued deposition of IgA and, in some instances, complement components. The precise pharmacologic mechanism of action of sulfapyridine and dapsone in this disease remains an intriguing mystery.

Skin manifestations of lupus erythematosus are seen in both the systemic and the chronic discoid forms of the disease. The clinical and immunologic manifestations of SLE have been described elsewhere in this chapter. The characteristic skin lesions of chronic discoid lupus consist of a sharply circumscribed scaling erythematous dermatitis (Fig. 20–56) in which follicular plugging, telangiectasia, and atrophy are common features (Fig. 20–57). In both SLE and discoid lupus, immunoglobulins and complement components are found in a granular deposition at the dermal-epidermal junction (Fig. 20–58). In SLE, however, the deposition is seen in both involved and uninvolved areas

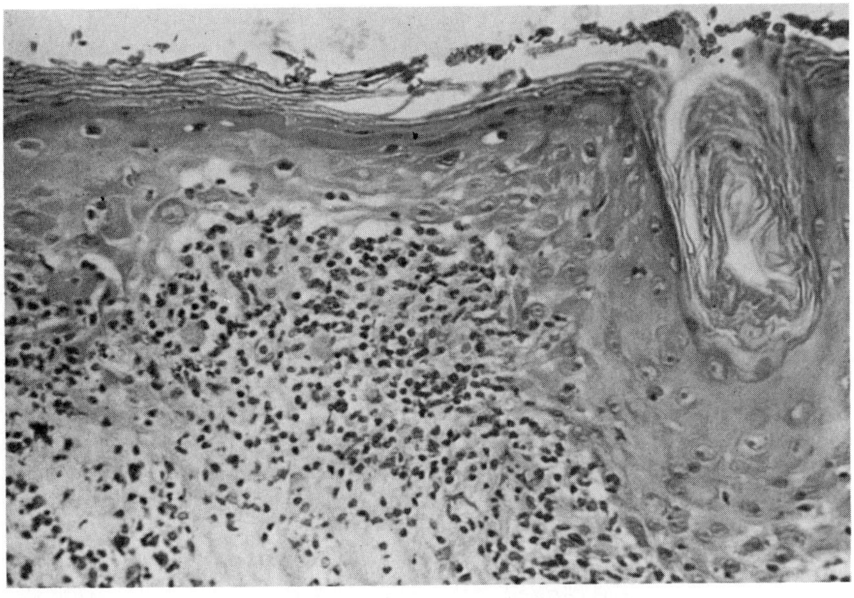

Figure 20–57. Photomicrograph of a skin lesion of chronic discoid lupus erythematosus showing the characteristic atrophy of skin, follicular plugging, and cellular infiltrate. (Courtesy of Dr. Thomas T. Provost.)

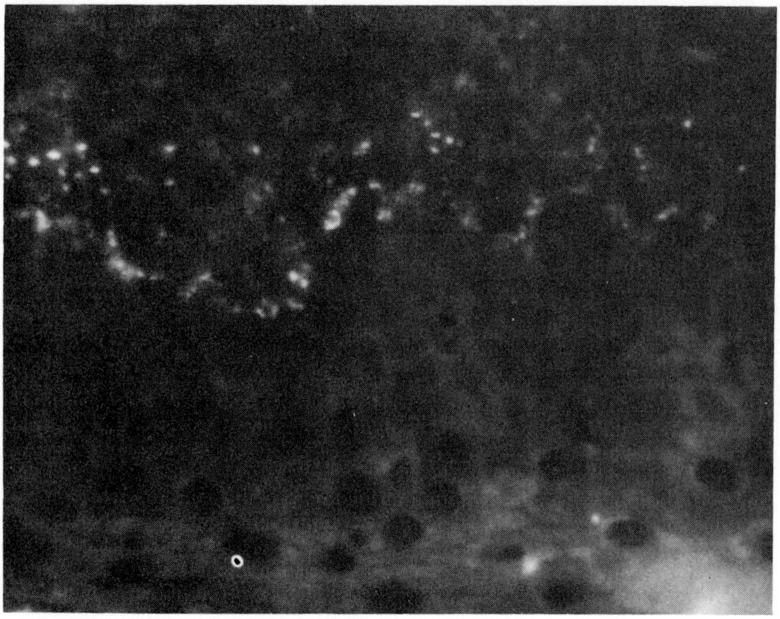

Figure 20–58. Photomicrograph of skin of a patient with chronic discoid lupus erythematosus, showing a characteristic lupus band with granular deposition of IgG at the dermal-epidermal junction involving only the affected skin. (Courtesy of Dr. Thomas T. Provost.)

of skin, whereas in chronic discoid lupus, the deposition of the immune reactants appears to be confined to the involved areas of skin.

Bullous pemphigoid is a disease characterized by an onset in the fifth and sixth decades of life. The skin lesions are characterized by tense subepidermal blisters that may arise on normal as well as inflamed skin (Fig. 20–59). The lesions have a predilection for flexural areas of the body, including the neck, the axillae, and the inguinal area. The disease is a generally benign, self-limited entity that usually responds to steroid therapy within four to six months with complete resolution. Recurrences after therapy occur in approximately 10 to 15 per cent of cases. The characteristic immunopathologic findings in skin include a linear homogeneous IgG deposition along the basement membrane zone, detected by direct immunofluorescence (Fig. 20–60). All classes of immunoglobulins and early and late complement components are seen, as well as fibrin. Approximately 80 per cent of patients demonstrate in their serum an IgG anti–basement membrane antibody that can be detected by indirect immunofluo-

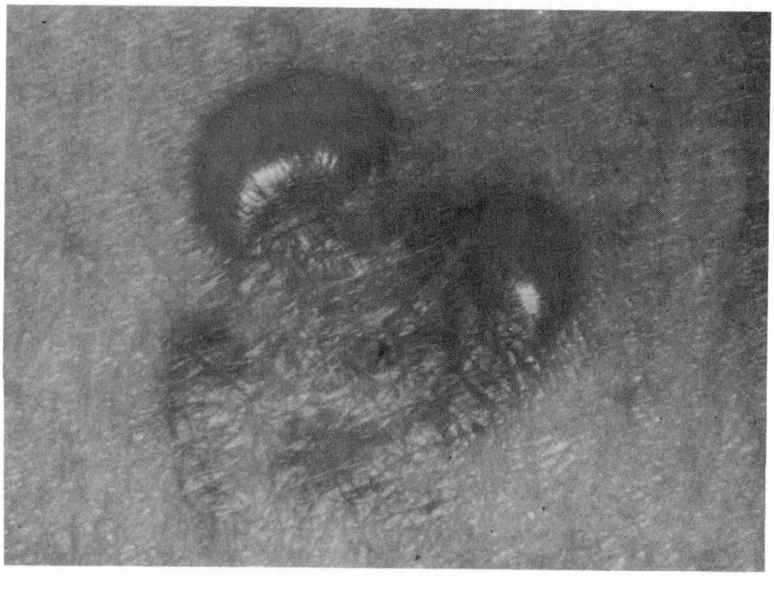

Figure 20–59. Photograph of a patient with pemphigus vulgaris, illustrating the large flaccid blisters characteristic of the disease. (Courtesy of Dr. Thomas T. Provost.)

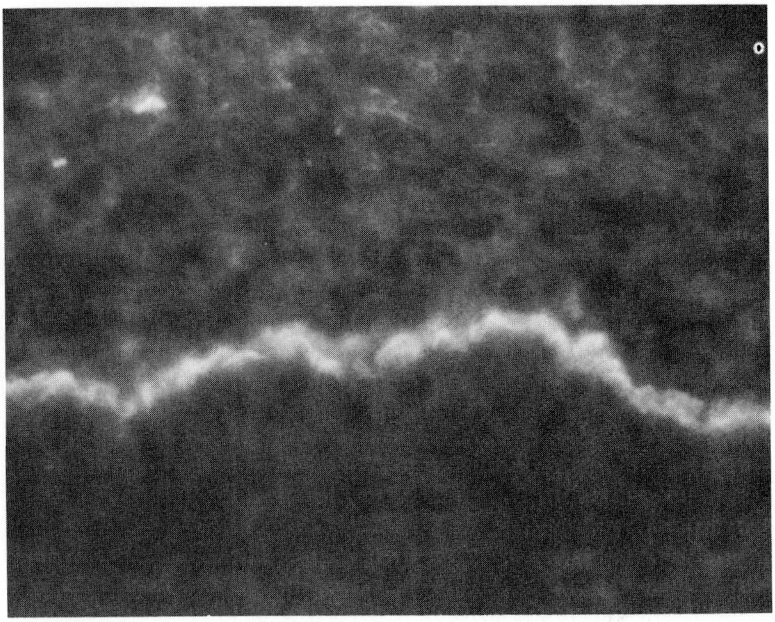

Figure 20–60. Photomicrograph of skin of a patient with bullous pemphigoid, illustrating the characteristic linear homogeneous IgG deposition along the basement membrane zone detected by direct immunofluorescence. (Courtesy of Dr. Thomas T. Provost.)

rescence (Table 20–38). With treatment, the serum autoantibody and the tissue deposition of immunoglobulins and complement disappear.

Pemphigus vulgaris is a blistering disease characterized by the presence of flaccid bullae arising in the mouth and scalp but rapidly disseminating over the entire body. Its striking feature is interepidermal blister formation that occurs with destruction of normal intercellular bridges (Fig. 20–61). Upon pressure, the lesions rapidly extend their margins (Nikolsky's sign). Although it was previously associated with a predilection for those of Jewish origin, recent reports indicate that the disease occurs in all racial and ethnic groups. This serious blistering disease carried with it a significant mortality rate prior to the era of steroids, with approximately 50 per cent of patients dying within 12 to 15 months after initial diagnosis. The disease can be controlled with steroids or with a combination of steroids and immunosuppressive agents (e.g., cyclophosphamide) (Chapter 25). Direct im-

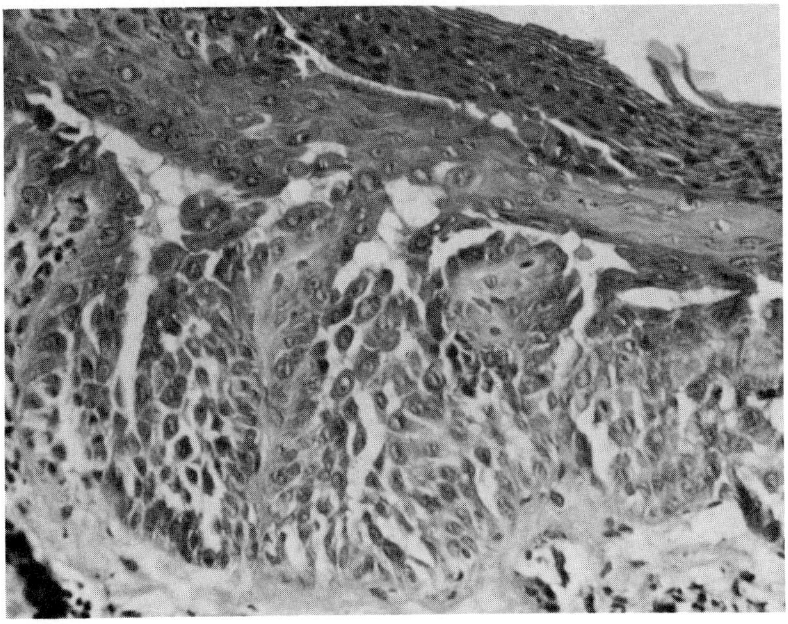

Figure 20–61. Photomicrograph of the skin lesion of pemphigus vulgaris, showing the characteristic interepidermal edema formation associated with destruction of normal intercellular bridges. (Courtesy of Dr. Thomas T. Provost.)

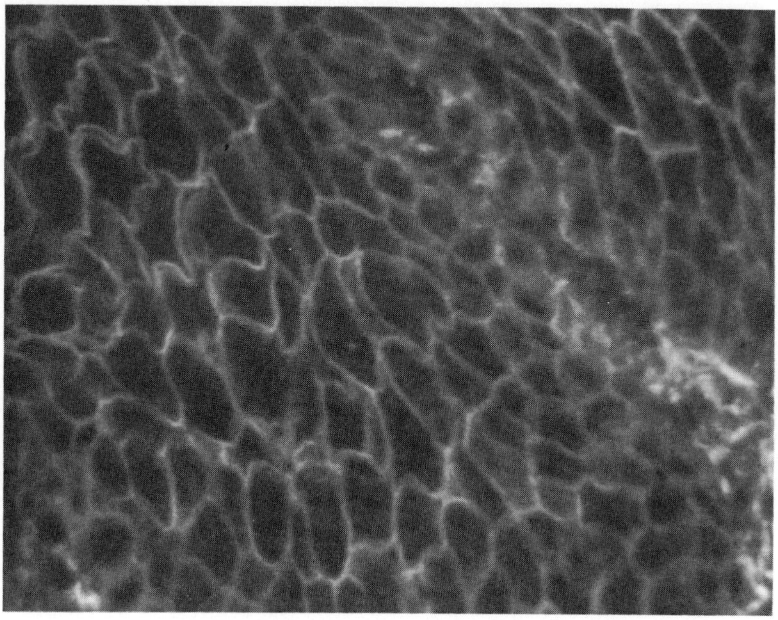

Figure 20–62. Photomicrograph of an indirect immunofluorescent examination of a monkey esophagus that has been layered with the serum of a patient with pemphigus vulgaris, illustrating the presence of circulating autoantibody to intercellular squamous epithelium detected by indirect immunofluorescence. (Courtesy of Dr. Thomas T. Provost.)

munofluorescence of perilesional skin lesions of patients with pemphigus vulgaris has demonstrated IgG, C1q, C3, properdin, and properdin factor B in the squamous intercellular spaces. In addition, in about 90 per cent of patients, the presence of circulating autoantibody to intercellular squamous epithelium has been demonstrated by indirect immunofluorescence (Table 20–38 and Fig. 20–62).

Eye

The eye is isolated anatomically and contains a variety of antigens that normally are not in contact with the circulation (sequestered antigens). Autoimmune phenomena have been implicated in three diseases of the eye: (1) phacogenic uveitis (lens), (2) sympathetic ophthalmia (uvea), and (3) autoimmune reaction involving the lacrimal gland (Sjögren's syndrome).

The release of lens protein into the circulation due to trauma or surgery may result in a sequence of immunologic events leading to inflammation and destruction of the lens. Both inflammatory and immunologic events are triggered. Inflammatory cells are found within the lesions and antilens antibody is found within the circulation and aqueous humor of the affected individual.

Sympathetic ophthalmia results from a perforating wound of the eye. Following trauma to one eye (exciting eye), there is secondary involvement of the other (sympathizing eye). Antiuveal antibodies have been detected in the serum.

SUMMARY

The autoimmune diseases represent a collection of poorly defined, incompletely understood groups of disorders that have in common the manifestation of antibody or delayed hypersensitivity to body constituents (autoimmune phenomena). They are commonly grouped into those disorders that involve multiple systems (multisystemic disorders) and those that are confined or restricted to one organ (organ-specific). The relationship of the autoimmune phenomena to the disease is not understood. A frequent finding in many of these disorders has been an abnormal sex ratio, usually with a female predominance. Although the cause of these diseases is unknown, evidence suggests that they are under genetic control and that they represent disorders of regulation (suppression) of the lymphoid system.

Suggestions for Further Reading

General Textbooks and Monographs

Middleton, E., Jr., Reed, C. E., and Ellis, E. F., (eds.): Allergy: Principles and Practice. St. Louis, C. V. Mosby Co., 1983.

Parker, C. W. (ed.): Clinical Immunology. Philadelphia, W. B. Saunders Co., 1980.

Patterson, R. (ed.): Allergic Diseases: Diagnosis and Management. Philadelphia, J. B. Lippincott Co., 1980.
Salvaggio, J. E. (ed.): Primer on Allergic and Immunologic Disease. JAMA, *248*:2579–2772, 1982.

Immunologically Mediated Disease Involving Exogenous Antigens (Allergy)

Austen, K. F., and Lichtenstein, L. M.: Asthma: Physiology, Immunopharmacology and Treatment. New York, Academic Press, Inc., 1973.
Bates, D. V., Macklem, P. T., and Christie, R. V.: Respiratory Function in Disease. 2nd ed. Philadelphia, W. B. Saunders Company, 1971.
Bellanti, J. A.: Biologic significance of the secretory γA globulins. Pediatrics, *48*:715, 1971.
Casale, T. B., and Marom, Z.: Mast cells and asthma: The role of mast cell mediators in the pathogenesis of allergic asthma. Ann. Allergy, *51*:2, 1983.
Claman, H. M.: How corticosteroids work. J. Allergy Clin. Immunol., *55*:145, 1975.
Dale, D. C., Fauci, A. S., and Wolff, S. M.: Alternate-day prednisone: Leukocyte kinetics and susceptibility to infections. N. Engl. J. Med., *291*:1154, 1974.
Fauci, A. S., Dale, D. C., and Balow, J. E.: Glucocorticosteroid therapy: Mechanisms of action and clinical considerations. Ann. Intern. Med., *84*:304, 1975.
Frank, M. M., Gelfand, J. A., and Atkinson, J. P.: Hereditary angioedema: The clinical syndrome and its management. Ann. Intern. Med., *84*:580, 1976.
Gell, P. G. H., Coombs, R. R. A., and Lachmann, P. J.: Clinical Aspects of Immunology. Oxford, Blackwell Scientific Publications, Ltd., 1975.
Gleich, G. J., and Dunnette, S. L.: Comparison of procedures for measurement of IgE protein in serum and secretions. J. Allergy Clin. Immunol., *59*:377, 1977.
Hubscher, T. T.: Immune and biochemical mechanisms in the allergic disease of the upper respiratory tract; role of antibodies, target cells, mediators and eosinophils. Ann. Allergy, *38*:83, 1977.
Ishizaka, T., and Ishizaka, K.: Biology of immunoglobulin E: Molecular basis of reaginic hypersensitivity. Prog. Allergy, *19*:60, 1975.
Kaplan, A. P., Gray, L., Schaff, R. E., et al.: In vivo studies of mediator release in cold urticaria and cholinergic urticaria. J. Allergy Clin. Immunol., *55*:395, 1975.
Lefkowitz, R. J.: β-adrenergic receptors: Recognition and regulation. N. Engl. J. Med., *295*:323, 1976.
Levine, B. B.: Genetic factors in hypersensitivity reactions to drugs. Ann. N.Y. Acad. Sci., *151*:988, 1968.
Lichtenstein, L. M., Ishizaka, K., Norman, P. S., et al.: IgE antibody measurements in ragweed hayfever: Relationship to clinical severity and results of immunotherapy. J. Clin. Invest., *52*:472, 1973.
Lopez, M., and Salvaggio, J.: Hypersensitivity pneumonitis: Current concepts of etiology and pathogenesis. Annu. Rev. Med., *27*:453, 1976.
Marom, Z., and Casale, T. B.: Mast cells and their mediators. Ann. Allergy, *50*:367, 1983.
Middleton, E., Reed, C., and Ellis, E. (eds.): Allergy: Principles and Practice. St. Louis, C. V. Mosby Company, 1978.
Parker, C. W.: Drug allergy, N. Engl. J. Med., *292*:51, 732, 957, 1975.
Patterson, R.: Allergic Diseases: Diagnosis and Management. Philadelphia, J. B. Lippincott Company, 1972.
Patterson, R., Mellies, C. J., and Roberts, M.: Immunologic reactions against insulin: II. IgE anti-insulin, insulin allergy and combined IgE and IgG immunologic insulin resistance. J. Immunol., *110*:1135, 1973.
Pepys, J.: Hypersensitivity Diseases of the Lungs Due to Fungi and Organic Dusts. Basel, S. Karger, 1969.
Platts-Mills, T. A. E., von Mauer, R. K., Ishizaka, K., et al.: IgA and IgG anti-ragweed antibodies in nasal secretions. J. Clin. Invest., *57*:1041, 1976.
Rosenow, E. C.: The spectrum of drug-induced pulmonary disease. Ann. Intern. Med., *77*:977, 1972.
Salvaggio, J. E. (ed.): Primer on allergic and immunologic diseases. JAMA, *248*:2579, 1982.
Samter, M.: Immunological Diseases. Boston, Little, Brown & Company, 1971.
Tada, T., Taniguchi, M., and Takemori, T.: Properties of primed suppressor T cells and their products. Transplant. Rev., *26*:106, 1975.
Zweiman, B., Mishkin, M. M., and Hildreth, E. A.: An approach to the performance of contrast studies in contrast material-reactive persons. Ann. Intern. Med., *83*:159, 1975.

Immunologically Mediated Disease Involving Homologous Antigens

Gell, P. G. H., Coombs, R. R. A., and Lachmann, P. J.: Clinical Aspects of Immunology. Oxford, Blackwell Scientific Publications, Ltd., 1975.
Mollison, P.: Blood Transfusion in Clinical Medicine. Philadelphia, F. A. Davis Company, 1968.
Race, R. R., and Sanger, R.: Blood Groups in Man. Philadelphia, F. A. Davis Company, 1969.
Rapaport, F. T., and Dausset, J.: Human Transplantation. New York, Grune & Stratton, Inc., 1968.
Russell, P. S.: Transplantation, I, II, III. N. Engl. J. Med., *282*:786, 848, 896, 1970.
Witebsky, E., Rubin, M. I., Engasser, L., et al.: Studies on erythroblastosis fetalis. II. Investigation on detection of sensitization of red blood cells of newborn infants with erythroblastosis fetalis. J. Lab. Clin. Med., *32*:1339, 1947.
Zmijewski, C. M.: Immunohematology. New York, Appleton-Century-Crofts, 1968.

Organ Transplantation

Belzer, F. O., et al.: Is HL-A typing of clinical significance in cadaver renal transplantation? Lancet, 775, 1976.
Braun, W. E., Banowsky, L. H., et al.: Lymphoceles associated with renal transplantation. Report of cases and review of the literature. Am. J. Med., *57*:714, 1974.
Calne, R. Y., and Williams, R.: Orthotopic liver transplantation: The first 60 patients. Br. Med. J., *1*:471–476, 1977.
Cochrum, S., et al.: Mixed lymphocyte reaction and graft survival. Ann. Surg., 1974.
Friedman, B. A., Wenglin, B. D., Hyland, R. N., et al.: Roentgenographically atypical *Pneumocystis carinii* pneumonia. Am. Rev. Respir. Dis., *111*:89, 1975.
Gallis, H. A., et al.: Fungal infections following renal transplantation. Arch. Intern. Med., *135*:1163, 1975.
Kiser, W. S., Hewitt, C. B., and Montie, J. E.: The surgical complications of renal transplantation. Surg. Clin. North Am., *51*:1133, 1971.
Maher, J. F.: A logical approach to the diagnosis of renal transplant rejection. Immunologic, ischemic, and inflammatory impairment of renal function. Am. J. Med., *56*:275, 1974.

Matthew, T. H., Mathews, D. C., Hobbs, J. B., et al.: Glomerular lesions after renal transplantation. Am. J. Med., *59*:177, 1975.

Merrill, J. P.: New perspective on pathogenesis and treatment of rejection in kidney transplantation. Kidney Int., 7:S318, 1976.

Myerowitz, R. L., Medeiros, A. A., and O'Brien, T. F.: Bacterial infection in renal homotransplantation recipients. A study of 53 bacteremic episodes. Am. J. Med., *53*:308, 1972.

Rifkind, D., Marchioro, T. L., et al.: Infectious diseases associated with renal homotransplantation. JAMA, *189*:397, 402, 1964.

Suwansirikul, S., Ho, M., et al.: The transplanted kidney as a source of cytomegalovirus infection. N. Engl. J. Med., *293*:1109, 1975.

Van Bekkum, D. W., Fritz, H. B., et al.: A report from histocompatible allogeneic donors for aplastic anemia. A report from the ACS/NIH Bone Marrow Transplant Registry. JAMA, *236*(10):1131, 1976.

Immunologically Mediated Disease Involving Autologous Antigens

Asherson, G. L.: The role of microorganisms in autoimmune responses. Prog. Allergy, *12*:192, 1968.

Burnet, F. M.: Autoimmune disease: Some general principles. Postgrad. Med., *30*:91, 1961.

Carpenter, C. B.: Immunologic aspects of renal disease. Annu. Rev. Med., *21*:1, 1970.

Churg, J., and Grishman, R.: Ultrastructure of glomerular disease: A review. Kidney Int., *7*:254, 1975.

Cupps, T. R., and Fauci, A. S.: The Vasculitides. Philadelphia, W. B. Saunders Company, 1981.

Dawson, R. B.: HLA Typing. Washington, D. C., Am. Assoc. Blood Banks, 1976.

Gelfand, M. C., Shin, M. L., Nagle, R. B., et al.: The glomerular complement receptor in immunologically mediated renal glomerular injury. N. Engl. J. Med., *295*:10, 1976.

Koffler, D.: Immunopathogenesis of systemic lupus erythematosus. Annu. Rev. Med., *25*:149, 1974.

Krakauer, R. S., Strober, W., Rippeon, D. L., et al.: Prevention of autoimmunity in experimental lupus erythematosus by soluble immune response suppressor. Science, *196*:56, 1977.

Lehman, D. H., Wilson, C. B., and Dixon, F. J.: Extraglomerular immunoglobulin deposits in human nephritis. Am. J. Med., *58*:765, 1975.

McLean, R. H., and Michael, A. F.: Activation of the complement system in renal conditions in animals and man. Prog. Immunol., *5*:69, 1974.

Mikkelsen, W. M., Bunch, T. W., Calabro, J. J., et al.: Twenty-fourth rheumatism review: Review of the American and English literature for the years 1977 and 1978. Arthritis Rheum., *24*:113, 1981.

Mullin, B. R., Levinson, R. E., Friedman, A., et al.: Delayed hypersensitivity in Graves' disease and exophthalmos: Identification of thyroglobulin in normal human orbital muscle. Endocrinology, *110*:351, 1977.

Otaka, Y.: Immunopathology of Rheumatic Fever and Rheumatoid Arthritis. Tokyo, Igaku Shoin, Ltd., 1976.

Samter, M.: Immunological Diseases. Boston, Little, Brown & Company, 1978.

Sharp, G. C., Irwin, W. S., Tan, E. W., et al.: Mixed connective tissue disease. An apparent distinct rheumatic disease syndrome associated with a specific antibody to an extractable nuclear antigen (ENA). Am. J. Med., *52*:148, 1972.

Shearn, M.: Rheumatic diseases. Med. Clin. North Am., *61*:203, 1977.

Solomon, D. H., Chopra, I. J., Chopra, U., et al.: Identification of subgroups of euthyroid Graves' ophthalmopathy. N. Engl. J. Med., *296*:181, 1977.

Strober, W.: Gluten-sensitive enteropathy. Clin. Gastroenterol., *5*:429, 1976.

Svejgaard, A., Friis, J., Morling, N., et al.: HLA in rheumatology. J. Rheumatol., *8*:541, 1981.

Volpé, R., Farid, N. R., von Westarp, C., et al.: The pathogenesis of Graves' disease and Hashimoto's thyroiditis. Clin. Endocrinol (Oxf.), *3*:239, 1974.

Wilson, C. B., and Dixon, F. J.: Anti-glomerular basement membrane antibody induced glomerulonephritis. Kidney Int., *3*:74, 1973.

Wilson, C. B., and Dixon, F. J.: Renal response to immunological injury. *In* Brenner, B. M., and Rector, F. C., Jr. (eds.): The Kidney. Philadelphia, W. B. Saunders Company, 1976.

Chapter 21

Neoplasms of the Immune System

A. Monoclonal Gammopathies

George M. Bernier, M.D.

Several diseases of man, including some of the most devastating human malignancies, are characterized by abnormal proliferation of those cells that normally are the mediators of specific immunity: lymphocytes and plasma cells. When such proliferation involves cells that usually synthesize and secrete immunoglobulin, the disorder may be associated with excessive production of immunoglobulins. The nature of the immunoglobulins produced may indeed be characteristic of the disorder.

The immunoproliferative disorders discussed in this chapter are multiple myeloma, macroglobulinemia, cryoglobulinemia, and heavy-chain disease. These four disorders are often called the monoclonal gammopathies and will be described as a unit. The lymphomas and lymphocytic leukemias may be considered as examples of lymphoproliferative diseases in which immunoglobulin aberration is less readily apparent or nonexistent and in which distinctive features are often found in the proliferative cells themselves. These will be described in Chapter 21B.

CONCEPT

The immunoglobulins produced in response to the myriad antigens to which man is exposed are an extremely heterogeneous group of molecules. This heterogeneity undoubtedly reflects those variations in primary sequence related to antibody specificity and may be readily demonstrated by immunoelectrophoresis of serum (Fig. 21–1). The IgG fraction of serum is dispersed over a wide electrophoretic range, in contrast to the albumin and transferrin that migrate as discrete components. In a similar fashion, but to a less striking degree, the other immunoglobulins (IgA, IgM, IgD, and IgE) are electrophoretically heterogeneous or polydisperse. An individual plasma cell produces immunoglobulins that are homogeneous in terms of antibody specificity, light- and heavy-chain composition, genetic factors, and electrophoretic charge. The heterogeneity of immunoglobulins must therefore be the result of a heterogeneous cell population. Thus, for each of 10^8 to 10^{10} possible antibodies, there exists a different cell line or clone capable of producing that antibody. If one cell out of the many different cell lines or clones were selected for abnormal uncontrolled proliferation, and if it retained the ability to synthesize its immunoglobulin, a great excess of a homogeneous immunoglobulin could be expected to result (Fig. 21–2). When such situations occur, they are viewed as abnormalities of the immune, or gamma, system ("gammopathies"), arising in a single disordered clone of cells. They are called "monoclonal gammopathies" (Table 21–1). The protein elaborated is often called a monoclonal immunoglobulin or an M-component. When monoclonal immunoglobulins occur, they may be of any class (IgG, IgA, IgM, IgD, or IgE) or type (κ or λ). They are usually recognized as an increased homogeneous serum globulin. In many instances, patients with serum monoclonal immunoglobulins also have detectable amounts of free light chains. Light chains of either κ or λ type may be produced in excess of heavy

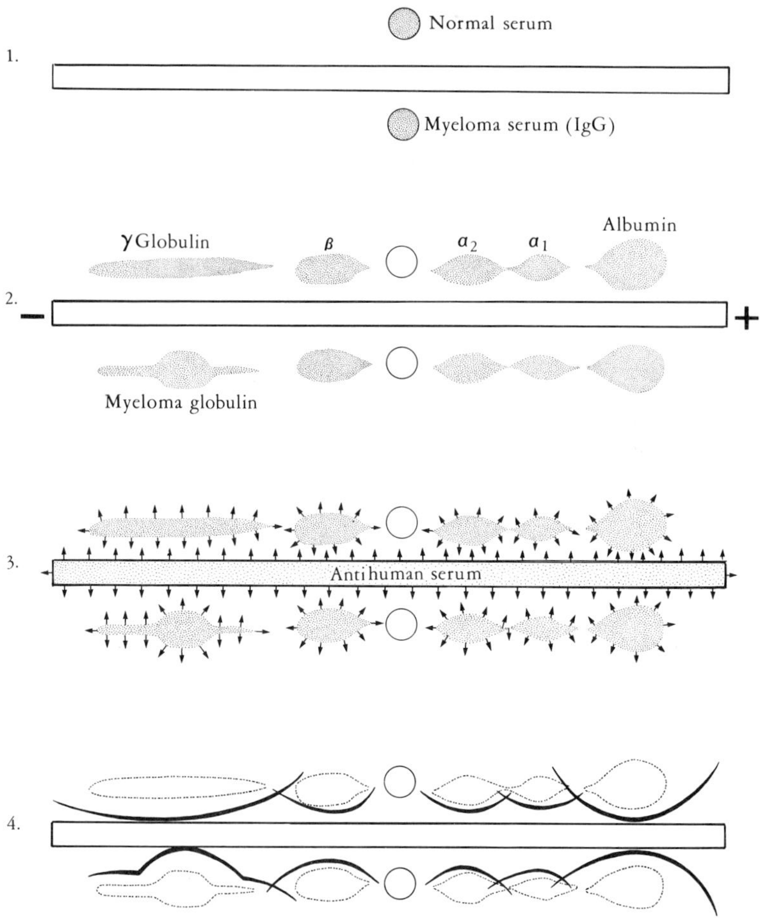

Figure 21–1. Schematic representation of immunoelectrophoresis of normal and myeloma serum.

Step 1: The sera are applied to wells punched out of agar slides.

Step 2: The agar slide is placed in an electric field, and the proteins migrate—albumin to the anode (+) and γ globulin to the cathode (−). Note that the myeloma globulin is restricted in its mobility to a portion of the γ globulin fraction.

Step 3: Antisera to human serum proteins are applied in the central trough and the antibodies diffuse into the agar toward the serum proteins, which also diffuse into the agar.

Step 4: Where serum proteins and their homologous antibodies meet, precipitation arcs develop. The arc has a characteristic position and shape for the particular protein. In this diagram, the serum is depicted as being composed of only five components, whereas most antisera detect at least 25 components. The normal IgG forms a long sweeping arc. Note that the IgG arc formed by the myeloma serum is distorted with a localized antigenic excess forming a "blister" on the IgG arc.

chains and may circulate as free homogeneous light chains. Because of their small size (a dimer of light chains has a molecular weight of 45,000 daltons), they are excreted rapidly in the urine. Free light chains in the monoclonal gammopathies are usually detected as electrophoretically homogeneous urinary proteins bearing the κ or λ antigenic determinants. Free light chains have unusual thermal solubility properties, which were first described by H. Bence Jones in 1847, and are often called Bence Jones proteins. They may be detected by appropriately heating the urine (see later). In approximately 20 per cent of myeloma patients, the affected clone of cells secretes only free light chains.

Table 21–1. Monoclonal Gammopathies

Disorder	Class of Protein	Light Chain
Multiple myeloma	IgG, IgA, IgD or IgE	κ or λ
Macroglobulinemia	IgM	κ or λ
Heavy-chain disease	IgG, IgA or IgM	None

Multiple Myeloma

Multiple myeloma, a malignant proliferation of plasma cells, is the most common of the malignant monoclonal gammopathies. In a pathophysiologic sense, the various features of the disorder may be viewed as consequences of the following: (1) the expansion of the cell mass; (2) the elaboration of the proteins by cells; and (3) the associated suppression of normal antibody synthesis. In its full-blown expression, the disease involves the skeletal system, the bone marrow, the kidneys, and the nervous system and has a profound suppressive effect upon the immune system.

BONE

The skeletal problems are extraordinarily troublesome and range from multiple osteolytic lesions and pathologic fractures to diffuse osteoporosis and painful compression fractures (Fig. 21–3). As progressive verte-

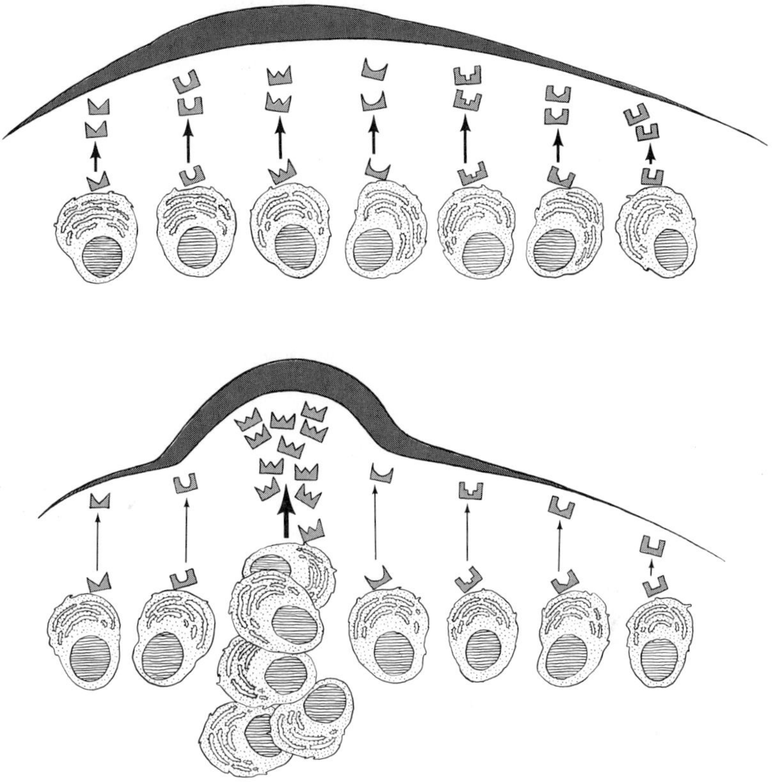

Figure 21–2. Diagrammatic illustration of the monoclonal immunoglobulin concept. Normal individuals *(top)* have many populations or clones of plasma cells, each producing immunoglobulins of differing electrophoretic mobility, indicated as molecules of differing shapes. The wide extremes of electrophoretic mobility give rise to a long, polydisperse immunoelectrophoretic arc. In contrast, if one clone or population were to be selected for proliferation *(bottom),* its product would be greatly increased. In association with this, the products of the other clones are decreased. This gives rise to an immunoglobulin of restricted mobility and the characteristically distorted immunoelectrophoretic arc.

bral collapse occurs, marked diminution in the patient's height may result. Spinal cord transection and paraplegia are uncommon tragic consequences of vertebral column compression fractures. The multiple individual osteolytic lesions of bone (myelomas) are readily explained as being due in part to plasma cell growth, but the mechanics of the diffuse osteoporosis is less well understood. Myeloma cells elaborate a low molecular weight factor that selectively stimulates *osteoclasts* (osteoclast activating factor), and this factor plays a role in both osteolytic and osteoporotic lesions. A direct consequence of the skeletal problems is disturbed calcium balance. During the course of their disease

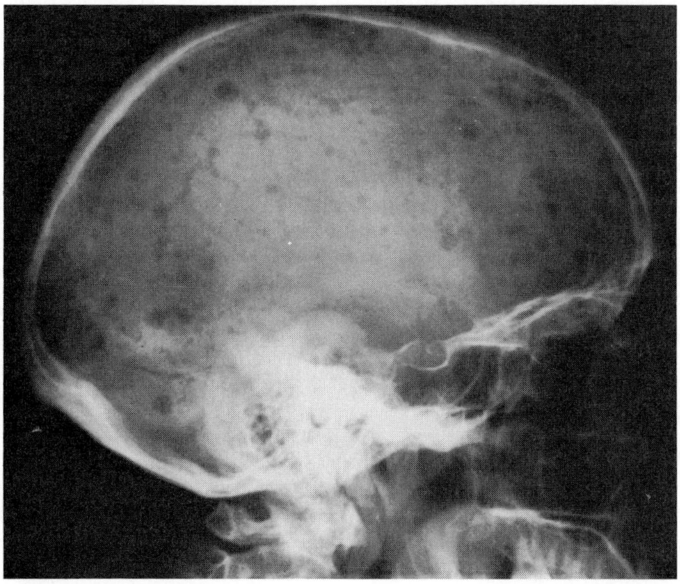

Figure 21–3. Skull x-ray of a myeloma patient showing many well-demarcated osteolytic lesions in the calvarium.

or even before it has been diagnosed, patients with multiple myeloma may have hypercalcemia of life-threatening degree. Symptoms of polyuria, constipation, lethargy, confusion, and stupor may occur. Unlike the case in hypercalcemia due to hyperparathyroidism or metastatic carcinoma, serum alkaline phosphatase activity is usually normal. It is important to point out that the immobilization of a myeloma patient for any reason predisposes to the development of hypercalcemia. For this reason, activity is to be encouraged to maintain the normal stress on the skeletal system.

BONE MARROW EFFECTS

The effect upon the bone marrow is, in part, related to the replacement of normal marrow elements with malignant plasma cells (Fig. 21–4). Some depression of normal cellular development occurs in instances in which extensive replacement is not evident, however, and less direct mechanisms of bone marrow suppression have to be postulated.

Anemia of some degree is remarkably common in multiple myeloma. In the early stages of the disease, the anemia may be slight. With progression of the disease, reduction of hematocrit to the 20 to 30 range is common. The anemia is usually normochromic and normocytic, but many instances of macrocytic anemia have been described. Leukopenia and thrombocytopenia occur but are less constant features. The anemia is the result of many factors, including infection, renal failure, blood loss, decrease in production due to bone marrow replacement by plasma cells, and a reduced red cell life span.

Bone marrow aspiration performed for the evaluation of anemia is sometimes the first clue to the presence of myeloma. Whereas normal bone marrow contains approximately 1 per cent plasma cells, myeloma is evidenced by increased numbers of plasma cells, often in clusters or sheets. In addition, myeloma cells appear to mature in an abnormal fashion; nuclear maturation lags behind that of the cytoplasm. For instance, when the cytoplasm has reached the developmental stage of synthesizing and secreting immunoglobulin, the nucleus may still be very primitive and retain its ability to divide (Fig. 21–5).

Occasionally, plasma cells are found in the circulating blood. In a form of plasmacytic proliferation called plasma cell leukemia, the number of plasma cells in the peripheral blood may reach 100,000 per mm^3.

KIDNEY INVOLVEMENT

Renal failure is a common cause of death in multiple myeloma. This is often associated with marked Bence Jones proteinuria. The kidney appears to have a dual relationship with Bence Jones protein. Free light chains are normally catabolized by the kidney, probably after a process of glomerular filtration and reabsorption. Impaired renal function interferes with the ability of the kidney to catabolize free light chains, and therefore the serum and urinary concentrations of Bence Jones protein increase. In turn, the large amounts of Bence Jones protein appear to have deleterious effects on the kidney: Proteinaceous casts may form, urine flow through the kidney may be impeded, and abnormalities of renal function, such as renal tubular acidosis, may occur.

Other ways in which the kidney may suffer in multiple myeloma are through plasma cell infiltration of the renal parenchyma, through associated amyloidosis of the kidney (which may produce a nephrotic syndrome picture), and through hypercalcemia and hyperuricemia. It is not surprising, therefore, that the diagnosis of multiple myeloma is frequently established through the investigation of unexplained proteinuria or azotemia in a patient.

Because a number of myeloma patients (mostly with Bence Jones proteinuria) have developed acute renal failure following intravenous pyelography, much caution must be exercised when using this procedure in patients with obscure renal failure. The dehydration that usually accompanies the procedure is surely responsible in part for the problem. In addition, interaction between the x-ray contrast dye and light chains has been implicated in the production of intratubular deposits.

NERVOUS SYSTEM

The brain, spinal cord, and peripheral nerves may all be affected in myeloma. It is easiest to demonstrate a causal relationship when the spinal cord is involved. Plasmacytomas, or masses of extramedullary plasma cells, may surround the cord, constrict the blood supply to it, and thus produce the signs and symptoms of transection.

Unexplained peripheral neuropathies also occur in multiple myeloma and have been variously attributed to protein deposits in the peripheral neural sheaths and to antibody

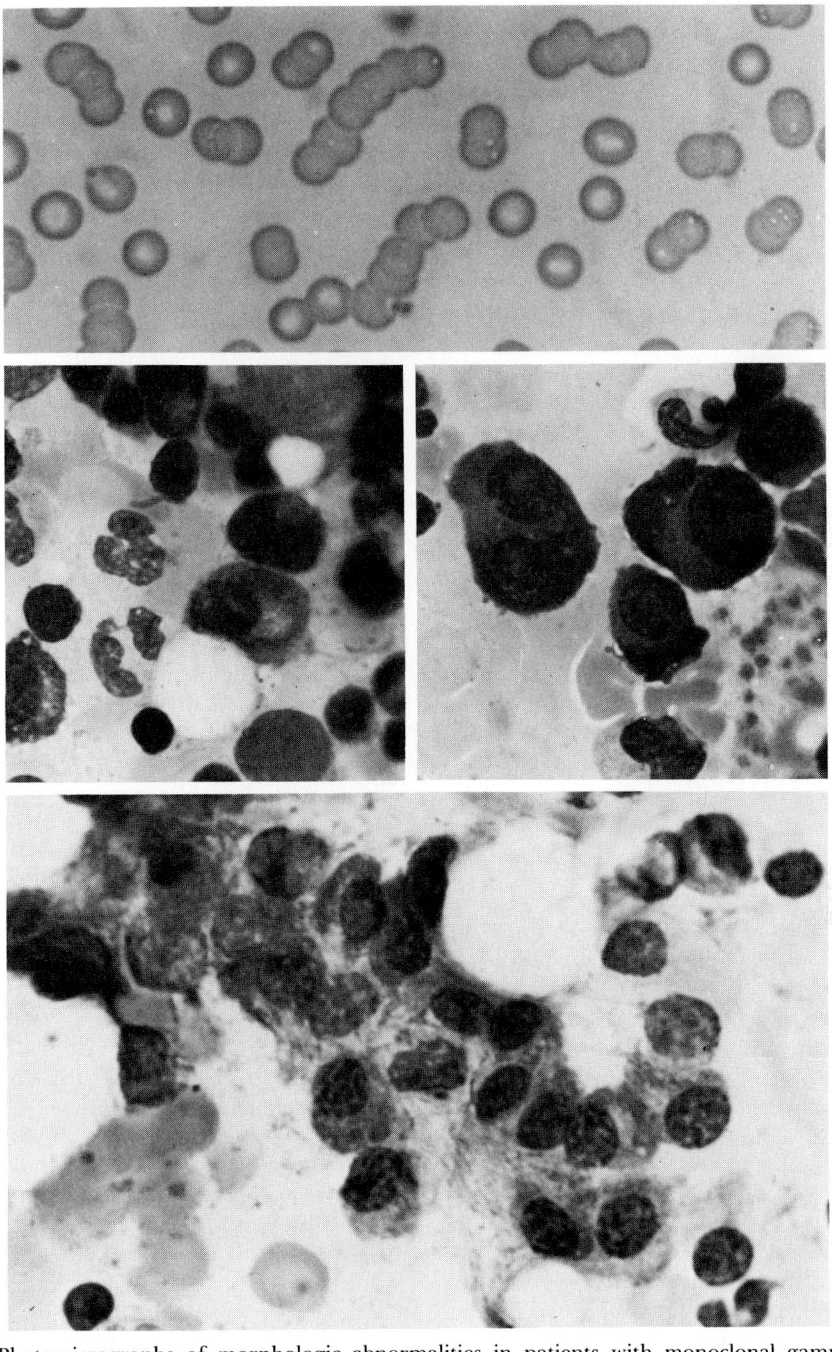

Figure 21–4. Photomicrographs of morphologic abnormalities in patients with monoclonal gammopathies. *Top,* Peripheral blood smear showing rouleaux (side-to-side stacking of red blood cells) and diffuse staining of the background, indicating high protein content. Smear is from a patient with IgA myeloma. *Middle,* Comparison of marrow from a patient with reactive plasmacytosis (left) and one with myeloma (right). The reactive cells have condensed nuclear chromatin and mature cytoplasms, markers of developed cells. The myeloma cells show large, primitive nuclei in the presence of well-developed cytoplasms (nuclear-cytoplasmic asynchrony). *Bottom,* Bone marrow from patient with macroglobulinemia showing cells of the lymphocytic-plasmacytic type.

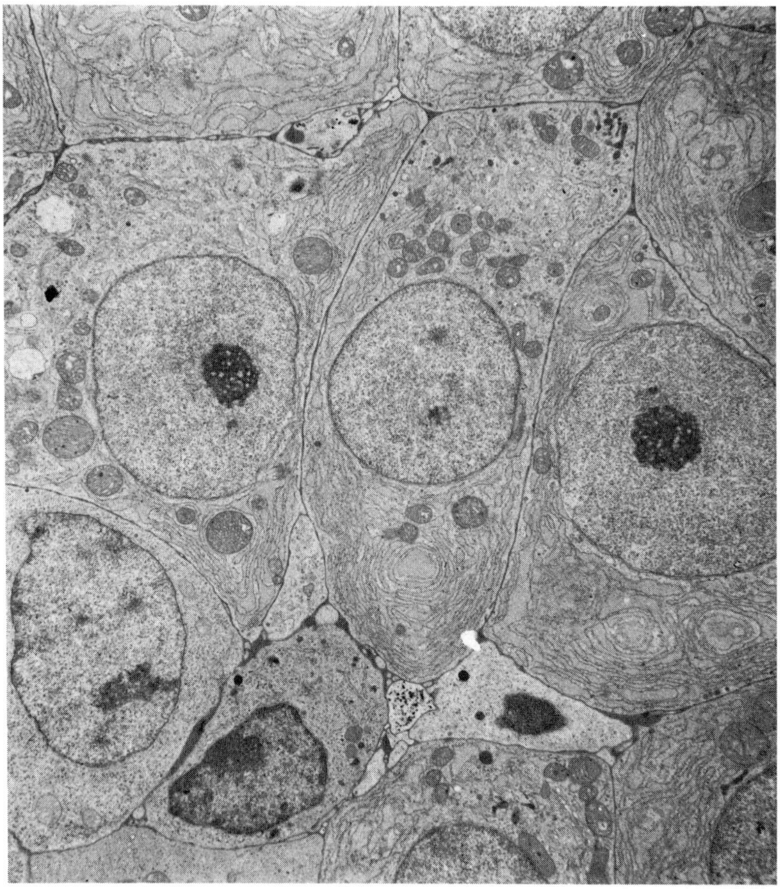

Figure 21–5. Electron micrograph of bone marrow plasma cells from a patient with advanced multiple myeloma. Shown are a cluster of asynchronous plasma cells showing primitive nuclei (little or no chromatin condensation) and very mature cytoplasms featuring well-developed endoplasmic reticulum (× 5000). (Courtesy of Dr. Richard C. Graham, Jr.)

activity of the myeloma protein directed against neural tissue. Amyloidosis may cause compression of the median nerve as it passes beneath the tenaculum at the wrist, resulting in "carpal tunnel syndrome."

Central nervous system symptoms of lethargy, stupor, and coma may be brought on by extreme blood viscosity due to the massive amounts of protein in the serum, by hypercalcemia, or by advanced renal failure.

For all the varied manifestations of the disease, the most common presenting complaint is low back pain. The most common finding of routine laboratory tests is anemia. Since these symptoms are common to many diseases, a high degree of suspicion is necessary in establishing the diagnosis.

PROTEINS IN MULTIPLE MYELOMA

M-Components. A virtual hallmark of multiple myeloma is the monoclonal immunoglobulin, which is present in more than 99 per cent of myeloma patients (Fig. 21–6). This M-component abnormality may be either a serum myeloma globulin (IgG, IgA, IgD, or IgE) or a Bence Jones protein (free κ chains or free λ chains), or both. The frequency of these manifestations in several large series of myeloma patients is indicated in Table 21–2. The most common finding is a serum myeloma globulin by itself. Bence Jones protein with a serum myeloma globulin and Bence Jones protein alone are somewhat less common. In fewer than 1 per cent of myeloma patients, a monoclonal gammopathy cannot be demonstrated, even though the rest of the clinical picture is entirely consistent with multiple myeloma. In many of these cases, the cells synthesize an immunoglobulin but fail to secrete it. In other cases, neither extracellular nor intracellular immunoglobulin can be detected by the highly sensitive techniques used, and one must conclude that the cells are making "blanks." Great care must be taken to test for the presence of very small amounts of Bence Jones protein by concentration and electrophoresis of the urine. Methods of detection are described later.

Bence Jones Proteins. Bence Jones proteins, which are homogeneous free light

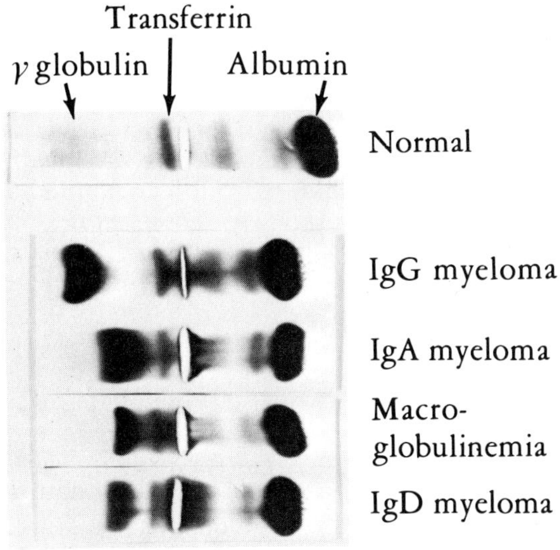

Figure 21–6. Agar gel electrophoresis of human sera. At the top is a normal serum with the albumin, transferrin, and gamma globulin fractions indicated. The four sera below are from patients with monoclonal gammopathy, and the type of monoclonal immunoglobulin is indicated at the right.

chains, were first recognized almost 140 years ago and have provided a valuable tool in the diagnosis of multiple myeloma. These urinary proteins have peculiar heat precipitability properties. When the urine is heated at pH 5, most Bence Jones proteins will precipitate at temperatures in the range of 48° to 56°C and will redissolve on boiling. When the urine is allowed to cool, the proteins reprecipitate.

Immunologic and electrophoretic techniques are usually employed in the detection of Bence Jones protein and, at present, provide the definitive test for this entity. An electrophoretically homogeneous urinary protein that reacts with antiserum to κ chains or λ chains and does not react with antiserum to the heavy chain of any immunoglobulin is, by present-day criteria, a Bence Jones protein.

Approximately 50 per cent of myeloma patients are found to have detectable Bence Jones proteinuria if the added precaution of concentrating the urine is taken. Under some conditions, particularly in the presence of renal failure, Bence Jones proteins may be found in the serum.

Table 21–2. Frequency of Various M-Components in Multiple Myeloma

Finding	Per Cent Occurrence
Serum myeloma globulin alone	48
Serum myeloma globulin plus Bence Jones protein	31
Bence Jones protein alone	20.5
No monoclonal immunoglobulin	0.5

IMMUNOGLOBULIN DEFICIENCY IN MULTIPLE MYELOMA

Quite commonly in multiple myeloma, the concentration of normal immunoglobulins is sharply reduced, and a functional hypogammaglobulinemia may be present. This can be seen when quantitative measures of serum immunoglobulins are made. Frequently, the concentrations of IgA and IgM globulins are subnormal when an IgG myeloma globulin is present, and IgG and IgM globulin levels are often low when IgA myeloma globulin is present. For all practical purposes, if one could remove the monoclonal immunoglobulin from the electrophoretic pattern, a deficiency of its class would be present as well.

This phenomenon of paucity in the midst of plenty is a major contributor to defective antibody formation and repeated bacterial infections. At least two mechanisms for the decreased serum levels of immunoglobulin exist—a decrease in the number of normal immunoglobulin-producing cells and accelerated catabolism of normal antibodies. Decreased numbers of normal plasma cells may reflect an inhibitor substance (*chalone*) released by the myeloma cells or an increased number of suppressor cells (T-lymphocytes or monocytes). Hypercatabolism of nonmyelomatous IgG occurs in patients with large amounts of monoclonal IgG of the IgG1, IgG2, or IgG4 subclass. Whatever the mechanism, the patient with antibody deficiency is uniquely susceptible to repeated infections with encapsulated organisms, particularly of the pneumococcal type. To date, treatment of this immune deficiency with exogenous γ-globulin has not been particularly effective.

FREQUENCY DISTRIBUTION OF MYELOMA GLOBULINS

As previously indicated, a myeloma globulin may be of either light-chain type or the IgG, IgA, IgD, or IgE globulin class. The IgM class by definition is associated with macroglobulinemia, but on rare occasions, patients with classic multiple myeloma have been found to have an IgM paraprotein. A close parallel exists between the serum concentration of an immunoglobulin class or type in normal individuals and the frequency of that class or type in a population of myeloma globulins. Of the many thousands of myeloma globulins that have been classified, IgG and IgA myeloma are the most common. IgD myeloma has been detected approximately 250 times, and IgE myeloma less than 10. The ratio of IgG to IgA myeloma globulins is approximately 3:1. A similar finding is true for light-chain type. In the normal individual, the ratio of κ chains to λ chains is 60:40, and the same distribution is observed in populations of myeloma globulins. As indicated earlier, individual plasma cells appear to produce only a single kind of light chain. The ratio of κ-producing cells to λ-producing cells is the same ratio as is found in normal serum and in large surveys of myeloma globulins (approximately 60:40). Therefore, it seems reasonable to conclude that the cellular population at risk in the genesis of multiple myeloma is in proportion to its normal frequency distribution.

In terms of prognostic factors, it would appear that patients with "light-chain myeloma" do least well (those with λ type worse than κ type), and patients with IgA myeloma probably do more poorly than those with IgG. IgD myeloma appears to occur in a younger age group than the other forms of myeloma and, curiously, is almost always of λ type and associated with excretion of Bence Jones protein.

TREATMENT

A number of therapeutic measures are used in the treatment of multiple myeloma. The need for ambulation, activity, braces, and other general supportive measures is stressed by many physicians in order to prevent acceleration of osteoporosis. Sodium fluoride has been used to increase the strength of bone, but its efficacy has been questioned. High fluid intake is important in forestalling renal complications and in treating hypercalcemia. Localized bone pain due to osteolytic lesions is often relieved by x-ray treatment. Testosterone has been used as an anabolic steroid and as a stimulator of erythropoiesis. Diphosphonates and mithramycin have been useful in controlling hypercalcemia.

Chemotherapy. Use of the alkylating agents cyclophosphamide and phenylalanine mustard has produced subjective and objective signs of improvement in a significant percentage of myeloma patients. Improvement in some patients has been dramatic. Intermittent high doses of phenylalanine mustard combined with prednisone have had the best reported results, with as high as 60 per cent of patients so treated having a favorable response. More recently, doxorubicin, vincristine, and high-dose dexamethasone have been used with some success in treating patients who are refractory to alkylating agents. Major toxic side effects of cyclophosphamide have been bone marrow depression, alopecia, and hemorrhagic cystitis. Phenylalanine mustard has bone marrow suppression, notably thrombocytopenia, as its major toxic effect. A significant number of myeloma patients treated for prolonged periods (years) with alkylating agents have developed acute granulocytic leukemia. Whether this is drug-induced or the "natural history" of myeloma remains conjectural.

Immunotherapy. With advances in knowledge about specific suppressor cells and the development of monoclonal antibodies of mouse and human origin, it is likely that attempts to treat myeloma with biologically active agents will occur in the present decade. Interferon, a potent biologic modifier, has had inconsistent but occasionally dramatic therapeutic effects in myeloma patients.

Macroglobulinemia

In 1944, on the basis of ultracentrifugation studies, Waldenström identified a group of hyperglobulinemic patients as having excessive amounts of high molecular weight protein in their serum. The clinical picture could be distinguished from more classic multiple myeloma in symptomatology and pathologic findings. The protein was called macroglobulin, and the condition has been known as Waldenström's macroglobulinemia. The clinical disturbance seen in this disorder is in part a result of the abnormal cellular proliferation and in part a result of the abnormal protein produced by the cells.

ABNORMALITY AND SYMPTOMATOLOGY

The abnormal protein in this condition is an electrophoretically homogeneous IgM globulin that is of high molecular weight (approximately 900,000) and has the chemical and immunochemical characteristics of the IgM globulin class. Because of the high intrinsic viscosity of the IgM globulin, large amounts of this protein may result in a marked increase in the viscosity of the patient's serum that, in turn, can lead to sluggish blood flow, thromboses, central nervous system disturbances, and bleeding. The most common bleeding sites are the skin, nasal mucosa, and gastrointestinal tract. Sluggish blood flow in the retinal vessels is particularly striking, with segmental disturbances in blood flow ("sausage links"), and may eventuate in retinal vein thrombosis and blindness. Coating of the red blood cells, the polymorphonuclear leukocytes, and particularly the platelets may result in impaired survival or function of these elements. Frequently, the hyperproduction of IgM globulin is accompanied by a decreased production of the other immunoglobulins. This functional hypogammaglobulinemia, in concert with the impaired white cell function and granulocytopenia, leads to repeated severe bacterial infections. Approximately one in ten macroglobulinemia patients has demonstrable Bence Jones proteinuria, and this may have adverse effects on the kidney, as described in the preceding section.

In addition to the protein, the cells engaged in the synthesis of the macroglobulin may produce abnormalities (see Fig. 21–4). Proliferation of the lymphoid tissue in lymph nodes, liver, and spleen is often excessive and can result in clinically detectable enlargement of these organs. On occasion, marked lymphocytosis may be present, and the condition may be indistinguishable from chronic lymphocytic leukemia. Total replacement of the bone marrow may occur. An increased number of tissue mast cells are often found in the bone marrow, but their significance is not known. The patients with this condition differ from myeloma patients in that most are spared the debilitating bone disease, presumably because the abnormal cells in macroglobulinemia do not secrete osteoclast activating factor.

Many patients with macroglobulinemia produce detectable amounts of low molecular weight macroglobulin (7S IgM). This monomer IgM contains two heavy chains and two light chains that are not linked to form the usual pentamer of IgM globulin (see Chapter 5), and it does not possess the viscosity properties of the pentamer.

If the monoclonal IgM has antibody activity, it may produce further symptoms by virtue of this property. Many cases are known in which monoclonal IgM protein is produced with an antibody specificity directed against the I antigen of the red blood cell. This results in a chronic hemolytic anemia and is called high-titer cold agglutinin syndrome. Another antibody activity that has been found for some IgM globulins is that against IgG globulin, in which circulating antigen-antibody complexes occur and arthritis and glomerular lesions ensue. Such macroglobulins usually are cryoglobulins as well, and produce problems of local blood flow.

TREATMENT

The management of macroglobulinemia involves treatment of the cellular proliferation and treatment of the effects produced by the protein. Alkylating agents, particularly chlorambucil, have been useful in keeping the mass of lymphocytes reduced and the level of macroglobulin low. In the patient population we have treated, intermittent high-dose phenylalanine mustard and prednisone treatment for approximately one year has led to a substantial number of long-term stable remissions. In the acute treatment of the hyperviscosity syndrome, however, more immediate measures are necessary to remove the protein. In such instances, plasmapheresis (removal of whole blood with reinfusion of cells) using manual techniques or a cell separator may be lifesaving.

Heavy-Chain Disease

In 1965, a different kind of proliferative disorder of immunoglobulins was described by Franklin. The cardinal feature of this disorder was the elaboration of a monoclonal protein of relatively low molecular weight that was present in both serum and urine. By immunologic analysis, it was seen that the protein possessed the antigenic determinants of IgG but lacked light-chain antigenic determinants. Chemical analysis (amino acid composition, peptide mapping, carbohydrate content) indicated that the protein was very similar to the Fc fragment of IgG that is produced by partial hydrolysis with papain (Chapter 5), and the disorder was termed heavy-chain disease. Amino acid sequence analysis of heavy-chain disease proteins demonstrated that the sequence of the heavy chains began with a normal amino terminal sequence, followed by an extensive deletion of most of the Fd fragment, and resumption of the normal sequence at position 216 in the hinge region. The extent of the deletion has varied, but the place where the normal sequence is resumed appears rather constant.

The size of the protein (approximately 55,000 daltons) is somewhat greater than that of Bence Jones protein and accounts for the fact that appreciable concentrations of the protein have often been found in both serum and urine of affected patients. Since the same protein occurs in serum and in urine, the presence of a homogeneous protein of beta-globulin mobility in these body fluids should alert the clinician to the possibility of heavy-chain disease. The diagnosis of gamma heavy-chain disease rests upon the demonstration of a protein with the antigenic characteristics of IgG and no light-chain component.

To date, approximately 30 cases of this disorder have been recognized, and the common features (in addition to the protein elaborated) have been repeated bacterial infections, enlargement of the lymphoid organs, anemia, eosinophilia, and edema of the palate, secondary to involvement of Waldeyer's ring, the lymphoid tissue of the pharnx. A varied pathologic picture has been present, with histologic features of lymphoma ranging from Hodgkin's disease to diffuse histiocytic lymphoma. Bone marrow examination has shown mixtures of lymphocytes and plasma cells.

The most frequent cause of death has been infection, a direct consequence of the profound impairment of antibody production that appears to be an integral part of the disorder.

Heavy-chain disease of the IgA system has quite predictably involved the gastrointestinal tract and the respiratory tree. Most of the cases of alpha-chain disease have occurred in association with intestinal lymphoma in patients living in the Mediterranean area. Cases outside that area have been recorded, and at least two instances of alpha heavy-chain disease have occurred in persons with lymphoma of the respiratory tract. The abnormal protein in alpha chain disease has not been characterized as extensively as the gamma heavy-chain disease proteins, but, in general, the protein is not detected in the urine. It has a tendency to polymerize and has a rapid and polydisperse electrophoretic mobility, usually in the $alpha_2$ globulin region.

IgM heavy-chain disease is quite rare and has occurred in patients with the unusual clinical picture of chronic lymphocytic leukemia and osteolytic bone disease. Unlike the other heavy-chain diseases, free light chain has been produced as well as the heavy chain, and indeed both chains arise in the same cell —plasma cells with large vacuoles. Obviously, there is a failure of heavy- and light-chain link-up, and a defect in the hinge region has been postulated.

Although IgD and IgE heavy-chain diseases should be expected to occur, to date no cases have been observed. This is in keeping with the relative rarity of myelomas of these classes.

A few instances of other "defective" molecules have been observed in the malignant immunoproliferative disorders. Half molecules (one heavy, one light chain) of IgG and IgA have been described, and in at least one case of "IgA/2" a deletion of the carboxyl-terminal domain has been observed. Similar deletions of the carboxyl-terminal domain have occurred in the IgM class.

As more unusual monoclonal proteins have been scrutinized, more and more "defective" molecules have been identified. Whether these molecules have "normal" counterparts has not been clearly established.

Cryoglobulinemia

A striking property of some monoclonal immunoglobulins is a markedly reduced solubility at temperatures lower than normal core body temperature. When the insolubility is of such a degree that aggregation or precipitation may take place within the vascular space, severe impairment of normal physiologic processes may result. The term "cryoglobulin" is applied to those immunoglobulins that are very insoluble in the cold. The clinical condition that results from their presence is termed cryoglobulinemia.

The symptomatology of cryoglobulinemia is directly related to the abnormal protein. Blood with high concentrations of cryoglobulin will encounter severe restrictions in flow through those portions of the skin where exposure to cold is high. The regions chiefly affected are the digits, shins, nose, and ears. Vasculitis, painful ischemia of these areas, even infarction of the tissues, may result from prolonged cold exposure; ulceration and purpura of the extremities can also occur.

At least three different mechanisms have been found to account for the protein abnormalities in monoclonal cryoglobulinemia.

Monoclonal proteins with an antibody specificity directed against IgG may cause cryoprecipitation of serum. These are commonly of the IgM class, but IgG and IgA monoclonal antibodies have been observed. A second mechanism, which is represented in Figure 21–7, is spontaneous crystallization of the monoclonal protein in the cold. We have observed an additional mechanism in two patients in whom monoclonal IgG proteins possessed antibody activity against human albumin, and the IgG-albumin complex underwent crystallization.

Not all kinds of cryoglobulinemia are associated with monoclonal proteins. In some instances, antibodies of a polyclonal nature can combine with a circulating antigen and produce a cold precipitable complex.

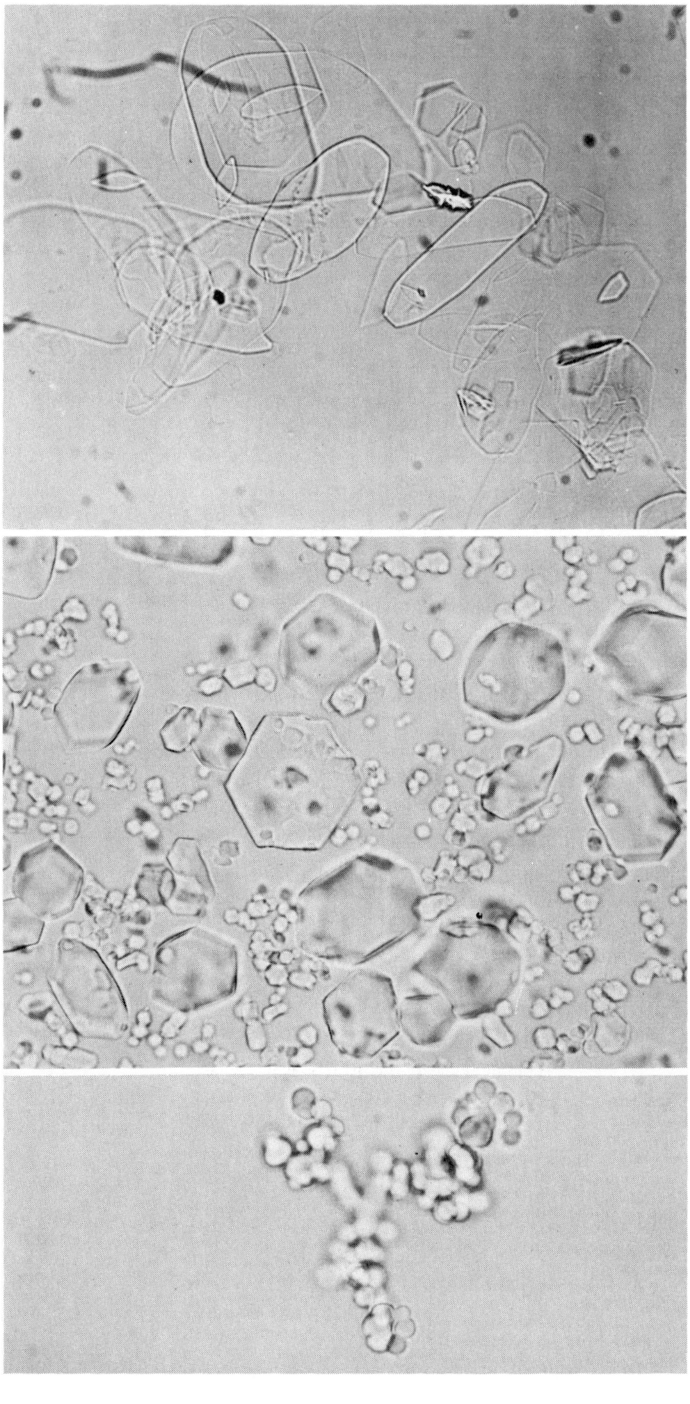

Figure 21–7. Photomicrographs of crystalline cryoglobulins (magnified ×250) from three patients with cryoglobulinemia. In each case, the protein is an IgG globulin with κ-type light chains. The protein at the bottom forms amorphous crystals, whereas the other two specimens have more definite structure.

Pyroglobulinemia

As the name implies, pyroglobulins are proteins sensitive to heat. They are monoclonal serum immunoglobulins that are precipitated when the serum is heated to 56°C. Often the phenomenon is explained by the presence of significant amounts of Bence Jones protein in the serum. Since free light chains precipitate at 56°C, they may confer this property. At the present state of our knowledge, this heat precipitability imparts no functional or pathologic significance to the protein but is merely a laboratory curio.

Amyloidosis

One way in which products of the plasma cell tumor may affect the patient is seen in the disorder called primary amyloidosis. Amyloid is a proteinaceous substance that is deposited in tissues and exhibits birefringence when stained with dyes such as Congo red. The so-called secondary form of the disease occurs in patients with chronic infectious processes such as tuberculosis and leprosy and affects chiefly liver, spleen, and kidneys. In primary amyloidosis, infiltration of organs such as skin, skeletal muscle, tongue, and heart causes severe compromise of these organs. This disorder is usually associated with the presence of monoclonal immunoglobulin (particularly free light chains). Elegant studies by Glenner and associates have shown a causal link between immunoglobulin and amyloidosis. They have demonstrated that free monoclonal immunoglobulin light chains from patients with amyloidosis can be cleaved by proteases or heat into variable and constant halves, and that the variable halves will undergo polymerization into amyloid substance. Hence, the protein by-product of plasma cell proliferation can and does cause problems by itself.

Benign Monoclonal Gammopathy

As serum protein electrophoresis has become an extremely common procedure in clinical laboratories, an increasing number of individuals have been found to have serum monoclonal immunoglobulins but none of the other stigmata of multiple myeloma. Although this condition is termed benign monoclonal gammopathy, the true nature of the condition is not known. Some of these patients have been observed for at least 20 years without detectable change occuring in their clinical condition. In some instances, patients have died of unrelated causes, and at post mortem examination, no evidence of myeloma has been found in the tissues. On the other hand, occasional patients have developed classic pictures of multiple myeloma as long as 18 years after detection of the monoclonal immunoglobulin. More extensive follow-up of affected patients will be necessary before one can fully evaluate this entity, but it is likely that the vast majority of patients diagnosed as having benign monoclonal gammopathy do not develop myeloma. Clearly, the "benign" designation refers to the cellular base of the condition, since the patient might have severe problems if the protein were cold precipitable (a cryoglobulin) or were "amyloidogenic."

Criteria used to distinguish benign from malignant monoclonal gammopathies include amount of monoclonal protein, degree of plasmacytosis, presence or absence of asynchronous plasma cell maturation, bone involvement, degree of anemia, and presence of Bence Jones proteinuria.

The Problems of Diagnosis of Myeloma

When the full spectrum of abnormalities associated with multiple myeloma is present, the diagnosis and the need for the treatment are evident. A problem on both counts is presented by the patient with minimal evidence of multiple myeloma, since chemotherapy has been neither curative nor uniformly successful and has its own hazards. The difficulty can be illustrated by the three following case histories.

Case 1. A 49-year-old man presented with cough, fever, and signs of right upper lobe pneumonia. The etiologic organism was identified as pneumococcus, and the patient improved after treatment with penicillin. He had a history of low back pain and generalized fatigue for the past six months. The hematocrit (28 per cent) and the white blood count (3700) were low, the blood calcium and urea nitrogen were elevated, and the serum phosphorus and alkaline phosphatase were normal. The urine showed 3′ protein, and free κ-chains were present. Total protein was 9 gm per 100 ml. Electrophoresis and immunoelectrophoresis of the serum showed a monoclonal IgG to be present at a concentration of 6 gm per 100 ml. X-rays showed a right upper lobe infiltrate, collapse of the lumbar spine, and multiple osteolytic lesions of skull and long bones. Bone marrow aspirate revealed sheets of plasma cells.

Case 2. A 60-year-old woman was seen by her physician for mild low back pain. X-rays showed moderate diffuse osteoporosis but no other abnormality. The hematocrit was slightly reduced (34 per cent). Total serum protein was 7.8 gm per 100 ml, and a monoclonal IgA was present (concentration 1.5 gm per 100 ml). Other blood and urine studies were normal. Bone marrow aspirate showed 7 per cent plasma cells.

Case 3. An asymptomatic 52-year-old man was discovered to have a monoclonal gammopathy during the laboratory portion of a routine physical examination. The M-component was determined to be an IgG (concentration 0.6 gm per 100 ml). X-rays, blood counts, blood chemistries, bone marrow examinations, and urine examinations were all within normal limits.

The first of the three patients presented with a great many symptoms and signs of multiple myeloma. He was severely ill and in need of treatment. The third patient was asymptomatic, and his disorder generally fit the criteria of benign monoclonal gammopathy. Few physicians would elect to do anything other than follow the patient.

The second case illustrates the problems associated with diagnosis and indication for therapy. A diversity of opinion would be encountered regarding which label ("multiple myeloma," "smoldering myeloma," or "benign monoclonal gammopathy") should be applied to this case at this time and whether chemotherapeutic measures should be begun. Until such time as uniformly successful therapy is available, such cases will probably remain a subject for disagreement and a problem for the physician involved in their care.

Etiology

As is the case with most forms of neoplasia, the cause of the malignant monoclonal gammopathies remains obscure, but several etiologic theories have been advanced. Separate lines of experimentation have suggested an environmental cause. In some instances, virus-like particles have been observed in myeloma cells and this has fostered a viral theory of the disease. An inbred strain of mice (Balb C) has been found to form plasmacytomas with paraprotein production in response to immunization with oil adjuvants. Such tumors are transplantable to other mice within the strain. Other species, including dogs and horses, less commonly and less constantly have been noted to develop monoclonal gammopathy. Of particular interest are monoclonal antibodies to streptococcal antigens arising in rabbits immunized with these proteins.

An ever-growing number of human monoclonal immunoglobulins have been found to possess antibody specificities against antigens ranging from such simple chemicals as dinitrophenol to such complex antigens as human lipoproteins. It is likely, therefore, that all human monoclonal immunoglobulins represent antibodies formed in response to antigenic stimulation and that the control of cellular proliferation is the major defect. Since monoclonal gammopathy is not an absolute requirement for myeloma (approximately 0.5 per cent of myeloma patients lack a monoclonal immunoglobulin), it is difficult to assign to it a central role in the pathogenesis of multiple myeloma.

Cellular Basis of Disease

The elegant studies of Salmon and coworkers have provided an example of how the basic information of immunology can be applied to an understanding of a human disease. They showed that very accurate estimates of tumor cell mass may be made in myeloma patients by measuring (1) the *in vitro* rate of synthesis of immunoglobulin per cultured myeloma cell; (2) the rate of catabolism of myeloma globulin *in vivo*; and (3) the total body mass of myeloma globulin. If the rate of catabolism of the myeloma protein and the rate at which cells produce myeloma globulin are known, the number of cells present in the patient may be calculated. Sequential measurements of the cell mass in myeloma patients have been used to provide objective estimates of rate of tumor growth and response to chemotherapeutic agents. As a derivative of these observations, an approximation of the tumor burden may be made by factoring in such variables as degree of anemia, presence of lytic lesions, and amount of myeloma protein. This approach has been useful in staging myeloma patients in chemotherapy trials.

POLYCLONAL GAMMOPATHY

In contrast to the relatively few disorders characterized by homogeneous increases in immunoglobulins, many diseases of man are associated with heterogeneous increases of immunoglobulins. Such disorders are termed polyclonal gammopathies, a term that implies that multiple cell lines are involved in the immunoglobulin increase. In most instances, increases occur in the three major classes of immunoglobulins and in both kinds of light chains. The disorders that are frequently associated with polyclonal gammopathies include inflammatory, infectious, and neoplastic diseases. Chief among these are rheumatoid arthritis, lupus erythematosus, cirrhosis of the liver, tuberculosis, leishmaniasis, and metastatic carcinoma. Lymphomas of the T-helper cell variety may induce polyclonal B-cell proliferation and hypergammaglobulinemia. A recently recognized pseudoneoplastic process, immunoblastic lymphadenopathy, is also associated with striking polyclonal increase in immunoglobulins. Although it is possible to demonstrate increases in the immunoglobulins in such diseases, it is impossible to identify an antibody role for a major percentage of the increase. For instance, many antibodies directed against normal tissue or serum antigens are found in lupus erythematosus, but these antibodies constitute only a small percentage of the immunoglobulin increase. In at least one instance (the original case of heavy-chain disease), transition from a polyclonal gammopathy to a monoclonal gammopathy has been observed.

Suggestions for Further Reading

Barlogie, B., Smith, L., and Alexanian, R.: Effective treatment of advanced multiple myeloma refractory to alkylating agents. N. Engl. J. Med., *310*(2):1353, 1984.

Durie, B. G. M., and Solmon, S. E.: A clinical staging system for multiple myeloma. Cancer, *36*:842, 1975.

Frangione, B., and Franklin, E. G.: Heavy-chain diseases: Clinical features and molecular significance of the disordered immunoglobulin structure. Semin. Hematol., *10*:53, 1973.

Glenner, G. G.: Amyloid deposits and amyloidosis. N. Engl. J. Med., *302*:1283, 1333, 1980.

Graham, R. C., Jr., and Bernier, G. M.: The bone marrow in multiple myeloma: Correlation of plasma cell ultrastructure and clinical state. Medicine, *54*:225, 1975.

Kyle, R. A.: Monoclonal gammopathy of undetermined significance: Natural history in 241 cases. Am. J. Med., *64*:814, 1978.

McIntyre, O. R.: Multiple myeloma. N. Engl. J. Med., *301*:193, 1979.

B. Lymphomas and Leukemias

Jeffrey Cossman, M.D.

Lymphomas and leukemias are malignant proliferations of cells whose normal counterparts are the cellular components of the immune system. Collectively, they are relatively frequent (50,000 new cases annually in the United States) and afflict persons of all ages. Although always fatal if untreated, they are nonetheless clinically heterogeneous and include a broad spectrum of disease, ranging from among the slowest to the most rapidly proliferative of all human cancers. Remarkable progress in the therapy of these disorders has been seen during the past 20 years. Now properly applied combinations of chemotherapy and radiation therapy result in eradication of disease and long-term survival in many lymphomas and leukemias, including Hodgkin's disease, acute lymphoblastic leukemia (ALL), Burkitt's lymphoma, and large cell lymphoma. Paradoxically, these disorders, particularly the latter three, are considered clinically "high-grade," for without therapy they quickly kill the patient. Indeed, Burkitt's lymphoma cells are the most rapidly dividing of all human cancers and double every 24 hours *in vitro*. At present, the non-Hodgkin's lymphomas and lymphocytic leukemias that are most amenable to elimination by therapy are naturally rapidly dividing. Because DNA synthesis assumes such a major role in their life span, these cells are more sensitive to toxic drugs or radiation that interrupt cell division. Other less proliferative processes such as follicular lymphoma, chronic lymphocytic leukemia, and hairy cell leukemia can be only partially controlled by chemotherapy. These are slow-growing accumulations of lymphocytes that gradually collect over many years in the bone marrow, liver, and other sites and are almost never eradicated by chemotherapy.

By definition, leukemias arise from stem cells in the bone marrow and are usually blood-borne, whereas lymphomas grow as isolated tumorous masses, often in lymph nodes and other lymphatic tissues. In certain situations the distinction is arbitrary, since leukemia cells can collect as masses in tissue and lymphomas can circulate in the blood. Traditionally, they have been subdivided on the basis of morphologic appearance into categories with the intent of predicting prognosis to allow selection of appropriate therapy. Lymphomas are subdivided into two main categories: Hodgkin's disease and non-Hodgkin's lymphomas. Leukemias are classified by their resemblance to normal cells: granulocytic, lymphocytic, erythroid, and so forth. Nearly all non-Hodgkin's lymphomas are neoplasms of lymphocytes, while the cell of origin of Hodgkin's disease is not yet known.

Techniques for the identification and characterization of the normal cellular elements of the immune system can be similarly applied to lymphomas and leukemias. Armed with this technology we now can precisely define, in nearly every case, the normal cell counterpart and classify the disorders according to cell type and presumed cell of origin. Cell types are distinguished from one another by the presence of intracellular, surface membrane–bound, and secreted products specifically made by only one cell type. A notable example of such a cell-derived product is immunoglobulin, the hallmark of B-cells. Detection methods for these products must be both sensitive and specific. Most useful here is a large battery of available antibodies raised in animals, which bind to antigenic determinants of cell-associated molecules and are visualized by fluorescence or other staining methods. For example monoclonal antibodies (hybridoma-derived) raised against human leukocytes can not only distinguish T-cells from B-cells but can also be used to identify functional subsets, such as helper or suppressor T-cells (Chapters 5 and 7). Furthermore, several antibodies (including T1, T6, B1, BA-1, and many others) have allowed for the identification of previously unrecognized cellular molecules (usually proteins) whose expression appears to be developmentally regulated. Although the exact function of these molecules is not yet known, their expression provides a phenotypic "fingerprint" of a cell and indicates its relative degree of differentiation or maturation.

Additional insight into the differentiation of B-lymphocytes has been attained through analysis of the configuration of their immunoglobulin genes (Fig. 21–8). During the early differentiation of the B-cell, structural genetic rearrangements occur that bring together previously separated DNA coding regions of the genes for the variable (V), diversity (D), and joining (J) regions of immunoglobulin heavy chains and V and J regions of light chains. Diversity of antibody specificity is generated by this mechanism, since a very great number of combinations is possible. By molecular analysis of the immunoglobulin genes, the genetic reorganizations that have taken place can be identified in both normal and neoplastic B-cell populations.

When one turns to the malignant lymphomas and leukemias, it is clear that these tumors more than just resemble normal cells. Most remarkably, the neoplastic cells express a phenotype that relates them to a level of differentiation beyond which they apparently cannot mature. Presumably a progenitor cell proliferates as a single clone, and the daugh-

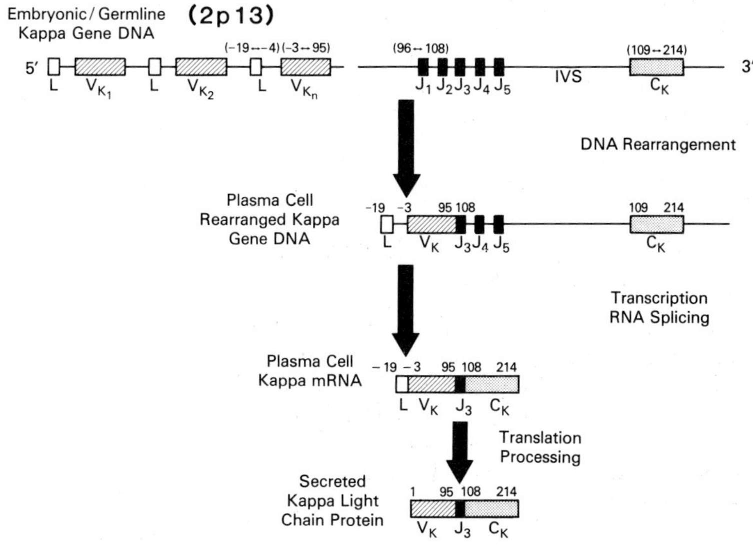

Figure 21–8. Diagram of the configurations of the immunoglobulin kappa chain gene. During the early stages of differentiation of a B-cell and prior to the onset of immunoglobulin synthesis, portions of the DNA are excised and only one of many variable (V_κ) region genes is annealed to one of five joining (J) genes to produce a rearranged immunoglobulin gene. The remaining noncoding regions, or intervening sequences (IVS), are excised from the transcribed mRNA to bring the V, J, and constant (C) regions together. Finally, an immunoglobulin kappa chain having a potentially unique variable region is synthesized. (From Korsmeyer, S. J., and Waldman, T. A.: Immunoglobulins II: Gene Organization and Assembly. *In* Stites, D. P., et al. (eds.): Basic and Clinical Immunology. 4th ed. Los Altos, Lange Medical Publications, 1982.

ter cells accumulate at a "frozen" stage of differentiation. As an example, in multiple myeloma (plasma cell malignancy) Dr. Max Cooper and associates have identified pre-B cells in the bone marrow that share an idiotypic determinant with the neoplastic plasma cells that compose the bulk of the tumor. The pre-B cells may be the proliferative cells giving rise to differentiated progeny that accumulate at the terminal or plasma cell stage of B-differentiation.

The relative stage of differentiation achieved by the malignant cells can determine whether the cell will carry out normal functions. For example, terminal differentiation status could result in immunoglobulin secretion by a B-cell neoplasm (e.g., multiple myeloma) or helper function and polyclonal gammopathy in a T-cell neoplasm (e.g., Sézary's syndrome). As we shall see, early and intermediate levels of normal lymphocyte differentiation are also represented by various lymphocytic (non-Hodgkin's) lymphomas and leukemias, so that for most known stages of leukocyte differentiation a corresponding malignancy has been identified.

B-CELL NEOPLASMS

The majority of non-Hodgkin's lymphomas and lymphocytic leukemias are derived from B-cells. This broad array of clinical disorders covers an extraordinary range of differentiation and proliferative capacity. Because of the advances in the phenotypic and genotypic characterization of B-cells the list of B-cell malignant neoplasms is now virtually complete. We have only recently learned that the majority of "histiocytic" lymphoma (large cell lymphoma or reticulum cell sarcoma), hairy cell leukemia, and common, acute lymphoblastic ("non-T, non-B") leukemia are monoclonal B-cell proliferations.

Early B-Cell Differentiation

COMMON, ACUTE LYMPHOBLASTIC LEUKEMIA

The most frequent malignant disorder in children is acute lymphoblastic leukemia (ALL). It is a rapidly progressive accumulation of primitive lymphoid cells in the bone marrow and peripheral blood that can eventually spread to the gonads and central nervous system. If not treated properly, ALL kills the patient by replacement of normal hematopoietic elements in the marrow, resulting in hemorrhage from thrombocytopenia (decreased platelets) or infection from leukopenia (decreased white blood cells). Improvements in combination chemotherapy have led to a dramatic increase in the number of patients (60 to 80 per cent) who are rid of their disease and apparently cured. Since the mid-1970's it has been known that approximately 20 per cent of these cases were derived from T-cells (Table 21–3). However, the cell lineage of the remaining 80 per cent of cases (common ALL) was not known. Although lymphocytic by morphology, the cells of common ALL expressed no surface membrane determinants that would mark them as either T- or B-cells. They were noted to bear Ia (HLA-DR) antigens, the "common, acute lymphoblastic leukemia antigen" (CALLA) and intranuclear terminal deoxynucleotidyl transferase (TdT). This latter enzyme is a maker of early T- and B-cell differentiation and may serve a function in gene reorganization. Common ALL was phenotypically neither T- nor B-cell. Subsequently, careful immunofluorescence studies carried out by Vogler and his colleagues indicated a scant amount of immunoglobulin μ heavy chain in the cytoplasm of 20 per cent of common ALL cases. Since normal primitive or pre-B cells also contained intracytoplasmic immunoglobulin, it was concluded that a subset of common ALL was B-cell–derived and could be related to the pre–B cell stage of B-cell differentiation (Table 21–3). The derivation of the remaining 60 per cent of common ALL continued to be a mystery until the production of human immunoglobulin gene probes and molecular analysis of DNA from the leukemia cells. Using cloned segments of human immunoglobulin DNA derived in the laboratory of Dr. Phillip Leder, Dr. Stanley Korsmeyer found that cells from all cases of common ALL had rearranged immunoglobulin genes, indicating their B-cell lineage (Fig. 21–9). Furthermore, the identical immunoglobulin gene reorganization was detected among all cells within each given case, thus demonstrating that each leukemia was monoclonal, i.e., derived from a single stem cell. So even though the majority of common ALL cells lack detectable immunoglobulin protein, they are bona fide B-cells and represent the very earliest stages of B-cell differentiation (Fig. 21–10). These events were discussed in Chapter 2 (Fig. 2–26).

Table 21–3. Lymphoblastic Malignancy: Distribution of Immunologic Phenotype and Predominant Cell Markers of Acute Lymphoblastic Leukemia (ALL) and Lymphoblastic Lymphoma (LBL)

Immunotype	% of ALL	% of LBL	E	cIg	Ia	CALLA	TdT
T	20	80	+	−	−	−	+
Pre-B	20	10	−	+	+	+	+
"Non-T, Non-B" (common ALL)	60	10	−	−	+	+	+

E: Sheep erythrocyte rosette formation. cIg: Intracytoplasmic immunoglobulin (usually μ heavy chain). Ia: HLA-DR. CALLA: Common ALL antigen. TdT: Terminal deoxynucleotidyl transferase activity.

Although "frozen" at this early stage *in vivo,* common ALL cells retain the capacity for further differentiation under appropriate conditions *in vitro.* In our laboratory we found that common ALL cells that were genetically committed to B-cell differentiation could be induced by a tumor promoter, tetra-decanoyl-phorbol-acetate (TPA), to synthesize cytoplasmic and surface immunoglobulin corresponding to the heavy and light chain predicted by the already rearranged immunoglobulin genes (Fig. 21–9). The mechanisms by which these cells were restrained from differentiation *in vivo* are not known but may well be associated with the cause of the leukemia.

Intermediate B-Cell Differentiation

BURKITT'S LYMPHOMA

Burkitt's lymphoma was first identified in central Africa, where it is endemic and often occurs as facial masses among children aged 2 to 12 years. In nonendemic areas, such as North America and Europe, the disease is less common, affects a slightly older age group, and usually presents itself as an abdominal mass growing in the wall of the intestine or in the ovaries. Soon after its identification it became evident that Burkitt's lymphoma was exquisitely sensitive to che-

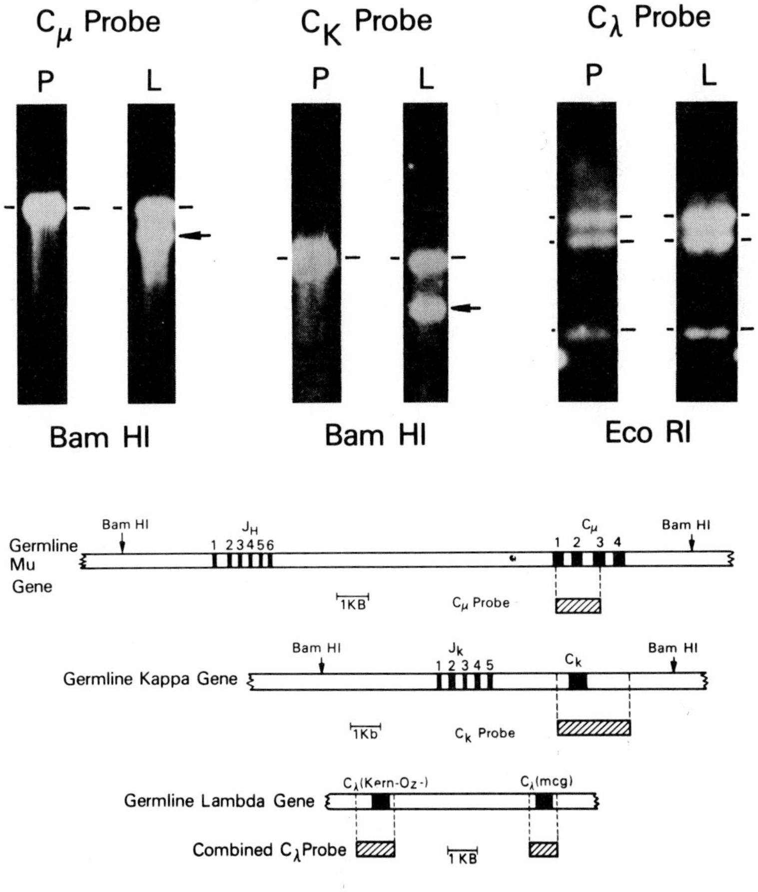

Figure 21–9. Immunoglobulin gene rearrangement in common ALL detected by Southern blot analysis. To determine if immunoglobulin gene rearrangement had occurred, DNA was extracted from leukemia lymphocytes (L) and compared with germline DNA from placenta (P). DNA was digested with the restriction endonucleases BamH1 or EcoR1. The DNA fragments were electrophoresed through a gel, blotted onto filter paper, and hybridized with cloned, radiolabeled DNA probes to the constant regions of human μ (C_μ), κ (C_κ), and λ (C_λ) genes (hatched boxes, below). Arrows indicate rearranged alleles for C_μ and C_κ. Fragments hybridized with C_λ are all germline (placental configuration, dash marks) and therefore are not rearranged. Cells from this case of common (precursor B-cell) ALL did not synthesize immunoglobulin *in vivo* but, when stimulated with the phorbol ester TPA, *in vitro* produced both cytoplasmic and surface IgMK. (From Cossman, J., Neckers, L. M., Arnold, A., et al.: Induction of differentiation in a case of common acute lymphoblastic leukemia. N. Engl. J. Med., *307*:1251, 1982.)

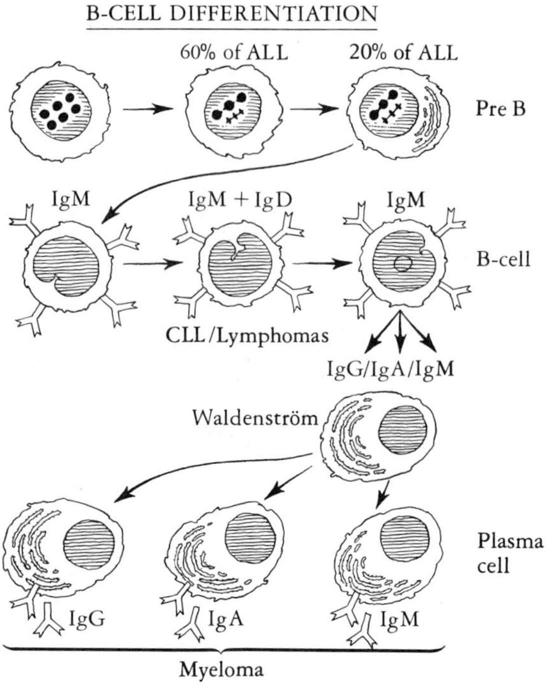

Figure 21–10. B-cell differentiation—position of B-cell neoplasms. In the pre–B cell stage, the immunoglobulin genes rearrange (shown as compressed blocks within the nucleus) and subsequently scant intracytoplasmic μ immunoglobulin (shown as cytoplasmic dots) is synthesized. Most cases of ALL resemble early B-cells during these early stages. Most B non-Hodgkin's lymphomas and leukemias resemble the intermediate stage, at which B cells attain a mature phenotype and express surface immunoglobulin. Immunoglobulin secretion is the hallmark of the plasma-cell stage, and the B-cell processes associated with a paraprotein correspond to this terminal differentiation stage.

motherapeutic agents that disrupt DNA and protein synthesis. Combination chemotherapy can now produce long-term disease-free remissions (probable cures) in more than 75 per cent of patients in the United States.

Tumor cells from African patients nearly always contain the Epstein-Barr virus (EBV), a DNA virus known to induce proliferation in normal B-cells and the clinical disorder infectious mononucleosis. Nonendemic Burkitt's lymphoma is rarely associated with EBV. In the African cases a cell surface receptor for EBV is found in close association with a receptor for the C3d fragment of complement, whereas neither receptor is detectable in most nonendemic cases. If EBV is an etiologic agent in African Burkitt's lymphoma, it may play a role in the initiation of proliferation.

Exciting new findings have focused considerable attention on the cause of Burkitt's lymphoma. In 1982 several investigators (including Drs. Carlo Croce and P. Leder) independently discovered a relationship between the immunologic phenotype and genetic abnormalities characteristic of Burkitt's lymphoma. The B-cell lineage of all cases of Burkitt's lymphoma was well established by immunofluorescence studies that showed the presence of surface membrane–bound immunoglobulin (sIg). Within an individual case the sIg was of a single heavy- and light-chain type, usually κ, indicating a single genetic clone. Also known from karyotyping (cytogenetic) studies were nonrandom chromosomal translocations. Most frequent was an exchange from the long arm of chromosome 8 (8q). This piece was usually translocated to the long arm of the fourteenth chromosome (8q−, 14q+) or, less commonly, to chromosomes 2 (8q+, 2p−) or 22 (8q−, 22q+). It was then discovered that the locations of the immunoglobulin genes were 14q for the heavy chains, 2p for κ light chain, and 22q for λ light chain. This latter observation becomes more intriguing because the cases of Burkitt's lymphoma that involved 2p expressed κ light chain sIg, whereas λ sIg occurred when the translocation was 8q−, 22q+. With the use of molecular probes, the identity of this fragment in 8q was shown to be c-myc, a normal cellular sequence of DNA that corresponds to the retrovirus (RNA tumor virus) v-myc, known to cause B-cell lymphomas in birds. The normal function of c-myc may occur during embryogenesis and early differentiation. When translocated to 14q in Burkitt's lymphoma, it inserts upstream from most of the immunoglobulin heavy-chain gene sequences and perhaps its gene expression is activated in this aberrant circumstance. These findings have shown us a glimpse of the complex events leading to the development of Burkitt's lymphoma. Perhaps these or similar mechanisms provide a proliferative advantage to cells and result in carcinogenesis of other cell types as well.

FOLLICULAR (NODULAR) LYMPHOMA

In contrast to common ALL and Burkitt's lymphoma, most B-cell neoplasms occur exclusively in adults. Follicular lymphomas are monoclonal B-cell proliferations that usually disseminate widely throughout lymph nodes, liver, spleen, and bone marrow. Patients can live for many years with follicular lymphoma but unfortunately stand little chance of eliminating the disease by therapy.

The nodular growth pattern of follicular lymphomas imparts a morphologic resemblance to physiologically hyperplastic (normal) germinal centers (B-cell zones) of normal lymph nodes. Biologic studies have corroborated this resemblance and reveal many features common to both normal germinal center cells and follicular lymphoma. Both are composed of B-lymphocytes with surface membrane complement and IgG-Fc receptors, abundant sIg (heavy and light chains), and scant cytoplasmic immunoglobulin. The essential immunologic difference is the pattern of immunoglobulin light-chain expression. The cells of a follicular lymphoma express a single immunoglobulin light-chain type (usually κ), in contrast to normal germinal centers, in which an admixture of κ- and λ-bearing cells are found. As in all B-cell malignancies, a monoclonal proliferation from an individual B-cell can, like a normal B-cell, make only one light-chain type. Indeed, the immunoglobulin protein molecule produced by a lymphoma is unique to that tumor because it contains a unique variable region or idiotype. If anti-idiotype antibody could be generated in the laboratory, it would be tumor-specific and useful for diagnosis of recurrence, radionuclide-tagged scans, and injection for immunotherapy. Dr. Ronald Levy and his colleagues have successfully treated a patient with follicular lymphoma using a murine monoclonal (hybridoma) anti-idiotype antibody. This approach may have general applicability in the therapy of otherwise incurable B-cell tumors.

Does the host respond to follicular lymphoma? Most lymph nodes involved by follicular lymphoma also contain many T-lymphocytes that appear normal by morphology and have a helper: suppressor ratio by phenotypic analysis (antibody staining) of approximately 4:1. Follicular lymphoma cells rarely secrete abundant immunoglobulin. This might be due to a host response in which suppressor T-cells limit the synthesis and secretion of immunoglobulin by the lymphoma cells. To date, this lack of immunoglobulin secretion remains unexplained.

WELL-DIFFERENTIATED LYMPHOCYTIC LYMPHOMA AND CHRONIC LYMPHOCYTIC LEUKEMIA

Two closely related B-cell disorders that occur in adults are the so-called well-differentiated lymphocytic lymphoma (WDL) and chronic lymphocytic leukemia (CLL). The leukemia cells themselves have little proliferative capacity, and prolonged survival without cure is the rule. The cells express sIg with a single light-chain type in a given case and bear complement receptors specific for C3d. In only 10 per cent of cases is immunoglobulin secreted into the serum at readily detectable levels. CLL cells can be induced by TPA to secrete immunoglobulin *in vitro*. Thus, these cells are capable of recapitulating terminal B-cell differentiation *in vitro* but are unable to do so in the patient. Processes that govern their differentiation *in vivo* may result in the massive accumulation of the clone at a preterminal differentiation stage. Clearly, elucidation of these mechanisms is an important focus of investigations in leukemogenesis.

A lymphoma similar to WDL is so-called intermediately differentiated lymphocytic lymphoma (IDL). The cells of this B-cell neoplasm, by immunologic analysis, appear to be "intermediate" between follicular lymphoma and WDL.

HAIRY CELL LEUKEMIA (LEUKEMIC RETICULOENDOTHELIOSIS)

The cell of origin of this slowly proliferative leukemia of adults remained controversial until recently, when it was definitively proved to be a B-cell process. Cells synthesize monoclonal immunoglobulin, express B-cell–associated antigens (e.g., B1), and have rearranged immunoglobulin heavy- and light-chain genes.

LARGE CELL LYMPHOMA ("HISTIOCYTIC" LYMPHOMA, "RETICULUM CELL SARCOMA")

It is now clear that greater than 95 per cent of these cases are lymphocytic neoplasms (approximately 55 per cent B-cell, 40 per cent T-cell, and <5 per cent true "histiocytes"). These rapidly growing tumors occur at all ages and are found in lymph nodes as well as in extranodal sites. Results with combination chemotherapy are encouraging, and disease can be eliminated in as many as 70 per cent of patients. Some cases arise from a pre-existing slowly proliferative B-cell neoplasm, such as follicular lymphoma or chronic lymphocytic leukemia (resulting in Richter's syndrome). When such conversion occurs, the malignant cells change morphology and divide more rapidly but continue to express the same sIg type. Perhaps an aberrant cell with enhanced proliferative potential springs from the clone. Alternatively, host mechanisms that previously governed proliferation and/or differentiation of the entire cell population may be interrupted.

Late B-Cell Differentiation

MULTIPLE MYELOMA, WALDENSTRÖM'S MACROGLOBULINEMIA

B-cell neoplasms of terminal differentiation are characterized by an extracellular monoclonal immunoglobulin in the serum and/or urine (see Chapter 21A). Although immunoglobulin secretion occurs in other B-cell neoplasms, the quantity secreted rarely is sufficient for detection by routine clinical laboratory methods. The abundant immunoglobulin secretion in multiple myeloma or Waldenström's macroglobulinemia is indicative of a highly differentiated B-cell. Morphologically, the tumor cells resemble plasma cells and plasmacytoid lymphocytes and, like plasma cells, the cytoplasm is rich in immunoglobulin.

Interrelationships of B-Cell Neoplasms

We have seen malignant B-cell proliferations that cover a broad spectrum of clinical behavior, growth potential, and differentiation status. The one feature common to all these disease processes is their commitment to B-cell differentiation, at least at the gene level. In most there is resemblance to normal B-cells at specific differentiation stages, and, taken together, the classes of B-cell malignancy appear to sequentially recapitulate the normal B-cell differentiation pathway. The relationships among the various clonal B-cell disorders can be further appreciated by the capacity of some to transform to more aggressive, rapidly proliferative, or more differentiated types during the clinical course. Most compelling are the immunologic genotypes and phenotypes of the lymphomas diagrammed in Figure 21–10. Here the sequence of B-cell differentiation is divided into three successive stages: pre–B cell, B-cell, and plasma cell. Within each stage the corresponding lymphoma or leukemia is shown. The extremes of B-cell differentiation are clearly represented by "common" and pre-B ALL (pre-B stage) and Waldenström's macroglobulinemia and myeloma (plasma-cell stage). Less clear, however, are the positions of the neoplasms within the B-cell stage. Perhaps there is a hierarchy of differentiation of follicular lymphoma, IDL, and WDL/CLL. The expression of several B-cell–associated surface membrane antigens, namely sIg, B1, and BA-1, diminishes (fewer sites per cell) as normal B-cells mature into plasma cells. Similarly, these markers are less intensively expressed as one proceeds from follicular lymphoma to IDL to WDL/CLL (Fig. 21–11). The relative positions of the highly proliferative B-cell–stage neoplasms, Burkitt's lymphoma and large cell lymphoma, are not yet known. They may be the counterparts of rapidly dividing cells, such as immunoblasts, and some germinal center cells that are activated by antigens to proliferate prior to plasma cell differentiation.

T-CELL NEOPLASMS

Malignant T-cell processes occur at all ages and represent a spectrum of leukemias and lymphomas.

Early T-Cell Differentiation

T-CELL ACUTE LYMPHOBLASTIC LEUKEMIA AND LYMPHOBLASTIC LYMPHOMA

Approximately 20 per cent of the predominant leukemia of children, ALL, and 30 per cent of all childhood non-Hodgkin's lymphomas are proliferations of primitive T-lymphocytes (Table 21–3). The leukemic and lymphomatous forms of primitive T-cell malignancy are closely related and are probably different manifestations of the same entity. Most frequently they are seen in adolescents, who often have thymic masses. If there is bone marrow infiltration and an elevated white blood count, it is referred to as ALL. Alternatively, if the lymph nodes are involved and the marrow and blood are involved only to a small extent, the disease is termed lymphoblastic lymphoma. These diseases are rapidly progressive and must be treated with multiple chemotherapeutic agents to attain remission.

Like virtually all normal T-cells, these malignant cells express an antigen identified by monoclonal antibody 3A1 and bind sheep erythrocytes (E-rosettes) through a cell sur-

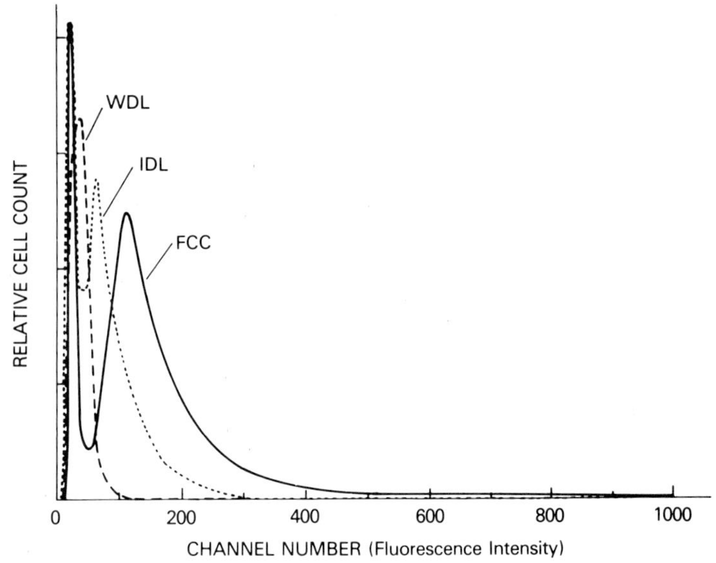

Figure 21–11. Fluorescence-activated cell sorter (FACS) analysis of B-cell lymphoma surface immunoglobulin. Lymphoma cells were stained with fluorescein-tagged anti-human immunoglobulin antibodies and analyzed by the FACS. Histograms of cell number versus fluorescence intensity show an increase from well-differentiated lymphocytic lymphoma (WDL), intermediately differentiated lymphocytic lymphoma (IDL), and follicular center-cell lymphoma (FCC). Surface immunoglobulin densities may indicate distinct maturational stages achieved by the lymphoma cells. (From Cossman, J., Neckers, S. M., Hsu, S. M., et al.: Low grade lymphomas: Expression of developmentally regulated B cell antigens. Am. J. Pathol., *115*:117, 1984.)

face receptor (whose normal function is unknown). The malignant cells uniformly contain intranuclear TdT, thus indicating their early lymphoid cell differentiation status. They bear cell surface markers usually seen on normal cortical thymocytes rather than mature T-cells from the peripheral blood or lymph nodes (Fig. 21–12). These markers, defined by murine monoclonal antibodies, are T6 and simultaneous expression of T4 (Leu 3) and T8 (Leu 2). These latter two antibodies react with two distinct populations of mature T-cells that usually have helper cell function (T4) or suppressor cell function (T8). Most normal cortical thymocytes and T-ALL cells express both antigens, lack T-

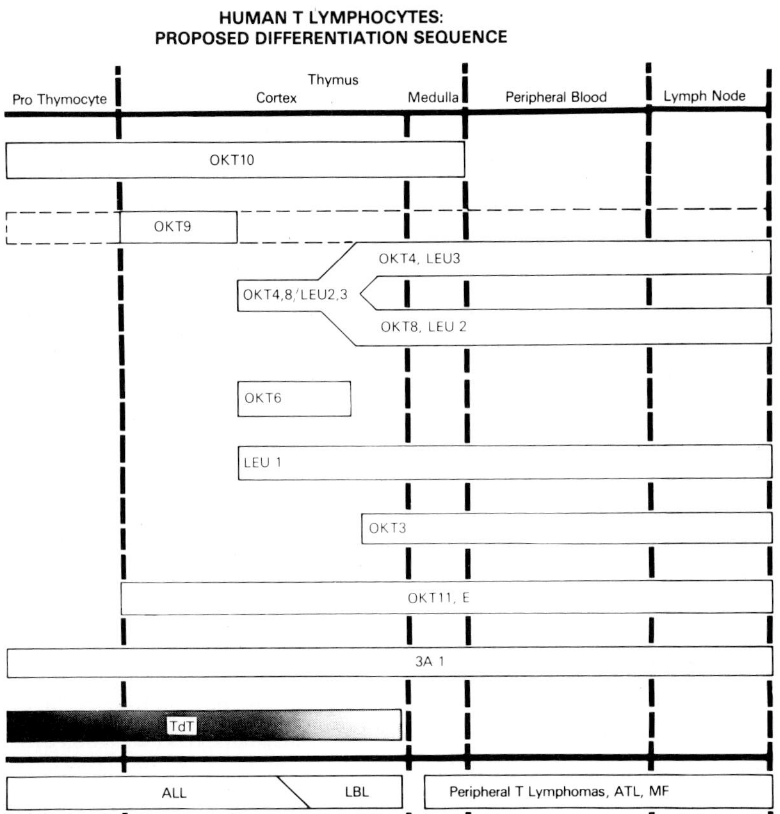

Figure 21–12. T-lymphocyte differentiation and position of T-cell neoplasms. With the use of various murine monoclonal antibodies, the stages of normal T-cell differentiation can be distinguished. The relationship of the T-cell malignancies is indicated in the bottom row. ALL: acute lymphoblastic leukemia; LBL: lymphoblastic lymphoma; ATL: adult T-cell leukemia; MF: mycosis fungoides. (From Cossman, J., Chused, T. M., Fisher, R. I., et al.: Diversity of immunological phenotypes of lymphoblastic lymphoma. Cancer Res., *43*: 4486, 1983.)

cell–associated functional activity, and are presumably precursors of the mature "helper" and "suppressor" T-cells but not yet committed to either arm. T-lymphoblastic lymphoma cases appear to be somewhat more mature than most T-ALL cases, since T4 and T8 are not simultaneously expressed. Like B-cell neoplasms, these malignancies may sometimes be capable of further differentiation *in vitro,* such as an instance of T-ALL that was induced to function as a suppressor cell only after activation in culture.

Mature T-Cell Differentiation

As a group, most mature T-cell malignancies resemble normal T-lymphocytes from blood and peripheral lymphoid tissue and may carry out some normal T-cell functions. Tumor cells lack TdT and T6 reactivity but express the T-cell–associated antigens detected by antibodies T3 (Leu 4), T4, T8, T11 (E-rosette receptor), and 3A1. Their position relative to T-cell differentiation, as determined by immunologic phenotype and functional studies, is shown in Figure 21–12. Chronic lymphocytic leukemia of T-cells, *T-CLL,* is a very rare accumulation of cells that may function *in vitro* in some cases as suppressor cells and in others as helper cells. *Mycosis fungoides* is a slowly growing lymphoma of T-cells that infiltrates the skin, particularly the epidermis. Occasionally the cells populate the blood, and this leukemic picture is then called *Sézary's syndrome.* Cells from most cases of mycosis fungoides and Sézary's syndrome that have been carefully studied have been shown to serve as helper cells and to express the antigen identified by T4. Indeed, the serum of some patients may contain elevated total immunoglobulin levels (polyclonal gammopathy) indicative of *in vivo* tumor cell helper function. Although their resemblance to normal helper T-cells is strong, these cutaneous T-cell lymphoma cells often do not express the cell surface determinant reactive with antibody 3A1.

Even excluding mycosis fungoides, approximately 40 per cent of clinically aggressive non-Hodgkin's lymphomas in adults are T-cell type. These are referred to as *peripheral T-cell lymphomas* in contrast to the central, or thymic, lymphoblastic lymphomas. The surface membrane phenotype usually corresponds to normal helper T-lymphocytes.

Recently, a retrovirus (RNA tumor virus) was isolated from the malignant cells in certain cases of mature T-cell lymphoma/leukemia. This virus, human T-cell leukemia virus (HTLV), was first characterized in the laboratory of Dr. Robert Gallo. By testing for serum antibody to virally coded proteins or direct identification of viral DNA in tumor cells, it has been shown that as many as 90 per cent of cases of so-called *adult T-cell leukemia/lymphoma (ATL)* in southern Japan are associated with infection by HTLV. Also, a small cluster of clinically similar HTLV-associated cases has been observed in native-born Caribbean Islanders. This is a clinically high-grade malignancy with only brief survival despite chemotherapy. The disease appears to be exceedingly rare outside these geographic areas, and despite intensive search, fewer than ten native-born North Americans have been found to have an HTLV-associated neoplasm. Integration of HTLV-coded DNA into the host's genome may require a genetic predisposition. Since retroviral infection can lead to lymphoid malignancy in animals, HTLV is a good candidate for an etiologic agent in this unusual T-cell process. Tumor cells from many of these cases bear receptors for T-cell growth factor (TCGF or interleukin-2) as identified by anti-TAC monoclonal antibody. Whether these cells, or any other malignant T-cells, require TCGF for maintenance of growth *in vivo* is not known. Most T-cell malignancies unassociated with HTLV lack the receptor and presumably proliferate efficiently without this particular growth factor. Paradoxically, functional assays of Japanese cases of HTLV-infected malignant T-cells have shown suppressor function despite a "helper" phenotype, T4+.

NEOPLASMS OF HISTIOCYTES

Histiocytes (macrophages or reticulum cells) are phagocytic cells residing in tissues and derived from monocytes. Before the advent of immunologic marker studies it was thought that many, if not most, aggressive lymphomas were derived from histiocytes—hence the names "histiocytic lymphoma" and "reticulum cell sarcoma." We now realize that more than 95 per cent of these tumors are actually derived from either B-lymphocytes (55 per cent) or T-lymphocytes (40 per cent). Accordingly, they are now called large cell lymphomas or peripheral T-cell lymphomas.

Less than 5 per cent of lymphomas with the morphologic classification of "large cell" have surface membrane and functional characteristics of histiocytes. Such cells lack markers of lymphocytes but stain with antibodies reactive with normal monocytes and macrophages. They also contain the same lysosomal enzyme activity of mononuclear phagocytes.

MYELOID LEUKEMIA

Acute and *chronic myelogenous leukemias* (AML and CML, respectively) are neoplasms of the granulocytes. Morphologically, immunologically, and functionally AML cells are the more primitive, whereas CML cells resemble maturing granulocytes. Clinically, AML is extremely aggressive and few patients survive, whereas patients can live many years with CML. In CML we have been provided with a model of hematopoietic differentiation. Here the leukemia cells, but not the patient's normal cells, display a specific nonrandom chromosomal abnormality; the Philadelphia chromosome, in which a fragment of chromosome 9, containing an oncogene, C-abl, is translocated to chromosome 22. Again, this "oncogene" is a component of the normal human genome but its function is unknown. This translocation apparently affords a proliferative advantage to a hematopoietic stem cell whose progeny differentiate along the myeloid series, where all maturation stages can be seen simultaneously. In about 25 per cent of cases a "blast crisis" ensues, in which an otherwise indolent clinical course is interrupted by a sudden outpouring of primitive "blast" cells, resulting in a picture of acute leukemia. In many instances the leukemia blast cells remain myeloid (AML), but 40 per cent of blast crises are lymphoid (ALL), and some are even erythroid (red cell precursor) or megakaryoblastic (platelet precursor). Although any arm of hematopoiesis can be produced, the leukemia cells retain the Philadelphia chromosome. Thus, an uncommitted hematopoietic stem cell can produce widely differing progeny and associated types of leukemia. Recently, it has been determined that cells from nearly all lymphoid blast crisis cases contain rearranged immunoglobulin genes and are therefore B-cells. These are primitive B-cells, however, since they usually do not make immunoglobulin protein but do contain intranuclear TdT.

HODGKIN'S DISEASE

Hodgkin's disease is a malignant process usually involving lymph nodes. A number of peculiarities distinguish Hodgkin's disease from the non-Hodgkin's lymphomas: (1) In most cases the bulk of the involved lymph node is composed of normal-appearing inflammatory cells such as lymphocytes, plasma cells, eosinophils, and histiocytes. The large cells characteristic of Hodgkin's disease (Reed-Sternberg cells and their variants), which are generally considered to be the malignant components, are in the minority. (2) The disease spreads by anatomic contiguity from one lymph node site to the next one adjacent. Radiotherapeutic strategies are based on this pattern of dissemination, and now the disease can be eliminated in most patients with radiotherapy or chemotherapy or both. (3) Cases have been observed in "clusters" within communities. Perhaps a transmissible agent plays a role in etiology. (4) The most common form grows in a nodular pattern, so that the involved lymph node contains multiple spheres of Hodgkin's disease that are separated by dense scarlike fibrous bands. This is called nodular sclerosing Hodgkin's disease. Unlike other lymphomas, it is more frequent in women than in men, usually striking women in their twenties. (5) In contrast to most of the disease processes covered in this chapter, the normal cell counterpart of the malignant cells of Hodgkin's disease is not known. (6) Hodgkin's disease patients frequently have functional abnormalities in their cell-mediated immune responses even after the disease has been eradicated by therapy.

It has been difficult to study the biology of Hodgkin's cells because the cells in tissue lack markers that might define their derivation. Only recently have long-term cultures of Hodgkin's cells been established. Preliminary studies suggest that these cells may be related to histiocyte-like antigen-presenting cells from lymph nodes. However, until more cell lines are obtained and common functional and phenotypic features are uncovered, the derivation of Hodgkin's cells will remain an enigma.

FUTURE DIRECTIONS

Because malignant lymphomas and leukemias so often mirror their normal cell counterparts they serve as monoclonal models for the study of differentiation and cell function. For example, the immunoglobulin genes were cloned from plasma cell neoplasms, which led to the discoveries that immunoglobulin gene rearrangements generate antibody diversity and that this must occur before normal B-cells can synthesize immunoglobulin. The lymphomas and leukemias serve as models of human oncogenesis, and great advances can now be made with regard to the cause of such malignancies as Burkitt's lymphoma and adult T-cell lymphoma/leukemia.

Despite great strides in the treatment of these disorders there is much room for progress. Passive immunotherapy with "tailor-made" anti-idiotypic antibodies may cure patients with low-grade B-cell lymphomas. As the tools of molecular biology become refined, perhaps a control of expression of endogenous oncogenes or retroviruses can be obtained. Novel approaches such as these offer great promise in the investigation of the cause and control of neoplasms of the immune system.

Suggestions for Further Reading

General

Magrath, I. T.: Lymphocyte differentiation: An essential basis for the comprehension of lymphoid neoplasia. J. Natl. Cancer Inst., *67*:501, 1981.

B-Cell Neoplasms

Klein, G.: Specific chromosomal translocation and the genesis of B cell derived tumors in mice and men. Cell, *32*:311, 1983.

Korsmeyer, S. J., Arnold, A., Bakhshi, A., et al.: Immunoglobulin gene rearrangement and cell surface antigen expression in acute lymphocytic leukemias of T cell and B cell precursor origins. J. Clin. Invest., *71*:301, 1983.

Lynch, R. G., Rohrer, J. W., Odermatt, B., et al.: Immunoregulation of murine myeloma cell growth and differentiation: A monoclonal model of B cell differentiation. Immunol. Rev., *48*:45, 1979.

Miller, R. A., Maloney, D. G., Warnker, R., et al.: Treatment of B cell lymphoma with monoclonal anti-idiotype antibody. N. Engl. J. Med., *306*:517, 1982.

Totterman, T. H., Nilsson, K., and Sundstrom, C.: Phorbol ester–induced differentiation of chronic lymphocytic leukemia cells. Nature, *288*:176, 1980.

T-Cell Neoplasms

Broder, S., Edelson, R. L., Lutzner, M. A., et al.: The Sézary syndrome: A malignant proliferation of helper T cells. J. Clin. Invest., *58*:1297, 1976.

Broder, S., Uchiyama, T., Muul, L., et al.: Activation of leukemic prosuppressor cells to become suppressor-effector cells: Influence of cooperating normal T cells. N. Engl. J. Med., *304*:1382, 1981.

Gallo, R. C., Kalyanaraman, V. S., Sarngadharan, M. G., et al.: Association of the human type C retrovirus with a subset of adult T-cell cancers. Cancer Res., *43*: 3892, 1983.

Greaves, M F., Delia, D., Sutherland, R., et al.: Expression of the OKT monoclonal antibody defined antigenic determinants in malignancy. Int. J. Immunopharmac., 3:283, 1981.

Reinherz, E. L., Kung, P. C., Goldstein, G. C., et al.: Discrete stages of human intrathymic differentiation: Analysis of normal thymocytes and leukemic lymphoblasts of T-cell lineage. Proc. Natl. Acad. Sci., *77*:1588, 1980.

Myeloid Neoplasms

Bakhshi, A., Minowada, A., Arnold, J., et al.: Lymphoid blast crises of chronic myelogenous leukemia represent B-cell precursor stages of development. N. Engl. J. Med., *309*:826, 1983.

Klein, A., Kessel, A. G. V., Grosveld, A., et al.: A cellular oncogene is translocated to the Philadelphia chromosome in chronic myelocytic leukemia. Nature, *300*:765, 1982.

Nowel, P. C., and Hungerford, D. A.: Chromosome studies on normal and leukemic leukocytes. J. Natl. Cancer Inst., *25*:85, 1960.

Hodgkin's Disease

Schwab, U., Stein, H., Gerdes, J., et al.: Production of a monoclonal antibody specific for Hodgkin's and Sternberg-Reed cells of Hodgkin's disease and a subset of normal lymphoid cells. Nature, *299*:65, 1982.

Chapter 22

Immune Deficiency Disorders

Joseph A. Church, M.D., and Robert J. Schlegel, M.D.

Immune deficiency disorders are the clinical sequelae of impaired function in one or more components of the immune system, including phagocytic cells, complement, B-lymphocytes, and T-lymphocytes. This basic class of human disease was first fully described in 1952 by Colonel Ogden Bruton of the U.S. Army Medical Corps. In studying the reasons why a young child hospitalized at the Walter Reed Army Hospital was suffering from repeated and life-threatening infections, he found that the child was unable to synthesize specific antibodies and, later, that the child's serum lacked gamma globulin. Further, the child's susceptibility to infection was reversed by immune serum globulin administration. Bruton's discoveries represented a fine example of clinical research and heralded the current explosive development of learning to be detailed in the remainder of this chapter.

CLINICAL SETTING

The clinician who would manage problems of immune deficiency bears a dual responsibility. First, there is the necessity of mastering a rapidly evolving technology and applying it to the treatment of patients in a safe and efficacious manner. Second, there is the need to consider the impact of a chronic, severe disease upon the patient's psychologic and social conditions. Affected individuals may incur depression, an undue dependence upon clinical facilities, and disruption of normal child development. Acute anxiety may be evoked by repeated bouts of sickness or painful treatments, and cosmetic defects may result from the primary disease or from attempts at therapy. Little is accomplished by enhancing immune responses if the person afflicted by one of these conditions is denied the opportunity to mature as a thinking, caring, and contributing individual.

Recognition of immune deficiency in most instances continues to be based on the clinical hallmark of a propensity to unusual or recurrent infections (Table 22–1). However, in recent years, a growing number of cases are being detected because of predilection to neoplasia or autoimmunity, because of clustered congenital malformations, or because of an inborn error of metabolism known to affect one or more of the systems that confer immunity. Further, as in other fields of clinical medicine, initial descriptions of dramatic diseases have given way to the elucidation of disorders having more subtle manifestations.

Since the clinical features of immune deficiency are not highly specific, it can be difficult to decide when to investigate a particular patient for confirmatory evidence of one of these disorders. For example, relatively few children who present only with recurrent viral respiratory infections, otitis media, or bronchitis will be found to have a primary defect of immunity. Therefore, the first step in deciding whether or not to evaluate a child immunologically is a detailed screening for more common explanations of the clinical findings. At the Children's Hospital of Los Angeles, 35 per cent of all children referred for suspected immune deficiency are found to have bronchial asthma, allergic rhinitis, or atopic dermatitis. In other medical centers, the majority of such referrals are accounted for by children having an increased exposure to viral respiratory pathogens in day care centers or in unusual home living arrangements. Clearly, these individuals can be screened by skillful primary care physicians.

Even when immune deficiency does seem likely, it is important to remember that acquired forms are far more common than are the primary immune deficiencies; examples

Table 22–1. **Characteristic Infections of the Primary Immunodeficiencies**

Component	Primary Organisms	Primary Sites	Clinical Examples
Phagocytic cell	*Staphylococcus aureus* *Escherichia coli* *Pseuodomonas* *Klebsiella*	Lung Skin Regional lymph nodes	Chronic granulomatous disease
Complement	*Pneumococcus* *Streptococcus* *Klebsiella* *Neisseria* species	Lung Upper respiratory tract CNS Skin	C3 deficiency Late component deficiencies
B-Lymphocyte	*Pneumococcus* *Streptococcus* *Hemophilus*	Lung Upper respiratory tract Skin CNS	Agammaglobulinemia Dysgammaglobulinemia
T-Lymphocyte	Viruses Fungi Mycobacteria Protozoa	Nonspecific	DiGeorge syndrome Mucocutaneous candidiasis

of these secondary deficiencies will be noted following the description of each class of primary immune deficiency. In addition to the management of the specific immune deficiency, special considerations arise regarding more general medical procedures in newly diagnosed patients. For example, in many of these conditions it is unsafe to administer conventional immunizing agents or blood products. Even a simple procedure such as lancing the skin for a routine blood test may lead to fatal septicemia in the neutropenic neonate.

Although most of these patients are managed in tertiary care settings, it is essential that the field of immune deficiencies not become too far removed from primary care medicine. Early recognition depends upon the clinical expertise of physicians engaged in everyday practice. Also, the primary care physician may be in the best position to help families adjust emotionally and intellectually to the burden of rearing a child afflicted by immune deficiency.

DEVELOPMENTAL BACKGROUND

Because many of the congenital immune deficiency syndromes result from abnormalities in cellular maturation, a brief summary of the ontogenetic development of the immune system is in order. The postnatal bone marrow provides stem cells that progressively differentiate to form three immunologically significant cell types: (1) phagocytic cells, (2) thymic-dependent or T-cells, and (3) bursa-dependent or B-cells (Fig. 22–1).

Mononuclear phagocytic cells migrate to lung, liver, spleen, and peripheral lymph nodes to form the reticuloendothelial system. These cells are responsible for antigen trapping, processing, and presentation for lymphocytic responses.

Uncommitted lymphoid stem cells may be influenced by hormonal factors from two sources. In the first, exposure to thymic factors results in the progressive differentiation of cells to form functional T-cells. These are recognized by their specific immunologic activities, such as binding to sheep red blood cells and proliferating in response to mitogens, antigens, or allogeneic cells. T-cells also may be recognized by identification of specific membrane proteins defined by monoclonal antibodies. It has been determined that the surface proteins of maturing T-cells change with the stage of development (Chapter 2). For example, membrane proteins characteristic of a common thymocyte appear and then disappear as the cell matures from a stem cell product to a fully developed T-lymphocyte. In addition, two functionally distinct populations of mature T-cells can be recognized using the same techniques; helper T-cells have been shown to possess surface proteins that are different from those of suppressor T-cells (Chapter 2).

The second source of factors that influence B-lymphocyte development is unknown in mammalian systems. In the chicken, the organ responsible for the development of antibody-producing cells is the bursa of Fabricius. Its mammalian counterpart accordingly is known as the bursa-equivalent, and its cellular products are B-cells. B-cell differentiation also may be described in terms of cell surface proteins, including the immunoglobulins that they synthesize. Pre–B cells have no surface immunoglobulins but

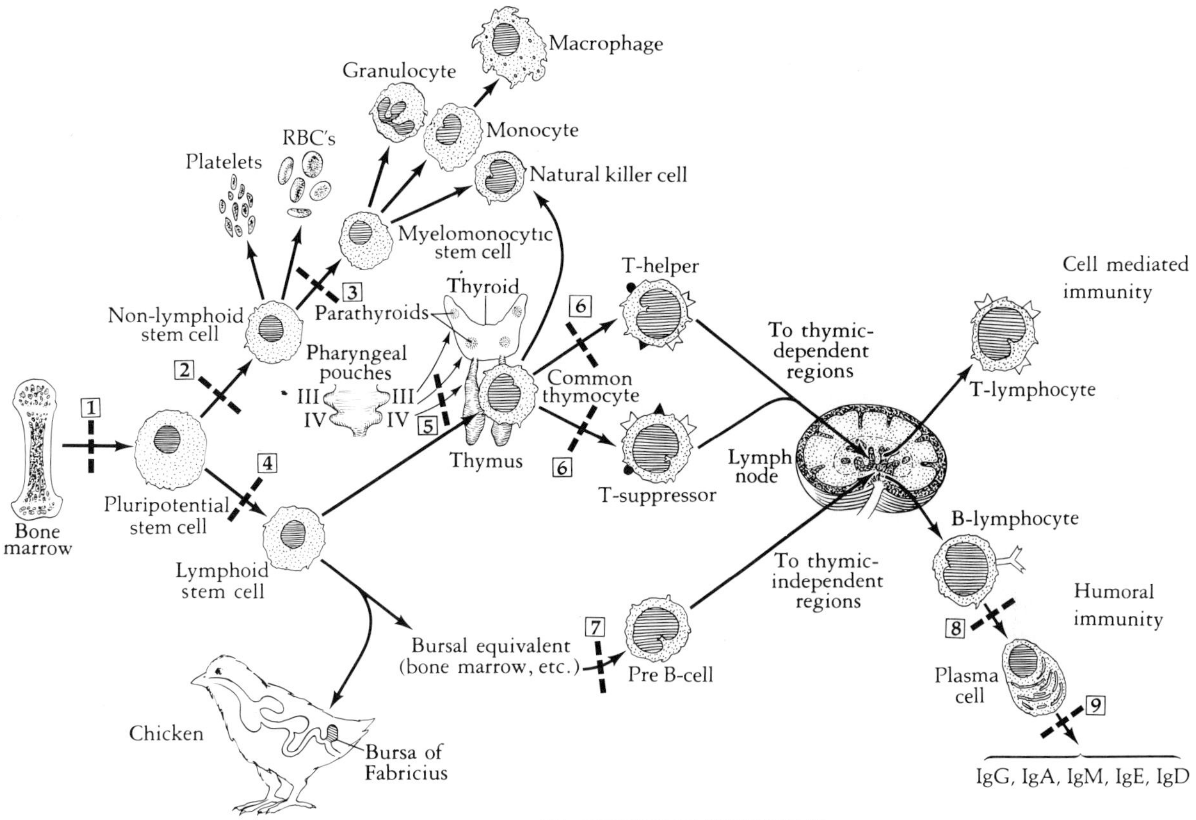

1 RETICULAR DYSGENESIS
2 APLASTIC ANEMIA
3 CHRONIC GRANULOMATOUS DISEASE, MYELOPEROXIDASE DEFICIENCY
4 SEVERE COMBINED IMMUNE DEFICIENCY
5 DIGEORGE SYNDROME
6 ABNORMAL T-HELPER AND SUPPRESSOR CELL FUNCTION
7 CONGENITAL AGAMMAGLOBULINEMIA
8 COMMON VARIABLE IMMUNODEFICIENCY
9 SELECTIVE IMMUNOGLOBULIN CLASS OR SUBCLASS DEFICIENCY

Figure 22–1. Schematic representation of points in immunologic development at which dysfunction or deficiency might occur.

1. Reticular dysgenesis
2. Aplastic anemia
3. Chronic granulomatous disease, myeloperoxidase deficiency
4. Severe combined immune deficiency
5. DiGeorge syndrome
6. Abnormal T-helper and suppressor cell function
7. Congenital agammaglobulinemia
8. Common variable immunodeficiency
9. Selective immunoglobulin class or subclass deficiency

may be recognized by the presence of other marker proteins. The earliest B-cells produce IgM, while cells capable of synthesizing the other immunoglobulins develop sequentially from these (Chapter 2).

Lymphocytes are compartmentalized in the lymph nodes, in which cortical and pericortical regions have separate though interrelated functions (Fig. 22–2). Both germinal centers in the cortex and medullary cords are responsible for antibody synthesis. Interposed between these two areas are the thymic-dependent regions that control cell-mediated and immunoregulatory events. While these spatial arrangements no doubt bear on peripheral tissue interactions between macrophages, T-cells, and B-cells in producing coordinated immune responses, there is much to be learned about this subject.

In animal systems, removal of the bursa or thymus during the early stages of development produces characteristic immunologic defects. Removal of the bursa results in deficient antibody production. If the thymus is excised, profound deficiencies in cell-mediated immunity occur. If both organs are removed, a combined immune deficiency results. Many of the congenital B-cell and T-

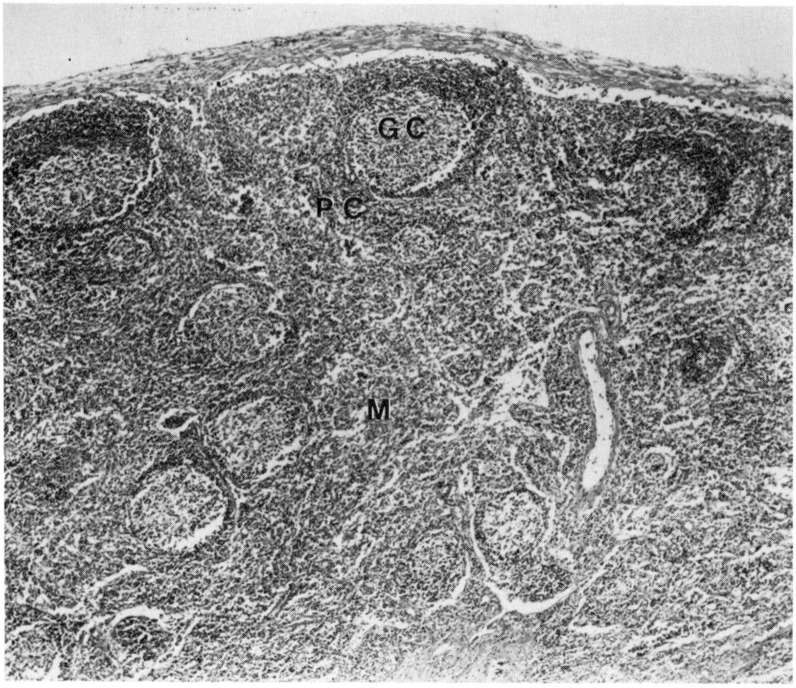

Figure 22–2. Histology of a normal lymph node stimulated by an infection. Note the germinal centers (GC) in the cortex and the medullary (M) cords, regions that contain B-cells; the paracortical (PC) region, interposed between these regions, contains T-cells. Hematoxylin and eosin stain, × 120.

cell deficiencies of man may be viewed as counterparts of these experimentally induced states.

Very recently, cells have been identified that are difficult to place in the standard developmental scheme of phagocytic cells, T-cells, and B-cells. Natural killer (NK) cells are large, granular lymphocytes found in both blood and peripheral lymphoid organs of normal humans. These elements share some surface membrane characteristics with both T-lymphocytes and monocytes. NK cells are defined by their ability to kill tumor cells *in vitro* without first being immunologically sensitized to the tumor. This "natural" killing may be profoundly important in immunosurveillance against cancer (Chapter 19) and in early responses to acute viral infection (Chapter 16).

Under normal conditions, the ultimate product of these developmental cellular interactions is an integrated system of cells and humoral components that provides a highly discriminatory mechanism for the detection of foreignness and, thereby, host protection. From a practical standpoint, immune deficiency syndromes may be classified according to the cell types or substances they affect: (1) phagocytic cells, (2) natural killer cells, (3) the complement system, (4) B-lymphocytes, (5) T-lymphocytes, and (6) B-lymphocytes and T-lymphocytes combined.

ABNORMALITIES OF PHAGOCYTIC CELLS

Cells of the phagocytic system include circulating monocytes and fixed-tissue macrophages of the mononuclear system as well as circulating polymorphonuclear leukocytes, particularly neutrophils. Disorders of number as well as intrinsic functional defects may occur in either of these systems (Table 22–2).

Disorders of Phagocytic Cell Number

HYPOSPLENISM

Although liver Kupffer cells provide the greater part of the body's fixed-tissue macrophages, quantitative defects of the macrophage system usually are due to changes in the spleen (Table 22–3). Abnormalities of splenic function occur in congenital aplasia, surgical removal, and hyposplenism secondary to hemolytic states. Splenectomy in children under five years of age and autosplenectomy (disease-induced alteration of the spleen) in those having sickle cell anemia have been associated with an increased risk of severe or even fatal bacterial septicemia.

Phagocytosis of blood-borne bacteria in the spleen initiates early antibody production

Table 22–2. **Disorders of Phagocytic Cells**

Quantitative deficiencies of phagocytic cells
Hyposplenism
Neutropenias
Disorders of neutrophil adherence
Disorders of neutrophil phagocytosis
Disorders of phagocytic cell chemotaxis
Disorders of bacterial killing
Chronic granulomatous disease
G-6-PD deficiency
Myeloperoxidase deficiency
Chédiak-Higashi syndrome
Complex phagocytic cell disorders
Malakoplakia
Hidradenitis suppurativa
Hyper-IgE syndrome

and results in protection against encapsulated organisms such as *Streptococcus pneumoniae* and *Hemophilus influenzae*. Laboratory investigation in rats has shown that removal of more than 50 per cent of the spleen results in a markedly diminished primary antibody response to intravenously administered antigens. It is the loss of this early antibody response to hematogenous antigens that is the likely cause of susceptibility to overwhelming infection.

Management of splenectomized patients requires immediate treatment of febrile episodes with antibiotics. Pneumococcal vaccine and continuous antibiotic prophylaxis (e.g., penicillin) are useful measures but cannot be relied upon to be 100 per cent effective. In patients with traumatic injury, surgical preservation of at least 50 per cent of the spleen will likely result in normal splenic immune responses.

NEUTROPENIA

Neutropenia is defined as an absolute granulocyte count in the peripheral blood below 1500 per cu mm. This may result from decreased production in bone marrow, increased destruction or clearance from the circulation, or simultaneous operation of both mechanisms. Neutropenia may be classified into either a primary or an acquired form, the former generally being ascribed to inherited factors and the latter to other diseases or toxins.

Table 22–3. **Disorders of the Spleen Associated with Immune Defects**

Type	Example
Congenital	Congenital absence of the spleen
Acquired	Splenectomy
	Functional splenectomy with hemolytic diseases (sickle cell disease)

The Primary Neutropenias. Cyclic neutropenia usually begins in childhood and is characterized by periods of well-being of approximately three weeks that are interrupted by one-week episodes of neutropenia, fever, malaise, aphthous stomatitis, and furunculosis. Bone marrow examination at the time of the neutropenia demonstrates a marked decrease in mature granulocytes. Studies of bone marrow morphology, myelopoiesis, and neutrophil kinetics have shown that cyclic neutropenia is primarily a disease of abnormally regulated neutrophil production. Treatment is with antibiotics, careful oral and dental care, and education of the patient. Although severe infections are rare, they may be seen (particularly when the neutropenia is associated with immunoglobulin deficiency states, as it is in some cases). Recent studies have indicated a beneficial effect of steroids.

Chronic granulocytopenia of childhood occurs in autosomal recessive or dominant inherited forms as well as in sporadic forms. These disorders are associated with diminished bone marrow production of mature granulocytes. The clinical course of these disorders is variable and generally dependent upon the degree of neutropenia. Some patients follow a relatively benign course with long-term survival, whereas others experience recurrent severe infection and early death.

Pancreatic insufficiency with bone marrow dysfunction (Shwachman syndrome) is characterized by exocrine pancreatic insufficiency, neutropenia, and failure to thrive in young children. This disorder may be confused with cystic fibrosis because of the associated infections and malabsorption syndrome. However, sweat chloride concentrations are normal. Treatment with pancreatic preparations may improve the gastrointestinal symptoms, but it does not affect the neutropenia.

The Acquired Neutropenias. Drug-induced neutropenia is caused by several mechanisms. Some drugs (e.g., chemotherapeutic agents) induce a profound suppression of myeloid cell formation. Others induce immunologic responses that destroy mature granulocytes. The list of drugs and substances known to be associated with neutropenia is ever-increasing and includes analgesics, antithyroid medications, anticonvulsants, antihistamines, antimicrobial agents, and tranquilizers. Furthermore, as man's environment is increasingly polluted with chemical toxins, additional causes of neutropenia are likely to be found.

Other immunologic disorders are sometimes associated with neutropenia. Neutropenia is found in X-linked agammaglobulinemia and other dysgammaglobulinemias. In a recent case, a seven-year-old girl experienced cyclic neutropenia and hypogammaglobulinemia. The neutropenia became chronic and severe, eventually evolving into aplastic anemia with a fatal outcome. Neutropenia may be found in classic autoimmune diseases, such as lupus erythematosus, rheumatoid arthritis, and Felty's syndrome (neutropenia, splenomegaly, and arthritis). Most recently, specific autoantibodies against neutrophil antigens have been reported in patients having otherwise unexplained chronic neutropenia.

Neutropenia occurs during or after infection with a variety of gram-negative and gram-positive bacteria, or viruses (influenza, rubella, measles, hepatitis B, Epstein-Barr). In some cases, it is difficult to determine whether an infection is the cause or the result of the neutropenia. Generally, when a decreased granulocyte number is the result of an infection, white cell concentrations will return to normal following clinical recovery.

Transient neutropenia may result from direct bone marrow suppression, from peripheral destruction, or from a combination of these mechanisms. Further, neutropenia may be caused by replacement of normal bone marrow elements with neoplastic tissue (myelophthisis), which is a common complication of acute leukemia. Increased destruction of neutrophils may occur in disorders associated with hypersplenism, including Gaucher's disease, primary splenic neutropenia, and congestive splenomegaly secondary to portal or splenic vein hypertension (Banti's syndrome).

Clinical Features of Neutropenia. Bacterial infections are characteristic complications of both primary and acquired forms of neutropenia. The clinical spectrum of these infections varies from relatively minor to life-threatening, depending on the etiology and degree of leukopenia. Causative infectious agents include *Staphylococcus aureus, Pseudomonas* species, *Streptococcus pneumoniae,* and gram-negative enteric organisms.

Pyoderma, otitis media, and pneumonitis are the most frequently encountered infections in patients with chronic neutropenia. Others include gingivostomatitis, sinusitis, peritonsillar and retropharyngeal abscesses, and enteritis. Septicemia is particularly common in granulocytopenic cancer patients and is responsible for approximately 20 per cent of febrile episodes in this population.

Congenital granulocytopenia in young children has a guarded prognosis. However, resistance to infection improves if children survive infancy. This presumably reflects compensatory development of antibody and cell-mediated responses, both of which are functionally intact in most of these patients.

Diagnosis. It is usually possible to distinguish primary neutropenias from acquired varieties by considering age of onset, history of exposure to toxic substances or drugs, family history, and blood and bone marrow analysis. In patients who are suspected of cyclic variations, peripheral neutrophil counts twice weekly for two months will reveal the characteristic pattern of periodic neutropenia. Bone marrow examination is essential for evaluating maturational characteristics of granulocyte precursors, destructive change, or replacement by other cell types.

Immunologically mediated neutropenia may be better established by determining the presence of serum leukoagglutinins or specific antineutrophil antibody. Such measurement also is useful in evaluating neonatal neutropenia in which it is difficult to distinguish primary neutropenia from the transient variety that is due to maternally acquired antineutrophil antibody. In the latter, the granulocyte count will begin to rise and leukoagglutinin titers decrease after the first month of life. A thorough search for underlying autoimmune disorders is indicated in selected cases of idiopathic neutropenia in children and adults.

Treatment. In acquired neutropenia, suspected drugs should be discontinued and environmental toxins avoided. In all patients, treatment is directed at preventing infection by limiting exposure to known sources of contagion and by rapidly attending to minor abrasions or other integumental insults. A more disturbing feature of infection in the neutropenic host is the tendency to rapid and potentially lethal dissemination. Although antimicrobial prophylaxis generally is not indicated, immediate attention must be given to febrile episodes. Broad-spectrum antibiotic coverage is an essential feature of management, and white blood cell transfusion may be helpful in the acute management of the critically ill patient. Effective prevention of the inherited neutropenias rests on genetic counseling.

Abnormalities of Phagocytic Cell Function

The syndromes associated with phagocytic cell abnormalities generally are characterized by recurrent sepsis and disseminated pyogenic lesions. However, as more sensitive assays of cellular function are developed, defects with less striking clinical presentations are being found. Primary disorders of cellular function include abnormalities of adhesion, phagocytosis, directed movement toward foreign matter (chemotaxis), and intracellular destruction of ingested pathogens. Many of these disorders are familial.

Yet, in one very commonly encountered example, the human newborn, diminished neutrophil and monocyte function is "normal." Studies reveal that cellular adherence and chemotaxis are markedly decreased relative to adult values. Further, examination of neutrophils from newborns stressed by infection or respiratory compromise reveals diminished oxidative and bactericidal responses. In addition, acquired defects of phagocytosis are induced by a variety of infections, metabolic disorders, nutritional deficiencies, and drugs. These secondary phagocytic cell dysfunctions result in predisposition to infection similar to that seen in the intrinsic defects.

DEFECTS IN NEUTROPHIL ADHESION AND PHAGOCYTOSIS

Primary cellular defects in adhesion have been identified only recently. Neutrophils from a five-year-old boy with recurrent *Pseudomonas* infection failed to adhere normally to plastic surfaces. This resulted in grossly impaired chemotaxis and moderately impaired phagocytosis. The absolute granulocyte count in the peripheral blood was strikingly elevated, over 100,000 cells per cu mm. This functional defect was associated with a missing cell membrane glycoprotein (GP 180). We have seen one six-month-old boy with recurrent staphylococcal abscesses, a white blood cell count of 200,000 per cu mm, abnormal chemotaxis, and impaired phagocyte adherence to nylon wool and glass. Yet another child, an eight-year-old boy who had recurrent infections, was shown to have a different, selective defect of phagocytosis. Chemotactic responses in this child were normal, and detailed studies revealed deficiency in another membrane protein (GP 150). In these three patients, intracellular bacterial killing was normal, and family studies suggested a variable genetic basis.

DEFICIENCIES OF PHAGOCYTIC CELL CHEMOTAXIS

Many different clinical disorders have been associated with abnormal phagocytic cell chemotactic responses. In most of these conditions, abnormal chemotaxis is a secondary phenomenon, although a number of patients (mostly children) have been described who have intrinsic cellular defects. Some primary adherence defects are associated with impaired chemotaxis, as noted previously. A possibly related disorder, primary neutrophil actin dysfunction, has been noted in an infant with recurrent bacterial infections. His neutrophils exhibited abnormal locomotion, ingestion, and degranulation. In the lazy leukocyte syndrome, findings include abnormal locomotion and ingestion along with peripheral neutropenia.

In glycogen storage disease (GSD) 1b, neutropenia is one feature, but chemotaxis is also impaired. Neutrophils from affected patients show normal *in vitro* phagocytosis and bacterial killing. The cells appear to possess the appropriate structural requirements for normal function. It appears that an alteration in metabolic pathways that are not involved in primary bacterial killing results in the defective chemotaxis.

INTRACELLULAR DEFECTS OF BACTERIAL KILLING

Chronic Granulomatous Disease (CGD). This disorder is the most common of the syndromes associated with defective bactericidal activity. In most cases, it is inherited as an X-linked trait, although autosomal recessive forms are known. The underlying defect is impaired generation of superoxide and hydrogen peroxide due to a variety of enzymatic defects, most commonly involving the NADPH oxidase system.

Clinical Features. Symptoms usually begin during the first few years of life with the advent of recurrent, disseminated abscesses or pneumonias (Fig. 22–3). These are accompanied in many instances by lymphadenopathy, hepatosplenomegaly, suppurative adenitis, and chronic dermatitis. Prominent etiologic agents include microorganisms normally found on the skin and in the gut. *Staphylococcus* is the predominant species, although *Klebsiella-Aerobacter, Escherichia coli, Serratia marcescens,* and *Pseudomonas* species are frequently encountered. *Candida* and *Aspergillus* species also can be troublesome agents in these patients.

In contrast to other immune deficiencies, the infectious agents found in CGD are of low virulence in normal individuals and are characteristically catalase-positive. Certain catalase-negative organisms, such as *S. pneumoniae* and *S. pyogenes,* also produce hydrogen peroxide. Since they do not often infect these patients, it is postulated that the alternative source of hydrogen peroxide produced by these organisms partially corrects the intracellular short supply found in CGD cells.

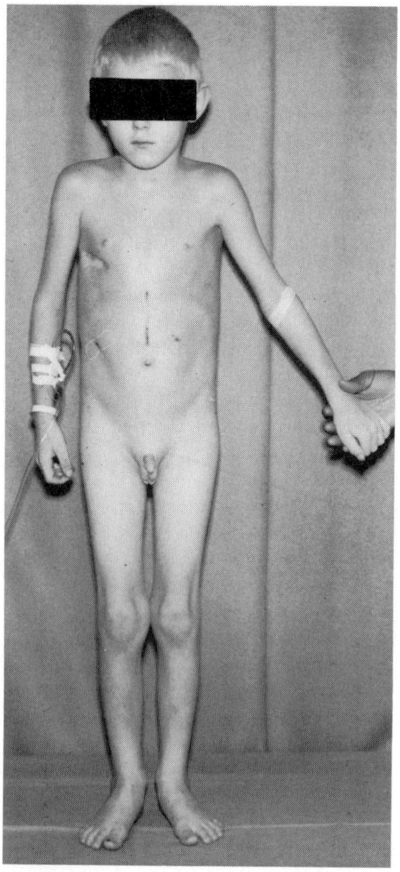

Figure 22–3. Photograph of a nine-year-old boy with chronic granulomatous disease. Note thoracotomy and laparotomy scars at sites of prior therapeutic procedures to drain abscesses of lung and liver.

Characteristic suppurative granulomas are scattered throughout the body in bone, lung, liver, and spleen. The granuloma consists of inflammatory cells surrounding a necrotic core (Fig. 22–4), superficially resembling mycobacterial lesions.

Diagnosis. CGD should be anticipated in a newborn when the diagnosis has been made in other family members. Because the more common inherited pattern is X-linked recessive, male children in affected families are particularly at risk. The characteristic infectious agents and clinical picture usually suggest the diagnosis in older children. However, exceptions to the classic picture are being found. In one family, four males were not diagnosed until their adult years. Although they experienced frequent infections as children, these markedly decreased in frequency after approximately 25 years of age. In another reported case, a 27-year-old man's first suspicious infection was *Mycobacterium fortuitum* pneumonia. We have recently diagnosed CGD in three unusual clinical situations. A two-month-old boy presented with *Candida lusitaniae* meningitis. Post-mortem examination revealed suspicious granulomatous lesions in lung and liver. This child's identical twin was found to have CGD. Presenting with her first major infection, a 12-year-old girl with multiple staphylococcal liver abscesses was found to have CGD. In another female, a 13-month-old child, mild pneumonia and asymptomatic splenomegaly were the initial findings. Clearly, a high degree of suspicion for CGD is essential if such patients are to be diagnosed and treated properly.

Infections may be heralded by prolonged fever of unknown cause without localizing signs. Chronic anemia is frequent and often exacerbated during hyperpyrexia. Elevated white blood cell counts, usually 20,000 to 30,000 per cu mm, are common, and hyperimmunoglobulinemia is usually present, presumably owing to stimulated antibody synthesis by chronic infection. Morphologically, peripheral blood neutrophils and monocytes appear normal by light and electron microscopy.

Laboratory analysis of phagocytic cell activity is necessary to document the diagnosis of CGD. Although peripheral blood neutrophils are the easiest cells to study, similar func-

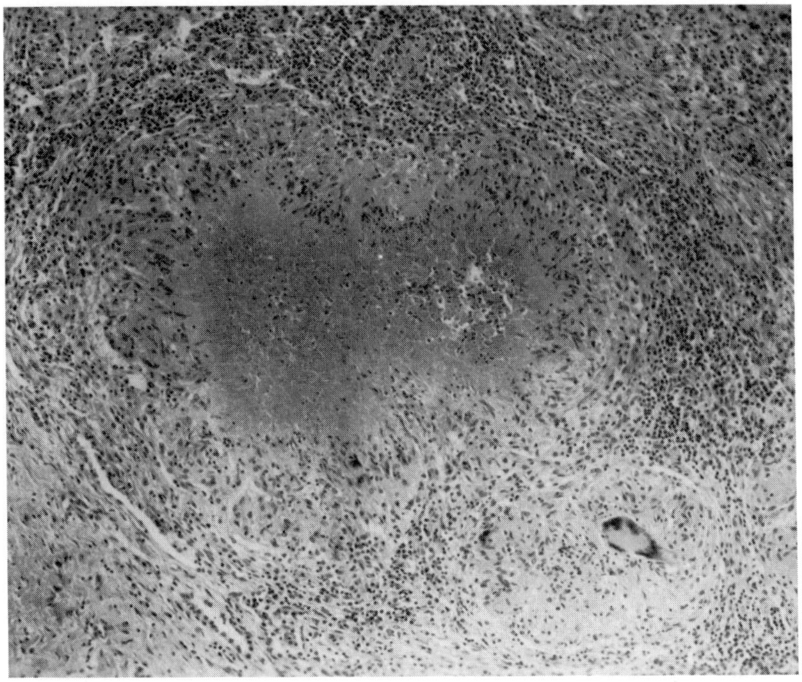

Figure 22–4. Photomicrograph of a granuloma seen in chronic granulomatous disease. Note the central area of necrosis surrounded by inflammatory cells and a multinucleated giant cell to the lower right. Hematoxylin and eosin stain, × 120.

tional and metabolic abnormalities can be detected in peripheral blood monocytes and in alveolar macrophages. Phagocytic cells from CGD patients respond normally to chemotactic stimuli and ingest bacteria and fungi adequately. However, bactericidal assays show that these cells are relatively ineffective in killing the bacteria and fungi that are responsible for clinical disease.

A variety of assays that measure disturbances in the metabolic response to phagocyte stimulation are available. Superoxide and hydrogen peroxide generation and oxygen consumption during respiratory burst activity may be measured directly with complex biochemical methods. The nitroblue tetrazolium (NBT) dye reduction test measures production of these metabolites indirectly. Activated normal neutrophils reduce the clear, pale yellow NBT to blue granular formazan, which may be assayed by simple colorimetric techniques. Chemiluminescence is another test of respiratory burst activity that has been used in a number of laboratories. CGD cells characteristically fail to produce superoxide and hydrogen peroxide when stimulated. Similarly, marked impairment of NBT dye reduction and chemiluminescence is noted in activated CGD cells.

White blood cells from newborns yield lower than normal values in these tests but not as low as those in CGD. Fetal neutrophils can now be studied using these same techniques, making possible the prenatal diagnosis of CGD.

Pathogenesis. The process of phagocytosis initiates a variety of metabolic responses in neutrophils. In brief, these include increased glucose utilization and ATP consumption, a surge of oxidative activity (the respiratory burst), and activation of the hexose monophosphate shunt pathway of glucose metabolism. In CGD cells, oxygen-dependent mechanisms of bacterial killing are primarily affected. Hydrogen peroxide (H_2O_2) and superoxide production in response to a phagocytic stimulus is markedly impaired. The lack of infections with H_2O_2-producing bacteria in CGD patients suggests the importance of oxygen radicals and the H_2O_2-myeloperoxidase-halide system in normal neutrophil killing.

CGD represents the common clinical end point of a number of different enzymatic deficiencies. Defective NADPH oxidase activity has been found in most patients with CGD in whom this activity has been measured. Enzyme activity is similar in normal and CGD cells in the resting state. However, CGD neutrophils fail to generate the increased NADPH oxidase activity seen in normal cells following phagocytosis. Additional laboratory analysis suggests that NADPH oxidase is present in the cells of some CGD patients but is not activated under physiologic conditions. Recent experience with a female CGD patient is of interest in this regard. *In vitro* generation of H_2O_2 and superoxide by her neutrophils was markedly defective when the usual particulate stimuli were employed to activate her neutrophils. However, in the presence of nonphysiologic lectins her cells were able to generate up to 30 per cent of a normal response, suggesting that the enzymatic defect of her cells is relative and not absolute.

Other metabolic defects have been described in patients with CGD. Severe glucose-6-phosphate dehydrogenase (G-6-PD) deficiency that affects both leukocytes and red blood cells has been associated with a clinical picture of recurrent granulomatous infections and chronic hemolytic anemia. Accelerated decay of G-6-PD activity has also been found in patients with CGD, although this may be a secondary phenomenon. Initially reported as a cause of CGD in females, leukocyte glutathione peroxidase deficiency may be one cause of CGD in selected male patients. Neutrophil-specific granule deficiency has been reported in several patients with recurrent infections similar to those seen in CGD. Morphologically, these neutrophils had bilobed nuclei and cytoplasm that appeared nearly devoid of granules. In specific granule deficiency, bactericidal activity, stimulated oxygen metabolism, and chemotactic responses are abnormal.

Treatment. The long-term prognosis of patients affected by CGD has greatly improved in recent years. Most infections are successfully eradicated by early and aggressive intervention with antibiotics and surgery. Continuous antibiotic prophylaxis may be of value in selected patients, as suggested by recent reports. However, the development of allergic reactions and the emergence of antibiotic-resistant organisms limit the effectiveness of this regimen. Further, infections with *Candida* and *Aspergillus* species are not prevented, and may be precipitated, by this approach in some individuals.

During acute infection, subjective clinical benefit has been noted following transfusions with donor white blood cells. The limited half-life of infused phagocytes and the unproven efficacy and considerable cost of such procedures restrict the use of this modality to life-threatening situations.

Pharmacologic enhancement of the phagocytic activity has been attempted. *In vitro* sulfisoxazole was reported to improve the bactericidal activity of CGD neutrophils, although not to normal levels. Trimethoprim-sulfa has resulted in similar improvement. The clinical usefulness of these approaches has yet to be defined, however. Ascorbic acid does not improve the bactericidal activities of CGD leukocytes.

At present, bone marrow transplantation offers the only hope for a true cure of CGD, and this has been accomplished in one reported case. However, the complications of this procedure and the recent improvements in prognosis in most patients with CGD limit its applicability.

Myeloperoxidase Deficiency. Very recent findings have indicated that myeloperoxidase (MPO) deficiency is the most common primary neutrophil defect, although it is associated only rarely with an increased susceptibility to serious infection. The incidence of partial or complete MPO deficiency approximates 50 per 100,000 in several large population studies. Since, in most cases, there seems to be no predilection to recurrent infection, alternative intracellular killing mechanisms appear to be protective. Most of the symptomatic subjects have also had diabetes mellitus and have experienced systemic infections with *Candida* species. The diagnosis of MPO deficiency may be established with histochemical techniques (Fig. 22–5*A*), and laboratory assessment of bacterial killing reveals a quantitative dysfunction that is much less severe than that seen in chronic granulomatous disease.

Chédiak-Higashi Syndrome (CHS). This autosomal recessive disorder is characterized by an unusual oculocutaneous albinism, a high incidence of lymphoreticular neoplasms, and recurrent pyogenic infections. Defective pigment distribution and abnormal neutrophil functions appear to be related to abnormal lysosomes in many cell types, including skin and phagocytic cells (Fig. 22–5*B*). The hair of an affected individual appears steel gray in color, and microscopic examination reveals abnormal melanin distribution. Neutrophils and monocytes may contain giant cytoplasmic granules. These cells are functionally defective with impaired chemotactic responses, bacterial killing, and degranulation, yet recurrent bacterial infections are not consistently found. Many patients develop an accelerated phase of the disease that is characterized by an aggressive lymphoma-like process with hepatosplenomegaly, lymphadenopathy, and pancyto-

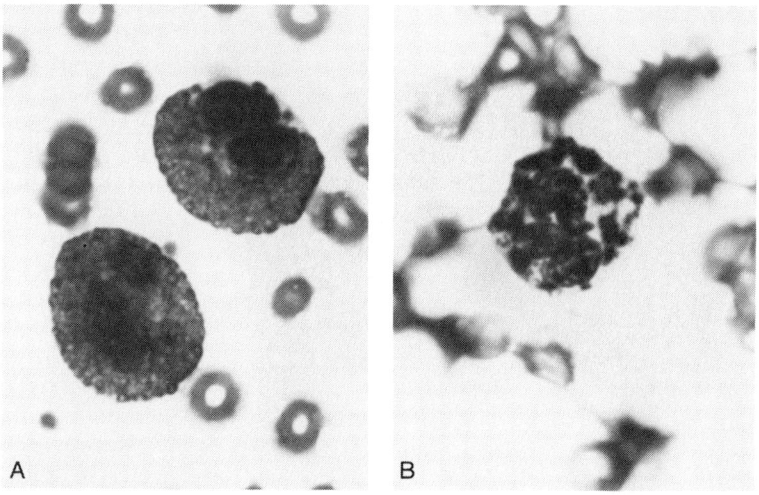

Figure 22–5. Normal (*A*) and Chédiak-Higashi (*B*) polymorphonuclear leukocytes that have been histochemically stained for myeloperoxidase. Note the numerous fine, peroxidase-positive granules in the normal cells compared with the bizarre, oversized granules in the cell from the patient with Chédiak-Higashi syndrome.

penia. The relationship of this process to a recently demonstrated deficiency of natural killer cell activity in CHS remains to be determined.

The impairments of leukocyte function in CHS have been attributed to several abnormalities, including abnormal lysosomal enzyme levels, microtubule dysfunction, increased membrane fluidity, specifically defective lysosome membranes, and abnormal lysosome membrane-microtubule interaction. Additional studies show that cyclic nucleotide metabolism, particularly excess accumulation of cyclic adenosine monophosphate (cAMP), is involved. Ascorbic acid has been shown to reduce the elevated intracellular cAMP concentrations and to improve *in vitro* chemotactic and bactericidal responses. These impressive results have been questioned by some investigators, and the long-term efficacy of ascorbic acid for preventing infection and the accelerated phase of CHS has yet to be documented. Ascorbic acid does not improve the pigment disturbance in these patients.

Malakoplakia and Hidradenitis Suppurativa. Malakoplakia, a rare acquired inflammatory granuloma, is characterized by the collection of large mononuclear cells called Hansemann macrophages. An infectious origin is suspected, and defective macrophage digestion of phagocytized bacteria is postulated. In one affected patient, monocyte cyclic guanosine monophosphate (cGMP) levels were found to be low and bacterial killing was impaired. Treatment with bethanechol, a cholinergic agonist, corrected the monocyte abnormality and led to control of the patient's infection. Very similar findings were noted in a patient with hydradenitis suppurativa. These two disorders indicate the importance of cyclic nucleotide metabolism in the regulation of phagocytic cell functions.

Hyperimmunoglobulinemia E with Recurrent Infections. Originally reported in 1966 as Job's syndrome, hyperimmunoglobulinemia E with recurrent infections (the hyper-IgE syndrome) is a complex disorder of undetermined etiology. Both sexes and all racial groups have been affected. From early infancy, patients experience severe infections of the skin and lung, including cold abscesses, adenitis, pneumonia, and lung abscess formation. *Staphylococcus aureus* has caused infections in all reported cases. *C. albicans, H. influenzae,* and *S. pyogenes* are also frequently encountered as pathogens. Enteric organisms may become secondary invaders as the disease progresses. Respiratory allergic symptoms are not regularly found. An atypical eczematoid dermatitis with a predilection for intertriginous areas is present frequently and may become exacerbated during periods of acute infection. Coarse facial features are common, and unrelated patients may resemble each other (Fig. 22–6). The hyper-IgE syndrome may have a genetic basis, and a number of families having multiple affected members have been recorded. The pattern of inheritance in these families has been interpreted as that of autosomal dominant with variable penetrance.

Diagnosis. Recurrent pyogenic infections without associated marked inflammatory responses ("cold" abscesses) are features of this disorder, although not found in all patients. Laboratory evaluation reveals marked elevation in serum IgE concentration (2000 to

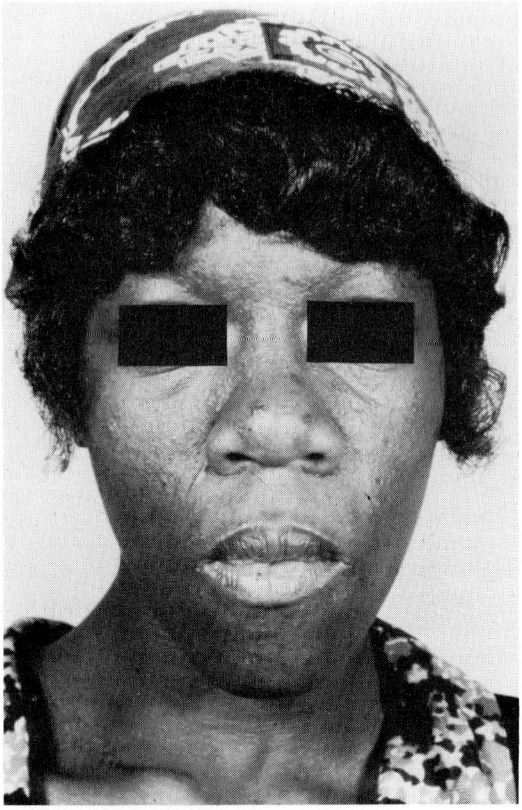

Figure 22–6. A patient with hyper-IgE syndrome, showing coarse facial features. Scar from surgical drainage procedure is noted in the right supraclavicular area.

50,000 U per ml), increased levels of other serum immunoglobulins, and peripheral blood eosinophilia. Although abnormal neutrophil and monocyte chemotaxis is often found, this is not seen in all cases, and other measures of phagocytic cell function are normal. Similarly, defective cell-mediated immunity is a variable finding.

Pathogenesis. The cause of this syndrome is unknown, although recent findings allow construction of a theoretical framework. Patients with the hyper-IgE syndrome appear to have a primary deficiency of T-suppressor cells, allowing overproduction of IgE that is specific for staphylococcal antigens. When a patient encounters staphylococcal organisms, the result is a vigorous allergic reaction rather than an ordered, protective response. Local tissue breakdown occurs, and other inflammatory mediators may result in secondary phagocytic cell dysfunction.

Treatment. Acute infections are treated aggressively with antibiotics and surgical drainage. The frequency of severe infections may be reduced by the use of prophylactic antibiotics. Levamisole, a common anthelmintic drug, has been shown to correct the phagocytic cell abnormalities in patients with hyper-IgE syndrome. In a recent study, however, levamisole was associated with an increased infection rate in hyper-IgE patients, suggesting that leukocyte dysfunction is not the primary cause of this disease.

Secondary Phagocytic Cell Defects. Myriad drugs as well as infections, metabolic alterations, and other clinical conditions have been shown to induce abnormal phagocytic cell function. Selected examples of these are presented in Table 22–4. Adherence and chemotaxis appear to be more vulnerable to extrinsic influences than is bacterial killing.

Recent investigations suggest a possible role for a unique high molecular weight glycoprotein, fibronectin, in the secondary abnormalities of phagocyte adhesion and chemotaxis. In addition to its involvement in platelet aggregation, fibronectin appears to be necessary for adherence of staphylococci to human neutrophils. Since severe infection in human subjects is associated with decreased plasma fibronectin levels, it is possible that at least some of the secondary leukocyte dysfunctions seen in sepsis may be due to fibronectin depletion.

NATURAL KILLER (NK) DEFICIENCY

As noted previously, natural killer cells compose a distinct population of large granular lymphocytes with cytotoxic activity against certain tumor cell lines. Although their role in host defenses remains to be clarified, NK cell deficiency has been described in a number of patients. Most notably, patients with Chédiak-Higashi syndrome have profoundly dysfunctional NK cells, although the cells are normal in number. The relationship of this abnormality to the development of the lymphoma-like accelerated phase in these patients is of great interest because of the postulated role of these cells in tumor surveillance. Diminished NK activity also has been reported in two patients with pure T-cell deficiency, suggesting that maturation of natural killer function is dependent upon normal T-cell development. Most recently, depressed NK cell activity has been noted in infants with protein calorie malnutrition, in patients receiving azathioprine, and in hyperthermia *in vitro.* Given the current level of interest, it is likely that the number of disorders found to be associ-

Table 22–4. Selected Pharmacologic Agents and Diseases Adversely Affecting Phagocytic Cell Function

Adherence/ Phagocytosis	Drugs: ethanol, steroids, aspirin, tetracycline Cigarette smoke (alveolar macrophages) Sepsis
Chemotaxis	Drugs: adrenergic agents, I.V. lipid emulsions, colchicine, D-penicillamine, amphotericin B Diabetes mellitus Down's syndrome Infections: sepsis, measles Severe allergic disorders Sickle cell crisis Thermal injury Surgical trauma Cancer Cirrhosis Kwashiorkor
Killing	Adrenergic agents Radiation therapy Down's syndrome Sepsis Cancer Vitamin B_{12}, iron deficiency

ated with NK cell deficiency will increase rapidly.

DEFICIENCIES OF THE COMPLEMENT SYSTEM

The complement system is a complex array of highly integrated proteins that interact in sequential fashion. Activation of this system may occur either through the classic pathway involving C1, C4, and C2 or through the alternative pathway involving factors P (properdin), D, and B. Both pathways result in cleavage of C3 and subsequent activation of the late components with production of chemotactic factors, anaphylatoxins, and other mediators of inflammation. The interaction of the early components is enzymatic, while that of components C5b, C6, C7, C8, and C9 involve noncovalent chemical bonding.

Reported abnormalities of the complement system include primary deficiencies of each of the components of the classic pathway and of the major regulatory proteins: C1 esterase inhibitor and C3b inactivator (Table 22–5). Early component deficiencies are often associated with collagen vascular disorders. C3 deficiency results in recurrent pyogenic infections similar to those seen in hypogammaglobulinemia. *Neisseria* species infections may complicate late component deficiencies; primary C1 esterase inhibitor deficiency results in hereditary angioedema.

C1 Deficiency. C1q deficiency has been found in association with combined immune deficiency, hypogammaglobulinemia, and glomerulonephritis in children. Cutaneous vasculitis has occurred in an adult patient. The mode of inheritance is unknown, except in one family in which an autosomal codominant pattern was noted. C1r and C1s deficiencies have been found in patients having lupus erythematosus–like syndromes.

C4 Deficiency. This disorder occurs as an autosomal recessive trait in guinea pigs. In man, C4 deficiency has been observed in a few patients with systemic lupus erythema-

Table 22–5. Complement Component Deficiencies

Component Deficiency	Clinical Features	Inheritance
C1q	SCID, cutaneous vasculitis, hypogammaglobulinemia	?, ACD
C1r	SLE, glomerulonephritis	ACD
C1s	SLE	?
C4	SLE	AR
C2	Normal, SLE, vasculitis, juvenile rheumatoid arthritis, dermatomyositis, recurrent bacterial infections	ACD
C3	Recurrent bacterial infections clinically similar to hypogammaglobulinemia; nephritis	ACD
C5	SLE, *Neisseria* infections	ACD
C5 dysfunction (?)	Leiner's disease	?
C6	Normal, *Neisseria* infections	ACD
C7	Normal, Raynaud's phenomenon, nephritis, *Neisseria* infections	ACD
C8	Normal, *Neisseria* infections, SLE, Xeroderma pigmentosum	ACD
C9	Normal	
C1 esterase inhibitor	Hereditary angioedema	AD
C3b inactivator	Recurrent bacterial infections	?

? = undetermined; ACD = autosomal codominant; AR = autosomal recessive; AD = autosomal dominant.

tosus. An autosomal recessive mode of inheritance was found in an affected family.

C2 Deficiency. The most common hereditary deficiency of classic pathway components involves C2. Homozygous and heterozygous C2 deficiency states have been found in asymptomatic individuals and in others with a variety of collagen vascular disorders. C2 deficiency also has been found in several patients who had recurrent severe pyogenic infections.

C3 Deficiency. Deficiency of C3 may result from a defect in the synthesis of C3, which is inherited as an autosomal codominant trait. Affected patients experience recurrent bacterial infections similar to those seen in hypogammaglobulinemia. Chronic glomerulonephritis may complicate the clinical course. C3 deficiency may also result from hypercatabolism associated with C3b inactivator deficiency. An increased susceptibility to bacterial infections is seen in these patients.

C5 Deficiency. Autosomal codominantly inherited C5 deficiency has been associated with systemic lupus erythematosus in one patient and recurrent meningococcemia in others.

Leiner's Disease (C5 Dysfunction?). This syndrome of young infants is characterized by failure to thrive, chronic diarrhea, recurrent infections, and severe seborrheic dermatitis. It has been limited to breast-fed neonates. Defective serum opsonization of baker's yeast particles has been reported and related to C5 "dysfunction." The relationship of Leiner's disease to C5 dysfunction is questionable, however, since the patients with C5 deficiency opsonize yeast normally; C5 levels are normal in patients with Leiner's disease, and patients having Leiner's disease are not subject to fungal infections. Infusion of fresh frozen plasma has resulted in clinical improvement, and complete resolution of this disorder generally has occurred by two months of age.

C6 Deficiency. Individuals with autosomal codominant C6 deficiency may be asymptomatic. Others have had recurrent meningococcal meningitis or gonococcal arthritis.

C7 Deficiency. Several families have been reported with autosomal codominant deficiency of C7. Patients may be asymptomatic or may present with Raynaud's phenomenon, chronic nephritis, or recurrent *Neisseria* infection.

C8 Deficiency. This variably inherited disorder has been found in asymptomatic individuals and in others afflicted with lupus, xeroderma pigmentosum, or recurrent *Neisseria* infections.

C9 Deficiency. C9 deficiency has been noted in a single individual who had no history of recurrent infection or evidence of collagen vascular disease. Family studies revealed autosomal codominant inheritance.

Hereditary Angioedema. This disorder is due to an autosomal dominant deficiency of an alpha$_2$-globulin that normally controls C1 esterase activity. C1 esterase inhibitor (C1 INH) is also a major regulatory factor for other humoral inflammatory systems (Fig. 22–7). Two genetic variants exist: one in

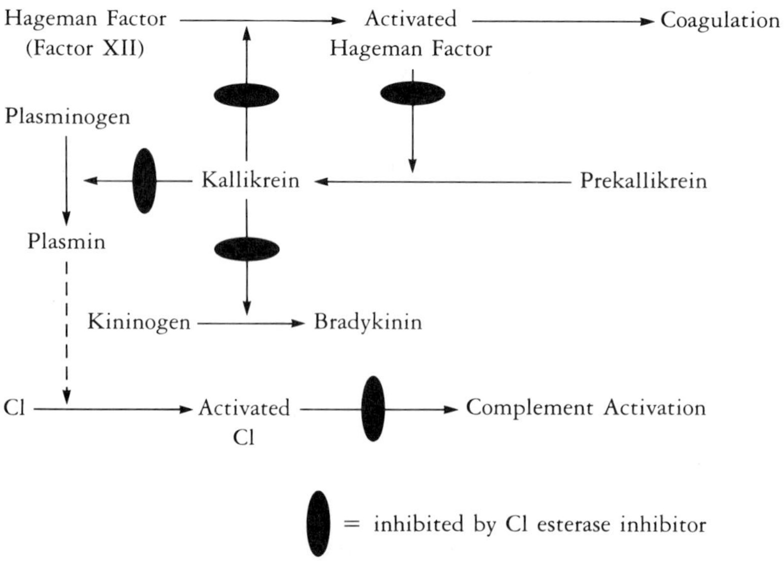

Figure 22–7. Inflammatory mediator pathways controlled by C1 esterase inhibitor.

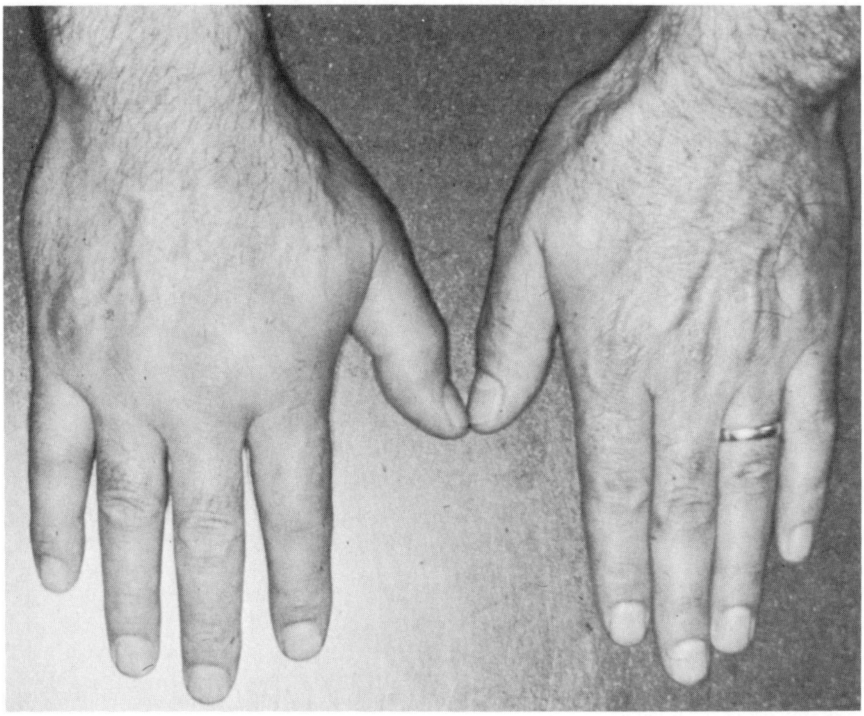

Figure 22–8. Photograph of the hands of a patient with hereditary angioedema, showing swelling of the dorsum of the right hand during an attack. (Courtesy of Dr. Fred S. Rosen.)

which no protein is produced, and another in which a nonfunctional protein is synthesized.

Hereditary angioedema (HAE) may present at any age, but it usually appears during late adolescence or early adulthood. It manifests as recurrent attacks of edema involving the gastrointestinal tract, skin, and respiratory mucosa (Fig. 22–8). Many individuals experience years of repeated bouts of acute abdominal pain before a diagnosis is suggested by the development of classic symptoms. The edema is nonpitting, nonpruritic, and unaccompanied by urticaria. Episodes may occur spontaneously or following trauma or emotional stress—hence the old term for this disease: angioneurotic edema.

Laboratory studies confirm the diagnosis. C2 and C4 levels are invariably low during acute episodes. C1 INH protein may be present in normal amounts (15 per cent of cases) or may be decreased (85 per cent of cases). C1 INH enzymatic activity is markedly diminished in all patients.

In the past, antifibrinolytic agents (epsilon-aminocaproic acid and tranexamic acid) were useful in reducing the number of attacks. More recently, two anabolic steroids (danazol and oxymetholone) have been shown to be highly effective in this regard. These drugs induce the synthesis of functional C1 INH in patients with either type of inhibitor abnormality. This phenomenon is of particular interest since it implies that other disorders of regulatory gene function may be amenable to pharmacologic intervention.

C1 INH deficiency with angioedema occurs also as an acquired disorder. In a recent review, 15 cases were reported in which secondary deficiency of C1 INH occurred as a complication of different underlying disorders, including lymphoreticular malignancies, systemic lupus erythematosus, autoimmune hemolytic anemia, and rectal carcinoma.

Clinical States Associated with Low Complement Levels. In infants, complement component concentrations and total complement activity are characteristically low relative to adult values. A number of diseases are associated with secondarily diminished complement levels (Table 22–6). Many are characterized by circulating immune complexes, and the magnitude of complement suppression in these conditions frequently is related to the activity of the primary disease state. In

Table 22–6. Clinical States Associated with Low Complement Levels

Newborn infancy
Collagen vascular disease
Serum sickness
Glomerulonephritis (variable)
Autoimmune hemolytic anemia
Endotoxic shock
Hepatitis B virus infection
Hemodialysis
Radiocontrast-induced anaphylaxis (variable)
Cirrhosis

yet other disorders (for example, severe liver disease) depressed complement levels reflect impaired synthesis of selective components.

PRIMARY DISORDERS OF THE B-LYMPHOCYTE SYSTEM

Antibody Deficiency Syndromes

The development of a specific antibody response requires the cooperation of several cell types. Macrophages process the antigen. T-lymphocytes recognize the antigen as "foreign" and program B-lymphocyte maturation to plasma cells. These synthesize and secrete antigen-specific immunoglobulin molecules. Impaired antibody responses may result from a defect in any of these elements but most often reflect a primary deficiency or dysfunction of the B-lymphocytes themselves (Table 22–7).

Generally, antibody deficiency is manifested by recurrent bacterial infections or chronic gastrointestinal tract complaints. These may begin at any age and may involve one or more of the immunoglobulin classes or subclasses. Quantitative serum immunoglobulin determinations are essential in suspected cases, since serum protein electrophoresis may not reveal a selective deficiency. Further, normal immunoglobulin levels do not necessarily indicate normal antibody function. To fully assess the competence of the B-cell system, measurement of functional antibody production must be undertaken.

Table 22–7. Lymphocyte Defects in Selected Primary Immune Deficiency Syndromes

	Affected Lymphocyte Populations		
	B-Cells	T-Cells	Mode of Inheritance
Disorders mainly affecting B-cells			
Congenital hypogammaglobulinemia (Bruton type)	Yes	No	X-linked
Congenital hypogammaglobulinemia	Yes	No	AR
Immunodeficiency with Hyper-IgM	Yes	No	X-linked
Common variable immunodeficiency	Yes	(Yes)*	?, Familial
IgA deficiency	Yes	No	Sporadic, AR, AD
IgM deficiency	Yes	No	Sporadic
IgG and IgG subclass deficiencies	Yes	No	Sporadic, AR
Disorders mainly affecting T-cells			
DiGeorge syndrome	No	Yes	Sporadic, familial
Chronic mucocutaneous candidiasis	No	Yes	Sporadic, AR
Combined B-cell and T-cell deficiencies			
Severe combined immunodeficiency	Yes	Yes	X-linked, AR
Immunodeficiency with abnormal immunoglobulins (Nezelof's syndrome)	Yes	Yes	Familial, X-linked, AR
Immunodeficiency with short-limbed dwarfism	Yes	Yes	AR
Immune Deficiency–Enzyme Deficiency Syndromes			
Ecto-5′-nucleotidase deficiency	Yes†	No	X-linked, AR, sporadic
Adenosine deaminase deficiency	Yes	Yes	AR
Nucleoside phosphorylase deficiency	No	Yes	AR
Biotin-dependent carboxylase deficiency	(Yes)	(Yes)	Sporadic
Complex Immunodeficiencies			
Wiskott-Aldrich syndrome	Yes	Yes	X-linked
Ataxia-Telangiectasia	(Yes)	Yes	AR
Immunodeficiency with thymoma	Yes	Yes	Sporadic
X-linked lymphoproliferative syndrome	(Yes)	(Yes)	X-linked
Acquired immunodeficiency syndrome	No	Yes	Sporadic

*Parentheses indicated that defect is variable or selective.
†Ecto-5′-nucleotidase is a marker for mature B-cells.
AR = autosomal recessive; ? = undetermined; AD = autosomal dominant.

① Administer antigens and see what happens.
Must use a new one though (he may have been immunozized earlier).

Immunizing agents used for this purpose include typhoid vaccine, pneumococcal vaccine, tetanus toxoid, keyhole-limpet hemocyanin, and bacteriophage ΦX-174. The Schick test employs intradermal injection of a small amount of diphtheria toxin. A local inflammatory reaction that evolves over two to five days indicates a lack of protective antidiphtheria antibodies. This test is a useful screening procedure for the presence of specific antibodies in individuals who have received routine immunizations.

At birth, infants are endowed with transplacentally acquired IgG, while serum IgA and IgM levels are markedly reduced relative to normal adult concentrations. During the first three to six months of life, serum IgG declines and thereafter increases, while IgA and IgM levels rise slowly from birth. Assessment of serum immunoglobulin levels in a child, without reference to age-adjusted normal values, may result in an inappropriate diagnosis of antibody deficiency.

CONGENITAL AGAMMAGLOBULINEMIA

Hypogammaglobulinemia was the first recognized immunodeficiency disease. The clinical manifestations of Bruton's initial case (Fig. 22–9) are typical of the illnesses that these patients experience. Although X-linked agammaglobulinemia (Bruton's type) is most frequently encountered, congenital immunoglobulin deficiency may occur sporadically or as an autosomal recessive trait.

Clinical Features. Typically, infants with this disorder do well during the first few months of life. Maternally acquired IgG provides adequate protection during this time. As maternal IgG is catabolized, the child begins to experience repeated infections. In exceptional cases, the condition may remain undetected for years.

Characteristic infections include otitis media, sinusitis, pneumonia, meningitis, and septicemia. An important clue to the diagnosis is a unique susceptibility to infection with encapsulated pyogenic organisms, including *S. pneumoniae, S. pyogenes, H. influenzae,* and *P. aeruginosa.* This phenomenon probably reflects a requirement for specific opsonization of these bacteria before efficient phagocytic cell ingestion is possible. Nonencapsulated organisms, mycobacteria, and fungi are not usually encountered as causes of infection in this clinical state.

Resistance to most viral infections (e.g., rubella, rubeola, and herpes), which gener-

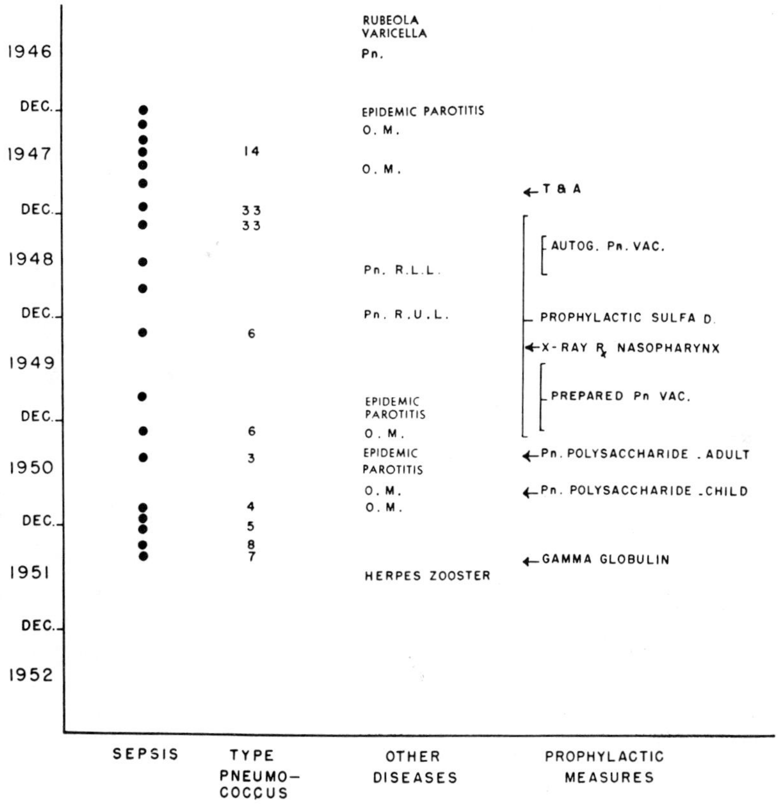

Figure 22–9. Chart published by Bruton showing his original observations of infection due to the same type of pneumococcus as in his case of agammaglobulinemia. (From Bruton, O. C.: Agammaglobulinemia. Pediatrics, *9*:722, 1952.)

Figure 22–10. Immunoelectrophoresis of serum. *Top,* Congenital agammaglobulinemia. Note complete absence of IgM, IgA, and IgG bands. *Bottom,* Normal serum showing normal amounts of IgM, IgA, and IgG. (Courtesy of Dr. Fred S. Rosen.)

ally depends upon intact T cell–mediated immunity, is usually normal. However, patients with congenital hypogammaglobulinemia are prone to viral central nervous system infections with the enteroviruses, and several patients have succumbed to chronic meningoencephalitis due to echoviruses or vaccine-related polioviruses.

Long-term pulmonary complications include the development of restrictive lung disease, cylindrical bronchiectasis, and (rarely) lymphoid interstitial pneumonitis. Gastrointestinal tract involvement is manifested by recurrent giardiasis, nodular lymphoid hyperplasia, and chronic malabsorption. Patients with immunoglobulin deficiency have an increased incidence of autoimmune disorders, including rheumatoid arthritis and dermatomyositis.

Physical findings are related to recurrent infection. Failure to thrive is common. Sparse lymphoid and tonsillar tissue is usual. Hearing loss may be associated with chronic ear disease. Signs and symptoms of bronchitis with obstructive or restrictive lung disease are often apparent.

Diagnosis. The diagnosis may be suggested by serum immunoelectrophoresis that reveals deficiency of one or more of the major immunoglobulin classes (Fig. 22–10). However, quantitation of serum immunoglobulin levels with radial immunodiffusion (Fig. 22–11) or kinetic nephelometry is the procedure of choice. In most instances, an IgG level of less than 200 mg per dl and depressed values for IgA, IgM, IgD, and IgE are apparent. IgA is absent from secretions, and specific antibody activity is undetectable.

Immunology. Most, but not all, patients with congenital hypogammaglobulinemia lack immunoglobulin-bearing (mature) B-lymphocytes. Lymphoid tissue, respiratory mucosa, and intestinal mucosa are devoid of plasma cells. It appears that these patients are deficient in the mammalian equivalent of the bursa of Fabricius, the organ responsible for B-cell maturation in the chicken. Recent studies confirm the presence of B-lymphocyte precursors in some patients with X-linked agammaglobulinemia, while in others suppression of the maturation process at later stages of differentiation seems likely.

Inborn errors in purine metabolism have been found in immunoglobulin deficiency (Fig. 22–12). Lymphocytes from patients with congenital agammaglobulinemia have reduced ecto-5′-nucleotidase activity when compared with normal lymphocytes. It is likely, however, that level of activity is a biochemical marker for mature B-lymphocytes, and that the deficiency seen in immunoglobulin deficiency syndromes is merely

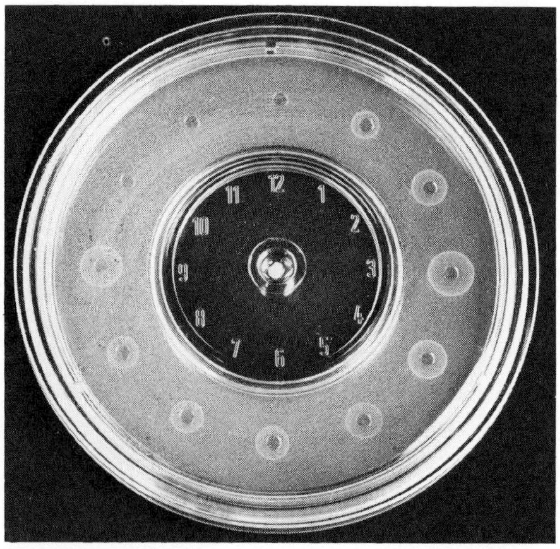

Figure 22–11. Radial immunodiffusion plate for IgG quantitation. Wells 1, 2, and 3 contain standard concentrations of IgG against which test sera are compared. Wells 10, 11, and 12 contain sera from patients with severe IgG deficiency.

PATHWAYS OF PURINE METABOLISM

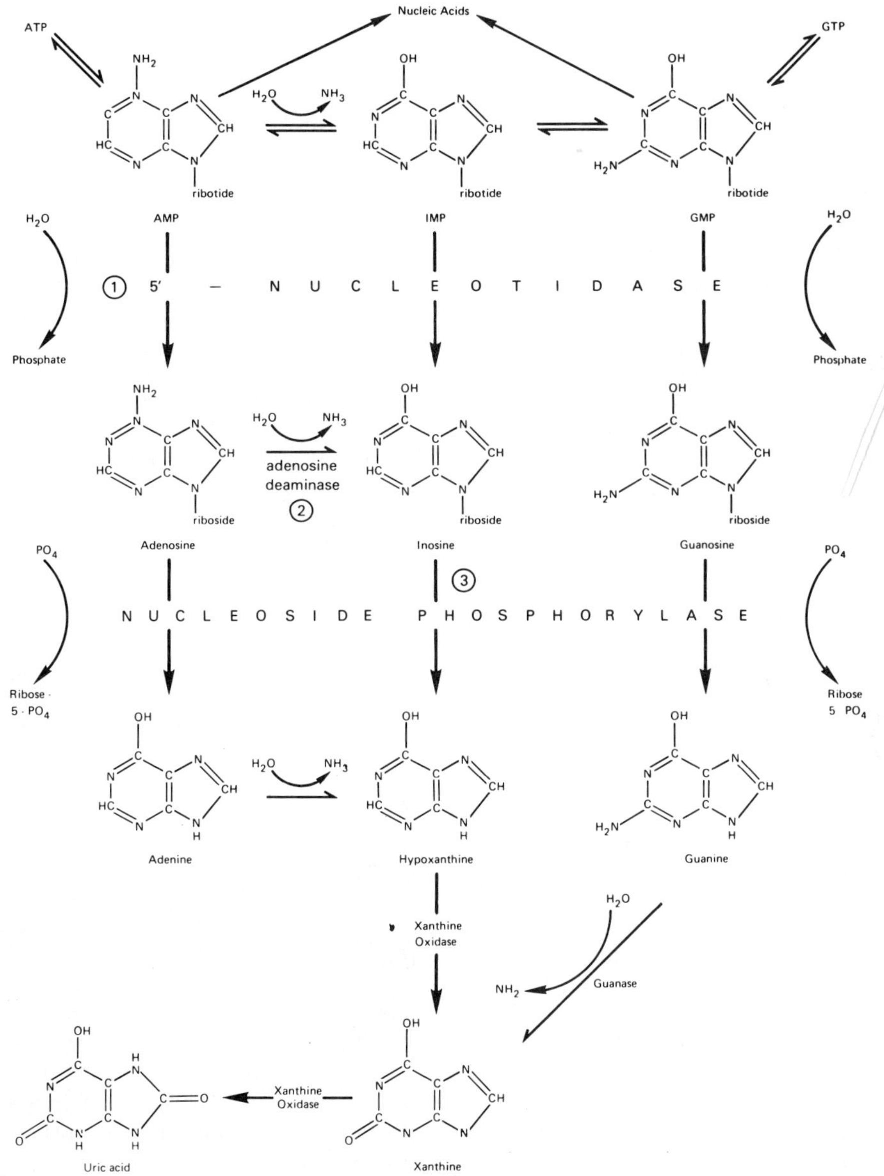

Figure 22–12. Pathways of purine catabolism in humans. Three immune deficiency syndromes have been associated with enzymatic defects in these pathways. ① Lymphocytes from patients with common variable immunodeficiency deficient in 5′-nucleotidase. ② Deficiency of adenosine deaminase occurs in some cases of combined immunodeficiency. ③ Nucleoside phosphorylase deficiency has been found in some patients with deficient T-cell functions.

secondary to the reduced number of B lymphocytes, rather than a cause of this condition.

Treatment. Replacement of circulating immunoglobulins may be accomplished with a variety of preparations. Immune serum globulin (0.6 ml per kg) may be injected intramuscularly or infused subcutaneously. As an alternative, intravenous infusion of compatible plasma (15 ml per kg) may be given. Hepatitis is a major risk of this procedure, but the risk can be minimized by using plasma from a limited number of regular volunteer donors. Very recently, an immune serum globulin has been modified for intravenous use by chemical reduction and alkylation and formulation of a 5 per cent solution in 10 per cent maltose. This preparation is available for clinical use and is administered over two to three hours in a dose of 2 ml per kg. As with any blood product that is infused intravenously, anaphylactoid reactions may complicate the procedure. All replacement preparations must be given every three to four weeks and the dosage modified by clinical assessment.

Unfortunately, none of these products replaces secretory immunoglobulin, so chronic respiratory or gastrointestinal symptoms may persist. The frequent or continuous use of antibiotics remains a major supportive measure in management. Importantly, live virus vaccines are contraindicated because they can result in fatal infections.

X-LINKED IMMUNODEFICIENCY WITH HYPER-IGM

This syndrome presents with recurrent pyogenic infections similar to those seen in congenital agammaglobulinemia. Neutropenia and autoimmune phenomena are more common complications in these patients. Laboratory investigation reveals decreased or absent serum IgG, IgA, and IgE but normal or elevated levels of IgM. T-lymphocytes are normal, and IgM-bearing B-cells are present. The defect appears to be intrinsic to B-cells that fail to switch from IgM to IgG synthesis.

TRANSIENT HYPOGAMMAGLOBULINEMIA OF INFANCY

This syndrome presents in early infancy with infections characteristic of antibody deficiency, but the diminished immunoglobulin levels eventually normalize by 12 to 36 months of age. Diminished IgG concentrations in the range of 150 to 300 mg per dl are found. Normal IgA and IgM concentrations and circulating T- and B-lymphocyte numbers are present. Recent studies indicate that a transient numerical and functional deficiency in helper T-cells underlies the diminished IgG production. Some children may require replacement therapy until severe infectious complications diminish.

ANTIBODY DEFICIENCY WITH NORMAL IMMUNOGLOBULINS

Rarely, antibody deficiency has been found to occur in the presence of normal or elevated immunoglobulin concentrations. Clinically, patients are indistinguishable from those with congenital immunoglobulin deficiencies. However, T- and B-lymphocyte numbers and serum immunoglobulin levels are normal. The diagnosis is documented by assessing antibody responses to various immunizing agents. Management of these patients follows the same basic principles as those outlined previously.

COMMON VARIABLE IMMUNODEFICIENCY (ACQUIRED HYPOGAMMAGLOBULINEMIA, ADULT-ONSET IMMUNODEFICIENCY)

These terms refer to a heterogeneous group of disorders that is characterized by the late development of recurrent pyogenic infections, decreased serum immunoglobulin levels, and variable T-cell dysfunction. Typically, sinopulmonary infections begin in the second or third decade, although patients may present before ten years of age. A sprue-like malabsorption syndrome often occurs that may be associated with giardiasis and hyperplasia of intestinal lymphoid tissue. A similar process may affect the lungs as lymphoid interstitial pneumonitis. A high degree of susceptibility to neoplasia, especially lymphoreticular malignancies and gastric carcinoma, has been noted.

Diagnosis. As in other forms of hypogammaglobulinemia, the diagnosis of common variable immunodeficiency is made by quantitation of serum immunoglobulins and antibody responses. As a rule, patients are deficient in all immunoglobulin classes, although levels may be higher than in the congenital deficiencies. We have observed three children with this disorder who maintained detectable isohemagglutinin titers despite repeated infections characteristic of severe antibody deficiency. T-cell function, as measured with delayed hypersensitivity skin tests and *in vitro* mitogen responses, is diminished in some patients.

Immunology. Most patients with common variable immunodeficiency have immunoglobulin-bearing B-cells in their blood and lymphoid tissue but lack mature plasma cells. In contrast to B-cells from normal subjects, patients' cells do not respond *in vitro* to stimulation with pokeweed mitogen or Epstein-Barr virus by secreting immunoglobulins. In most patients studied in this way, a primary defect in B-cell maturation has been demonstrated. However, this primary defect may be associated with other *in vitro* abnormalities. Some patients' T-cells provide inadequate helper function for normal B-cells; other patients' T-cells may actively suppress normal B-cell secretion of immunoglobulin. These observations suggest that abnormalities arise in the regulation of immunoglobulin synthesis as well as in the maturation of the B-lymphocyte population. Reports of familial occurrence indicate a genetic predisposition in some patients. It is clear from these studies that "common variable immunodeficiency" is not a single entity.

Treatment. Replacement therapy is indicated for patients experiencing repeated infections. The large doses of immune serum globulin or plasma that are required for treatment of adult patients make their management more difficult. Improved management awaits clarification of the primary causes of acquired B-cell dysfunction.

SELECTIVE IgA DEFICIENCY

This is the most common of the "dysgammaglobulinemias," a term applied when there are selective deficiencies of one or more, but not all, immunoglobulin classes. Estimates of the incidence of selective IgA deficiency range from 1 in 700 to 1 in 500. Many patients with this abnormality are completely asymptomatic, while others experience allergic disease, repeated infections, autoimmune phenomena, or an increased risk for neoplasm. IgA deficiency most often occurs sporadically but may be inherited as either an autosomal dominant or a recessive trait. It has been shown recently that many children with IgA deficiency have a transient defect that resolves over several years.

Clinical Features. Up to 50 per cent of affected patients have severe atopic disease, and the incidence of IgA deficiency in atopic subjects may be as high as 1 in 200. Further, transient IgA deficiency in children has been shown to predispose to the development of IgE-mediated allergy. IgA deficiency in the respiratory and intestinal tracts may allow absorption of intact allergenic proteins with subsequent stimulation of IgE production. In support of this, IgG antibodies to bovine proteins (cow's milk and cow, sheep, and goat serum) are often found in the serum of IgA-deficient subjects.

Sinusitis, pneumonia, and otitis media may complicate selective IgA deficiency. Gastrointestinal disturbances include chronic diarrhea, gluten-sensitive enteropathy, ulcerative colitis, regional enteritis, and giardiasis.

IgA deficiency has been associated with almost all of the major autoimmune diseases. Autoantibodies to a variety of antigens, including DNA, smooth muscle, mitochondria, and basement membrane, have been found in up to 50 per cent of patients. The incidence of IgA deficiency in systemic lupus erythematosus and rheumatoid arthritis (up to 1 in 100) seems too high to be merely coincidental.

Transfusion reactions of the anaphylactoid type are disturbingly common. It has been found that as many as 40 per cent of IgA-deficient patients have anti-IgA antibodies. Most of these patients have not received blood previously and are suspected of being sensitized as a consequence of breast feeding, absorption of bovine IgA, or inappropriate gamma globulin injections.

Diagnosis. The diagnosis is confirmed by demonstrating serum IgA levels of less than 5 mg per dl. Since IgA plays a major role in local immunity of the respiratory and gastrointestinal tracts, it is pertinent to measure IgA in respiratory secretions in some instances. A few cases have been described in which secretory IgA is present although serum IgA is diagnostically low. Conversely, at least two patients have been found who have had normal serum IgA levels but reduced IgA and secretory component in respiratory secretions.

Immunology. Previously, it was believed that selective IgA deficiency was not accompanied by abnormalities of T-cell function. Subsequent studies have revealed varying degrees of impaired T-cell function in some patients. These have included reduced total

T-cell numbers and reduced lymphocyte responses to T-cell mitogens. These findings suggest that selective IgA deficiency may reflect subtle T-cell dysfunction in these and other cases.

Most patients with IgA deficiency have B-lymphocytes with surface membrane α chains. *In vitro* stimulation of these cells, however, fails to induce secretion of IgA antibody. This indicates that in most patients with selective IgA deficiency, IgA B-cell maturation is arrested at an early stage of differentiation. The cause of this is unknown, although a few patients possess T-cells that suppress IgA synthesis *in vitro*.

Very recently, coexisting IgG2 deficiency has been found in some patients with symptomatic IgA deficiency but not in healthy subjects with IgA deficiency. The implication of this finding for the management of these patients remains to be determined.

Treatment. Immunoglobulin replacement therapy using current preparations is of no value in selective IgA deficiency. These contain little IgA, the serum half-life of infused IgA is brief (seven days), and IgA given parenterally does not enter into secretions. Further, the small amount of IgA in commercial immune serum globulin is sufficient to sensitize patients against IgA present in other blood products. Should the patient ever require such products, the likelihood of acute reaction is increased. When blood transfusions are required in an IgA-deficient patient, the likelihood of reactions can be minimized by the use of autologous frozen blood, blood from a matched IgA-deficient donor, or washed red blood cells.

Bacterial infections are treated with aggressive antibiotic therapy. Human colostrum, which is rich in secretory IgA, has been given orally to treat infectious complications of the gastrointestinal tract in selected individuals.

SELECTIVE IgM DEFICIENCY

This disorder has been defined as a serum IgM level of less than two standard deviations below the normal mean. The incidence of selective IgM deficiency using this criterion is 1 in 1000, making it the second most common selective immunoglobulin deficiency. However, many individuals so diagnosed have had serious underlying illnesses, which may have resulted in a secondary IgM deficiency. With a more conservative definition, a serum IgM level less than 20 mg per dl with normal IgG and IgA levels, selective IgM deficiency is a rare entity.

Clinically, IgM deficiency is manifested by recurrent infections, including sudden overwhelming sepsis. Other associated disorders include splenomegaly, atopy, and hemolytic anemia. The differential diagnosis includes Wiskott-Aldrich syndrome, in which IgM deficiency is a regular feature.

The cause of selective IgM deficiency is not known. Approximately half the patients studied have normal B-cells with surface μ heavy chains, while in others these cell numbers are reduced. In either case, the underlying defect appears to occur after the development of the other immunoglobulin-producing cell lines during fetal life.

Acute infections require prompt antibiotic therapy. The use of prophylactic plasma infusion for IgM replacement is limited by the short biologic half-life of infused IgM. However, plasma infusion for treatment of life-threatening infection may be useful.

SELECTIVE IgG DEFICIENCY

At least two children with this disorder have been reported. Both suffered from chronic pyogenic infections. Serum IgG concentrations were markedly reduced, while IgA and IgM levels were elevated. In one patient, *in vitro* lymphocyte study revealed two defects: a lack of IgG B-cell maturation and an IgG-specific T-suppressor cell. Treatment consists of immunoglobulin replacement therapy.

SELECTIVE IgG SUBCLASS DEFICIENCY

Deficiencies have been described in one or more of the four subclasses of IgG (IgG1, IgG2, IgG3, IgG4). These patients have repeated infections of the lung, ears, and upper respiratory tract caused by encapsulated bacterial pathogens such as *S. pneumoniae* and *H. influenzae*. Selective IgG4 deficiency has been associated with this clinical picture, although a significant number of asymptomatic individuals also appear to lack this particular IgG subclass. Satisfactory responses to immunoglobulin replacement have been noted in selected cases.

ANTIBODY DEFICIENCY WITH TRANSCOBALAMIN II DEFICIENCY

Transcobalamin II is a serum protein involved in the transport of vitamin B_{12} (cobalamin). Deficiency of transcobalamin II is an autosomal recessive disorder characterized by failure to thrive, diarrhea, megaloblastic anemia, and agammaglobulinemia. Vitamin B_{12} levels, phagocytic cell functions, and T-lymphocyte functions are normal. Treatment with high doses of vitamin B_{12} results in complete clinical and immunologic recovery.

SECONDARY ANTIBODY DEFICIENCIES

Diminished immunoglobulin levels and antibody activities may occur as complications of other clinical states (Table 22–8). For example, immunoglobulin loss may occur through the gastrointestinal and urinary tracts as a result of increased membrane permeability. Surgical or functional splenectomy results in decreased serum IgM levels. In multiple myeloma, mononuclear phagocytic cells actively suppress nonmyeloma immunoglobulin synthesis. IgA deficiency may result from enhancement of T-suppressor function by phenytoin (Dilantin). D-penicillamine therapy and protein calorie malnutrition both can cause low IgA levels in serum and secretions. Severe immunoglobulin deficiency has been noted in patients with congenital rubella, although high titers of anti–rubella virus antibody are more common.

In all of these conditions, the secondary antibody deficiency may result in frequent or overwhelming infections.

PRIMARY DISORDERS IN T-LYMPHOCYTE–DEPENDENT IMMUNITY

Patients having defective T-cell function may not have an accompanying antibody deficiency. This is somewhat unexpected, since optimal antibody responses by B-cells generally depend upon normal T-cell cooperation. Despite this, several selective T-cell deficiencies have been described.

Table 22–8. States Associated with Secondary Antibody Deficiency

Protein-losing enteropathy
Nephrotic syndrome
Splenectomy
Multiple myeloma
Phenytoin administration
D-Penicillamine administration
Congenital rubella

In contrast to the encapsulated bacterial pathogens commonly seen in antibody-deficiency states, viruses such as cytomegalovirus, fungi such as *Candida albicans,* and *Pneumocystis carinii* characteristically infect patients with cellular immunodeficiency. In addition, these patients are susceptible to fatal complications of live virus or bacterial vaccines and to the development of graft-versus-host disease following blood product transfusion.

THE DIGEORGE SYNDROME (III–IV PHARYNGEAL POUCH SYNDROME)

In the fully expressed form, this disorder is characterized by neonatal hypocalcemia with tetany, congenital abnormalities of the aortic arches and heart, and absence or hypoplasia of the thymus. Cardiac lesions include interrupted aortic arch, truncus arteriosus, and tetralogy of Fallot. Additional congenital defects affecting facial and midline structures include low-set, notched, or folded ears; hypertelorism; anti-mongoloid slant to the eyes; a small, fish-like mouth; and absent philtrum. Although DiGeorge syndrome generally arises sporadically, familial occurrences have been reported.

Clinical Features. Most patients present with intractable hypocalcemia or severe cardiac disease in the first few weeks of life. The classic facial appearance is not always apparent at birth but may develop in time (Fig. 22–13). The clinical expression of immune

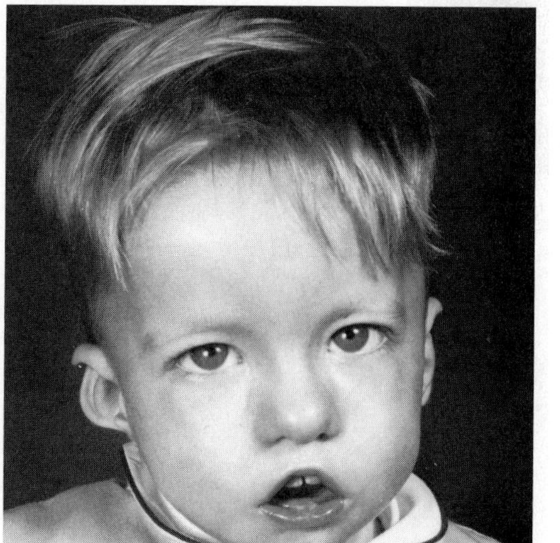

Figure 22–13. A child with DiGeorge syndrome. Note the dysplasia of the ears and mouth and the hypertelorism. (Courtesy of Dr. Fred S. Rosen; from Kretschmer, R., et al.: Congenital aplasia of the thymus gland. N. Engl. J. Med., *279*:1295, 1968.)

deficiency is similar to that of other syndromes with subnormal T-cell function and includes failure to thrive, resistant oral candidiasis, and chronic diarrhea. Interstitial pneumonia, exfoliative dermatitis, and cutaneous candidiasis have also been noted. The prognosis depends largely on the severity of the cardiovascular malformation or the hypocalcemia.

Diagnosis. Diagnosis of the complete form of DiGeorge syndrome requires demonstration of hypoparathyroidism with depressed parathormone levels and hypocalcemia, along with congenital heart disease and diminished T-cell immunity. The latter is manifested by T-lymphopenia and deficient *in vitro* responses to mitogens and antigens. B-lymphocyte responses are difficult to measure in young infants and, rarely, may be abnormal. Sequential study has revealed that spontaneous resolution of the immune deficiency occurs in some patients, while progressive loss of immune function is seen in others. Complete immunologic evaluation and close monitoring are clearly indicated in suspected cases.

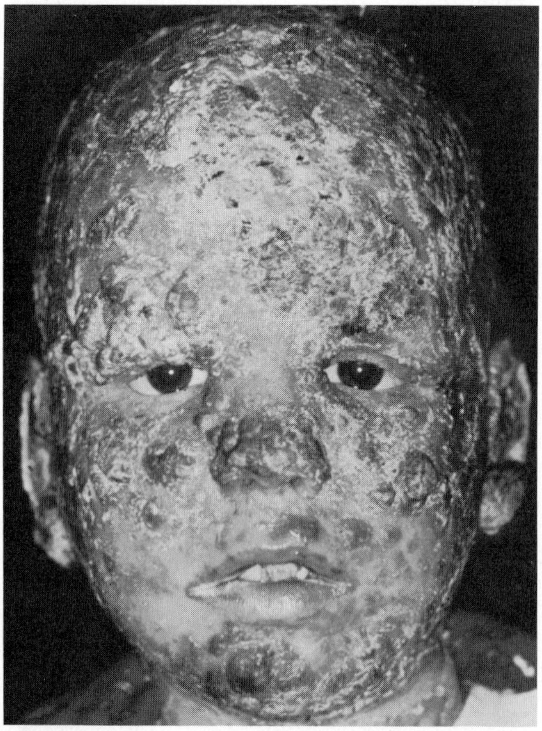

Figure 22–14. A nine-year-old boy with chronic mucocutaneous candidiasis who was found to be deficient in cell-mediated immunity. (From Schlegel, R. J., et al.: Severe candidiasis associated with thymic dysplasia, IgA deficiency, and plasma antilymphocyte effects. Pediatrics, *45*:926, 1970.)

Immunology. The DiGeorge syndrome results from abnormal embryogenesis of the pharyngeal pouches during the sixth to tenth weeks of gestation. The recent association of DiGeorge syndrome with partial monosomy of chromosome 22 indicates that at least some cases may arise from specific chromosomal deletions. Immunologic manifestations vary. The degree of thymic hypoplasia is known to differ from one patient to another; humoral factors that induce cell maturation might be passed transplacentally from mother to fetus; and thymic atrophy or hypertrophy might occur after birth. The latter two possibilities have not been documented definitely, so that much remains to be learned about the pathogenesis of this syndrome.

Treatment. Management of the immunologic aspects of DiGeorge syndrome is complicated by the spontaneous recovery of T-cell function that some patients experience. In cases in which recovery is unlikely, fetal thymus transplantation (either as free fragments or enclosed in a Millipore chamber) is recommended. Other measures that have met with limited success include injections of thymosin and transplantation of cultured thymic epithelium.

CHRONIC MUCOCUTANEOUS CANDIDIASIS (CMC)

Chronic mucocutaneous candidiasis is a selective cellular immunodeficiency characterized by chronic infections of the skin, nails, and mucous membranes with *Candida* species, usually *C. albicans.* The presentation varies, and CMC is sometimes associated with endocrinopathies. Although it most often occurs sporadically, autosomal recessive forms of the syndrome have been reported.

Clinical Features. Severe cases present with persistent thrush or diaper rash during the first month of life. Typically, the infection spreads from the perineal and circumoral areas over the extremities, scalp, and face, usually involving fingernails and toenails. Candidal laryngitis and esophagitis are common, yet there is little predisposition to other parenchymal involvement. *Candida* is readily cultured from infected sites.

Chronic *Candida* infection may be seen in patients with more extensive immunologic compromise. For example, severe candidiasis has been noted in a patient with IgA deficiency and impaired cell-mediated immunity (Fig. 22–14). In another patient with generalized T-cell dysfunction, mucocutaneous candidiasis and severe interstitial pneumonia were noted. These patients should not be considered to have CMC, but more severe immunologic compromise. CMC may present later in life but then is usually mild and often limited to the nails or buccal mucosa.

Endocrine dysfunction appears at any age, although it usually begins during childhood. Endocrinopathy, usually hypothyroidism, may affect 50 per cent of patients with the severe, early-onset form of CMC. Other glands affected include the adrenals, parathyroids, and gonads.

Immunology. Chronic mucocutaneous candidiasis represents a highly specific disorder of T-cell function. Overall, T-cell numbers and their responses to nonspecific mitogens are normal. In contrast, the cells of affected patients fail to respond to *Candida* antigens when studied by proliferation or lymphokine assays. Delayed hypersensitivity skin tests to *Candida* are negative, and tests using other antigens are variable. *Candida* responses do not develop even when the primary infection is controlled, indicating that the T-cell defect is primary and not caused by the presence of chronic infection.

Immunoglobulin concentrations and antibody responses to *Candida* antigens are normal or high. Similarly, granulocyte candidacidal activities are normal while defective monocyte killing of *Candida* organisms is seen in some patients.

Patients with endocrinopathy often have serum antibodies that react with a variety of endocrine tissues. To explain the association of CMC with endocrinopathy, it has been proposed that this disorder reflects a generalized autoimmune process affecting all endocrine glands, including the thymus. Alternatively, a subtle, primary defect of thymic function could result in a predisposition to fungal infections and the emergence of autoimmune disease.

Previously, amphotericin B was the only effective antifungal agent for the treatment of severe *Candida* infection. Nephrotoxicity associated with the use of this drug stimulated the search for effective modes of immunologic enhancement. Transfer factor and leukocyte transfusions were tried, with variable success. Topical therapy with nystatin and gentian violet, while helpful, does not control severe infections. The development of imidazole derivatives for topical and oral use has altered the management of chronic mucocutaneous candidiasis dramatically. One drug in particular, ketoconazole, is relatively nontoxic, orally absorbed, and highly effective in the treatment of chronic mucocutaneous candidiasis caused by *C. albicans*. Control of infection is rapid and often complete. Administration must be continued indefinitely, since relapses occur shortly after the drug is stopped.

COMBINED ANTIBODY (B-CELL) AND CELL-MEDIATED (T-CELL) IMMUNE DEFICIENCIES

The combined immune deficiency diseases form a heterogeneous group of disorders in which the common feature is abnormal function of B- and T-lymphocyte systems. These give rise to severe symptoms during early infancy with increased susceptibility to a broad spectrum of infectious agents.

RETICULAR DYSGENESIS

In this rare congenital condition there is a failure of differentiation of an early hematopoietic stem cell. Reticular dysgenesis has been fatal in all reported cases, most patients dying in the first three weeks of life. Bone marrow transplantation from an appropriately matched donor should cure the condition if accomplished soon after birth.

SEVERE COMBINED IMMUNODEFICIENCY (SCID)

The conditions discussed under this designation share the common features of severely impaired T- and B-cell function. Severe combined immunodeficiency occurs in X-linked recessive, autosomal recessive, and sporadic forms.

Clinical Features. Initial clinical findings often reflect the T-cell abnormalities, since newborn infants are protected in part by maternal IgG. Often the first infection is resistant oral candidiasis. Patients are also highly susceptible to sepsis and pneumonia. Infections are caused by viruses such as cytomegalovirus and parainfluenza virus, by low-grade pathogenic bacteria, or by *Pneumocystis carinii*. Failure to thrive, chronic diarrhea, and sparse lymphoid tissue are regular findings.

A clinical picture similar to that found in infantile histiocytosis X has been noted in some SCID patients. These children present

15% under immuno suppression get it

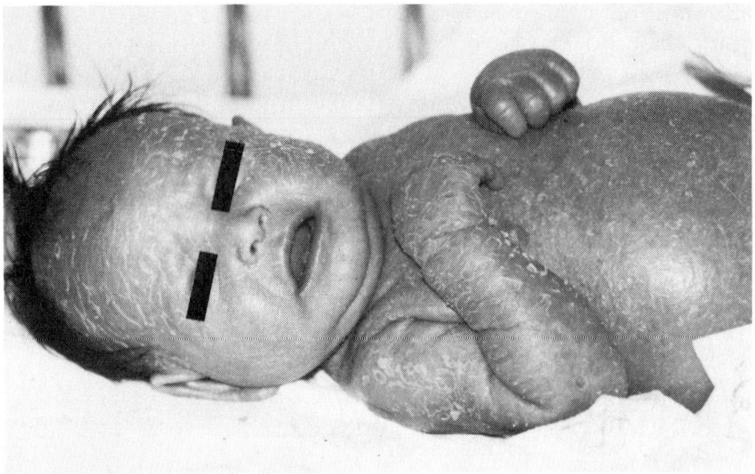

Figure 22–15. An infant with severe combined immune deficiency. Note generalized exfoliative dermatitis and abdominal organomegaly.

with exfoliative dermatitis, hepatosplenomegaly, lymphadenopathy, and wasting during the first few weeks of life (Fig. 22–15). Serum IgE levels are sometimes markedly elevated, although other immunoglobulin concentrations are diminished. Graft-versus-host disease secondary to engraftment of maternal lymphocytes has been proposed as a possible mechanism for this process.

Diagnosis. Lymphopenia with reduced B- and T-cell numbers is common but not invariable. Immunoglobulin concentrations may appear adequate because maternal IgG is present and serum IgA and IgM are low in normal infants under six months of age. However, peripheral blood lymphocytes fail to respond to mitogens or allogeneic cells in proliferation or lymphokine assays, and specific antibody responses do not develop. The thymus, in contrast to that of normal subjects (Fig. 22–16), shows poor differentiation and no Hassall's corpuscles (Fig. 22–17).

Immunology. There are several different causes of severe combined immunodeficiency. Severe thymic dysplasia is a constant feature of the disease, and direct demonstration of thymic dysfunction has been made in some patients. However, thymus transplantation has often failed to correct the deficiency. A defect in the generation of lymphoid stem cells has been postulated and is supported by reports of successful reconstitution of immune functions with stem cell grafts from fetal liver and bone marrow. Intrinsic lymphocyte defects (e.g., due to abnormalities in calcium transport) may result in severe combined immunodeficiency.

Treatment. The goal of treatment is complete reconstitution of immune function. Transfer factor and thymic hormones have been given to some patients, with limited success. Similarly, results have been inconsistent with transplantation of fetal liver, fetal thymus, and cultured thymic epithelium. Bone marrow transplantation from genotypically matched donors is most likely to affect long-term therapeutic success (Table 22–9). Unfortunately, the risk of graft-versus-host disease, even with apparently ideal matches, is high, and matched donors are often not available. Current efforts, utilizing monoclonal antibodies, are directed toward eliminating the cells in donor bone marrow that cause graft-versus-host disease while retaining those that reconstitute immune functions.

CELLULAR IMMUNODEFICIENCY WITH ABNORMAL IMMUNOGLOBULINS (NEZELOF'S SYNDROME)

This is a variant form of combined immune deficiency in which T-cell and antibody functions are abnormal but immunoglobulins are present. Normal concentrations of all immunoglobulin classes are seen in some patients, while selective immunoglobulin deficiencies are apparent in others. In most cases, there is poor antigen-specific antibody production. The mode of inheritance of Nezelof's syndrome may be autosomal recessive, X-linked recessive, undefined familial, or sporadic.

Clinical Features. Failure to thrive, pulmonary infection, oral or cutaneous candidiasis, and chronic diarrhea are common. The onset of symptoms may be gradual, and prolonged survival without specific therpeutic intervention is sometimes seen.

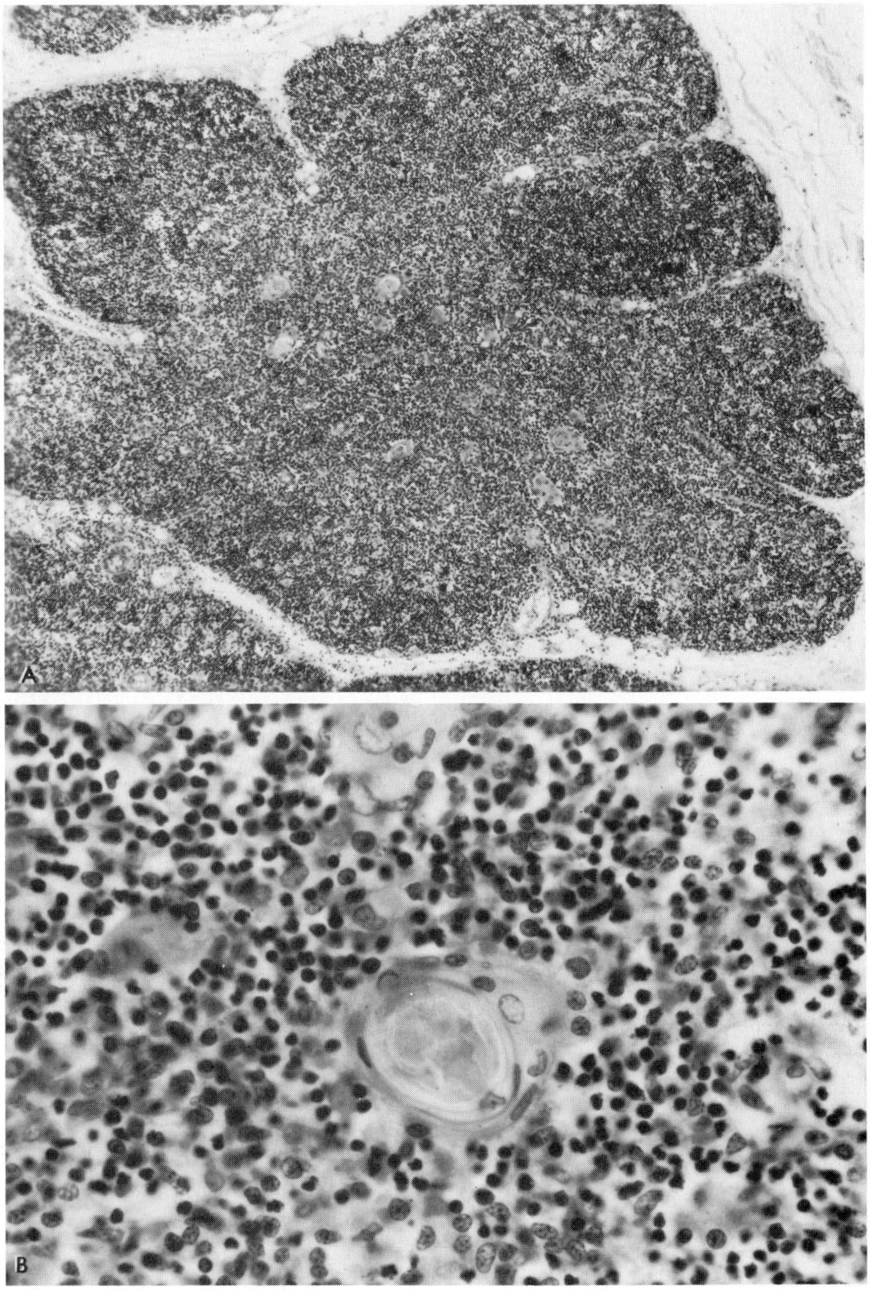

Figure 22–16. Histology of a normal thymus. *A,* Note the clearly defined structure of the thymus gland with numerous Hassall's corpuscles and the clear delineation of cortex and medulla of thymic lobules. *B,* A higher magnification of the thymus gland showing a Hassall's corpuscle.

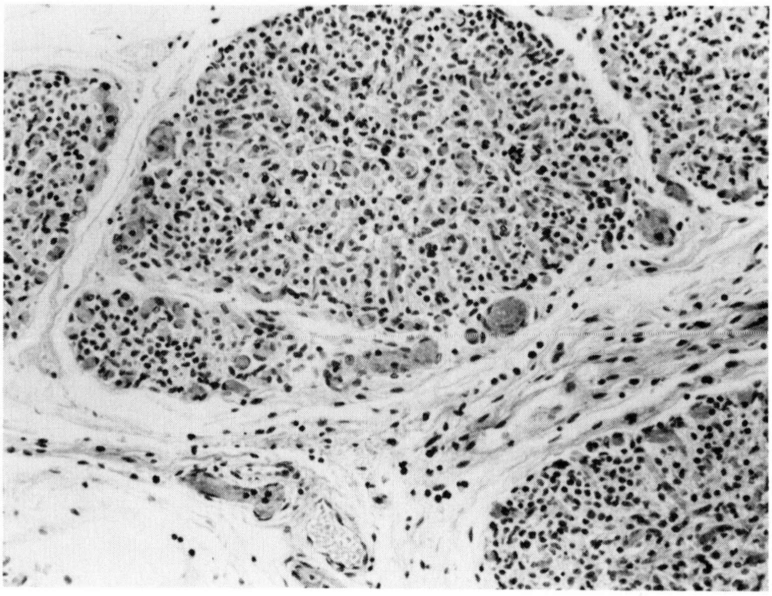

Figure 22–17. Histology of the thymus gland from a child with severe combined immune deficiency. The gland is fibrotic and lacks Hassall's corpuscles and a normal lymphocyte population.

Diagnosis. Depressed T-cell numbers and impaired T cell–mediated immune responses are found. Although quantitative immunoglobulin deficiency is not always apparent, specific antibody responses are often defective.

Treatment. Aggressive antibiotic therapy and immunoglobulin replacement are indicated. Bone marrow or thymus transplantation has benefited some patients.

IMMUNODEFICIENCY WITH SHORT-LIMBED DWARFISM

The immunodeficiency in this syndrome is variable. Most affected patients (90 per cent) have a selective deficiency of T-cell immunity. Others have selective antibody deficiency or combined immunodeficiency. The disorder is inherited as an autosomal recessive trait. Cartilage-hair hypoplasia is a variant of short-limbed dwarfism in which T-cell dysfunction is progressive. Susceptibility to viral infections, especially varicella, is common.

Clinical Features. Patients have short stature, pudgy hands and feet, redundant skin folds over the extremities and neck, and short arms and legs. In contrast to some other syndromes of dwarfism, the head size is normal. X-rays show irregular, scalloped metaphyseal ends of the long bones. In cartilage-hair hypoplasia, the hair is fine, is light-colored, and lacks a central pigmented core.

Infants with combined immune deficiency may succumb to early overwhelming infection. For most patients, however, the prognosis is better than for other severe T-cell deficiencies, and many survive into the fourth or fifth decade.

Immunology. T-cell immunity is diminished as evidenced by decreased peripheral blood T-cell numbers; impaired lymphocyte proliferative responses to mitogens, antigens, and allogeneic cells; and cutaneous anergy. T-cell functions deteriorate further over time. Immunoglobulin levels and antibody responses are usually normal, but abnormalities have been noted in a few patients.

Table 22–9. **Results of Reconstitutive Therapy of SCID**

Histocompatibility Group	Number of Patients	Survivors: 6 Months	Moderate or Severe GVH Disease*
Genotypic identity of HLA-A, HLA-B, and HLA-D	16	10 (63%)	5/14
Identity at HLA-D; HLA-A and HLA-B are either identical or nonidentical	13	5 (38%)	6/11
Nonidentity at HLA-D; HLA-A and HLA-B are either identical or nonidentical	19	1 (5%)	7/10
Fetal tissues (liver or thymus)	21	9 (21%)	4/13

*Not every patient could be scored for GVH. Data from Bortin, M. M. and Rihm, A. A.: JAMA *238*:591, 1977.

Further, some patients experience chronic neutropenia with maturational arrest of granulocyte precursors.

Treatment. The approach to the treatment of an individual patient is dependent upon the extent of immune dysfunction and the clinical course.

IMMUNODEFICIENCY–ENZYME DEFICIENCY SYNDROME

Deficiencies of either B- or T-lymphocyte systems and combined immune deficiencies have been associated with biochemical abnormalities. Most often these involve enzymes in purine nucleotide metabolism (see Fig. 22–12). The clinical features resemble those previously described for B- and T-cell disorder having other causes. It is important to differentiate these inborn errors of metabolism from the other causes of immune dysfunction because alternative modes of treatment may be useful and prenatal diagnosis is particularly reliable.

ADENOSINE DEAMINASE (ADA) DEFICIENCY

The immune defect caused by ADA deficiency affects both T- and B-lymphocyte functions. It is inherited as an autosomal recessive trait.

Clinical Features. Some infants present in the first weeks of life with the infections typically associated with immune deficiency. Others are seen after several months as their immunologic functions show progressive deterioration. A peculiar chondro-osseous dysplasia may be seen on x-ray as flaring and cupping of the costochondral junctions of the ribs. Severe lymphopenia is a common finding.

Diagnosis. Low levels of red blood cell and lymphocyte adenosine deaminase activity are diagnostic. Fibroblasts cultured from amniotic fluid may be studied for prenatal diagnosis.

Immunology. Unlike other causes of severe immunodeficiency, ADA deficiency does not result from a primary defect in thymic function or lymphocyte differentiation. The inability to catabolize adenosine results in the accumulation of adenosine metabolites, most notably deoxyadenosine. Deoxyadenosine is markedly toxic to lymphocytes, T-lymphoblasts being killed by lower concentrations than are B-lymphoblasts. The selective nature of this toxicity is reflected in the marked depletion of lymphocytes in blood and peripheral lymphoid tissue (Fig. 22–18) while other tissues are generally intact.

Treatment. Adenosine deaminase deficiency may be partially corrected with repeated transfusions of irradiated red blood cells, a rich source of adenosine deaminase. Although not uniformly effective, this treatment may allow clinical stabilization while definitive measures are undertaken. Bone marrow transplantation provides lymphoid stem cells and partially corrects the metabolic defect. In successfully transplanted patients,

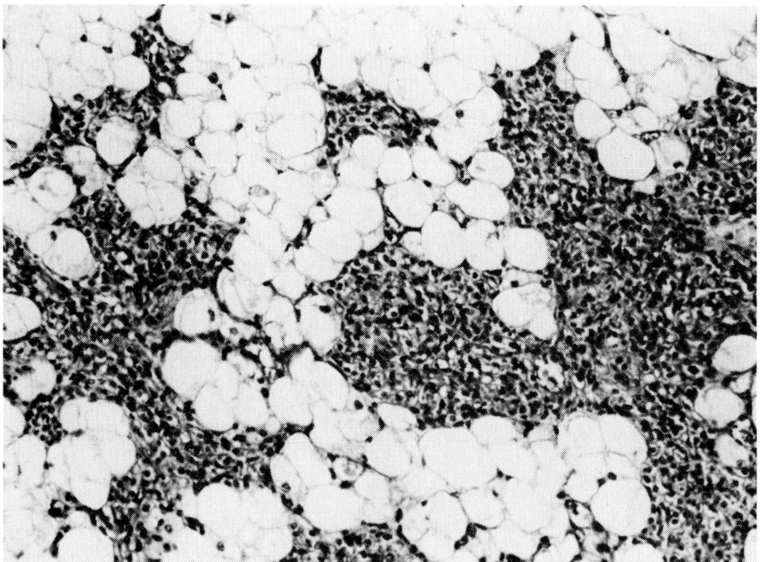

Figure 22–18. Histology of the thymus gland from a patient with adenosine deaminase deficiency. Fatty degeneration has taken place. Lymphocytes are absent, and the only cellular elements are epithelioid cells and macrophages.

abnormal adenosine metabolites are reduced (although not to normal levels) and immune functions are significantly improved.

NUCLEOSIDE PHOSPHORYLASE DEFICIENCY

Deficiency of the enzyme purine nucleoside phosphorylase (NP) causes a severe, selective T-lymphocyte dysfunction. Autosomal recessive inheritance has been shown in several families.

Clinical Features. Children having nucleoside phosphorylase deficiency may present later than those with combined immunodeficiency, and at least one affected child has been asymptomatic. All patients studied have had a severe lymphopenia and defective cell-mediated immunity. Recurrent infections and diarrhea are common, and autoimmune hemolytic anemia is seen in some children.

Diagnosis. Red blood cell and lymphocyte nucleoside phosphorylase activity is markedly diminished. Prenatal diagnosis is possible by measuring cultured fibroblast enzyme activity.

Immunology. Accumulation of the nucleoside phosphorylase substrate deoxyguanosine may play a major role in the pathogenesis of the clinical syndrome. This is analogous to the role proposed for deoxyadenosine in patients with ADA deficiency. In tissue culture, T-lymphoblasts are extremely sensitive to deoxyguanosine, while B-lymphoblasts are relatively resistant. This may explain the selective loss of T-cell function in these patients.

Treatment. In some patients, erythrocyte infusions have been used as enzyme replacement therapy, with improvement in biochemical and immunologic status. Bone marrow transplantation is the treatment of choice.

BIOTIN-DEPENDENT CARBOXYLASE DEFICIENCY

Biotin-responsive multiple carboxylase deficiency has been associated with variable defects in T-cell and B-cell immunity.

Clinical Features. Biotin deficiency presents in early infancy with alopecia, rash, keratoconjunctivitis, hypotonia, and metabolic acidosis. Seizures, developmental regression, *Candida* dermatitis, and pneumonia also have been seen in some instances.

Immunology. The immune deficiency is variable, and some patients with biotin deficiency have normal immune functions. In others, selective IgA deficiency, poor responses to pneumococcal vaccine, absent skin test reactions, and diminished *in vitro* T-cell studies have been measured. Recent *in vitro* studies indicate that biotin is essential for the development of normal cytotoxic T-cell responses.

Diagnosis. The condition is characterized by an abnormal urine amino acid pattern and restoration of normal clinical and metabolic findings following dietary biotin supplementation.

Treatment. Oral biotin, 10 mg per day, is the recommended treatment.

COMPLEX IMMUNE DEFICIENCIES

WISKOTT-ALDRICH SYNDROME (WAS)

An X-linked disorder, WAS is characterized by thrombocytopenia with bleeding, eczema, and immunodeficiency with recurrent infections.

Clinical Features. Petechiae or bleeding episodes occur within the first six months of life. Eczema appears within the first year and is indistinguishable from typical atopic eczema (Fig. 22–19). Chronic otitis media with draining ears and pneumonia then develop. Patients are also susceptible to herpes simplex, cytomegalovirus, *Pneumocystis carinii*, and varicella virus infections. Nephropathy has been noted in several patients and may be accentuated by transfer factor therapy. Malignancy develops in over 10 per cent of the cases, and the overall risk for this complication is greater than 100 times that of the general population. Lymphoreticular tumors and leukemias account for over 80 per cent of the cancers in WAS. Variant forms of this syndrome have been noted, and recurrent infections or eczema may not be present in every case.

Diagnosis. The disease is recognized as the triad of thrombocytopenia, eczema, and recurring infection in a male child. Serum immunoglobulin determinations disclose low IgM, normal or elevated IgA and IgG, and markedly elevated IgE. Specific antibody responses to polysaccharide antigens, such as blood group substances and bacterial capsular antigens, are poor. Thus, patients have low isohemagglutinin titers and markedly diminished responses to immunizations with

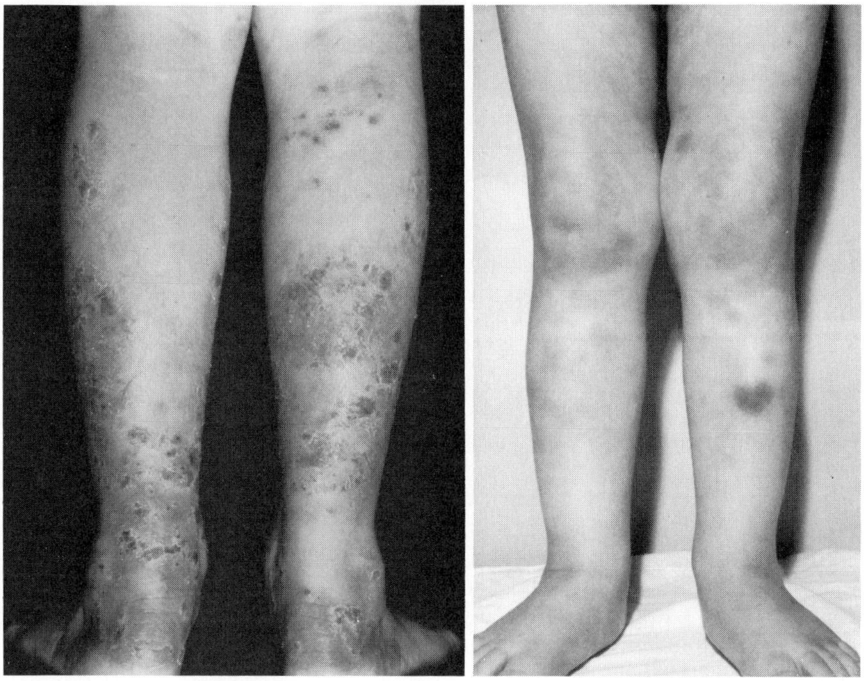

Figure 22–19. Wiskott-Aldrich syndrome. *A,* Eczematoid lesions in a four-year-old boy. *B,* Purpuric lesions in a six-year-old boy.

agents such as pneumococcal vaccine. In contrast, antibody responses to protein antigens are generally normal.

Abnormal cell-mediated immune responses have been noted in some patients. Absolute T-lymphocyte number and proliferative responses to antigens and allogeneic cells may be reduced, while similar assays employing phytohemagglutinin are normal. Cutaneous anergy is common. Young patients may have normal immunoglobulin levels and T-cell functions that show attrition with advancing age.

Small platelet size, half-normal, is found almost exclusively in the thrombocytopenia of WAS and may be helpful in early diagnosis. Other hematologic abnormalities include anemia, eosinophilia, and progressive lymphopenia.

The carrier state of WAS has been detected by measurement of platelet agglutination following metabolic stress induced with 2-deoxy-D-glucose, an inhibitor of glycolysis.

Immunology. The mechanism underlying this complex immune deficiency has not been defined. Hypercatabolism contributes to the low levels of immunoglobulins, but the cause of this is unknown. The inability to respond to polysaccharide antigens focused attention on the macrophage at one time, but investigations of mononuclear phagocytic cell function have been unrewarding.

Recent studies have revealed cell membrane glycoprotein abnormalities in patients with WAS. From these findings, it has been suggested that the absence of specific glycoproteins in both T-cells and platelets might be the primary defect in this disorder.

Treatment. The eczema in WAS responds to topical steroid therapy and local skin care. Severe thrombocytopenia may require platelet transfusions, but corticosteroids should be avoided, as they will enhance the susceptibility to infection. Splenectomy corrects the thrombocytopenia and normalizes platelet size. Splenectomy also markedly increases the risk of overwhelming septicemia. If this procedure is required, continuous administration of prophylactic antibiotics is indicated.

Treatment of the immunodeficiency yields less predictable results. Transfer factor has been used in a number of patients, and subjective improvement has been observed in approximately 50 per cent. Conversion of immunologic reactivity is correlated with clinical benefit and prolonged survival. A few patients have received bone marrow transplants, with long-lasting benefits.

ATAXIA-TELANGIECTASIA (AT)

This autosomal recessive syndrome is characterized by progressive cerebellar ataxia, ocular and cutaneous telangiectasia, chronic sinopulmonary infection, endocrine abnormalities, and a predisposition to malignancy.

Clinical Features. Ataxia usually begins in early childhood and progresses to incapacitation by adolescence. Mentation is normal early on, but development reaches a plateau at about ten years. Telangiectasia initially involving the bulbar conjunctivae (Fig. 22–20) develops within the first few years and may progress to affect other tissues. Repeated infection occurs in the lungs and sinuses and is caused by both bacterial and viral agents. During adolescence, endocrine abnormalities, including growth failure, gonadal hypoplasia, and insulin-dependent diabetes, may develop. Patients with AT have a marked predilection to develop malignancies, especially lymphoma and acute lymphocytic leukemia, and over 10 per cent die of cancer.

Diagnosis. Varying degrees of immunodeficiency are seen. T-cell number and mitogen responses may be normal initially and then diminish with advancing age. Serum IgA is absent in approximately one half of patients, and IgE deficiency is very common. Recent evidence points to a high incidence of immunoglobulin subclass deficiencies in AT. Undetectable or low IgG2 or IgG4 levels are often seen, and IgA2 deficiency is usually found in patients when IgA is present at all. Defects in neutrophil chemotaxis have also been reported.

Immunology. The underlying cause of AT is not known. There seems to be a primary defect in tissue differentiation, since elevated serum concentrations of alpha-fetoprotein and carcinoembryonic antigen are present. Complement-dependent cytotoxic antibodies to brain and thymus tissue have been described recently in affected patients, suggesting that autoimmune phenomena may play a role in the pathogenesis of this complex condition. Cells from ataxia-telangiectasia patients are extremely sensitive to radiation; an abnormal number of chromosome breaks occur when these cells are exposed to *in vitro* radiation, raising the possibility that a defect in DNA repair is the underlying cause.

Treatment. Thymus transplantation, thymosin, and transfer factor have been used, with little evidence of sustained success. Recurrent infection may result as much from IgG subclass deficiency as from IgA deficiency, and immune serum globulin replacement may be helpful.

IMMUNODEFICIENCY WITH THYMOMA (GOOD'S SYNDROME)

This is a combined B- and T-cell immunodeficiency state that is associated with a primary benign or malignant thymic tumor. Patients are over 40 years of age and the male-to-female ratio is 1:2. Complications include sinopulmonary infections, septicemia, urinary tract infections, chronic diarrhea, dermatitis, and aplastic anemia. Panhypogammaglobulinemia and deficient cell-mediated immunity are found in most patients.

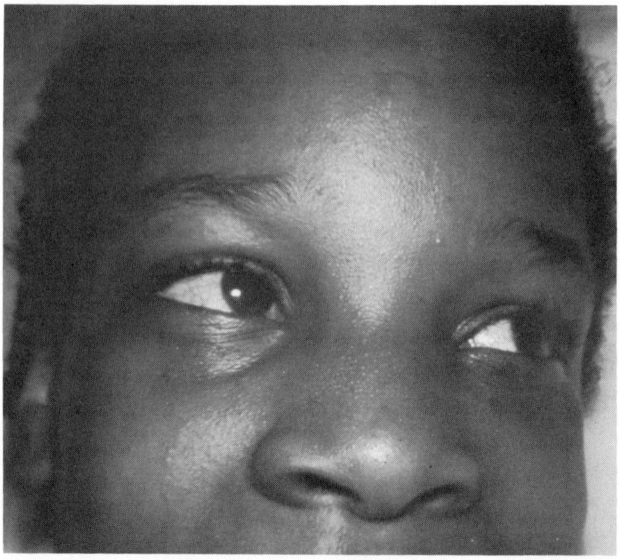

Figure 22–20. A 12-year-old girl with ataxia-telangiectasia, showing the ocular telangiectasia of the conjunctivae. (Courtesy of Dr. Sanford Leiken.)

Removal of the thymoma does not improve the immunodeficiency. Therapy is directed at the primary tumor and immunoglobulin deficiency, but the prognosis is poor.

X-LINKED LYMPHOPROLIFERATIVE SYNDROME (XLP)

Initially reported in six boys from a single family (the Ducan kindred), XLP is characterized by immune deficiency, particularly to Epstein-Barr virus (EBV), and a susceptibility to fatal infectious mononucleosis, acquired hypogammaglobulinemia, and lymphoma.

Clinical Features. The age of onset in reported cases has varied from 5 months to 22 years. Fatal infectious mononucleosis is the presentation in over 50 per cent of patients. Survivors develop agranulocytosis, aplastic anemia, or a combined immune deficiency of variable severity.

Diagnosis. Immunologic studies of XLP patients reveal the following: evidence for chronic EBV infection, transient or incomplete EBV-specific antibody response, progressive deterioration of cell-mediated immunity, abnormal T-helper and suppressor cell subsets, and defective natural killer cell activity. Maternal carriers exhibit abnormally elevated titers of EBV antibodies.

Immunology. XLP may result from an inherited deficiency in the specific immune response to EBV. An intrinsic B-cell defect may be responsible for the poor antibody responses and the susceptibility to abnormal B-cell proliferation. Alternatively, abnormal T-cell regulation of B-cell responses or a primary defect in natural killer cell immunosurveillance may be responsible for the syndrome.

Treatment. Successful treatment for the underlying immune deficiency has not been reported. The prognosis is poor, with a mean survival time of one and one-half years from diagnosis. However, early diagnosis could provide an opportunity for immune or antiviral therapy to be effective.

ACQUIRED IMMUNODEFICIENCY SYNDROME (AIDS)

The acquired immunodeficiency syndrome is a disease that has been recognized since 1981. It is characterized by a severe acquired immunodeficiency affecting certain recognized risk groups. It is defined by the Centers for Disease Control (CDC) as the presence of a reliably diagnosed disease that is at least moderately indicative of an underlying defect in cell-mediated immunity; for example, Kaposi's sarcoma in an individual who is less than 60 years of age, *Pneumocystis carinii* pneumonia, or other life-threatening opportunistic infections. Critical to the definition of AIDS is the absence of known causes of underlying immune deficiency and of any other host defense defects reported to be associated with the disease, such as iatrogenic immunosuppression or lymphoreticular malignancies.

Epidemiology. AIDS is seen in four major risk groups: (1) homosexual or bisexual males (71 per cent), (2) intravenous drug users (17 per cent), (3) Haitians with no admitted history of homosexuality or intravenous drug abuse (5 per cent), and (4) hemophiliacs (0.8 per cent). Recently, cases of AIDS have been described in infants of mothers with AIDS or at risk for AIDS, or who have received blood products, e.g., transfusions. Fewer than 6 per cent of patients fall into no apparent risk group. As of October 1983 there were approximately 2500 reported cases of AIDS. Although the disease was first seen almost exclusively in New York City, San Francisco, and Los Angeles, it has now been reported from more than 40 states and more than 20 countries. The incidence of the disease has been approximately doubling every six months. The major source of spread is through sexual contact and blood or blood products. It is generally felt that the disease will remain confined to the aforementioned major risk groups; casual contact does not seem to spread this disease.

Etiology. Although the etiology is unclear, it is generally well accepted that this is a transmissible disease most likely due to an infectious agent, particularly a viral agent. A number of hypotheses exist, foremost among which is the possibility that the disease is due to a lymphocytotropic virus that infects T-lymphocytes. Foremost among the suspects are the retrovirus group, particularly the human T-cell leukemia virus (HTLV). However, it must be emphasized that at this time the agent has not been definitively identified.

Clinical Features. Full-blown AIDS is characterized by opportunistic infections with or without unusual neoplasms such as Kaposi's sarcoma. The most common opportunistic infection is *Pneumocystis carinii* pneumonia; it is seen in the absence of Kaposi's sarcoma in 50 per cent of patients, and together with Kaposi's sarcoma in an additional 8 per cent of patients. Twenty-six per cent of patients have Kaposi's sarcoma without *Pneumocystis carinii* pneumonia, and another 15 per cent of patients have other opportunistic infections without Kaposi's sarcoma or *Pneumocystis carinii* pneumonia. Among the other opportunistic infections are included *Mycobacterium avium intracellulare, Cryptococcus neoformans* meningitis, *Candida albicans* esophagitis and thrush, disseminated cytomegalovirus infection, progressive *herpes simplex* virus infection of the mucocutaneous area, *Toxoplasma gondii* infection (particularly of the central nervous system), and cryptosporidiosis. The Kaposi's sarcoma is of the epidemic form and is unlike the usually indolent Kaposi's sarcoma, which is generally seen in older individuals of Mediterranean origin. Other neoplastic processes that are seen are non-Hodgkin's lymphoma of the Burkitt's type, particularly primary central nervous system lymphoma.

A large number of male homosexuals have what has been termed the lymphadenopathy syndrome, which is characterized by chronic persistent lymphadenopathy of unknown etiology involving two or more extrainguinal sites. Following biopsy, nodes reveal nonspecific lymphoid hyperplasia. The relationship between this syndrome and full-blown AIDS is unclear at present, although some feel that it may be a prodrome of the classic syndrome.

Immunology. The common denominator of AIDS is an acquired cellular immune defect that seems to be quite selective. The patients develop a lymphocytopenia that is predominantly of the T4 lymphocyte subset, which phenotypically defines the helper or inducer T-cell population. The number of T8 or suppressor cells is variable in AIDS but is normal for the most part. The selective depletion of the T4 subset leads to a reversal of the T4:T8 ratio. Although it has been stated that the B-cell limb of the immune response is normal, these patients do indeed have B-lymphocyte abnormalities in that they have hyperactivity of the B-cell limb with hypergammaglobulinemia, immune complex formation, and spontaneous secretion of immunoglobulin by individual B-cells. In addition, the patients have a defect in both natural killer cell (NK) activity and cell-mediated cytotoxicity against viral infected targets.

Diagnosis. AIDS is a diagnosis made on both epidemiologic and clinical grounds. Patients who fall into the CDC empirical definition of an opportunistic infection and/or an unusual neoplasm in the setting in which there is no explanation for an acquired cell-mediated immune defect are diagnosed as having AIDS. Although the lymphocyte abnormalities described are characteristic of AIDS, these are not specific and are by no means diagnostic. Therefore, the diagnosis is made by the constellation of clinical findings in an individual who has no recognizable reason for an immunologic defect.

Treatment. Although several of the opportunistic infections can be adequately treated, they often relapse upon cessation of therapy. At the present time there have been no cases of either spontaneous or induced reversal of the profound immunologic defect. A number of therapies have been tried, including treatment with lymphokines, such as alpha interferon and gamma interferon as well as interleukin-2. There has been a report of some remissions in Kaposi's sarcoma secondary to treatment with recombinant alpha interferon. However, long-term reversals of the underlying defect have not been reported. At present, there is no effective therapy for the underlying defect in AIDS.

Prognosis. Although the published mortality for this disease is approximately 40 per cent, it is likely that it will be much higher, even approaching 90 or 100 per cent, since very few patients who have contracted AIDS two to three years ago are alive at the present time. Therefore, it stands to be a disease with an extraordinarily poor prognosis once the patient has exhibited the full-blown manifestations of the syndrome, such as opportunistic infection, unusual neoplasm, or both.

CONDITIONS ASSOCIATED WITH SECONDARY T-CELL OR COMBINED T-CELL AND B-CELL IMMUNODEFICIENCY

Many clinical conditions are associated with secondarily depressed cell-mediated immunity (Table 22–10). In some instances, such as pregnancy and certain systemic viral infections, this immunosuppression serves a protective role by limiting host responses. In other conditions, such as malnutrition and malignancy, the secondary immune deficiencies directly contribute to the morbidity of the primary disorder.

The mechanisms responsible for these processes are variable. The newborn state and systemic fungal infections are associated with an increased number of T-suppressor cells. Pregnancy is accompanied by hormonal changes and a decreased number of T-helper

Table 22–10. Conditions Associated with Secondary T-Cell or Combined T-Cell and B-Cell Immunodeficiency

Pregnancy
Normal newborn infancy
Congenital infections: rubella virus, cytomegalovirus
Fetal alcohol syndrome
Down's syndrome
Intestinal lymphangiectasia
Systemic infections: fungal, mycobacterial, viral
Malignancies
Stress: surgical, emotional
Malnutrition: protein, calorie, iron, zinc
Aging

cells. Dietary zinc deficiency produces a striking but reversible involution of the thymus. Intestinal lymphangiectasia results in loss of lymphocytes and immunoglobulins from the gastrointestinal tract. Physical and emotional stress may alter cyclic nucleotide concentrations in immunoreactive cells. The further elucidation of these processes will have important implications for all areas of clinical medicine.

CONCLUSION

Study of the primary immune deficiency states has advanced the care of affected patients. Early diagnosis has allowed avoidance of harmful transfusions and immunizations, and the known spectrum of infectious agents peculiar to each of these various diseases has permitted a more appropriate initial selection of antimicrobial therapy. Family counseling has been improved by accurate estimation of genetic risks and, in some situations, prenatal diagnosis. Experimental advances have occurred in specific treatment since the initial discovery that immune serum globulin limited serious infections in IgG deficiency. Bone marrow transplantation has restored immune responses, in patients with severe combined immune deficiency, and transplants with fetal thymus have corrected the cell-mediated immune deficiency in DiGeorge syndrome. Thymosin and transfer factor have been used successfully in selected cases of more subtle T-cell dysfunction. It is likely that the prognosis for these patients will improve further as existing treatments are refined and new modes are developed. In addition to these direct benefits, investigations of immune defects have enhanced the understanding of normal immune responses and have directed the application of new knowledge to other clinical conditions.

Suggestions for Further Reading

General

Bergman, D., Good, R. A., Finstad, J., et al.: Immunodeficiencies in Man and Animals. National Foundation–March of Dimes Original Article Series. Sunderland, Mass., Sinauer Associates, 1975.

Fudenberg, H. H., Stites, D. P., Caldwell, J. L., et al.: Basic and Clinical Immunology. Los Altos, Calif., Lange, 1980.

Horowitz, S. D., and Hong, R.: The Pathogenesis and Treatment of Immunodeficiency. New York, S. Karger, 1977.

Stiehm, E. R., and Fulginiti, V. A.: Immunologic Disorders in Infants and Children. Philadelphia, W.B. Saunders Company, 1980.

Clinical Setting

Allen, J. C.: Infection and the Compromised Host. Baltimore, The Williams & Wilkins Company, 1976.

Miller, M. E.: The child with recurrent infection. Pediatr. Clin. North Am., *24*:1, 1977.

Spector, B. D., Perry, G. S., and Kersey, J. H.: Genetically determined immunodeficiency diseases (GDID) and malignancy: report from the immunodeficiency-cancer registry. Clin. Immunol. Immunopathol., *11*:12, 1978.

Development

Foon, K. A., Schroff, R. W., and Gale, R. P.: Surface markers on leukemia and lymphoma cells: recent advances. Blood, *60*:1, 1982.

Gelfand, E. W., and Dosch, H.: Biological Basis of Immunodeficiency. New York, Raven Press, 1980.

Abnormalities of Phagocytic Cell Number

Dale, D. C., DuPont, G., Wewerka, J. R., et al.: Chronic neutropenia. Medicine, *58*:128, 1979.

Pearson, H. A.: Splenectomy: its risks and its roles. Hosp. Pract., *15*(8):85, 1980.

Pincus, S. H., Boxer, L. A., and Stossel, T. P.: Chronic neutropenia in childhood. Am. J. Med., *61*:849, 1976.

Trigg, M. D.: Immune function of the spleen. South. Med. J., *72*:593, 1979.

Weetman, R. M., and Boxer, L. A.: Childhood neutropenia. Pediatr. Clin. North Am., *27*:361, 1980.

Abnormalities of Phagocytic Cell Function

Abdou, N. I., NaPombejara, C., Sagawa, A., et al.: Malakoplakia: evidence for monocyte lysosomal abnormality correctable by cholinergic agonist in vitro and in vivo. N. Engl. J. Med., *297*:1413, 1977.

Arnaout, M. A., Pitt, J., Cohen, H. J., et al.: Deficiency of a granulocyte-membrane glycoprotein (gp 150) in a boy with recurrent bacterial infections. N. Engl. J. Med., *306*:693, 1982.

Bellanti, J. A., and Dayton, D. H.: The Phagocytic Cell in Host Resistance. New York, Raven Press, 1975.

Blume, R. S., and Wolff, S. M.: The Chédiak-Higashi syndrome: studies in four patients and a review of the literature. Medicine, *51*:247, 1972.

Boxer, L. A., Hedley-Whyte, T., and Stossel, T. P.: Neutrophil actin dysfunction and abnormal neutrophil behavior. N. Engl. J. Med., *291*:1093, 1974.

Buchanan, M. D., Crowley, C. A., Rosin, R. E., et al.: Studies on the interaction between GP-180–deficient neutrophils and vascular endothelium. Blood, *60*:160, 1982.

Buckley, R. H., Wray, B. B., and Belmaker, E. Z.: Extreme hyperimmunoglobulinemia E and undue susceptibility to infection. Pediatrics, *49*:59, 1972.

Crowley, C. A., Curnutte, J. T., Rosin, R. E., et al.: An inherited abnormality of neutrophil adhesion. N. Engl. J. Med., *302*:1163, 1980.

Davis, S. T., Schaller, J., and Wedgwood, R. J.: Job's syndrome. Lancet, *1*:1013, 1966.

Dilworth, J. A., and Mandell, G. L.: Adults with chronic granulomatous disease of "childhood." Am. J. Med., *63*:233, 1977.

Gallin, J. I.: Disorders of phagocytic chemotaxis. Ann. Intern. Med., *92*:520, 1980.

Gallin, J. I., Fletcher, M. P., Seligmann, B. E., et al.: Human neutrophil-specific granule deficiency: a model to assess the role of neutrophil-specific granules in the evolution of the inflammatory response. Blood, *59*:1317, 1982.

Geha, R. S., Reinherz, E., Leung, D., et al.: Deficiency of suppressor T cells in the hyperimmunoglobulin E syndrome. J. Clin. Invest., *68*:783, 1981.

Miller, M. D., Oski, F. A., and Harris, M. B.: Lazy-leukocyte syndrome. Lancet, *1*:665, 1971.

Parry, M. D., Root, R. K., Metcalf, J. A., et al.: Myeloperoxidase deficiency: prevalence and clinical significance. Ann. Intern. Med., *95*:263, 1981.

Quie, P. G., Mills, E. L., McPhail, L. C., et al.: Phagocytic defects. Springer Semin. Immunopathol., *1*:323, 1978.

Schopfer, K., Baerlocher, K., Price, P., et al.: Staphylococcal IgE antibodies, hyperimmunoglobulinemia E and *Staphylococcus aureus* infections. N. Engl. J. Med., *300*:835, 1979.

Tauber, A. I.: Current views of neutrophil dysfunction. Am. J. Med., *70*:1237, 1981.

Natural Killer Cell

Herberman, R. B.: Natural killer cells. Hosp. Pract., *17*(4):93, 1982.

Rager-Zisman, B., and Bloom, B. R.: Natural killer cells in resistance to virus-infected cells. Springer Semin. Immunopathol., *4*:397, 1982.

Sirianni, M. C., Fiorilli, M., Pandolfi, F., et al.: Natural killer activity and lymphocyte subpopulations in patients with primary humoral and cellular immunodeficiencies. Clin. Immunol. Immunopathol., *21*:12, 1981.

Complement Deficiency Disorders

Agnello, V.: Complement deficiency states. Medicine, *57*:1, 1978.

Frank, M. M.: Hereditary angioedema: the clinical syndrome and its management. Ann. Intern. Med., *84*:580, 1976.

Gelfand, J. A., Sherins, R. J., Alling, D. W., et al.: Treatment of hereditary angioedema with danazole. N. Engl. J. Med., *295*:1444, 1976.

Gelfand, J. A., Boss, G. R., Conley, C. L., et al.: Acquired C1 esterase inhibitor deficiency and angioedema: a review. Medicine, *58*:321, 1979.

Johnston, R. B., and Stroud, R. M.: Complement and host defense against infection. J. Pediatr., *90*:169, 1977.

Lint, T. T., Zeitz, H. J., and Gewurz, H.: Inherited deficiency of the ninth component of complement in man. J. Immunol., *125*:2252, 1980.

Müller-Eberhard, H. J.: Complement abnormalities in human disease. Hosp. Pract., *13*(12):65, 1978.

Antibody Deficiency Disorders

Ammann, A. J., Ashman, R. F., Buckley, R. H., et al.: Use of intravenous gamma-globulin in antibody deficiency: results of a multicenter controlled trial. Clin. Immunol. Immunopathol., *22*:60, 1982.

Ashman, R. F., Saxon, A., and Stevens, R. H.: Profile of multiple lymphocyte functional defects in acquired hypogammaglobulinemia, derived from in vitro cell recombination analysis. J. Allergy Clin. Immunol., *65*:242, 1980.

Beck, C. S., and Heiner D. C.: Selective immunoglobulin G4 deficiency and recurrent infections of the respiratory tract. Am. Rev. Respir. Dis., *124*:94, 1981.

Berger, M., Cupps, T. R., and Fauci, A. S.: Immunoglobulin replacement therapy by slow subcutaneous infusion. Ann. Intern. Med., *93*:55, 1980.

Chipps, B. E., Talamo, R. C., and Winkelstein, J. A.: IgA deficiency, recurrent pneumonias and bronchiectasis. Chest, *73*:519, 1978.

Church, J. A., Isaacs, H., Saxon, A., et al.: Lymphoid interstitial pneumonitis and hypogammaglobulinemia in children. Am. Rev. Respir. Dis., *124*:491, 1981.

Cooper, M. D., Lawton, A. R., Prud'homme, J. L., et al.: Primary antibody deficiencies. Springer Semin. Immunopathol., *1*:265, 1978.

Geha, R. S., Schneeberger, E., Merler, E., et al.: Heterogeneity of "acquired" or common variable agammaglobulinemia. N. Engl. J. Med., *291*:1, 1974.

Hermans, P. E., Diaz-Buxo, J. A., and Stobo, J. D.: Idiopathic late-onset immunoglobulin deficiency. Am. J. Med., *61*:221, 1976.

Hitzig, W. H., Dohmann, U., Pluss, H. J., et al.: Hereditary transcobalamin II deficiency: clinical findings in a new family. J. Pediatr., *86*:622, 1974.

Østergaard, P. A.: Clinical and immunological features of transient IgA deficiency in children. Clin. Exp. Immunol., *40*:561, 1980.

Oxelius, V., Laurell, A., Lindquist, B., et al.: IgG subclasses in selective IgA deficiency. N. Engl. J. Med., *304*:1476, 1981.

Rothbach, C., Nagel, J., Rabin, B., et al.: Antibody deficiency with normal immunoglobulins. J. Pediatr., *94*:250, 1979.

Schur, P. H., Borel, H., Gelfand, E. W., et al.: Selective gamma-G globulin deficiencies in patients with recurrent pyogenic infections. N. Engl. J. Med., *283*:631, 1970.

Schur, P. H., Rosen, F., and Norman, M. E.: Immunoglobulin subclasses in normal children. Pediatr. Res., *13*:181, 1979.

Stiehm, E. R.: Standard and special human immune serum globulins as therapeutic agents. Pediatrics, *63*:301, 1979.

Strober, W., Krakauer, R., Klaeveman, H. L., et al.: Secretory component deficiency. N. Engl. J. Med., *294*:351, 1976.

Taylor, B., Norman, A. P., Orgel, H. A., et al.: Transient IgA deficiency and pathogenesis of infantile atopy. Lancet, *2*:111, 1973.

Tiller, T. L., and Buckley, R. H.: Transient hypogammaglobulinemia of infancy: review of the literature, clinical and immunologic features of 11 new cases, and long-term follow-up. J. Pediatr., *92*:347, 1978.

Deficiencies of Cell-Mediated Immunity

Barrett, D. J., Ammann, A. J., Wara, D. W., et al.: Clinical and immunologic spectrum of the DiGeorge syndrome. J. Clin. Lab. Immunol., *6*:1, 1981.

Conley, M. E., Beckwith, J. B., Mancer, J. F. K., et al.: The spectrum of the DiGeorge syndrome. J. Pediatr., *94*:883, 1979.

Feigin, R. D., Shackelford, P. G., Eisen, S., et al.: Treatment of mucocutaneous candidiasis with transfer factor. Pediatrics, *53*:63, 1974.

Rosenblatt, H. M., Byrne, W., Ament, M. E., et al.: Successful treatment of chronic mucocutaneous candidiasis with ketoconazole. J. Pediatr., *97*:657, 1980.

Combined B-cell and T-cell Immunodeficiencies

Ammann, A. J., Sutliff, W., and Millinchick, E.: Antibody-mediated immunodeficiency in short-limbed dwarfism. J. Pediatr., *84*:200, 1974.

Church, J. A., and Uittenbogaart, C.: Partial immunologic reconstitution and hyperimmunoglobulinemia-E in neonatally acquired graft-versus-host disease. Ann. Allergy, *44*:212, 1980.

Hitzig, W. H., and Martin, D. W.: Severe combined immunodeficiency diseases. Springer Semin. Immunopathol., *1*:283, 1978.

Lawlor, G. J., Ammann, A. J., Wright, W. C., et al.: The syndrome of cellular immunodeficiency with immunoglobulins. J. Pediatr., *84*:183, 1974.

Ownby, D. R., Pizzo, S., Blackmon, L., et al.: Severe combined immunodeficiency with leukopenia (reticular dysgenesis) in siblings: immunologic and histopathologic findings. J. Pediatr., *89*:382, 1976.

Schlegel, R. J., Bernier, G. M., Bellanti, J. A., et al.: Severe candidiasis associated with thymic dysplasia, IgA deficiency, and plasma antilymphocyte effects. Pediatrics, *45*:926, 1970.

Immunodeficiency–Enzyme Deficiency Syndromes

Cowan, M. J., Packman, S., Wara, D. W., et al.: Multiple biotin-dependent carboxylase deficiencies associated with defects in T-cell and B-cell immunity. Lancet, *2*:115, 1979.

Giblett, E. R., Anderson, J. E., Cohen, F., et al.: Adenosine-deaminase deficiency in two patients with severely impaired cellular immunity. Lancet, *2*:1067, 1972.

Giblett, E. R., Ammann, A. J., Sandman, R., et al.: Nucleosidephosphorylase deficiency in a child with severely defective T-cell immunity and normal B-cell immunity. Lancet, *1*:1010, 1975.

Hirschhorn, R.: Defects of purine metabolism in immunodeficiency diseases. *In* Schwartz, R. S. (ed.): Progress in Clinical Immunology. Vol. 3. New York, Grune & Stratton, 1977, pp. 67–83.

Mitchell, B. S., and Kelley, W. N.: Purinogenic immunodeficiency disease: clinical features and molecular mechanisms. Ann. Intern. Med., *92*:826, 1980.

Thompson, L. F., Boss, G. R., Spiegelberger, H. L., et al.: Ecto-5′-nucleotidase activity in T and B lymphocytes from normal subjects and patients with congenital X-linked agammaglobulinemia. J. Immunol., *123*:2475, 1979.

Complex Immunodeficiencies

Case Records of the Massachusetts General Hospital (Ataxia-Telangiectasia). N. Engl. J. Med., *292*:1231, 1975.

Gottlieb, M. S., Schroff, R., Schanker, H. M., et al.: *Pneumocystis carinii* pneumonia and mucosal candidiasis in previously healthy homosexual men: evidence of a new acquired cellular immunodeficiency. N. Engl. J. Med., *305*:1425, 1981.

Hamilton, J. K., Paquin, L. A., Sullivan, J. L., et al.: X-linked lymphoproliferative syndrome registry report. J. Pediatr., *96*:669, 1980.

Lum, L. G., Tubergen, D. G., Corash, L., et al.: Splenectomy in the management of the thrombocytopenia of the Wiskott-Aldrich syndrome. N. Engl. J. Med., *302*:892, 1980.

Marx, J. L.: Research news: New disease baffles medical community. Science, *217*:618, 1982.

Ochs, H. D., Slichter, S. J., Harker, L. A., et al.: The Wiskott-Aldrich syndrome: studies of lymphocytes, granulocytes, and platelets. Blood, *55*:243, 1980.

Oxelius, V., Berkel, A. I., and Hanson, L. A.: IgG2 deficiency in ataxia-telangiectasia. N. Engl. J. Med., *306*:515, 1982.

Perry, G. S., Spector, B. D., Schuman, L. M., et al.: The Wiskott-Aldrich syndrome in the United States and Canada (1892–1979). J. Pediatr., *97*:72, 1980.

Purtilo, D. T., DeFlorio, D., Hutt, L. M., et al.: Variable phenotypic expression of an X-linked recessive lymphoproliferative syndrome. N. Engl. J. Med., *297*:1077, 1977.

Purtilo, D. T., Bhawan, J., Szymanski, I., et al.: Epstein-Barr virus infections in the X-linked recessive lymphoproliferative syndrome. Lancet, *1*:798, 1978.

Purtilo, D. T., Sakamoto, K., Barnabei, V., et al.: Epstein-Barr virus–induced diseases in boys with the X-linked lymphoproliferative syndrome (XLP): update on studies of the Registry. Am. J. Med., *73*:49, 1982.

Rivat-Peran, L., Buriot, D., Salier, J., et al.: Immunoglobulins in ataxia-telangiectasia: evidence for IgG4 and IgA2 subclass deficiencies. Clin. Immunol. Immunopathol., *20*:99, 1981.

Spitler, L. E.: Transfer factor therapy in the Wiskott-Aldrich syndrome: results of long-term follow-up in 32 patients. Am. J. Med., *67*:59, 1979.

Acquired Immunodeficiency Syndrome (AIDS)

Fauci, A. S., Macher, A. M., Longo, D. L., et al.: NIH Conference: Acquired Immunodeficiency Syndrome: Epidemiologic, Clinical, Immunologic, and Therapeutic Considerations. Ann. Intern. Med., *100*:92, 1984.

Gottlieb, M. S., Groopman, J. E., Weinstein, W. M., et al.: The acquired immunodeficiency syndrome. Ann. Intern. Med., *99*:208, 1983.

Lane, H. C., Masur, H., Edgar, L. C., et al.: Abnormalities of B-cell activation and immunoregulation with the acquired immunodeficiency syndrome. N. Engl. J. Med., *309*:453, 1983.

Scott, G. B., Buck, B. E., Leterman, J. G., et al.: Acquired immunodeficiency syndrome in infants. N. Engl. J. Med., *310*:76, 1984.

Chapter 23

Immunoprophylaxis: The Use of Vaccines

Joseph A. Bellanti, M.D., and John B. Robbins, M.D.

The use of vaccines, or immunoprophylaxis, to prevent infectious diseases developed from the observations that individuals who had recovered from a specific infectious disease did not contract that disease again. Vaccination with inactivated or attenuated organisms or their products has been shown to be an effective method for increasing host resistance and ultimately has led to the eradication of certain common and serious infectious diseases. As Edsall so aptly put it, "Never in the history of human progress has a better and cheaper method of preventing illness been developed than immunization at its best" (Fig. 23–1).

One of the most successful efforts in the field of immunoprophylaxis evolved from a series of observations leading to the development of vaccines that ultimately resulted in eradication of smallpox. Variolation, the intradermal application of powdered smallpox scabs, which was practiced in the Middle East for centuries, was brought to the Western world by Lady Mary Wortley Montagu (Chapter 1). The practice was not without its difficulties, however, since some subjects who received the intracutaneous injection developed full-blown smallpox that was often fatal. Nonetheless, the practice was adopted in England because the mortality and morbidity of smallpox contracted by variolation was considerably lower than from the natural route. Subsequently, Jenner observed that milkmaids who came in contact with cattle infected with a virus related to smallpox, i.e., cowpox, were solidly protected against smallpox. Since Jenner's discovery of the resistance of smallpox after cowpox infection (vaccination) (Fig. 23–2), many other vaccines and various modes of application have been developed that are based on the principles and mechanisms of immunology described in Sections One and Two.

During the last century, increasing emphasis was placed on the development of both viral and bacterial vaccines in the hope of eliminating disease (Figs. 23–3 to 23–5). The subsequent effective use of chemotherapy and antibiotics seemed to diminish the necessity for the further development of bacterial vaccines. Since these therapeutic agents were not effective against viral diseases, the major emphasis of vaccine development centered on antiviral vaccines. However, the emergence of antibiotic-resistant bacteria gradually assumed widespread clinical significance and resulted in a resurgence of interest in the development of new bacterial vaccines.

The prevention of viral diseases by vaccines represents one of immunology's greatest triumphs, e.g., the eradication of certain fatal and crippling diseases of man, such as poliomyelitis. This overall progress in vaccine development, however, has not been without cost, since for almost every new vaccine that has been developed an adverse reaction has also been described. Thus, although modern vaccines are extremely safe and effective, they are neither perfectly safe nor perfectly effective. The goal of vaccine development is to achieve the highest degree of protection with the lowest rate of untoward effects.

Physicians must continue to be aware of existing as well as new vaccines and to observe the results of vaccination in subjects for both efficacy, i.e., *"immunogenicity,"* and safety, i.e., *"reactogenicity."* Any deviation from expected efficacy or any untoward reaction should be carefully observed and a detailed description of the occurrence recorded and transmitted to responsible public health authorities and to the manufacturer of the vaccine. Thus,

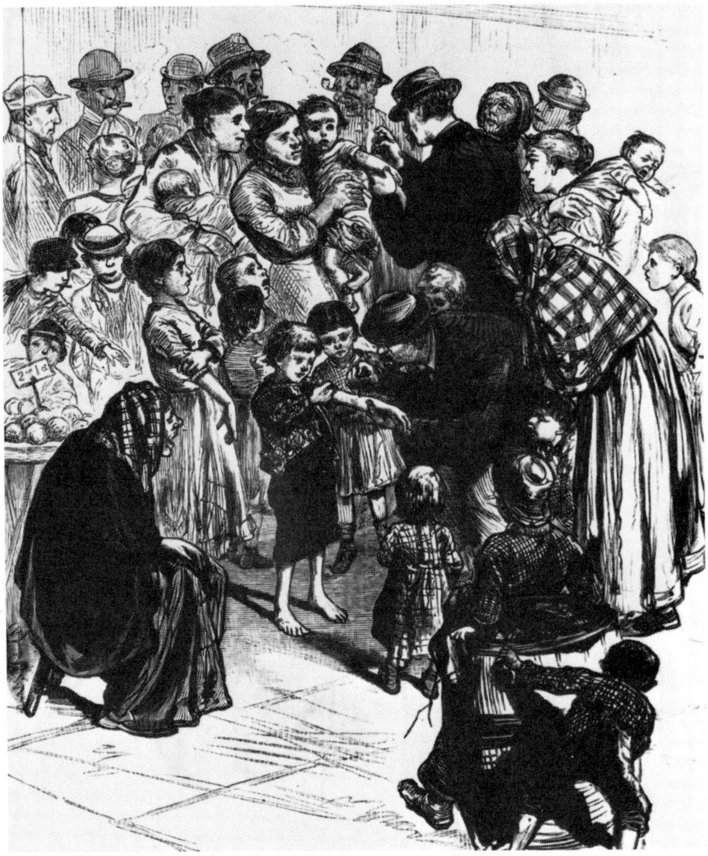

Figure 23–1. Compulsory public vaccination against smallpox. (Courtesy of National Library of Medicine.)

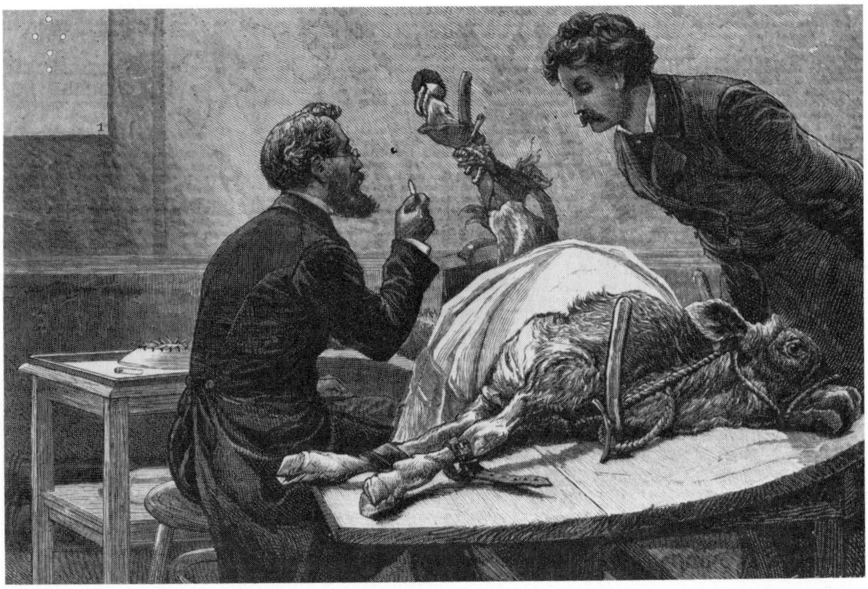

Figure 23–2. Early scene showing preparation of smallpox vaccine. (Courtesy of National Library of Medicine.)

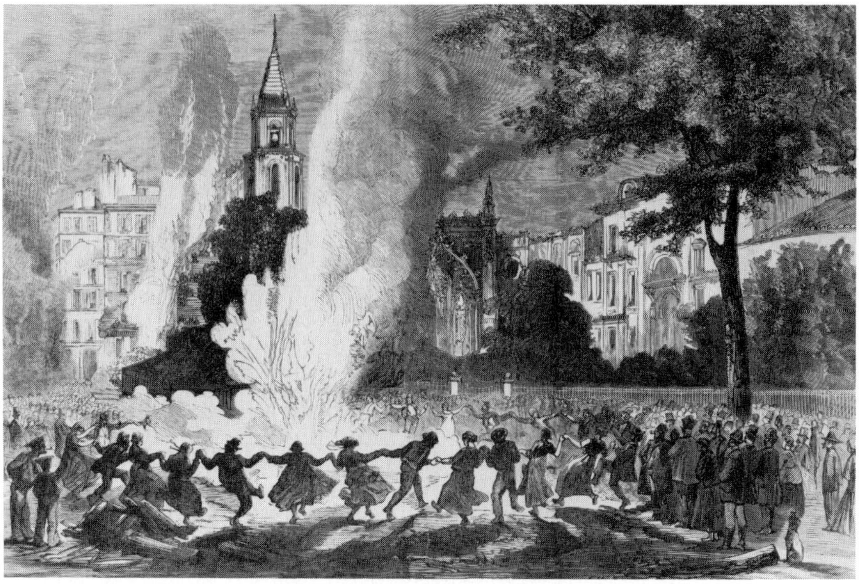

Figure 23–3. Early scene at Marseilles showing folklore ritual in an attempt at cholera eradication by dancing and fire. (From Harper's Weekly, *9*:724, 1865; courtesy of National Library of Medicine.)

the physician must be ever cognizant not only of the principles of immunology that are the basis of vaccines and their adverse effects but also of the broader societal, ethical, and legal issues surrounding their use.

PRINCIPLES OF ACTIVE IMMUNIZATION

The use of vaccines is based on the stimulation of the specific immune response within a host (active immunization); this is in contrast to the transfer of preformed antibody (passive immunization) (Chapter 24). The meaning of the term "vaccine" (*vacca:* L., cow), referring to jennerian vaccination with cowpox, has been broadened to include any biologic product prepared from microorganisms or other biologic substances, e.g., allergens or tumor products, that is useful in the prevention or treatment of disease. The term *toxoid* refers to a toxin preparation that has

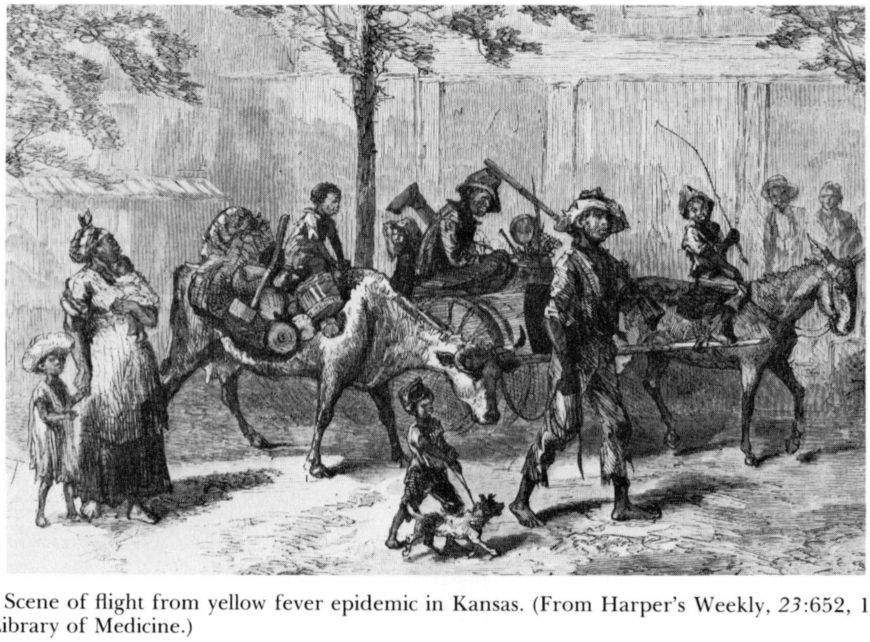

Figure 23–4. Scene of flight from yellow fever epidemic in Kansas. (From Harper's Weekly, *23*:652, 1879; courtesy of National Library of Medicine.)

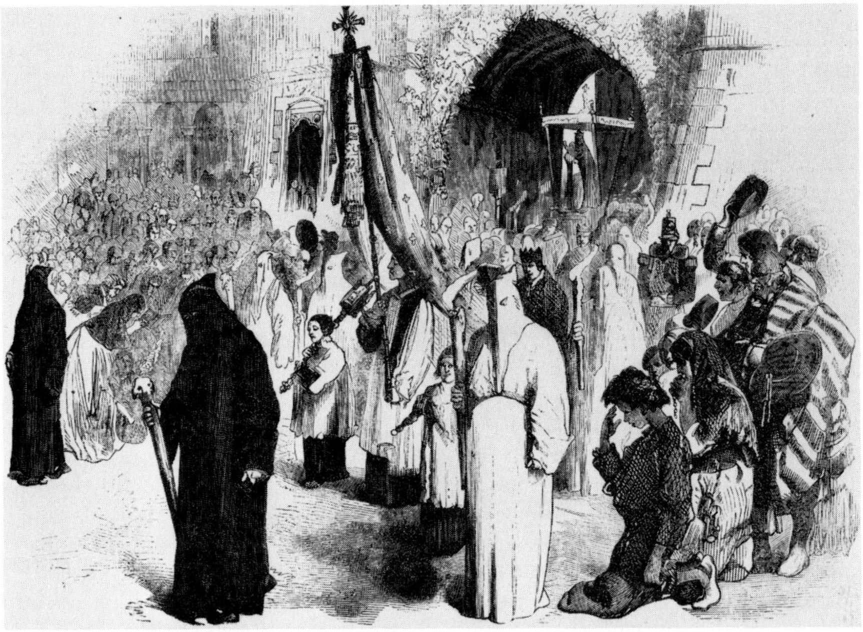

Figure 23–5. Penitential procession during a yellow fever epidemic in Lisbon, Portugal. (From Harper's Weekly, *2*:109, 1858; courtesy of National Library of Medicine.)

been rendered nontoxic but still retains its immunogenic properties and is therefore useful as a vaccine. Although active and passive immunization procedures have been applied for the most part to infectious diseases, they are being tested in other areas, such as the prevention and treatment of malignant disorders (Chapter 19), the prevention of hemolytic disease of the newborn, and the neutralization of certain drugs, e.g., digoxin (Chapter 24).

General Principles

The effectiveness of a vaccine is generally determined by the degree of protection afforded an immunized host after challenge. This determination is usually made in a field study in which vaccinated and unvaccinated individuals selected at random are exposed to the same disease risk. The assessment of protection is made by calculating the incidence of disease in both groups. A vaccine is considered effective if it significantly reduces the disease incidence in the immunized group compared with that in the control group. *It should be stressed that the effectiveness of a vaccine is not determined by the induction of serum antibody alone, but rather by the demonstration of enhanced protection against disease.*

A knowledge of the pathogenesis of the disease is essential in the use of vaccines. Infections may be divided into two major groups: (1) *localized,* which exert their effects at the portal of entry by local replication of the microorganism and inflammatory changes; and (2) *generalized,* in which after a limited period of replication at a local site the organism (bacterium or virus) or its products (toxin) are widely disseminated (Table 23–1).

Table 23–1. **Characteristics of Infectious Diseases**

	Group 1 (Localized)	Group 2 (Generalized)
Site of pathology	Portal of entry	Systemic
Examples	Respiratory viral infections (influenza)	Diphtheria, measles, poliomyelitis
Incubation period	Relatively short	Relatively long
Presence of blood-borne phase	Negative	Positive
Duration of immunity	Short or unknown	Usually lifelong
Immunity mechanism	Local antibody (IgA); local CMI	Humoral antibody (IgG, IgM); systemic CMI

Localized infections, as illustrated by those produced by respiratory viruses, are surface infections involving primarily the tissues at the portal of entry. In general, the latent period between exposure and appearance of symptoms is short (days). Blood-borne dissemination of organisms or toxin is unusual, in spite of any generalized symptoms. Since the local tissues seem to be the primary sites of inflammation, local factors of immunity appear to be of major importance, e.g., local IgA and local cell-mediated immunity (CMI).

Systemic infections include diseases, such as diphtheria and the childhood exanthems, that are associated with relatively longer incubation periods. Since these diseases involve a more complex pathogenesis, with passage of the organisms or toxins through the blood stream, the primary immunity mechanism appears to be mediated by serum antibody of the IgG, IgM, and IgA varieties as well as systemic cell-mediated immunity (CMI).

In general, the most effective vaccines are those that most closely simulate the recovery or protective mechanisms seen following convalescence from the natural disease. For example, protection in many respiratory viral infections has been shown to correlate better with the presence of IgA-associated antibody in the respiratory tract than with that of serum IgG antibody. Vaccines effective in localized viral infections are those that stimulate the local immune responses. On the other hand, the presence of serum IgG diphtheria antitoxin following active immunization has been shown to be correlated with clinical protection from this generalized disease.

Duration of Protection

The most important advantage of active immunization over passive immunization is its longer duration of protection. The host is protected after an appropriate time lapse (latent period), following which immunity is detected (Chapter 7). This protection is associated with many of the factors of immunity (cellular and humoral) but is usually measured in vitro by the presence of serum antibody. Unlike the case in passive immunity, in which the protective levels of serum antibody are maintained for relatively short periods, active immunization elicits protected levels of antibody for years.

The response associated with the initial encounter with vaccine is referred to as *primary immunization.* The initial immunoglobulin responses detected in serum are of the IgM class; later, IgG antibody is found. The IgA class of antibody seems to appear as an intermediate phase between IgM and IgG (Chapters 7 and 16).

Following subsequent exposure of the immunized host to the same or a similar antigen in the form of a vaccine or natural disease, antibody production occurs much sooner, involves a shorter latent period, and attains much higher levels of antibody. This response is referred to as an *anamnestic, secondary,* or *booster response* (Chapter 7). During this secondary response, the major antibody component in serum is of the IgG variety; the IgM is present but in diminished amount.

It is important to stress that the ability to demonstrate this recall phenomenon occurs after stimulation not only with the same antigen but also with closely related antigens. For example, certain strains of influenza change antigenically and are responsible for recurring epidemics (Chapter 16). This changed antigenicity may involve new antigenic specificities while retaining antigens found in earlier strains. Thus, upon encounter with an influenza variant, an individual may elicit a primary response to the new antigenic determinants of previous strains, i.e., the doctrine of "original antigenic sin" proposed by Francis. This booster effect is one explanation of enhanced resistance and accelerated antibody production seen in older persons who had prior antigenic experience with related strains, e.g., following the extensive immunization with "swine flu" vaccines.

A critical level of immunity, such as the concentration of serum antibody, is necessary to ensure that the vaccinated individual remains protected against disease. The action of vaccines to achieve this goal is varied. In the case of bacterial toxoids, e.g., tetanus, the levels of antibody achieved after initial immunization may decline to nonprotective levels after five to ten years. Thus, in a patient with deep wound infections, e.g., burns or war injuries, the levels of tetanus antitoxin may be inadequate. This slow decline of vaccine-induced antibodies is the rationale for booster immunization with tetanus every ten years. Moreover, immunization with tetanus toxoid is recommended for individuals considered at risk, such as armed forces recruits and veterinarians. Tetanus also continues to be a problem in certain underdeveloped nations where routine immunization with tetanus toxoid is not routinely practiced. There are as many as 1 in 10 to 1 in 100 infants born in these countries who succumb to neonatal tetanus caused by neonatal infection via the umbilical cord. For this reason, immunization of women of childbearing age with tetanus toxoid is recommended in these countries to provide levels of tetanus antitoxin to the neonate.

Status of Antigen

Another principle underlying the use of active immunization is the status of the immunogen itself (Chapter 4). In general, vaccines that contain virulent, attenuated, or "live" organisms are more effective than inactivated or killed preparations. This enhanced effect is manifested by a greater degree of initial protection and a longer duration of immunity. After the use of inactivated influenza vaccine, for example, protection may be noted, but influenza can occur in immunized individuals. Infections with yellow fever, on the other hand, are generally prevented in individuals receiving the live yellow fever vaccine. The reasons for this enhanced efficacy of live vaccines are unclear but may be related to destruction of critical antigens during the preparation of inactivated vaccine, e.g., neuraminidase of swine influenza virus vaccine. Another explanation is that duration of immunity seems to be favored by antigens that persist. Live vaccines contain antigens capable of sustained persistence and prolonged immunogenic effect. Shown in Table 23–2 are some examples of the characteristics of immunization responses based upon the status of the antigen.

Immunization with certain types of inactivated vaccines (measles and respiratory syncytial virus vaccines) can also be followed by serious untoward responses seen after subsequent exposure to virus in nature. These reactions are tertiary manifestations of the immune response due to prior sensitization with killed vaccine that result in hypersensitivity rather than protective immunity and are described in detail below.

Simultaneous Administration of Vaccines

Another principle that has practical relevance to whether vaccines may be administered simultaneously is the phenomenon of interference. If a live viral vaccine is given and a different live vaccine is administered thereafter, the second immunization may be inhibited. This effect appears to be mediated by the antiviral mechanism of interferon (Chapter 16). Interference has been demonstrated in the human with measles, smallpox, and poliovirus vaccines. For example, if one administers smallpox vaccine to an individual immediately after administering measles vaccine, there will be a reduction in the number of successful immunizations. Similarly, successful immunization with live oral poliovirus vaccine may be inhibited if immunization is carried out during community epidemics of enterovirus infections. Because of this problem of interference, immunization with live viral vaccines should be postponed if significant intercurrent infections exist. Although the simultaneous administration of live virus vaccines was not recommended previously

Table 23–2. Characteristics of Immunization Responses Related to Status of Antigens

	Nonreplicative (Killed or Inactivated Vaccines)	Replicative (Live, Attenuated Vaccines)
Example	Bacterial (DPT) Some viral (poliovirus, measles, influenza)	Viral (yellow fever, vaccinia, rubeola, rubella, mumps, and poliovirus)
Immunization principle	Preformed antigenic mass	Self-replicative
Effect of passive antibody	No inhibitory effect	May prevent successful immunization
Duration of immunity	Relatively short; requires "boosters"	Relatively long (mimic natural infection); do not usually require boosters
Prime immunity mechanism	Humoral IgG	Humoral IgG; local IgA

because of this problem of virus interference, more recent studies have indicated that combined virus vaccines given at the same or separate sites are as effective as administration of individual vaccines. From a practical standpoint, therefore, the phenomenon of interference does not appear to present a major obstacle in the design of vaccine programs, and several viral vaccines may be administered simultaneously with good efficacy, e.g., measles, mumps, and rubella (MMR) vaccine. In addition, inactivated vaccines (e.g., bacterial vaccines) can be administered simultaneously at different sites. It should be pointed out, however, that when vaccines that individually have side effects are combined, the adverse effects of the combination may be accentuated.

Routes of Administration

Most vaccines are administered by the parenteral route regardless of their natural portal of entry (Table 23–3). There are notable exceptions to this general statement. For example, live, oral poliovirus vaccine is given via the enteric route and yellow fever vaccine is given by the parenteral route—the natural portal of entry of the respective pathogens.

In addition to those listed in Table 23–3, new approaches to immunoprophylaxis are being introduced, such as the local application of antigen in the respiratory tract. Intranasal immunization has been shown to stimulate local IgA immune mechanisms. These applications are currently being investigated in the case of influenza, rubella, and respiratory syncytial virus vaccines. Thus, a more durable immunity that is similar to the responses seen following natural infection may be attained.

Table 23–3. **Route of Administration of Vaccine**

Example of Vaccine	Vaccine Route*	Natural Portal of Entry
Rubeola	I.M.	Respiratory tract
Rubella	I.M.	
Influenza	I.M.	
Poliovirus (Sabin)	P.O.	Gastrointestinal tract
Poliovirus (Salk)	I.M.	
Smallpox	I.D.	Respiratory tract
Rabies	I.M.	Skin (neural)
Yellow fever	I.M.	Skin (bloodborne)

*I.M. = intramuscular
I.D. = intradermal
P.O. = oral

Immunologic Status of the Host

Another important principle guiding immunization procedures is the immunologic competence and reactivity of the host. The significance is apparent when the developmental immaturity of the young infant and the clinical entities in which underlying immunologic or physiologic deficiencies exist (Chapter 22) are considered.

Previously, infants were believed to be incapable of eliciting an immune response; this was attributed to physiologic or immunologic immaturity of the young host. This widely held view led to the tacit assumption that small infants could not be immunized successfully. Fortunately, this fallacy was corrected as a result of many studies that clearly demonstrated the immunologic responsiveness of the young infant (Fig. 23–6). There are, however, quantitative and qualitative differences from adult responses. A pattern of prolonged or exclusive macroglobulin synthesis was shown to be the hallmark of the immature immunologic response and is seen after immunization of the young infant and after intrauterine infections of the fetus (rubella, cytomegalovirus infection, toxoplasmosis, and syphilis). This pattern of prolonged IgM antibody synthesis lasts for varying intervals and is different from the IgG response characteristic of the adult.

The inhibitory effect of passively acquired antibody is another example of the effect of the host's immunologic reactivity to subsequent immunization procedures (Chapter 10). Passively acquired antibody can be obtained through (1) transplacental transfer of maternal IgG antibody, (2) passive immunization by serum gamma globulin through immunoprophylaxis, or (3) transfer of antibody in breast milk.

The placental transfer of maternal IgG globulins to the infant occurs readily and provides the newborn with a rich source of preformed antibodies from the maternal circulation. There is great variability, however, in the types of antibodies obtained in this manner (Table 23–4). This is in part reflective of the quantity and molecular size of antibody in the maternal circulation. For example, the low molecular weight IgG anti-

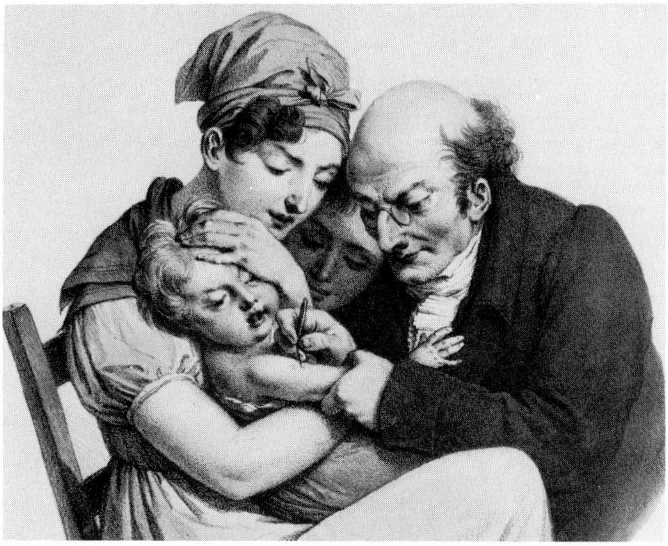

Figure 23–6. Vaccination of an infant with smallpox vaccine. (From L. L. Boilly, 1827; courtesy of National Library of Medicine.)

bodies (e.g., rubeola antibody) present in high concentration in maternal serum are readily transferred; IgG antibodies present in lower concentration (e.g., antibody to *Bordetella pertussis*) are poorly transferred; and IgM anti-LPS antibodies are excluded.

In addition to providing the newborn with protection, these passively acquired IgG antibodies may interfere with active antibody synthesis following certain immunization procedures. This observation is relevant to the design of immunization schedules for infants, particularly with regard to certain live viral vaccines. From a practical standpoint, the effectiveness of beginning immunization procedures with killed vaccines, e.g., diphtheria, pertussis, and tetanus (DPT), in infants two to three months old does not appear to be appreciably inhibited by passive antibody. The passively acquired antibody can inhibit successful immunization of infants with parenteral live virus vaccines; therefore, such live virus immunization procedures should be delayed until the age of 15 months. Since oral poliovirus vaccines are given by the enteric route, they are not inhibited by serum IgG poliovirus antibody and therefore can be effectively administered to infants at two to four months of age.

Another situation in which passively acquired antibody may interfere with active antibody synthesis is in the case of "natural" immunity acquired by the newborn from breast milk. Although not absorbed, this IgA antibody may provide local immunity to many enteric pathogens. Large quantities of this local antibody present in the gastrointestinal tract may neutralize virus; however, breast-fed infants have recently been shown to be capable of successful immunization with oral poliovirus vaccines while receiving breast milk.

The status of the immune response not only affects the success of the primary immunization procedures but also may contribute to adverse effects. These adverse effects are seen primarily following the use of live vaccines and predominantly in those individ-

Table 23–4. Relationship of Antibody Type with Transplacental Transfer

Good Passive Transfer	Poor Passive Transfer	No Passive Transfer
Diphtheria antitoxin	*Hemophilus influenzae*	Enteric somatic (0) antibodies (salmonella, shigella, *E. coli*)
Tetanus antitoxin	*Bacillus pertussis*	Skin-sensitizing antibody
Antierythrogenic toxin	Dysentery	Heterophil antibody
Antistaphylococcal antibody	Streptococcus MG	Wassermann antibody
Salmonella flagella (H) antibody		
Antistreptolysin		
All the antiviral antibodies present in maternal circulation (rubeola, rubella, mumps, poliovirus)		

uals with depressed immune function, and are described below.

Physicochemical State of The Antigen

There are several other factors that determine the overall immunogenicity of a vaccine, including the size and complexity of the antigen and its physical state (Chapter 4). The larger and more complex the molecule is, the greater is its immunogenicity. In general, soluble proteins are poorer immunogens than those rendered insoluble or those enhanced through the use of adjuvants (Chapter 10).

THE USE OF VACCINES

Indications for Use

Immunization should be instituted in those population groups that have (1) the least protection, (2) the highest rates of exposure to a given pathogen, and (3) the greatest risk of disease or its complications. For the most part, immunization procedures are used to prevent diseases in situations for which there are no other satisfactory means of treatment, e.g., viral diseases. The population groups at greatest risk to disease are determined by the following factors.

AGE

In general, the population groups that are at greatest risk and have the least protection are at either end of the age spectrum—the very young and the very old. The very young are susceptible by virtue of their immunologic immaturity; the old are vulnerable because of waning immunity or secondary degenerative diseases that predispose them to illness, e.g., cardiac disease.

ECOLOGY

Certain population groups are at greater risk by virtue of their environment. These groups include (1) *institutionalized individuals,* in whom there is greater risk of hepatitis, influenza, and respiratory diseases; and (2) *military recruits,* who are predisposed to acute respiratory diseases. Individuals are also placed at increased risk by virtue of travel to foreign countries where they may have a greater exposure to new and exotic pathogens, such as those producing cholera, plague, and dysentery. Environmental pollutants that are directly deleterious or function as chronic irritants (e.g., smog) also place the host at greater risk of infection.

STATUS OF THE HOST

Physiologic states, such as pregnancy, increase the risk of contracting diseases such as influenza and poliomyelitis. Individuals with chronic diseases of the lungs or heart (e.g., cystic fibrosis or congenital heart disease) are predisposed to serious complications of respiratory viral infections. Because of their increased risk, these groups should be adequately immunized.

Preparations and Immunization Schedules

The commonly used vaccines and their optimal time of administration are listed in Table 23–5; the primary immunization of infants and children is given in Table 23–6. The currently available vaccines (Table 23–7) may be categorized as follows: (1) whole-cell bacterial vaccines (e.g., pertussis), (2) toxoids (e.g., diphtheria, tetanus), (3) viral vaccines, and (4) capsular polysaccharide vaccines.

WHOLE-CELL BACTERIAL VACCINES

These are vaccines composed of bacterial cells that have been inactivated with formalin or other agents. Although these vaccines are effective, they are often associated with significant side reactions. These are due for the most part to the presence of adventitious bacterial components not related to the specific protective effect but associated with inflammation and fever.

Pertussis vaccine exemplifies the problems of whole-cell vaccines. Vaccines for the prevention of pertussis, a disease caused by *Bordetella pertussis,* were developed in the 1930's, when the pathogenesis of this common and serious respiratory disease of infants and children was poorly understood.

Whooping cough or, as it is more accurately termed, pertussis, is a highly communicable disease transmitted by droplet infection via the respiratory route. The disease begins as an upper respiratory infection with nonspecific symptoms

Table 23–5. Commonly Used Vaccines

	Preparation	Comments
Bacterial		
Diphtheria, Pertussis, Tetanus	Inactivated	Infancy and childhood
Pneumococcal, Meningococcal, *H. influenzae*	Polysaccharide	Used only under certain circumstances
BCG	Live	
Cholera, Salmonella, Plague	Inactivated	
Viral		
Smallpox	Live—calf lymph	Recommended in infants and children
Poliomyelitis	Live—Sabin (OPV); Salk (IPV)	
Rubeola	Live	
Rubella	Live	
Mumps	Live	
Hepatitis B	Inactivated	Used only under special circumstances
Rabies	Inactivated	
Influenza	Inactivated	
Yellow fever	Live	
Adenovirus	Inactivated	
	Live (not licensed, used only in military)	
Rickettsial		
Typhus	Inactivated	Used only under special circumstances
Rocky Mountain spotted fever	Inactivated	

and progresses in intensity until the third or fourth week when the characteristic paroxysmal cough, often ending in a respiratory stridor (whoop), commences. It has been known for years that in the early stages of the disease the organisms are readily isolated from the nasopharynx. Nonetheless, when the distinctive symptoms of pertussis appear at three to four weeks, the organism becomes increasingly difficult to isolate. Even at the end of two to three months, when the disease symptoms may be still manifest, it is not possible to isolate the organism. Recently, Pittman proposed that the pathologic features of the disease are mediated by a toxin, termed pertussis toxin, which appears to be of immunologic interest for the following reasons: (1) It has a structure and enzymatic function similar to cholera toxin. This toxin within a narrow dosage range acts as an adjuvant for both antibody formation and induction of cell-mediated immunity. (2) This toxin

Table 23–6. Recommended Schedule for Active Immunization and Tuberculin Testing for Normal Infants and Children*

2 months	DTP—Trivalent OPV
4 months	DTP—Trivalent OPV
6 months	DTP—Trivalent OPV
15 months	Tuberculin test—live measles, mumps, rubella vaccine
18 months	DTP—Trivalent OPV
4–6 years	DTP—Trivalent OPV
14–16 years	Td
Thereafter	Td every 10 years

*From the Report of the Committee on Infectious Diseases. 19th ed. American Academy of Pediatrics, 1982.

Table 23–7. Classification of Commonly Used Vaccines

Category of Vaccine	Example
Whole-cell bacterial	Pertussis vaccine Typhoid vaccine BCG
Toxoids	Tetanus Diphtheria
Viral	Poliomyelitis Measles Rubella
Capsular polysaccharide	Pneumococcal Meningococcus *H. influenzae* Type b

protein is capable of expanding the lymphoid cell population differentiated to produce IgE (reaginic) antibody. (3) Pertussis toxin is responsible for the remarkable peripheral blood lymphocytosis seen in the disease. The peripheral lymphocytes do not appear to be newly formed. Rather, they are released from pre-existing stores. Pertussis toxin, which has also been referred to as lymphocytosis-promoting factor, is responsible for this unusual effect upon lymphoid cells. (4) In addition, pertussis toxin can affect glucose regulation by its action upon pancreatic islet cells, leading to an inhibitory effect of the insulin response to changes in blood glucose. Pittman has postulated that both symptoms of and immunity to pertussis are mediated by this toxin and that an effective pertussis vaccine may, in the future, be developed from this toxin after it has been rendered nontoxic (i.e., toxoid).

At the present time, pertussis vaccine is composed of whole bacterial cells. The lipopolysaccharide (LPS) of this gram-negative organism, in addition to the minute quantities of pertussis toxin, appears to contribute to the side reactions caused by the vaccine. Pertussis vaccine may be cited as an example of a whole-cell bacterial vaccine containing a complex mixture of adventitious components of the bacterium in addition to the protective moiety. In order to develop a more effective vaccine, well-defined components of *B. pertussis* need to be developed with fewer side effects. An intensive search for new pertussis vaccines is currently under way, and it is entirely conceivable that a more effective vaccine, derived from purified proteins of the organism, will be soon developed.

Typhoid vaccine is another example of a whole bacterial vaccine useful in the prevention of typhoid fever, a disease caused by *Salmonella typhi.* Although *S. typhi* is an enteric microorganism, typhoid fever is characterized by septicemic and not primarily by diarrheal manifestations. The organism is encapsulated and contains a polysaccharide called the Vi antigen. In addition to other bacterial components, the typhoid vaccine contains LPS, which may be responsible for some of the adverse effects of the vaccine (e.g., fever, myalgia). The precise mechanism of protection of the vaccine is not completely understood, and there is controversy in the literature concerning the role of the Vi capsular polysaccharide as a protective antigen. In the United States, typhoid vaccine consists of an acetone-inactivated suspension of *S. typhi* organisms. Since the efficacy of this vaccine is only between 50 and 70 per cent, a search for new vaccines has been made. Recently, a mutant strain of *S. typhi,* Ty-21A, has been developed by mutagenesis of the wild-type organism. The bacterial mutants have no epimerase enzyme capable of converting glucose to galactose, the latter being an essential component of the polysaccharide side chain of its LPS. The mutation thus results in deficient biosynthesis of LPS, which is an essential component of the outer membrane. The defective bacteria grow poorly in the small intestine and rapidly succumb to both the host's natural defenses and their own intrinsic impaired metabolism. During its brief sojourn in the intestinal tract, this attenuated organism is capable of inducing a protective immune response and yet incapable of producing disease. This newly attenuated bacterial strain is under clinical evaluation, but early studies indicate a degree of protection greater than 90 per cent, which appears to be long-lasting with no significant side reactions. The mutant strain is administered by orally feeding the organism with sodium bicarbonate, which neutralizes gastric acidity and permits the vaccine strain to survive in the small intestine, where it elicits a protective immune response. At present, only the inactivated whole-cell typhoid vaccine is available in the United States; its use is recommended for those who may be at risk for typhoid fever, e.g., individuals traveling to areas where typhoid fever is still endemic.

The bacillus Calmette-Guérin (BCG) is an attenuated bovine strain used to immunize humans against tuberculosis. The vaccine is injected subcutaneously, and after several weeks, acquired cellular immunity is evident by the appearance of delayed-type hypersensitivity in a significant proportion of vaccinates. BCG is not used routinely in the United States but is used in those parts of the world where tuberculosis is still endemic. In addition to its specific immune response, BCG vaccine exerts an effect upon lymphoid cells and macrophages. The use of BCG in experimental immunotherapy of malignancy is described in Chapter 19.

TOXOIDS

A group of infectious diseases, e.g., diphtheria and tetanus, are expressions of the biochemical actions of specific toxins. Antibodies that react with these toxins by combining with the molecular sites of the proteins responsible for their tissue binding neutralize the effect of these toxins. Therefore, the prevention of toxin-mediated diseases is accomplished by the induction of antitoxin antibodies (Chapter 15). Bacterial toxin is inactivated with chemical agents, e.g., formalin, which react with the protein to form a modified compound termed toxoid. This toxoid can no longer exert its toxic actions on the native protein but is still capable of inducing neutralizing antibodies to the toxin.

Diphtheria and tetanus toxoids are usually combined with pertussis vaccine and adsorbed onto aluminum salts (DTP vaccine) as a combined vaccine for use in primary immunization of infants and children less than six years of age. Both the aluminum salts and the pertussis component exert an adjuvant effect on the antibody response to the diphtheria and tetanus toxoids. The *B. pertussis* microorganism contains at least two substances with adjuvant activity: (1) lipopolysaccharide (LPS) and (2) pertussis toxin. Diphtheria and tetanus toxoids are also available for immunization of adults either as tetanus and diphtheria toxoids (dT) or as tetanus toxoid (TT) alone. The small "d" denotes a lowered amount of diphtheria toxoid in the adult preparation, since the higher dose used for infants elicits local adverse reactions in a significant number of adult recipients. The latter adult toxoid preparations are given as booster immunizations; the pertussis component is not included since pertussis is not usually a serious disease in the older child and adult.

There are new approaches to eliciting antitoxin antibodies. These include the preparation of mutants of the wild-type bacteria that produce protein molecules that are antigenically identical to the toxin but that have lost their toxic properties. One of the most successful examples of this approach has been the characterization of mutants of *Corynebacterium diphtheriae* that have a change in the amino acid composition of the A or toxic portion of the diphtheria toxin protein. The resultant protein retains all the antigenic properties of the native molecule but has lost its ability to interfere with host protein synthesis because it can no longer enzymatically bind ADP ribose to the elongation factor involved in protein synthesis. These new experimental approaches promise to provide even more effective immunogens for the induction of antitoxin antibodies.

VIRAL VACCINES

Several experimental approaches have provided vaccines for the prevention of viral diseases. A classic example of how more than one approach may achieve the same therapeutic effect is illustrated by poliomyelitis. Poliomyelitis is caused by the destructive action of the virus on the anterior motor neurons of the spinal cord. There are three antigenic variants of poliovirus (1, 2, 3) that may infect the gastrointestinal tract, where the virus undergoes multiplication. The virus may escape into the blood stream (viremia) in a small proportion of infected humans and invade the motor neurons, causing their destruction with eventual loss of innervation of the peripheral nerves. The first successful poliovirus vaccine was composed of three antigenic variants of poliovirus inactivated with formalin (Salk vaccine). The resultant formalin-inactivated polioviruses were no longer infectious and, when injected subcutaneously, elicited the formation of serum antibodies that inactivated the blood-borne stages of viral disease. The first formalin-inactivated poliovirus vaccines had several drawbacks. First, the virus was difficult to cultivate to provide sufficient antigenic mass to elicit the formation of antibodies in virtually all recipients. Second, the degree of inactivation of the virus preparation was difficult to control. During the early stages of development one batch of incompletely inactivated vaccine, i.e., Type III poliovirus, was the cause of paralytic polio in some of its recipients. Subsequently, Sabin and his associates developed attenuated strains of all three polio antigenic variants. These attenuated strains could be administered orally. Viral multiplication then occurred within the gastrointestinal tract with subsequent induction of local immunity in the intestinal tract and serum antibody. These viral strains were excreted in the stool, which resulted in a more widespread immunization of the population, i.e., herd immunity. Both types of viral vaccines have been used successfully. In the United States, virtually all poliovirus vaccines have been of the Sabin attenuated viral type. These attenuated poliovirus vaccines have two deficiencies: (1) Rarely, they will cause paralytic disease when administered to an infant or child with as yet an undiagnosed immune deficiency; and (2) the attenuated strains of virus may fail to induce immunity in recipients with active gastrointestinal infection. This latter complication is most often observed in undeveloped areas, where intestinal parasitosis and bacterial infections are common. In the United States, there are approximately 6 to 12 cases annually of paralytic poliomyelitis per 3 million vaccinates caused by attenuated viral vaccines. Almost all have been undiagnosed cases of immunodeficiency.

Two new areas of research have developed in this field. The first is the more effective cultivation of poliovirus using newer tissue culture techniques and viral purification. Vaccines prepared with these newer techniques have considerably greater amounts of formalin-inactivated virus and induce higher levels of antibodies for more prolonged periods than either the previous Salk type formalin-inactivated vaccines or the later Sabin attenuated poliovirus vaccines. Thus, these new formalin-inactivated viral preparations have the advantage of being more resistant to changes in temperature and climate and are capable of inducing protective antibodies in virtually all recipients regardless of their current state of gastrointestinal health. Another approach has been to clone the genes responsible for the synthesis of the capsid proteins of poliovirus. Employing recombinant DNA technology, cloned genes of poliovirus have veen transferred to *E. coli,* where the synthesis of capsid proteins is greatly increased and the possibility of infectious virus is eliminated.

Another advance in the field of viral vaccines is illustrated by vaccines developed for the prevention of rubeola (measles). Measles, a member of the paramyxo group, caused disease in almost every infant and child in the United States prior to the advent of vaccines in the 1960's. Measles is acquired by droplet spread, and the virus multiplies and spreads via the blood stream through the body. The prevention of measles by immunization was stimulated by two complications associated with this disease. The first was the incidence of postmeasles encephalitis (1 in 1000), including subacute sclerosing encephalitis (SSPE). This was a serious complication with a high rate of morbidity and mortality. The second was the accompanying bacterial complications of measles infection. It was known for many years that passive immunization with pooled gamma globulin administered to susceptible individuals who had been in contact with recent patients could prevent clinical measles. Therefore, the first vaccines were formalinized inactivated virus preparations designed to elicit serum antibodies. These initial vaccines were successful in preventing measles, but their effectiveness was less than optimal. Moreover, some individuals who had been vaccinated with inactivated virus vaccine developed atypical and serious cases of measles several years later when exposed to natural measles. Soon thereafter, the first attenuated viral vaccines were developed from the Edmonston strain of rubeola. These first attenuated strains caused clinical symptoms in a large proportion of recipients and accordingly were administered simultaneously with low doses of gamma globulin. The results were not completely satisfactory since the effectiveness was not close to 90 per cent. Further attenuated measles virus vaccines were then developed that induced a high rate of seroconversion and whose duration of immunity has been lifelong. The mechanisms of immunity induced by attenuated strains of vaccine have been postulated to be mediated by both serum-neutralizing antibody and cell-mediated immunity. The nature of the cell-mediated immunity seems to be the development of specific lymphocytes that recognize host cells that have been infected by measles virus.

More recently, Choppin and his colleagues have provided evidence that the lesser protective effect of the formalin-inactivated measles virus was due in part to the reduction of the immunogenic potential of the F glycoprotein of measles. The F glycoprotein of paramyxoviruses, including rubeola, is responsible for cell fusion, hemolysis, and virus penetration into cell membranes of the host. The F protein of measles virus, therefore, is a critical protective antigen. The use of formalin to inactivate the measles virus resulted in a significant reduction in the immunogenicity of this protein.

The outstanding success of the attenuated measles virus vaccine in preventing clinical measles is well documented. Outbreaks of measles that have been reported in the United States occur in individuals who have not been vaccinated, or who have been vaccinated with earlier measles vaccine, or who have been vaccinated before they were 12 months old. Rubeola is one of the diseases that seems to be exclusively confined to humans, and it has been proposed that the use of measles vaccine throughout the world could potentially result in complete eradication of this disease. DNA recombinant technology with the F glycoprotein of measles gene transferred to *E. coli* or other bacteria has been used for protein production in order to provide a less expensive and equally effective vaccine for the prevention of rubeola.

New vaccines have been developed for the prevention of viral infections and include the hepatitis B vaccine that has been recently licensed. Current vaccines are prepared from pools of human plasma containing hepatitis B antigen. Although there has been some concern regarding the source of this material, i.e., the possibility of AIDS, there have been no reported incidents of transmission of AIDS by the use of these vaccines. Nonetheless, there is a major effort to develop new sources of antigen for vaccines. These include (1) the use of recombinant DNA technology for a new source of material; (2) the vaccinia model, which uses live immunizing vaccines as the vehicle to insert other antigens both viral and bacterial; and (3) synthetic polypeptides.

CAPSULAR POLYSACCHARIDE VACCINES

Encapsulated bacteria, including *Streptococcus pneumoniae* (pneumococci), *Neisseria meningitidis* (meningococci), *Hemophilus influenzae* Type B, *Escherichia coli* K1, and the Group B beta-hemolytic streptococci, are the most commonly encountered bacteria that cause invasive disease in individuals otherwise considered to be healthy. This property of invasiveness is due to the capsular material of the microorganisms, which is composed of polysaccharides and serves as a virulence factor(s) by interfering with the action of complement upon bacterial surfaces. Complement can be activated to induce protective effects directly by the lipopolysaccharide of gram-negative bacteria and the teichoic acid of gram-positive bacteria (Chapter 6). Unencapsulated variants of the aforementioned species are rapidly inactivated by complement-enhanced phagocytosis (Chapter 15). However, the presence of some capsular polysaccharides of these species interferes with the effective action of complement and thus impairs effective phagocytosis. Immunity to diseases caused by these bacteria therefore requires the presence of antibody to activate complement on the bacterial surface with its resultant protective activities, which include bacteriolysis and opsonization (Chapter 6). Although the overall physical and chemical properties of bacterial capsular polysaccharides are similar, there is a high degree of specificity related to their property of invasiveness (Chapter 14). Thus, of the 83 known pneumococcal capsular types, most infections are caused by only 15 to 20 of these. Similar relationships exist in the case of the meningococcus. Of the ten capsular polysaccharide types identified, Groups A, B, and C bacteria cause over 90 per cent of cases of meningococcal meningitis, with the remainder caused almost exclusively by Groups Y and W135. Similarly, although there are six capsular polysaccharide types of *Hemophilus influenzae,* virtually all cases of meningitis are caused by organisms with the Type b capsule.

Vaccines composed of the highly purified capsular polysaccharides of meningococcus Groups A, C, W135, and Y are now licensed in the United States. These tetravalent preparations are indicated for use in preventing meningitis due to meningococcus in individuals over two years of age who might be at risk for contracting the disease. These include members of the armed forces and individuals in intimate contact with meningitis patients.

A pneumococcal vaccine composed of the 23 most common types associated with invasive disease is also available. Vaccination is recommended for individauls over 50 years of age who might be at risk for contracting pneumococcal infection as well as for other individuals with decreased resistance, such as those in institutions and those with chronic debilitating disease, e.g., alcoholism or diabetes mellitus. The vaccine is also suggested for individuals older than two years of age who have impaired resistance to pneumococcal infection, including those with splenectomy or functional asplenia, e.g., hemolytic anemia, sickle cell anemia, or hereditary spherocytosis.

A polysaccharide vaccine composed of a capsular antigen of *Hemophilus influenzae* Type b will be licensed for children over the age of two years. It is likely that a recommendation will be made for its use in children who attend day care nurseries and day care centers. In addition, Indian children on reservations and Eskimo children in Alaska, who have an unusually high rate of this serious disease, will probably be candidates for the vaccine. The mode of its protective action is the induction of serum antibodies of the IgG and IgM isotypes. These antibodies have been shown to activate complement on the surface of bacteria, resulting in the protective actions that have been described previously. The importance of complement in the participation of immunity to diseases caused by encapsulated bacteria is illustrated also by the repeated infections caused by pneumococci, meningococci and *Hemophilus influenzae* Type b in individuals with complement protein deficiencies, e.g., C2, C4, C3, C5, C6, C7, and C8 (Chapter 6). In these individuals, the presence of serum antibody to the capsular polysaccharides may be insufficient for protection against diseases caused by these encapsulated organisms.

The vaccines are composed of purified capsular polysaccharides of the organisms and are stored in the freeze-dried state. A subcutaneous injection of a saline solution of either 25 or 50 μg of each capsular polysaccharide induces serum antibodies of at least five to ten years' duration in young adults. Although the pneumococcal vaccines contain 23 antigenically distinct capsular polysaccharides, it is of interest that the presence of these components with similar overall physicochemical characteristics does not interfere with the immune response to each antigenically distinct component.

Capsular polysaccharide vaccines have at least two limitations that have interfered with their use on a routine basis. First is a distinct age-related response to these capsular polysaccharides. In general, those capsules associated with the highest incidence of invasive disease in infants and children are not immunogenic in infants less than two years of age. Second, these capsular polysaccharide vaccines are T cell–independent (Chapter 4). The term refers to the fact that reinjection of these capsular polysaccharides does not result in the "booster" or anamnestic response so characteristic of protein and viral vaccines. Thus, the vaccines do not induce protective immune responses in infants and young children, the age group with the highest incidence of disease caused by these invasive bacteria. Nonetheless, there are some exceptions. Pneumococcus Type 3, the cause of invasive disease in infants, induces a protective immune response in infants as young as two to three months of age. A second injection of meningococcus Group A polysaccharide in infants and children up to three years of age results in a booster response. This booster response is of sufficient intensity to lead to a protective immunity vaccine against epidemic meningitis in the infant and young child age group. The second exception is that of Group B meningococcus and *Escherichia coli* K1 polysaccharide antigens. These two capsular polysaccharides are identical and are composed of a linear homopolymer of *N*-acetyl neuraminic acid (alpha 2-8 linked sialic acid). This polysaccharide antigen is of unusual interest since it is susceptible to rapid degradation by mammalian neuraminidase and since gangliosides, present in normal human tissues, contain terminal sialic acid residues of identical linkage. Thus, it is probable that the Group B *Escherichia coli* K1 polysaccharide represents a "self-antigen" and that this may explain the failure of this polysaccharide to induce IgG antibodies in humans. The subject is under intensive investigation.

Interest in preventing diseases caused by these encapsulated bacteria has also been stimulated by the fact that antibiotic resistance among these bacterial species is increasing at a significant rate. Thus, resistance to ampicillin, the most effective antibiotic agent for the treatment of *H. influenzae* Type b meningitis, which is the most common form of bacterial meningitis in children, now ranges from 10 to 30 per cent of isolates from patients. Strains of pneumococci resistant to penicillin and other commonly used antibiotics also are being observed with increasing frequency. In addition, although chemotherapeutic agents are now available for the treatment of bacterial meningitis caused by these organisms, the mortality rate continues to be significant, ranging from 3 to 10 per cent, with a morbidity characterized by fixed central nervous system deficits being quite common among patients "cured" by antibiotics.

The immunogenicity of capsular polysaccharides has been increased by devising methods for the covalent attachment to T cell–dependent proteins. Intensive investigations are now under way to examine the immune responses elicited by the semi-synthetic vaccines composed of polysaccharides and proteins (usually diphtheria or tetanus toxoid) and the capsular polysaccharides of *H. influenzae* type b, meningococcal Groups A and C, and pneumococcal types 3 and 6 polysaccharides. The immune response to the capsular polysaccharides of these complex molecules has been shown to resemble that of the T cell–dependent protein component. In addition, these conjugates have been shown to elicit antibodies in infant lab-

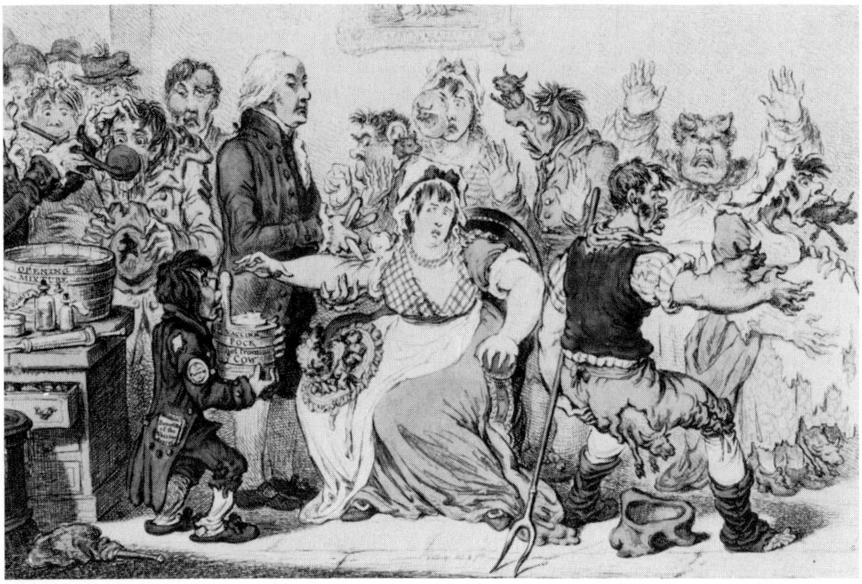

Figure 23–7. Fantasy depicting the side effects of vaccination with cowpox by John Gillray. (Courtesy of National Library of Medicine.)

oratory animals in contrast to the inability of the purified polysaccharides to elicit immune responses in control subjects.

COMPLICATIONS OF ACTIVE IMMUNIZATION

A number of vaccine side effects are being reported with increasing frequency (Fig. 23–7). This is due to the increase in number of vaccines available to the physician; also, the complications of a vaccine can be adequately evaluated only after several years have elapsed. The decision to use a vaccine therefore must be made by weighing the risk of complications from the vaccine against the morbidity and mortality of the disease itself. Routine smallpox vaccination has been discontinued in the United States because it now appears that the disease is virtually eradicated here; moreover, the incidence of complications from the vaccine is higher than the risk of contracting smallpox (Fig. 23–8). The wis-

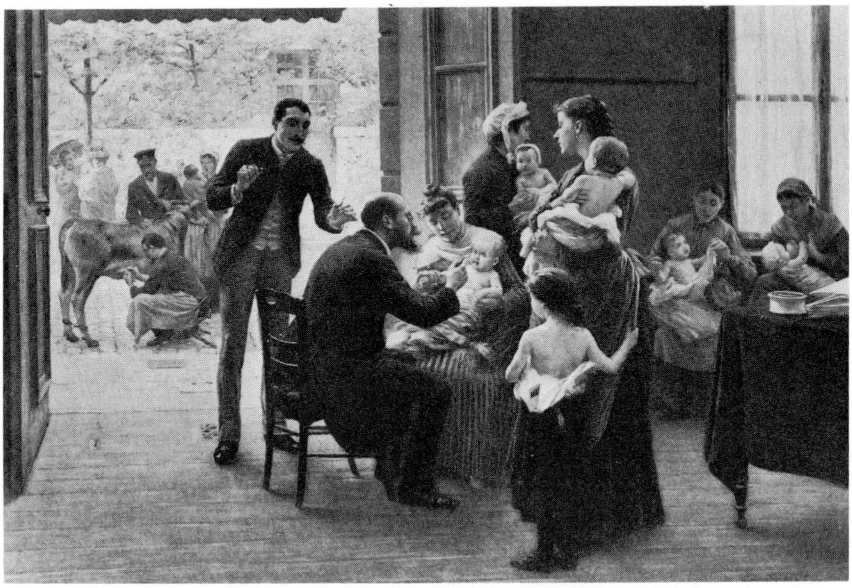

Figure 23–8. Administration of live smallpox vaccine by Scalbert. (Courtesy of National Library of Medicine.)

Table 23–8. **Adverse Effects of Vaccines**

Type	Example	Example of Vaccine	Pathogenetic Mechanism(s)
Nonimmunologic effects			
Host response	Localized reactions: swelling	DPT	
	Generalized reactions: pyrogenic or febrile reactions	DPT	Toxins and other contaminating materials
	Eczema vaccinatum	Smallpox	Break in integrity of skin; (?) T-cell defect
Vaccine response	Adventitious agents; potential oncogenic effect of SV-40	Salk (IPV)	Constituents of vaccine
	Paralytic poliomyelitis	Sabin (OPV)	Reversion of virulence; lack of sufficient attenuation; higher incidence in children with hypogammaglobulinemia
Immunologic effects			
Immunologically compromised hosts	Progressive vaccinia	Smallpox	Primary or secondary immunodeficiency, e.g., T-cell
	Disseminated BCG	Bacille Calmette-Guérin (BCG)	
	Infection of fetal tissues following immunization in pregnancy	Smallpox Rubella (? not proved)	Diminished CMI during pregnancy; greater susceptibility of fetal tissues to infection; immunologic immaturity of the fetus
Allergic (atopic) hosts	Anaphylaxis due to egg sensitivity	Influenza	Contamination of vaccine with egg proteins leading to Type I immunologic injury
Normal hosts (effects related to nature of antigen or route of administration)	Postinfectious or postvaccinal encephalomyelitis	Rabies, smallpox, mumps, measles	Type IV (cell-mediated ?)
	Urticaria or Arthus reaction	Tetanus toxoid	Type I or III
	Atypical measles	Killed measles	Type III, Type IV (?) injury
	RSV bronchiolitis	Killed RSV vaccine	Type I, III, IV
Normal hosts (?)	Arthritis	Rubella	Unknown
	Thrombocytopenia	Rubella, rubeola	Unknown
	SSPE	Rubeola, rubella (?)	Unknown
	Stevens-Johnson syndrome	Smallpox	Unknown
	Erythema multiforme	Smallpox	Unknown
	Guillain-Barré syndrome	Swine influenza	Unknown

dom of this decision will require the passage of time.

Many vaccines that have been introduced are accompanied by both *immunologic* and *nonimmunologic* complications. These are given in Table 23–8.

Nonimmunologic Complications

Nonimmunologic complications are related to *host response* or to properties of the *vaccine*.

HOST RESPONSE

Perhaps the most common complication seen following immunization is a local reaction occurring at the site of inoculation. It consists of localized swelling and tenderness and may be accompanied by systemic symptoms (fever) that are usually seen within the first 24 hours and seem to be related to the toxic properties of the vaccine itself. In the case of a small infant, these signs may be associated with high fever and sometimes with convulsions. Febrile convulsions occur so frequently in infants with cerebral damage that immunization procedures in such patients should be postponed for one year.

Rarely, in infants under one year of age, a poorly understood encephalopathy occurs following the use of pertussis vaccine. This is usually seen within a few days after the first inoculation and is manifested by convulsions and coma. The precise mechanism of this entity is not understood: The findings are compatible with the effects of hypoglycemia and/or hypoxia resulting from uncontrolled seizures. If high fever, somnolence, or convulsions occur after a DPT injection, the pertussis component should be omitted for all subsequent injections. In this case, DT should be used.

Another type of nonimmunologic complication related to host response is that of vaccinial spread to the lesions of eczema (eczema vaccinatum). Infants with eczema or other breaks in the continuity of the skin (burns) should not be immunized with smallpox vaccine because of the danger of spread. Furthermore, siblings of infants with eczema should not be vaccinated unless they can be physically removed from the patient for several days. The use of vaccinia immune globulin (VIG) has been recommended for this complication of eczema vaccinatum (Chapter 24).

PROPERTIES OF THE VACCINE

A continual examination of vaccines is essential (Table 23–8). Since viral vaccines are grown in tissue culture or eggs, there is an opportunity for viruses indigenous to the tissue to contaminate the vaccine. Such an occurrence was described in 1960, when a monkey virus (simian virus-40 [SV-40]) was found to contaminate many lots of monkey kidney tissue used to produce inactivated and attenuated poliovirus vaccines. Since SV-40 had been shown to induce tumors in newborn hamsters, potential danger lay in the fact that millions of people in the United States and abroad had received this virus during the course of poliovirus vaccination. Fortunately, there have been no recognized problems with human neoplasms to date. This experience, however, has caused a greater awareness of the potential complications related to vaccine quality.

A more serious problem was observed in 1962, shortly after the licensure of Type III oral poliovirus vaccine, when a number of cases of paralytic poliomyelitis occurred in temporal association with administration of live poliovirus vaccine. A formal report issued by the Surgeon General of the Public Health Service, based on the findings of his advisory committee, revealed that a small but significant number of cases were due to the vaccine itself. The mechanism of this response appeared to be related to a reversion of the attenuated virus vaccine to a more neurovirulent form. This complication continues to occur in both the immunized subject and the household contacts of infants fed oral poliovirus vaccines. Most of the cases occurred in older individuals. It is currently recommended, therefore, that immunization with live oral poliovirus vaccines not be routinely performed in individuals over the age of 18 years. Recently, infants and children with hypogammaglobulinemia were shown to be at particular risk of developing vaccine-associated paralytic disease, with an incidence estimated to be 10,000 times greater than that of normal children (Chapter 22).

Immunologic Complications

The immunologic complications that follow the use of vaccines are those occurring in either immunologically deficient hosts or those with normal immune mechanisms in whom immunologic factors play a role (Table 23–8). For ease of discussion, the adverse effects to vaccines may be divided into (1) those effects that are seen in immunologically compromised hosts, (2) those hypersensitivity reactions that are seen predominantly in allergic (atopic) individuals, (3) those effects that are seen in normal hosts and appear to be related to the nature of the antigen or the route of administration, and (4) those effects that are seen in normal hosts and whose pathogenesis is unclear but may have an immunologic basis.

ADVERSE EFFECTS SEEN IN IMMUNOLOGICALLY COMPROMISED HOSTS

Not only does the status of the immune response affect the success of primary immunization, but it also may contribute to its adverse effects. These are usually seen after the use of live vaccines and predominantly in individuals with depressed immune function. For example, progressive vaccinia (vaccinia necrosum or vaccinia gangrenosa) has been observed in children with defects in the thymic-dependent limb of immunity, such as severe combined immunodeficiency (Fig. 23–9*A*). This rare but highly fatal complication of smallpox immunization consists of a failure of the primary lesion to heal normally, with progressive spread to adjacent areas of skin (Fig. 23–9*B* and *C*). With necrosis of tissue, new lesions develop over a period of months, often involving metastatic lesions to other parts of the body, such as bone and viscera. This complication carries a high mortality and has been observed predominantly in children with immunologic deficiency of the thymic- (T-) dependent type (Chapter 22). It has also been seen in secondary immunologic deficiency, e.g., in leukemia, in lymphoma, and in patients receiving immu-

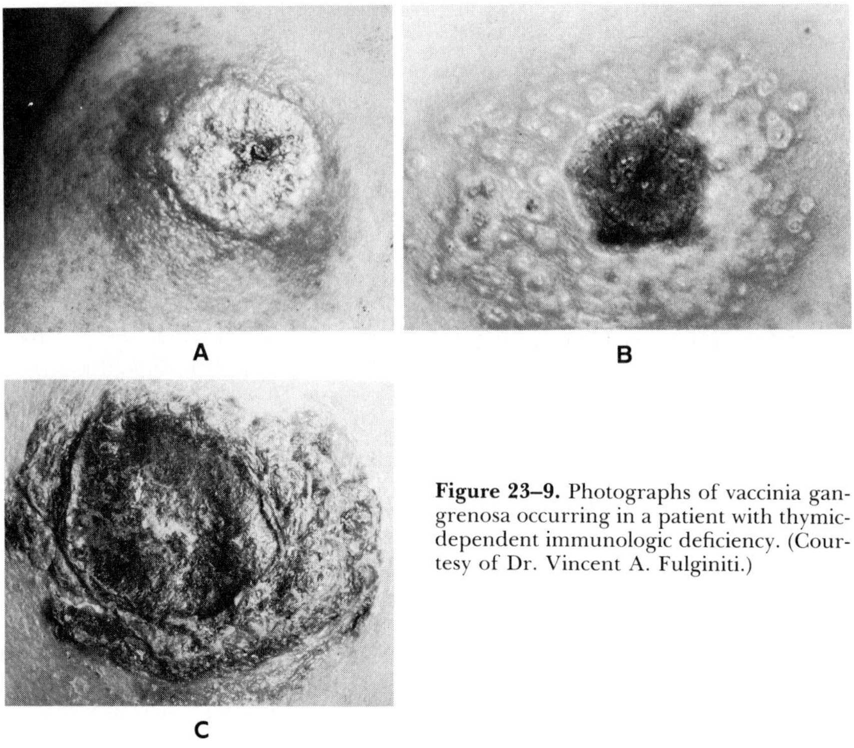

Figure 23–9. Photographs of vaccinia gangrenosa occurring in a patient with thymic-dependent immunologic deficiency. (Courtesy of Dr. Vincent A. Fulginiti.)

nosuppressive therapy. The basis for this tragic complication appears to be a specific deficiency of the immune system, particularly of cell-mediated immunity. The recommended treatment with vaccinia immune globulin (VIG) alone, therefore, is not totally satisfactory, and immunologic reconstitution through transplantation of immunocompetent cells or transfer factor may be more effective (Chapter 24).

Another example of a vaccine complication related to an underlying immunologic deficiency is the fatal giant cell (Hecht cell) pneumonia reported in children exposed to measles or receiving live measles vaccine. This has been described in children with primary immunodeficiency diseases and in malnourished children, particularly in the developing countries of the world. These children fail to develop the rash of measles and specific measles-neutralizing antibody and subsequently die. Although these children appear to be deficient in both cell-mediated and humoral immunity, the deficiency in cellular immunity

Table 23–9. Commercially Available Viral Vaccines

Vaccine	Strain	Source	Manufacturer	Brand Name
Influenza	Varies from year to year	Chick embryo	Parke/Davis	Fluogen
			Connaught Labs	Fluozone
Mumps	Jeryl-Lynn	Chick embryo	Merck, Sharp & Dohme	Mumpsvax
Poliovirus	Salk (killed)	Monkey kidney	Connaught Labs	Poliomyelitis vaccine (purified)
	Sabin (live)	Monkey kidney	Lederle	Orimune
Rabies		Human diploid (WI-38) cell culture	Merieux Institute, Inc.	Imovax
		Human diploid (WI-38) cell culture	Wyeth	Wyvac
Rubella	Wistar RA 27/3	Human diploid (WI-38) cell culture	Merck, Sharp & Dohme	Meruvax
Rubeola (measles)	Enders-Edmonston (further attenuated strain)	Chick embryo	Merck, Sharp & Dohme	Attenuvax
Vaccinia		Calf lymph tissue	Wyeth	Dryvax
Hepatitis B		Human plasma	Merck, Sharp & Dohme	Hepatavax-B

appears to be of more frequent occurrence and of greater import in these reactions.

Pregnancy also constitutes an altered physiologic state in which the use of certain live vaccines, such as smallpox or rubella, is contraindicated because of the possibilities of infection of the fetus and a more severe spread of virus. In the case of rubella immunization, exposure of the immunized pregnant woman to wild virus has been associated with the finding of wild virus shedding in the recipient, but no reports of congenital rubella syndrome in infants delivered by a previously vaccinated woman have been verified. The general status of cell-mediated immunity has been shown to decrease during pregnancy, particularly with respect to certain viruses, such as rubella and cytomegalovirus, which may account for the increased susceptibility of the pregnant female to certain live viral vaccines.

It is apparent from these unfortunate experiences that individuals with impaired immunologic reactivity, on the basis of either *primary* or *acquired* causes, should not receive live vaccines. Descriptions of overwhelming viral infections in patients receiving antilymphocyte serum add another example to the list of the "right treatment for the wrong patient."

ADVERSE HYPERSENSITIVITY REACTIONS SEEN PREDOMINANTLY IN ALLERGIC (ATOPIC) INDIVIDUALS

Since many vaccines are grown in tissue culture or eggs, e.g., viral vaccines, there is an opportunity for them to be contaminated with heterologous tissues, proteins, or other foreign substances that can lead to immunologically mediated reactions.

The possible allergens in viral vaccines that could give rise to allergic reactions include (1) those of the host cells in which the virus is grown, (2) those of the medium or its additive, and (3) those foreign antigens that may be added during the preparation and purification of the vaccine, e.g., antibiotics. Most hypersensitivity reactions are seen in atopic individuals and are associated with egg proteins or antibiotics, e.g., penicillin.

Newer techniques in vaccine preparation, such as zonal centrifugation and the use of avian tissue cell culture, appear to have reduced the incidence of severe anaphylactic reactions. Nonetheless, allergic reactions continue to occur, and the physician should be aware of the tissue cultures in which vaccines are grown in order to prevent certain allergic reactions in atopic individuals. Table 23–9 contains a listing of commercially available viral vaccines and the tissue cultures in which they are prepared. Individuals sensitive to eggs may also be allergic to vaccines grown in chick embryo. Screening by history of ability to eat eggs without adverse effects is a reasonable way to identify those individuals possibly at risk of reaction to egg-grown vaccines. Furthermore, if individuals who are allergic to eggs need protection against influenza, for example, a scratch test with the vaccine as antigen can be used as a screening procedure.

ADVERSE EFFECTS OF VACCINES SEEN IN NORMAL HOSTS THAT APPEAR TO BE RELATED TO THE NATURE OF THE ANTIGEN OR THE ROUTE OF ADMINISTRATION

Postinfectious or postvaccinal encephalomyelitis is the classic example of a disease mediated by cell-mediated hypersensitivity resulting from the use of vaccines or natural infection (Chapter 20C). This disease was originally shown to follow the use of rabies vaccine (Pasteur vaccine) and later was seen following the use of smallpox, measles, and mumps vaccines. Natural viral infections have also been associated with postinfectious encephalitis. The pathogenesis of the encephalitis is believed to be similar to that of experimental allergic encephalitis (EAE) (Chapter 20C). Evidence now supports the view that this type of reaction is related to a delayed hypersensitivity phenomenon mediated by sensitized T-lymphocytes. Sensitization by these viral vaccines may occur because most viruses associated with this complication contain a lipid envelope. During maturation these viruses are released from infected tissues at cell surfaces (steady-state viruses) (Chapter 16). This virus-host interaction may provide a pathogenetic mechanism of "alteration of self" at the host's cell surface, with the resulting induction of a delayed hypersensitivity reaction. With rare exceptions, efforts to recover virus from the brain of an individual with postvaccinal encephalitis have been unsuccessful. However, in light of the recovery of measles virus from the brain biopsy material from patients with subacute sclerosing panencephalitis (SSPE), the possibility of the so-called slow viruses

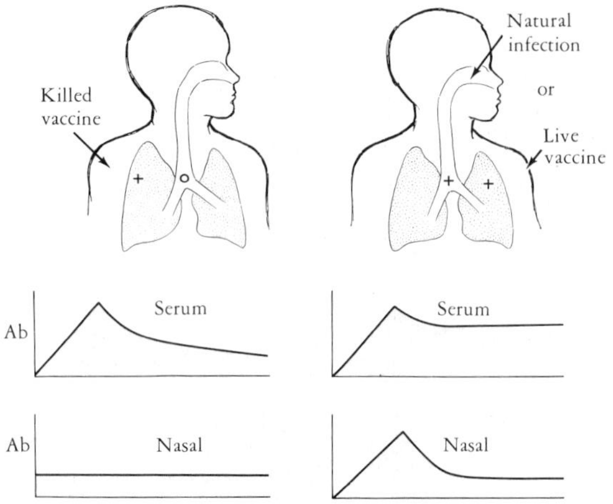

Figure 23–10. Schematic representation of development of nasal and serum antibody after immunization with live and killed measles vaccine and natural infection. Note the absence of development of nasal antibody after administration of killed vaccine.

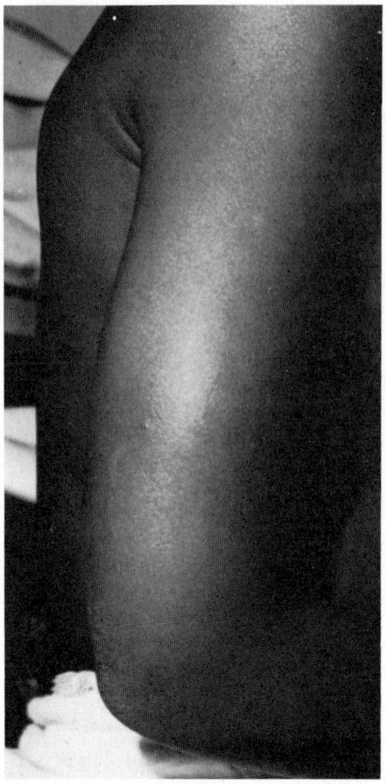

Figure 23–12. Arthus reaction occurring at the site of a subsequent live measles vaccination in a child previously immunized with inactivated measles vaccine.

being present in masked form in other entities exists. This possibility may prove to be of importance in the pathogenesis of postvaccinal encephalitis.

Immunologic complications associated with hypersensitivity phenomena mediated by humoral factors occurring in otherwise normal individuals represent another category (Table 23–8). These reactions range from immediate Type I (reaginic) hypersensitivity phenomena, associated with localized urticaria occurring within a few minutes after immunization, to the Arthus or immune-complex type of hypersensitivities (Type III), seen after a more prolonged interval. For example, localized reactions at the site of immunization have been noted in individuals receiving tetanus toxoid. These reactions consist of localized tenderness, redness, and swelling and are believed to be of the Arthus type, induced by antigen-antibody complexes (Chapter 13). Because of these adverse reactions and because protective serum tetanus antitoxin is detectable for as long as ten years after immunization, it is now recommended that booster injections of tetanus toxoid not be given more often than every ten years.

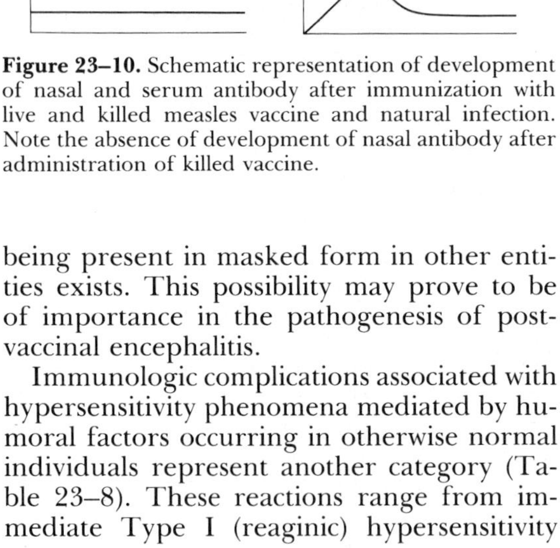

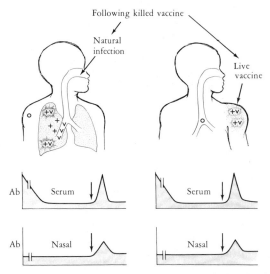

Figure 23–11. Schematic representation of the development of immune complex–type injury due to deposition of virus-antibody complexes in the respiratory tract (generalized) after exposure to natural measles and in the skin (localized) after subsequent immunization with live measles vaccine.

Another more serious complication of killed virus vaccines is the atypical responses seen in children who have received inactivated viral vaccines, such as killed measles virus vaccine (Chapters 16 and 20A). When these children are later exposed to wild virus in nature, an atypical illness is observed that is significantly more severe and more toxic than the disease that occurs in unimmunized children. Following immunization with inactivated vaccine, there appears to be a selective stimulation of serum antibody but little IgA antibody in the respiratory tract (Fig. 23–10). Immunization with either live vaccine or natural infection, however, stimulates both serum and local antibody levels (Fig. 23–10). Following immunization with inactivated measles virus vaccine, therefore, the respiratory tract is not fully immunized. There is produced the anomalous situation of compartmentalization with selective immunization of the humoral compartment without immunization of the secretory IgA antibody (immunologic imbalance) (Chapter 2). After this compartmentalized immunization, natural infection leads to replication of virus in the respiratory tract and an accelerated response of serum antibody (Fig. 23–11). Thus, favorable conditions exist for immune-complex formation within the lung, with subsequent tissue injury mediated by an immune-complex reaction. Similar mechanisms have been proposed (1) for the altered reactivity to respiratory syncytial virus (RSV) seen in children previously immunized with inactivated RSV vaccine and (2) in the pathogenesis of respiratory tract disease of early infancy due to RSV in immunized infants. It is believed that in both situations a compartmentalization occurs in which there is a selective serum IgG antibody in the absence of respiratory tract IgA antibody. After the individual is exposed to wild virus, conditions for the resultant complex formation between serum antibody and RSV antigen in the lungs occur, with immunologic injury as the result.

Localized Arthus-type reactions have been observed in children who were previously immunized with killed measles vaccine and who subsequently receive live measles virus immunization. Swelling, tenderness, and erythema occur at the site of the live measles virus vaccination (Fig. 23–12). Recently, histopathologic and immunofluorescent evidence has been obtained for an Arthus-type hypersensitivity in the pathogenesis of these lesions (Fig. 23–13 through 23–18). In addition to Type III injury, IgE-mediated (Type I) and delayed-hypersensitivity (Type IV) mechanisms have been implicated in the pathogenesis of these reactions (Table 23–8).

ADVERSE EFFECTS OF VIRAL VACCINES SEEN IN NORMAL HOSTS, THE PATHOGENESIS OF WHICH IS UNCLEAR BUT WHICH IS THOUGHT TO HAVE AN IMMUNOLOGIC BASIS

A number of other adverse effects of vaccines have been described that are similar to those seen after natural disease and whose pathogenesis may be immunologic in nature. These complications include the occurrence of joint manifestations and neuropathy observed in association with natural rubella in-

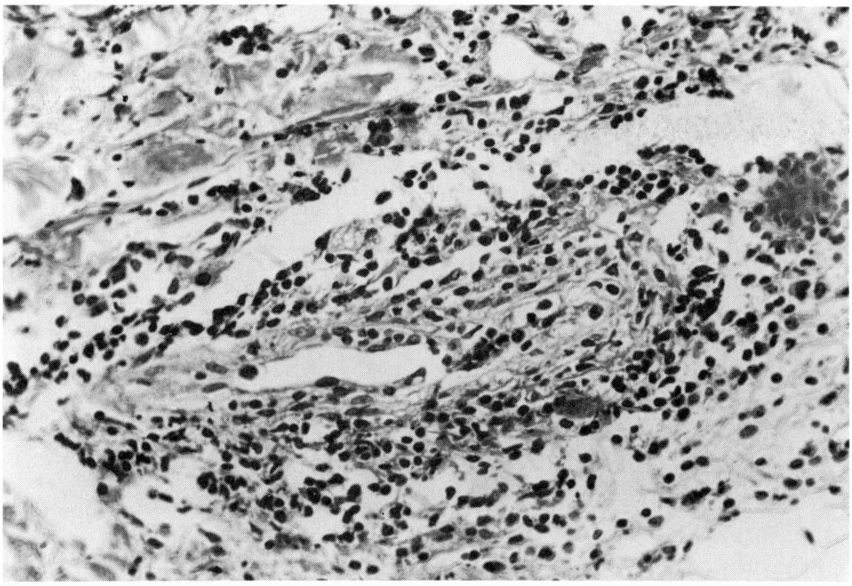

Figure 23–13. Histologic section of localized measles reaction (24 hours) showing a mixed cellular infiltration consisting of lymphocytes, monocytes, and neutrophils. Hematoxylin and eosin stain, × 100. (From Bellanti, J. A.: Biologic significance of the secretory γA immunoglobulins. Pediatrics, *48*:715, 1971.) (Courtesy of Dr. Peter A. Ward.)

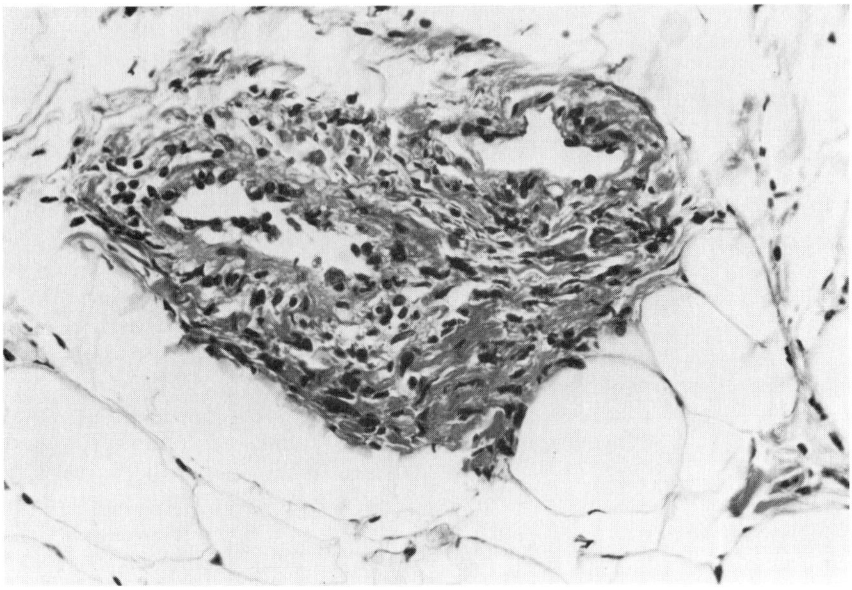

Figure 23–14. Histologic section of localized measles reaction consisting predominantly of neutrophils. Hematoxylin and eosin stain, × 100. (From Bellanti, J. A.: Biologic significance of the secretory γA immunoglobulins. Pediatrics, *48*:715, 1971.) (Courtesy of Dr. Peter A. Ward.)

fection and, to a lesser extent, with rubella vaccines. In 20 to 40 per cent of adults receiving the live rubella vaccine, arthralgia and arthritis have been observed. The implications of these responses in immunologically mediated disease were described in Chapter 20C. In addition, thrombocytopenia has been observed following the use of rubella or rubeola vaccines, sometimes severe enough to be associated with purpura. Of perhaps greater clinical significance are recent reports of the possible association of subacute scle-

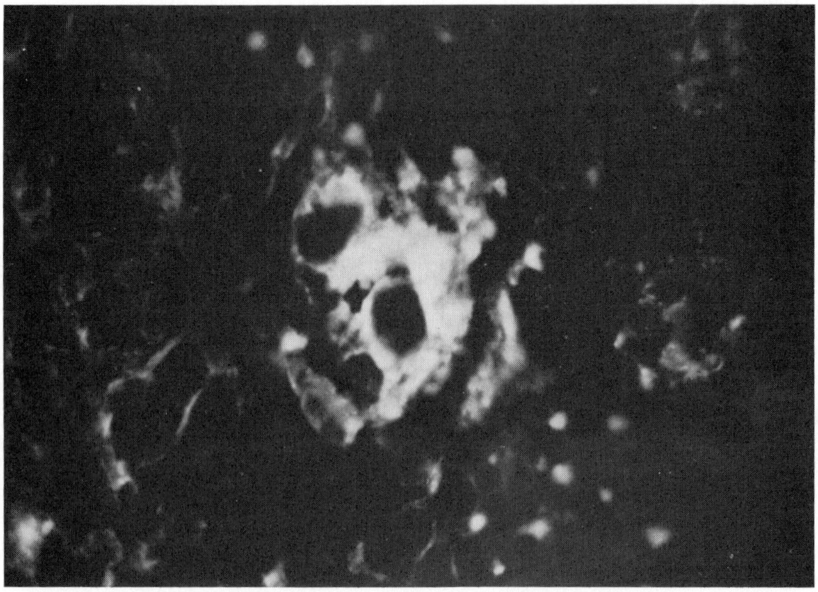

Figure 23–15. Immunofluorescent examination of biopsy from localized measles reaction showing deposition of IgG globulin. (From Bellanti, J. A.: Biologic significance of the secretory γA immunoglobulins. Pediatrics, *48*:715, 1971.) (Courtesy of Dr. Peter A. Ward.)

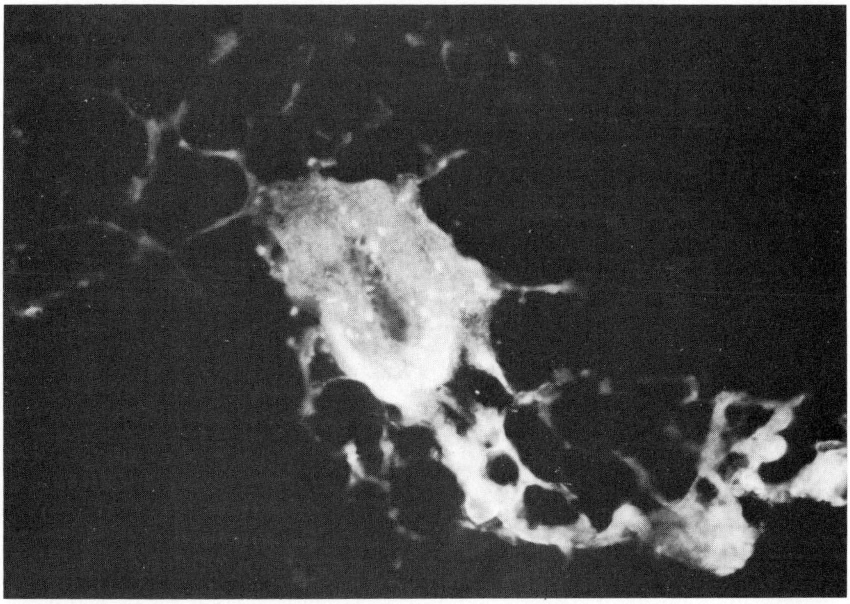

Figure 23–16. Immunofluorescent examination of biopsy from localized measles reaction showing C3 deposition within blood vessel wall. (From Bellanti, J. A.: Biologic significance of the secretory γA immunoglobulins. Pediatrics, *48*:715, 1971.) (Courtesy of Dr. Peter A. Ward.)

rosing panencephalitis (SSPE) with rubeola vaccine. The number of cases of SSPE associated with natural rubeola virus disease has been decreasing, and an upward trend has been observed in association with rubeola vaccine. However, recent reports suggest no significant increase in the number of SSPE cases associated with rubeola vaccine. Other complications are listed in Table 23–8, the most recent being the occurrence of the Guillain-Barré syndrome in recipients of the swine influenza virus vaccine.

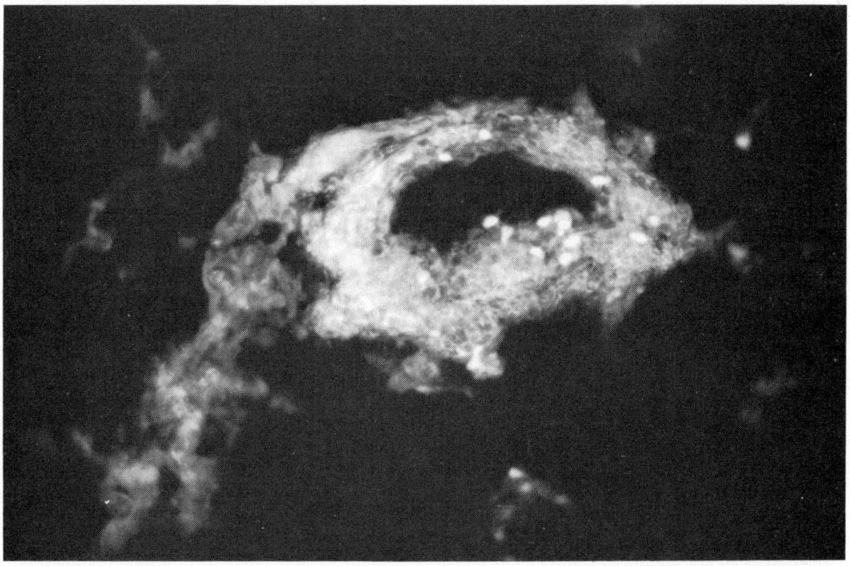

Figure 23–17. Immunofluorescent examination of biopsy from localized measles reaction showing fluorescence of measles antigen. (From Bellanti, J. A.: Biologic significance of the secretory γA immunoglobulins. Pediatrics, *48*:715, 1971.) (Courtesy of Dr. Peter A. Ward.)

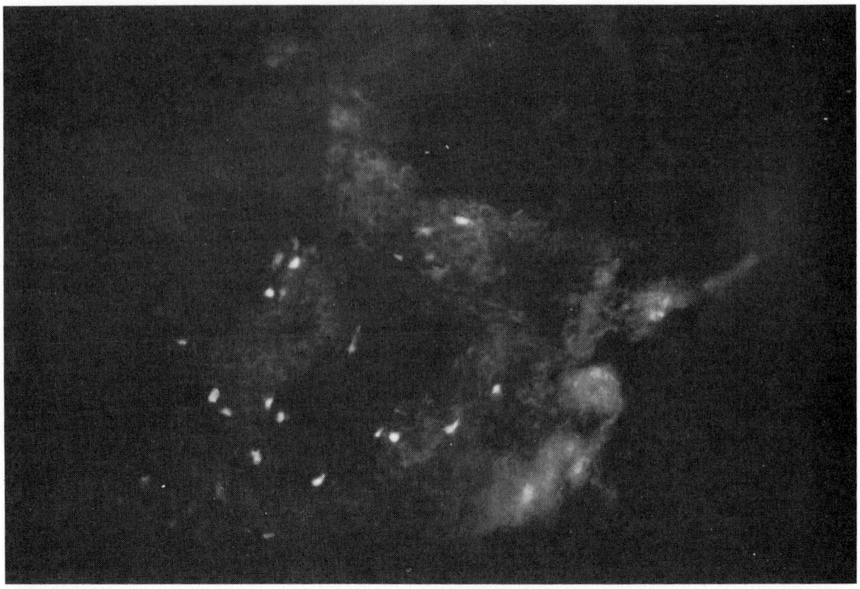

Figure 23–18. Immunofluorescent examination of biopsy from localized measles reaction showing negative fluorescence for IgA globulin. (From Bellanti, J. A.: Biologic significance of the secretory γA immunoglobulins. Pediatrics, *48*:715, 1971.) (Courtesy of Dr. Peter A. Ward.)

Thus, in using vaccines for the stimulation of protective immunity, the physician must be constantly aware of the undesirable complications. These may take the form of nonimmunologic as well as immunologic reactions. Since more vaccines will be developed and undoubtedly introduced in the future, the physician must be alert to known complications as well as future, as yet unknown, complications. All physicians would be well advised to keep in mind the warning, "Primum non nocere!" ("First do no harm!")

Suggestions for Further Reading

Asano, Y., Nakayama, H., Yazaki, T., et al.: Protective efficacy of vaccination in children in four episodes of natural varicella and zoster in the ward. Pediatrics, *59*:8, 1977.

Asano, Y., Nakayama, H., Yazaki, T., et al.: Protection against varicella in family contacts by immediate inoculation with live varicella vaccine. Pediatrics, *59*:3, 1977.

Bellanti, J. A.: The biologic significance of the secretory γ A immunoglobulin. Pediatrics, *48*:715, 1971.

Bellanti, J. A., and Frenkel, L. D.: Adverse reactions to immunizing agents. *In* Middleton, F., Reed, C., and Ellis, E. (eds.): Allergy: Principles and Practice. St. Louis, C. V. Mosby Company, 1978.

Chu, C., Schneerson, R., Robbins, J. B., et al.: Further studies on the immunogenicity of *Hemophilus influenzae* type b and pneumococcal type 6A polysaccharide-protein conjugates. Infect. Immun., *40*:245, 1983.

Fulginiti, V. A., and Clyde, W. A. (eds.): Workshop on bronchiolitis. Pediatr. Res., *11*:209, 1977.

Gold, R., and Lepow, M. L.: Present status of polysaccharide vaccines in the prevention of meningococcal disease. Adv. Pediatr., *23*:71, 1976.

Immunization Against Disease. United States Department of Health, Education and Welfare, Public Health Service, October 1970.

John, T. J., Devarajan, L. V., Luther, L., et al.: Effect of breast-feeding on seroresponse of infants to oral poliovirus vaccination. Pediatrics, *57*:47, 1976.

Krugman, S.: Present status of measles and rubella immunization in the United States: A medical progress report. J. Pediatr., *90*:1, 1977.

Modlin, J. F., Jabbour, J. T., Witte, J. J., et al.: Epidemiologic studies of measles, measles vaccine, and subacute sclerosing panencephalitis. Pediatrics, *59*:505, 1977.

Report on the Control of Infectious Diseases. American Academy of Pediatrics, 1974.

Reports and Recommendations of the National Immunization Work Groups, submitted to the Office of the Assistant Secretary for Health, Department of Health, Education and Welfare, Public Health Service, March 15, 1977.

Robbins, J. B., Hill, J. C., and Sadoff, J. C. (eds.): Bacterial Vaccines, Vol. 4, Seminars in Infectious Diseases. New York, Thieme-Stratton, 1982.

Chapter 24

Immunotherapy: The Use of Passive Immunization

Joseph A. Bellanti, M.D., and John B. Robbins, M. D.

Classically, immunotherapy referred to passive immunization, i.e., the use of serum or gamma globulin in the treatment or prevention of infectious diseases by transferring to one host antibodies actively produced in another. A specialized application of immunotherapy is its use in immunosuppression and prevention of isoimmunization (Chapter 10). Recently, the meaning of immunotherapy has been broadened to include the use of immunopotentiators, agents used in the treatment of cancer (Chapter 19) and in hyposensitization therapy of allergy (Chapter 20A). The complexity of the term has been increased by the extension of its meaning to include the replacement not only of antibody but also of immunocompetent lymphoid tissues, e.g., bone marrow and thymus, or their products, e.g., thymosin and transfer factor (Chapters 10 and 22). This chapter will deal primarily with those applications of immunotherapy that pertain to the more classic uses of serum or gamma globulin therapy in the prevention and therapy of infectious diseases.

The first uses of antitoxin in the therapy of infectious diseases, such as diphtheria and tetanus, were seen during the early part of this century (Fig. 24–1). The early dramatic successes obscured the preferable prevention of infectious diseases by active immunization through the use of vaccines (Chapter 23). Nevertheless, passive immunization is still needed for protection against those diseases for which vaccines are not available, e.g., botulism, and in the treatment of individuals incompletely immunized. Newer applications of immunotherapy include the prevention of Rh_0 sensitization and immunosuppression during tissue transplantation. In some situations, such as severe burns, the patients may have a limited period of severe acquired immune deficiency that requires immunotherapy to prevent serious and sometimes life-threatening infection. A fundamental understanding of the principles underlying immunotherapy is, therefore, necessary for the student and for the modern-day practitioner so that they can use passive immunization properly and evaluate applications that will inevitably appear in the future.

PRINCIPLES OF PASSIVE IMMUNIZATION

General Principles

There has been some confusion of terminology in the areas of active and passive immunization. The term *vaccine* should be reserved solely for those antigenic substances that result in a state of active immunity; such terms as serum, antitoxin, and gamma globulin refer to *antibody preparations*. The uses of antibody preparations in immunotherapy are shown schematically in Figure 24–2 and include such antimicrobial activities as *toxin neutralization*, *viral neutralization*, and *antibacterial* effects due to lysis or opsonization and phagocytosis. In addition, immunosuppressive activity with antibody preparations has been successful in the prevention of maternal Rh_0 isoimmunization and in immunosuppression during tissue transplantation.

The basic principle of passive immunization is the injection of antibodies from an immune host into a nonimmune host to achieve a desired prophylactic or therapeutic effect. Today, in most cases, passive immunization is achieved with immunoglobulin derived from pooled human plasma. In indus-

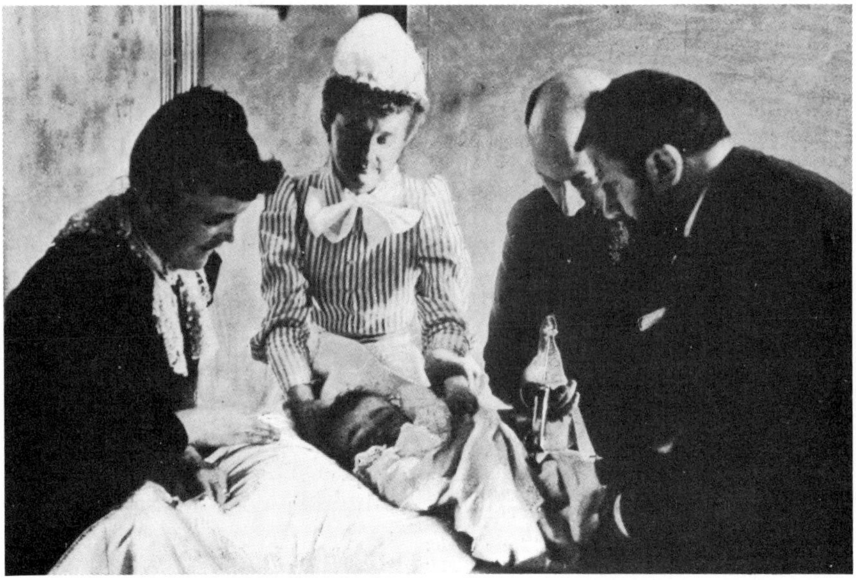

Figure 24–1. Photograph showing early use of diphtheria antitoxin in immunotherapy of diphtheria. (Courtesy of National Library of Medicine.)

trialized countries, virtually all such material is derived from human plasma or serum. In other parts of the world where the cost of such materials is prohibitive or where the facilities for their production are not yet available, globulins or sera from animal sources, mostly equine, are also used. Antibodies of human origin are preferred because these proteins do not elicit an immune response that could have an adverse effect, e.g., serum sickness, as is seen following the use of gamma globulins of animal origin.

Immediacy of Action

The most important reason for the use of passive immunization is its "immediacy of action"—the ability of preformed antibody to exert its effect immediately on interaction with an antigen (Fig. 24–2). The delay of the *latent period* required by an active immune response is thereby avoided. The obvious advantage, therefore, is that passive immunization procedures can be used in emergency situations when there is insufficient time to achieve an active immune response or when vaccine is unavailable. In general, the efficacy of passive immunization is related to the length of time between exposure to the pathogen and administration of the antibody, i.e., the shorter the interval, the greater the likelihood of prevention of the disease or of its successful treatment. In some instances, the antibody may be given prior to exposure, as in the use of gamma globulin for prevention of hepatitis A (infectious hepatitis) in individuals traveling to high-risk areas. In addition, passive immunization has important advantages for individuals who have primary or acquired (secondary) deficiencies of antibody synthesis (Chapter 22).

Metabolism of Gamma Globulin

Also important in the use of passive immunization are the factors that govern the metabolism of the antibody preparation (Chapter 7). It is now generally accepted that once antibody molecules are synthesized, they, like all other protein molecules, have a limited biologic half-life. There is continual loss and replacement of these molecules in a dynamic state that is referred to as *turnover.* By the very nature of the passive immunization procedure, the introduction of preformed antibody into a host ensures that in the absence of any active synthesis the duration of antibody activity will be finite. For example, if human (homologous) IgG immunoglobulin is administered to a healthy human, the biologic half-life ($t\frac{1}{2}$) will be 20 to 30 days. More rapid rates of degradation are observed with other isotypes, e.g., IgA $t\frac{1}{2}$ = four to eight days and IgM $t\frac{1}{2}$ = two to four days. The half-life of horse (heterol-

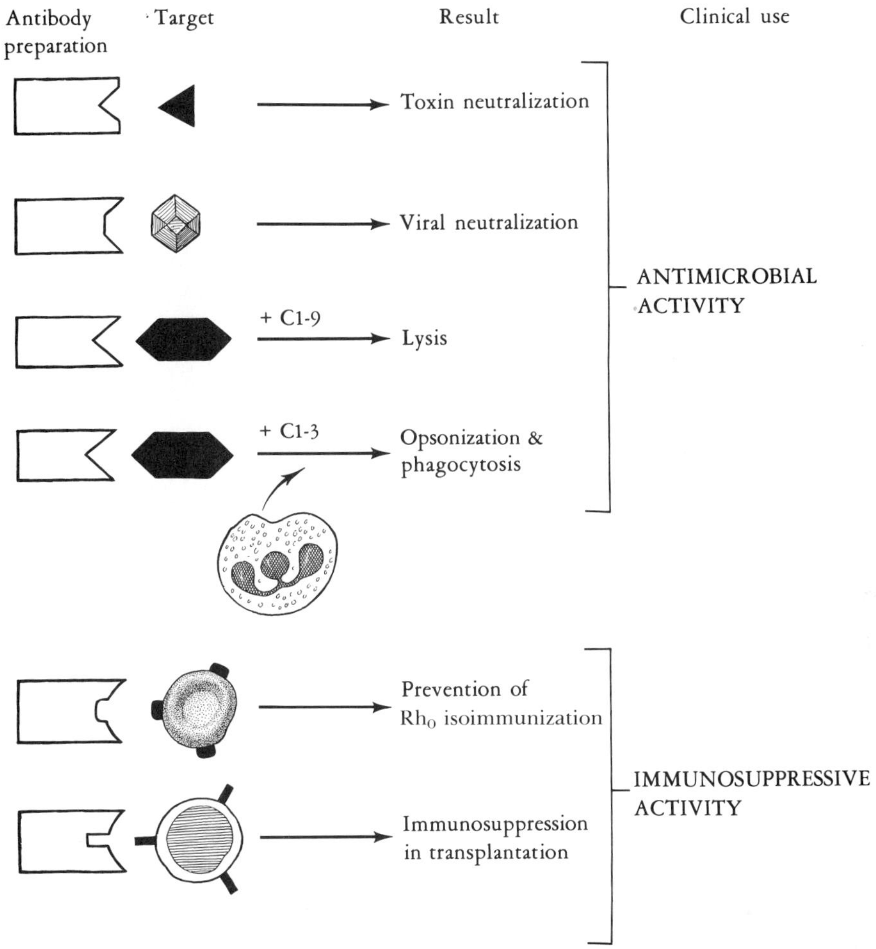

Figure 24–2. Schematic representation of the uses of antibody preparations in immunotherapy.

ogous) immunoglobulin administered to humans, on the other hand, is considerably shorter. In the latter case, in addition to the degradation governed by the biologic properties of the preparation, the recognition of foreign horse gamma globulin by the human results in an active immune response leading to antibody-mediated enhanced catabolism or immune elimination (Chapter 7). These events are represented schematically in Figure 24–3. For immunoglobulins of animal origin, this degradation process may vary. Antitoxins of equine origin, such as diphtheria or tetanus globulins, have been treated with pepsin to remove as much of the Fc fragment as possible. The pepsin-digested antibodies are catabolized quite rapidly, with an approximate half-life of two to eight days. Thus, although passive immunization can result in the rapid and predetermined rise of antibodies, the duration of such protection is finite and is determined by both the amount and the type of immunoglobulin administered.

The pattern of elimination of gamma globulin (antibody) administered intravenously to an animal occurs in three phases (Fig. 24–3). Phase 1 is a period of redistribution or equalization between vascular and extravascular spaces that results in a striking drop in peak titer shortly after administration of the antibody. Phase 2 is a slower, steady drop in serum levels due to the metabolic (catabolic) half-life of the gamma globulin. These diminutions in serum levels apply to both homologous and heterologous gamma globulins. Phase 3 is an accelerated period of degradation, occurring only in the case of heterologous gamma globulin, that takes place simultaneously with the development of antibody of the foreign gamma globulin. This third phase is referred to as *immune elimination.*

These metabolic properties of gamma

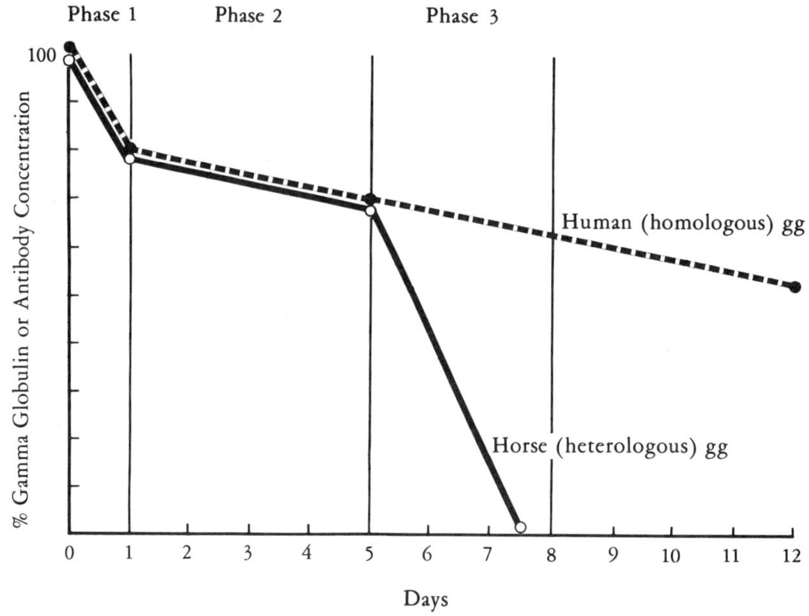

Figure 24–3. Schematic comparison of the catabolism of homologous and heterologous antibody (gg) preparations in the human.

globulin also have relevance to the passive immunization that occurs as a natural event in every human—the transplacental transfer of homologous IgG immunoglobulins from mother to fetus (Chapter 2). There is a gradual degradation and diminished concentration of IgG immunoglobulins following birth (physiologic hypogammaglobulinemia).

Variability of Preparations

A third principle governing the use of passive immunization is the great variability of biologic effectiveness seen with different preparations of gamma globulin. The use of immunotherapy is highly effective for some diseases, particularly when antibody is called on to neutralize the effect of extracellular toxin, e.g., tetanus toxin, or in certain viral diseases, e.g., measles. In other instances, the effectiveness of immunotherapy is less than optimal, but its use continues nevertheless. For example, the use of immunotherapy in hepatitis A does not necessarily prevent the disease, but it may convert a clinical disease into a subclinical one. In still other situations, the value of passive immunization is uncertain, highly questionable, and often controversial. For example administering gamma globulin to a pregnant female exposed to rubella in the first trimester may prevent clinical rubella in the mother, but a subclinical disease may occur. This may be followed by the full-blown congenital rubella syndrome in the infant.

The reason for the disparity in efficacy between various gamma globulin preparations employed in immunotherapy is not entirely apparent. The following factors appear to be of importance: (1) The *time of administration* of the preparation. Optimally, an antibody preparation should be given immediately after exposure to an infectious agent. (2) The *differences in pathogenesis* of the various disease entities. Those infectious agents that have a blood-borne phase will be more effectively neutralized by the use of gamma globulin than those that are localized. (3) The *content of specific antibody* in any given preparation. Because of variations in antibody content in serum and to ensure an adequate level of antibody, gamma globulin preparations are obtained preferably from hyperimmune sera.

Inhibition of Primary Immune Response

A fourth important principle is the application of immunotherapy in the suppression of the immune response (Chapter 10). The passive administration of specific antibody will inhibit active production of antibody by means of negative feedback inhibition. Thus, if red cells from an Rh_0-positive individual are coated with incomplete anti-Rh_0 antibody prior to injection into an Rh_0-negative individual, the formation of anti-Rh_0 antibodies is prevented. This use of antibody immunosuppression apparently affects the "afferent" limb of the immune system by preventing the production of antibody (Fig. 24–4). The use of antilymphocyte sera (ALS), on the other hand, appears to inhibit the primary immune response by interfering with the "efferent" limb of immunity (Fig. 24–4).

TYPES OF PREPARATIONS

The various preparations commonly available for use in immunotherapy are listed in Table 24–1. The official titles of these products are taken from Establishments and Products, licensed under section 351 of the Public Health Service Act, U.S. Department of Health and Human Services, Publication No. (FDA)-83-9003, July 1983.

Immune Serum Globulin (ISG)

Immune serum globulin (human), also called gamma globulin, is derived from the blood, plasma, or serum of human donors and contains most of the antibodies found in whole blood. The amounts of specific antibody vary in different preparations. The ISG preparation (usually derived from placental blood) contains a concentration of antibodies approximately 25 times that found in blood. Final concentration of the preparation contains 165 mg of gamma globulin per milliliter. Each lot of immune serum globulin represents a pooling of not fewer than 1000 donors, which provides a wide spectrum of antibody but also increases the risk of sensitization after prolonged usage. These preparations contain primarily IgG immunoglobulins, with lesser amounts of IgM antibodies important in bacterial defense. Although there are IgA immunoglobulins in commercial gamma globulin, these proteins are poorly transmitted to mucosal surfaces, sites where the secretory IgA globulins normally provide defense.

The advantages of gamma globulin preparations over whole serum are as follows: (1) Gamma globulin is free from hepatitis virus B; (2) it is concentrated, permitting the administration of a large amount of antibody in a small volume; and (3) it is stable during long-term storage.

There are disadvantages to the use of concentrated ISG preparations. All preparations have a tendency to aggregate into large 11S polymers. These aggregates account for the occasional anaphylactic reactions seen follow-

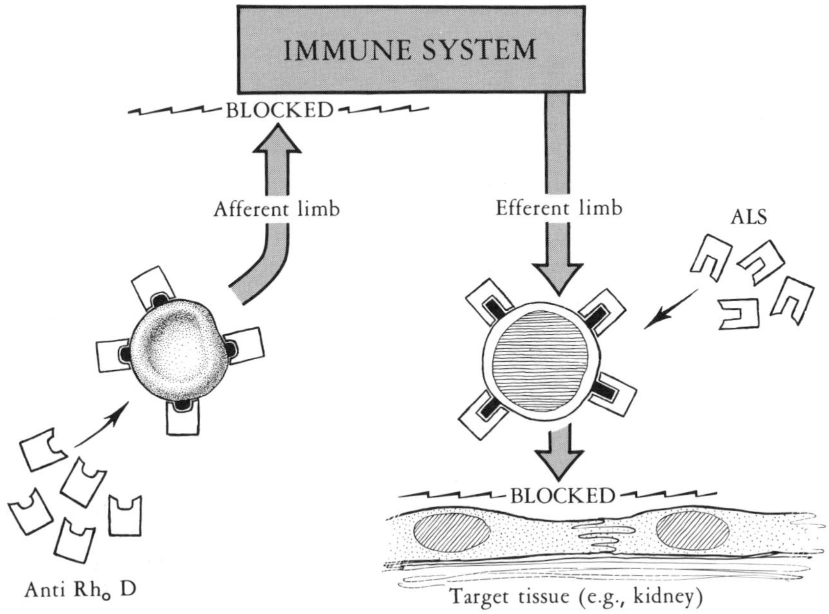

Figure 24–4. Schematic representation of the modes of immunosuppression by specific anti-Rh_0 antibody and by antilymphocyte sera (ALS).

Table 24–1. **Preparations in Common Use for Immunotherapy**

Preparation	Source	Comments
Immune serum globulin (ISG)	Human	Rubeola, hepatitis A, congenital agammaglobulinemia
Immune globulin intravenous		Indications same as ISG for intravenous use
Specific immune serum globulin (SIG)	Human	Prepared from hyperimmune sera; use established
Pertussis immune globulin		
Rabies immune globulin		
Tetanus immune globulin		
Vaccinia immune globulin		
Varicella-zoster immune globulin		
Rh_0 (D) immune globulin		
Hepatitis B immune globulin		
Therapeutic immune sera		
Antirabies serum	Animal	Not established or produce untoward complications, e.g., serum hepatitis or sensitization
Antilymphocyte sera		
Lymphocyte immune globulin, antithymocyte globulin	Equine	
Antitoxins (animal)		
Antivenins	Animal	
Botulism	Animal	
Diphtheria	Animal	

ing prolonged usage. The frequency of these reactions is far too high for ISG to be administered via the intravenous route; therefore, the intact preparation should not be given intravenously. Since each lot represents a pool of many donors, the likelihood of sensitization is increased with continued usage. Isoimmunization against the Gm factors of gamma globulin has been reported after prolonged administration in immunologically normal individuals and in children with acquired agammaglobulinemia.

The value of immune serum globulin (human) has been demonstrated unequivocally in only three situations: (1) prevention of rubeola, (2) prevention of hepatitis A, and (3) replacement therapy in congenital agammaglobulinemia of the Bruton type. Although it has not been proved, ISG may be useful in preventing three other infectious diseases: (1) rubella in the first trimester of pregnancy, (2) varicella in exposed patients on immunosuppressive therapy, and (3) posttransfusion hepatitis. One reason for the lack of effectiveness in these latter diseases may be the lack of sufficient specific antibody in ordinary ISG preparations.

Any uses of immune serum globulin other than those listed previously constitute misuses or abuses of the preparation. There is no justification for the use of gamma globulin in children with repeated upper respiratory tract infections due to viruses. Similarly, there is no indication for its use in asthma, tonsillitis, or chronic pyelonephritis. In the interpretation of possible immunoglobulin deficiencies in children, the level of serum gamma globulin must be age-adjusted because of the developmental immunologic immaturity of the young infant and child (Chapters 22 and 26).

Recently, gamma globulin preparations for intravenous use have been developed. These materials are prepared by enzymatic or chemical treatment of intact gamma globulin in order to render them suitable for intravenous use. Although the indications for the use of these preparations are essentially similar to those of the intramuscular ISG preparations, they have the advantage of obviating the local reactions that follow intramuscular injection in the older child or adult.

Specific Immune Serum Globulin (SIG)

Specific immune serum globulins (SIG) are prepared from the sera of convalescent individuals or those who are hyperimmunized to a given material (Table 24–1). Since such preparations contain a higher content of specific antibody to the agent in question than that found in ISG, they are preferable to the latter.

The more commonly used specific immune globulins are listed in Table 24–1. The World Health Organization has also recommended human sources for specific immune globulins that are currently unavailable or in short supply, e.g., zoster immune globulin (ZIG).

Therapeutic Immune Sera and Antitoxins

The antisera and antitoxins listed in Table 24–1 are produced in animals and should be used only in clinical situations in which human sources of immune globulin are not available, because they present the problem of possible hypersensitivity reactions (serum sickness) (Chapter 20A).

Rh_0(D) Immune Globulin

This material consists of IgG–anti-Rh_0(D) prepared from pooled human sera. This preparation has been used in the prevention of Rh_0 isosensitization and has received several thousand clinical trials.

Antilymphocyte Sera (Horse)

This material is produced by active immunization of horses with human thymocytes for use in immunosuppression in transplantation. Although it is a licensed product, the use of this material in humans is confined primarily to the pretreatment of transplant recipients as described below.

USES OF PASSIVE IMMUNIZATION

The classic use of passive immunization has been and continues to be its application in the prevention or treatment of infectious diseases, including those associated with bacteria or their products (toxins), viruses, and certain protoza (malaria). However, new applications of passive immunization in the suppression of the primary immune response are now being included. Applications of passive immunization are given in Table 24–2. The uses of passive immunization form two major categories: *replacement therapy* and *suppression* of the primary immune response. Replacement therapy is used in cases in which gamma globulin is congenitally deficient, e.g., agammaglobulinemia, or in which there is an absence of specific antibody, e.g., unimmunized individuals. The use of passive immunization in suppressing the immune response includes the prevention of Rh_0 isoimmunization and immunosuppression in tissue transplantation.

Replacement Therapy

This type of therapy employs either immune serum globulin (ISG) or specific immune globulins (SIG).

IMMUNE SERUM GLOBULIN (ISG)

Immunologic Deficiency Syndromes. The use of gamma globulin therapy in the immunologic deficiency syndrome is described in Chapter 22. Its greatest efficacy is seen in the disorders involving the thymic-independent types of immune deficiency, such as the Burton type of congenital agammaglobulinemia and acquired types of hypogammaglobulinemia. Since ISG has a high content of specific antibody against those organisms that commonly infect agammaglobulinemic patients, this type of replacement therapy is highly effective. However, since immune serum globulin contains predominantly IgG antibodies, these patients may continue to have localized infections, particularly of the respiratory and gastrointestinal tracts.

Table 24–2. **Applications of Passive Immunization**

Indication	Application	Type of Preparation
Replacement therapy	Immunologic deficiency syndrome	Immune serum globulin (ISG)
	Prevention or treatment of certain infectious diseases (rubeola, mumps, hepatitis, and tetanus)	ISG, Serum immune globulin (SIG)
Suppression of primary immune response	Prevention of Rh_0 isoimmunization	Rh_0 (D) immunoglobulin
	Immunosuppression in transplantation	Antilymphocyte sera (ALS)

Patients with agammaglobulinemia are subject to repeated episodes of bacterial infection, especially those due to pneumococci and *Hemophilus influenzae* Type B. Passive immunization with pooled immunoglobulin, approximately every three weeks, has been shown to confer a high degree of immunity on such patients. Unfortunately, passive immunization with immune serum globulin does not result in sufficiently high levels of antibodies into external secretions such as secretions of the middle ear, lacrimal fluid of the eye, or intestinal secretions. Accordingly, although such therapy is effective in preventing diseases whose pathogenesis is involved with invasion of the blood stream (generalized infections), it is less satisfactory for diseases that are characterized by involvement of external secretory tissues (localized infections), such as otitis media. Until recently, most patients were treated with intramuscular injections of gamma globulin. For older children, this may have involved injection of 10 to 20 ml of immunoglobulin at intramuscular sites. Such therapy was often painful and in many cases difficult with individuals who were ill. Immune serum globulin, prepared by the Cohn fractionation procedure, had to be given intramuscularly because of the serious episodes of hypotension and/or shock that were observed after intravenous use. The best explanation for the toxicity of immune serum globulin, prepared by Cohn fractionation, when given intravenously is that these materials contain, in addition to immunoglobulins, other aggregates and serum proteins involved with coagulation and release of vasoactive peptides as generated by the kallikrein system (Chapter 13). This toxicity of immune serum globulin, when administered intravenously, has been overcome by the use of sophisticated methods of preparing serum proteins, including ion exchange and absorption chromatography followed by enzymatic and chemical treatment of the purified gamma globulin. The resultant products contain considerably reduced amounts of other serum proteins and, when administered intravenously under controlled conditions, have proved to be safe and effective. Although these products are at present more expensive than the materials prepared by column fractionation, their use is rapidly expanding. Therapeutic levels of antibodies can be achieved more rapidly and discomfort to the patient can largely be avoided by the use of intravenous immune serum globulin.

Prevention of Certain Infectious Diseases. In addition to its use in replacement therapy for individuals who have a primary or secondary deficiency of antibody synthesis, immune serum globulin has been successful in the prevention of certain specific viral diseases. Nonimmune individuals who have been exposed to patients with rubeola or hepatitis A can be effectively treated with immune serum globulin. The reason is that the prevention of these infectious diseases requires only small amounts of antibody. Pooled immunoglobulin, obtained from individuals who have had measles or hepatitis A as children, has a sufficient amount of antibodies to prevent these viral diseases. Thus, adults who have never been immunized with measles vaccine and who did not have measles in their childhood should be treated with immune serum globulin if they have a known contact with a case of rubeola. Immunization with measles vaccine can then be instituted several weeks later.

Individuals who travel or who are sent to countries where hepatitis A is prevalent may wish to be passively immunized with immune serum globulin (Table 24–3). This protection may last as long as two to three months, depending upon the dose of the immunoglobulin injected. Less substantiated is the efficacy of immune serum globulin in the prevention of hepatitis B, which is often transmitted by intimate contact with blood or blood products from an infected donor. However, there are now preparations of immunoglobulin, taken from individuals immunized with hepatitis B vaccine, that have substantially higher titers of antibodies than that of immune serum globulin. This material has been only newly manufactured, and its cost is high. However, its therapeutic effectiveness has been established and its use is to be preferred over that of immune serum globulin, if possible.

Immune serum globulin has also been advocated by some for mumps and rubella. However, its effectiveness in the prevention of mumps, especially in sexually mature men or in pregnant women, has never been established and immune serum globulin is not licensed for these therapeutic objectives in the United States.

SPECIFIC IMMUNE GLOBULINS

One of the most significant recent advances in passive immunization was the development

Table 24–3. Guidelines for Prophylaxis of Hepatitis A

Weight (lbs)	ISG Dose (ml)
Up to 50	0.5
50–100	1.0
> 100	2.0

of a human source of tetanus immune globulin. The most commonly used specific immune globulin is tetanus immune globulin that is prepared from donors who are immunized with tetanus toxoid. Tetanus immune globulin is the treatment of choice for the prevention of tetanus in individuals who have had deep wound, crushing, or burn injuries or in those whose immunization status is unknown. Its effectiveness in the treatment of established tetanus is less clear, but its use in this case is recommended in the unlikely circumstance that human globulin is unavailable. The equine product, horse antitetanus toxin, is a pepsin-digested globulin taken from horses repeatedly immunized, initially with tetanus toxoid and then with whole *Clostridium tetani* culture filtrates. The amount of antibodies in this preparation is extraordinarily high. The prophylactic effectiveness of this product has been established, and it is used throughout the world where tetanus immune globulin is not available.

Hardegree and her associates have noted that equine antitetanus toxin contains antibodies both to the B fragment of tetanus toxin responsible for binding to the tissue receptor and (in contrast to tetanus immune globulin) to the toxic or A fragment of tetanus toxin. Antibodies to the B polypeptide chain of tetanus toxin can effectively neutralize these toxic proteins by locking their interaction with the host cells. However, it is generally thought that the tetanus toxin, once fixed to the host cells, internalizes and then passes on to the synaptic junction of the neuron, and is no longer accessible to the neutralizing effect of antibodies. This is why tetanus immune globulin has little or no effect in the treatment of established tetanus. Some investigators have claimed, however, that large doses of equine antitetanus toxin, injected intravenously and/or directly into the spinal fluid, may have a therapeutic effect on established tetanus. In this case, antibodies to the toxic fragment may exert a therapeutic action upon the tissue-fixed toxin. The subject is under investigation at this time.

Diphtheria Antitoxin. To date in the United States and throughout the world, only equine antidiphtheria toxin antibodies are available. Equine diphtheria antitoxin antibodies are an integral part of the treatment of diphtheria. The effectiveness of this product is directly related to the timing of administration in relation to the stage of disease. If antitoxin is administered in appropriate doses early in the course of the disease, it can effectively inhibit the tissue fixation of diphtheria toxin. However, if the disease has been established and symptoms present for at least three or four days, the therapeutic effectiveness of the diphtheria antitoxin antibodies is extremely limited. Owing to the widespread and effective use of diphtheria toxoids, diphtheria is now a rare disease. However, cases are encountered, and the use of antitoxin, in addition to antibiotics, is indicated in the treatment of diphtheria. The problem of acute hypersensitivity reactions, such as anaphylaxis, must be considered. The present practice is to try to assess the sensitivity state of the recipient by injecting highly diluted equine diphtheria antitoxin intracutaneously as described in the package insert of the product. If acute wheal and flare reactions occur with highly diluted materials, then a gradual process of desensitization must be undertaken before the therapeutic dose of the immune globulin can be administered (Chapter 3). Since the dose of the diphtheria antitoxin antibody is related to the duration of the clinical disease, an estimate must be made of the number of days that clinical diphtheria has been established. Active immunization with diphtheria toxoid should commence as soon as possible.

Vaccinia. The production of a vaccinia immune globulin (VIG) has been made possible through the American National Red Cross and the Armed Forces. It is prepared from the pooled plasma of 1000 or more volunteers. This material has been recommended for use in the catastrophic complications of smallpox vaccination, including those that occur in eczema (eczema vaccinatum) and certain of the immunologic deficiency syndromes (Chapters 22 and 23). It is recommended in infants suffering from eczema who have been inadvertently vaccinated or exposed to recently vaccinated individuals, in infants with other breaks in the continuity of the skin, e.g., burns, and in infants with eczema who are required to have a smallpox vaccination prior to overseas travel. The use of VIG has not been shown to be beneficial in the prevention or treatment of postvaccinial encephalitis. The use of the preparation is also recommended in the prevention of smallpox in close contacts of patients with the disease. The dose for prophylaxis is 0.3 ml per kilogram and the dose for treatment is 0.6 ml per kilogram intramuscularly. Although the use of VIG is recommended in the treatment of progressive vaccinia, its efficacy is doubtful, since many of these children have been shown to be deficient predominantly in the thymic-dependent, cell-mediated limb of immunity. The basic defect, therefore, does not appear to be correctable by VIG alone.

Zoster Immune Globulin (ZIG). An innovative approach and specialized series of immunologic events have permitted the preparation of a useful immunoprophylactic and therapeutic reagent called ZIG (zoster immune globulin). Individuals who have recovered from herpes zoster neuritis (shingles) have a brief period of high-titered antibodies to it and varicella virus (chickenpox). Plasma extracted from such convalescent patients has been prepared (ZIG) for use in the prevention or treatment of varicella in susceptible or infected individuals, such as those with acquired immunodeficiency states. Especially susceptible are adults with treated or advanced chronic lymphatic leukemia or Hodgkin's disease. At this time, the availability of this material is conditioned by the availability of donors (convalescent patients) and funds for the manufacture of ZIG.

OTHER APPLICATIONS OF PASSIVE IMMUNIZATION

An interesting and potentially useful application of immunologic principles has been the development of antibodies to drugs. It is a medical emergency when digoxin is taken in an excessive dose, either by deliberate action of a patient or by inadvertent administration to a patient. By a clever combination of the properties of this commonly used compound with our new knowledge of immunoglobulins, a therapeutic preparation of antidigoxin antibodies has been successfully used for treatment of overdosage with this agent. Digoxin is a glycone trisaccharide and is not immunogenic by itself. By chemical attachment to a protein, specific antibodies to this compound may be raised in rabbits and goats. These digoxin-specific antibodies may be purified from the antisera by use of affinity resins. The specific antibody is further treated with pepsin to selectively remove the Fc fragment without loss of antibody activity. The Fab fragment has two unusual properties that give it greater therapeutic effectiveness than that of the intact antidigoxin antibodies. The first is that the catabolic rate of the Fab fragments is markedly greater than that of the intact immunoglobulin. Thus, the almost instantaneous combination of the Fab fragment with the hapten (digoxin) results in inactivation of the cardiotoxicity and rapid excretion of the antigen-antibody complex in the urine. Second is the decreased immunogenicity of the Fab fragment as compared with the intact immunoglobulin. Thus, the Fab anti-intoxicant has the specificity and combining activity of the intact antibody but has a more rapid excretion and lesser immunogenicity. The limitations of this therapeutic approach are the need for the immunochemist to produce high-binding antibodies and the relation between the amount of hapten (potential toxin) and the amount of antibody-derived Fab protein required for a therapeutic effect. The success of this approach for intoxication with digoxin and related molecules will inspire scientists to seek preparations for the treatment of other conditions caused by small molecules with intoxicant activities at comparatively low concentrations.

Immunosuppression

Rh_0 PREVENTION

The use of specific anti-Rh_0(D) globulin has been shown to be effective in preventing Rh_0 isoimmunization by preventing transplacentally acquired fetal erythrocytes from reacting with maternal immunologically competent cells. The production of anti-Rh_0 antibody is therefore "blocked" (Fig. 24–4). The recommended dose of the preparation is 1.0 ml administered within 72 hours of delivery in cases in which an Rh_0-positive baby is born to an Rh_0-negative mother (Chapter 10). The use of this preparation represents one of the most exciting new applications of immunotherapy.

IMMUNOSUPPRESSION BY ALS

Recently, the administration of antilymphocyte sera has been shown to be effective in immunosuppression in animals. Similar immunosuppressive approaches using this preparation have been used in man. The sera are produced in animals such as the horse by the injection of suspensions of lymphocytes with Freund's adjuvant. The sera are then administered to recipients of transplants, usually in conjunction with other forms of immunosuppressive therapy (Chapter 25). The precise mechanism of action of ALS is unknown. The most plausible therory is that the preparation is reacting with critical receptors on the surface of lymphocytes, coating them, and making the lymphocyte unavailable for its interaction with target cells (Fig. 24–4). ALS has been shown to be a potent inhibitor of cell-mediated immunologic events and may be a possible adjunct in transplantation immunology. However, there are several undesirable features of ALS: (1) the lack of standardized preparations, (2) the problem of reactions with heterologous horse sera, (3) the recent demonstration that ALS enhances viral replication *in vitro* and *in vivo*, leading to overwhelming viral infections in man, and (4) the enhancement of tumor development following its use (Chapter 19).

THE HAZARDS OF IMMUNOGLOBULIN THERAPY

Millions of doses of gamma globulin have been administered to humans over the past 25 years. With this increased usage and experience, a number of reactions and hazards have become apparent. Prior to considering immunotherapy, therefore, the physician must critically evaluate the indications for its use. The problems associated with immunoglobulin therapy are related to properties of the *preparation* as well as to the *host's response* to the gamma globulin.

The properties of the preparation that are of clinical importance include the following: (1) Commercial gamma globulin is prepared from many foreign genetic types of gamma globulin, and therefore the likelihood of sensitization is great, particularly after prolonged usage; (2) the preparation contains mainly IgG; and (3) preparations from placental sources are contaminated with A and B blood group substances. Another important property of the gamma globulin is that all commercial preparations have a tendency to aggregate into large 11S biopolymers. These aggregates are of clinical importance, since they may be responsible for severe reactions, particularly when given intravenously. These polymers can lead to sensitization and upon standing tend to fragment, with subsequent loss of antibody content (Table 24–4).

The clinical reactions to gamma globulin are given in Table 24–4. Standard gamma globulin cannot be given intravenously, since severe pyrogenic and cardiovascular reactions have occurred that are believed to be related to the presence of aggregates in the preparation. The reactions are believed to be nonimmunologic in nature and can occur in individuals receiving intravenous gamma globulin for the first time. The use of plasmin digests of gamma globulin has been shown to be clinically effective, and plasmin digests appear to eliminate the problem of aggregates. These preparations are still biologically active and can be given intravenously.

Table 24–4. Clinical Reactions After Immunoglobulin Therapy

Reaction	Mechanism
Cardiovascular shock, fever after intravenous use	Aggregates
Loss of antibody activity	Fragmentation
Sensitization	Sensitization due to: (1) Anti-Gm (2) Antibody to aggregates (3) Anti-IgA antibody
Development of anti-A and anti-B	A and B contamination of placental sources

In addition to this type of reaction, the repeated use of gamma globulin can lead to sensitization in normal persons and even in patients with various types of immunologic deficiencies. At least three types of sensitization have been described (Table 24–4). The first of these is caused by antibody to the Gm determinant and is seen after prolonged gamma globulin usage. A second type of sensitization to the aggregated gamma globulin itself may occur. The development of precipitating antibody to aggregated but not native gamma globulin was demonstrated in children with acquired agammaglobulinemia who had been receiving gamma globulin. This was associated with "anaphylactic shock" after intramuscular administration. A third type of sensitization to gamma globulin is the development of anti-IgA antibodies. This was first described in patients with ataxia-telangiectasia with IgA deficiency but has been subsequently described in normal persons with normal IgA levels. Patients with IgA deficiency develop anti-IgA with broad class specificity; normal persons develop anti-IgA of a more restricted specificity (Chapter 5).

All these antigammaglobulin antibodies of the IgG class are able to fix complement and may be associated with hypersensitivity reactions mediated by antibody (Chapter 13). They all appear to be important in nonhemolytic transfusion reactions, particularly the anti-IgA antibodies (Chapter 20B).

A final complication of the use of gamma globulin is the development of isohemagglutinins of anti-A and anti-B specificity in individuals receiving gamma globulin. This is primarily true of gamma globulin prepared from placental sources that appears to be contaminated by the blood group substances. This complication may be of particular significance in women receiving anti-Rh_0(D) globulin for the prevention of Rh_0 disease.

PROJECTIONS FOR THE FUTURE USE OF IMMUNOTHERAPY

At least two new approaches for passive immunization of infectious diseases are under active investigation. The first is the preparation of monoclonal antibodies derived from hybridoma cultures (Chapter 5). These hybridoma cultures may be composed of mouse cells exclusively or of human cells, or they may be a mixture of human and mouse cells. At present there is no licensed product derived from hybridoma cultures for prevention or treatment of infectious diseases. This is because the oncogenic potential of products of malignant cell type(s) is not known. Yet, the potential for preparing antibodies of defined specificity for the treatment of diseases already mentioned and for other bacterial infections is enormous. There are several advantages to this technique. First, virtually all the protein in monoclonal antibodies is of a desired antibody specificity. This would provide materials with highly specific activity for passive immunization—incomparably higher than even specific immune globulin. Thus, the amount of antibodies that could be administered would be substantially greater. A second advantage is that immunoglobulins of various isotypes, such as IgM and IgA, could be administered. To date, immunoglobulin preparations of either intramuscular or intravenous type contain almost exclusively IgG antibodies. It is hoped that monoclonal antibodies of specific isotypes will provide more widespread therapeutic effects, such as in the immunodeficiency states. The other aspect of passive immunization that has attracted a great deal of research activity is the possibility of preventing or treating hospital-acquired (nosocomial) infections, which constitute the most common infectious diseases in clinical medicine today. Approximately 80,000 to 100,000 individuals undergo bacteremic infection annually. Almost all of these are associated with the effects of modern therapy, including cancer chemotherapy and extensive surgery. Although the causes of hospital-acquired infections are numerous, the most common etiologic agents are gram-negative bacteria, including *Escherichia coli, Klebsiella pneumoniae, Pseudomonas aeruginosa,* and other species. *Staphylococcus aureus* constitutes most of the gram-positive organisms. The antigenic diversity of these bacterial species has discouraged the use of passive immunoglobulins for treating these diseases. For instance, *Escherichia coli* associated with hospital-acquired infections include approximately 50 capsular polysaccharide and about 70 lipopolysaccharide antigens. There are approximately 60 *Klebsiella* capsular polysaccharides associated with invasive infection.

An innovative experimental approach to this problem has been advocated by Ziegler and Braude. These investigators have pointed out that the general structure of lipopolysaccharides of all gram-negative bacteria share some structural characteristics. In addition to their O-specific side chain, which determines the antigenic diversity of lipopolysaccharide, and the lipid A, which is inaccessible to any therapeutic effect of antibodies since it is buried in the lipid layer of the outer membrane, there is a "core region" that is exposed to antibodies and is widely shared by gram-negative organisms. Antibodies to this core region can be deliberately induced in animals. Such "core antibodies," directed against mutant bacteria with this region exposed, e.g., *E. coli* J5 strain, exert a protective effect in experimental animals to infections caused by numerous gram-negative bacterial species. Ziegler and Braude have demonstrated that immune plasma taken from adults immunized with heat-killed *E. coli* J5 (a mutant bacterium with an exposed core region in its LPS) confers a protective effect against both infection and shock caused by gram-negative bacteria in hospitalized patients.

Other investigators have prepared specific immune globulins from plasma of volunteers injected with pneumococcal, *Hemophilus influenzae* type b, and meningococcal vaccines. These plasmas have been screened so that those responding with the highest levels of antibodies are used for the preparation of the globulin. The resulting product contains as high as 300 to 400 times the level of these anticapsular polysaccharide antibodies as does immune serum globulin. Such globulins could be used for passive immunization of infants who are at risk for invasive diseases due to these encapsulated bacteria, such as those with sickle cell anemia and splenectomy or those from such high-risk groups as Alaskan Eskimos and Navajo Indians. In addition, these investigators plan to use such products for passive immunization of patients with severe impairment of their lymphoid function such as occurs in individuals with Hodgkin's disease who had been splenectomized and received prolonged chemotherapy and/or radiation.

The prophylactic or therapeutic effect of pertussis immune globulin (PIG) has never been verified, and its use has been under review by the Food and Drug Administration. One explanation for the failure of these preparations, taken from adults immunized with pertussis vaccine, is that their level of antipertussis toxin antibodies was low. The availability of highly refined components of pertussis, including detoxified pertussis toxin, appears imminent, and it is hoped that the effectiveness of such preparations can be improved.

An extension of immunotherapy is the replacement not of gamma globulin but of the immunocompetent lymphoid tissues. The transplantation of thymus or bone marrow has now been successfully accomplished in restoring immunocompetence to children with immune deficiencies (Chapters 20B and 22). The successful use of transfer factor in the reconstitution of such individuals has also been reported. This form of immunotherapy has the obvious advantage over gamma globulin replacement of permanency. As better methods of histocompatibility matching become available, this form of immunotherapy will become increasingly useful in the restoration of immunologic function.

Suggestions for Further Reading

Alving, B. M., and Fintayson, J. S. (eds.): Immunoglobulins: Characteristics and Uses of Intravenous Preparations. Washington, D.C., U.S. Department of Health and Human Services, PHS, FDA, DHHS, Publication No. (FDA)-80-9005, 1979.

Ambrosino, D., Schreiber, J. R., Daum, R. S., et al.: Efficacy of human hyperimmune globulin in prevention of *Hemophilus influenzae* type b in infant rats. Infect. Immun., *39*:709, 1983.

Brunell, P. A., Ross, A., Miller, L. H., et al.: Prevention of varicella by zoster immune globulin. N. Engl. J. Med., *280*:1191, 1969.

Edsall, G.: Passive immunization. Pediatrics, *32*:599, 1963.

Fudenberg, H., Good, R. A., Goodman, H. C., et al.: Primary immunodeficiencies. Pediatrics, *47*:927, 1971.

Krugman, S.: The clinical uses of gamma globulin. N. Engl. J. Med., *269*:195, 1963.

Merler, E. (ed.): Immunoglobulins: Biologic Aspects and Clinical Usage. Washington, D.C., National Academy of Sciences, 1970.

Nydegger, V. F. (ed.): Immunohemotherapy: A Guide to Immunoglobulin Prophylaxis and Therapy. London, Academic Press, 1981.

Pollack, W., Gorman, J. G., and Freda, V. J.: Prevention of Rh_0 hemolytic disease. Progr. Hematol., *6*:121, 1969.

Ziegler, E. J., McCutchan, A., Fierer, J., et al.: Treatment of gram negative bacteremia and shock with human antiserum to a mutant *Escherichia coli.* N. Engl. J. Med., *307*:1225, 1982.

Chapter 25

Clinical Aspects of Immunosuppression: Use of Cytotoxic Agents and Corticosteroids

Anthony S. Fauci, M.D.

Immunosuppression is the negative control or regulation of immunologic reactivity (Chapter 10). There are several major categories of immunosuppressive agents, including x-irradiation, antilymphocyte globulin, cytotoxic agents, and corticosteroids. Radiation therapy is used predominantly for its cytocidal effects on certain types of neoplastic cells; the major use of antilymphocyte globulin has been in the prevention of organ transplant rejection. Certain categories of cytotoxic agents (usually in very high doses) have been used in a variety of neoplasms. As with radiation therapy, the desired effect has been cytocidal for tumor cells. However, in recent years cytotoxic agents have been used with increasing frequency solely for their immunosuppressive effects in immunologically mediated diseases. Although corticosteroids are used in certain neoplasms, particularly of the lymphoid, reticuloendothelial, and hematopoietic organs, their major use has been as anti-inflammatory or immunosuppressive agents.

In this chapter we will not attempt to encompass the entire scope of immunosuppression but will be concerned predominantly with the mechanisms of action and clinical considerations in the use of cytotoxic agents and corticosteroids in man. We will focus on the use of these agents in the treatment of diseases characterized by inflammatory or immunologically mediated phenomena (Chapter 20).

CYTOTOXIC AGENTS

Clinical Usage

Although a variety of classes of cytotoxic agents have been used in immunologically mediated diseases, the most commonly used agents have been cyclophosphamide (an alkylating agent), azathioprine (a purine analog antimetabolite), and methotrexate (a folic acid antagonist). These agents have been used mainly in diseases in which corticosteroid therapy was attempted but was unsuccessful in controlling the aberrant inflammatory or immunologic reactivity.

Depending on the disease in question, cyclophosphamide generally appears to be the most efficacious of these agents for chronic use in man because it results in a high degree of immunosuppression without great cost in adverse side effects. For example, it results in striking remissions in certain diseases, such as Wegener's granulomatosis and corticosteroid-resistant nephrotic syndrome, at doses that cause relatively few side effects. Cyclophosphamide therapy has also been shown to be extremely effective in the severe systemic necrotizing vasculitides. In addition, it has been used with some success in severe cases of certain collagen vascular diseases. It is for this reason that cyclophosphamide and, to a lesser extent, azathioprine are often considered the prototypes in discussions of mechanisms of action and clinical effects of cytotoxic agents in immunologically mediated diseases.

However, regardless of the cytotoxic agents employed or the disease in question, it is essential that one understand the general mechanisms of the immunosuppressive effects of these agents and appreciate the delicate balance between the therapeutically desirable suppression of aberrant immune reactivity and the potentially dangerous suppression of normal host defense mechanisms against infections, in addition to being aware of the spectrum of other adverse side effects of these agents.

Mechanisms of Action of Cytotoxic Agents

Since the pathogenesis of many of the immunologically mediated diseases that are treated with cytotoxic agents is unclear, it is difficult to delineate the precise mechanisms whereby cytotoxic agents cause clinical improvement in a particular disease. It is possible that clones of autoreactive or aberrantly reactive lymphoid cells are selectively eliminated by the drug. In a less specific manner, the general anti-inflammatory and immunosuppressive effects may control the abnormal immune reactivity until the stimulus is removed or until a state of tolerance ensues naturally. It is also possible that the drug directly induces a state of tolerance to the stimulus in question. These potential mechanisms are outlined in Table 25–1.

Cytotoxic agents, particularly cyclophosphamide at extremely high doses, have been shown to have profound effects on practically every aspect of cell-mediated and humoral immune responses. These effects vary with the immunizing antigen, the dose of administered drug, and the temporal relationship between drug administration and immunization. Different cytotoxic agents have been shown in one study or another to suppress all parameters of immune reactivity, to selectively inhibit one or more limbs of the immune response, to cause enhancement of responses by selectively eliminating suppressor cells, and to induce tolerance by eliminating immune-reactive clones of cells. Although these studies are important in elucidating the scope of the mechanisms of action of these agents and in providing information regarding cellular requirements and interactions in different stages of the immune response, they may not all be directly applicable to the clinical situation. In the treatment of immunologically mediated diseases, cytotoxic agents are almost always administered to suppress an ongoing immunologic process. Low to moderate doses are usually administered over long periods of time (up to several years). Under these circumstances, it appears that the major mechanism of the immunosuppressive effect of these agents is a quantitative one of absolute lymphocytopenia. The mechanism of cell death varies with the particular cytotoxic agent used. For example, cyclophosphamide causes cross linkage of DNA, and although it is most effective in depleting rapidly dividing cells, it is also effective against resting cells. Hence, a dramatic absolute lymphocytopenia of all identifiable lymphocyte populations occurs, despite the fact that several subpopulations of lymphocytes have relatively long half-lives. In this regard, it has been demonstrated in animal studies that cyclophosphamide has a selective effect against B-lymphocytes, which in general have shorter half-lives than T-lymphocytes. This selective effect on B-cells occurs with brief courses of high-dose therapy. In chronic dosage regimens used in human immunologically mediated diseases, cyclophosphamide therapy has been shown to deplete all lymphocyte classes. However, there is indeed a relatively selective decrease in the functional capability of the surviving B-cells.

The well-documented immunosuppressive effects of cyclophosphamide administered chronically to man in dosages of 1 to 2 mg per kg per day are listed in Table 25–2. It should be pointed out that many of the tests of cell functional capability are carried out *in vitro* in the absence of drug. In addition, these tests are often relatively unsophisticated and most likely do not truly reflect the complex functional interactions occurring *in vivo*. Hence, to what degree functional impairment of *in vivo* immunologic parameters occurs is still unclear.

Table 25–1. Potential Mechanisms Whereby Cytotoxic Agents Are Efficacious In Immunologically Mediated Diseases

Elimination of autoreactive or aberrantly reactive lymphoid clones
General suppression of aberrant immunologic reactivity
Nonspecific anti-inflammatory effects
Induction of tolerance to the underlying stimulus

Table 25–2. Immunosuppressive Effects of Chronic Cyclophosphamide Therapy

Absolute lymphocytopenia of both T- and B-cells with early preferential depletion of B-cells
Suppression of *in vitro* lymphocyte blastogenic responses to specific antigenic stimuli
Selective suppression of *in vitro* B-cell function
Reduction of elevated serum immunoglobulin levels
Suppression of antibody response and cutaneous delayed hypersensitivity to a new antigen with relative sparing of established cutaneous delayed hypersensitivity

In recent years, a wide range of lymphocyte functional capabilities has been delineated in connection with both the afferent and the efferent limbs of immunologic reactivity. Although immunologic reactions in their final manifestations are often attributed to a single type or class of lymphoid cell, it is clear that practically all reactions in either their inductive or their effector phases require complex interactions with other cell types and various mediators. Cytotoxic agents can potentially exert their immunosuppressive effects by a direct functional impairment of one or more of these cell types, by an actual depletion of the cells, or by a combination of these two mechanisms. These effects are illustrated in Figure 25–1. The clinical situation in which both of these effects are clearly seen is during massive-dose therapy, usually in neoplastic diseases and usually with combined chemotherapy. The major goal in this setting is to eliminate neoplastic cells. Severe leukopenia and even bone marrow aplasia, which are usually reversible, ensue. The functional capabilities of lymphoid cells during these inductions of therapy are almost always severely suppressed, either because the cells are dying and will soon be cleared from the circulation or because their metabolic capabilities are severely compromised. As mentioned previously, however, the most obvious effect of cytotoxic agents used chronically in relatively low doses that can be correlated with therapeutic efficacy is absolute lymphocytopenia and not a dramatic impairment of the functional capabilities of surviving cells, except for the decreased B-cell function seen with chronic cyclophosphamide therapy. This has obvious practical clinical relevance, since lymphocyte counts can easily be monitored.

It is desirable to reduce the lymphocyte count as much as possible while maintaining the total leukocyte count (particularly the neutrophil count) above a certain critical level, which in effect is that level above which there is no significant risk of infection. It is often erroneously assumed that patients receiving cytotoxic agents are at an extremely high risk of infection because of their immunosuppressed state, regardless of the level of their granulocyte count. Indeed, it has been demonstrated in patients treated solely with cytotoxic agents such as cyclophosphamide that there is virtually no increased risk of bacterial infection if the drug dosage is carefully monitored to maintain the leukocyte count at a level no lower than 3000 per mm^3. This point deserves emphasis, since such therapeutic regimens can thus lend themselves not only to close monitoring of the immunosuppressive effects but also to a realistic appraisal of the general host defense status of the patients.

A point should be made regarding the kinetics of the leukopenia associated with administration of cytotoxic agents such as cyclophosphamide. When using the drug regimens described above, specifically chronic administration of 1 to 2 mg per kg per day, a significant decrease in lymphocyte count is usually seen at approximately the fourteenth day of therapy. At about this time a noticeable clinical response usually occurs; a decrease in neutrophil count occurs almost

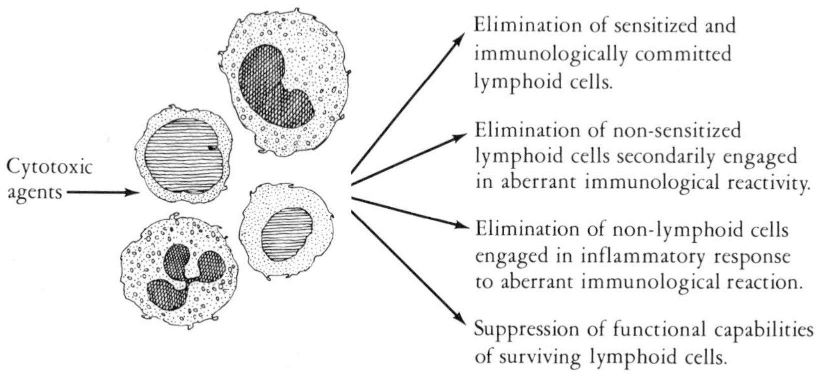

Figure 25–1. Various mechanisms of action of cytotoxic agents on inflammatory and immunological responses.

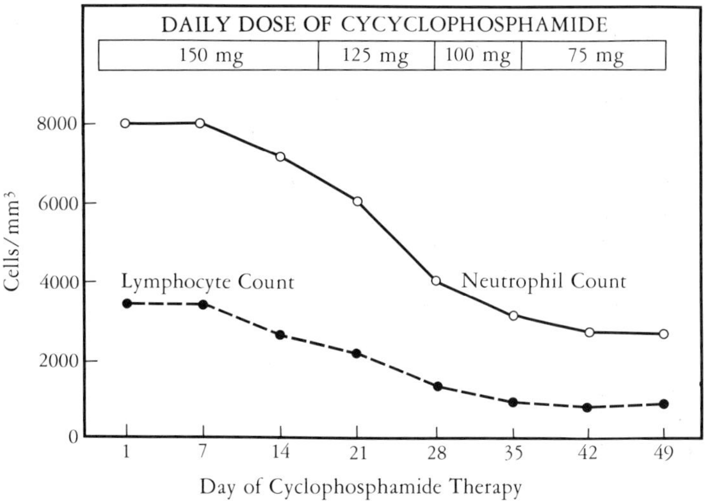

Figure 25–2. Kinetics of cyclophosphamide-induced leukopenia. This patient with Wegener's granulomatosis was started on 1.5 mg per kg per day of cyclophosphamide. A typical kinetic pattern of drug-induced leukopenia is shown. Within 10 to 14 days of initiation of therapy, a gradual but progressive leukopenia of neutrophils and lymphocytes ensues that requires adjustment of dosage until a plateau is reached. Maintenance of high-dose therapy during leukopenia usually results in a disproportionate further decrease, more in neutrophils than in lymphocytes.

simultaneously with the lymphocytopenia. At this point, the slope of decline of the leukocyte count must be determined and the drug dose eventually adjusted so that the total leukocyte count "levels off" at more than 3000 per mm^3. The neutrophil count is usually 1500 per mm^3 or greater at this point, and the lymphocyte count will probably be as low as it feasibly can be. Any attempt to further decrease the lymphocyte count or to further suppress the functional capabilities of the remaining cells usually results only in a disproportionately greater decrease in the neutrophil count. A typical kinetic pattern of leukopenia with cyclophosphamide administration is shown in Figure 25–2.

Another important observation made with cytotoxic regimens is the progressive decrease in bone marrow reserve that occurs with chronic administration of these agents. In other words, most patients can tolerate progressively less drug while maintaining an adequate leukocyte count after months or years of therapy. The same degree of leukopenia (of all leukocyte classes) can be maintained with lower doses of drug. Therefore, reasonably frequent monitoring of the leukocyte count must be done, despite the fact that the disease is stable and the count appears stable.

Complications of Treatment with Cytotoxic Agents

As mentioned earlier, one of the most important complications of treatment with cytotoxic agents is increased risk of infection, which is usually directly related to neutropenia. As a rule, the infections are bacterial and the organisms frequently are gram-negative rods such as *Pseudomonas aeruginosa,* which is the most common bacterial infection associated with the neutropenic state. For patients who are mildly neutropenic owing to cytotoxic agents, but whose leukocyte counts are within the range recommended above, there is relatively little increased risk of mycobacterial, fungal, parasitic, or viral infection unless there are other factors involved, such as corticosteroid therapy or some underlying host defense defect. The exception to this rule is the increased risk of *herpes zoster* infection seen in patients receiving chronic cyclophosphamide therapy even if their leukocyte count is within normal range. The zoster does not, however, viscerally disseminate and serious complications seldom occur.

Another complication of cytotoxic therapy is decreased immune surveillance and subsequent development of malignant disorders. This has been seen most commonly in renal transplant patients receiving chronic azathioprine therapy. In this group there has been a strikingly large percentage of histiocytic lymphomas involving the central nervous system.

There are other complications with cytotoxic agents that are too numerous to list and beyond the scope of this discussion, since many of them are specific for a given agent. However, the immunosuppressive doses of a cytotoxic agent such as cyclophosphamide that are commonly used in immunologically mediated diseases only infrequently result in serious or life-threatening side effects. Gonadal dysfunction and variable degrees of alopecia are rather consistent findings with chronic cyclophosphamide therapy. Hemorrhagic cystitis and bladder fibrosis also occur. In addition, other less well documented findings such as pulmonary fibrosis have been reported. Finally, leukemia as a secondary oncogenic complication of chronic cyclophosphamide therapy has been reported.

Cytotoxic drugs clearly hold an important place as immunosuppressive agents in the treatment of immunologically mediated diseases. No doubt, new agents will be developed with even greater efficacy and specificity, and thus their use will increase. It must be re-emphasized that at doses commonly employed clinically, most of the effects of cytotoxic agents related to immunosuppression and suppression of host defense are predictable and quantifiable. Appreciation of this will allow intelligent and confident use of these agents when indicated, with appropriate respect for the hazards involved.

Finally, it should be pointed out that, above all, controlled clinical trials of these agents are mandatory in order to firmly establish their degree of efficacy in various diseases and to ensure their appropriate clinical use, guided by the principles outlined above.

CORTICOSTEROIDS

Clinical Usage

Corticosteroids are clearly the most widely used agents in the treatment of inflammatory and immunologically medicated diseases. Their beneficial effects are often dramatic, and their efficacy has been clearly established in several disease states. A partial list of diseases in which corticosteroid therapy frequently results in clinical improvement is shown in Table 25–3. However, the hazards and side effects of these agents are numerous and must always be considered when therapeutic régimens are undertaken.

Corticosteroids, as anti-inflammatory and immunosuppressive agents, differ greatly from the cytotoxic drugs discussed previously. The prototype of corticosteroids is cortisol, an endogenous hormone in man that is essential for proper physiologic and metabolic function of virtually every organ system. Administration of this hormone or its analogs in pharmacologic doses not only results in anti-inflammatory and immunosuppressive effects but also has profound effects on a variety of metabolic functions. The mechanisms of action of these agents are also clearly quite different from those of cytotoxic drugs. In order to gain maximal therapeutic benefit from these agents, it is essential both to appreciate their real and potential mechanisms of action in suppressing the inflammatory and immune responses and to understand the delicate interrelationships between the pharmacologic concentrations of these agents and the normal physiologic and endocrinologic functions of the patient.

Table 25–3. Diseases Commonly Treated With Corticosteroid Therapy

Connective tissue diseases: systemic lupus erythematosus, rheumatoid arthritis, acute rheumatic fever, polymyositis, dermatomyositis, scleroderma, and so forth
Inflammatory bowel diseases: ulcerative colitis and regional enteritis
Hypersensitivity or allergic states: allergic vasculitis and severe drug reactions
Renal disease: idiopathic nephrotic syndrome and various nephritides
Immunologically mediated hematologic diseases: autoimmune hemolytic anemia
Organ transplantation rejection
Severe asthma
Noninfectious granulomatous diseases: sarcoidosis
Dermatologic diseases: contact dermatitis, pemphigus, and so forth
Ophthalmologic diseases: uveitis, allergic blepharitis, and so forth

Mechanisms of Action of Corticosteroids

It has been known for many years that corticosteroid administration results in the destruction of lymphoid tissue in certain animal species, with subsequent shrinkage of spleen and lymph nodes and reduction in thymic weight and circulating lymphocytopenia.

The precise mechanism whereby corticosteroids cause destruction of lymphoid tissue in these animal species is not known at present. However, it is felt that most of the tissue and cellular responses to corticosteroids are mediated by intracellular corticosteroid receptors. In a series of complex events, hormone binds to intracytoplasmic corticosteroid receptors and forms steroid-receptor complexes that migrate to and become associated with the cell nucleus. Synthesis of specific mRNA, which directs new protein synthesis, follows. This new protein may be inhibitory. Indeed, it has been shown that corticosteroid-induced RNA and protein synthesis is associated with the earliest detectable inhibitory effect on lymphoid cells, which is inhibition of glucose uptake. This is followed by inhibition of protein and nucleic acid metabolism, inhibition of growth, and cell lysis.

There is a fundamental difference between man and several animal species with regard to lymphoid-cell lysis as a major mechanism of immunosuppression. Certain animal species, such as the mouse, rat, and rabbit, are "corticosteroid-sensitive"; destruction of lymphoid tissue as described above is a major mechanism of action of this hormone on the immune system. On the other hand, man, as well as the monkey and guinea pig, is "corticosteroid-resistant." Pharmacologic concentrations of corticosteroids *in vivo* and even suprapharmacologic concentrations *in vitro* do not result in lysis of normal lymphocytes in man. It is true that in certain malignancies of lymphoid tissue in man, corticosteroid administration results in rapid shrinkage of enlarged nodes. This is most likely due, at least in part, to cell lysis. However, it should be pointed out that these lymphocytes are abnormal, and in certain lymphoid neoplasms they have been shown to contain a high density of corticosteroid receptors that are not found on normal lymphocytes and that render them susceptible to corticosteroid-induced lysis. Hence, cell lysis is not a major mechanism of corticosteroid-induced immunosuppression in inflammatory or immunologically mediated diseases in man. The mechanisms of action in man involve an overlap of pure anti-inflammatory effects with true immunosuppressive effects.

It is very difficult to clearly and distinctly separate anti-inflammatory from immunosuppressive effects, since the inflammatory response can function in both the afferent and the efferent limbs of the immune response. However, it has recently been possible to separate some of these effects while maintaining an appreciation of the natural overlap. Table 25–4 lists some of these effects, several of which will be described in detail below.

It is important to emphasize again that much of the information regarding the effect of corticosteroids on various cell types originates from animal studies in which the species employed was not comparable to man in degree of corticosteroid sensitivity. In addition, in most *in vitro* studies with human cells, the concentrations of *in vitro* corticosteroids used are clearly suprapharmacologic and unattainable *in vivo*. Practically every functional capability of leukocytes can be suppressed if a high enough concentration of corticosteroids is added to cultures. It is important to separate laboratory phenomena from true anti-inflammatory and immunosuppressive effects of *in vivo* corticosteroids in concentrations that can feasibly be administered to patients. This will be pointed out in the following discussions.

Table 25–4. Anti-Inflammatory and Immunosuppressive Effects of Corticosteroids

I. Anti-inflammatory effects
   1. Stabilization of vascular bed with decrease in leakage of fluid and cells into inflammatory sites
   2. Decreased granulocyte and monocyte accumulation in inflammatory loci
   3. Impairment of various granulocyte and monocyte functional capabilities
   4. Suppression of various steps in immediate hypersensitivity reactions

II. Immunosuppressive effects
   1. Decrease in circulating lymphocytes and monocytes
   2. Decrease in certain lymphocyte and particularly monocyte functional capabilities
   3. Decrease in immunoglobulin and complement levels

It is convenient to divide the effects of corticosteroids on various leukocyte classes into effects on (1) cell movement (traffic, kinetics, and circulatory capabilities), and (2) cell functional capabilities.

EFFECTS ON CELL MOVEMENT

Perhaps the major mechanism whereby corticosteroids exert their anti-inflammatory effects in man is simply by preventing the accumulation of neutrophils at inflammatory sites. This can be accomplished with reasonable pharmacologic doses of drug, whereas suppression of such functional capabilities as phagocytosis, enzyme release, and intracellular killing of microbes requires concentrations of drug that for all practical purposes are unattainable *in vivo*. The effects of corticosteroids on neutrophil movement are complex and multifaceted. They cause a release of young neutrophils from the bone marrow into the circulation; this is the basis for the use of these agents to determine bone marrow reserves. In addition, they cause an increase in neutrophil circulating half-life. The combination of these two effects results in the well-recognized corticosteroid-induced neutrophilia. Finally, these agents cause a decrease in migration and accumulation of neutrophils in inflammatory sites. Neutrophils adhere to vascular endothelium following an inflammatory stimulus and subsequently migrate into the inflammatory site. Corticosteroids prevent this action by impeding the initial adherence. In this regard, it has been clearly demonstrated that corticosteroid administration significantly decreases the normal neutrophil adherence to nylon-wool columns. Similar phenomena have recently been demonstrated with eosinophil adherence. The various effects of corticosteroids on neutrophil kinetics are illustrated in Figure 25–3.

The striking degree of eosinopenia seen following corticosteroid administration is felt to be due not to a destruction of cells, but to a redistribution of circulating eosinophils from the intravascular space into other body compartments. Hence, the effect of corticosteroids on circulating eosinophils is at least twofold: They impede cell adherence and subsequent migration into inflammatory sites, and they cause an eosinopenia by redistribution of cells.

Corticosteroid administration also has profound effects on lymphocyte and monocyte traffic and circulatory kinetics. There are marked but transient lymphocytopenia and monocytopenia that are maximal at four to six hours after oral or parenteral administration of the drug, with a return to normal counts by 24 hours. This phenomenon is reproducible after each dose of corticosteroids (Fig. 25–4). In addition, the effects are not cumulative over months and years of drug administration. This is particularly evident in patients who are receiving a single daily dose or a single dose on alternate days of a corticosteroid preparation such as prednisone. Before each dose the lymphocyte count returns to a normal level, only to decrease dramatically four to six hours after drug administration.

It is noteworthy that the lymphocytopenia is selective; i.e., T-lymphocytes are preferentially depleted from the circulation to a greater extent than are B-lymphocytes. In addition, there is a selective depletion of certain T-cell subpopulations, as determined by phenotypic markers as well as by functional capabilities. Of interest is the fact that at the point of maximal lymphocytopenia, after doses of prednisone in the range of 60 to 80 mg, there is very little, if any, suppression of the functional capabilities of the lymphocytes left in the circulation, as measured by various *in vitro* functional parameters. In other words, one of the major effects of corticosteroids on lymphoid cells in doses commonly used in inflammatory and immunologically mediated diseases is not a qualitative functional suppression but a quantitative depletion of lymphocytes from the circulation, thus making them less readily available to the tissue involved in the immunologic reaction. There also appears to be a

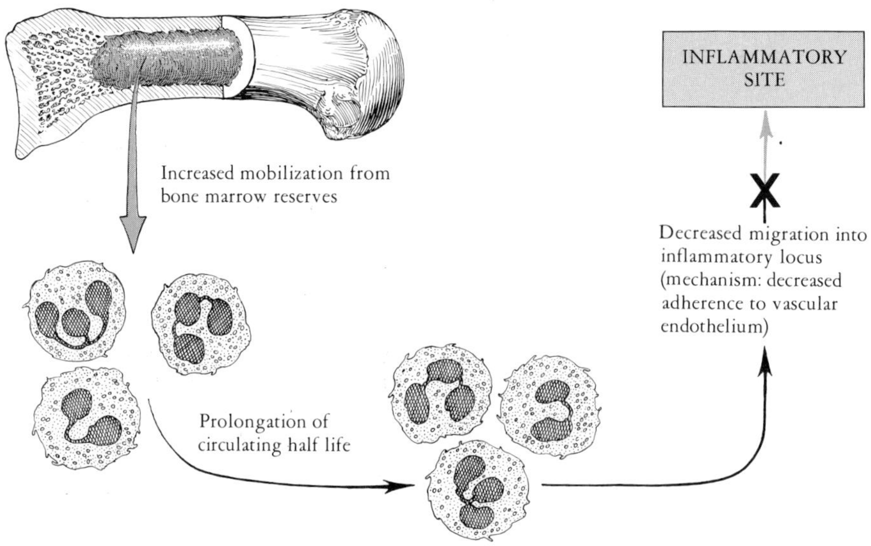

Figure 25–3. Effect of corticosteroid therapy on neutrophil kinetics. Corticosteroids affect neutrophil kinetics by increasing mobilization of cells from bone marrow reserves, by prolonging the circulating half-life of the neutrophil, and by decreasing migration of neutrophils into inflammatory loci.

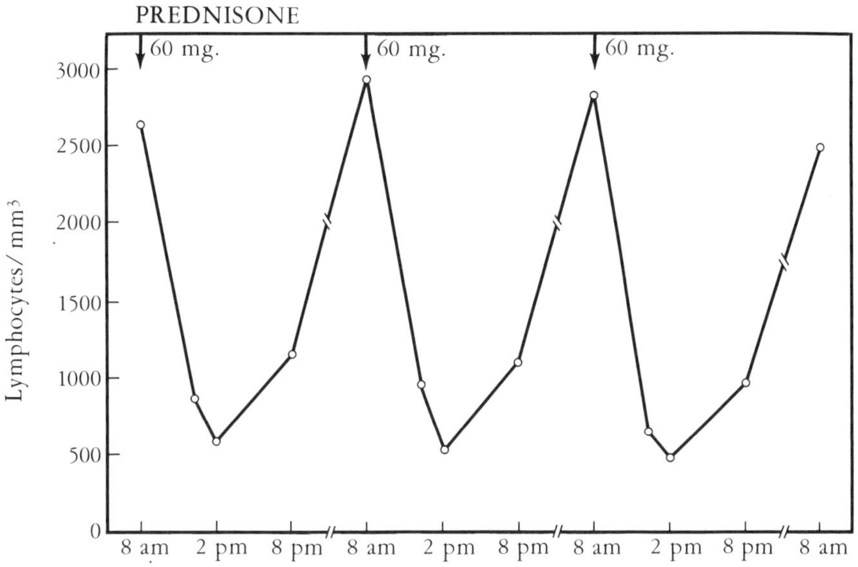

Figure 25–4. Effect of corticosteroid administration on circulating lymphocytes. This patient was given 60 mg per day of prednisone orally in a single dose. A marked, but transient, lymphocytopenia was seen four to six hours after each dose of drug, with a return to normal counts by the next morning.

lower limit of lymphocytopenia beneath which even massive doses of corticosteroids cannot push the lymphocyte count. In fact, the degree and kinetics of lymphocytopenia that follows a wide range of doses of corticosteroids from approximately 20 mg of prednisone to as high as 1 gm of methylprednisolone are strikingly similar. The increase in immunosuppressive effects at these higher doses of corticosteroid is due much less to a quantitative effect of a greater degree of lymphocytopenia than to a qualitative effect on functional capabilities of cells, which will be discussed below. The effects of corticosteroid administration on leukocyte movement and kinetics in man are summarized in Table 25–5.

One can best understand the mechanisms whereby corticosteroid administration causes a lymphocytopenia in man by appreciating the fact that intravascular lymphocytes comprise two major pools, as summarized in Table 25–6. Corticosteroids cause a depletion of cells predominantly from the intravascular recirculating pool. The depletion is caused by a redistribution of cells out of the circulation from the intravascular to the extravascular recirculating pool. This phenomenon is illustrated schematically in Figure 25–5. Corticosteroids thus cause a depletion in the intravascular space of predominantly long-lived T-cells, which are part of a large total-body recirculating pool of cells that under normal circumstances have relatively free access into and out of the intravascular space. The drug acts by affecting the traffic of these cells and temporarily altering this constant equilibrium in the direction of the lymphocytopenic state.

The precise mechanisms whereby corticosteroids cause this redistribution are unclear at present. The drug may act directly or indirectly on the microvasculature, or it may affect the lymphocyte itself, or a combination of the two may occur. *In vitro* treatment of lymphocytes with various enzymes that affect

Table 25–5. Effects of Corticosteroid Administration on Leukocyte Movement and Kinetics in Man

1. Neutrophilia resulting from a mobilization of bone marrow reserves and prolongation of circulating half-life
2. Decrease in accumulation of neutrophils in inflammatory loci by a decrease in cell adherence to vascular endothelium
3. Eosinopenia by redistribution of cells out of the circulation and decrease in accumulation of eosinophils in inflammatory loci by decrease in adherence to vascular endothelium
4. Circulating lymphocytopenia with a selectively greater depletion of T-lymphocytes than of B-lymphocytes by a redistribution of cells out of the circulation
5. Circulating monocytopenia, probably resulting from a redistribution phenomenon, and decrease in accumulation of monocytes in inflammatory loci

Table 25–6. Intravascular Pools of Circulating Lymphocytes

1. *Recirculating Pool:* makes up approximately 70 per cent of intravascular lymphocyte pool; comprises mostly long-lived T-lymphocytes; in constant equilibrium with and has free access to the vastly larger extravascular portion of the recirculating lymphocyte pool contained in the lymph nodes, spleen, thoracic duct, and bone marrow
2. *Nonrecirculating Pool:* makes up approximately 30 per cent of intravascular lymphocyte pool; comprises mostly short-lived non–T-lymphocytes; cells do not normally have free access into and out of the circulation; either live out their life span and become effete or are activated and leave the intravascular space

the cell-surface molecular configuration causes modifications of circulation patterns upon reinfusion similar to that seen with *in vivo* corticosteroids. Thus, it is likely that corticosteroid-induced modification of the lymphocyte surface plays a major role in the mechanisms of redistribution. Similar effects on cell-surface molecular configuration may explain the corticosteroid effects on monocyte circulation and on adherence properties of neutrophils and eosinophils.

EFFECTS ON CELL FUNCTION

As mentioned previously, it is possible to interfere with virtually every functional capability of the different classes of leukocytes by using sufficiently high concentrations of *in vitro* corticosteroids. Probably very few of these suppressive effects are relevant to pharmacologic concentrations of *in vivo* corticosteroids used in patients, however. For example, *in vitro* corticosteroids have been shown to suppress phagocytosis and microbicidal functions of neutrophils. When used in suprapharmacologic concentrations they stabilize granulocyte lysosomal membranes and can potentially alter all functional capabilities, as well as decrease inflammatory responses by blocking the release of lysosomal enzymes. In addition, the responses of granulocytes to chemotactic factors have been suppressed by high concentrations of *in vitro* corticosteroids. However, it appears that the major neutrophil-related effect of corticosteroids at pharmacologic *in vivo* concentrations is to block cells from reaching the inflammatory site, with a relative sparing of actual functional capabilities.

It is noteworthy that monocytes are more sensitive to the effects of corticosteroids than are neutrophils. Corticosteroids not only

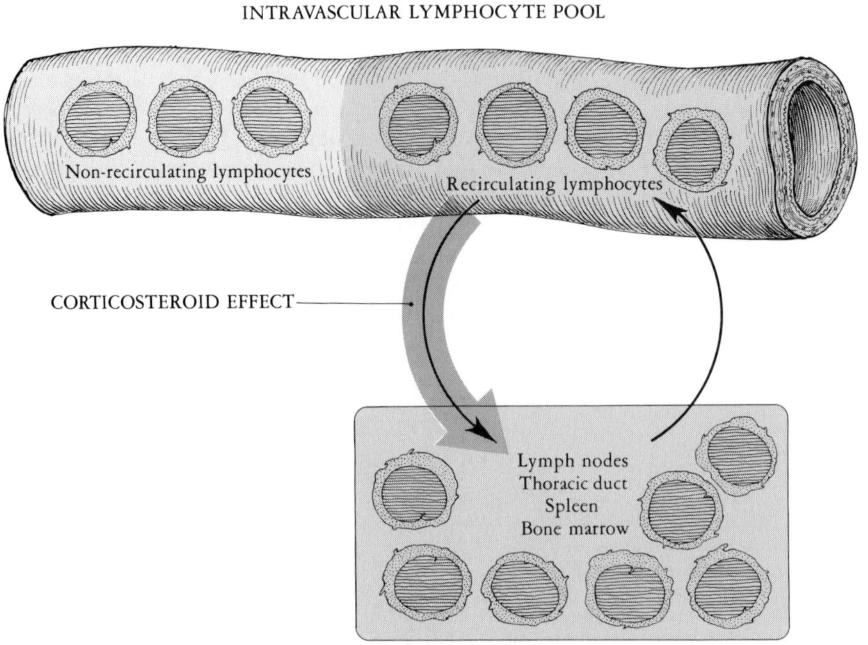

Figure 25–5. Corticosteroid-induced redistribution of recirculating lymphocytes from the intravascular to the extravascular pool. Recirculating lymphocytes are normally in equilibrium between these pools, and corticosteroids redirect traffic of these cells in the direction of the extravascular pool, resulting in a transient lymphocytopenia.

cause monocytopenia and decreased migration of monocytes into inflammatory sites, but also inhibit microbicidal activity of human monocytes at concentrations of drug that are attainable *in vivo*. The inability of monocytes to respond normally to macrophage migration inhibitory factor (MIF) produced by sensitized lymphocytes may well explain the suppression of cutaneous delayed hypersensitivity seen during daily corticosteroid therapy.

Monocyte-macrophages are the cells that are transformed into epithelioid cells and multinucleated giant cells in the formation of granulomatous reactions. Thus, this high degree of monocyte sensitivity to corticosteroids may explain the dramatic response of certain hypersensitivity granulomatous diseases to corticosteroid therapy as well as the breakdown of granulomas that contain dormant mycobacteria, leading to the reactivation of tuberculosis in some patients receiving corticosteroid therapy.

Practically all aspects of lymphocyte function, ranging from antigen processing and lymphocyte activation through proliferation, differentiation, and a whole host of effector functions, can be suppressed by high enough concentrations of *in vitro* corticosteroids. There is much conflicting evidence in the area of corticosteroids and lymphocyte function, relating in part to the fact that in some studies drug was given *in vivo* and *in vitro* functions were measured, and in other studies drug was placed *in vitro* and the cell suspension was assayed. Moreover, most phenomena related to cell-mediated, as well as humoral, immunity represent a complexity of cellular interactions and cooperations ranging from a balance of helper and suppressor effects to the cumulative effects of multiple cooperating cell types involved in the effector limb of the immune response. Interference with the functions or availability of a given cell type may impede the entire immunologic reaction. Corticosteroids have the potential to directly suppress the functional capability of lymphocytes and monocytes or interfere with their availability to the immunologic reaction, or both. As mentioned previously, certain monocyte functions are quite sensitive to corticosteroids. From a practical standpoint, however, most of the lymphocyte functional capabilities, such as mediator production and release, cytotoxic effector activity, and even proliferative responses, are relatively resistant to pharmacologically attainable concentrations of corticosteroids. However, recent studies have indicated that activated lymphocytes, such as those that are present in immunologically mediated disease states, are selectively sensitive to corticosteroids with regard to sensitivity to lysis and suppression of functional capabilities. It should be mentioned that although immunoglobulin production in man can be suppressed somewhat by high doses of corticosteroids, specific antibody production, particularly in secondary IgG responses, is quite resistant to corticosteroid therapy. Thus, it appears that the major mechanism whereby pharmacologic concentrations of corticosteroids exert their effects on lymphoid cells is by interfering with their availability to the immunologic reaction.

Therapeutic Regimens

The major goal in designing or choosing a therapeutic regimen is to obtain the maximal anti-inflammatory and immunosuppressive effects balanced with the least adverse side effects. It is clear, however, that the most effective immunosuppressive regimen, namely high-dose, divided-dose, daily therapy, is associated with the most severe side effects. A list of some of the adverse side effects associated with corticosteroid therapy is given in Table 25–7. As the total dose of drug is lowered, and, more importantly, as one goes from divided daily doses to a single daily dose or preferably to a single dose on alternate days, there are relatively few side effects. It has been shown that alternate-day corticosteroid regimens cause significantly less

Table 25–7. Adverse Side Effects Associated with Daily Corticosteroid Therapy

Diabetes mellitus
Osteoporosis
Psychologic disorders
Hypertension
Electrolyte disturbances
Increased susceptibility to infections
Suppression of normal hypothalamic-pituitary-adrenal axis
Cushingoid body habitus
Retardation of growth in children
Cataracts
Glaucoma
Aseptic necrosis of bone
Pancreatitis
Intracranial hypertension
Panniculitis
Poor wound healing
Exacerbation of peptic ulcer
Hypercatabolism

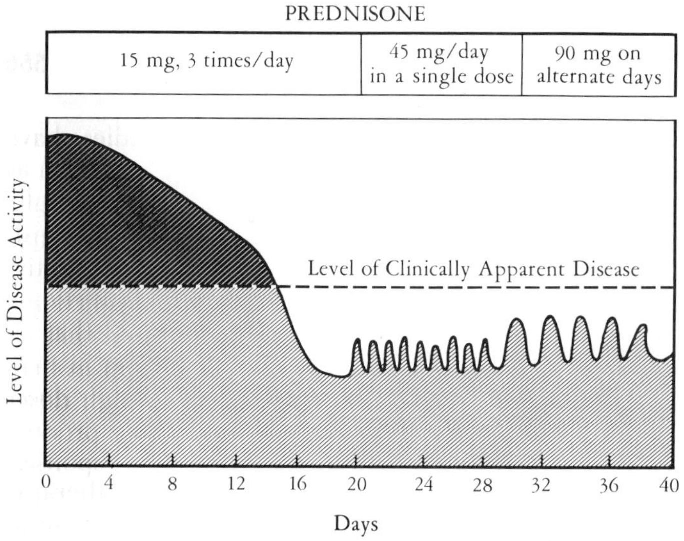

Figure 25–6. Effect of various regimens of corticosteroid therapy on disease activity in inflammatory and immunologically mediated diseases. During flagrant disease activity, daily divided dose therapy is usually necessary to bring the disease process under control and to a state of clinically inapparent activity. Once this is achieved, one can gradually convert to a single daily dose or alternate-day dose. This type of regimen can usually maintain the disease process in remission with slight fluctuations in activity related to the drug administration but within the subclinical or clinically inapparent area.

growth retardation in children and result in relatively little suppression of the normal pituitary-adrenal axis. In addition, there is a marked reduction, if not disappearance, of most of the other adverse side effects listed in Table 25–7.

The preferable approach in serious active inflammatory or immunologically mediated diseases is to initiate therapy with high (45 to 80 mg of prednisone) divided daily doses until the disease activity is brought under control. At this point, attempts should be made to convert to a single daily dose of drug and then gradually to a single-dose alternate-day regimen.

With alternate-day corticosteroid regimens, for the entire "off day" and part of the "on day," monocyte and lymphocyte counts, proportions of lymphocyte subpopulations, various functional capabilities of cells, and all other measurable parameters are normal. This explains the intact cutaneous delayed hypersensitivity and the lack of increased susceptibility to infections in patients under alternate-day corticosteroid regimens. Such regimens are quite effective, in certain diseases, in maintaining a state of remission, despite the fact that inflammatory and immunologic reactivity are normal for at least half the time. This is due to the fact that full expression of inflammatory activity in most immunologically mediated diseases requires several days to accelerate in order to be clinically detectable. The intermittent suppression of the mechanisms of inflammatory or immunologic reactivity is sufficient to keep the disease process from reaccelerating, and hence it remains at a subclinical level. However, as mentioned above, induction of disease remission usually requires "semi-continuous" administration of drug in daily divided doses until disease activity is brought to the clinically inapparent level, where it can be maintained with alternate-day therapy. This therapeutic approach is illustrated in Figure 25–6. Likewise, when a disease relapses on alternate-day therapy, it is usually necessary to revert temporarily to daily single-dose or divided-dose therapy until the disease activity is brought to a point at which it can again be maintained in remission by an alternate-day regimen. Such an approach should provide the optimal necessary immunosuppressive effect with minimal adverse side effects, which is the major objective in the treatment of immunologically mediated diseases with corticosteroids.

Suggestions for Further Reading

Baxter, J. D., and Forsham, P. H.: Tissue effects of glucocorticoids. Am. J. Med., *53*:573, 1972.

Baxter, J. D., and Harris, A. W.: Mechanisms of glucocorticoid action: General features with reference to steroid-mediated immunosuppression. Transplant. Proc., 7:55, 1975.

Calabresi, P., and Parks, R. E., Jr.: Alkylating agents, antimetabolites, hormones, and other antiproliferative agents. *In* Goodman, L. S., and Gilman, A. (eds.): The Pharmacological Basis of Therapeutics. 6th ed., London, The Macmillan Company, 1981.

Claman, H. N.: Corticosteroids and lymphoid cells. N. Engl. J. Med., *287*:388, 1972.

Cupps, T. R., and Fauci, A. S.: Corticosteroid-mediated immunoregulation in man. Immunol. Rev., *65*:133, 1982.

David, D. S., Grieco, M. H., and Cushman, P., Jr.: Adrenal glucocorticoids after twenty years. A review of their clinically relevant consequences. J. Chronic Dis., *22*:637, 1970.

Fauci, A. S., Dale, D. C., and Balow, J. E.: Glucocorticosteroid therapy: Mechanisms of action and clinical considerations. Ann. Intern. Med., *84*:304, 1976.

Fauci, A. S., Dale, D. C., and Wolff, S. M.: Cyclophosphamide and lymphocyte subpopulations in Wegener's granulomatosis. Arthritis Rheum., *17*:355, 1974.

Gabrielsen, A. E., and Good, R. A.: Chemical suppression of adaptive immunity. Adv. Immunol., *6*:91, 1967.

Steinberg, A. D., Plotz, P. H., Wolff, S. M., et al.: Cytotoxic drugs in treatment of nonmalignant diseases. Ann. Intern. Med., *76*:619, 1972.

Thompson, E. B., and Lippman, M. E.: Mechanisms of action of glucocorticoids. Metabolism, *23*:159, 1974.

Thorn, G. W.: Clinical considerations in the use of corticosteroids. N. Engl. J. Med., *274*:775, 1966.

Chapter 26

Diagnostic Applications of Immunology

Joseph A. Bellanti, M.D., and Stephen M. Peters, Ph.D.

Immunologic testing is used in conjunction with other laboratory procedures in the assessment of immunologic function and the diagnosis of disease states. The following series of appendices is grouped into two major categories: *(1) immunologic techniques used in the diagnosis of diseases in which altered immunologic function occurs* and *(2) immunologic techniques employed in the diagnosis of nonimmunologic diseases.*

This section includes the use and interpretation of the basic tests of immunologic function. For further details the reader is referred to the *Manual of Clinical Immunology.**

TESTS OF IMMUNOLOGIC FUNCTION

The tests that may be used in assessing immunologic function are shown in Table 26–1. For ease of discussion, these are classified according to an arbitrary scheme (presented in Chapter 20) as *nonspecific (primary), specific (secondary),* and *tissue-damaging (tertiary)* immune responses.

Tests of Nonspecific (Primary) Immune Function

The tests of nonspecific immune function measure one or more aspects of the *inflammatory response* and *phagocytic cell function* and reflect the body's nonspecific responses to encounter with a foreign configuration (Chapter 2).

TESTS OF INFLAMMATORY RESPONSE

The white blood cell and differential count, sedimentation rate, C-reactive protein, complement activity, Rebuck skin window technique, and chemotactic assay are all useful in assessing whether an inflammatory response is in progress as well as in determining the functional integrity of the phagocytic cell system. In general, they all are increased during the phase of acute inflammation, and the sedimentation rate is elevated in more protracted (chronic) inflammatory responses.

Complement. Measurement of serum complement activity is a useful test in several clinical situations. Either total serum complement or individual complement components may be measured (Chapter 6). C3 (β_1C globulin) is the major component of complement in serum and is easily measured by radial immunodiffusion or, more recently, by automated nephelometric techniques. The complement system is evaluated to detect deficiencies resulting from (1) inborn deficiencies of the complement components, e.g., hereditary angioedema (HAE), or the presence of inhibitors of complement activity (Chapters 6 and 22) or (2) increased complement utilization resulting from ongoing inflammatory processes, e.g., systemic lupus erythematosus (SLE) (Chapter 20C).

The primary role of the inflammatory response and phagocytosis in the body economy is the localization and removal or destruction of foreign substances, such as bacteria. For ease of discussion, the tests of inflammatory response and phagocytic cell function can be divided into the sequential steps described in Chapter 2 that measure (1) cell movement (motility), (2) phagocytosis (attachment and ingestion), (3) metabolic events associated with phagocytosis, and (4) antimicrobial mechanisms.

*Rose, N. R., and Friedman, H. (eds.): Manual of Clinical Immunology. 2nd ed. Washington, D.C., American Society for Microbiology, 1980.

Table 26–1. **Tests of Immunologic Function**

Nonspecific (Primary) Immune Response	Specific (Secondary) Immune Response	Tissue-Damaging (Tertiary) Immune Response
Tests of Inflammatory Response and Phagocytic Cell Function WBC count and differential Sedimentation rate C-reactive protein Complement activity Rebuck skin window technique Quantitative or histochemical NBT test Chemiluminescence Chemotactic assay Phagocytic index Bactericidal activity Phagocytic cell adherence Measurement of specific WBC enzymes	**Enumeration of B Lymphocytes** (EA and EAC rosettes, SMIg, monoclonal antibodies) **Enumeration of T Lymphocytes and subsets** (E rosettes, monoclonal antibodies) **Tests of Humoral (Antibody) Function** Quantitation of immunoglobulins and IgG subclasses Specific antibody responses: prior sensitization, isohemagglutinins (IgM), DPT, poliovirus, or measles (IgG) Schick and Dick tests (IgG) Specific antibody responses: *de novo* sensitization, *Salmonella* O (IgM); H (IgG) **Tests of Cell-Mediated (Delayed Hypersensitivity) Function** *In vivo* Skin tests (prior sensitization), *Candida, Trichophyton* Skin tests (*de novo* senitization), DNCB Skin grafts *In vitro* Lymphocyte stimulation: nonspecific (PHA); specific (antigen) Measurement of effector molecules (MIF) Mixed lymphocyte culture (MLC) Natural killer (NK) cell activity Antibody-dependent cellular cytotoxicity (ADCC) or killer (K) cell activity **Lymph Node Biopsy**	**Tests of Reagin (IgE) Hypersensitivity** Direct measurement of total IgE globulins (PRIST) IgE specific antibody (RAST) Immediate-hypersensitivity skin tests Histamine release **Tests of Cytotoxic Injury** Red cell agglutinins Antiglobulin test (Coombs') **Tests of Ag-Ab Complex Injury** Rheumatoid factor (RF) Antinuclear factor (ANF) Serum complement (C1q, C3, C5) Tissue biopsy (localization of IgG and C components by immunofluorescence) **Tests of Injury Due to Delayed Hypersensitivity** Tissue biopsy, infiltration of lymphocytes in areas of injury Skin tests (patch) in contact hypersensitivity

TESTS OF CELL MOVEMENT

Rebuck Skin Window Technique. A classic *in vivo* method for the study of inflammation is the "skin window" technique of Rebuck. A sterile coverslip is placed over a superficially abraded area of skin; several hours later, the coverslip is removed and the number of leukocytes is counted. Within three to four hours, over 90 per cent of the cellular composition consists of polymorphonuclear leukocytes. After 12 hours, they are replaced by mononuclear cells, and at 24 hours, well over 50 per cent of the cells are monocytes and macrophages. The technique may also be used to study the response to both antigenic and nonantigenic stimuli. Its use is indicated in defects of chemotaxis, in complement deficiencies, and in other conditions that affect the inflammatory response, such as alcoholism, steroid administration, and diabetes as well as developmental and nutritional immaturity. Although the technique is semiquantitative and may not be truly measuring chemotaxis, it provides some useful information regarding *in vivo* cell movement.

In Vitro **Tests of Cell Movement.** The movement of phagocytic cells can be either *random* or *directed* (chemotaxis). Random motility of leukocytes is commonly performed by the measurement of leukocyte migration in the absence of a chemoattractant. Patients with the lazy leukocyte syndrome have been described as demonstrating abnormalities of random migration in conjunction with defective chemotaxis and neutropenia (Chapter 22).

The technique most widely used today for *in vitro* examination of chemotaxis is the one introduced by Boyden and modified by several investigators that employs plastic chambers separated into two parts by filters of known porosity, e.g., Millipore filter. Leukocyte suspensions are introduced on one side of the chamber, and fluids containing chemoattractants are placed on the other side. After a variable interval, the filters are removed and stained and the number of leukocytes that have migrated through are determined (Fig. 26–1). More recently, an alternative technique has been developed that employs the measurement of chemotaxis under agarose. Attractants used in these assays can be derived from several sources, including bacterial extracts; products of the complement system, e.g., C5a; synthetic pep-

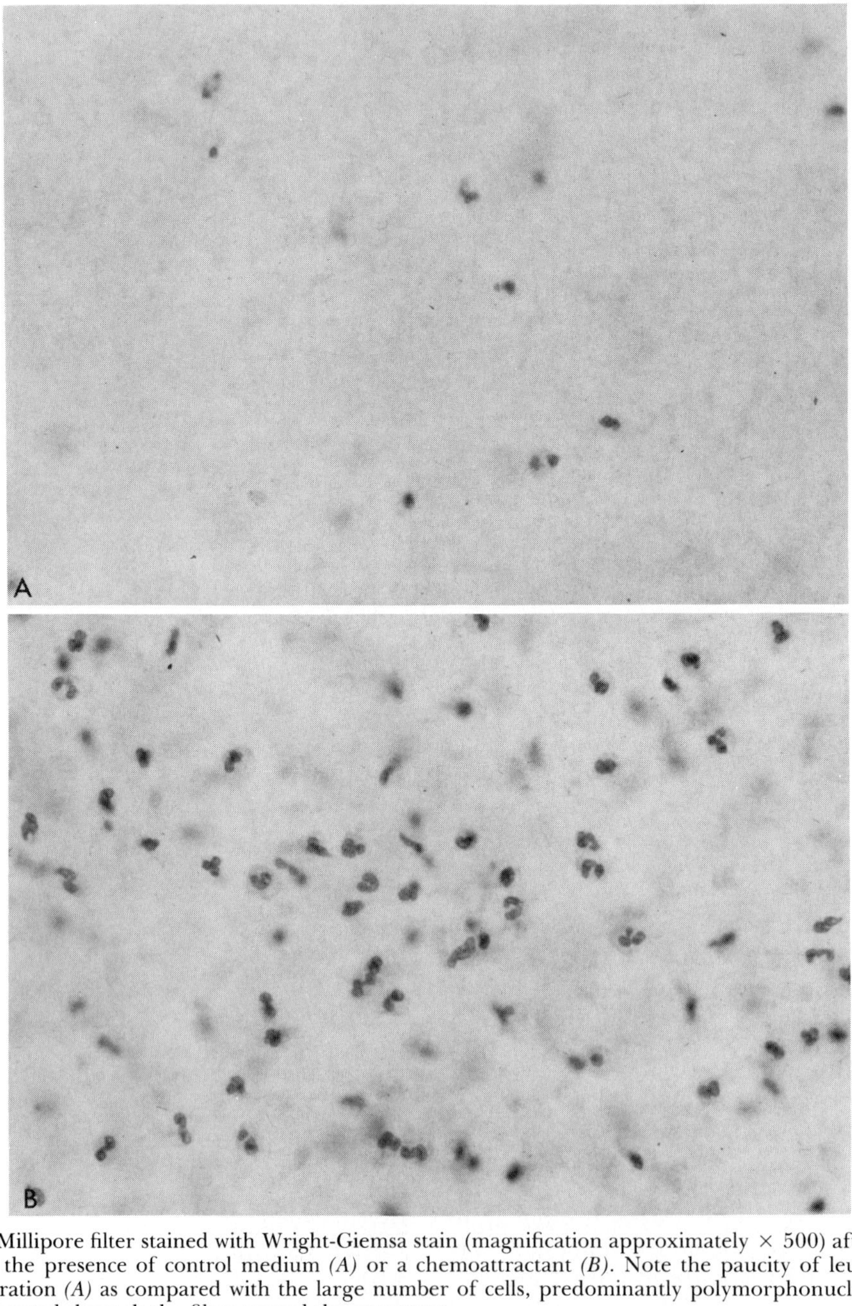

Figure 26–1. Millipore filter stained with Wright-Giemsa stain (magnification approximately × 500) after 30 minutes' incubation in the presence of control medium *(A)* or a chemoattractant *(B)*. Note the paucity of leukocytes in the control preparation *(A)* as compared with the large number of cells, predominantly polymorphonuclear leukocytes, that have emigrated through the filter toward the attractant.

tides; arachidonic acid metabolites, e.g., leukotrienes; or leukocytic products or products of the lymphoid cells, e.g, lymphokines. Assays of chemotaxis most frequently involve the functional assessment of blood neutrophils and monocytes, however, since these cells are the ones most importantly involved in the inflammatory response.

Chemotactic defects are found most commonly in patients with chronic recurrent bacterial infections that can be due to either *intracellular defects,* e.g., Chédiak-Higashi syndrome, or defects in the generation of *extracellular* chemotactic factors, e.g., C3 deficiency (Chapter 22).

TESTS OF PHAGOCYTOSIS (ATTACHMENT AND INGESTION)

These tests of phagocytosis measure the capacity of the phagocytic cell to take up particles, e.g., polystyrene; microorganisms, e.g., bacteria; or immunoglobulin-coated erythrocytes. Since internalization of these particles may require the presence of opsonins (complement or antibody), the tests are usually performed in the presence of fresh serum, either the patient's serum, which will test its opsonic ability, or pooled human serum. After an appropriate incubation under specified conditions, not only is the number of cells that are phagocytic determined but also the number of particles ingested per phagocytic cell. These tests measure the ability of the phagocyte to ingest particles but not necessarily its ability to degrade them intracellularly. However, modifications of these tests, employing either supravital stains or fluorochromes, have made it possible to combine tests of phagocytic function with those measuring intracellular digestion. Tests of phagocytosis are commonly performed in patients suspected of having disorders of the phagocytes, such as the neutrophil dysfunction syndrome, or defects in complement- or antibody-mediated opsonization (Chapter 22).

TESTS MEASURING METABOLIC EVENTS ASSOCIATED WITH PHAGOCYTOSIS

Following the stimulation of a phagocytic cell membrane by particulate substances, e.g., bacteria, or soluble substances, e.g., C5a, a series of biochemical events is initiated (Chapter 2). Primarily these events include the stimulation of the arachidonic acid pathway, the glycolytic pathways, and the hexose monophosphate (HMP) shunt ("respiratory burst"); the release of lysosomal enzymes into the phagosome ("degranulation"); and the generation of H_2O_2 and several activated forms of oxygen, e.g., superoxide radical that can be measured by chemiluminescence (Chapter 2). Although a number of sophisticated biochemical reactions can be measured, two assays have received attention in clinical immunology laboratories: the nitroblue tetrazolium dye reduction (NBT) test and chemiluminescence.

A quantitative NBT test has been developed that is based on the increased metabolic activity of the phagocyte that occurs following phagocytic cell stimulation. The release of electrons during activation of the HMP is measured colorimetrically by the reduction of the nitroblue tetrazolium dye to a blue formazan pigment or by emission of light through chemiluminescence. These tests are markedly depressed in cases in which there is an impairment in metabolic activity of leukocytes, such as in chronic granulomatous disease (CGD).

A number of more rapid and less expensive histochemical tests for NBT dye reduction that measure the number of cells reducing the dye *in situ* have been developed. These tests may also measure the relative degree of dye reduction by resting (unstimulated) leukocytes as well as those that have been stimulated by the ingestion of particles or by exposure to endotoxin. The NBT test is a good initial screening test for the diagnosis of chronic granulomatous disease.

TESTS MEASURING ANTIMICROBIAL MECHANISMS

The ultimate test of phagocytic cell function is its microbicidal activity. These tests are usually performed with bacteria and measure the ability of the phagocytic cell to ingest (phagocytose) and subsequently kill the organism. Phagocytic activity involves a multiphasic act requiring the integrity of both extracellular factors (complement and antibody), cell surface receptors, and intracellular factors (intact metabolic integrity of the cell). The test is usually performed by mixing a suspension of leukocytes with bacteria in the presence of serum containing adequate opsonic activity, e.g., C3b and specific antibody. After an appropriate length of time, the amount of viable bacteria remaining within the cells is measured by direct culture technique, fluorescence, or supravital stains. Although *Staphylococcus aureus* is commonly used, the test should also include the infectious organism obtained from the patient as well as other microorganisms, e.g., catalase-negative bacteria, which may be helpful in the final diagnosis of CGD (Chapters 2 and 22) (Fig. 26–2). These tests are indicated in the diagnosis of neutrophil dysfunction and in deficiencies of specific antibody or complement.

QUANTITATIVE MEASUREMENT OF SPECIFIC LEUKOCYTE ENZYMES

It is now apparent that a number of causes of recurrent infections are related to selective enzyme deficiencies, as seen in the neutrophil dysfunction syndrome. These specific enzyme deficiencies include leukocyte NADH-oxidase, NADPH-oxidase, glucose-6-phosphate dehydrogenase (G-6-PD), glutathione peroxidase, leukocyte myeloperoxidase (MPO), and lactoferrin (Chapter 22). These assays are not currently performed in most clinical laboratories but may be considered when defects of microbicidal activity are detected.

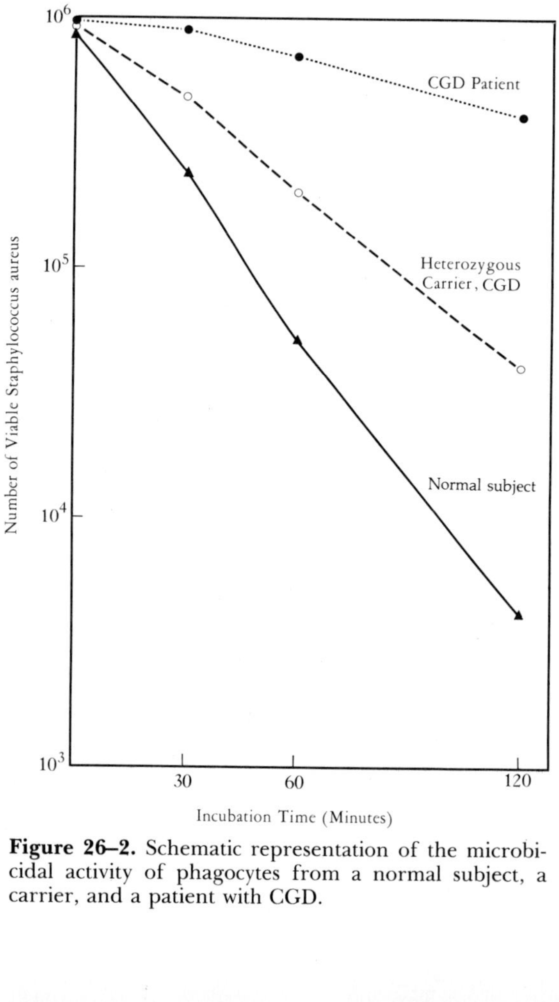

Figure 26–2. Schematic representation of the microbicidal activity of phagocytes from a normal subject, a carrier, and a patient with CGD.

Tests of Specific (Secondary) Immune Function

These tests measure those functions associated with humoral (B-lymphocyte–mediated) immunity or with cell-mediated (T-lymphocyte–mediated) immunity (Table 26–1).

ENUMERATION OF LYMPHOCYTE POPULATIONS

Diagnostic studies should begin with a white blood cell and differential count to assess the total and the relative number of lymphocytes in the peripheral blood. The absolute lymphocyte count is usually greater than 2500 cells per cubic millimeter, and a count below 1500 per cubic millimeter is suggestive of a *primary* immune deficiency that could occur at the stem cell, B-cell, or T-cell level, or of any of a number of *secondary* immune deficiencies that result in the diminution of the total numbers of circulating lymphocytes (Chapter 22).

The next step in the immunologic evaluation is the determination of relative numbers of B- and T-lymphocytes. It is important to stress that these techniques are in a rapid state of flux as better methods of purification and identification of lymphocyte populations and subpopulations have become available. Therefore, the clinician should be aware of these changes and be prepared to avail himself of new techniques and their interpretations as they are evolving. These tests are based upon the principles of lymphocyte characteristics described in Chapter 7.

Human peripheral blood lymphocytes are commonly classified into B, T, or null cell types on the basis of certain surface characteristics. Shown in Table 26–2 are some of the more commonly used methods of enumeration of these cells. The tests are commonly performed on blood mononuclear cells separated by ficoll-hypaque gradients; approximately 30 per cent of these cells consist of monocytes, the remainder being predominantly lymphocytes. Approximately 80 per cent of the lymphocytes are identified as

Table 26–2. **Methods of Identifying B-, T-, and Null Cells**

Marker	Method	Cells B	T	Null	Per Cent Mean* ± 1 SD (Range)
Rosette formation with sheep erythrocytes	E-rosette test	0	+	0	85 ± 6 (72–93)
Surface membrane IgM and IgD	SMIg test	+	0	0	11.4 ± 4.5 (4–21)
Presence of membrane receptor for Fc of IgG	EA test	+	±	±	16 ± 5.1 (6–27)
Presence of surface receptor for complement (C3b) employing IgM antibody	EAC test	+	0	±	16.5 ± 5.1 (6–28)

*After Ross, G. D., and Winchester, R. J.: Methods for enumerating lymphocyte populations. *In* Rose, N. R., and Friedman, H. (eds.): Manual of Clinical Immunology. 2nd ed. Washington, D.C., American Society for Microbiology, 1980.

T-lymphocytes on the basis of their ability to form rosettes with sheep erythrocytes; from 10 to 15 per cent are B-cells on the basis of surface immunoglobulins detected by direct immunofluorescence, and the remainder are null cells that lack both surface Ig and the ability to form rosettes with sheep erythrocytes. Moreover, B-cells contain two additional receptors that have facilitated their identification. These include surface receptors for the C3b component of complement and the Fc portion of immunoglobulin molecules (Table 26–2).

Recently, characterization of T-cells has been greatly facilitated by the availability of monoclonal antibodies (Chapter 5) directed against specific T-cell antigenic determinants or "markers" (Chapter 2). These have not only permitted the characterization of human T-cells during intrathymic differentiation but have also provided potent reagents for the enumeration and immunologic function of lymphoid cells in circulation and in tissues. Shown in Table 26–3 are more recent methods of identifying T-lymphocytes and subsets, their immunologic function, and their older nomenclature.

PERFORMANCE OF ASSAYS FOR B- AND T-CELL ENUMERATION

E-Rosette Test (T-Cells). This technique is derived from the observation that T-lymphocytes form spontaneous but weak rosettes with sheep erythrocytes, which provides one of the simplest biologic markers for identifying T-lymphocytes. Although several modifications of the test have appeared in the older literature, some purporting to measure "active E-rosettes" that correlated better with cell-mediated immunity, the major current use of the test is for enumerating total numbers of T-lymphocytes. The mean value of E-rosettes is 85 ± S.D. 6 per cent with a range of 72 to 93 per cent (Table 26–2).

Surface Membrane Immunoglobulin (SMIg) (B-Cells). This test is performed by a direct immunofluorescence assay, and lymphocytes bearing surface immunoglobulins are detected by antibody labeled with fluorochrome. It is important in these determinations that the surface immunoglobulin be shown to be synthesized by the lymphocyte and not exogenously adsorbed. The predominant immunoglobulins on the surface of the

Table 26–3. **Methods of Identifying T-Cell Subsets Employing Monoclonal Antibodies to Specific Surface Markers, the Immunologic Function, and Nomenclature**

Surface Marker	Older Nomenclature	Immunologic Function	Per Cent of Peripheral T-Cell Population
T3, T11	E-rosette	Total T-cell population	> 95
T4	$T\mu$	Helper/inducer	65
T5/T8	$T\gamma$	Suppressor/cytotoxic	35

peripheral blood B-lymphocytes are the IgD and IgM (Table 26–2). Anti-Fab′2 reagents are commonly used in these assays, since the use of anti-whole immunoglobulin or aggregated immunoglobulin will lead to factitiously elevated values owing to binding to the Fc receptor–bearing cells, e.g., T-lymphocytes and monocytes. The mean value for SMIg is 11.4 ± S.D. 4.5 per cent with a range of 4 to 21 per cent (Table 26–2).

Tests for Membrane Receptor for Fc Receptor (Primarily on B-Cells). These tests commonly employ immune complexes tagged with fluorochrome or rosette formation with IgG or IgM antibody-coated erythrocytes (EA-rosette test). Originally described to differentiate T-helper (Tμ) from T-suppressor (Tγ) lymphocytes using IgM-coated erythrocytes and IgG-coated erythrocytes, respectively, these tests have been replaced by assays that employ monoclonal antibody to specific antigenic receptors as described above. The Fc receptors of IgG are detected primarily on B-cells but to a lesser extent on T- and null cells. The mean value for EA rosette–forming cells is 16 ± S.D. 5.1 per cent with a range of 6 to 27 per cent (Table 26–2).

Tests for Surface Receptor for Complement (C3b) (Primarily on B-Cells). Human lymphocytes also contain two types of complement receptors, including (1) the immune adherence receptor C3b, and (2) the C3d receptor. These are found predominantly on B-cells but also to a lesser extent on null cells. Complement receptor–bearing lymphocytes are detected by rosette formation with sheep erythrocytes coated with IgM-associated antibody and complement (EAC) (Chapter 7). The mean value for EAC rosette–forming cells is 16.5 ± S.D. 5.1 per cent with a range of 6 to 28 per cent (Table 26–2).

Interpretation and Significance of Test Results. According to the results of these tests, B-lymphocytes account for 4 to 21 per cent of circulating blood lymphocytes and T-cells for approximately 72 to 93 per cent. The nature of the cell population composing the remainder, i.e., the null population, is unclear, but it appears to be a heterogenous collection of other lymphocytes and mononuclear cells, including killer (K) cells that participate in antibody-dependent cellular cytotoxicity (ADCC) reactions, natural killer (NK) cells, and other null cells that contain no detectable surface markers (Chapter 9).

Clinical Indications for Performing Tests of Lymphocyte Enumeration. Currently, the enumeration of B- and T-lymphocytes by surface markers is receiving increasing clinical application for both the diagnosis and the management of many disease processes with immunologic features. These include their use in the diagnosis of lymphoproliferative diseases in which there are abnormal collections of B-cells (e.g., chronic lymphatic leukemia) or of T-cells (e.g., Sézary syndrome) or in the differentiation of various forms of leukemia and lymphoma (Chapter 21B). They are used as well in the immune deficiencies in which there are deficiencies of B-cells (e.g., X-linked agammaglobulinemia) or of T-cells (e.g., DiGeorge syndrome) or a common variable immune deficiency in which there may be elevated quantities of suppressor T-cells (Chapter 22). These tests also have application in the area of immunologically mediated diseases, e.g., allergy, autoimmune disease (Chapter 20), and immune deficiencies associated with malignant disorders (Chapter 19). The most recent and clinically relevant application of these assays has been seen in the diagnosis of the acquired immune deficiency syndrome (AIDS), in which the enumeration of T-cells and their subsets by monoclonal antibodies directed to T-cell antigenic determinants has been widely employed. The reversal of the T4/T8 (helper-inducer/suppressor-cytotoxic) ratio has been shown to be most useful in the diagnosis of AIDS (Chapter 22).

FUNCTIONAL TESTS OF LYMPHOCYTES

Tests of Humoral (B Lymphocyte–Mediated) Immune Function. The most commonly used test is the quantitation of the individual gamma globulins. The test is available in most clinical laboratories and is most commonly performed by radial immunodiffusion in agar, using plates impregnated with specific antisera to each of the individual immunoglobulins (Fig. 26–3). It is preferred to quantitation by paper or cellulose acetate electrophoresis, which lacks the sensitivity and specificity of the immunochemical techniques. Immunoelectrophoresis of immunoglobulins in serum or urine frequently provides additional information, e.g., multiple myeloma. In addition, newer and more sensitive techniques have been developed for the quantitation of immunoglobulins, including (1) automated immune precipitation (AIP), (2) electroimmunoassay (EIA), also called the Laurell rocket technique, and (3) a wide variety of methods based on antigen-antibody

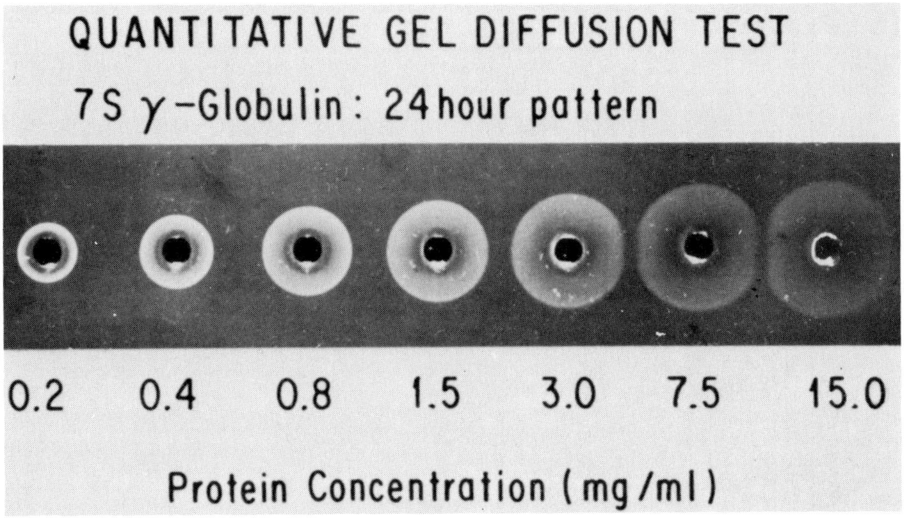

Figure 26–3. Photograph of radial-immunodiffusion method of quantification of the immunoglobulins. Note the gradually increasing diameters of rings of precipitation, which are proportional to the concentration of gamma globulin. (Courtesy of Dr. John L. Fahey; from Fahey, J. L., and McKelvey, E. M.: Quantitative determination of serum immunoglobulins in antibody-agar plates. J. Immunol., *94*:84, 1965.)

interactions employing fluorescent, nephelometric, enzymatic, or radioactive markers (Chapter 8). These tests are indicated in the assessment of patients with immunologically mediated diseases (Chapter 20), and with immunoproliferative diseases (Chapter 21), and in the immunologic deficiency states (Chapter 22).

The postnatal development of the individual gamma globulins proceeds at different rates, and interpretations of gamma globulin levels must be made with reference to age-adjusted normal values (Chapter 2). This is particularly important in the diagnosis of immunologic deficiency in infancy and childhood. Because of difficulty in standardizing normal values between laboratories, it has been suggested that control values be established for each laboratory before immunoglobulin concentrations are assessed. Currently, through the WHO and the IUIS, standards and reference sera are available for the quantitation of immunoglobulins. In addition, since prior gamma globulin administration may alter the results of these studies, gamma globulin administration therapy should be withheld for at least six to eight weeks before the true levels of gamma globulin are determined. Shown in Tables 26–4 and 26–5 are age-adjusted values for immunoglobulins.

Tests of Specific Antibody Responses: Prior Sensitization. The patient's ability to produce specific antibody is measured in one of two ways: (1) measurement of antibody that occurred as a consequence of natural exposure or prior immunization, e.g., isohemagglutinins, poliovirus, and measles antibody; or (2) measurement of *de novo* antibody synthesis following the use of specific vaccines, e.g., tetanus toxoid and salmonella vaccines. These functional tests of antibody are sometimes used in the assessment of immune deficiencies involving the humoral limb of immunity, e.g., hypogammaglobulinemia (Chapter 22).

In addition to these *in vitro* studies, the Schick and Dick tests are *in vivo* procedures that measure circulating IgG-associated diphtheria and erythrogenic antitoxin activity, respectively.

Tests of Cell-Mediated (T Lymphocyte–Mediated) Immune Function. The patient's ability to elicit cell-mediated immunity can be measured by *in vivo* or *in vitro* tests (Table 26–1). The *in vivo* tests, e.g., delayed-hypersensitivity skin testing, measure either prior sensitization or *de novo* sensitization. Since it is known that over 80 per cent of individuals have delayed-hypersensitivity responses to common skin test antigens, e.g., Candida and Trichophyton, these antigens provide convenient *in vivo* test vehicles for delayed hypersensitivity. In addition, if it is known that a patient has had a prior fungal infection or tuberculosis, delayed-hypersensitivity reactions to these organisms can be tested. Furthermore, in a patient known to be previously reactive to these antigens who no longer displays this reactivity (anergy), suspicion of

Table 26–4. **Levels of Immune Globulins in Sera of Normal Subjects at Different Ages***

Age	Number of Subjects	Level of IgG† mg/dl (Range)	Level of IgG† % of Adult Level	Level of IgM† mg/dl (Range)	Level of IgM† % of Adult Level	Level of IgA† mg/dl (Range)	Level of IgA† % of Adult Level	Level of Total Ig-Globulin† mg/dl (Range)	Level of Total Ig-Globulin† % of Adult Level
Newborn	22	1031 ± 200 (645–1244)	89 ± 17	11 ± 5 (5–30)	11 ± 5	2 ± 3 (0–11)	1 ± 2	1044 ± 201 (660–1439)	67 ± 13
1–3 months	29	430 ± 119 (272–762)	37 ± 10	30 ± 11 (16–67)	30 ± 11	21 ± 13 (6–56)	11 ± 7	481 ± 127 (324–699)	31 ± 9
4–6 months	33	427 ± 186 (206–1125)	37 ± 16	43 ± 17 (10–83)	43 ± 17	28 ± 18 (8–93)	14 ± 9	498 ± 204 (228–1232)	32 ± 13
7–12 months	56	661 ± 219 (279–1533)	58 ± 19	54 ± 23 (22–147)	55 ± 23	37 ± 18 (16–98)	19 ± 9	752 ± 242 (327–1687)	48 ± 15
13–24 months	59	762 ± 209 (258–1393)	66 ± 18	58 ± 23 (14–114)	59 ± 23	50 ± 24 (19–119)	25 ± 12	870 ± 258 (398–1586)	56 ± 16
25–36 months	33	892 ± 183 (419–1274)	77 ± 16	61 ± 19 (28–113)	62 ± 19	71 ± 37 (19–235)	36 ± 19	1024 ± 205 (499–1418)	65 ± 14
3–5 years	28	929 ± 228 (569–1597)	80 ± 20	56 ± 18 (22–100)	57 ± 18	93 ± 27 (55–152)	47 ± 14	1078 ± 245 (730–1771)	69 ± 17
6–8 years	18	923 ± 256 (559–1492)	80 ± 22	65 ± 25 (27–118)	66 ± 25	124 ± 45 (54–221)	62 ± 23	1112 ± 293 (640–1725)	71 ± 20
9–11 years	9	1124 ± 235 (779–1456)	97 ± 20	79 ± 33 (35–132)	80 ± 33	131 ± 60 (12–208)	66 ± 30	1334 ± 254 (966–1639)	85 ± 17
12–16 years	9	946 ± 124 (726–1085)	82 ± 11	59 ± 20 (35–72)	60 ± 20	148 ± 63 (70–229)	74 ± 32	1153 ± 169 (833–1284)	74 ± 12
Adults	30	1158 ± 305 (569–1919)	100 ± 26	99 ± 27 (47–147)	100 ± 27	200 ± 61 (61–330)	100 ± 31	1457 ± 353 (730–2365)	100 ± 24

*From Stiehm, E. R., and Fudenberg, H. H.: Serum levels of immune globulins in health and disease: A survey. Pediatrics, *37*:715–727, 1966.
†Mean ± 1 SD.

Table 26–5. **Normal Serum IgE Values as Determined by Radioimmunoassay**

Age	Number of Subjects	Paper Radioimmunosorbent Test (PRIST)* Geometric Mean U/ml	Geometric Mean ± 1 SD U/ml
Newborn	37	0.53	0.27–1.04
1–11 months	51	2.45	0.51–11.75
1 year	22	2.74	0.50–15.08
2 years	26	6.18	1.33–28.66
3 years	33	11.83	4.05–34.54
4 years	27	7.44	1.69–32.71
5 years	30	21.00	7.90–55.84
6 years	31	15.79	2.62–95.10
7 years	30	13.97	2.22–87.82
8 years	32	18.84	4.97–71.38
9 years	35	16.52	3.12–87.53
10 years	40	28.48	7.41–109.51
11–14 years	98	26.89	6.53–110.76
15–19 years	50	24.23	6.08–96.48
20–30 years	52	14.37	3.52–58.67
31–50 years	52	19.38	4.74–79.27
51–80 years	34	11.79	2.88–48.24

65% of healthy individuals < 20 U/ml; atopic genesis not probable.
1% of healthy > 100 U/ml; atopic genesis highly probable.
2% of allergic individuals < 20 U/ ml; atopic genesis not probable.
63% of allergic individuals > 100 U/ml; atopic genesis highly probable.

*Pharmacia Diagnostics, 1981.

underlying disease, such as sarcoidosis or lymphoma, is aroused.

In vivo tests that demonstrate *de novo* sensitization include the use of dinitrochlorobenzene (DNCB) sensitization, in which delayed responses are tested by applying a challenging dose that is followed 10 to 14 days later by a sensitizing dose. This test measures not only the ability of an individual to manifest a cell-mediated (delayed-hypersensitivity) phenomenon but also the afferent and efferent limbs of the thymic-dependent (T-lymphocyte) system. Although allogeneic skin grafts have been used to test this phenomenon, their use is rare. They may lead to isoimmunization and carry the additional hazard of graft-versus-host reactions in immunologically deficient individuals, as well as the problem of transmission of the hepatitis B virus.

With the increasing use of immunopotentiators, e.g., *C. parvum* and levamisole (Chapter 10), delayed-hypersensitivity skin testing has been of assistance in monitoring the efficacy of these agents. In addition, changes in the course of a disease process can be assessed by means of delayed-hypersensitivity skin testing.

Lymphocyte Stimulation. These tests are based on the transformation, proliferation, and replication responses of normal lymphocytes to stimulation *in vitro* by nonspecific stimulants (e.g., phytohemagglutinin [PHA]), foreign cells, or specific antigen. Although most of the mitogens stimulate both B- and T-lymphocytes, some exhibit a selectivity (Chapter 7) for certain classes of lymphocytes. The end point of the reaction is measured by blast transformation, a mitotic index, or the incorporation of radioactive precursors into DNA (tritiated thymidine) or RNA (tritiated uridine). It is believed that these techniques measure one parameter of the cell-mediated response, i.e., the afferent limb. Other parameters may be measured by the release of effector molecules, such as migration inhibitory factor (MIF) (Chapter 9). It should be pointed out that there are dissociations of lymphoproliferative responses and elaboration of lymphokines. For example, a normal MIF response can be seen with a deficient response to PHA. A number of other immunologic tests of T-cell activity have been described, e.g., leukocyte inhibition factor (LIF) and lymphocytotoxicity. Nonetheless, their clinical significance is poorly understood at present. The tests of effector molecules will undoubtedly assume greater clinical significance when the complete array has been identified. The procedures covered in this section are helpful in diagnosing the primary and secondary deficiencies in cell-mediated immunity (Chapter 22).

Measurement of Lymphocyte Enzymes. It is now apparent that several enzyme deficiencies have been associated with certain forms of immune deficiency in the human, e.g., deficiencies of either B- or T-lymphocyte systems as well as severe combined immune deficiency (SCID). These enzyme deficiencies include adenosine deaminase (ADA) deficiency, nucleoside phosphorylase deficiency, and biotin-dependent carboxylase deficiency (Chapter 22). Tests are currently available to measure these enzymes in the erythrocytes of patients with these disorders.

Tests of Tissue-Damaging (Tertiary) Immune Function

Tests of tissue-damaging immune function measure immune responses that cause disease manifestations through immunologic injury (Chapters 13 and 20). Examples of these are shown in Table 26–1 and are grouped according to four mechanisms of tissue injury. These include (1) measurement of specific reagins (IgE) by *in vivo* immediate-hypersensitivity skin testing and *in vitro* testing by RAST or histamine release or direct measurement of IgE globulins by PRIST (Chapters 8 and 22), (2) Coombs' test, (3) rheumatoid factor (RF) test, and (4) LE cell phenomenon and tissue biopsy (Chapter 20C). These are indicated when manifestations of immunologically mediated diseases are present (Chapter 20).

Suggestions for Further Reading

Tests of Nonspecific (Primary) Immune Function

Baehner, R. L.: The growth and development of our understanding of chronic granulomatous disease. *In* Bellanti, J. A., and Dayton, D. H. (eds.): The Phagocytic Cell in Host Resistance. New York, Raven Press, 1975, p. 173.

Baehner, R. L., and Karnovsky, M. L.: Deficiency of reduced nicotinamide-adenine dinucleotide oxidase in chronic granulomatous disease. Science, *162*:1277, 1968.

Baehner, R. L., and Nathan, D. G.: Quantitative nitroblue tetrazolium test in chronic granulomatous disease. N. Engl. J. Med., *278*:971, 1968.

Bellanti, J. A., Cantz, B. E., and Schlegel, R. J.: Accelerated decay of glucose-6-phosphate dehydrogenase activity in chronic granulomatous disease. Pediatr. Res., *4*:405, 1970.

Bellanti, J. A., and Dayton, D. H. (eds.): The Phagocytic Cell in Host Resistance. New York, Raven Press, 1975.

Boyden, S.: The chemotactic effects of antibody and antigen on polymorphonuclear leukocytes. J. Exp. Med., *115*:453, 1962.

Gallin, J. I.: Abnormal chemotaxis, cellular and humoral components. *In* Bellanti, J. A., and Dayton, D. H. (eds.): The Phagocytic Cell in Host Resistance. New York, Raven Press, 1975, p. 227.

Gallin, J. I., and Wolff, S. M.: Leucocyte chemotaxis: Physiological considerations and abnormalities. Clin. Haematol., *4*:567, 1975.

Gewurz, H., and Suyehira, L. A.: Complement. *In* Rose, N. R., and Friedman, H. (eds.): Manual of Clinical Immunology. 2nd ed. Washington, D.C., American Society for Microbiology, 1980, p. 163.

Hohn, D. C., and Lehrer, R. I.: NADPH oxidase deficiency in X-linked chronic granulomatous disease. J. Clin. Invest., *55*:707, 1975.

Holmes, B., Park, B. H., and Malawista, S. E.: Chronic granulomatous disease in females. N. Engl. J. Med., *283*:217, 1970.

Mastuda, I., Oka, Y., Taniguchi, N., et al.: Leukocyte glutathione peroxidase deficiency with chronic granulomatous disease. J. Pediatr., *88*:581, 1976.

Ochs, H. G., and Igo, R. P.: The NBT slide test: A simple screening method for detecting chronic granulomatous disease and female carriers. J. Pediatr., *83*:77, 1973.

Quie, P. G., White, J. G., and Holmes, B.: *In vitro* bactericidal capacity of human polymorphonuclear leukocytes: Diminished activity in chronic granulomatous disease of childhood. J. Clin. Invest., *46*:668, 1967.

Ruddy, S., and Austen, K. F.: Complement and its components. *In* Cohen, A. S. (ed.): Laboratory Diagnostic Procedures in the Rheumatic Diseases. Boston, Little, Brown & Company, 1974, p. 131.

Rutenberg, W. D., Yang, M. C., Doberstyn, B. D., et al.: Multiple leukocyte abnormalities in chronic granulomatous disease: A familial study. Pediatr. Res., *11*:158, 1977.

Sites, D. P., Stobo, J. D., Fudenberg, H. H., et al. (eds.): Basic and Clinical Immunology, 4th ed. Los Altos, Calif., Lange Medical Publications, 1982.

Southam, C. M., and Levin, A. G.: A quantitative Rebuck technique. Blood, *27*:734, 1966.

Stossel, T. P.: Phagocytosis. *In* Rose, N. R., and Friedman, H. (eds.): Manual of Clinical Immunology. 2nd ed. Washington, D.C., American Society for Microbiology, 1980, p. 309.

Ward, P. A., and Maderazo, E. G.: Leukocyte chemotaxis. *In* Rose, N. R., and Friedman, H. (eds.): Manual of Clinical Immunology. 2nd ed. Washington, D.C., American Society for Microbiology, 1980, p. 261.

Tests of Specific (Secondary) Immune Function

Aisenberg, A. C.: Studies on delayed hypersensitivity in Hodgkin's disease. J. Clin. Invest., *41*:1964, 1962.

Alford, C. A.: Immunoglobulin determinations in the diagnosis of fetal infection. Pediatr. Clin. North Am., *18*:99, 1971.

Fahey, J. L., and McKelvey, E. N.: Quantitative determination of serum immunoglobulins in antibody-agar plates. J. Immunol., *94*:84, 1965.

Fudenberg, H., Good, R. A., Goodman, H. C., et al.: Primary immunodeficiencies. Pediatrics, *47*:927, 1971.

Hobbs, J. R.: Primary immune paresis. *In* Adinolfi, M. (ed.): Immunology and Development. London, William Heinemann Medical Books, Ltd., 1969.

Hong, R.: Immunodeficiency. *In* Rose, N. R., and Friedman, H. (eds.): Manual of Clinical Immunology, 2nd ed. Washington, D.C., American Society for Microbiology, 1980, p. 833.

Jackson, A. L., and Davis, N. C.: Quantitation of immunoglobulins. *In* Rose, N. R., and Friedman, H. (eds.): Manual of Clinical Immunology. 2nd ed. Washington, D.C., American Society for Microbiology, 1980, p. 109.

Johnston, R. B., Jr., and Janeway, C. A.: The child with frequent infections: Diagnostic considerations. Pediatrics, *43*:596, 1969.

Kochwa, S.: Electrophoretic and immunoelectrophoretic characterization of immunoglobulins. *In* Rose, N. R., and Friedman, H. (eds.): Manual of Clinical Immunology. 2nd ed. Washington, D.C., American Society for Microbiology, 1980, p. 121.

Mancini, G., Vaerman, J. P., Carbonara, A. O., et al.: A single-radial diffusion method for the immunological quantitation of proteins. *In* Peeters, H. (ed.): XI Colloquium on Protides of the Biological Fluids. Amsterdam, Elsevier, 1964, p. 370.

Spitler, L. E.: Delayed hypersensitivity skin testing. *In* Rose, N. R., and Friedman, H. (eds.): Manual of Clinical Immunology. 2nd ed. Washington, D.C., American Society for Microbiology, 1980, p. 200.

Stiehm, E. R., and Fulginiti, V. A. (eds.): Immunologic Disorders in Infants and Children. Philadelphia, W. B. Saunders Company, 1973.

Ross, G. D., and Winchester, R. J.: Methods for enumerating lymphocyte populations. *In* Rose, N. R., and Friedman, H. (eds.): Manual of Clinical Immunology. 2nd ed. Washington, D.C., American Society for Microbiology, 1980, p. 213.

Tests of Tissue-Damaging (Tertiary) Immune Function

Adkinson, N. F., Jr.: Measurement of total serum immunoglobulin E and allergen specific immunoglobulin E antibody. *In* Rose, N. R., and Friedman, H. (eds.): Manual of Clinical Immunology. 2nd ed. Washington, D.C., American Society for Microbiology, 1980, p. 794.

Agnello, V.: Methods for detection of immune complexes utilizing C1q or rheumatoid factors. *In* Rose, N. R., and Friedman, H. (eds.): Manual of Clinical Immunology. 2nd ed. Washington, D.C., American Society for Microbiology, 1980, p. 178.

Norman, P. S.: Skin testing. *In* Rose, N. R., and Friedman, H. (eds.): Manual of Clinical Immunology. 2nd ed. Washington, D.C., American Society for Microbiology, 1980, p. 789.

Siraganian, R. P., and Hook, W. A.: Histamine release and assay methods for the study of human allergy. *In* Rose, N. R., and Friedman, H. (eds.): Manual of Clinical Immunology. 2nd ed. Washington, D.C., American Society for Microbiology, 1980, p. 808.

Theofilopoulos, A. N., Pereira, A. B., Eisenberg, R. A., et al.: Assays for detection of complement-fixing immune complexes (Raji cell, conglutinin, and Anti-C3 assay). *In* Rose, N. R., and Friedman, H. (eds.): Manual of Clinical Immunology. 2nd ed. Washington, D.C., American Society for Microbiology, 1980, p. 186.

APPROACH TO THE PATIENT WITH IMMUNOLOGIC DISEASE

Appendix 1

Problem: Repeated Infections in the Young Infant

CLINICAL EVALUATION

A. History

Age of onset (the earlier the onset, the more severe the defect)
Site of infection (pyodermas, otitis media, pneumonia, abscesses, sepsis, meningitis)
Type of organism (viruses and fungi: consider thymic-dependent defects; bacteria, high-grade virulence: consider agammaglobulinemia; bacteria, low-grade virulence: consider neutrophil dysfunction [e.g., chronic granulomatous disease]; protozoa [*Pneumocystis carinii*] common in all immunologic deficiencies)
Family history (similar familial infections; other infant deaths, particularly males; polyendocrinopathy: thyroid, parathyroid, adrenal; allergies; collagen-vascular diseases; malignant diseases; diabetes; *draw pedigree*)
Dietary history (unusual reactions to foods or other ingestants)
History of medications (prior gamma globulin administration, antibiotics)
History of unusual reactions to vaccines (vaccinia necrosum) or to allergens (if patient had poison ivy dermatitis, his cell-mediated responses are probably intact)
Associated findings (spruelike disorders)

B. Physical Examination

Growth and development (severe defects, e.g., thymic dysplasia, product physical underdevelopment)
Skin and appendages (evaluate skin and subcutaneous tissues for signs of infection: staphylococcal, monilial; eczema [Wiskott-Aldrich syndrome, hyper-IgE syndrome]; telangiectasis [e.g., ataxia-telangiectasia]; clubbing; cyanosis [chronic pulmonary or cardiac disease])
Ears (otitis media; shape of ears, e.g., notching in DiGeorge syndrome)
Chest (chronic emphysematous changes; bronchiectasis)
Cardiovascular (murmurs, cardiomegaly; congenital heart disease can also present with repeated infections)
Abdomen (hepatomegaly, splenomegaly)
Lymph nodes (evaluate for lymphadenopathy)
Neurologic (ataxia: consider ataxia-telangiectasia)

UNDERLYING IMMUNOLOGIC PROBLEM

In the evaluation of the child with repeated infections, the physician must decide whether an immunologic problem exists. In general,

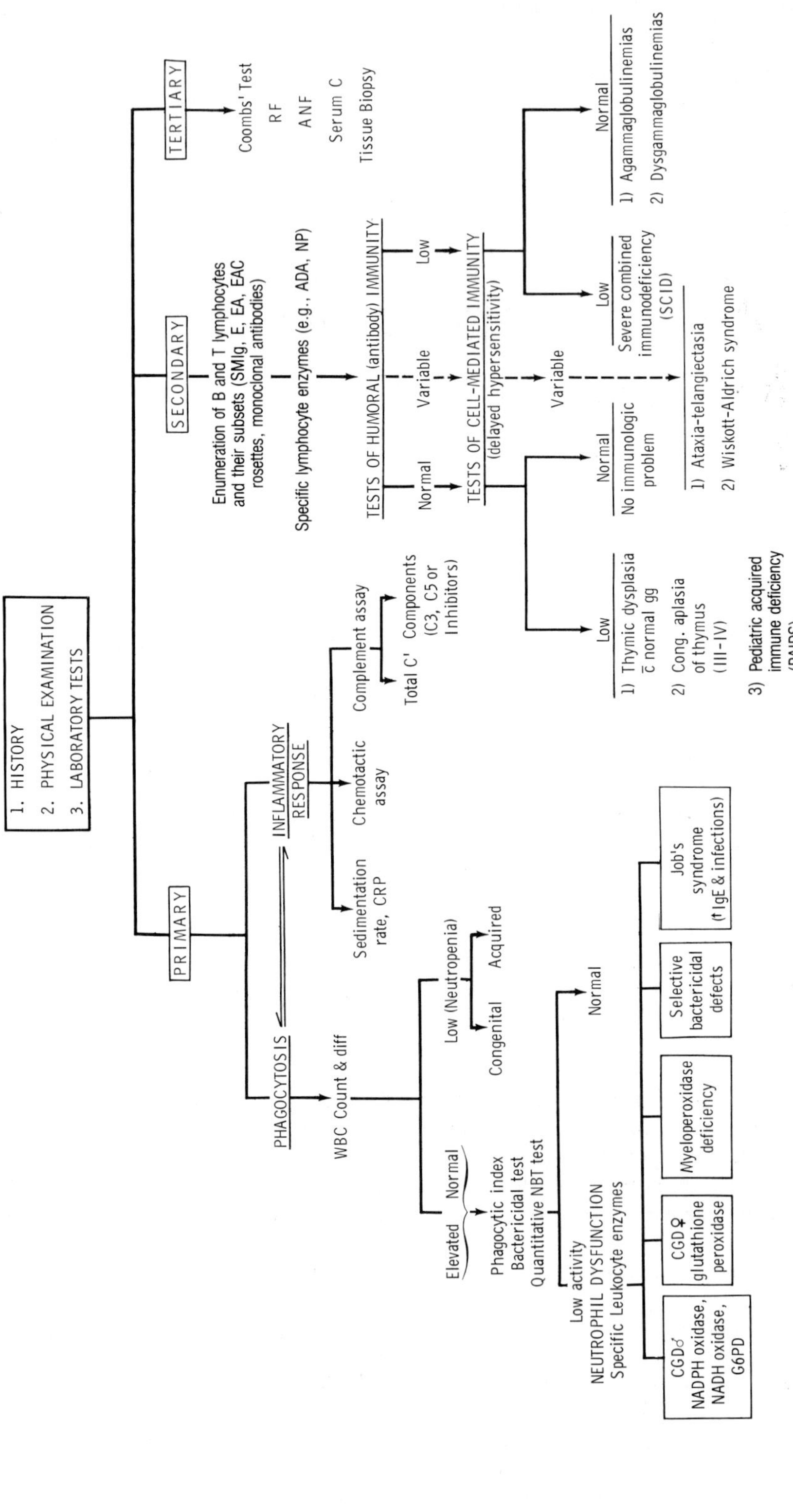

Figure 26–4. Scheme of approach in the investigation of the infant who presents with repeated infections.

there are four cardinal features suggestive of an immunologic defect: (1) repeated infections caused by bacteria of high-grade virulence, e.g., *D. pneumoniae,* (2) recurrent infections caused by bacteria of low-grade virulence, e.g., paracolon and bizarre organisms (Serratia), (3) recurrent fungal infections, e.g., Candida, and (4) unusual reactions to live vaccines, e.g., progressive vaccinia. The history of repeated respiratory viral infections commonly seen in clinical practice does not usually constitute an indication of underlying immunologic deficiency but rather results from increased exposure to infected individuals (e.g., common colds).

Other conditions that predispose to repeated infections must be considered and are easily excluded by appropriate testing. Examples of these include congenital cardiac disease, asthma, and cystic fibrosis. In those situations in which derangement of an underlying immunologic mechanism is suspected, specialized tests are required, e.g., sweat test.

Recently, the description has appeared of a pediatric form of acquired immune deficiency syndrome resulting from vertical transmission from a high-risk mother (prostitute, IV drug user) or from neonatal transfusions (Chapter 22).

LABORATORY TESTS

A rational approach to the diagnosis of immune deficiency is given in Figure 26–4. In this scheme, the history and physical findings are crucial in establishing the diagnosis. Although it is apparent that many of these procedures can be performed only in specialized centers, the provisional diagnosis can be established in most cases by procedures that are performed in the physician's office.

The choice of laboratory procedure will depend on the clinical expression of the recurrent infection and the availability of the test. The first step in identifying the underlying disorder rests with the identification of the infecting organism. The physician is well advised to identify the organism by appropriate cultures in order to determine the nature of the infection.

For example, patients with impaired phagocytic functions will present with recurrent infections caused by bacterial organisms of low-grade virulence, such as *Serratia marcescens.* The tests indicated include a complete blood count and differential, which may show an elevated white count with leukocytosis. Impaired bactericidal activity and a low quantitative NBT test will establish the diagnosis of neutrophil dysfunction syndrome, e.g., chronic granulomatous disease. The use of pedigree and leukocyte enzyme tests can further differentiate one dysfunction from another.

Recurrent infections may also be a manifestation of impaired inflammatory response resulting from a lack or inhibition of certain complement components (Fig. 26–4). These children present with recurrent infections caused by gram-negative organisms or *Staphylococcus aureus.* Determination of chemotactic activity and the individual complement components would be indicated. If the infecting organism is identified as one producing high-grade fulminating infections, e.g., *D. pneumoniae,* the physician must differentiate between a quantitative lack of phagocytes (neutropenia) and a lack of opsonizing antibody (e.g., agammaglobulinemia). The former can be established by history and complete blood count. Enumeration of lymphocyte populations together with tests of humoral (antibody function) and quantitative immunoglobulin determination will establish the diagnosis of humoral deficiency or dysgammaglobulinemia (see Table 26–1 and Fig. 26–4).

Repeated infections due to certain viruses, e.g., vaccinia, and fungi, e.g., *Candida albicans,* may indicate a thymic-dependent lesion. Affected children will have normal primary immune functions (phagocytosis and inflammatory response) but will show striking deficiencies in tests of cell-mediated function. Tests of humoral immunity would differentiate severe combined immunodeficiency (SCID) from those defects restricted to the thymus. The associated finding of hypocalcemia tetany should raise a consideration of the III–IV pharyngeal pouch syndrome (DiGeorge syndrome).

Appropriate tests of teritary function are indicated when hemolytic anemia, rheumatoid arthritis, or systemic lupus erythematosus is present.

Appendix 2

Problem: Repeated Infections in the Adult Patient

CLINICAL EVALUATION

A. History

Age of onset (the expression of recurrent infections in the adult varies with underlying disorders)
Site of infection (similar to those seen in the child)
Type of organism (viruses, fungi, bacteria, protozoa)
Occupation (certain pneumoconioses predispose to infection)
Family history (allergy, diabetes mellitus, autoimmune diseases)
History of medications (immunosuppressive drugs, steroids, gamma globulin, antibiotics)
Associated findings (weight loss, malaise, polydipsia, bone pain, spruelike illness)

B. Physical Examination

General appearance
Skin (pallor, purpura, and cyanosis)
Extremities (clubbing)
Eyes (retinopathy, e.g., diabetes)
Chest (emphysema)
Cardiovascular (murmurs, cardiomegaly)
Abdomen (hepatosplenomegaly seen in lymphomas, chronic liver disease that may present with frequency of infections)
Lymph nodes (node enlargement, e.g., lymphoma)
Neurologic (paraplegia, muscular weakness)

UNDERLYING IMMUNOLOGIC PROBLEM

The cause of repeated infections in the adult include the many etiologies of immu-

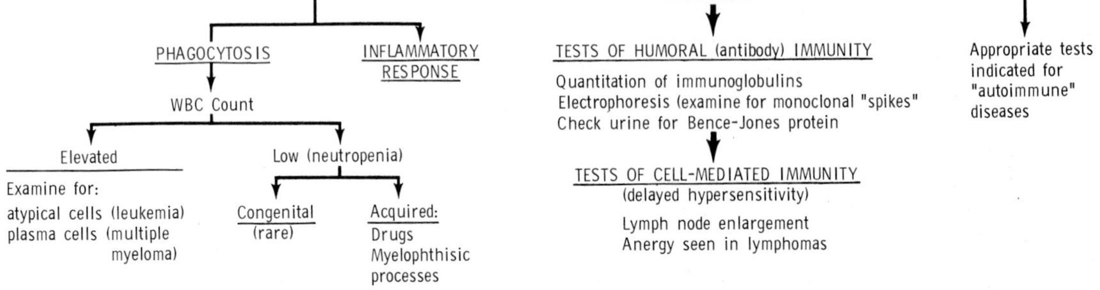

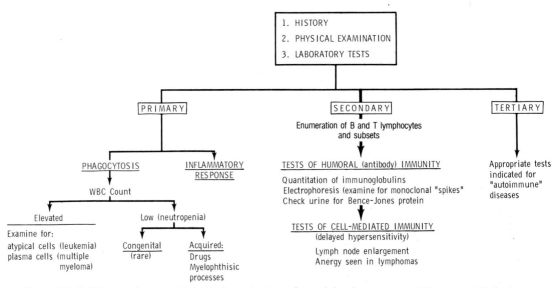

Figure 26–5. Scheme of approach in the investigation of an adult who presents with repeated infections.

nologic deficiency seen in the child (Appendix 1). In general, the severe primary immune defects are seen much earlier. The most frequent causes of increased susceptibility to infections in the adult are those related to underlying diseases, e.g., cardiac disease, respiratory disease, allergy, and diabetes. The immunologic causes for repeated infections in the adult are mainly secondary immunologic deficiencies, including those secondary to lymphoproliferative diseases, the autoimmune diseases, immunosuppressive therapy, and malignant diseases.

The widespread epidemic of acquired immune deficiency syndrome (AIDS) is a new addition to the secondary immunologic deficiencies (Chapter 22).

LABORATORY TESTS

The laboratory tests used in the diagnosis of recurrent infections in the adult are shown in Figure 26–5. The choice of laboratory tests will be determined by the history and clinical presentation of the disease.

Although the underlying cause may differ from that seen in chidren, the same general approach should be used. For example, neutropenia that is drug-induced would require the same diagnostic test of primary immune function described in Appendix 1. In the adult, the most useful procedures include tests of secondary immune function: enumeration of lymphocyte populations, quantification of immunoglobulins, examination of serum electrophoresis for monoclonal peaks, and analysis of the urine for Bence Jones protein. These would substantiate the diagnosis of lymphoproliferative disease, e.g., multiple myeloma. Lymph node enlargement with loss of delayed hypersensitivity (anergy) would suggest a diagnosis of lymphoma. Those tertiary tests of immune function should be performed in cases in which autoimmune disease is suspected (Table 26–1).

Appendix 3

Problem: Approach to Patient with "Allergic" (Hypersensitivity) Disease

CLINICAL EVALUATION

A. History

Age of onset (can occur at any age)
History of environmental exposure and occupational hazards (foods, contactants, inhalants, pets, and other environmental exposures)
Site of involvement (skin, gastrointestinal tract, respiratory tract)
Type of disease expression (atopic eczema, contact dermatitis, hives, diarrhea and vomiting, rhinitis, wheezing)
Family history (obtain a pedigree because of the marked tendency of atopy to occur within families)
History of medication (important in the assessment of drug hypersensitivity)
Associated findings (anemia, weight loss, malaise)

B. Physical Findings

Growth and development (physical underdevelopment may occur in certain forms of chronic allergic diseases in children)
Skin (evaluate the type of eruption, its distribution, and its localization)
Mucous membranes (evaluate the extent and degree of congestion or pallor of the mucous membranes, polyps)
Chest (evaluate emphysema, respiratory distress)
Extremities (evaluate clubbing and cyanosis)
Cardiovascular (evaluate the heart for murmurs, cardiomegaly; i.e., rheumatic fever can present with skin and other hypersensitivity manifestations)
Neurologic (paresthesias and muscle weakness are sometimes seen in hypersensitivity diseases of the CNS)

UNDERLYING IMMUNOLOGIC PROBLEM

The IgE reagin-mediated (Type I) responses form the basis of most allergic diseases of man and are characterized by heightened responses to many exogenous antigens (Chapter 20A). In addition, cytotoxic (Type II) responses, immune-complex (Type III) reactions, and delayed hypersensitivity (Type IV) reactions may also be present. In many cases of hypersensitivity, infection commonly enters into the differential diagnosis. At times it may be the precipitating event, and at other times it may complicate the clinical picture.

The diagnosis of hypersensitivity disease is made after a careful history has been taken and a thorough physical examination has been done. After this, a combined regimen of antigen elimination and appropriate immunologic testing should be performed to establish the diagnosis.

LABORATORY TESTS

The laboratory tests that are commonly used in the diagnosis of hypersensitivity diseases of man are listed in Figure 26–6. An elevated leukocyte count and leukocytosis may provide important clues to bacterial infection. Blood eosinophilia and nasal eosinophilia are commonly seen in atopic diseases. In the pulmonary hypersensitivity diseases,

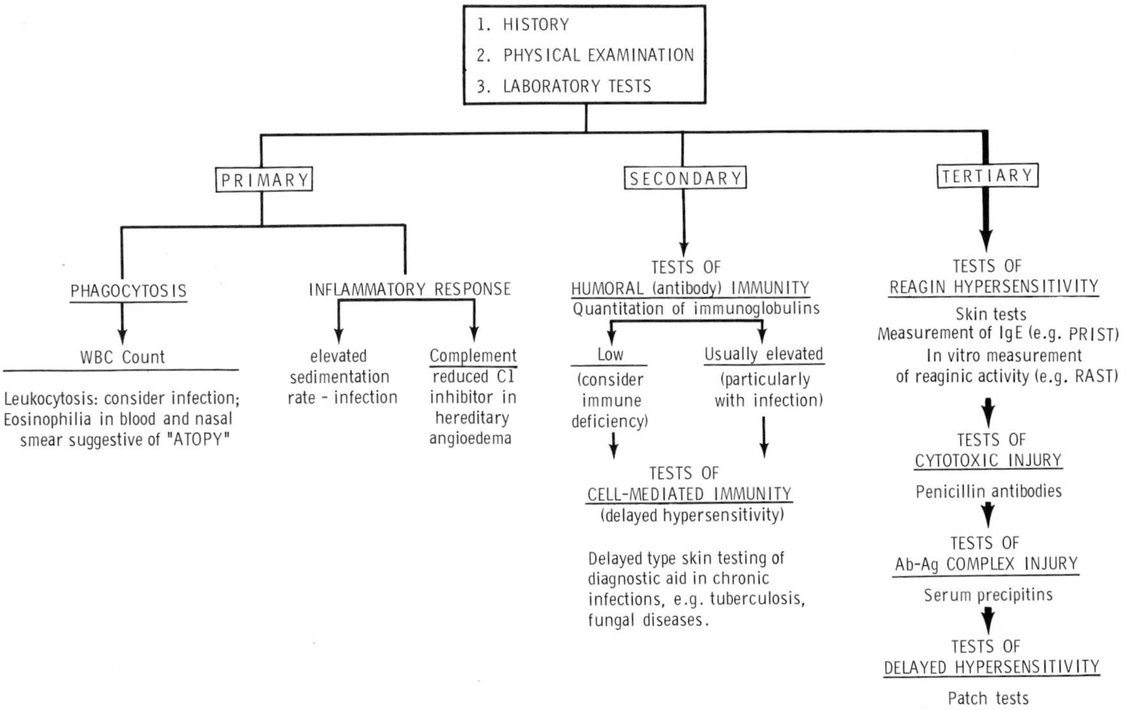

Figure 26–6. Scheme of approach in the investigation of the patient who presents with allergic (hypersensitivity) diseases.

the examination of sputum for eosinophils or aspergillus and of serum for precipitins and IgE may be helpful (Chapter 20A). Other tests of primary immune function include the measurement of complement activity, which would help to establish some of the other hereditary causes of allergy, e.g., hereditary angioedema (Chapter 20A).

The measurement of total gamma globulins is often indicated to exclude underlying immunologic deficiency. Tests of delayed hypersensitivity may be helpful in cases in which chronic infection is suspected, e.g., tuberculosis. Since most of the allergic diseases are mediated through the IgE reaginic response, most test procedures center on measurement of these activities (Table 26–1). These include tests of immediate hypersensitivity, skin testing, the PRIST and RAST tests, and *in vitro* tests of histamine release. In certain cytotoxicity-mediated reactions, such as pencillin hypersensitivity, antibodies to penicillin may be measured. In cases in which a Type III immune-complex reaction is suspected (e.g., extrinsic allergic alveolitis, milk allergy), the measurement of serum-precipitating antibody can be performed. Finally, in cases of contact hypersensitivity, the mechanism of delayed hypersensitivity can be detected through the use of patch tests.

Appendix 4

Problem: Approach to Immunologic Diseases in the Newborn (Isoimmunization and Immunologic Problems in the Mother Affecting the Infant)

CLINICAL EVALUATION

A. History

Previous isoimmunization in mother (due to pregnancy or transfusions [Rh_0, ABO] or gamma globulin administration)

Previous diseases in mother (autoimmune diseases, e.g., SLE, thyroiditis, myasthenia gravis, idiopathic thrombocytopenic purpura)

History of medications in mother (quinine, quinidine, apronalide [Sedormid])

History of infections during pregnancy (rubella, cytomegalic inclusion disease, toxoplasmosis, syphilis, herpes simplex; although nonimmunologic, these intrauter-

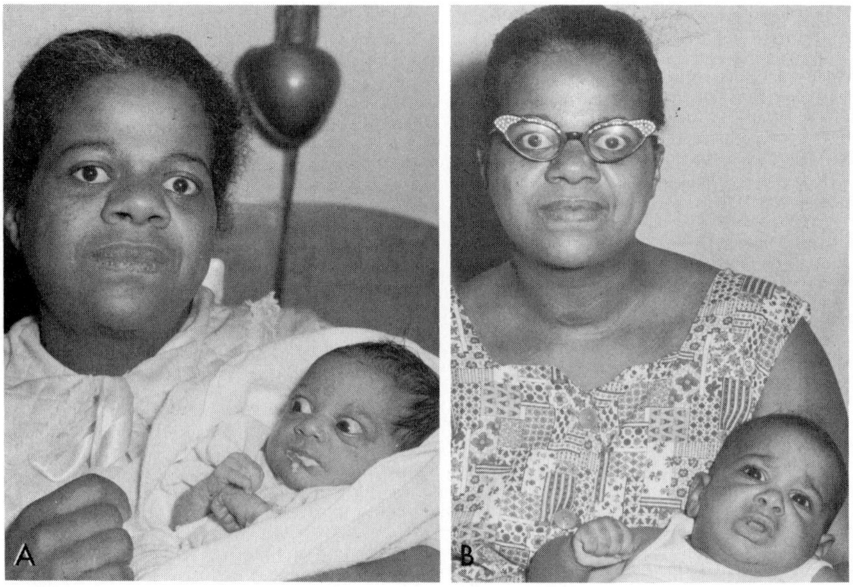

Figure 26–7. *A*, Photograph of a mother and her three-day-old daughter, illustrating exophthalmos in both due to transplacental transfer of LATS. *B*, Photograph of the same mother and her five-month-old daughter, showing exophthalmos only in the mother. (From Martin, M. M., and Matus, R. N.: Neonatal exophthalmos with maternal thyrotoxicosis. Am. J. Dis. Child., *111*:545, 1966.)

Table 26–6. Maternal Antibodies That Can Lead to Harmful Effects in the Infant

Maternal Disease	Antibodies	Effect on Newborn
Hyperthyroidism	LATS	Transient hyperthyroidism (exophthalmos)
Idiopathic thrombocytopenia	Platelet antibodies	Transient thrombocytopenia
Isoimmunization (platelets, neutrophils, red blood cells)	Platelet, neutrophil, isohemagglutinins, or $RH_0(D)$ antibodies	Transient thrombocytopenia, neutropenia, anemia
Lupus erythematosus	Autoantibodies to blood elements (LE cell factor, Coombs' test, platelet)	Transient LE cell phenomenon, neutropenia, thrombocytopenia

ine infections must be considered, since they may occur because of immunodeficiency of the fetus or mother). Additionally, the occurrence of AIDS in infants of mothers with AIDS or at risk of AIDS, e.g., drug abusers, should be considered (Chapter 22).

B. Physical Examination

General appearance (assess degree of activity: hyperactivity, consider hyperthyroidism, passive transfer of LATS; hypoactivity or muscle weakness, consider myasthenia gravis with transfer of maternal antibodies directed to muscle; purpura, consider thrombocytopenia due to the passive transfer of antibodies to platelets)
Skin (jaundice in the first 24 hours; petechiae are characteristic of isoimmunization, e.g., erythroblastosis fetalis)
Eyes (exophthalmos due to LATS)
Chest (pneumonitis seen in many intrauterine infections)
Cardiovascular (evaluate murmurs for congenital heart disease)
Abdomen (hepatosplenomegaly: seen in severe erythroblastosis fetalis and in congenital intrauterine infections)
Extremities (note deformities and other birth defects)
Neurologic (convulsions, weakness)

UNDERLYING IMMUNOLOGIC PROBLEMS

Several clinical conditions must be evaluated in the assessment of the newborn, including congenital infections and congenital abnormalities, all of which could present with similar clinical expressions of immunologic disease. However, it is the laboratory findings that will reveal the immunologic basis of these diseases.

In all these entities, the newborn is affected by the passive transfer of maternal IgG antibody, which is deleterious to the infant (Fig. 26–7). These antibodies arise in the mother either as a consequence of isoimmunization due to previous pregnancies or transfusions or through diseases in which antibodies are found in the maternal circulation (Chapters 2 and 20B). Listed in Table 26–6 are some examples of the harmful effects of transplacentally acquired antibodies that have been associated with disease in the infant.

On the basis of the history and physical examination, the physician should be alerted to the possibilities of these abnormal immunologic responses in the newborn infant and order appropriate tests.

LABORATORY TESTS

Since the basic mechanism of injury involves the transfer of IgG antibody, detection is readily made by measurement of these antibodies in maternal and infant sera (Table 26–6). Congenital intrauterine infections can also be excluded by appropriate history, physical examination, and cultures and through the use of tests that measure IgM responses characteristic of intrauterine infections (Appendix 6).

Appendix 5

Problem: Approach to Patient with Musculoskeletal ("Autoimmune") Disorders

CLINICAL EVALUATION

A. History

Age of onset (usually occur in young adults and in children, e.g., juvenile rheumatoid arthritis)
Site of involvement (skin rashes, malar eminences, joints [arthralgia], muscle complaints [myalgia], kidney [hematuria])
Type of involvement (transient and migratory [e.g., SLE] or protracted and crippling [e.g., rheumatoid arthritis]; also assess degree of inflammation)
History of medications (drugs giving rise to serum sickness–like illnesses, e.g., penicillin; drugs giving rise to false positive LE phenomena, e.g., hydralazine)
Associated findings (malaise, weakness, fever)

B. Physical Findings

Growth and development (physical underdevelopment in childhood, e.g., juvenile rheumatoid arthritis)
Skin (rashes on malar eminence or on pressure points, dystrophic changes)
Hair (alopecia)
Eyes (episcleritis, keratitis, funduscopic changes in many of the multisystem diseases)
Nails (periungual necrotic lesions)
Muscle (define areas of weakness, tenderness, or swelling)
Joints (localize and identify areas of joint involvement, degree of inflammation, joint effusions. If present, joint fluid should be withdrawn and tested)
Neurologic (evaluate neuropathies; footdrop)

UNDERLYING IMMUNOLOGIC PROBLEMS

Vasculitis seems to form the backbone of this group of multisystem disorders (Chapter 20C). In rheumatoid arthritis, synovial proliferation may occur with or without vasculitis. The presence of immune complexes may contribute to the pathologic changes in the joints. In systemic lupus erythematosus, immune-complex injury due to DNA–anti-DNA complexes is believed to account for the vasculitis and the kidney involvement.

On the basis of the history and physical examination, the physician must decide whether a multisystem disease is present. Since many of these entities are preceded by infection, the physician should decide whether an infectious disease is also present. The degree of multisystem involvement, together with the chronicity of the clinical course, is helpful in suggesting the diagnosis.

LABORATORY TESTS

The laboratory tests useful in the diagnosis of the autoimmune diseases are shown in Figure 26–8. Tests of primary immune function should include a complete blood count and differential. An elevated white blood count provides the first laboratory clue in all the multisystem diseases, with the exception of systemic lupus erythematosus in which leukopenia is seen in approximately 80 per cent of the cases. An elevated sedimentation rate is another useful finding in all the autoimmune diseases, with the exception of dermatomyositis in which it may be normal in approximately half of the cases.

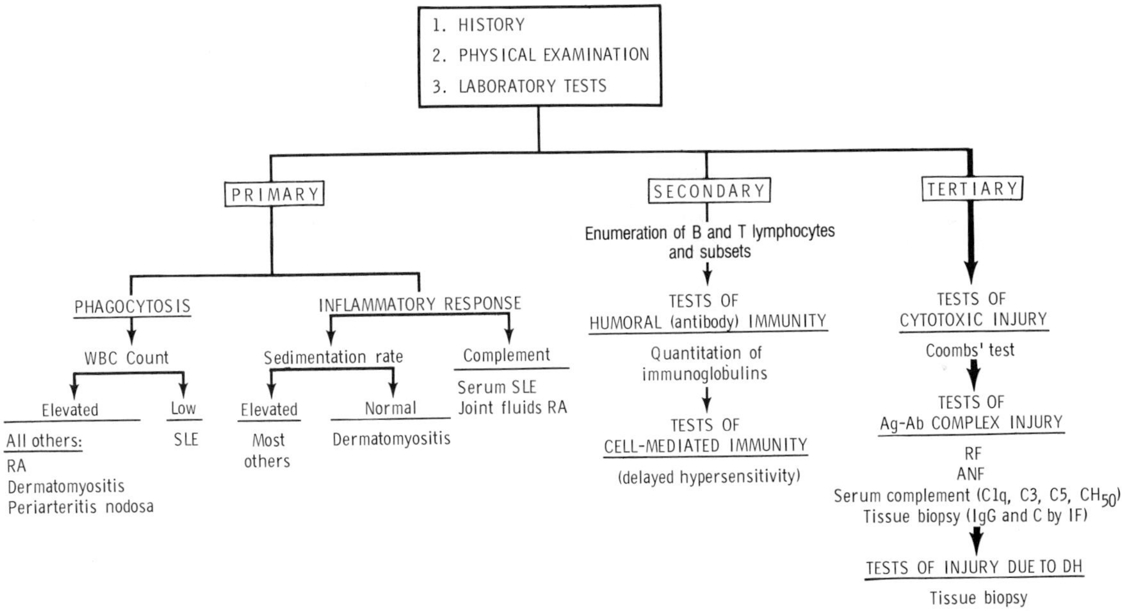

Figure 26–8. Scheme of approach in the investigation of the patient who presents with musculoskeletal (autoimmune) disorders.

Other tests that should be performed include tests of humoral (antibody) function, such as the quantification of the immunoglobulins, which usually reveals a diffuse polyclonal hypergammaglobulinemia.

Tests of tertiary immune function should be performed and should form the backbone of all laboratory testing procedures. These include the Coombs' test, antinuclear factors, rheumatoid factor, ENA, LE cell preparations, and serum complement levels. When indicated, specimens for tissue biopsy may be obtained from appropriate tissues, e.g., muscle and kidney.

From these studies and the history and physical examination, a diagnosis can often be established. For example, in a patient with multiple joint involvement, elevated sedimentation rate, leukocytosis, and positive rheumatoid factor, a diagnosis of rheumatoid arthritis would be most likely. If joint fluid is available, the additional finding of a lowered complement, a polymorphonuclear leukocyte response, and an increased protein in this fluid would establish the diagnosis. On the other hand, in a patient presenting with transient arthritis, elevated sedimentation rate, leukopenia, positive antinuclear factor, and lowered complement, a diagnosis of systemic lupus erythematosus should be considered. If joint fluid is available, it would classically show a lowered complement, fewer cells, and lowered protein. In some cases, tissue biopsy is required for additional substantiation of the diagnosis. For example, in periarteritis nodosa, the diagnosis would be established by a muscle, nerve, or blood vessel biopsy, particularly in a male patient. In dermatomyositis, a biopsy of skin and muscle, in addition to enzyme studies and electromyography, would help establish the diagnosis. The discovery of associations of HLA types with certain autoimmune diseases (Chapters 3 and 20C) suggests that histocompatibility typing may provide another diagnostic aid, e.g., ankylosing spondylitis.

Appendix 6

Problem: Use of Immunology in Diagnosis of Infectious Diseases

Many immunologic tests are available to the physician that aid in the diagnosis of infectious diseases. Listed in Table 26–7 are examples of immunologic techniques that are commonly used. These consist of (1) determination of antibodies, which can be used either to identify an organism in the laboratory or to demonstrate an infection in the patient through a rise in serum antibody titer and (2) demonstration of delayed-hypersensitivity skin tests, which are particularly useful in the diagnosis of chronic bacterial, fungal, and some viral diseases (Table 26–7).

In addition to these tests, there are a number of other laboratory procedures that rely on serologic cross reactivity or heterogenetic responses (Chapter 4). These are listed in Table 26–8 with examples of each.

The prominent macroglobulin response characteristic of the fetal and newborn immune responses has been used in the diagnosis of intrauterine and perinatal infections. Both the direct measurement of IgM immunoglobulins and the measurement of IgM-associated antibodies have been useful in this regard. These are shown in Table 26–9.

References

Alford, C. A., Jr.: Immunoglobulin determinations in the diagnosis of fetal infection. Pediatr. Clin. North Am., *18*:99, 1971.

Overall, J. C., Jr., and Glasgow, L. A.: Virus infections of the fetus and newborn infant. J. Pediatr., 77:315, 1970.

Sever, J. L.: Immunologic responses to perinatal infections. J. Pediatr., Vol. 75, Part 2, December 1969.

Table 26–7. **Types of Immunologic Procedures That Are Used in Diagnosis of Infectious Diseases**

Type of Infection	Antibody		Skin Test		
	Assay Procedure	Example	Immediate	Delayed	Other
Bacterial	Agglutination Precipitation (flocculation) Complement fixation Fluorescent antibody	Salmonella O & H agglutinins Kahn Wassermann Streptococcal		Tuberculosis Infections with atypical mycobacteria	Toxin neutralization (Schick test) Erythrogenic toxin (Dick test)
Viral	Neutralization Complement fixation Hemagglutination inhibition Fluorescent antibody ELISA	Poliovirus Mumps Rubella Variola Herpes (simplex) hominis		Mumps	
Fungal	Precipitation (flocculation) Agglutination Complement fixation Fluorescent antibody	Histoplasma Coccidioides Blastomyces Actinomyces	Skin test in cases of atopic disease caused by fungi, e.g., aspergilli	Histoplasmosis Coccidioidomycosis Blastomycosis	
Parasitic	Precipitation Complement fixation Hemagglutination Fluorescent antibody ELISA	Trichinella Leishmania Amoeba Toxoplasma Schistosoma	Trichinella		

Table 26–8. Serologic Procedures in Diagnosis of Infectious Diseases Based Upon Serologic Cross Reactivity

Disease	Nonspecific Tests	Specific Tests
Primary atypical pneumonia	Cold agglutinins (anti-I)	*M. pneumoniae* antibody (CF, growth inhibition)
Rocky Mountain spotted fever (RMSF)	Weil-Felix (OXK, OX19) agglutinins	RMSF CF test
Infectious mononucleosis	Heterophil antibody	Epstein-Barr (EB) fluorescent antibody
Syphilis	Wassermann, VDRL	Fluorescent *Treponema* antibody test (FTA)

Table 26–9. Serologic Procedures for Diagnosis of Intrauterine and Perinatal Infections Based on Prominent IgM Responses

Disease	Tests
Toxoplasmosis	Specific fluorescent IgM antibody Quantitation of immunoglobulins
Syphilis	Fluorescent *Treponema* antibody test (FTA) Quantitation of immunoglobulins
Rubella	Specific fluorescent IgM antibody Quantitation of immunoglobulins
Cytomegalic inclusion disease	Specific fluorescent IgM antibody Quantitation of immunoglobulins
Herpes simplex	Specific fluorescent IgM antibody Quantitation of immunoglobulins
Acute bacterial infections	Quantitation of immunoglobulins Tests of specific IgM antibody
Hepatitis A	Tests of specific IgM antibody, e.g., radioimmunoassay
Hepatitis B	Tests for HB_SAg or HB_SAb, e.g., radioimmunoassay or ELISA

Index

Note: Page numbers in *italic* type indicate illustrations; page numbers followed by (t) refer to tables.

The illustration on the facing page is an adaptation of a figure that appears in Chapter 9, "Cell-mediated Reactions." The intent is to indicate the complexity of the immune response and the interrelationships and interdependencies of various cellular and humoral components of the immunoregulatory network. It also illustrates the pivotal role of the T-lymphocyte in this immunoregulatory network and in the various expressions of cell-mediated and humoral immune responses.